PHARMACOLOGY

GET CONNECTED

To Content Updates, Study Tools, and More!

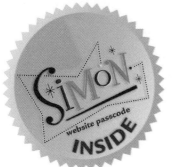

Meet SIMON   Your free online website companion

sign on at:

http://www.wbsaunders.com/SIMON/KeeHayes/
pharmacology/

what you'll receive: Whether you're a student or an instructor, you'll find information just for you. Things like:
- Content updates ● Links to related publications
- Author information . . . and more

plus:

WebLinks

LIFT HERE

PASSCODE INSIDE

Use this passcode to access hundreds of active websites keyed specifically to the contents of this book. The WebLinks are updated continually, with new ones added as they develop.

If passcode tab is removed, this textbook cannot be returned to W.B. Saunders

KEEP YOUR KNOWLEDGE TOP-OF-THE-LINE
with our *Simon* on-line resource for Kee & Hayes: PHARMACOLOGY: A NURSING PROCESS APPROACH, 3e. Sign on now to stay ahead of the game with:

- drug updates to keep you current on new drugs, dosages, forms, precautions and interactions released by the FDA
- case study exercises to test your skills in applied knowledge
- quick reference charts
  on Therapeutic Drug Monitoring, Drugs that Cause Fever, and Drugs that Discolor Bodily Secretions
- the 2000 Recommended Childhood Immunization Schedule
- web links to state poison control centers

W.B. SAUNDERS COMPANY

PHARMACOLOGY

A Nursing Process Approach

Third Edition

Joyce LeFever Kee, MS, RN

Associate Professor Emerita
College of Health and Nursing Sciences
University of Delaware
Newark, Delaware

Evelyn R. Hayes, PhD, RN, CS-FNP

Professor
College of Health and Nursing Sciences
Department of Nursing
University of Delaware
Newark, Delaware

W.B. Saunders Company

An Imprint of Elsevier Science

Philadelphia London New York St. Louis Sydney Toronto

W.B. SAUNDERS COMPANY
An Imprint of Elsevier Science

The Curtis Center
Independence Square West
Philadelphia, Pennsylvania 19106

Library of Congress Cataloging-in-Publication Data

Kee, Joyce LeFever.
    Pharmacology : a nursing process approach / Joyce LeFever Kee, Evelyn R.
Hayes.—3rd ed.

      p. cm.

    Includes bibliographical references and index.

    ISBN 0–7216–8299–5

    1. Pharmacology.   2. Nursing.   I. Hayes, Evelyn R. II. Title.
    [DNLM: 1. Pharmacology nurses' instruction. 2. Drug Therapy nurses' in-
struction. QV 4 K26p 2000]
    RM301.K44 2000   615.5'8—dc21

    DNLM/DLC   98-50608

PHARMACOLOGY: A Nursing Process Approach   ISBN 0–7216–8299–5

Printed in the United States of America.

Last digit is the print number: 9   8   7   6   5

In Loving Memory of My Parents
Esther B. and Samuel H. LeFever

Joyce LeFever Kee

To My Parents
Margaret and Justin Hayes
for their ever-present love and confidence

Evelyn R. Hayes

NOTICE

Pharmacology is an ever changing field. Standard safety precautions must be followed, but as new research and clinical experience broaden our knowledge, changes in treatment and drug therapy become necessary or appropriate. The editors of this work have carefully checked the generic and trade names and verified drug dosages to assure that the dosage information in this work is accurate and in accord with the standards accepted at the time of publication. Readers are advised, however, to check the product information currently provided by the manufacturer of each drug to be administered to be certain that changes have not been made in the recommended dose or in the contraindications for administration. This is of particular importance in regard to new or infrequently used drugs. It is the responsibility of the treating physician or health care provider, relying on experience and knowledge of the client, to determine dosages and the best treatment for their client. The editors and publisher cannot be responsible for misuse or misapplication of the information in this work.

To the Reader

Consult the product information contained in the package insert of each drug before administering the medication.

Abbott Laboratories
American Regent
Apothecon Laboratories
Bristol-Myers Squibb Company
DuPont/Merck Pharmaceuticals
Eli Lilly and Company
Elkins-Sinn, Inc.
Glaxo-Wellcome, Inc.
Marion Merrell Dow, Inc.
Mead Johnson Pharmaceuticals

Merck and Co., Inc.
McNeil Consumer Products Co.
Mylan Pharmaceuticals, Inc.
Parke-Davis
SmithKline Beecham Pharmaceuticals
E. R. Squibb and Sons, Inc.
Summit Pharmaceuticals/Ciba-Geigy
    Pharmaceuticals
Warner-Lambert Consumer Health Products
Wyeth-Ayerst Laboratories

Contributors

Helene S. DeHaan, MSN, FNP-C
Family Nurse Practitioner
Bridgeton, New Jersey
Chapter 6

Linda Goodwin, RNC, MEd
Clinical Faculty
Department of Maternal and Child Nursing
University of Washington
Manager, Family Birthplace and Family Beginnings
Group Health Hospitals
Seattle and Redmond, Washington
Chapters 47, 48, 49

Kathleen J. Jones, RN, MS, ANP
Adult Nurse Practitioner
Oncology Clinic
Walter Reed Army Medical Center
Washington, DC
Chapters 50, 51

Robert Kizior, RPh
Education Coordinator
Department of Pharmacy
Alexian Brothers Medical Center
Elk Grove Village, Illinois
Chapter 31

Anne E. Lara, RN, MS, OCN, CS
Adjunct Faculty, Department of Nursing
University of Delaware
Administrative Director
Department of Radiation Oncology
Christiana Health Services
Newark, Delaware
Chapter 34

Linda Laskowski-Jones, RN, MS, CS, CCRN, CEN
Trauma Program Coordinator/Clinical Nurse Specialist
Christiana Hospital
Newark, Delaware
Chapter 52

Patricia S. Lincoln, BSN, RN
Education Coordinator
HIV Infectious Disease Clinic and Mid Atlantic
    AIDS Education Training Center
Christiana Care Health Systems
Newark, Delaware
Chapter 31

Larry D. Purnell, PhD, RN
Professor
College of Health and Nursing Services
University of Delaware
Newark, Delaware
Professor
University of Panama
Republic of Panama
Chapter 6

Nancy C. Sharts-Hopko, RN, PhD
Professor
Villanova University
Villanova, Pennsylvania
Chapters 50, 51

Jane Purnell Taylor, RN, MS
Associate Professor
Department of Nursing
Neumann College
Aston, Pennsylvania
Chapters 47, 48, 49

Lynette M. Wachholz, MSN, RN
Clinical Faculty
School of Nursing
University of Washington
Seattle, Washington
Pediatric Nurse Practitioner and Lactation Consultant
The Everett Clinic
Everett, Washington
Chapter 32

Consultants

Heidi Hartenstein Benoit, MS, RN
School of Health Sciences
Lafayette General Medical Center
Lafayette, Louisiana

Donita D'Amico, EdM, RN
Assistant Professor
RN Program Coordinator
Department of Nursing
William Paterson University
Wayne, New Jersey

Dianne Endres, EdD, MS
Baylor University School of Nursing
Dallas, Texas

Jane M. Hartsock, MA, RN, AOCN, CNS
Trinity College of Nursing
Moline, Illinois

Karen Hill, PhD, MN, RN
School of Nursing
Southeastern Louisiana University
Hammond, Louisiana

Kimberly Mathai, MS, RD
Nutritional Consultant
Nutrition By Design
Seattle, Washington

Nancy O'Donnell, MSN, RN
Associate Professor
J. Sargeant Reynolds Community College
Richmond, Virginia

Christine E. Reilly, PhD, RN
College of Health and Nursing Sciences
University of Delaware
Newark, Delaware

Leslie Robbins, MSN, RNCS
Assistant Professor
Doña Ana Branch Community College
Las Cruces, New Mexico

Donna Roddy, MSN, RN
Chattanooga State Technical Community College
Chattanooga, Tennessee

Martha Shemin, MSN, RN
Holy Name Hospital School of Nursing
Teaneck, New Jersey

Sharon P. Shipton, PhD, MSN, AS
Youngstown State University
Youngstown, Ohio

Wanda Staab, MSN, CCRN
Ursuline College
Pepper Pike, Ohio

Diane M. Tomasic, EdD, RN
Nursing Division
West Liberty State College
West Liberty, West Virginia

Patricia P. Wickham, MSN, RN
Practical Nursing Program
Center for Arts and Technology
Brandywine Campus
Coatesville, Pennsylvania

Preface

This unique clinical pharmacology textbook presents complex pharmacologic principles in a student-friendly and comprehensive manner. *Pharmacology: A Nursing Process Approach,* Third Edition, focuses on the understanding of pharmacologic principles, the administration of medications, and the evaluation of client responses. These foci are essential to the foundations of professional nursing practice. The textbook is designed for students in a variety of nursing programs, for NCLEX review and preparation, and for nurses practicing in a variety of settings.

Organization

The textbook is organized into 14 units and 52 chapters. The first unit presents an overview of pharmacologic principles. Chapter 4 presents a comprehensive review of drug dosage calculations for adults and children. The chapter consists of six sections: Systems of Measurement with Conversion, Methods for Calculation, Calculations of Oral Dosages, Calculations of Injectable Dosages, Calculations of Intravenous Fluids, and Calculations of Pediatric Dosages. Throughout this chapter, we added colorful new photographs of the equipment used to deliver medications. We also use clinical practice problems and real drug labels in full color for practicing dosage calculations. With its variety and number of practice problems using different health care settings, this chapter eliminates the student's need to purchase a separate dosage calculation textbook. The accompanying Student Guide provides additional practice problems with answers and a basic math review.

The rest of the units in this textbook present all the drug families. Each chapter provides an outline, objectives, key terms, drug pharmacokinetics and pharmacodynamics, and the nursing process. Pharmacology is at the forefront of the knowledge explosion. Thus, we added several new chapters in this edition, such as Chapter 6, Cultural Considerations; Chapter 8, Herbal Therapy and Nursing Implications; Chapter 10, Medication Administration in Community Settings; Chapter 31, HIV-Related Agents; and Chapter 32, Vaccines.

Features

Throughout this textbook, we use a variety of features to teach students the fundamental principles of pharmacology and to illustrate the role of the nurse in drug therapy.

- **Prototype Drug Charts.** This edition contains about 100 charts that illustrate basic and comparative data for prototype drugs in selected categories. Students can see how different steps of the Nursing Process correlate to different aspects of drug information and therapy.
- **Nursing Process.** We integrated the Nursing Process throughout the textbook. The Nursing Process presented in each chapter includes Assessment, Nursing Diagnoses, Planning, Nursing Interventions, and Evaluation.
- **Client Teaching.** Under Nursing Interventions, we include Client and Family Teaching information in color type. We have expanded this section and now suggest helpful teaching tips that relate to general information, self-administration, diet, and side effects.
- **Cultural Considerations.** In addition to a new chapter discussing general cultural considerations during drug therapy, we have added a section for Cultural Considerations under Nursing Interventions. These sections provide information when it is relevant for the nurse to consider cultural implications during drug administration.
- **Critical Thinking in Action.** Each chapter concludes with a clinical scenario, followed by a series of critical thinking questions. These exercises challenge students to carefully consider the scenario, and apply their knowledge and analysis skills to respond to the situations.

- **Study Questions.** At the end of each chapter, a series of Study Questions provides students with an immediate review and reinforces the objectives of the chapter. Students can scan the content of the chapter to confirm their answers.
- **Drug Tables.** The comprehensive drug tables found in the therapeutic chapters provide drug names (generic, brand, and Canadian), dosages, uses and considerations, pregnancy categories, and pharmacokinetics.

Other New Features

- A **colorful** design and new illustrations and photographs, including innovative technology for medication administration.
- Expanded Unit introductions with illustrated **overviews of anatomy and physiology.**
- Updated drug information, including the **latest FDA-approved drugs** in all categories.
- Internet sites of interest are listed on the front inside cover.
- **Selected Drug Interactions** listed on the last page of the textbook.

Teaching and Learning Resources

Pharmacology: A Nursing Process Approach, Third Edition, is accompanied by ancillary resources to provide pharmacology instructors and students with a complete teaching/learning package. These resources include:

- **Study Guide.** It provides application of the nursing process to clinical situations through a variety of formats. In addition to multiple choice and completion questions, the student guide offers labeling exercises, matching exercises, word searches, and critical thinking case studies. Answers are provided.
- **Instructor's Electronic Resource CD-ROM.** This CD-ROM provides three instructor's resources. The **Online Instructor's Manual** contains objectives, outlines, and teaching strategies to promote critical thinking. The Instructor's Manual also provides a basic math test and answers. Instructors receive this resource in both Microsoft Word and WordPerfect. Instructors can incorporate their own materials or simply print chapters out as is. The **ExaMaster** electronic test bank consists of more than 900 questions. The ExaMaster program allows instructors to generate tests, incorporate their own questions, and maintain a grade book. Finally, the CD-ROM also includes an **Electronic Image Collection,** featuring more than 40 colorful illustrations from the textbook. These images can be imported into any electronic lecture presentation or printed on transparency acetates. This valuable CD-ROM is available only to schools that adopt *Pharmacology: A Nursing Process Approach*, Third Edition.

It is our hope that nursing students will enhance their knowledge of pharmacology and their roles in drug therapy through this textbook and its accompanying resources.

Joyce LeFever Kee
Evelyn R. Hayes

Acknowledgments

We wish to extend our sincere appreciation to the many professionals who assisted in the preparation of *Pharmacology: A Nursing Process Approach,* Third Edition, by reviewing chapters and offering suggestions.

We wish to especially thank the authors of the new chapters, and the original authors and those who updated the established chapters: Larry D. Purnell, PhD, RN, Patricia S. Lincoln, BSN, RN, Robert Kizior, RPh, Lynette M. Wachholz, MSN, RN, Anne E. Lara, RN, MS, OCN, CS, Jane Purnell Taylor, RN, MS, Linda Goodwin, RNC, EdD, Nancy C. Sharts-Hopko, RN, PhD, Kathleen J. Jones, RN, MS, ANP, and Linda Laskowski-Jones, RN, MS, CS, CCRN, CEN.

Of course, we are deeply indebted to the many clients and students we have had throughout our many years of professional nursing practice. From them we have learned many fine points about the role of therapeutic pharmacology in nursing practice.

Our deepest appreciation goes to pharmaceutical companies for permission to use their drug labels. Pharmaceutical companies that extended their courtesy to this book include:

Abbott Laboratories
American Regent
   Luitold Pharmaceuticals
Astra Pharmaceuticals
Bristol-Myers Squibb Co.
   Apothecon Laboratories
   Mead Johnson Pharmaceuticals
   E. R. Squibb and Sons, Inc.
DuPont/Merck Pharmaceuticals
Eli Lilly and Company
Elkins-Sinn, Inc.
   A subsidiary of A. H. Robins

Glaxo-Wellcome, Inc.
Marion Merrell Dow, Inc.
McNeilab, Inc.
   McNeil Consumer Products Co.
   Ortho-McNeil Pharmaceutical
Merck and Co., Inc.
Mylan Pharmaceuticals Inc.
SmithKline Beecham Pharmaceutical
Warner-Lambert Consumer Health
   Products
   Parke-Davis
Wyeth-Ayerst Laboratories

We extend our sincere thanks to the companies and publishers who gave us permission to use photographs, illustrations, and other materials in the text. These include:

American Association of Critical-Care
   Nursing
Appleton & Lange
Baxter Healthcare Corp.
Becton-Dickinson Division
Ciba-Geigy Pharmaceuticals
Mosby-Year Book

F. A. Davis
IMED Corporation
Medical Letter, Inc.
Pyxis System
W.B. Saunders Co.
Wyeth-Ayerst Laboratories

Our sincere and deepest thanks to the staff at W.B. Saunders, especially Maura Connor, former Senior Editor, Nursing Books; Kevin Law, former Senior Developmental Editor, Nursing Books; Linda R. Garber and Frank Polizzano, Senior Production Managers; Edna Dick, Copy Editor; Victoria Legnini, Assistant Developmental Editor; Frances Murphy, Developmental Editor Assistant; and Sharon Iwanczuk, Illustrator, for their suggestions and assistance. Also thanks to Don Passidomo, librarian at the Department of Veterans Affairs, Wilmington, Delaware, for his help with library research.

Appreciation and love go out to my husband, Edward D. Kee (JLK), and to my parents, Margaret K. and Justin F. Hayes (ERH), for their support.

Joyce L. Kee
Evelyn R. Hayes

Contents

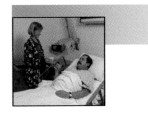

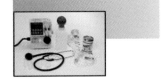

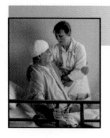

Unit IV

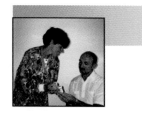

Unit V

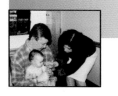

Unit VI

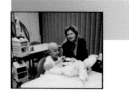

Unit VII

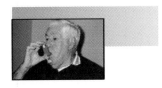

Unit VIII

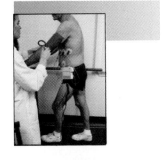

Unit IX

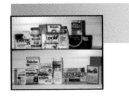

Unit X

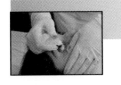

Unit XI

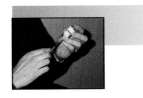

Unit XII

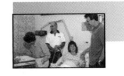

Unit XIII

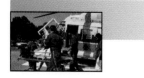

Unit XIV

Emergency Agents   976

Unit I

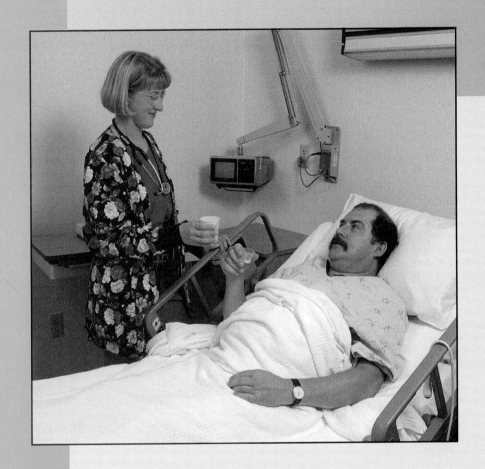

A Nurse's Perspective of Pharmacology

Assessing a client's response to drug therapy is an ongoing nursing responsibility. To adequately assess, plan, intervene, and evaluate drug effects, the nurse needs to have knowledge of the pharmaceutic, pharmacokinetic, and pharmacodynamic phases of drug action. A drug chart—see Introduction to Drug Chart Use—organizes specific drug data needed for preparation and application of the nursing process. Client teaching is essential to promote client and family adherence to the drug regimen and therapy.

Along with understanding the three phases of drug action, nursing process, and client teaching, applying of principles of drug administration and calculating drug doses are important functions in nursing practice. Chapter 3, Principles of Drug Administration, contains basic learning material for the administration of medications. It describes the "ten rights" in drug administration, drug orders, drug distribution, drug charting, guidelines for drug administration, and routes for drug administration with illustrated parenteral sites.

Chapter 4, Medications and Calculations, provides practice in drug calculation for adult and child dosages. This chapter could be assigned as an overall review of drug calculation. Chapters 3 and 4 may be used for drug administration and calculation in place of a nursing fundamentals text or a drug calculation text.

Drug Action: Pharmaceutic, Pharmacokinetic, and Pharmacodynamic Phases

Outline

Objectives

- Define the three phases of drug action.
- Identify the two processes that occur before tablets are absorbed into the body.
- Describe the four processes of pharmacokinetics.
- Explain the meaning of pharmacodynamics, the receptor, and nonreceptors in drug action.
- Define the terms *protein-bound drugs, half-life, therapeutic index, therapeutic drug range, side effects, adverse reaction,* and *drug toxicity.*
- Check drugs for half-life, percentage of protein-binding effect, therapeutic range, and side effects in a drug reference book.

Terms

active absorption	high therapeutic index	pharmacokinetic
adverse reactions	ligand-binding domain	pinocytosis
agonists	loading dose	placebo effect
antagonists	low therapeutic index	protein-binding
bioavailability	metabolism	rate limiting
creatinine clearance	nonselective drug response	receptor
disintegration	nonspecific drug response	side effects
dissolution	onset of action	tachyphylaxis
distribution	passive absorption	therapeutic index
duration of action	peak action	therapeutic window
elimination	peak level	therapeutic range
first-pass effect	pharmaceutic phase	time–response curve
free drugs	pharmacodynamic	toxicity
half-life	pharmacogenetics	trough level

INTRODUCTION

A drug taken by mouth goes through three phases—pharmaceutic (dissolution), pharmacokinetic, and pharmacodynamic—in order for drug action to occur. In the pharmaceutic phase, the drug goes into solution so that it can cross the biologic membrane. When the drug is administered parenterally by subcutaneous, intramuscular, or intravenous routes, there is no pharmaceutic phase. The second phase, the pharmacokinetic, is made up of four processes: absorption, distribution, metabolism (or biotransformation), and excretion. In the pharmacodynamic phase, a biologic or physiologic response results.

PHARMACEUTIC

Approximately 80% of drugs are taken by mouth. The **pharmaceutic** (dissolution) is the first phase of drug action. In the gastrointestinal (GI) tract, drugs need to be in solution to be absorbed. A drug in solid form (tablet or capsule) must disintegrate into small particles to dissolve into a liquid, a process known as dissolution. Drugs in liquid form are already in solution. Figure 1–1 displays the pharmaceutic phase of a tablet.

Tablets are not 100% drug. Fillers and inert substances, generally called excipients, are used in drug preparation to allow the drug to take on a particular size and shape and to enhance dissolution of the drug. Some additives in drugs, such as the ions potassium (K) and sodium (Na) in penicillin potassium and penicillin sodium, increase the absorbability of the drug. Penicillin is poorly absorbed from the GI tract because of gastric acid. By making the drug a potassium or sodium salt, penicillin can be absorbed. An infant's gastric secretions have a higher pH (alkaline) than those of adults, so babies absorb more penicillin.

Disintegration is the breakdown of the tablet into smaller particles. **Dissolution** is the dissolving of the smaller particles in the gastrointestinal fluid before absorption. **Rate limiting** refers to the time it takes the drug to disintegrate and dissolve to become available for the body to absorb it. Drugs in liquid form are more rapidly available for GI absorption than are solids. Generally, drugs disintegrate faster and are absorbed faster in acidic fluids that have a pH of 1 or 2 than in alkaline fluids. The young and the elderly have less gastric acidity, so drug absorption is generally slower for those drugs absorbed primarily in the stomach.

Enteric-coated drugs resist disintegration in the gastric acid of the stomach, so disintegration does not occur until the drug reaches the alkaline environment in the small intestine. Enteric-coated tablets can remain in the stomach for a long time; therefore, their effect may be delayed in onset. Enteric-coated tablets or capsules and sustained-release (beaded) capsules *should not be crushed.*

Food in the GI tract may interfere with the dissolution and absorption of certain drugs. However, food can enhance absorption of other drugs; thus, some drugs should be taken with food. Some drugs are irritating to the gastric mucosa, so fluids or food may be necessary to dilute drug concentration and act as protectants.

PHARMACOKINETICS

Pharmacokinetics is the process of drug movement to achieve drug action. The four processes are absorption, distribution, metabolism (or biotransformation), and excretion (or elimination).

By using the knowledge of the four pharmacokinetic processes of the make-up of the drug, the prescriber promotes safety of drug therapy. The nurse needs to be alert to possible adverse drug effects that can result from the pharmacokinetics of the drug and to report promptly such findings.

Absorption

Absorption is the movement of drug particles from the GI tract to body fluids by passive absorption, active absorption, or pinocytosis. Most oral drugs are absorbed into the surface area of the small intestine through the action of the extensive mucosal villi. If the villi are decreased in number because of disease, drug effect, or removal of small intestine, absorption is reduced. Protein-based drugs, such as insulin and growth hormones, are destroyed in the small intestine by digestive enzymes. **Passive absorption** occurs mostly by diffusion (movement from higher concentration to lower concentration). With the process of diffusion, the drug does not require energy to move across the membrane. **Active absorption** requires a carrier such as an enzyme or protein to move the drug against a concentration gradient. Energy is required for active absorption. **Pinocytosis** is a process by which cells carry drug across their membrane by engulfing the drug particles (Fig. 1–2).

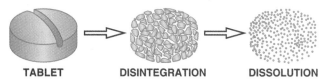

TABLET   DISINTEGRATION   DISSOLUTION

Figure 1–1
The two pharmaceutic phases are disintegration and dissolution.

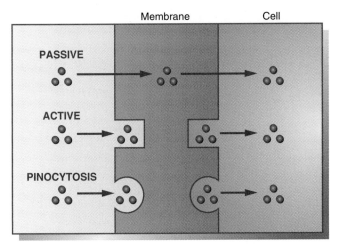

Membrane   Cell

PASSIVE

ACTIVE

PINOCYTOSIS

Figure 1–2
The three major processes for drug absorption through the gastrointestinal membrane are passive absorption, active absorption, and pinocytosis.

The GI membrane is composed mostly of lipid (fat) and protein, so drugs that are lipid soluble pass rapidly through the GI membrane. Water-soluble drugs need a carrier, either enzyme or protein, to pass through the membrane. Large particles pass through the cell membrane if they are nonionized (no positive or negative charge). Weak acid drugs, such as aspirin, are less ionized in the stomach, and they pass through the stomach lining easily and rapidly. Hydrochloric acid destroys some drugs, such as penicillin G; therefore, a large oral dosage of penicillin is needed to offset the partial dose loss.

REMEMBER: Drugs that are lipid soluble and nonionized are absorbed *faster* than water-soluble and ionized drugs.

Drug absorption is affected by blood flow, pain, stress, hunger, fasting, food, and pH. Poor circulation resulting from shock, vasoconstrictor drugs, or disease hampers absorption. Pain, stress, and foods that are solid, hot, and fatty can slow gastric emptying time, so the drug remains longer in the stomach. Exercise can decrease blood flow by causing more blood to flow to the peripheral muscle, decreasing blood circulation to the GI tract.

Drugs given intramuscularly can be absorbed faster in muscles that have more blood vessels, such as the deltoid, than those that have fewer blood vessels, such as the gluteal. Subcutaneous tissue has fewer blood vessels, so absorption is slower in such tissue.

Some drugs do *not* go directly into the systemic circulation following oral absorption but pass from the intestinal lumen to the liver via the portal vein. In the liver, some drugs may be metabolized to an inactive form, which may then be excreted, thus reducing the amount of active drug. Some drugs do not undergo metabolism at all in the liver, and others may be metabolized to drug metabolite, which may be equally or more active than the original drug. The process in which the drug passes to the liver first is called the **first-pass effect,** or hepatic first pass. Examples of drugs with first-pass metabolism are warfarin (Coumadin) and morphine. Lidocaine and some nitroglycerins are *not* given orally, because they have extensive first-pass metabolism and the majority of the dose would be destroyed.

Bioavailability is a subcategory of absorption. It is the percentage of the administered drug dose that reaches the systemic circulation. For the oral route of drug administration, bioavailability occurs after absorption and hepatic drug metabolism. The percentage of bioavailability for the oral route is always less than 100%. Bioavailability for the intravenous route is usually 100%. Oral drugs that have a high first-pass hepatic metabolism may have a bioavailability of 20% to 40% upon entering systemic circulation. To obtain desired drug effect, the oral dose could be three to five times larger than the drug dose for intravenous use.

Factors that alter bioavailability include (1) the drug form (tablet, capsule, sustained-release, liquid, transdermal patch, rectal suppository, inhalation), (2) route of administration (oral, rectal, topical, parenteral), (3) GI mucosa and motility, (4) food and other drugs, and (5) changes in liver metabolism caused by liver dysfunction or inadequate hepatic blood flow. A decrease in liver function or a decrease in hepatic blood flow can increase the bioavailability of a drug, but only if the drug is metabolized by the liver. Less

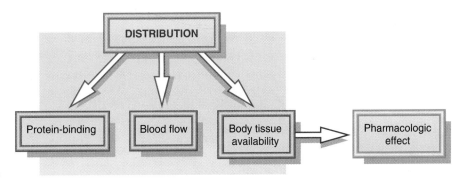

DISTRIBUTION

Protein-binding   Blood flow   Body tissue availability   Pharmacologic effect

Figure 1–3
Drug distribution.

drug is destroyed by hepatic metabolism in the presence of liver disorder.

With some oral drugs, rapid absorption increases the bioavailability of the drug and can cause an increase in drug concentration. Drug toxicity may result. Slow absorption can limit the bioavailability of the drug, thus causing a decrease in drug serum concentration.

Distribution

Distribution is the process by which the drug becomes available to body fluids and body tissues. Drug distribution is influenced by blood flow, its affinity to the tissue, and **protein-binding** effect (Fig. 1–3).

As drugs are distributed in the plasma, many are bound to varying degrees (percentages) with protein (primarily albumin). Drugs that are greater than 89% bound to protein are known as highly protein-bound drugs; drugs that are 61% to 89% bound to protein are moderately highly protein-bound; drugs that are 30% to 60% bound to protein are moderately protein-bound; and drugs that are less than 30% bound to protein are low protein-bound drugs. Table 1–1 lists selected highly protein-bound drugs and moderately highly protein-bound drugs. The portion of the drug that is bound is inactive because it is not available to receptors, and the portion that remains unbound is free, active drug. Only **free drugs** (drugs not bound to protein) are active and can cause a pharmacologic response. As the free drug in the circulation decreases, more bound drug is released from the protein to maintain the balance of free drug.

When two highly protein-bound drugs are given concurrently, they compete for protein-binding sites, thus causing more free drug to be released into the circulation. Drug accumulation and possible drug toxicity can result in this situation. Also, a low protein level decreases the number of protein-binding sites and can cause an increase in the amount of free drug in the plasma. Drug overdose may then result. Drug dose is prescribed according to the percentage in which the drug binds to protein.

With some health conditions that result in a low serum protein level, excess free or unbound drug goes to nonspecific tissue binding sites until needed and excess free drug in the circulation would not occur.

Some drugs bind with a specific protein component such as albumin or globulin. Most anticonvulsants bind primarily to albumin. Some basic drugs such as antidysrhythmics (lidocaine, quinidine) bind mostly to globulins.

Clients with liver or kidney disease or who are malnourished may have an abnormally low serum albumin level. This results in fewer protein-binding

Table 1–1
Protein-Binding Percentage and Half-Life of Specific Drugs

DRUG	PROTEIN-BOUND (%)	HALF-LIFE (t½) (h)
HIGHLY PROTEIN-BOUND DRUGS (>89%)		
Amitriptyline	97	40
Chlorpromazine	95	30
Diazepam	98	30–80
Dicloxacillin	95	0.5–1
Digitoxin	90	8
Furosemide	95	1.5
Ibuprofen	98	2–4
Lorazepam	92	15
Piroxicam	99	30–86
Propranolol	92	4
Rifampin	89	2
Sulfisoxazole	85–95	4.5–7.5
Valproic acid	92	15
MODERATELY HIGHLY PROTEIN-BOUND DRUGS (61%–89%)		
Erythromycin	70	3
Nafcillin	86	2–20
Phenytoin	88	10–40
Quinidine	70	6
Trimethoprim	70	11
MODERATELY PROTEIN-BOUND DRUGS (30%–60%)		
Aspirin	49	0.25–2
Lidocaine	50	2
Meperidine	56	3
Pindolol	40	3–4
Theophylline	60	9
Ticarcillin	45–65	1–1.5
LOW PROTEIN-BOUND DRUGS (<30%)		
Amikacin	4–11	2–3
Amoxicillin	20	1–1.5
Atenolol	6–16	6–7
Cephalexin	10–15	0.5–1.2
Digoxin	25	36
Neostigmine bromide	15–25	1–1.5
Terbutaline sulfate	25	3–11
Timolol maleate	<10	3–4
Tobramycin sulfate	10	2–3

Key: >: greater than; <: less than; h: hour.

sites, which, in turn, leads to excess free drug and eventually to drug toxicity. The elderly are more likely to have hypoalbuminemia.

Checking the protein-binding percentage of all drugs administered to a client is important to avoid possible drug toxicity. The nurse should also check the client's plasma protein and albumin levels, because a decrease in plasma protein (albumin) decreases protein-binding sites, permitting more free drug in the circulation. Depending on the drug the result could be life-threatening.

Abscesses, exudates, body glands, and tumors hinder drug distribution. Antibiotics do not distribute well at abscess and exudate sites. In addition, some drugs accumulate in particular tissues, such as fat, bone, liver, eyes, and muscle.

Metabolism, or Biotransformation

The liver is the primary site of **metabolism.** Most drugs are inactivated by liver enzymes and are then converted or transformed by hepatic enzymes to inactive metabolites or water-soluble substances for excretion. A large percentage of drugs are lipid soluble; thus, the liver metabolizes the lipid-soluble drug substance to a water-soluble substance for renal excretion. However, some drugs are transformed into active metabolites, causing an increased pharmacologic response. Liver diseases, such as cirrhosis and hepatitis, alter drug metabolism by inhibiting the drug-metabolizing enzymes in the liver. When the drug metabolism rate is decreased, excess drug accumulation can occur, which can lead to toxicity.

The **half-life,** symbolized as $t^{1/2}$, of a drug is the time it takes for one-half of the drug concentration to be eliminated. Metabolism and elimination affect the half-life of a drug. For example, with liver or kidney dysfunction, the half-life of the drug is prolonged and less drug is metabolized and eliminated. When a drug is taken continually, drug accumulation may occur. Table 1–1 gives the half-life of selected drugs.

A drug goes through several half-lives before more than 90% of the drug is eliminated. If the client takes 650 mg (milligrams) of aspirin and the $t^{1/2}$ is 3 h (hours), then it takes 3 h for the first half-life to eliminate 325 mg, and the second half-life (at 6 h) for an additional 162 mg to be eliminated, and so on until the sixth half-life (or 18 h), when 10 mg of aspirin is left in the body (Table 1–2). A short half-life is considered to be 4 to 8 h and a long one is 24 h or longer. If the drug has a long half-life (such as digoxin: 36 h), it takes several days until the body completely eliminates the drug.

By knowing the half-life, the time it takes for the drug to reach a steady state of serum concentration can be computed. Administration of the drug for three to five half-lives saturates the biologic system to

Table 1–2
Half-Life of 650 mg of Aspirin

NUM-BER $t^{1/2}$	TIME OF ELIMINA-TION (h)	DOSAGE REMAIN-ING (mg)	PERCENT-AGE LEFT
1	3	325	50
2	6	162	25
3	9	81	12.5
4	12	40	6.25
5	15	20	3.1
6	18	10	1.55

the extent that the intake of drug equals the amount metabolized and excreted. An example is digoxin, which has a half-life of 36 h with normal renal function. It would take approximately 5 days to 1 week (three to five half-lives) to reach a steady state for digoxin concentration. Steady-state serum concentration is predictive of therapeutic drug effect. The half-life of drugs is also discussed in Pharmacodynamics.

Excretion, or Elimination

The main route of drug **elimination** is through the urine. Other routes include bile, feces, lungs, saliva, sweat, and breast milk. Free, unbound drugs, water-soluble drugs, and drugs that are unchanged are filtered by the kidneys. Protein-bound drugs cannot be filtered through the kidneys. Once the drug is released from the protein, it is a free drug and eventually is excreted in the urine. The lungs eliminate volatile drug substances and products metabolized to CO_2 and H_2O.

The urine pH influences drug excretion. Urine pH varies from 4.5 to 8. Acid urine promotes elimination of weak base drugs, and alkaline urine promotes elimination of weak acid drugs. Aspirin, a weak acid, is excreted rapidly in alkaline urine. If a person takes an overdose of aspirin, sodium bicarbonate may be given to change the urine pH to alkaline to help potentiate excretion of the drug. Large quantities of cranberry juice can decrease urine pH, causing an acid urine, thus inhibiting the elimination of the aspirin.

With a kidney disease that results in decreased glomerular filtration rate (GFR) or decreased renal tubular secretion, drug excretion is slowed or impaired. Drug accumulation with possible severe adverse drug reactions can result. A decrease in blood flow to the kidneys can also alter drug excretion.

The most accurate test to determine renal function is **creatinine clearance (CL_{cr}).** Creatinine is a metabolic byproduct of muscle that is excreted by the kidneys. Creatinine clearance varies with age and gender. Lower values are expected in elderly and female clients because of their decreased muscle mass. A decrease in renal GFR results in an increase in serum creatinine level and a decrease in urine creatinine clearance.

With renal dysfunction resulting from kidney disorders or in the elderly, drug dosage usually needs to be decreased. In these cases, the creatinine clearance needs to be determined to establish appropriate drug dosage. When the creatinine clearance is decreased, drug dosage may need to be decreased. Continuous drug dosing according to a prescribed dosing regimen could result in drug toxicity.

The creatinine clearance test consists of a 12- or 24-hour urine collection and a blood sample. Normal creatinine clearance is 85 to 135 mL/min. This rate decreases with age, because aging decreases muscle mass and results in a decrease in functioning nephrons. Elderly clients may have a creatinine clearance of 60 mL/min. For this reason, drug dosage in the elderly may need to be decreased.

PHARMACODYNAMICS

The study of the effect of a drug on cellular physiology and biochemistry and the drug's mechanism of action is known as **pharmacodynamics.** Drug response can cause a primary or secondary physiologic effect, or both. The primary effect is desirable and the secondary effect may be desirable or undesirable. An example of a drug with a primary and secondary effect is diphenhydramine (Benadryl), an antihistamine. The primary effect of diphenhydramine is to treat the symptoms of allergy, and the secondary effect is a central nervous system depression that causes drowsiness. The secondary effect is undesirable when the client drives a car, but at bedtime, it could be desirable by causing a mild sedation.

Onset, Peak, and Duration of Action

Onset of action is the time it takes to reach the minimum effective concentration (MEC) after a drug is administered. **Peak action** occurs when the drug reaches its highest blood or plasma concentration. **Duration of action** is the length of time the drug has a pharmacologic effect. Figure 1–4 illustrates the areas in which onset, peak, and duration of action occur.

Some drugs produce effects in minutes, but others may take hours or days. A **time–response curve** evaluates three parameters of drug action: the onset of drug action, peak action, and duration of action.

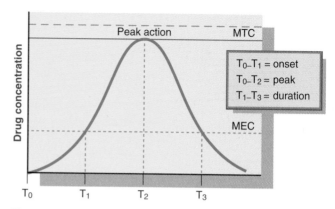

Figure 1–4
The time–response curve evaluates three parameters of drug action: (1) onset, (2) peak, and (3) duration. MEC: minimum effective concentration; MTC: minimum toxic concentration.

Figure 1–4 indicates these parameters by using T (time) with subscripts (e.g., T_0, T_1, T_2, T_3).

It is necessary to understand the time–response in relationship to drug administration. If the drug plasma or serum level decreases below threshold or MEC, adequate drug dosing is *not* achieved; too high a drug level, above the minimum toxic concentration (MTC), can result in toxicity.

Receptor Theory

Most **receptors,** protein in structure, are found on cell membranes. Drug-binding sites are primarily on proteins, glycoproteins, proteolipids, and at enzymes. Lehne (1998) states that there are four receptor families: (1) cell membrane–embedded enzymes, (2) ligand-gated ion channels, (3) G protein–coupled receptor systems, and (4) transcription factors. The term *ligand-binding domain* is the site on the receptor in which drugs bind.

- **Cell membrane–embedded enzymes.** The ligand-binding domain for drug binding is on the cell surface. The drug activates the enzyme (inside the cell) and a response is initiated.
- **Ligand-gated ion channels.** The drug spans the cell membrane and, with this type of receptor, the channel opens, allowing for the flow of ions into and out of the cells. The ions are primarily sodium and calcium.
- **G Protein–coupled receptor systems.** There are three components to this receptor response: (1) the receptor, (2) G protein that binds with guanosine triphosphate (GTP), and (3) the effector that is either an enzyme or an ion channel. The system works as follows:

$$drug \xrightarrow{activates} receptor \xrightarrow{activates} G\ protein \xrightarrow{activates} effector$$

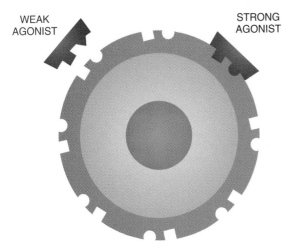

WEAK AGONIST   STRONG AGONIST

Figure 1–5
Two drug agonists attach to the receptor site. The drug agonist that has an exact fit is a strong agonist and is more biologically active than the weak agonist.

• **Transcription factors.** Transcription factors are on the DNA in the cell nucleus and not on the surface of the cell membrane. Activation of receptors through the transcription factors is prolonged. With the first three receptor groups, the activation of the receptors are rapid.

Drugs act through receptors by binding to the receptor to produce (initiate) a response or to block (prevent) a response. The activity of many drugs is determined by the ability of the drug to bind to a specific receptor. The better the drug fits at the receptor site, the more biologically active the drug is. It is similar to the fit of the right key in a lock. Figure 1–5 illustrates a drug binding to a receptor.

Drugs that produce a response are called **agonists,** and drugs that block a response are called **antagonists.** Isoproterenol (Isuprel) stimulates the beta$_1$ receptor, and so it is an agonist. Cimetidine (Tagamet), an antagonist, blocks the H$_2$ receptor, thus preventing excessive gastric acid secretion. The effects of an antagonist can be determined by the inhibitory (I) action of the drug concentration on the receptor site. I$_{50}$ indicates that the drug is effective in inhibiting receptor response in 50% of persons.

Almost all drugs, agonists and antagonists, lack specific and selective effects. A receptor produces a variety of physiologic responses, depending on where in the body that receptor is located. Cholinergic receptors are located in the bladder, heart, blood vessels, lungs, and eyes. A drug that stimulates or blocks the cholinergic receptors affects all anatomic sites of location. Drugs that affect various sites are considered to be **nonspecific** or have properties of nonspecificity. Bethanechol (Urecholine) may be prescribed for postoperative urinary retention to increase bladder contraction. This drug stimulates the cholinergic receptor located in the bladder, and urination occurs by

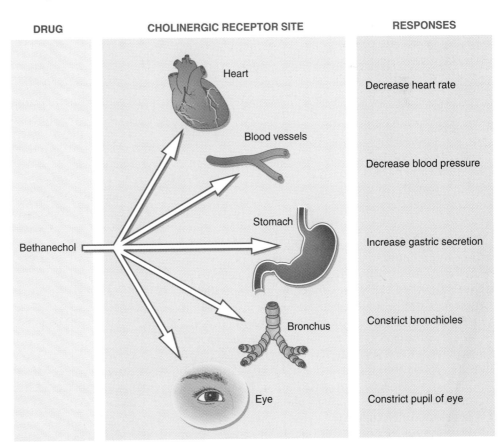

DRUG   CHOLINERGIC RECEPTOR SITE   RESPONSES

Heart   Decrease heart rate

Blood vessels   Decrease blood pressure

Bethanechol

Stomach   Increase gastric secretion

Bronchus   Constrict bronchioles

Eye   Constrict pupil of eye

Figure 1–6
Cholinergic receptors are located in the heart, blood vessels, stomach, bronchi, and eyes.

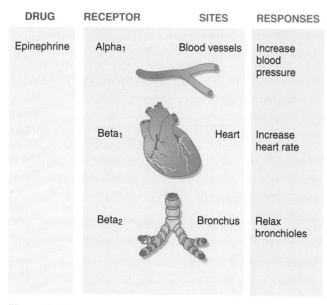

DRUG	RECEPTOR	SITES	RESPONSES
Epinephrine	Alpha$_1$	Blood vessels	Increase blood pressure
	Beta$_1$	Heart	Increase heart rate
	Beta$_2$	Bronchus	Relax bronchioles

Figure 1–7
Epinephrine affects three different receptors: alpha$_1$, beta$_1$, and beta$_2$.

strengthening bladder contraction. Because bethanechol affects the cholinergic receptor, other cholinergic sites are also affected. The heart rate decreases, blood pressure decreases, gastric acid secretion increases, the bronchioles constrict, and the pupils of the eye constrict (Fig. 1–6). These other effects may be desirable or may be harmful. Drugs that evoke a variety of responses throughout the body have a nonspecific response.

Drugs may act at different receptors. Drugs that affect various receptors are **nonselective** or have properties of nonselectivity. Chlorpromazine (Thorazine) acts on the norepinephrine, dopamine, acetylcholine, and histamine receptors, and a variety of responses result from action at these receptor sites (Fig. 1–7). Epinephrine acts on the alpha$_1$, beta$_1$, and beta$_2$, receptors.

Drugs that produce a response but do *not* act on a receptor may act by stimulating or inhibiting enzyme activity or hormone production.

The four categories of drug action include (1) stimulation or depression, (2) replacement, (3) inhibition or killing of organisms, and (4) irritation. In drug action that stimulates, the rate of cell activity or the secretion from a gland increases. In drug action that depresses, cell activity and function of a specific organ are reduced. Replacement drugs, such as insulin, replace essential body compounds. Drugs that inhibit or kill organisms interfere with bacterial cell growth (e.g., penicillin exerts its bactericidal effects by blocking the synthesis of the bacterial cell wall). Drugs also can act by the mechanism of irritation: laxatives can irritate the inner wall of the colon, thus increasing peristalsis and defecation.

Drug action might last hours, days, weeks, or months. The length of action depends on the half-life of the drug, so half-life is a reasonable guide for determining drug dosage intervals. Drugs with a short half-life, such as penicillin G (t ½ is 2 h), are given several times a day. Drugs with a long half-life, such as digoxin (36 h), are given once a day. If a drug with a long half-life is given twice or more times a day, drug accumulation in the body and drug toxicity are likely to result. If there is liver or renal impairment, the half-life of the drug increases. In these cases, high doses of the drug or too-frequent dosing can result in drug toxicity.

Therapeutic Index and Therapeutic Range (Therapeutic Window)

The safety of drugs is a major concern. The **therapeutic index** (TI) estimates the margin of safety of a drug by using a ratio that measures the effective (therapeutic or concentration) dose in 50% of persons or animals (ED$_{50}$) and lethal dose in 50% of animals (LD$_{50}$) (Fig. 1–8). The closer the ratio is to 1, the greater the danger of toxicity.

$$TI = \frac{LD_{50}}{ED_{50}}$$

In some cases the ED may be 25% (ED$_{25}$) or 75% (ED$_{75}$).

Drugs with a **low therapeutic index** have a narrow margin of safety (Fig. 1–9A). Drug dosage might need adjustment and plasma (serum) drug levels need to be monitored because of the small safety range between effective dose and lethal dose. Drugs with a **high therapeutic index** have a wide margin of safety and less danger of producing toxic effects (see Fig. 1–9B). Plasma (serum) drug levels do not need to be monitored routinely for drugs with a high therapeutic index.

The **therapeutic range (therapeutic window)** of a drug concentration in plasma should be between the minimum effective concentration (MEC) in the plasma

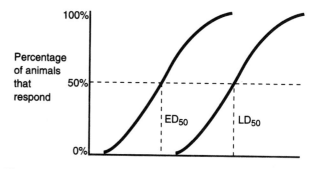

Figure 1–8
The therapeutic index measures the margin of safety of a drug. It is a ratio that measures the effective therapeutic dose and the lethal dose.

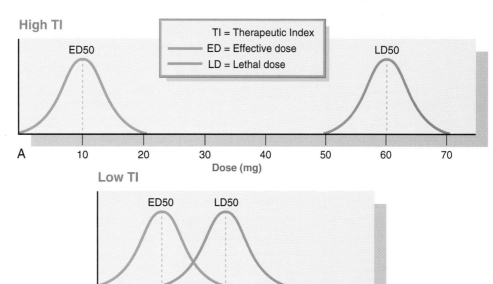

Figure 1–9
(A) A high therapeutic index drug has a wide margin of safety and carries less risk of drug toxicity. (B) A low therapeutic index drug has a narrow margin of safety, and the drug effect should be closely monitored. (Adapted from Swonger, A. K., and Matejski, M. P.: *Nursing Pharmacology*, 2/E. Philadelphia: JB Lippincott, p. 37, 1991.)

for obtaining desired drug action and the minimum toxic concentration (MTC), the toxic effect. When the therapeutic range is given, it includes both protein-bound and unbound portions of the drug. Drug reference books give many plasma (serum) therapeutic ranges of drugs. If the therapeutic range is narrow, such as for digoxin (0.5 to 2 ng/mL [nanograms per milliliter]), the plasma drug level should be monitored periodically to avoid drug toxicity. Monitoring the therapeutic range is not necessary if the drug is *not* considered highly toxic. Table 1–3 lists the therapeutic ranges and toxic levels for anticonvulsants.

Peak and Trough Levels

Peak drug level is the highest plasma concentration of drug at a specific time. If the drug is given orally, the peak time might be 1 to 3 h after drug administration. If the drug is given intravenously, the peak

time might occur in 10 min. A blood sample should be drawn at the proposed peak time, according to the route of administration.

The **trough level** is the lowest plasma concentration of a drug and measures the rate at which the drug is eliminated. Trough levels are drawn immediately before the next dose of drug is given, regardless of route of administration. Peak levels indicate the **rate of absorption** of the drug, and the trough levels indicate the **rate of elimination** of the drug. Peak and trough levels are requested for drugs that have a narrow therapeutic index and are considered toxic, such as the aminoglycoside antibiotics (Table 1–4). If either the peak or trough level is too high, toxicity can occur. If the peak is too low, no therapeutic effect is achieved.

Loading Dose

When immediate drug response is desired, a large initial dose, known as the **loading dose,** of drug is

Table 1–3
Anticonvulsants: Therapeutic Ranges and Toxic Levels

DRUG	THERAPEUTIC RANGE (μg/mL)	TOXIC LEVEL (μg/mL)
Carbamazepine	6–12	>12–15
Ethosuximide	40–80	>80–100
Phenytoin	10–20	>30
Primidone	5–10	>12–15
Valproic acid	50–100	>100

Table 1–4
Aminoglycoside Antibiotics: Peaks and Troughs

DRUG	PEAK (μg/mL)	TROUGH (μg/mL)	TOXIC PEAK LEVEL (μg/mL)	TOXIC TROUGH LEVELS (μg/mL)
Amikacin	15–30	5–10	>35	>10
Gentamicin	5–10	<2	>12	>2
Tobramycin	5–10	<2	>12	>2

given to achieve a rapid MEC in the plasma. After a large initial dose, a prescribed dosage per day is ordered. Digoxin, a digitalis preparation, requires a loading dose when first prescribed. *Digitalization* is the term used to achieve the MEC level for digoxin in the plasma within a short time.

Side Effects, Adverse Reactions, and Toxic Effects

Side effects are physiologic effects not related to desired drug effects. All drugs have side effects, desirable or undesirable. Even with a correct drug dosage, side effects occur and are predicted. Side effects result mostly from drugs that lack specificity, such as bethanechol (Urecholine). In some health problems, side effects may be desirable, such as the use of diphenhydramine HCl (Benadryl) at bedtime when its side effect of drowsiness is beneficial. At times, however, side effects are called adverse reactions. The terms *side effects* and *adverse reactions* might be used interchangeably. **Adverse reactions** are more severe than side effects. They are a range of untoward effects (unintended and occurring at normal doses) of drugs that cause mild to severe side effects, including anaphylaxis (cardiovascular collapse). Adverse reactions are always undesirable. Adverse effects must always be reported and documented, because they represent variances from planned therapy.

Toxic effects, or **toxicity,** of a drug can be identified by monitoring the plasma (serum) therapeutic range of the drug. However, for drugs that have a wide therapeutic index, the therapeutic ranges are seldom given. For those drugs with a narrow therapeutic index, such as aminoglycoside antibiotics and anticonvulsants, the therapeutic ranges are closely monitored. When the drug level exceeds the therapeutic range, toxic effects are likely to occur from overdosing or drug accumulation.

Pharmacogenetics

Pharmacogenetics is the effect of a drug action that varies from a predicted drug response because of genetic factors or hereditary influence. Because people have different genetic make-up, they do not always respond identically to a drug dosage or planned drug therapy. Genetic factors can alter the metabolism of the drug in converting its chemical form to an inert metabolite; thus, the drug action can be enhanced or diminished. Some persons are less or more sensitive to drugs and their drug actions because of genetic factors.

Tachyphylaxis

Drug tolerance to a frequently repeated administration of a certain drug is known as **tachyphylaxis.** Drug categories that can cause tachyphylaxis include narcotics, barbiturates, laxatives, and psychotropic agents. Prevention of tachyphylaxis should always be part of the therapeutic regimen.

Placebo Effect

A **placebo effect** is a psychologic benefit from a compound that may not have the chemical structure of a drug effect. The placebo is effective in approximately one-third of persons taking a placebo compound. Many of the clinical drug studies involve a group of subjects who receive a placebo.

SUMMARY

The phases of drug action are pharmaceutic, pharmacokinetic, and pharmacodynamic. Figure 1–10 illustrates these three phases for drugs given orally, but drugs given by injection are involved only in the pharmacokinetic and pharmacodynamic phases. Nurses should be aware that tablets must disintegrate and go into solution (the pharmaceutic phase) to be absorbed.

To avoid toxic effects, the nurse needs to know the half-life, protein-binding percentage, normal side effects, and therapeutic ranges of the drug. This information can be obtained from drug reference books.

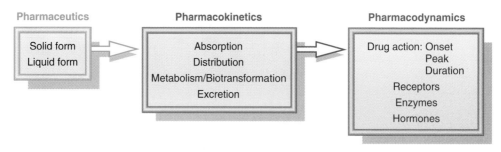

Figure 1–10
Three phases of drug action.

NURSING PROCESS

Assessment

- Recognize that drugs in liquid form are absorbed faster than those in solid form.
- Assess for signs and symptoms of drug toxicity when giving two drugs that are highly protein-bound. The drugs compete for protein-binding sites and displacement of drugs occurs. More free drug is in circulation because there are not enough protein-binding sites. Too much of a free drug can result in drug toxicity.
- Assess for side effects of drugs that are nonspecific (same receptor at different tissue and organ sites). For example, when atropine is the drug, assess for tachycardia, dry mouth and throat, constipation, urinary retention, and blurred vision. If nonspecific drugs are given in large doses or at frequent intervals, many side effects are likely to occur.
- Assess for side effects of drugs that are nonselective (drugs that affect different receptors).
- Check peak levels and trough levels of drugs that have a narrow therapeutic range, such as aminoglycosides. If the trough level is high, toxic effects can result.

Nursing Interventions

- Advise the client not to eat fatty food before ingesting an enteric-coated tablet, because fatty foods decrease absorption rate.
- Check the drug literature for the protein-binding percentage of the drug. Those drugs with a high protein-binding effect have a large portion of drug bound to protein, causing the drug to become inactive until it is released from the protein. The portion that is not bound to protein is free drug.
- Report to the health care provider if drugs with a long half-life (greater than 24 h) are given more than once a day. Some drugs with a long half-life, such as the anticoagulant warfarin (Coumadin), can be more dangerous than others and should be monitored frequently.
- Monitor the therapeutic range of drugs that are more toxic or have a narrow therapeutic range, such as digoxin.

Evaluation

- Evaluate the determinants affecting drug therapy according to Figure 1–11 on p. 14.

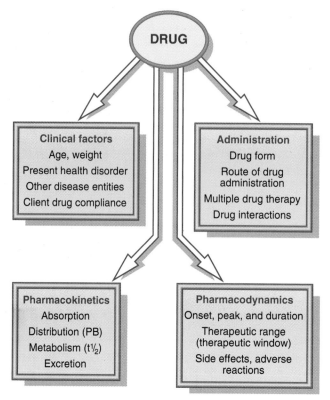

Figure 1–11
Determinants affecting drug therapy.

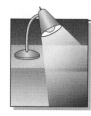

Study Questions

1. What are the three phases of drug action?

2. What are the two processes that a tablet undergoes before it is absorbed? Describe each process.

3. What is the purpose of pharmacokinetics? Name the four processes involved and describe each.

4. Explain the term *first-pass effect* or *hepatic metabolism* of the drug. What effect does first-pass have on drug bioavailability and activity?

5. What is the purpose of pharmacodynamics? What is the role of receptors in this phase? Of what importance is the location of the receptor? Differentiate between nonspecific and nonselective drug responses.

6. Define the following: bioavailability, protein-bound drugs, half-life, therapeutic index, therapeutic drug range, therapeutic window, side effects, adverse reaction, and toxicity. What are the implications of these terms to your nursing practice?

7. A drug that is 75% protein-bound is considered to be _____ protein-bound.

Nursing Process and Client Teaching

Outline

Objectives

- Identify the steps of the nursing process and their purpose in relation to drug therapy.
- Identify the components of a goal.
- State at least eight principles for health teaching related to drug therapy plans.

Terms

assessment

evaluation

goal setting

holistic nursing approach

implementation

nursing diagnosis

planning

INTRODUCTION

Nurses have a significant role in the management of drug therapy. Influences on this role include technology, increased longevity of the citizenry, and survival of those with multiple and varied bio-psychosocial needs. Variables in drug therapy are numerous and, at times, unknown. A **holistic nursing approach** to care is crucial to the success of drug therapy initiation, maintenance, and evaluation.

This chapter explores the use of the nursing process as it relates to drug therapy. Careful detail to each step of the process fosters the client's success with the prescribed medication regimen. Considerations in the use of over-the-counter (OTC) drugs and herbal remedies are explored in Chapters 7 and 8, respectively.

NURSING PROCESS

The steps of the nursing process are assessment (including nursing diagnosis), planning, implementation, and evaluation. Each step is discussed as it relates to health teaching in drug therapy.

Assessment

Assessment, the first step of the nursing process, is particularly important because the data provided by the assessment form the basis on which care is planned, implemented, and evaluated. Data collection involves both subjective and objective information.

Subjective Data

Current health history

Client symptoms as verbalized by client

Current medications
   Dosage, frequency, route, prescribing health care provider, if any
   Client knowledge about drug and its side effects, and for what diagnosis/symptoms the client is taking the drug
   Client expectation and perception of drug effectiveness
   Client compliance with regimen and reasons for deviations. Are deviations based on valid data/rationale and clinically sound?
   Drug allergies or reactions, both past and present; also food/dye intolerance and reactions
   OTC drugs
   Herbal remedies
   Street drugs—frequency of use

Past health history
   Past illnesses, major injuries, and drug therapy, including reactions
   Medications saved from previous use; how stored; expiration date
   Street drugs
Client's environment
   History of compliance with drug therapy as prescribed; i.e., were prescriptions filled and finished?
   Does client read and follow instructions from the health care provider and/or the pharmacy?
   Availability, willingness, and ability to administer or assist in the administration of medications. This information is essential for third-party payment for continued home visits or for admission to an extended care facility
   Household members, neighbors, friends, and their roles; ages of household members
   Activities of daily living (ADL) capabilities
   Dietary patterns, cultural and economic influences, safety
   Financial resources (drugs can be expensive)
   Mental status

REMEMBER: Clients, even those who do not intend to withhold information, do not always tell all about their medications. Therefore, in addition to asking about prescription drugs, ask specifically about vitamin, birth control, aspirin or acetaminophen, and antihistamine or decongestant use. Also identify caffeine and nicotine use. Ask to see the contents of the medicine chest at home (or other storage area for medications) and whether a pharmacist is used as a consultant.

Objective Data

Laboratory tests   } Baseline data for future
Diagnostic studies   }   comparisons
Physical assessment

Data collection should focus on symptoms and those organs most likely to be affected by drug therapy. For example, if a drug is nephrotoxic, the client's creatinine clearance would be assessed. Assess major body systems for any signs of reaction or interaction of drugs or ineffectiveness of therapy.

NURSING DIAGNOSIS

A **nursing diagnosis** is made based on the analysis of the assessment data. More than one applicable nursing diagnosis may be generated, and a nursing diagnosis may be actual or potential. The registered nurse formulates nursing diagnoses and uses them, with the assistance of others, to guide the care plans. A list of nursing diagnoses accepted by the North American Nursing Diagnosis Association (NANDA) is presented in Table 2–1.

Common nursing diagnoses related to drug therapy include the following:

• Knowledge deficit about drug action, administration, and side effects related to language difficulties
• Risk for injury related to side effects of drug, such as dizziness and drowsiness related to a cerebral vascular accident
• Alteration in thought processes related to forgetfulness, affecting whether the client takes medication as prescribed
• Ineffective management of therapeutic regimen

The benefit to the client of the nursing diagnosis is that it facilitates development of an optimal quality care plan.

Planning

The **planning** phase of the nursing process is characterized by **goal setting** or expected outcomes. Effective goal setting has the following qualities:

• Client-centered and clearly states the expected change
• Acceptable to both client and nurse (dependent on client decision-making ability)
• Realistic and measurable
• Shared with other health care providers
• Realistic deadlines
• Prescriptive for evaluation

Examples of a goal are (1) E. C. (client) will independently administer prescribed dose of insulin by the end of the fourth session of instruction; (2) D. Z. will prepare a medication recording sheet that correctly reflects prescribed medication schedule within 3 days.

Table 2–1
Nursing Diagnoses Accepted by NANDA 1997

Activity intolerance	Coping, ineffective community	Health maintenance, altered
Activity intolerance, risk for	Coping, defensive	Health-seeking behaviors (specify)
Adaptive capacity, decreased: intracranial	Coping, family: potential for growth	Home maintenance management, impaired
Adjustment, impaired	Coping, ineffective family: compromised	Hopelessness
Airway clearance, ineffective	Coping, ineffective family: disabling	Hyperthermia
Anxiety	Coping, ineffective individual	Hypothermia
Aspiration, risk for	Decisional conflict (specify)	Incontinence, bowel
Body image disturbance	Denial, ineffective	Incontinence, functional
Body temperature, altered, risk for	Diarrhea	Incontinence, reflex
Bowel elimination, altered	Disuse syndrome, risk for	Incontinence, stress
Bowel incontinence	Diversional activity deficit	Incontinence, total
Breastfeeding, effective	Dysreflexia	Incontinence, urge
Breastfeeding, ineffective	Energy field disturbance	Infant behavior, disorganized
Breastfeeding, interrupted	Environmental interpretation syndrome, impaired	Infant behavior, disorganized, risk for
Breathing pattern, ineffective	Family processes, altered	Infant behavior, organized, potential for enhanced
Cardiac output, decreased	Family processes, altered: alcoholism	Infant feeding pattern, ineffective
Caregiver role strain	Fatigue	Infection, risk for
Caregiver role strain, risk for	Fear	Injury, risk for
Comfort, altered	Fluid volume deficit (1)	Knowledge deficit (specify)
Communication, impaired verbal	Fluid volume deficit (2)	Loneliness, risk for
Confusion, acute	Fluid volume deficit, risk for	Management of therapeutic regimen (community), ineffective
Confusion, chronic	Fluid volume excess	
Constipation	Gas exchange, impaired	Management of therapeutic regimen (families), ineffective
Constipation, colonic	Grieving, anticipatory	
Constipation, perceived	Grieving, dysfunctional	Management of therapeutic regimen (individual), effective
Coping, community: potential for enhanced	Growth and development, altered	

Table continued on following page

Table 2–1 *Continued*
Nursing Diagnoses Accepted by NANDA 1997

Management of therapeutic regimen (individual), ineffective	Powerlessness	Sleep pattern disturbance
Memory, impaired	Protection, altered	Social interaction, impaired
Mobility, impaired physical	Rape-trauma syndrome	Social isolation
Noncompliance (specify)	Rape-trauma syndrome: compound reaction	Spiritual distress (distress of the human spirit)
Nutrition, altered: less than body requirements	Rape-trauma syndrome: silent reaction	Spiritual well-being, potential for enhanced
Nutrition, altered: more than body requirements	Relocation stress syndrome	Suffocation, risk for
Nutrition, altered: risk for more than body requirements	Role performance, altered	Swallowing, impaired
Oral mucous membrane, altered	Self-care deficit, bathing/hygiene	Thermoregulation, ineffective
Pain	Self-care deficit, dressing/grooming	Thought processes, altered
Pain, chronic	Self-care deficit, feeding	Tissue integrity, impaired
Parent/infant/child attachment, altered, risk for	Self-care deficit, toileting	Tissue perfusion, altered (specify type) (renal, cerebral, cardiopulmonary, gastrointestinal, peripheral)
Parental role conflict	Self-concept, disturbance in	Trauma, risk for
Parenting, altered	Self-esteem disturbance	Unilateral neglect
Parenting, altered, risk for	Self-esteem, chronic low	Urinary elimination, altered patterns
Perioperative positioning injury, risk for	Self-esteem, situational low	Urinary retention
Peripheral neurovascular dysfunction, risk for	Self-mutilation, risk for	Ventilation, inability to sustain spontaneous
Personal identity disturbance	Sensory/perceptual alterations (specify) (visual, auditory, kinesthetic, gustatory, tactile, olfactory)	Ventilatory weaning process, dysfunctional (DVWR)
Poisoning, risk for	Sexual dysfunction	Violence, risk for: directed at others
Post-trauma response	Sexuality patterns, altered	Violence, risk for: self-directed
	Skin integrity, impaired	
	Skin integrity, impaired, risk for	

Implementation

The **implementation** phase includes the nursing actions necessary to accomplish the established goals or expected outcomes. Client education and teaching are key nursing responsibilities during this phase. In most practice settings, administration of drugs and assessment of drug effectiveness are also important nursing responsibilities.

Client education is an ongoing process. Teaching is more effective in an environment free of distractions, and the information should be tailored to the client's interests and level of understanding. Assessment data suggest the complexity, number, and length of teaching sessions that may be required. Be sensitive to the client's motivation to learn, attention span, and level of frustration. Readiness to learn is paramount. Readiness should be assessed first, before information is presented to the client. Use a positive approach; for example, "This narcotic is usually effective in relieving the type of pain that you have." Be an *active* listener and observer.

The inclusion of a family member or friend in the teaching plan is an excellent idea. Provide simple written materials. Assessment data guide the nurse to the appropriate persons to be included. This other person may act as a psychological support, actually administer all or part of the drug therapy, observe the effectiveness and side effects of drug therapy, and implement other changes, such as doing the shopping or instituting new methods of food preparation. Health professionals should be available for the client to call with any questions or concerns.

Client teaching is a complex activity. As such, it might be helpful for the nurse to use an outline format. Suggested headings related to pharmacotherapeutics include the following:

• *General.* Instruct the client to take drug as prescribed. Compliance is of utmost importance, because discontinuing the drug before the course is completed may result in relapse or future ineffectiveness of the drug. Do not adjust dose, frequency, or time of day taken unless directed by the health care provider. Advise women contemplating pregnancy to check first with their health care provider before taking the antitubercular drugs ethambutol or rifampin. Advise clients to consult with their health care provider about laboratory tests such as liver enzymes, blood urea nitrogen (BUN), creatinine, and electrolytes, which should be monitored when taking drugs such as antifungal agents.

• *Self-administration.* Instruct the client on administration of drug according to prescribed route, such as eye or nose drops, subcutaneous insulin injections, suppositories, swish and swallow suspensions, and metered-dose inhalers with and without spacers. Include demonstration and return demonstration in the instruction when appropriate and give written instructions for the sighted client or audio instructions for the visually impaired. Instruct more than one person, when possible, because this aids in reinforcement and retention of information.

• *Diet.* Instruct clients about what foods to include in their diet and what foods to avoid. For example, advise clients to eat foods rich in potassium (e.g., bananas) when taking most diuretics, unless they are on a KCl supplement, and to avoid large amounts of green, leafy vegetables if taking warfarin (Coumadin) preparations.

• *Side effects.* Instruct the client to immediately report to the designated health care provider, usually a nurse, physician, or pharmacist, if he or she experiences unusual symptoms. Also, give the client instructions that help minimize any side effects, such as avoiding direct sunlight when there is risk of photosensitivity/sunburn. Inform the client of any expected changes in the color of urine or stool. Advise the client who has dizziness caused by orthostatic hypotension to rise slowly from a sitting to a standing position.

• *Cultural considerations.* Be alert to client/family cultural expectations. For example, *time* may not be viewed as important, thereby affecting the client's adherence to taking medications at specific time intervals during the day to ensure therapeutic blood levels of the medication.

A teaching plan with interventions that involve stimulation of several senses and active participation by the client enhances learning. Inclusion of return demonstrations by the client and others, when applicable, gives the nurse important feedback about the client's learning and gives the client confidence in carrying out the regimen or selected aspects of the regimen. Additional teaching tips include the following:

• Provide written instructions in addition to other teaching aids.
• Use colorful charts and graphs.
• Teach with audiocassette tapes; obtain a tape recorder.
• Encourage client and family questions; provide time for this. Do not rush.

• Use materials and language appropriate to the client's level of understanding.
• Space instruction over several sessions, if appropriate.
• Review community resources related to the client's nursing diagnosis.
• Support multiagency collaboration in mobilization of resources.

A client teaching session is shown in Figure 2–1. The use of teaching drug cards is helpful. These cards provide information about a specific drug or drug group. They may be developed by the health care provider or obtained from drug manufacturers. Cassette tapes and videos are available from many drug companies. Group classes are useful for clients with certain diagnoses or who require certain drugs. A variety of formats can be developed. Be creative! Helpful components include the following:

• Name of drug
• Reason you are taking drug
• Your dose is
• Specific times to take the drug
• What specific things you should or should not do while taking the medication; e.g., tablets may or may not be crushed, etc.
• Possible side effects of medication

In addition to the individualized component of the teaching drug card, there are some general helpful and healthful points to remember. These pointers are presented in Table 2–2.

Enhancing client compliance with the drug therapy regimen is an essential component of health teaching. The client and family response to the following three questions provides the nurse with critical information unique to each client's teaching situation.

1. What things help you take your medicine as you should?

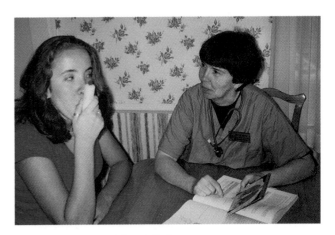

Figure 2–1
Client teaching session.

Table 2–2
Helpful and Healthful Points to Remember

1. Take medication as prescribed by your health care provider. If you have questions, call.
2. Keep medication in original labeled container and store as instructed.
3. Keep all medicines **out of reach** of children. Remind grandparents and visitors to monitor their purses and luggage when visiting.
4. **Before** using any OTC drugs, check with your health care provider. This includes use of aspirin, laxatives, and so on. Pharmacists are good resources to ask before buying or using a product.
5. Bring all medications with you when you visit the health care provider.
6. Know why you are taking each medication and under what circumstances to notify the health care provider.
7. Alcohol may alter the action and absorption of the medication. Use of alcoholic beverages is discouraged around the time you are taking your medications and is absolutely contraindicated with certain medications.
8. Smoking tobacco also alters the absorption of some medications (e.g., theophylline-type drugs, tranquilizers, antidepressants, and pain medications). Consult your health care provider/pharmacist for specific information.

2. What things prevent you from taking your medicine as you should?

3. What would you do or what do you do when you forget to take a medication?

Frequently cited factors for noncompliance include forgetfulness, knowledge deficit, side effects, low self-esteem, depression, lack of trust in the health care system, family problems, language barriers, high cost of medications, anxiety, value systems (religious and other), and lack of motivation.

Many people take multiple medications simultaneously several times each day, presenting a challenge to the client, his or her family, and the nurse. This complex activity can be segmented into several simple tasks, including the following:

• Preparation of 1 day's or 1 week's supply of medication. The day's medication can be put in one container. Sorting of a day's supply allows the client and the nurse to see at a glance what medications have and have not been taken. Keep in mind that a missing pill may have been dropped and not actually taken. A variation in accomplishing this task is to take a day's medication and sort or package the pills according to the time each is to be taken. Multicompartment dispensers (available at local drug or

variety stores) or an egg carton may help some clients sort their drugs.

• A recording sheet may be helpful. The client or a family member marks when each medication is taken. The sheet is designed to meet the client's individual needs; for example, the time can be noted by the client or could be entered before hand, with the client marking when each dose is taken. A generic format follows:

MEDICATION	DOSAGE (mg daily)	DAY OF WEEK S M T W T F S
Captopril (Capoten)	12.5	
Digoxin	0.25	
Furosemide (Lasix)	40	

Figure 2–2 shows a nurse reviewing recording of medications with her client. Alternatives to recording sheets are also available. Mechanical alarm reminder devices may be helpful to some clients.

• A combination of daily supply and recording may be helpful. Consider color coding. Visual acuity, manual dexterity, and mental processes have a major effect on which system works best for each client.

Throughout the teaching plan, the nurse promotes client independence. The nurse should not lose sight of the goals or outcomes and become immersed in the intervention process, for example, teaching a client with short-term memory loss. Table 2–3 presents suggestions for a checklist for health teaching in drug therapy.

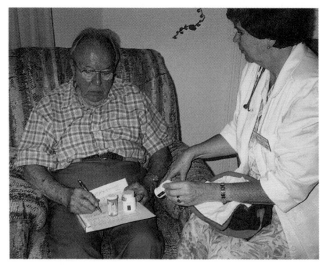

Figure 2–2
A client records his medications on a schedule sheet.

Table 2-3
Checklist for Health Teaching in Drug Therapy

- Comprehensive drug and health history
- Reason for medication therapy
- Expected results
- Side effects and adverse reactions
- When to notify physician, pharmacist, or health care provider
- Drug–drug, drug–food, drug–laboratory, drug–environment interactions
- Required changes in ADL
- Demonstration of learning; may take several forms, such as listening, discussing, or return demonstration of psychomotor skills (insulin administration)
- Medication schedule, associated with ADL and drug level of action as appropriate
- Recording system
- Discussion and monitoring of access to financial resources, medication, and associated equipment
- Development and support of back-up system
- Community resources

Evaluation

The effectiveness of health teaching about drug therapy and attainment of goals are addressed in the evaluation phase of the nursing process. The time at which the **evaluation** of a goal occurs is dependent on the time frame specified in the statement of a goal.

Evaluation should be ongoing and related to progress as well as to attainment of the final goal.

If goals are not met, the nurse needs to determine the reasons for this and revise the plan accordingly. This includes additional assessment data and the setting of new goals. If the goals are met, the plan of care has been completed.

To complete the care for any current client, follow these recommendations:

- Review with the client and family the need for follow-up care, if required.
- Encourage choices in ADL.
- Refer the client to community resources, as necessary.

Figure 2–3 shows a nurse meeting with a client and his spouse to review his therapeutic regimen.

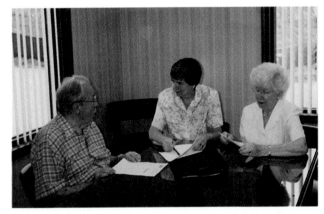

Figure 2-3
A nurse reviews the therapeutic regimen with a client and spouse.

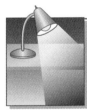

Study Questions

1. What are the steps of the nursing process and the primary purpose of each step?
2. Explain how the nursing process relates to administration of medications.
3. What are the essential components of a goal? Write a goal that incorporates all the essential components. How and when would you know if a goal or outcome is realistic for client?
4. What is the basis of a nursing diagnosis?
5. List at least five principles of health teaching about drug therapy regimens.
6. Identify at least two ways to suggest to organize multiple medications being taken on a daily basis.
7. List three ways to evaluate whether a client is compliant with a drug therapy regimen.

3

Principles of Drug Administration

Outline

Objectives

- Describe the "five plus five rights" of drug administration.
- List safety guidelines for drug administration.
- Identify factors modifying drug response.
- Describe routes of administration.
- Identify the various sites for parenteral therapy.
- Explain the equipment and technique used in parenteral therapy.
- Explain the method for charting medications.
- Describe the nursing interventions related to administration of medications by various routes.

Terms

absorption	metabolism	right route
buccal	metered-dose inhaler	right time
canister	parenteral	spacer
cumulative effect	pharmacogenetics	subcutaneous
distribution	right assessment	sublingual
informed consent	right client	suppositories
inhalation	right documentation	tolerance
instillation	right dose	topical
intradermal	right drug	toxicity
intramuscular	right to education	transdermal
intravenous	right evaluation	unit dose
meniscus	right to refuse	Z-track technique

INTRODUCTION

Administration of medications is a basic activity in nursing practice. As a result of the transition from hospital/institution to community-based services, an increasing number of nurses are practicing in a variety of settings. Nurses must be knowledgeable about the actual drugs, their administration, client response, and related resources.

Nurses are accountable for the safe administration of medications. Nurses must know all the components of a drug order and question those orders that are not complete or clear or that give a dosage outside the recommended range. Nurses are legally liable if they give a prescribed drug and the dosage is incorrect or the drug is contraindicated for the client's health status. In some health care settings, medical students write drug orders; these orders must be countersigned by an attending or staff physician or other prescribing health care provider before they are considered official. Once the drug has been administered, the nurse becomes liable for the predicted effects of that drug. Drug references, such as the *United States Pharmacopeia (USP), National Formulary (NF), Physicians' Desk Reference (PDR), and American Hospital Formulary* drug reference handbook, and human resources, such as pharmacists, must be consulted when the nurse is unsure about the expected therapeutic effect, contraindications, dosage, potential side effects, or adverse reactions of a medication.

This chapter describes selected, essential content related to administration of medications, a multifaceted activity. Selected content areas include the "rights" of drug administration, factors that modify drug response, guidelines for various routes of administration, and related nursing implications.

THE "FIVE PLUS FIVE RIGHTS" IN DRUG ADMINISTRATION

To provide safe drug administration, the nurse should practice the "rights" of drug administration. The traditional five rights are the right client, the right drug, the right dose, the right time, and the right route. Experience indicates that five additional rights are essential to professional nursing practice: the right assessment, the right documentation, the client's right to education, the right evaluation, and the client's right to refuse.

The **right client** can be assured by checking the client's identification bracelet and by having the client state her or his name. Some clients answer to any name or are unable to respond, so client identification should be verified *each* time a medication is administered. In the event of a missing identification bracelet, the nurse must verify the client's identity before any drug administration.

Nursing implications include

- Verify client by checking the identification band. Some facilities put the client's photo on his or her health record.
- Distinguish between two clients with the same last name; have warnings highlighted in bright color on identification (ID) tools, such as med cards, bracelet, or Kardex.

Where clients are not wearing ID bands (school, occupational health, outpatient departments, health care provider's office), the nurse also has the responsibility of accurately identifying the individual when administering a medication.

The **right drug** means that the client receives the drug that was prescribed. Medication orders may be prescribed by a physician (MD), dentist (DDS), podiatrist (DPM), or a licensed health care provider such as an advanced practice registered nurse (APRN) with authority from the state to order medications. Prescriptions may be written on a prescription pad and filled by a pharmacist at a drug store or hospital pharmacy (Fig. 3–1). For institutionalized clients, the drug orders may be written on "order sheets" and signed by the duly authorized person (Fig. 3–2). A telephone order (TO) or verbal order (VO) for medication must be cosigned by the health care provider within 24 h. The nurse must comply with the institution's policy regarding a telephone order, which sometimes requires that two licensed practitioners listen to and sign the order.

The use of computerized systems has added speed and a safety feature to the order process. Orders can be written from virtually any location and sent via modem. The computer will not "take" the order unless all the information is included. Also, there is no need to worry about illegible orders or signatures. The same benefits are available to nurses for recording the medications given or refused.

The components of a drug order are as follows:

- Date and time the order is written
- Drug name (generic preferred)
- Drug dosage
- Route of administration
- Frequency and duration of administration, such as times seven days, times three doses
- Any special instructions for withholding or adjusting dosage based on nursing assessment, drug effectiveness, or laboratory results
- Physician or other health care provider's signature or name if TO or VO
- Signatures of licensed practitioners taking TO or VO

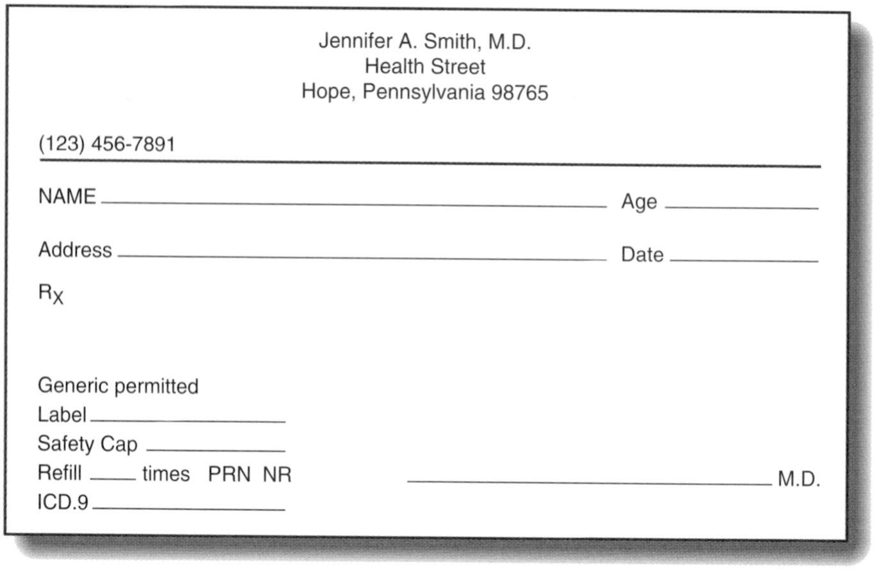

Jennifer A. Smith, M.D.
Health Street
Hope, Pennsylvania 98765

(123) 456-7891
_____

NAME _____ Age _____

Address _____ Date _____

R~X~

Generic permitted
Label _____
Safety Cap _____
Refill ____ times PRN NR   _____ M.D.
ICD.9 _____

Figure 3–1
Prescription pad medication order.

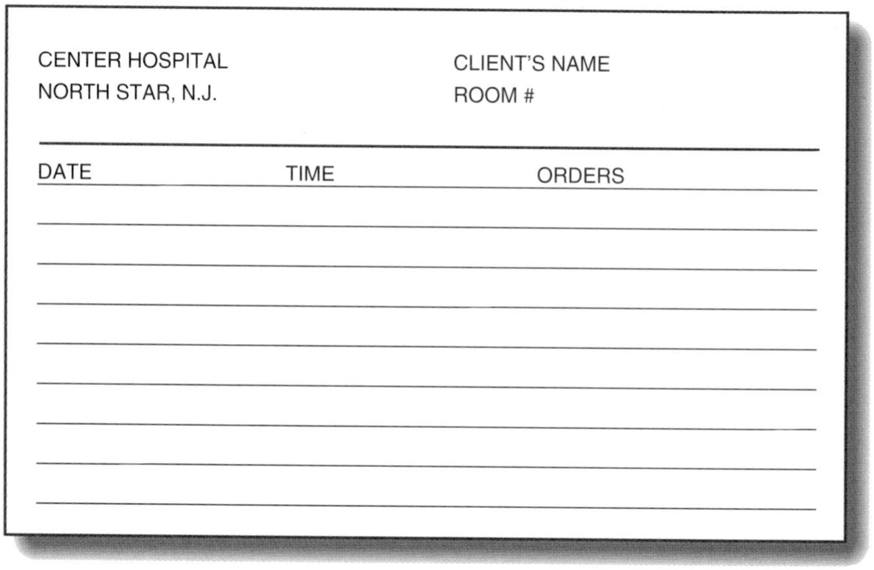

CENTER HOSPITAL   CLIENT'S NAME
NORTH STAR, N.J.   ROOM #
_____

DATE   TIME   ORDERS
_____
_____
_____
_____
_____
_____
_____
_____

Figure 3–2
Client's or-
ders.

Although the nurse's responsibility is to follow an appropriate order, if any one of the components is missing, the drug order is incomplete and the drug should not be administered. Clarification of the order must be done in a timely manner; the health care provider is usually contacted. The following is an example of a drug order and its interpretation: **6/4/99 10:10A Lasix 40 mg, PO, q.d. (signature)** (Give 40 mg of Lasix by mouth daily.)

To avoid drug error, the drug label should be read three times: (1) at the time of contact with the drug bottle or container, (2) before pouring the drug, and (3) after pouring the drug. The first dose, one-time, and PRN medication orders should be checked against original orders. Nurses should be aware that certain drug names sound alike and are spelled simi-

larly. Examples are digoxin and digitoxin; quinidine and quinine; Keflex and Kantrex; Demerol and dicumarol; and Percocet and Percodan. More specifically, Percocet contains oxycodone and acetaminophen, whereas Percodan contains oxycodone and aspirin. A client may be allergic to aspirin, so it is important that this client receive Percocet. **Read the labels carefully.**

Nursing implications include

• Check that the medication order is complete and legible. If the order is not complete or legible, notify the nurse manager and health care provider.
• Know the reason for which the client is receiving the medication.
• Check the drug label three times before administering the medication.

Table 3–1
Categories of Drug Orders

CATEGORY DESCRIPTION	EXAMPLES
STANDING ORDERS	
May be an ongoing order or may be given for a specific number of doses or days	Digoxin 0.2 mg PO q.d. Colace 100 mg PO q.d., PRN
May have special instructions to base administration on laboratory values	Digoxin, maintain blood level of 0.5–2.0 ng/mL
May include PRN orders	
ONE-TIME OR SINGLE ORDERS	
Given once and usually at a specific time	Versed 2 mg IM at 7 AM
PRN ORDERS	
Given at the client's request and nurse's judgment concerning need and safety	Tylenol 650 mg q3 to 4h PRN for headache
STAT ORDERS	
Given once, immediately	Morphine sulfate 2 mg IV STAT

• Med card/Kardex should include the date the medication was ordered and any last date; for example, for controlled substances and antibiotics, and for limited/specific number of doses. Some agencies have "automatic stop orders," which are generally facility specific. Examples of such orders include controlled drugs that need to be renewed every 48 hours, anticoagulants and antibiotics to be renewed after 7 days, and cancellation of all medications when the client goes to surgery.

There are four categories of drug orders:

1. Standing
2. One-time (single)
3. PRN
4. STAT

Table 3–1 summarizes the drug order categories with examples of each.

The **right dose** is the dose prescribed for a particular client. In most cases, this dose is within the recommended range for the particular drug. Nurses must calculate each drug dose accurately, considering the variables: drug availability and the prescribed drug dose. In selected situations, the client's weight range must also be considered, such as 3 mg/kg/day. Refer to Chapter 4A through 4F for drug calculations.

Before calculating a drug dose, the nurse should have a general idea of the answer based on a knowledge of the basic formula or ratios and proportions. Calculation of drug doses should be rechecked if a fraction of a dose or an extremely large dose has been calculated. Consultation with a peer or a pharmacist should occur whenever doubt exists.

The stock drug method and unit dose method are the two most frequently used methods of drug distribution. Table 3–2 describes these methods and the advantages and disadvantages of each.

In the traditional stock drug method, the drugs are dispensed to all clients from the same containers. In the **unit dose** method, drugs are individually wrapped and labeled for single doses. The unit dose method is popular in many institutions and community settings. Unit dosing has eliminated many drug dosage errors.

Automation of medication administration, introduced more than a decade ago, is promoted as saving time and decreasing costs associated with the administration of medications. Some features include a link to the pharmacy information system and current clinical client data. In addition, the ability to automati-

Table 3–2
Drug Distribution Methods

STOCK	UNIT DOSE
DESCRIPTION	
Drugs are stored on unit and dispensed to all clients from the same container	Drugs are packaged in doses for 24 h by the pharmacy
ADVANTAGES	
Always available, cost efficiency of large quantities	Saves time for nurse; no dose calculation required
	Billed for specific doses
	More accountability
	Less chance for contamination and error
DISADVANTAGES	
Drug errors are more prevalent with multiple "pourers"	Potential delay in receiving drug
More risk of abuse by health care workers	Not immediately replaceable if contaminated
Less accountability for amount used; unable to track usage	More expensive

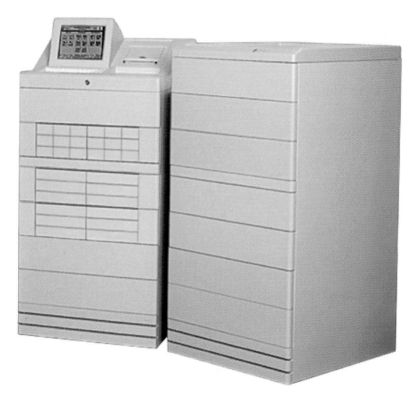

Figure 3–3
Computerized medication management system. (Courtesy of Pyxis Corp., San Diego, CA.)

cally collect information about charting and recording of medication is available. An activity report menu is a popular feature. Flexible dose modes are available, including single-dose, multi-dose, and multiple-medications. Pyxis is an example of automated medication dispensing technology (Fig. 3–3). It assists the nurse to correctly and quickly administer medications. Thus, this technology has the potential to improve client care by promoting accurate and quick access to medications.

The nursing implications include

• Calculate the drug dose correctly. When in doubt, the drug dose should be recalculated and checked by another nurse. In many settings, the first nurse to administer the particular drug to the client must calculate the dose according to the stated formulary doses and sign in the nurse's signature space once the safety parameter has been established.
• Check the *PDR, American Hospital Formulary*, drug package insert, or other drug references for recommended range of specific drug doses.

The **right time** is the time at which the prescribed dose should be administered. Daily drug dosages are given at specified times during a day, such as b.i.d. (twice a day), t.i.d. (three times a day), q.i.d. (four times a day), or q6h (every 6 h), so that the plasma level of the drug is maintained. When the drug has a long half-life (t½), the drug is given once a day. Drugs with a short half-life are given several times a

day at specified intervals (see Chapter 1). Some drugs are given before meals, and others are given with meals or with food.

Many nursing settings currently are using military time, a 24-hour clock. For examples, 2 AM is 0200; 2 PM is 1400; 6:10 AM is 0610; and 5:30 PM is 1730. AM hours correlate with the traditional clock; 12 hours are added for the PM hours (Fig. 3–4). Military time

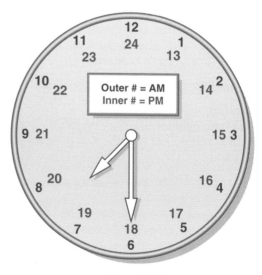

Figure 3–4
Military time.

has the advantages of reducing administration errors and decreasing documentation.

Nursing implications include

- Administer drugs at the specified times. Drugs may be given 0.5 h before or after the time prescribed if the administration interval is >2 h. Refer to agency policy.
- Administer drugs that are affected by foods, such as tetracycline, before meals.
- Administer drugs that can irritate the stomach (gastric mucosa), such as potassium and aspirin, with food.
- The drug administration schedule may sometimes be adjusted to fit schedule of client's lifestyle, activities, tolerances, or preferences.
- It is the nurse's responsibility to check whether the client is scheduled for any diagnostic procedures, such as endoscopy or fasting blood tests, that would contraindicate the administration of medications. Determine per policy if the medication should be given after test is completed.
- Check the expiration date. Discard the medication or return it to the pharmacy (depending on policy) if the date has passed.
- Antibiotics should be administered at even intervals (e.g., q8h rather than t.i.d.) throughout a 24-hour period in order to maintain therapeutic blood levels.

The **right route** is necessary for adequate or appropriate absorption. The more common routes of absorption include oral (by mouth): liquid, elixir, suspension, pill, tablet, or capsule; sublingual (under tongue for venous absorption); buccal (between gum and cheek); topical (applied to the skin); inhalation (aerosol sprays); instillation (in nose, eye, ear), suppository (rectal, vaginal); and four parenteral routes: intradermal, subcutaneous, intramuscular, and intravenous.

Nursing implications include

- Assess the client's ability to swallow before administering oral medications.
- Do not crush or mix medications in other substances before consulting a pharmacist.
- Use aseptic technique when administering drugs. Sterile technique is required with the parenteral routes.
- Administer the drugs at the appropriate sites.
- Stay with the client until oral drugs have been swallowed.

The **right documentation** requires that the nurse immediately record the appropriate information about the drug administered. This includes the *name* of the drug, the *dose,* the *route* (injection site if applicable), the *time* and *date,* and the nurse's *initials* or *signature.* Documentation of the client's response to the medica-

tion is required with a variety of medications, such as (1) narcotics (how effective was the pain relief?), (2) nonnarcotic analgesics, (3) sedatives, (4) antiemetics, and (5) unexpected reactions to the medication, such as gastrointestinal (GI) irritation or signs of skin sensitivity. Delay in charting could result in forgetting to chart the medication or in another nurse's administering the drug because she or he thought the drug was not given.

To assist in the accurate and timely recording of drugs administered, many health care facilities are using a graphic format (Fig. 3–5) or computerized systems.

The **right assessment** requires that appropriate data be collected before administration of the drug. Examples of assessment data may include measuring the apical heart rate before administering digitalis preparations or serum blood sugar levels before the administration of insulin.

The **right to education** requires that the client receive accurate and thorough information about the medication and how it relates to his or her particular situation. Client teaching also includes therapeutic purpose, possible side effects of the drug, any diet restrictions or requirements, skill of administration, and laboratory monitoring. This right is a principle of **informed consent,** which is based on the individual's having the knowledge necessary to make a decision.

The **right evaluation** requires that the effectiveness of the medication be determined by the client's response to the medication. Evaluation in this context asks, "Did the medication do for the client what it was supposed to do?" It is also appropriate to determine the extent of side effects and adverse reactions, if any.

The **right to refuse the medication.** Clients can and do refuse to take a medication. It is the nurse's responsibility to determine, when possible, the reason for the refusal and to take reasonable measures to facilitate the client's taking the medication. Explain the risk to the client of refusing to take the medication and reinforce the reason for the medication. When a medication is refused, this refusal must be documented immediately. The nurse manager, primary nurse, or health care provider should be informed when the omission may pose a specific threat to the client, such as with insulin. Follow-up is also required when a change is expected in the laboratory test values, such as with insulin and warfarin (Coumadin).

All medication errors are serious or potentially serious, A medication error may involve one or more of the following: administration of the wrong medication or IV fluid or the incorrect dose or rate; administration to the wrong patient, by the incorrect route, at the incorrect schedule interval; administration of known allergic drug or IV fluid; omission of dose,

UNIVERSITY HOSPITAL

CLIENT'S NAME

ROOM #

Nurse's Signature/Title	Initials
Evelyn Hayes RN	EH
Joyce Kee RN	JK
Rodney Brown LPN	RB
Jody Smith LPN	JS

Allergies:
                Codeine

Continuing Medical Record

Date Order	Stop Date	Medication/Dosage/Route/Frequency	Time	Date 8/14	8/15	Initials 8/16	8/17
8/14		Digoxin 0.125 mg po qd	0900	EH	EH	JK	
EH				AR=74	AR=70	AR=70	
8/14		Capoten 12.5 mg po bid	0900	EH	EH	JK	
EH			2100	RB	RB	RB	
8/15	8/22	Amoxicillin 250 mg po q6h	0600	✕	✕	JS	
EH	LD 0600	x7d	1200	✕	EH	JK	
1100			1800	✕	RB	RB	
			2400	✕	JS	JS	

One-Time/PRN/STAT Medications

Date	Medication/Dosage/Route/Frequency	Time/Initials	Reason	Result
8/14	Nitroglycerin 1/150 gr sublingual PRN	1600 EH	Chest pain	Relief of pain
	Chest pain			

Figure 3–5
Medication record.

or discontinuation of medication or IV fluid that was not discontinued.

MEDICATION SELF-ADMINISTRATION

Self administration of medication is a common practice in the home and in many community-based settings, such as the workplace. However, self-administration (SAM) is relatively new to clients and staff in institutional settings. In practical terms, SAM means that the nurse gives the client a packet of appropriate medications and instructions that are kept at the bedside and the client takes home on discharge. The client is responsible for taking the medications according to the instructions when she or he feels they are needed. The client has a key role in his or her care and exercises control associated with taking of selected medications. SAM helps clients to manage medications during the hospital stay and prepares them to keep as comfortable as possible at home. For example, refer to Chapters 47 and 48 for a thorough description of SAM for the maternity client.

SPECIAL CONSIDERATIONS: FACTORS THAT MODIFY DRUG RESPONSE

The pharmacologic response to a drug is complex. Nurses must be mindful of the number and variety of factors that influence an individual's response to a drug. (Refer to Chapters 7 and 9 for comprehensive information.) Examples of factors that modify drug responses include the following:

• **Absorption:** A major variable is the route of administration of the drug. Oral absorption takes place as drug particles move from the GI tract (stomach and small intestine) to body fluids. Any GI disturbances (e.g., vomiting or diarrhea) affect drug absorption.
• **Distribution:** Protein-binding is a major modifier of drug distribution in the body. Propranolol (Inderal) is 90% protein-bound. Another factor is the blood–brain barrier, which allows only lipid-soluble drugs, such as general anesthetics and barbiturates, to enter into the brain and cerebral spinal fluid. Compounds that are strongly ionized and poorly soluble in fat are barred from entry into the brain. Neoplastic agents are examples of drugs that do not cross the blood–brain barrier. The placental barrier is a membrane that, for the most part, keeps the blood of the mother and fetus separate. However, both lipid-soluble and lipid-insoluble drugs can diffuse across the placenta. Some drugs have teratogenic effects if taken during the first trimester of pregnancy; that is, they may induce aberrant development of fetal organs or body systems. This is especially true if the drugs are taken during the fourth through eighth weeks of gestation.
• **Metabolism, or biotransformation:** The liver is the primary organ for drug metabolism. All infants, especially neonates and low-birthweight infants, have immature liver and kidney function. Influences on liver function, such as the aging process, also affect the metabolism of a medication.
• **Excretion:** The main route of drug excretion is via the kidney. Through the normal aging process, there is a decrease in the functioning cells of the kidney with the result of decreased excretion of drugs. Bile, feces, respiration, saliva, and sweat are also routes of drug excretion.
• **Age:** Infants and the elderly are more sensitive to drugs. The elderly are hypersensitive to barbiturates and central nervous system (CNS) depressants. Such clients have poor absorption through the GI tract because of decreased gastric secretion. Infant doses are calculated based on weight in kilograms, rather than on biologic or gestational age.
• **Body weight:** Drug doses (e.g., of antineoplastics) may be ordered according to body weight. Obese people may need increased drug doses, and very thin persons may need decreased doses.
• **Toxicity:** This term refers to the *first adverse symptoms* that occur at a particular dose. Toxicity is more prevalent in those persons with liver or renal impairment and in the young and old.
• **Pharmacogenetics:** This term refers to the influence of genetic factors on drug response. If a parent has an adverse reaction to a drug, the child may also; some genetic factors are associated with ethnicity.
• **Route of administration:** Drugs administered intravenously act more rapidly than those administered orally.
• **Time of administration:** The presence or absence of food in the stomach can affect the action of some drugs.
• **Emotional factors:** Suggestive comments about the drug and its side effects may influence its effects.
• **Preexisting disease state:** Liver, kidney, heart, circulatory, and GI disorders are examples of preexisting states that can affect a response to a drug. For instance, diabetics should not be given elixirs or syrups that contain sugar.
• **Drug history:** The use of the same or different drugs may reduce or intensify the effects of the drug.
• **Tolerance:** The ability of a client to respond to a particular dose of a certain drug may diminish after days or weeks of repeated administration. A combination of drugs may be given to decrease or delay the development of tolerance for a specific drug.

- **Cumulative effect:** This occurs when the drug is metabolized or excreted more slowly than the rate at which it is being administered.
- **Drug-drug interaction:** The effects of a combination of drugs may be greater than, equal to, or less than the effects of a single drug. Some drugs may compete for the same receptor sites. An adverse reaction may lead to toxicity or complications, such as anaphylaxis.
- **Food-drug interaction:** The effects of selected foods may speed, delay, or prevent absorption of specific drugs.

Table 3–3
Guidelines for Correct Administration of Medications

PREPARATION

Wash hands before preparing medications.

Check for drug allergies; check the assessment history and Kardex.

Check medication order with health care provider's orders, Kardex, medicine sheet, and medicine card.

Check label on drug container three times.

Check expiration date on drug label, card, Kardex; use only if date is current.

Recheck drug calculation of drug dose with another nurse.

Verify doses of drugs that are potentially toxic with another nurse or pharmacist.

Pour tablet or capsule into the cap of the drug container. With unit dose, open packet at bedside after verifying client identification.

Pour liquid at eye level. Meniscus, lower curve of the liquid, should be at the line of desired dose (see Fig. 3–7).

Dilute drugs that irritate gastric mucosa (potassium, aspirin) or give with meals.

ADMINISTRATION

Administer only those drugs that you have prepared. Do not prepare medications to be administered by another. Identify the client by ID band or ID photo.

Offer ice chips to numb taste buds when giving bad-tasting drugs.

When possible, give bad-tasting medications first, followed by pleasant-tasting liquids.

Assist the client to an appropriate position, depending on the route of administration.

Provide only liquids allowed on the diet.

Stay with the client until the medications are taken.

Administer no more than 2.5–3 mL of solution intramuscularly at one site. Infants receive no more than 1 mL solution intramuscularly at one site and no more than 1 mL subcutaneously. *Never* re-cap needles (universal precautions).

When administering drugs to a group of clients, give drugs last to clients who need extra assistance.

Discard needles and syringes in appropriate containers.

Drug disposal is dependent on agency policy and state law. For example,
   Discard drugs in the sink or toilet, *not* in the trash can. Controlled substances must be returned to the pharmacy.
   Some disposals need signed witnesses.
   Discard unused solutions from ampules.

Appropriately store (some require refrigeration) unused stable solutions from open vials. Write date and time opened and your initials on label.

Keep narcotics in a double-locked drawer or closet. Medication carts must be locked at all times when a nurse is not in attendance.

Keys to the narcotics drawer must be kept by the nurse and *not* stored in a drawer or closet.

Keep narcotics in a safe place, out of reach of children and others in the home.

Avoid contamination of one's own skin or inhalation to minimize chances of allergy or sensitivity development.

RECORDING

Report drug error immediately to client's health care provider and to the nurse manager. Complete an incident report. Charting: record drug given, dose, time, route, and your initials.

Record drugs promptly after given, especially STAT doses.

Record effectiveness/results of medication administered, especially PRN medications.

Report to health care provider and record drugs that were refused with reason for refusal.

Record amount of fluid taken with medications on input and output chart.

Table 3–4
Behaviors to Avoid with Administration of Medication

Do *not* be distracted when preparing medications.

Do *not* give drugs poured by others.

Do *not* pour drugs from containers with labels that are difficult to read, or whose labels are partially removed or have fallen off.

Do *not* transfer drugs from one container to another.

Do *not* pour drugs into your hand.

Do *not* give medications for which the expiration date has passed.

Do *not* guess about drugs and drug doses. Ask when in doubt.

Do *not* use drugs that have sediment, are discolored, or are cloudy (and should not be).

Do *not* leave medications by the bedside or with visitors.

Do *not* leave prepared medications out of sight.

Do *not* give drugs if the client says he or she has allergies to the drug or drug group.

Do *not* call the client's name as the sole means of identification.

Do *not* give drug if the client states the drug is different from the drug he or she has been receiving. Check the order.

Do *not* re-cap needles. Use universal precautions.

Do *not* mix with large amount of food/beverage or foods that are contraindicated.

GUIDELINES FOR DRUG ADMINISTRATION

General guidelines for administering drugs are listed in Tables 3–3 and 3–4. These guidelines are summarized as the "dos" and "don'ts" of drug administration. Nurses should follow these guidelines to enhance safety when administering medications. Application of the nursing process to medication administration is presented later in this chapter.

FORMS AND ROUTES FOR DRUG ADMINISTRATION

There are a variety of forms and routes for the administration of medications, including oral (tablets, capsules, liquids, suspensions, elixirs); sublingual; buccal; transdermal; topical; instillation (drops and sprays); inhalations; nasogastric and gastrostomy

tubes; suppositories; and parenteral (Fig. 3–6). A brief description of each follows.

Tablets and Capsules

- Oral medications are *not* given to clients who are vomiting, lack a gag reflex, or who are comatose. Clients who gag may need a brief rest before proceeding with further intake of medications.
- Do not mix with a large amount of food/beverage or with contraindicated food. Clients may not be able to eat all the food and will not get the full dose of medication.
- Enteric-coated and timed-release capsules *must* be swallowed whole to be effective.
- Administer irritating drugs *with food* to decrease GI discomfort.
- Administer drugs on an empty stomach if food interferes with medication absorption.
- Drugs given **sublingually** (placed under tongue) or **buccally** (placed between cheek and gum) remain in place until fully absorbed. No food or fluids should be taken while the medication is in place.
- Encourage the use of child-resistant caps. The Consumer Public Safety Commission has ordered a redesign of these caps because the current caps are difficult for elderly clients. This has contributed to a safety hazard for children and others because many

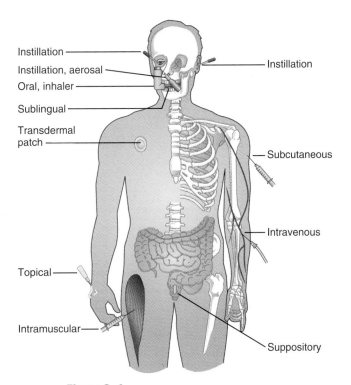

Figure 3–6
Some of the routes for medication administration

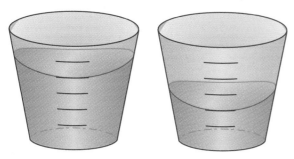

Figure 3–7
To read the meniscus, locate the lowest fluid mark.

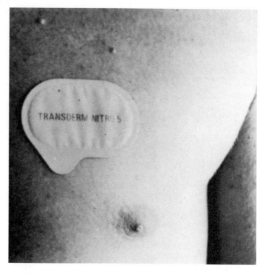

Figure 3–8
Transdermal nitroglycerin patch. (Courtesy of Summit Pharmaceuticals, Novartis, E. Hanover, NJ.)

people, in an effort to have easy access to their medications, leave the caps off. The new design requires a person to lightly squeeze the two side bottle tabs and turn the cap. Non–child-resistant caps are available on request.

Liquids

- There are several forms of liquid medication, including elixirs, emulsions, and suspensions.
- Read the labels to determine whether dilution or shaking is required.
- The **meniscus** is at the line of desired dose (Fig. 3–7).
- Many liquids require refrigeration once reconstituted.

Transdermal

- **Transdermal** medication is stored in a patch placed on the skin and absorbed through skin, thereby having systemic effect. There was widespread use of such patches beginning in the 1980s. Patches for cardiovascular drugs, neoplastic drugs, hormones, drugs to treat allergic reactions, and insulin are in production or being developed. Transdermal drugs provide more consistent blood levels and avoid GI absorption problems associated with oral products (Fig. 3–8).
- A common question is whether to cut the patches in half. Depending on the client's situation and the type of patch, it may be appropriate to cut the patch. If the drug is embedded in a *matrix patch* and diffuses into the skin (e.g., Climara, Vivelle, Nicotrol, Nitro-Dur, and Testoderm), the drug is spread over the entire surface of the patch and probably may be cut. Clients must be alert for underdosing or overdosing. The drug is pooled in a *reservoir patch* and is released via a semipermeable membrane (e.g., Catapres-TTS, Duragesic, Estraderm,

Transderm Scōp, Transderm-Nitro, and Androderm). These patches should not be cut because too much drug may be released. However, it is possible to peel back the protective layer half-way. Advise clients to secure the patch with tape, being careful not to apply it too tightly, which could alter the drug delivery. For legal and financial reasons, manufacturers do not recommend cutting the patches.

Topical

- **Topical** medications can be applied to the skin in a number of ways, such as with a glove, tongue blade, or cotton-tipped applicator. Never apply with one's own skin unprotected.
- Use appropriate technique to remove medication from container and apply to clean, dry skin, when possible. Do not contaminate medication in container; use gloves or an applicator.
- Observe sterile technique when the skin is broken. Take precautions to avoid medication stains.
- Use firm strokes if medication is to be rubbed in.

Instillations

Instillations are liquid medications usually administered as drops, ointment, or sprays in the following forms:

- Eye drops (Table 3–5, Fig. 3–9)
- Eye ointment (Table 3–6, Fig. 3–10)
- Ear drops (Table 3–7, Fig. 3–11)
- Nose drops and sprays (Table 3–8, Figs. 3–12 and 3–13)

Table 3–5
Administration of Eye Drops

WASH HANDS

Instruct client to lie or sit down and to look up toward the ceiling.

Gently draw skin down below the affected eye to expose the conjunctival sac.

Administer the prescribed number of drops into the center of the sac. Medication placed directly on the cornea can cause discomfort or damage. Do not touch eyelids or eye lashes with dropper. Self-administration of drops is enhanced with the use of Drop-eze, a cuplike device that holds the eyelids open.

Gently press on lacrimal duct with sterile cotton ball or tissue for 1–2 min after instillation to prevent systemic absorption through lacrimal canal.

Client should keep eyes closed for 1–2 min following application to promote absorption.

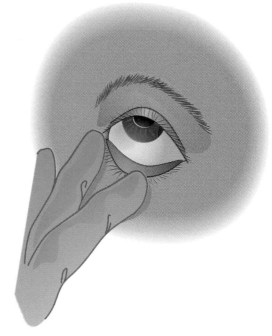

Figure 3–9
To administer eye drops, gently pull down the skin below the eye to expose the conjunctival sac.

Table 3–6
Administration of Eye Ointment

WASH HANDS

Instruct client to lie or sit down and to look up toward the ceiling.

Gently draw skin down below the affected eye to expose the conjunctival sac.

Squeeze strip of ointment (about ¼ inch unless stated otherwise) onto conjunctival sac. Medication placed directly on cornea can cause discomfort or damage.

Instruct client to close eyes for 2–3 min.

Instruct client to expect blurred vision for a short time. Apply at bedtime, if possible.

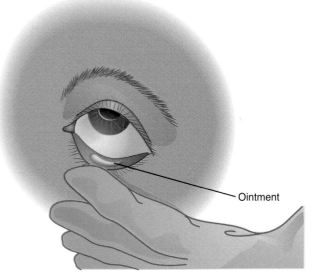

Ointment

Figure 3–10
To administer eye ointment, squeeze a 1/4-inch wide strip of ointment onto the conjunctival sac.

Table 3–7
Administration of Ear Drops

WASH HANDS

Medication should be at room temperature.

Client should sit up with head tilted slightly toward the unaffected side. To straighten the external ear canal for better visualization and to facilitate drops reaching the affected area, see Fig. 3–11.

   Child: pull down and back on auricle. After 3 years of age, same as adult.

   Adult: pull up and back on auricle.

Instill prescribed number of drops.

Take care not to contaminate dropper.

Have client maintain position for 2–3 min.

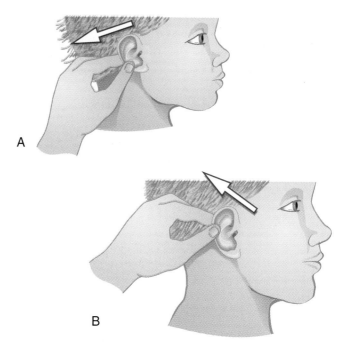

Figure 3–11
To administer ear drops, straighten the external ear canal by (A) pulling down on the auricle in children and (B) pulling up and back on the auricle in adults.

Table 3–8
Nose Drops and Sprays

Have client blow nose.

Have client tilt head back for drops to reach frontal sinus and tilted to affected side to reach ethmoid sinus.

Administer prescribed number of drops or sprays. Some sprays have instructions to close one nostril, tilt head to closed side, and hold breath or breathe through nose for a minute.

Have client keep head tilted backward for 5 min after instillation of drops.

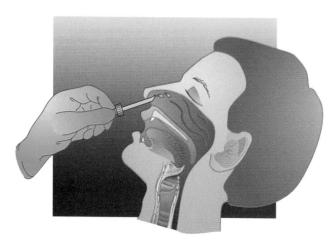

Figure 3–12
Administering nose drops.

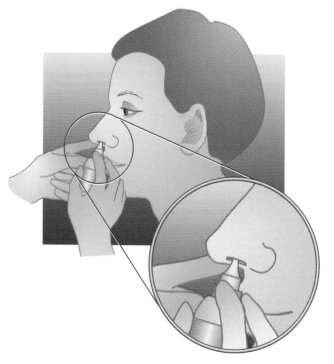

Figure 3–13
Administering nasal spray.

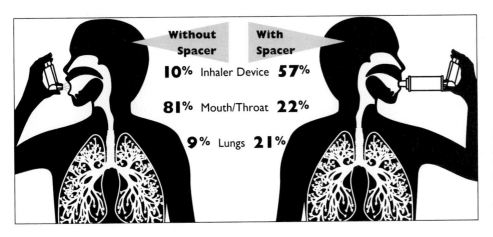

Figure 3–14
Distribution of medication with and without a spacer. (From American Lung Association: *Understanding Lung Medications: How They Work— How to Use Them.* New York, p. 5, 1993.)

Inhalations

- Hand-held nebulizers
- Hand-held metered-dose devices are a convenient method of administration of these medications. See Figure 3–14.
- **Spacers** are devices used to enhance the delivery of medications from the MDI. Figure 3–14 illustrates the distribution of medication with and without a spacer. AeroChamber (distributed by Forest Pharmaceuticals, St. Louis, MO) and Inspirease (distributed by Key Pharmaceuticals, Kenilworth, NJ) are examples of spacers available.
- Preferred client position is semi- or high Fowler's.
- Teach client correct use of equipment.
- Nebulizer (aerosol) changes a liquid medication into a fine mist.
- **Metered-dose inhaler** (MDI). See Table 3–9 for correct use of inhaler and Figure 3–15 to monitor amount of medication in **canister** (contains the medication).

Nasogastric and Gastrostomy Tubes

- Check for proper placement of tube.
- Pour drug into syringe without plunger or bulb, release clamp, and allow medication to flow in properly, usually by gravity.
- Flush tubing with 50 mL of water. (Refer to agency policy for exact amount.)
- Clamp tube and remove syringe.

Suppositories

RECTAL

- Medications administered as **suppositories** or enemas can be given rectally for both local and systemic absorption. The numerous small capillaries in the rectal area promote absorption.
- The foil around the suppository is removed, and the suppository may be lubricated before insertion.

When medications such as antipyretics and bronchodilators are given, the clients must be reminded to retain the medication and not to expel it.
- Suppositories tend to soften at room temperature and, therefore, need to be refrigerated.

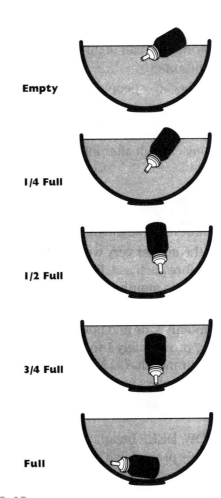

Empty

1/4 Full

1/2 Full

3/4 Full

Full

Figure 3–15
Testing a medication inhaler canister for the amount of medication remaining. (From American Lung Association: *Understanding Lung Medications: How They Work—How to Use Them.* New York, p. 4, 1993.)

Table 3-9
Correct Use of Metered Dose Inhaler

1. Insert the medication canister into the plastic holder.
2. Shake the inhaler well before using. Remove cap from mouthpiece.
3. Breathe out through the mouth. Open mouth wide and hold the mouthpiece 1–2 inches from the mouth. Do *not* put mouthpiece in the mouth unless using a spacer. Discuss techniques with the health care provider.
4. With mouth open, take slow, deep breath through mouth and at same time push the top of the medication canister once. Autohalers (e.g., Maxair) do not require coordination of pushing down top of canister and taking deep breath. With autohaler in upright position, raise lever and shake. Inhale deeply through mouthpiece with steady, moderate force, which triggers the release of medicine, making a click sound and puffing out the medicine. Continue to take deep breaths.
5. Hold breath for a few seconds; exhale slowly through pursed lips.
6. If a second dose is required, wait 2 min and repeat the procedure by first shaking the canister in the plastic holder with the cap on.
7. If the inhaler has not been used recently or when it is first used, "test spray" before administering the metered dose.
8. If a glucocorticoid inhalant is to be used with a bronchodilator, wait 5 min before using the inhaler containing the steroid.
9. Teach client to monitor pulse rate.
10. Caution against overuse, because side effects and tolerance may result.
11. Teach client to monitor amount of medication remaining in the canister (see Fig. 3–14). Advise the client to ask his or her health care provider or pharmacist to estimate when a new inhaler will be needed based on dosing schedule. A common practice of placing the canister in water to determine the amount of drug remaining is not appropriate for all inhalers.
12. Instruct client to avoid smoking.
13. Teach client to do daily cleaning of the equipment including: wash hands; take apart all washable parts of equipment and wash with warm water; rinse; place on clean towel and cover with another clean towel to air dry; store in clean plastic bag when *completely* dry. It is a good idea to have two sets of washable equipment to make this process easier.

• Explain the procedure to the client and provide for privacy.
• Use glove for insertion.
• Instruct client to lie on left side and breathe through the mouth to relax the anal sphincter.

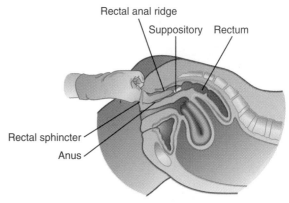

Figure 3–16
Inserting a rectal suppository.

• Apply a small amount of water-soluble lubricant to tip of the unwrapped suppository and gently insert the suppository beyond the internal sphincter (Fig. 3–16).
• Have the client remain on his or her side for 20 min after insertion.
• If indicated, teach the client how to self-administer suppositories and observe return demonstration for effectiveness.

VAGINAL

• Vaginal suppositories are similar to rectal suppositories. They are generally inserted into the vagina with an applicator (Fig. 3–17). Wear gloves. Client should be in lithotomy position. After insertion of medication, provide client with sanitary pad.

Parenteral

Safety is always a special concern with **parenteral** medication. Thus, manufacturers have responded with safety features in an effort to decrease or eliminate needle stick injuries and the possible transfer of bloodborne diseases, such as hepatitis and HIV.

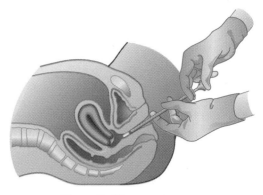

Figure 3–17
Inserting a vaginal suppository.

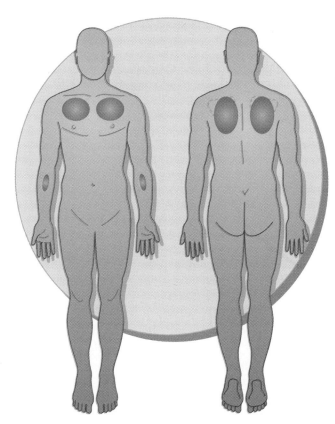

Figure 3–18
Common sites for intradermal injection.

There are multiple types of parenteral routes including **intradermal, subcutaneous, intramuscular, Z-track technique,** and **intravenous.** A description of each follows with special considerations noted for the pediatric client.

INTRADERMAL
Action

- Local effect
- Small amount is injected so that volume does not interfere with wheal formation or cause a systemic reaction.
- Used for observation of an inflammatory (allergic) reaction to foreign proteins. Examples include tuberculin testing, testing for drug and other allergic sensitivities, and some immunotherapy for cancer.

Sites
Locations are chosen so that an inflammatory reaction can be observed. Preferred areas are lightly pigmented, thinly keratinized, and hairless, such as ventral mid-forearm, clavicular area of chest; and scapular area of back (Fig. 3–18).

Equipment

- Needle: 26 to 27 gauge
  –Syringe: 1 mL calibrated in 0.01-mL increments
  –Usually 0.01- to 0.1-mL injected

Technique

- Cleanse area using circular motion; observe sterile technique.
- Hold skin taut.
- Insert needle, bevel up, at a 10- to 15-degree angle; outline of needle under skin should be visible (Fig. 3–19).
- Inject medication slowly to form a wheal (blister or bleb).
- Remove needle slowly.
- Do *not* massage area; instruct client not to do so.
- Mark area with pen and ask client not to wash it off until read by health care provider.
- Assess for allergic reaction in 24 to 72 h; measure diameter of local reaction. For tuberculin, measure only indurated area—do not include redness.

SUBCUTANEOUS
Action

- Systemic effect
- Sustained effect; absorbed mainly through capillaries. Usually slower in onset than with intramuscular route.
- Used for small doses of nonirritating, water-soluble drugs.

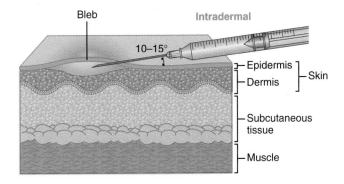

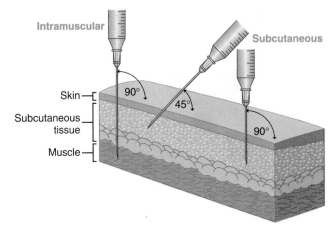

Figure 3–19
Needle–skin angle for intradermal, subcutaneous, and intramuscular injections.

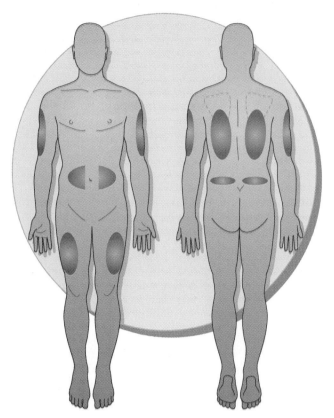

Figure 3–20
Common sites for subcutaneous injections.

Sites

Locations for subcutaneous injection are chosen for adequate fat-pad size and include the abdomen, upper hips, upper back, lateral upper arms, and lateral thighs (Fig. 3–20).

Equipment

- Needle: 25 to 27 gauge ½ to ⅝ inches in length
- Syringe: 1 to 3 mL
  –Usually 0.5- to 1.5-mL injected
- Insulin syringe measured in units for use with insulin only.

Technique

- Cleanse area with circular motion using sterile technique.
- Pinch the skin.
- Insert needle at angle appropriate to body size: 45 to 90 degrees (45 degrees for those with little SC tissue) (see Fig. 3–19).
- Release skin.
- Aspirate, except with heparin.
- Inject medication slowly.
- Remove needle quickly; do not re-cap.
- Gently massage area, unless contraindicated as with heparin.
- Apply Band-Aid if needed.

INTRAMUSCULAR
Action

- Systemic effect
- Usually more rapid effect of drug than with subcutaneous
- Used for irritating drugs, aqueous suspensions, and solutions in oils

Sites

Locations are chosen for adequate muscle size and minimal major nerves and blood vessels in the area. Locations include ventrogluteal, dorsogluteal, deltoid, and vastus lateralis (pediatrics) (Tables 3–10 through 3–13). A section on each site is shown in the diagrams of the sites (Figs. 3–21 through 3–24 and includes the volume of drug administered, needle size, angle of injection, client position, site location, advantages and disadvantages of site, and additional considerations, if any. Clients with low weight should be evaluated for sites with adequate muscle. The ventrogluteal is the preferred site for adults and infants older than 7 months.

Equipment

- Needle: 20 to 23 gauge; 18 gauge for blood products –1 to 1.5 inches in length

Technique

- Same as for subcutaneous injection, with two exceptions: flatten the skin area using the thumb and index finger, injecting between them; insert the needle at a 90-degree angle into the muscle (see Fig. 3–19).
- Syringe: 1 to 3 mL
  –Usually 0.5- to 1.5-mL injected

Preferred Intramuscular Injection Sites

- Ventrogluteal (Table 3–10, Fig. 3–21)
- Dorsogluteal (Table 3–11, Fig. 3–22)
- Deltoid (Table 3–12, Fig. 3–23)
- Vastus lateralis (pediatric Table 3–13, Fig. 3–24)

Z-TRACK INJECTION TECHNIQUE

Z-track technique prevents medication from leaking back into the subcutaneous tissue. It is frequently advised for medications that cause visible and permanent skin discolorations (e.g., iron dextran). The gluteal site is preferred. Following medication order policy and aseptic technique, draw up the medication. Replace the first needle with a second needle of appropriate gauge and length to penetrate muscle tissue and deliver the medication to the selected site. Removal of the first needle prevents the medication that is adhering to the needle shaft from being taken into the subcutaneous tissue. If removal is not possible, gently wipe needle with sterile source; this does present a chance for contamination and also for "self-

Table 3–10
Preferred Intramuscular Injection Site: Ventrogluteal

VOLUME OF DRUG ADMINISTERED
Usual: 1.0–4.0 mL
Maximum: 5.0 mL

COMMON NEEDLE SIZE
20–23 gauge, 1.25–2.5 inches

CLIENT POSITION
Supine lateral (with appropriate restraint, if pediatric)

LOCATE SITE
Place heel of hand on greater trochanter of femur (with thumb toward umbilicus), the index finger marks the anterosuperior iliac spine. The middle finger traces the iliac crest curvature. The space between index and middle finger (lower portion) is proper site for injection.

ANGLE OF INJECTION
Angle the needle slightly toward the iliac crest

SPECIAL CONSIDERATIONS
Serves as alternative to dorsogluteal and vastus lateralis for deep IM or Z-track injections. Considered secondary to vastus lateralis site for infants and children.

ADVANTAGES
Relatively free of major nerves and vascular branches

Well defined by bony anatomic landmarks

Thinner layer of fat than dorsogluteal site

Sufficient muscle mass for deep IM or Z-track injections

Readily accessible from several client positions

DISADVANTAGES
Should a hypersensitivity reaction occur, tourniquet cannot be applied to delay absorption

Health professional's unfamiliarity with site

Adapted from Tubex/Wyeth-Ayers: Intramuscular Injections, A Guide to Sites and Technique. *Philadelphia: Wyeth-Ayerst Laboratories, 1989. Permission granted.*

Table 3–11
Intramuscular Injection Site: Dorsogluteal

VOLUME OF DRUG ADMINISTERED
Usual: 1.0–3.0 mL
Maximum: 3.0 mL
5.0 mL gamma globulin

COMMON NEEDLE SIZE
18–23 gauge; 1.25–3.0 inches
Longer for obese clients

CLIENT POSITION
Prone

LOCATE SITE
Draw an imaginary line between posterior iliac spine and greater trochanter. Proper site for injection is at the midpoint and above this line.

ANGLE OF INJECTION
90-degree angle to flat surface, upon which client is lying prone

ADDITIONAL CONSIDERATIONS
Requires strict adherence to correct anatomic site location and injection technique

ADVANTAGES
Large muscle mass accommodates deep IM or Z-track injections. Injection not visible to client

DISADVANTAGES
Boundaries of the upper outer quadrant are arbitrarily selected and may exceed margin of safety

Danger of injury to major nerves and vascular structures if incorrect site or technique

Fat is often very thick; an injection intended for muscle may be subcutaneous

If hypersensitivity reaction occurs, tourniquet cannot be used

Difficult area to maintain antisepsis

Incision and drainage of abscesses complicated by proximity of large nerves and vascular structures

Adapted from Tubex/Wyeth-Ayerst: Intramuscular Injections, A Guide to Sites and Technique. *Philadelphia: Wyeth-Ayerst Laboratories, 1989. Permission granted.*

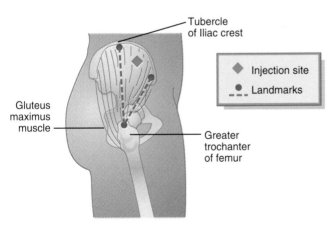

Figure 3–21
Ventrogluteal injection site.

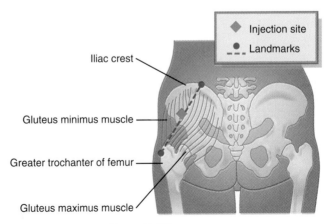

Figure 3–22
Dorsogluteal injection site.

Table 3–12
Intramuscular Injection Site: Deltoid

VOLUME OF DRUG ADMINISTERED

Usual:	0.5 mL
Maximum:	1.0 mL

COMMON NEEDLE SIZE

23–25 gauge, $\frac{5}{8}$–1.5 inches

CLIENT POSITION

Sitting, prone, supine, lateral

LOCATE SITE

Locate the acromion process of the scapula and the deltoid, a large muscle (shape of inverted tear drop) just below. Measure 2 to 3 finger breadths below acromion process on lateral midline of arm for proper site for injection.

ANGLE OF INJECTION

90-degree angle to skin surface (or angled slightly toward acromion)

ADDITIONAL CONSIDERATIONS

Preferred site for administration of vaccines in infants older than 7 months

ADVANTAGES

Easily accessible

General acceptance by client

In hypersensitivity reaction, tourniquet can be applied above

DISADVANTAGES

Small muscle mass relative to other sites

Close proximity to nerves and vascular structures; small margin of safety with any deviation from site

Not suitable for repeated or large-volume (>2.0 mL) injections

Adapted from Tubex/Wyeth-Ayerst: Intramuscular Injections, A Guide to Sites and Technique. *Philadelphia: Wyeth-Ayerst Laboratories, 1989. Permission granted.*

Table 3–13
Preferred Intramuscular Injection Site: Vastus Lateralis (Pediatric, Younger than 7 months)

VOLUME OF DRUG ADMINISTERED

Usual:	<0.5 mL infants
	1.0 mL pediatric
Maximum:	1.0 mL infants
	2.0 mL pediatric

COMMON NEEDLE SIZE

22–25 gauge; $\frac{5}{8}$–1 inch

CLIENT POSITION

Supine, sitting

LOCATE SITE

Vastus lateralis is the most lateral leg muscle; measure a hand's breadth below the greater trochanter and above the knee for the proper injection site.

ANGLE OF INJECTION

45-degree angle to frontal, sagittal, and horizontal planes of the thigh (directed toward the knee)

ADDITIONAL CONSIDERATIONS

IM site of choice for infants younger than 7 months

ADVANTAGES

Relatively large muscle mass at birth; suitable site for infants

Area of sufficient size for several injections

Free of major nerves and vascular branches

DISADVANTAGES

Use of long needle relative to small extremity may reach sciatic nerve or femoral vascular structures if improper technique is used

Adapted from Tubex/Wyeth-Ayerst: Intramuscular Injections, A Guide to Sites and Technique. *Philadelphia: Wyeth-Ayerst Laboratories, 1989. Permission granted.*

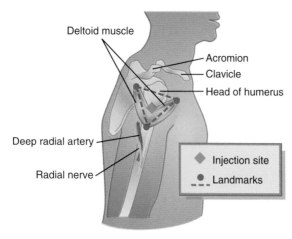

Figure 3–23
Deltoid injection site.

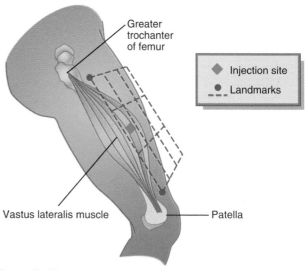

Figure 3–24
Vastus lateralis injection site in children.

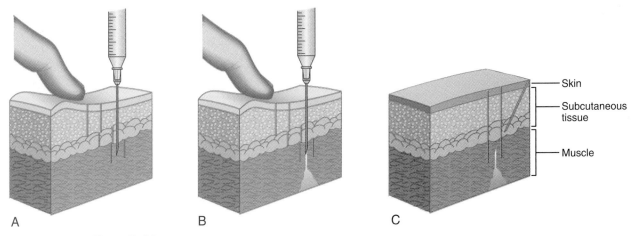

Figure 3–25
Z-track injection. (A) Pull skin to one side and hold; insert needle. (B) Holding skin to side, inject medication. (C) Withdraw needle and release skin. This technique prevents medication from entering the subcutaneous tissue.

sticks." Consider having medication prepared in the pharmacy.

Z-track injection technique is presented in Figure 3–25.

INTRAVENOUS
Action

- Systemic effect
- More rapid than IM or SC

Sites

Accessible peripheral veins (e.g., cephalic or cubital vein of arm; dorsal vein of hand) are preferred (Fig. 3–26). When possible, ask client for preference. Avoid needless restriction. In newborns, the veins of the feet, lower legs, and head may also be used after the previous sites have been exhausted.

Equipment

- Needle: 20 to 21 gauge; 1 to 1.5 inches
  - 24 gauge; 1 inch for infants
  - 22 gauge; 1 inch for children
  - Larger bore for viscous drugs, whole blood or fractions; large volume for rapid infusion
- Electronic intravenous delivery device, an infusion controller or pump

Technique

- Apply a tourniquet.
- Cleanse area using aseptic technique.
- Insert butterfly or catheter, and bend up into vein until blood returns. Remove tourniquet.
- Stabilize needle and dress site.
- Monitor flow rate, distal pulses, skin color and temperature, and insertion site.
- Consult agency policy regarding addition of medications to bottle or bag, piggyback technique, IV push, and so on.

NURSING IMPLICATIONS FOR ADMINISTRATION OF PARENTERAL MEDICATIONS

Sites

- Ventrogluteal site is preferred for IM injections in adults and infants older than 7 months.
- Do not use the dorsogluteal site for IM injections in children. For infants younger than 7 months, the vastus lateralis is preferred.

Equipment

- Use a needle size and syringe appropriate to the client's needs.
- Size of syringe should approximate volume of medication to be administered.
- Use tuberculin syringe for amounts <0.5 mL.
- Use filter needle to draw up medication from glass vial or ampule. Change the needle before adminis-

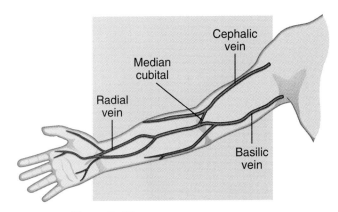

Figure 3–26
Common sites for intravenous administration.

tration to prevent tissue irritation from any medication left on the needle.

Technique

- Explain what you are going to do. Gain the client's cooperation. Allow the client time to cooperate.
- Demonstrate empathy and concern for every client, as well as using proper technique.
- Allay anxiety. Encourage expression of feelings.
- Position the client.
- Administer medication only via ordered route.
- Inspect skin before each injection.
- Inject medication slowly to minimize tissue damage.
- Do not administer injections if sites are inflamed, edematous, or lesioned (moles, birth marks, scars).
- Rotate injection site to enhance absorption of drug (e.g., insulin). Document injection site.
- Observe client for drug effectiveness. Report any untoward reactions immediately.

DEVELOPMENTAL NEEDS OF PEDIATRIC CLIENTS

Anticipate developmental needs. Examples of these needs associated with administration of medications include the following:

- Stranger anxiety (infant): Maintain a nonthreatening approach and move slowly.
- Hospitalization and illness/injury may be viewed as punishment (3 to 6 years old): Allow control where appropriate, obtain child's view of situation, encourage positive relationships and expression of feelings in acceptable manner and activities.
- Fear of mutilation (3 to 6 years old): Explain procedures carefully, use less intrusive routes whenever possible, such as oral medication, allow children to give "play injections" to a doll or stuffed animal.

NURSING PROCESS
OVERVIEW OF MEDICATION ADMINISTRATION

Assessment

- Obtain appropriate vital signs and relevant laboratory test results for future comparisons and evaluation of the therapeutic response.
- Obtain drug history, including drug allergies.
- Identify high-risk clients for reactions.
- Assess client's capability to follow therapeutic regimen.

Potential Nursing Diagnoses

- Risk for injury related to possible adverse reaction
- Risk for ineffective management of therapeutic regimen
- Risk for impaired home maintenance management

Planning

- Identify goals.
- Promote therapeutic response and prevent or minimize adverse reactions.
- Identify strategies to promote adherence.
- Identify interventions.

Nursing Interventions

- Prepare equipment and environment; wash hands.
- Check for allergies and other assessment data.
- Check drug label three times; check expiration date.
- Be certain of drug calculation; verify dose with another RN, as necessary.
- Pour liquids at eye level.
- Keep all drugs stored properly, especially related to temperature, light, and moisture.
- Avoid contact with topical and inhalation preparations.
- Verify client identification.
- Administer only drugs you have prepared.

Nursing Process continued on following page

NURSING PROCESS *Continued*
OVERVIEW OF MEDICATION ADMINISTRATION

- Assist client to desired position.
- Discard needles and syringes in "sharps" container.
- Follow policy related to discarding drugs and controlled substances.
- Report drug errors immediately.
- Record all appropriate information in a timely manner.
- Record effectiveness of drugs administered and reason for any drugs refused.

Client Teaching

General
- Client safety is of primary concern.
- Client's physical abilities require on going assessment.
- Keep or store medications in original labeled containers with child-safe caps when needed.
- Provide client or family with written instructions (audio instructions if sight impaired) about the drug regimen.
- Advise client or family about the expected therapeutic effect and length of time to achieve a therapeutic response from the medication and the expected duration of treatment.
- Advise client or family about possible drug–laboratory test interaction.
- Advise client of nonpharmacologic measures to promote therapeutic response.
- Advise client or family to have adequate supply of necessary medications available.
- Caution against the use of over-the-counter (OTC) preparations without *first* contacting the health care provider.
- Reinforce the importance of follow-up appointments with health care providers.
- Encourage clients to wear Medic-Alert band with medications or allergies indicated.
- Reinforce that community resources are available and need to be mobilized according to the client or family needs.

Diet
- Advise client or family about possible drug-food interactions.
- Advise client or family what foods are contraindicated.
- Advise regarding alcohol use.

Self-Administration
- Instruct client or family regarding drug dose and dosing schedule.
- Instruct client or family on all psychomotor skills related to the drug regimen.
- Provide client or family with contact person and telephone number for questions and concerns.

Side Effects
- Advise client or family about general side effects and adverse reactions of the medications.
- Advise when to notify health care provider.

Cultural Considerations
- Assess personal beliefs of clients or family.
- Modify communications to meet cultural needs of client or family.
- Communicate respect for client or family culture.

Evaluation

- Evaluate effectiveness of medications administered.
- Identify expected time frame of desired drug response; consider modification of therapy as needed.
- Determine client satisfaction with regimen.

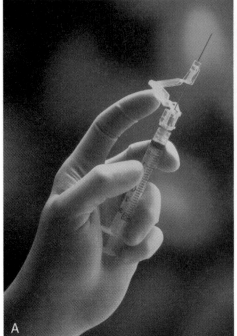
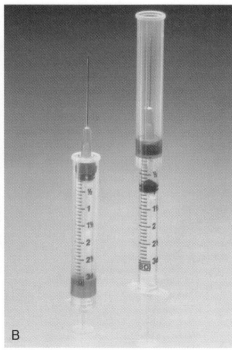

Figure 3-27
Safety needles. (Courtesy of Becton Dickinson and Company, Franklin Lakes, NJ.)

TECHNOLOGIC ADVANCES

Advances in parenteral therapy continue to enhance safety, increase accessibility to sites, promote client mobility, and improve client compliance. Examples of these advances include

- Safety needles and syringes, which help prevent accidental needle sticks (Fig. 3–27).
- Patient-controlled analgesia (PCA) systems, which allow clients to control the amount and frequency (within set limits) of narcotic analgesic administration (Fig. 3–28).
- EMLA (eutectic mixture of local anesthetics) cream, a local dermal anesthetic that relieves the pain associated with injection or catheter insertion and is especially useful for children (Fig. 3–29).
- An insulin "pen," a portable insulin delivery system that uses a prefilled cartridge and disposable needle to deliver a precise insulin injection.
- A portable syringe infusion system that allows a client to receive a continuous infusion while performing activities of daily living.

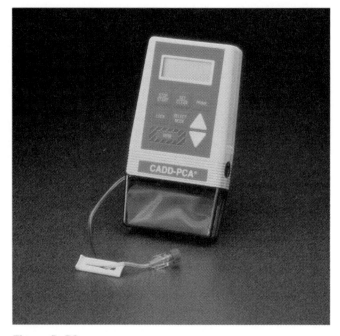

Figure 3-28
A patient-controlled analgesia (PCA) system. (Courtesy of SIMS Deltec, Inc., St. Paul, MN.)

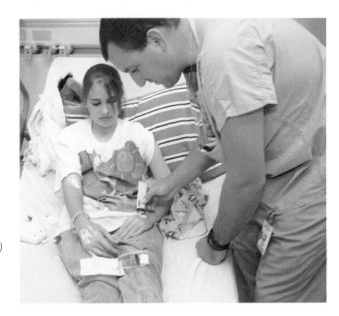

Figure 3–29
Applied to the skin at the site, EMLA (eutectic mixture of local anesthetics) cream reduces the pain of needle or catheter insertion and reduces the child's distress. (From Bowden, V., Dickey, S., & Greenberg, C. *Children and Their Families: The Continuum of Care*. Philadelphia: W.B. Saunders, 1998.)

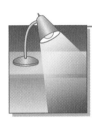

Study Questions

1. What is the meaning of the "rights" of medication administration to your nursing practice? What precautions must you take to ensure them?

2. List 10 safety guidelines for safe administration of medications.

3. What are the sites for administration of medication via parenteral routes? What factors influence the selection of the site?

4. What are the nursing implications for each route of medication administration?

5. What is the preferred angle of needle insertion for each type of parenteral injection?

6. What are the essential items to be charted for the administration of each medication? What do you record when an ordered medication is not given?

7. What do you need to do when a client refuses to take a medication?

8. Describe at least 10 factors that modify client response to a drug.

9. List at least three nursing interventions specific to the pediatric client associated with the administration of medications.

10. Describe the purpose of medication self-administration.

Medications and Calculations

OVERVIEW

This chapter on medications and calculations is subdivided into six sections: (A) systems of measurement, (B) methods for calculation, (C) calculations of oral doses, (D) calculations of injectable dosages; (E) calculations of intravenous fluids; and (F) pediatric drug calculations. The nurse may proceed independently through Sections A–F to practice and master calculation of drug doses during the fundamental nursing or pharmacology course. This chapter also serves as a review of drug calculation for nurses in practice settings.

Numerous drug labels are used in the drug calculation problems in order to familiarize the nurse with important information on a drug label. That information is then used in correctly calculating the drug dose.

There are four calculation methods explained; two are general methods (the nurse selects one of the methods), and the other two methods are used for individualizing drug dosing by body weight and body surface area. The drug calculation charts, Tables 4A–4 and 4B–1, may be used in the clinical setting. Abbreviations for drug dosing are found inside the front cover. The nurse might find it helpful to review Chapter 3, Principles of Drug Administration.

Keeping in mind that your goal is to prepare and administer medications in a safe and correct manner, we offer the following recommendations:

- **Think.** Focus on each step of the problem. This applies to simple as well as to difficult problems.
- **Read accurately.** Pay particular attention to the location of the decimal point and to the operation to be done, such as conversion from one system of measurement to another.
- **Picture the problem.**
- **Identify an expected range** for the answer.
- **Seek to understand the problem,** not merely the mechanics of how to do it. Ask for help when unsure of the calculation.

SECTION A

47

Systems of Measurement with Conversion

Outline

Objectives

- Name the three systems of measurement.
- Convert measurement within the metric system, larger units to smaller units, and smaller units to larger units.
- Convert measurements within the apothecary system, larger units to smaller units, and smaller units to larger units.
- Convert measurements within the household system, larger units to smaller units, and smaller units to larger units.
- Convert metric, apothecary, and household measurements among the three systems of measurement as appropriate.

Terms

apothecary system	household measurement	metric system
dram	liter	minim
grain	meter	ounce
gram		

INTRODUCTION

Three systems of measurement (metric, apothecary, and household) are used in measuring drugs and solutions. The metric system, developed in the late eighteenth century, is the internationally accepted system of measure. It is replacing the apothecary system, which dates back to the Middle Ages and had been used in England since the seventeenth century. Household measurement is commonly used in community and home settings in the United States.

METRIC SYSTEM

The **metric system** is a decimal system based on the power of 10. The basic units of measure are **gram** (g, gm, G, Gm) for weight; **liter** (l, L) for volume; and **meter** (m, M) for linear measurement, or length. Prefixes indicate the size of the units in multiples of 10. Table 4A–1 gives the metric units of measure in weight (gram), volume (liter), and length (meter), in larger and smaller units that are commonly used.

Table 4A–1
Metric Units of Measurements

UNIT	NAMES AND ABBREVIATIONS	MEASUREMENTS
Gram (weight)	1 kilogram (kg, Kg)	1000 g
	1 gram (g, gm, G, Gm)	1 g
	1 milligram (mg)	0.001 g
	1 microgram (μg, mcg)	0.000001 g
	1 nanogram (ng)	0.000000001 g
Liter (volume)	1 kiloliter (kL, KL)	1000 L
	1 liter (L, l)	1 L
	1 milliliter (mL)	0.001 L
Meter (length)	1 kilometer (km)	1000 m
	1 meter (m, M)	1 m
	1 centimeter (cm)	0.01 m
	1 millimeter (mm)	0.001 m

Note: 1 mL (milliliter) = 1 cc (cubic centimeter). Values are the same in drug and fluid therapy. 1 mg (milligram) = 1000 μg (micrograms).

Kilo is the prefix used for larger units (e.g., kilometer), and centi, milli, micro, and nano are the prefixes for smaller units (e.g., milligram). The prefix stands for a specific degree of magnitude; for instance, kilo stands for thousands, milli for one-thousandth, centi for one-hundredth, and so forth. Because the difference between degrees of magnitude is always a multiple of 10, converting from one magnitude to another is relatively easy.

Conversion Within the Metric System

The metric units most frequently used in drug notation are

> 1 g = 1000 mg
> 1 L = 1000 mL
> 1 mg = 1000 μg (mcg)

To be able to convert a quantity, one of the values must be known, such as gram or milligrams, liter or milliliters, and milligrams or micrograms. Gram, liter, and meter are larger units; milligram, milliliter, and millimeter are smaller units.

Metric Conversion

A. When converting *larger* units to smaller units in a metric system, move the decimal point one space to the **right** for each degree of magnitude change.
Note: It does not apply to micro and nano units.

Example

Change 1 gram to milligrams.
Grams are three degrees of magnitude **greater** than milligrams (see Table 4A–1). Move the decimal point three spaces to the right.

$$1 \text{ g} = 1.000 \text{ mg} \quad \text{ or } \quad 1 \text{ g} = 1000 \text{ mg}$$

B. When converting *smaller* units to larger units in the metric system, move the decimal point one space to the **left** for each degree of magnitude of change.

Change 1000 milligrams to grams.

Milligrams are three degrees of magnitude **smaller** than grams. Move the decimal point three spaces to the left.

$$1000 \text{ mg} = 1\underbrace{000.}\text{ g} \quad \text{or} \quad 1000 \text{ mg} = 1 \text{ g}$$

Remember: When changing larger units to smaller units, move the decimal point to the *right,* and when changing smaller units to larger units, move the decimal point to the *left.*

PRACTICE PROBLEMS

I. Metric Conversion

Larger to Smaller Units
1. Change 2 g to mg
2. Change 0.5 (½) g to mg
3. Change 2.5 L to mL

Smaller to Larger Units
4. Change 1500 mg to g
5. Change 3 g to kg
6. Change 500 mL to L

APOTHECARY SYSTEM

The **apothecary system** uses Roman numerals instead of ordinary Arabic numbers to express the quantity, and the Roman numeral is placed after the symbol or abbreviation for the unit of measure. The Roman numerals are written in lowercase letters; for example, gr x stands for 10 grains. The letters $\overline{ss}$ indicate one-half; for example, gr $\overline{ss}$ stands for ½ grain.

In the apothecary system, the unit of weight is the **grain** (gr), and the units of fluid volume are the **ounce** (fluidounce, or f℥), the **dram** (fluidram, or f℈), and the **minim** (♏, min). Drams are not used frequently.

In clinical practice, ounce and dram are more frequently used for measurement of fluid volume than for dry weights. Therefore, when writing fluid volume, the word fluid (f) in front of an ounce or dram is usually dropped. Table 4A–2 gives the apothecary equivalent of larger and smaller units of measure in drug weight and fluid volume.

Table 4A–2
Apothecary Equivalents in Weights and Fluid Volume

DRY WEIGHT		FLUID VOLUME*	
Larger Units	**Smaller Units**	**Larger Units**	**Smaller Units**
1 ounce (oz)	= 480 grains (gr)	1 quart (qt)	= 2 pints (pt)
1 ounce (oz)	= 8 drams (3)	1 pint (pt)	= 16 fluid ounces (fl oz or fl ℥)
1 dram (℈)	= 60 grains (gr)	1 fluid ounce	= 8 fluid dram (fl dr or fl 3)
1 scruple	= 20 grains (gr)	1 fluid dram	= 60 minims (♏, min)
		1 minim	= 1 drop (gt)

Fluid volume units are more commonly used than dry weight and should be remembered.

SECTION A

Apothecary Conversion

A. When converting a larger unit to a smaller unit, *multiply* the measurement that is requested by the basic equivalent value.

Examples

1. 3 Fluidounces (f℥, fl oz) = _____ fluid dram (f℥, fl dr).
   The equivalent value is 1 f℥ (1 fl oz) = 8 f℥ (8 fl dr)

$$3 \text{ f℥ (3 fl oz)} \times 8 \text{ f℥ (8 fl dr)} = \underline{24} \text{ f℥ (fl dr)}$$

B. When converting a smaller unit to a larger unit, *divide* the requested number by the basic equivalent value.

Examples

1. 8 fluidounces (f℥) = _____ pint (pt).
   The equivalent value is 1 pt = 16 f℥.

$$8 \div 16 = 0.5 \text{ pt, or } \tfrac{1}{2} \text{ pt}$$

Larger to Smaller Units	**Smaller to Larger Units**
1. Change 3 qt to pt	4. Change 3 pt to qt
2. Change 1.5 pt to f℥	5. Change 32 f℥ to qt
3. Change 2 f℥ to f℥	6. Change 4 f℥ to f℥

HOUSEHOLD SYSTEM

The household system of measurement is not as accurate as the metric system because of the lack of standardization of spoons, cups, and glasses. The measurements are approximate. A teaspoon (t) is considered to be equivalent to 5 mL according to the official USP. Milliliters (mL) is the same as cubic centimeters (cc) in value (Fig. 4A–1). Three teaspoons equal 1 tablespoon (T). Ounces are fluid ounces in the household measurement; the word "fluid" in front of ounce is usually not used.

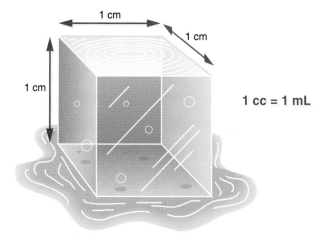

1 cc = 1 mL

Figure 4A–1
One cubic centimeter equals one milliliter.

One milliliter of water fills a cubic centimeter exactly.
Table 4A–3 gives the household equivalents in fluid volume. The measurements having asterisks are frequently used in drug therapy and should be remembered.

Table 4A-3
Household Equivalents in Fluid Volume

1 measuring cup	=	8 ounces (oz)
1 medium-size glass (tumbler size)	=	8 ounces (oz)
1 coffee cup (c)	=	6 ounces (oz) (varies with cup size)
1 ounce (oz)	=	2 tablespoons (T)
1 tablespoon (T)	=	3 teaspoons (t)
1 teaspoon (t)	=	60 drops (gtt)*
1 drop (gt)*	=	1 minim (Ⅲ, min)

Varies with viscosity of liquid and dropper opening.

Household Conversion

A. When converting larger units to smaller units within the household system, *multiply* the requested number by the basic equivalent value.

Example

Change 2 glasses of water to ounces.
The equivalent value is 1 medium-size glass = 8 oz.

$$2 \text{ glasses} \times 8 \text{ oz} = \underline{16} \text{ oz.}$$

PRACTICE PROBLEMS

III. Household Conversion

Remember: To change larger units to smaller units, *multiply* the requested number of units by the basic equivalent value. To change smaller units to larger units, *divide* the requested number of units by the basic equivalent value. Refer to Table 4A-3 as needed.

Larger to Smaller Units
1. Change 3 oz to T
2. Change 5 T to t
3. Change 3 coffee cups to oz

Smaller to Larger Units
4. Change 3 T to oz
5. Change 16 oz to a measuring cup
6. Change 12 t to T

PRACTICE PROBLEMS

IV. Summary: Metric, Apothecary, and Household Measurements

Metric System: Refer to Table 4A-1 as needed.

1. 2 g = _____ mg

2. 1.2 kg = _____ g

3. 5 mg = _____ μg

4. 2.5 L = _____ mL

5. 1.5 km = _____ m

6. 500 mg = _____ g

7. 10,000 μg = _____ mg

8. 2400 mg = _____ g

9. 1500 mL = _____ L

10. 1200 cm = _____ m

Apothecary System: Refer to Table 4A–2 as needed.

1. 5 qt = _____ pt
2. 2 pt = _____ f℥
3. f℥v = _____ f℈
4. f℈iiss (2½) = _____ ♍ (minims)
5. 1.5 pt = _____ f℥

6. 8 f℥ = _____ pt
7. 3 pt = _____ qt
8. 12 f℥ = _____ f℈
9. 32 f℥ = _____ qt
10. 5♍ = _____ gtt

Household System: Refer to Table 4A–3 as needed.

1. 5 glasses = _____ oz
2. 3 T = _____ t
3. 2 c = _____ oz

4. 4 oz = _____ T
5. 15 t = _____ T
6. 5 T = _____ oz

CONVERSION BETWEEN THE METRIC, APOTHECARY, AND HOUSEHOLD SYSTEMS

Drug doses are usually ordered in metric units (grams, milligrams, liters, or milliliters), but some health care providers still use the apothecary units of measurement (grain) when prescribing medication. To calculate drug doses, the same unit of measure (grams, milligrams, or grains) must be used. The nurse needs to be familiar with the three systems of measure and their equivalents (Table 4A–4). Note that the metric and apothecary equivalents are approximate; thus, the equivalents should be rounded off to a whole number, for example, 1 g = 15.432 gr, or 1 g = 15 gr.

SECTION A

Table 4A–4
Approximate Metric, Apothecary, and Household Equivalents

	METRIC SYSTEM		APOTHECARY SYSTEM	HOUSEHOLD SYSTEM
Weight	1 kg;	1000 g	2.2 lb	2.2 lb
	*1 g;	1000 mg	15 (16) gr	
	0.5 g;	500 mg	$7\frac{1}{2}$ gr	
	0.3 g;	300 (325) mg	5 gr	
	0.1 g;	100 mg	$1\frac{1}{2}$ gr	
	*0.06 g;	60 (65) mg	1 gr	
	0.03 g;	30 (32) mg	$\frac{1}{2}$ gr	
	0.01 g;	10 mg	$\frac{1}{6}$ gr	
		0.6 mg	$\frac{1}{100}$ gr	
		0.4 mg	$\frac{1}{150}$ gr	
		0.3 mg	$\frac{1}{200}$ gr	
Volume	1 L; 1000 mL (cc)		1 qt; 32 oz (f ℥)	1 qt
	0.5 L; 500 mL		1 pt; 16 oz (f ℥)	1 pt
	0.24 L; 240 mL		8 ℥ (f ℥)	1 glass
	0.18 L; 180 mL		6 ℥	1 c
	*30 mL		1 ℥; 8 3 (f ℥)	2 T; 6 t
	15 mL		$\frac{1}{2}$ ℥; 4 3	1 T; 3 t
	†5 mL			1 t
	4 mL		1 ℥; 60 ♍ (min)	1 t
	1 mL		15 (16) ♍	15–16 gtt
Height/Distance	2.54 cm		1 inch	1 inch
	25.4 mm		1 inch	1 inch

*Equivalents commonly used for computing conversion problems by ratio.
†5 mL = 1 t (teaspoon); Official USP measurement.
Key: g = gram; mg = milligram; gr = grain; L = liter; mL = milliliter; f ℥ = fluidounce; T = tablespoon; t = teaspoon; gtt = drops; ♍ = minim; kg = kilogram; cc = cubic centimeter; ℥ = dram.

Some authorities indicate that it is easier to convert to the unit used on the bottle or container. The answer is in the system of the drug to be dispensed. If the label on the bottle reads in milligrams and the order is in grains, the conversion should be from grains to milligrams.

Example

Order: Compazine spansule gr ¼.
Available: Compazine spansule 15 mg. Convert grains to milligrams, gr ¼ = 15 mg.

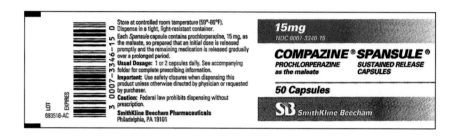

Metric, Apothecary, and Household Equivalents

Conversion to one unit of measure is essential in administering drugs. With discharge teaching for a client who requires liquid medication(s) at home, the nurse may find it necessary to convert metric to household measurements. Table 4A–4 gives the metric and apothecary equivalents by weight, and the metric, apothecary, and household equivalents by volume.

PRACTICE PROBLEMS

V. Metric, Apothecary, and Household Conversion

Change measurements by conversion. Refer to Table 4A–4 as needed.

1. 3 g to gr
2. 7½ gr (gr vii$\overline{\text{ss}}$) to g
3. 2.5 g to mg
4. 0.5 g to gr
5. 0.1 g to gr
6. 4 gr to mg
7. 3 gr to g
8. 7½ gr to mg
9. 150 gr to g
10. 10 mg to gr
11. 1.5 ℥ to mL
12. 15 mL to t
13. 2t to mL
14. 8 ℥ to mL
15. 60 mL to oz
16. 75 mL to T
17. 2 coffee cups to mL
18. 9 t to T
19. 3 oz to T
20. ½ oz to t

ANSWERS TO PRACTICE PROBLEMS

I. Metric Conversion

1. 2.0 g = 2.000 mg   or   2.0 g = 2000 mg

The gram is three degrees of magnitude greater than the milligram, so the decimal point is moved three spaces to the right.

2. 0.5 g = 0.500 mg   or   0.5 g = 500 mg

The gram is three degrees of magnitude greater than the milligram, so the decimal point is moved three spaces to the right.

3. 2.5 L = 2.500 mL   or   2.5 L = 2500 mL

The liter is three degrees of magnitude greater than the milliliter, so the decimal point is moved three spaces to the right.

4. 1500 mg = 1.500. g   or   1500 mg = 1.5 g

The milligram is three degrees of magnitude smaller (less) than the gram, so the decimal point is moved three spaces to the left.

5. 3 g = 003. kg   or   3 g = .003 kg

The gram is three degrees of magnitude smaller than the kilogram, so the decimal point is moved three spaces to the left.

6. 500 mL = 500. L   or   500 mL = 0.5 L

The milliliter is three degrees of magnitude smaller than the liter, so the decimal point is moved three spaces to the left.

II. Apothecary Conversion

1. 3 qt × 2 pt = 6 pt;
   the equivalent value is 1 qt = 2 pt
2. 1.5 pt × 16 = 24 f℥;
   the equivalent value is 1 pt = 16 f℥
3. 2 f℥ × 8 f℥ = 16 f℥;
   the equivalent value is 1 f℥ = 8 f℥
4. 3 pt = 1.5 qt;
   the equivalent value is 1 qt = 2 pt; 3 pt ÷ 2 = 1.5 qt
5. 32 f℥ = 2 pt or 1 qt;
   the equivalent values are 1 pt = 16 f℥ or 1 qt = 2 pt
6. 4 f℥ = 0.5 or ½ f℥;
   the equivalent value is 1 f℥ = 8 f℥; 4 f℥ ÷ 8 f℥ = 0.5 f℥

III. Household Conversion

1. 3 oz = 6 T;
   the equivalent value is 3 oz × 2 = 6 T
2. 5 T = 15 t;
   the equivalent value is 1 T = 3 t
3. 3c = 18 oz;
   the equivalent value is 1 c = 6 oz
4. 3 T = 1½ oz;
   the equivalent value is 3 T ÷ 2 = 1½ or 1.5 oz
5. 16 oz = 2 c;
   the equivalent value is 1 measuring cup = 8 oz
6. 12 t = 4 T;
   the equivalent value is 1 T = 3 t

Metric

1. 2000 mg

$$1\ g = 1000\ mg$$

$$2 \times 1000\ mg = 2000\ mg$$

or 2 000 mg

(three spaces to the right)

2. 1200 g
3. 5000 μg

$$1\ mg = 1000\ \mu g$$

4. 2500 mL
5. 1500 meters

6. 0.5 g

$$1000\ mg = 1\ g$$

$$500 \div 1000 = 0.5$$

or 500 g = 0.5 g

(three spaces to the left)

7. 10 mg
8. 2.4 g
9. 1.5 L
10. 1.2 m

Apothecary

1. 10 pt
2. 32 f℥
3. 40 f℥ v = 5 (Roman numeral)
4. 150 ♏
5. 24 f℥

6. ½ pt
7. 1½ qt
8. 1½ f℥
9. 1 qt
10. 5 gtt

Household

1. 40 oz
2. 9 t
3. 12 oz

4. 8 T
5. 5 T
6. 2 ½ oz

V. Metric, Apothecary, Household Conversion

1. 45 gr
2. 0.5 g
3. 2500 mg
4. 7½ gr
5. 1½ (1.5) gr
6. 240 mg
7. 0.2 g
8. 500 mg
9. 10 g
10. ⅙ gr

11. 45 mL
12. 3 t
13. 10 mL
14. 240 mL
15. 2 oz
16. 5 T
17. 360 mL
18. 3 T
19. 6 T
20. 3 t

SECTION 4B
Methods for Calculation

Outline

Objectives

- Select a formula, the basic formula or the ratio-and-proportion method, for calculating drug dosages.
- Convert all measures to the same system, and same unit of measure within the system, prior to calculating drug dosage.
- Calculate drug dosage using one of the general formulas.
- Calculate drug dosage according to body weight and body surface area.
- List meanings for abbreviations used in drug therapy.

Terms

INTRODUCTION

Two general methods for calculating drug doses are the basic formula and ratio and proportion. These methods are used for calculating oral and injectable drug doses. The nurse needs to select one of the methods to calculate drug doses and use that method consistently.

For drugs that require individualized dosing, calculation by body weight (BW) or by body surface area (BSA) may be necessary. In the past, these two methods have been used for calculating pediatric dosage and for drugs used in the treatment of cancer (antineoplastic drugs). Currently, we calculate by body weight and body surface area especially for those individuals whose body weight is low, who are obese, or who are older adults.

Before calculating drug doses, all units of measure must be converted to a single system (see Section 4A). It is most helpful to convert to the system used on the drug label. If the drug is ordered in grains (gr) and the drug label gives the dose in milligrams (mg), convert grains to milligrams, the measurement on the drug label, and proceed with the drug calculation. Table 4B–1 gives the metric and apothecary conversions most frequently used for dry and liquid measurements.

Table 4B–1
Metric and Apothecary Conversions

METRIC		APOTHECARY
Grams (g)	Milligrams (mg)	Grains (gr)
1	1000	15
0.5	500	$7\frac{1}{2}$
0.3	300 (325)	5
0.1	100	$1\frac{1}{2}$
0.06	60 (64)	1
0.03	30 (32)	$\frac{1}{2}$
0.015	15 (16)	$\frac{1}{4}$
0.010	10	$\frac{1}{8}$
0.0006	0.6	$\frac{1}{100}$
0.0004	0.4	$\frac{1}{150}$
0.0003	0.3	$\frac{1}{200}$

Liquid (approximate)
30 mL (cc) = 1 oz (fl ℥) = 2 tbsp (T) = 6 tsp (t)
15 mL (cc) = 0.5 oz = 1 T = 3 t
1000 mL (cc) = 1 quart (qt) = 1 liter (L)
500 mL (cc) = 1 pint (pt)
5 mL (cc) = 1 tsp (t)
4 mL (cc) = 1 fl dr (f ℥)
1 mL (cc) = 15 minims (♏) = 15 drops (gtt)

INTERPRETING ORAL AND INJECTABLE DRUG LABELS

The pharmaceutical companies usually label their drugs with the brand name of the drug in large letters and the generic name in smaller letters. The dose per tablet, capsule, or liquid (for oral and injectable doses) is printed on the drug label. Two examples of drug labels are given below, one for an oral drug and the second for an injectable drug.

Example 1: **Oral Drug**

Tagamet is the brand (trade) name, cimetidine is the generic name, and the dose is 200 mg/tablet.

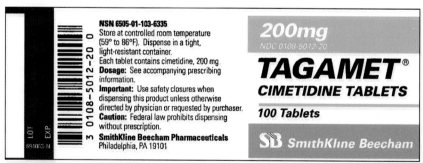

Example 2: **Injectable Drug**

Compazine is the brand (trade) name, prochlorperazine is the generic name, and the dose is 5 mg/mL injectable.

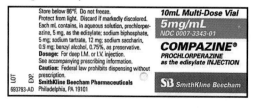

BASIC FORMULA

The **basic formula** is easy to recall and is most frequently used in calculating drug dosages. The formula is:

$$\frac{D}{H} \times V = A$$

where D is the desired dose: drug dose ordered by the physician,
H is the on-hand dose: drug dose on label of container (bottle, vial),
V is the vehicle: drug form in which the drug comes (tablet, capsule, liquid), and
A is the amount calculated to be given to the client.

Examples

1. Order: cefaclor 0.5 g PO b.i.d.
   Available:

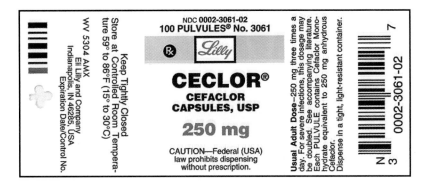

   a. The unit of measure that is ordered, grams, and the unit on the bottle, milligrams, are from the same system of measurement, the metric system. Conversion to the same unit is necessary to work the problem. Since the bottle is in milligrams, convert grams to milligrams.
   To convert grams (large value) to milligrams (smaller value), move the decimal point three spaces to the right (see Section 4A: Conversion Within the Metric System).

   $$0.5 \text{ g} = 0.500 \text{ mg or } 500 \text{ mg}$$

   b. $\dfrac{D}{H} \times V = \dfrac{500 \text{ mg}}{250 \text{ mg}} \times 1 \text{ capsule} = \dfrac{500}{250} = 2 \text{ capsules}$

2. Order: codeine gr i (1), PO, STAT
   Available:

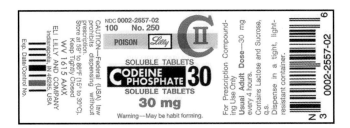

   a. Grains need to be converted to milligrams before you can calculate drug dose (see Table 4A–4 or 4B–1). 1 gr = 60 mg

   b. $\dfrac{D}{H} \times V = \dfrac{60 \text{ mg}}{30 \text{ mg}} \times 1 \text{ tablet} = \dfrac{60}{30} = 2 \text{ tablets}$

RATIO AND PROPORTION

The **ratio-and-proportion** method is the oldest method currently used in calculating drug dosage. The formula is:

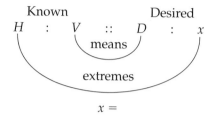

$$H \; : \; V \; :: \; D \; : \; x$$

Known — H : V   Desired — D : x

means (V :: D)

extremes (H ... x)

$$x =$$

where H is the drug on hand (available),
    V is the vehicle or drug form (tablet, capsule, liquid),
    D is the desired dose (as ordered),
    x is the unknown amount to give, and
    :: stands for "as" or "equal to."

Multiply the means and the extremes. Solve for x; x is the divisor.

Examples

1. Order: amoxicillin 100 mg PO q.i.d.
   Available:

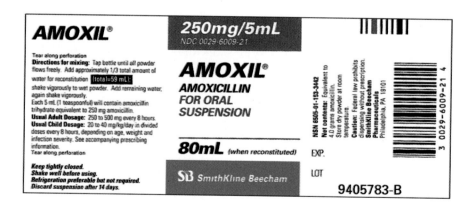

a. Conversion is not needed because both are expressed in the same unit of measure.
b. $H \quad : \quad V \quad :: \quad D \quad : \quad x$

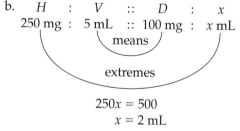

$$250 \text{ mg} \; : \; 5 \text{ mL} \; :: \; 100 \text{ mg} \; : \; x \text{ mL}$$

means

extremes

$$250x = 500$$
$$x = 2 \text{ mL}$$

Answer: amoxicillin 100 mg = 2 mL

2. Order: aspirin/ASA gr x, q4h, PRN
   Available: aspirin 325 mg/tablet
   a. Convert to one system and unit of measure. Change grains to milligrams (see Table 4A–4 or 4B–1).
   b.

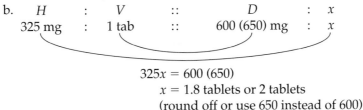

$$325x = 600 \ (650)$$
$$x = 1.8 \text{ tablets or 2 tablets}$$
$$(\text{round off or use 650 instead of 600})$$

Answer: Aspirin gr x = 2 tablets

BODY WEIGHT

The **body weight** method of calculating allows for individualizing the drug dose and involves three steps:

1. Convert pounds to kilograms if necessary (lb ÷ 2.2).
2. Determine drug dose per body weight by multiplying:

$$\text{Drug dose} \times \text{body weight} = \text{Client's dose per day}$$

3. Follow the basic formula or ratio-and-proportion method to calculate drug dosage.

Examples

1. Order: fluorouracil (5-FU), 12 mg/kg/day intravenously, not to exceed 800 mg/day. The adult weighs 132 lb.
   a. Convert pounds to kilograms by dividing the number of pounds by 2.2 (1 kg = 2.2 lb).

$$132 \div 2.2 = 60 \text{ kg}$$

   b. mg × kg = client's dose
      12 × 60 = 720 mg IV/day

Answer: fluorouracil 12 mg/kg/day = 720 mg

2. Order: cefaclor (Ceclor) 20 mg/kg/day in three divided doses. The child weighs 31 lb. Available:

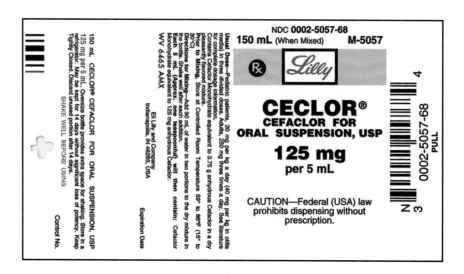

a. Convert pounds to kilograms.

$$31 \div 2.2 = 14 \text{ kg}$$

b. $20 \text{ mg} \times 14 \text{ kg} = 280 \text{ mg per day}$

$$280 \text{ mg} \div 3 \text{ divided doses} = 93 \text{ mg/dose}$$

c. $\dfrac{D}{H} \times V' = \dfrac{93}{125} \times 5 = \dfrac{465}{125} = 3.7 \text{ mL}$

or:

$$
\begin{array}{ccccccc}
H & : & V & :: & D & : & x \\
125 \text{ mg} & : & 5 \text{ mL} & :: & 93 \text{ mg} & : & x \text{ mL}
\end{array}
$$

$$125x = 465$$

$$x = \frac{465}{125} = 3.7 \text{ mL}$$

Answer: cefaclor 20 mg/kg/day = 3.7 mL per dose

BODY SURFACE AREA

The **body surface area** (BSA) method is considered to be the most accurate way to calculate the drug dose for infants, children, older adults, and clients who are on antineoplastic agents or whose body weight is low. The body surface area, in square meters (m^2), is determined by where the person's height and weight intersect the nomogram scale (Figs. 4B–1 [children] and 4B–2 [adults]). To calculate the drug dosage by the BSA method, multiply the drug dose ordered by the number of square meters.

$$100 \text{ mg} \times 1.8 \text{ m}^2 \text{ (BSA)} = 180 \text{ mg per day}$$

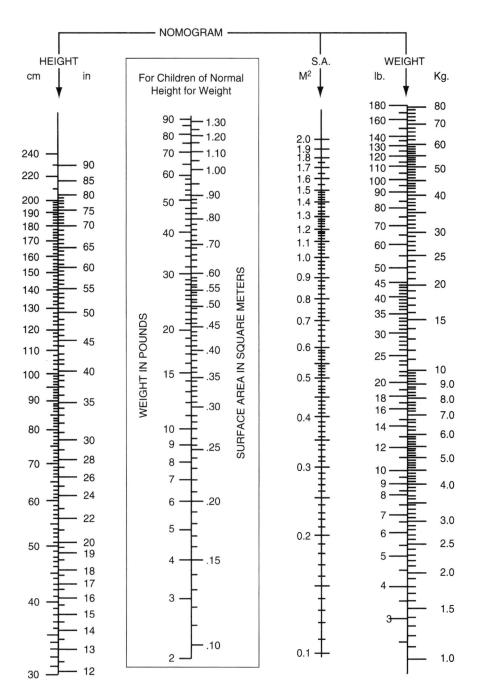

Figure 4B–1

West nomogram for infants and children. *Directions:* (1) Find height. (2) Find weight. (3) Draw a straight line connecting the height and weight. Where the line intersects on the S.A. column is the body surface area (m²). (Modified from data of E. Boyd and C. D. West. In Behrman, R. E., and Vaughan. V. C.: *Nelson Textbook of Pediatrics,* 14th ed. Philadelphia: WB Saunders, 1992.)

SECTION B

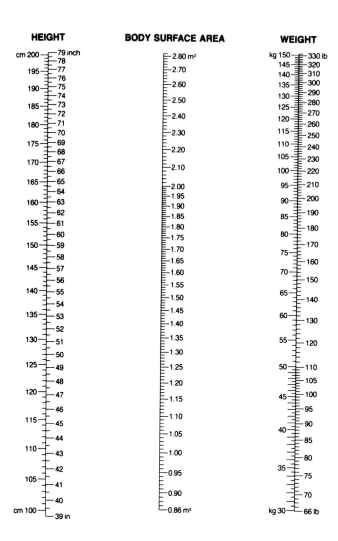

HEIGHT   **BODY SURFACE AREA**   **WEIGHT**

Nomogram of body surface area for adults. *Directions:* (1) Find height. (2) Find weight. (3) Draw a straight line connecting the height and weight. (4) Where the line intersects on the Body Surface Area column is the body surface area (m²). (Sources: Deglin, J. H., Vallerand, A. H., and Russin: *Davis's Drug Guide for Nurses,* 2nd ed. Philadelphia: F. A. Davis, 1991; Lentner, C. [ed.]: *Geigy Scientific Tables,* 8th ed. Vol. 1. Basle, Switzerland: Ciba-Geigy, pp. 226–227, 1981.)

Examples

1. Order: cyclophosphamide (Cytoxan) 100 mg/m²/day, IV.
   Available:

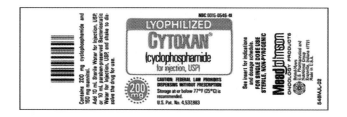

   Client is 5 ft 10 in. (70 in.) tall and weighs 160 lb.
   a. 70 in. and 160 lb intersect the nomogram scale at 1.97 m² (BSA).
   b. 100 mg × 1.97 = 197 mg.

Answer: Administer cyclophosphamide 197 mg or 200 mg/day.

2. Order: mephenytoin (Mesantoin) 200 mg/m² PO in three divided doses. The child is 42 in. tall and weighs 44 lb.
   a. 42 in. and 44 lb intersect the nomogram scale at 0.8 m².
   b. 200 mg × 0.8 = 160 mg/day or 50 mg (53) t.i.d. (three times a day).

Answer: Administer mephenytoin 50 mg t.i.d.

SECTION B

Additional practice problems are given in Sections 4C and 4D (orals and injectables).

I. Drug Dosage Using a General Formula

Solve the problem and determine the drug dose given the following:

1. Order: cimetidine (Tagamet) 0.4 g PO q6h (every 6 h).
   Available:

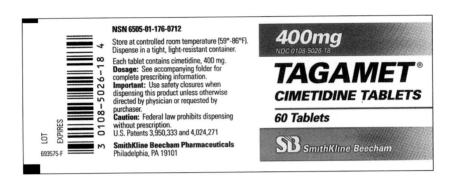

How many tablet(s) of Tagamet should the client receive? _____

2. Order: dexamethasone (Hexadrol) 1 mg PO q.d.
   Available: dexamethasone 0.5 mg tablet
   How many tablet(s) should the client receive? _____

3. Order: phenobarbital gr ½ PO t.i.d.
   Available: phenobarbital 15 mg tablet
   How many tablet(s) should the client receive? _____

4. Order: hydrochlorothiazide (HydroDIURIL) 25 mg PO q.d.
   Available:

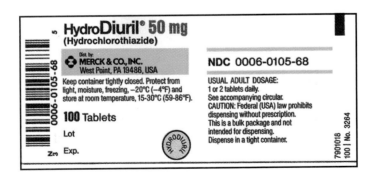

How many tablet(s) should the client receive? _____

5. Order: cefadroxil (Duricef) 500 mg PO b.i.d.
   Available:

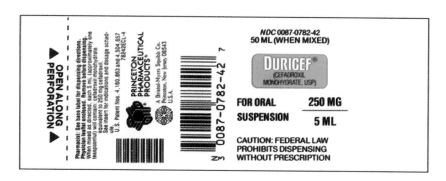

How many mL should the client receive? _____

6. Order: dicloxacillin 100 mg PO q8h
   Available: dicloxacillin 62.5 mg/5 mL
   How many mL should the client receive? _____

7. Order: meperidine (Demerol) 35 mg IM STAT
   Available:

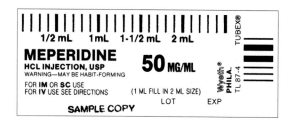

How many mL should the client receive? _____

8. Order: atropine sulfate gr 1/200 SC on call.
   Available (drug label): atropine sulfate 0.4 mg/1 mL

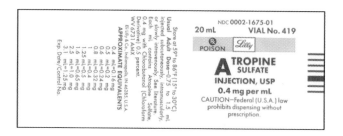

How many mL should the client receive? _____

II. Drug Dosage Using Body Weight

9. Order: phenytoin (Dilantin) 5 mg/kg/day P.O. in two divided doses.
   Client weighs 55 lb.
   How many milligrams (mg) should the client receive per day? _____
   Per dose? _____

10. Order: sulfisoxazole (Gantrisin) 50 mg/kg/day P.O. in four divided doses (q6h). Child weighs 44 lb.
    How many mg should the client receive per day? _____ Per dose? _____

11. Order: albuterol (Proventil) 0.1 mg/kg/day P.O. in four divided doses. Client weighs 86 lb.
    How many mg should the client receive per dose? _____

12. Order: cefprozil 15 mg/kg/day P.O. in two divided doses. Child weighs 33 lb.
    Available:

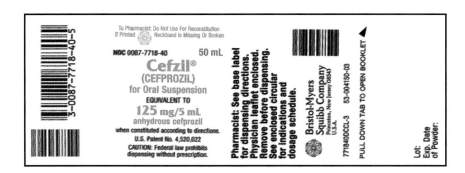

   a. How many milligrams should be given per day? _____
   b. How many milliliters should the child receive per dose? _____

III. Drug Dosage Using Body Surface Area

13. Client's height is 62 in. and weight is 130 lb. The BSA is _____

14. Order: bleomycin sulfate 20 Units/m^2 IV. Client is 70 in. tall and weighs 160 lb.
    How many unit(s) should the client receive? _____

15. Order: sulfisoxazole (Gantrisin) 2 g/m^2 in four divided doses. Child's height is 50 in. and weight is 60 lb.
    Available: sulfisoxazole 500 mg/5 mL.
    a. What is the child's BSA? _____
    b. How many gram(s) should the child receive per day? _____
    c. How many mL should the child receive per dose? _____

ANSWERS TO PRACTICE PROBLEMS

Drug Dosage Using a General Formula and Ratio and Proportion

1. a. Convert grams to milligrams by moving the decimal point three spaces to the right.

    0.4 g = 0.400 mg

   b. $\dfrac{D}{H} \times V = \dfrac{400 \text{ mg}}{400 \text{ mg}} \times 1$ tablet = 1 tablet

2. 2 tablets

    $$\dfrac{1 \text{ mg}}{0.5 \text{ mg}} = 0.5\,\overline{)1.0}^{\,2.0 \text{ tablets}}$$

3. a. Convert grains to milligrams. Table 4A–4 or 4B–1 gives 30 mg = ½ gr, or 60 mg = 1 gr 60 mg : 1 gr :: x mg : ½ gr

$x = 60 \times 0.5$ (½)

$x = 30$ mg

b. $\dfrac{D}{H} \times V = \dfrac{30}{15} \times 1 = 2$ tablets

4. ½ tablets

5. 10 mL

6. $\dfrac{D}{H} \times V = \dfrac{100}{62.5} \times 5 = \dfrac{500}{62.5} = 8$ mL

7. 0.7 mL

8. a. The drug label shows 0.4 mg = 1 ml. Change 1/200 gr to milligrams (see Table 4A–4 or 4B–1). $\frac{1}{200}$ gr = 0.3 mg

b. $\dfrac{D}{H} \times V = \dfrac{0.3}{0.4} \times 1$ mL $= 0.4\sqrt{0.3\underset{\curvearrowright}{.}0}\overset{0.75}{} = 0.75$ mL

Drug Dosage Using Body Weight

9. a. 55 lb ÷ 2.2 kg = 25 kg
   b. 5 mg × 25 kg = 125 mg/day, or 62.5 mg b.i.d.

10. a. 44 lb ÷ 2.2 kg = 20 kg
    b. 50 mg × 20 kg = 1000 mg/day
       1000 ÷ 4 times a day = 250 mg q.i.d., or q6h

11. a. 86 ÷ 2.2 = 39 kg
    b. 0.1 mg × 39 = 3.9 mg, or 4 mg
       4 ÷ 4 = 1 mg q6h

12. 33 ÷ 2.2 = 15 kg
    15 mg × 15 = 225 mg/day
    225 ÷ 2 times a day = 112.5 mg q12h per dose

$\dfrac{D}{H} \times V = \dfrac{112.5}{125} \times 5$ mL $= \dfrac{562.5}{125} = 4.5$ mL q12h

a. Administer cefprozil 225 mg/day
b. Administer 112.5 mg = 4.5 mL q12h

Drug Dosage Using Body Surface Area

13. 1.65 m²

14. a. Client's height and weight intersect the nomogram scale at 1.97 m².
    b. 20 U × 1.97 = 39.4 or 39 U

15. a. Height and weight intersect the nomogram scale at 0.98 m².
    b. 2 g × 0.98 = 1.96 g, or 2 g/day
    c. 5 mL (convert grams to milligrams. 0.5 g = 0.500 mg)

Calculations of Oral Dosages

4

Outline

Objectives

- Calculate oral dosages from tablets, capsules, and liquids with selected formula.
- Calculate oral medications according to body weight and body surface area (BSA).
- Calculate the amount of tube feeding solution needed for dilution according to the percentage ordered.

Terms

body surface area

capsule

drug parameters

enteric-coated

sustained-release

tablet

tube feeding

INTRODUCTION

Eighty percent of all drugs consumed are given orally. Oral drugs are available in tablet, capsule, powder, and liquid form. The written abbreviation for drugs given orally is P.O. or PO (per os, or by mouth). Oral medications are absorbed by the gastrointestinal tract, mainly from the small intestine.

Oral medications have the following advantages: the client frequently can take the drug without assistance, the cost of the drug is usually less than when given via other routes, e.g., parenteral, and it is easy to store. The disadvantages include variation in absorption as a result of food in the gastrointestinal (GI) tract and pH variation of GI secretions, irritation of the gastric mucosa by certain drugs (potassium chloride), and destruction or partial inactivation of the drugs by liver enzymes. Section 4C discusses oral dosages for adults, whereas Section 4F discusses oral dosages in pediatrics.

TABLETS, CAPSULES, AND LIQUIDS

Tablets come in different forms and drug strengths. Most tablets are scored, and thus can be readily broken when half of the drug amount is needed. **Capsules** are gelatin shells containing powder or timed-release pellets (beads). **Sustained-release** (pellet) capsules *should not* be crushed and diluted, because the medication will be absorbed at a much faster rate than indicated by the manufacturer. Many of the medications that are in tablet form are also available in liquid form. When the client has difficulty in taking tablets, the liquid form of the medication is given. The liquid form can be in a suspension, syrup, elixir, or tincture. Some liquid medications that are irritating to the stomach, such as potassium chloride, are diluted. The tincture form is always diluted.

Enteric-coated (hard shell) tablets *must not* be crushed, because the medication could irritate the gastric mucosa. Enteric-coated drugs pass through the stomach, with the coating being dissolved in the small intestine; thus, absorption takes place in the intestine. Oral drugs (tablets, capsules, liquids) that irritate the gastric mucosa should be taken with 5 to 8 oz of fluids or taken during mealtime. Figure 4C–1 shows the different forms of tablets and capsules.

Liquid medications are poured into a medicine cup that is calibrated in ounces, teaspoons, tablespoons, and milliliters. Figure 4C–2 shows the markings on a medicine cup.

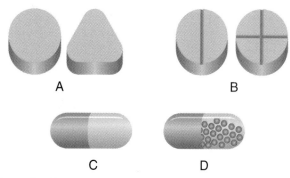

Figure 4C–1
Shapes of tablets and capsules. *A* and *B*: tablets; *C* and *D*: capsules.

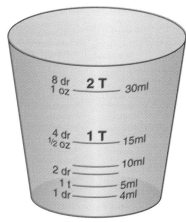

Figure 4C–2
Medicine cup for liquid measurement. (From Kee, J. L., and Marshall, S. M.: *Clinical Calculations*, 3rd ed. Philadelphia: WB Saunders, p. 99, 1996.)

INTERPRETING ORAL DRUG LABELS

The pharmaceutical companies usually label their drugs with the brand (trade) name of the drug in large letters and the generic name in smaller letters. The dose per tablet, capsule, or liquid is often printed under the drug name. Two examples of oral drug labels follow:

Example 1

Avapro is the brand (trade) name, and irbesartan is the generic name. The dose is 75 mg/tablet.

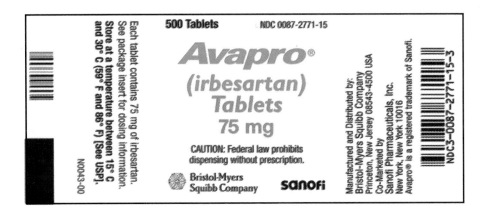

Example 2

Ceftin is the brand (trade) name, and cefuroxime axetil is the generic name. The dose is 125 mg/5 mL (oral suspension).

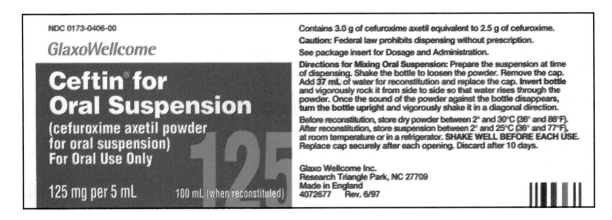

DRUG DIFFERENTIATION

Some drugs with similar names, such as quinine and quinidine, have different chemical drug structures. Extreme care must be exercised when administering drugs whose names look alike. Examine the following examples.

Example 1 — Percodan and Percocet

Percodan contains oxycodone and aspirin, and Percocet contains oxycodone and acetaminophen. A client may be allergic to aspirin or should not take aspirin because of a stomach ulcer; therefore, it is important that the client take Percocet. *Read the drug labels carefully.*

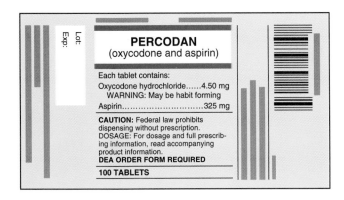

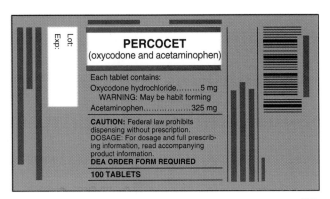

Example 2   **Hydroxyzine and Hydralazine**

Hydroxyzine is an antianxiety drug and hydralazine is an antihypertensive drug.

CALCULATION FOR TABLET, CAPSULE, AND LIQUID DOSES

When calculating oral dosages, choose one of the methods for calculation from Section 4B. Examples are given using the basic formula and the ratio-and-proportion methods.

Basic Formula

$$\frac{D}{H} \times V =$$

Ratio and Proportion

H : V :: D : x
on hand   vehicle   desired   unknown
                       dose

means

extremes

$x =$

Examples

1. Order: diltiazem (Cardizem) 60 mg PO b.i.d.
   Available:

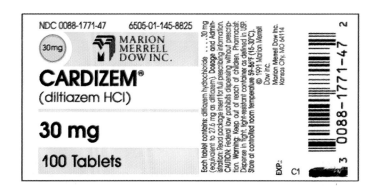

NDC 0088-1771-47   6505-01-145-8825

MARION
MERRELL
DOW INC.

CARDIZEM®
(diltiazem HCl)

30 mg

100 Tablets

0088-1771-47

   a. $\dfrac{D}{H} \times V = \dfrac{60}{30} \times 1 = 2$ tablets
   b. H : V :: D : x
      30 mg : 1 tab :: 60 mg : x tab

   $$30x = 60$$

   $$x = 2 \text{ tablets}$$

   Answer: diltiazem (Cardizem) 360 mg = 2 tablets

2. Order: codeine phosphate 1 gr PO STAT
   Available: Refer to the conversion tables 4A−4 or 4B−1.

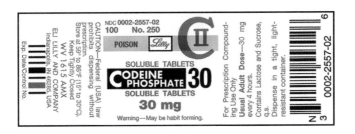

a. gr 1 = 60 mg

b.
$$\frac{D}{H} \times V = \frac{60}{30} \times 1 = 2 \text{ tablets}$$

$$
\begin{array}{ccccccc}
H & : & V & :: & D & : & x \\
30 \text{ mg} & : & 1 \text{ tab} & :: & 60 \text{ mg} & : & x \text{ tab}
\end{array}
$$

$$30x = 60$$

$$x = 2 \text{ tablets}$$

Answer: codeine 1 gr = 2 tablets

PRACTICE PROBLEMS

I. Tablets, Capsules, and Liquid

Solve the drug problems for *x*, the unknown amount of drug to be given. Refer to Sections 4A and 4B for the conversion tables, methods of conversion, and the method chosen to solve the drug problems:

1. Order: prednisone 5 mg PO b.i.d.
   Available: prednisone 2.5 mg tablet
   How many tablet(s) should the client receive per dose? _____

2. Order: grepafloxacin (Raxar) 0.4 g PO q.d.
   Available:

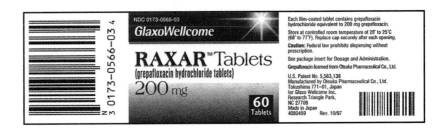

   How many tablet(s) should the client receive per dose? _____

3. Order: allopurinol (Zyloprim) 450 mg PO q.d.
   Available: allopurinol 300 mg tablet
   How many tablet(s) should the client receive? _____

4. Order: aspirin gr *x* STAT
   Available: aspirin 325 mg tablet
   How many tablet(s) of aspirin should the nurse give? _____

5. Order: digoxin (Lanoxin) 0.5 mg PO q.d.
   Available:

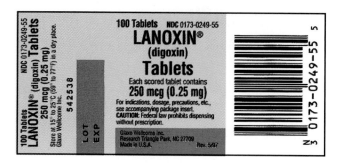

How many tablet(s) should the nurse administer? _____

6. Order: nitroglycerin ⅟₁₅₀ gr, sublingual, STAT
   Available:

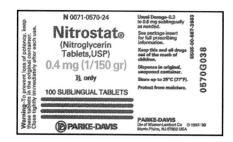

How many sublingual tablet(s) should the client take? _____

7. Order: bethanechol Cl (Urecholine) 20 mg PO t.i.d.
   Available:

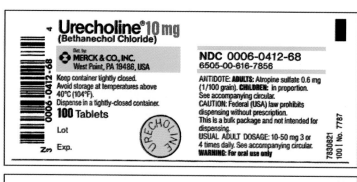

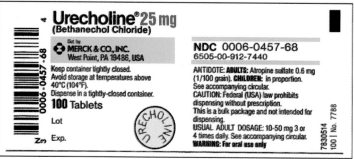

a. Which Urecholine bottle should the nurse select? _____
b. How many tablet(s) should the client receive per dose? _____

8. Order: Augmentin 500 mg PO b.i.d.
   Available:

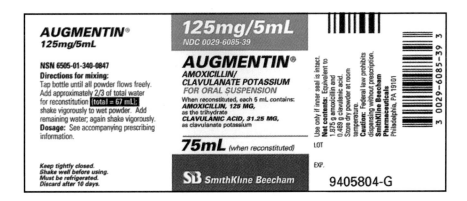

How many mL should the client receive per dose? _____

9. Order: nystatin (Mycostatin) 300,000 units, swish and swallow t.i.d.
   Available:

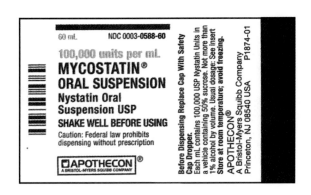

How many mL should the client receive per dose? _____

10. Order: Amoxicillin, 200 mg PO q6h
    Available:

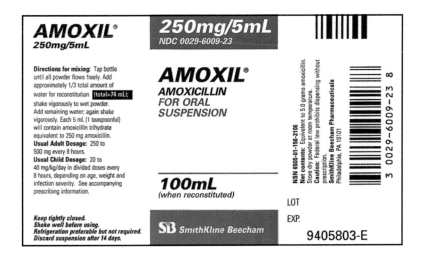

How many mL should the client receive per dose? _____

11. Order: potassium chloride (Kay Ciel) 30 mEq PO q.d.
    Available: potassium chloride 20 mEq/15 mL (cc)
    How many mL should the client receive per day? _____

12. Order: docusate sodium (Colace) 50 mg PO h.s.
    Available: Colace syrup 20 mg/5 mL
    How many mL should the client receive at bedtime? _____

13. Order: cefadroxil (Duricef) 500 mg PO b.i.d.
    Available:

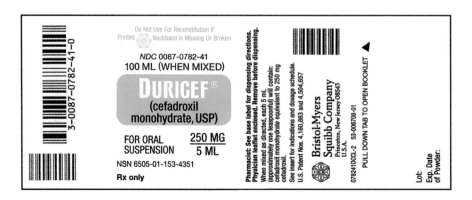

    How many mL should the client receive per dose? _____

14. Order: prazosin (Minipress) 10 mg PO q.d.
    Available: prazosin 1-mg, 2-mg, and 5-mg tablets
    Which tablet would you select and how much would you give? _____

15. Order: carbidopa–levodopa (Sinemet) 12.5–125 mg PO b.i.d.
    Available: Sinemet 25- to 100-, 25- to 250-, 10- to 100-mg tablets
    Which tablet would you select and how much would you give? _____

BODY WEIGHT AND BODY SURFACE AREA

Calculating the drug dosage for adults by body weight and body surface area is used mostly when administering drugs to treat cancer (antineoplastic drugs). These two individualized methods are used frequently in calculating drug dosage for children. Examples and practice problems for pediatrics are given in Section 4F.

To use the **body weight** method, convert the person's weight in pounds to kilograms (kg). To convert, divide pounds by 2.2 to equal kilograms. In using the **body surface area** method, the person's weight and height and a nomogram are needed. (See Section 4B and the pediatric section of 4F). Daily requirements are usually divided into two to four doses per day.

Example

Order: cyclophosphamide (Cytoxan) 2 mg/kg/day/PO
Client weighs 143 lb. How much does the client weigh in kilograms? How many milligrams (mg) should the client receive?

Answer:

$$143 \text{ lb} \div 2.2 = 65 \text{ kg}$$

$$2 \text{ mg} \times 65 = 130 \text{ mg of Cytoxan daily}$$

II. Body Weight

1. Order: valproic acid (Depakene) 8 mg/kg/day in four divided doses. Client weighs 165 lb. How much Depakene should be administered per dose?

2. Order: cyclophosphamide (Cytoxan) 4 mg/kg/day. Client weighs 176 lb. How much Cytoxan should the client receive per day?

PERCENTAGE OF SOLUTIONS

When clients are unable to take food or fluids by mouth, they may receive nutrients through a nasogastric (NG) tube. The nutrients that are administered through NG tubes are in solution form, and the process is usually called **tube feeding.** When tube feedings are initiated, they are usually diluted with water to prevent diarrhea that may result from the richness of the solution. Dilutions of tube feeding are ordered in percentage. Clients tolerate tube feedings better when the feedings are started at low strength and the concentration is incrementally increased over time. When a percentage strength of solution is ordered, the nurse calculates the amount of solution and water that are to be given.

The percentage of a solution indicates its strength. Tube feeding solutions, such as Ensure, Ensure Plus, Osmolite, Isomil, and others, are considered to be 100%. Fifty percent of the solution is 50% strength of the solution or 50/100. To determine the amount (mL) of tube feeding solution to give, the basic formula or ratio-and-proportion method can be used with the following changes:

D stands for the desired percentage.
H represents the on-hand strength, which is 100%.
V represents the desired total volume.
x stands for the unknown amount of solution.

Following the tube feeding, 30 mL (cc) of water should be given to clear the tubing. Usually the tube is clamped for 30 min after feeding to keep fluid content from backing out of the stomach into the tube. The client should remain with head elevated at a 30- to 90-degree angle after feeding for 30 minutes.

Example

Order: 250 mL (cc) of 30% solution, q4h × 6 feedings, via NG tube

Calculate how much Ensure and water is needed to make 250 mL of 30% solution.

Note: 30% solution is 30 in 100 parts.

a. $\dfrac{D}{H}\left(\dfrac{\text{Desired \%}}{\text{On-hand strength}}\right) \times V \text{ (Desired total volume)} =$

$$\frac{30}{100} \times 250 = \frac{7500}{100} = 75 \text{ mL of Ensure}$$

b.

H	:	V	::	D	:	
100	:	250	::	30	:	x

$$100x = 7500$$
$$x = 75 \text{ mL of Ensure}$$

How much water should be added?

$$\text{Total amount} - \text{Amount of tube feeding} = \text{Amount of water}$$

$$250 \text{ mL} - 75 \text{ mL} = 175 \text{ mL}$$

Answer: 75 mL of Ensure + 175 mL of water.

Oral medications can be administered through the nasogastric tube, but should *not* be mixed with the entire tube feeding solution. Mixing the medications in a large volume of tube feeding decreases the amount of drug the client receives for a specific time. The medication (**NOT** time-released or sustained-release capsules and psyllium hydrophilic mucilloid [Metamucil]) should be diluted in 1 oz, or 30 mL, of warm water unless otherwise instructed, administered through the tube, and followed with extra water to ensure that the drug reaches the stomach and is not left in the tube.

PRACTICE PROBLEMS

III. Percentage of Solutions

Refer to example as needed.

1. Order: 500 mL of 60% Ensure Plus solution three times a day through the nasogastric tube.
   How much Ensure Plus solution and water should be mixed to equal 500 mL?

2. Order: 250 mL of 70% Osmolite solution, q6h, via NG tube.
   How much Osmolite and water should be mixed to equal 250 mL?

3. Order: 400 mL of 40% Isomil solution, q6h, through the NG tube.
   How much Isomil and water should be mixed to equal 400 mL?

4. Order: 300 mL of 75% Ensure solution four times a day through the NG tube.
   How much Ensure and water should be mixed to equal 300 mL?

ANSWERS TO PRACTICE PROBLEMS

I. Oral Medications (a and b are the two methods of calculation)

1. 2 tablets

   a. $\dfrac{D}{H} \times V = \dfrac{5}{2.5} \times 1 = 2$ tablets

   b.
H	:	V	::	D	:	x
2.5 mg	:	1 tab	::	5 mg	:	x tab

   $$2.5x = 5$$
   $$x = \frac{5.0}{2.5} = 2 \text{ tablets}$$

2. 2 tablets
   Change grams to milligrams. Move decimal point three spaces to the right. Refer to Section 4A if necessary.

   $$0.400 \text{ g} = 400 \text{ mg}$$

3. 1½ tablets
4. Convert grains to milligrams. See Table 4A–4 or 4B–1.
   5 gr = 300, or 325 mg; thus 10 gr = 650 mg (approximate value)

   a. $\dfrac{D}{H} \times V = \dfrac{650}{325} \times 1 = 2$ tablets

   b.
H	:	V	::	D	:	x
325 mg	:	1 tab	::	650 mg	:	x tab

   $$325x = 650$$
   $$x = 2 \text{ tablets}$$

5. 2 tablets

   a. $\dfrac{D}{H} \times V = \dfrac{0.5}{0.25} \times 1 = 0.25\overline{\smash{\big)}0.50.0}\ \ 2.0 = 2$ tablets

   b.
H	:	V	::	D	:	x
0.25 mg	:	1 tab	::	0.5 mg	:	x tab

   $$0.25x = 0.5 = 2 \text{ tablets}$$

6. 1 sublingual tablet

   Convert grains to milligrams. $\frac{1}{150}$ gr = 0.4 mg

7. a. Select Urecholine 10 mg bottle.

   b. $\dfrac{D}{H} \times V = \dfrac{20 \text{ mg}}{10 \text{ mg}} \times 1 \text{ tab} = \dfrac{20}{10} = 2$ tablets

8. 20 mL of Augmentin suspension
9. 3 mL of Mycostatin
10. 4 mL

    a. $\dfrac{D}{H} \times V = \dfrac{200}{250} \times 5 = \dfrac{1000}{250} = 4 \text{ mL}$

    b.
H	:	V	::	D	:	x
250 mg	:	5 mL	::	200 mg	:	x mL

    $$250x = 1000 \qquad x = 4 \text{ mL of amoxicillin}$$

11. 22.5 mL or 4½ t

    a. $\dfrac{D}{H} \times V = \dfrac{30}{20} \times 15 = \dfrac{450}{20} = 22.5 \text{ mL}$

    b.
H	:	V	::	D	:	x
20 mEq	:	15 mL	::	30 mEq	:	x mL

    $$20x = 450 \qquad x = \dfrac{450}{20} = 22.5 \text{ mL of potassium chloride}$$

12. 12.5 mL (cc) of Colace syrup
13. 10 mL of cefadroxil

    a. $\dfrac{D}{H} \times V = \dfrac{500}{250} \times 5 = \dfrac{2500}{250} = 10 \text{ mL}$

    b.
H	:	V	::	D	:	x
250 mg	:	5 mL	::	500 mg	:	x mL

    $$250x = 2500 \qquad x = 10 \text{ mL}$$

14. Select 5-mg tablets. Give two tablets.
15. Select 25–250 mg strength. Give ½ tablet.

II. Body Weight

1. 150 mg/dose; 600 mg/day.
2. 320 mg/day

1. $\dfrac{D}{H} \times V = \dfrac{60}{100} \times 500 = \dfrac{30,000}{100} = 300$ mL of Ensure Plus

H	:	V	::	D	:	x
100	:	500	::	60	:	x

$$100x = 30,000$$
$$x = 300 \text{ mL of Ensure Plus}$$

Total amount $-$ Amount of tube feeding $=$ Amount of water

500 mL $-$ 300 mL $=$ 200 mL

300 mL of Ensure Plus $+$ 200 mL of water

2. 175 mL of Osmolite $+$ 75 mL of water
3. 160 mL of Isomil $+$ 240 mL of water
4. 225 mL of Ensure $+$ 75 mL of water

Calculations of Injectable Dosages

4

Outline

Objectives

- Describe the difference between vials and ampules.
- Describe the types of syringes and needles and their uses.
- Explain how to administer intradermal, subcutaneous, and intramuscular injections.
- Calculate dosage of drugs for subcutaneous and intramuscular injections.
- Identify the amount of insulin dosage using an insulin syringe.
- Explain the methods for mixing two insulins in one insulin syringe and for mixing two injectable drugs in one syringe.
- Describe the procedure for preparing and calculating medications in powdered form for injectable use.

Terms

ampule	insulin syringe	parenteral
bevel	intradermal	subcutaneous
diluent	intramuscular	tuberculin syringe
gauge	lumen	vial

INTRODUCTION

When medications cannot be taken by mouth because of an inability to swallow, a decreased level of consciousness, an inactivation of the drug by the gastric juices, or a desire to increase the effectiveness of the drug, the parenteral route may be the route of choice. **Parenteral** medications are administered intradermally (under the skin), subcutaneously (SC, into the fatty tissue), intramuscularly (IM, within the muscle), and intravenously (IV, in the vein).

Intravenous injectables are discussed in Section 4E. The injectables in this section include intradermal, subcutaneous (including insulin and heparin), and intramuscular from prepared liquid and reconstituted powder in vials and ampules. Prefilled drug cartridges (syringes) are also discussed.

This section is divided into five sections: (1) injectable preparations, (2) intradermal injections, (3) subcutaneous injections, (4) insulin injections, and (5) intramuscular injections. With the four latter groups, examples and practice problems to solve for the correct dosage are given.

INJECTABLE PREPARATIONS

The appropriate drug container (vial or ampule) and the correct selection of needle and syringe are essential when preparing the prescribed drug dose. The route of administration is part of the medication order.

VIALS AND AMPULES

Vials are usually small glass containers with a self-sealing rubber top. Some are multiple-dose vials, and when properly stored they can be used over time. **Ampules** are glass containers with a tapered neck for snapping open and are used only once. Drugs that deteriorate readily in liquid form are packaged in powder form in vials and ampules for storage. Once the dry form of the drug is reconstituted (usually with sterile water, bacteriostatic water, or saline), the drug is used immediately or must be refrigerated. Check the accompanying drug circular for specific storage length and other instructions. The person reconstituting the drug should write on the label when the drug is to be discarded and include her or his initials. Usually a vial should be used within 96 h to 1 week.

Drug labels on vials and ampules provide the following information: generic and brand name of the drug, drug dose in weight (milligrams, grams, milliequivalents) and amount (milliliters), expiration date, and directions about administration. If the drug is in powdered form, mixing instructions and dose equivalents (such as milligrams equal milliliters) may be given. Figure 4D–1 is a diagram of a vial and ampule.

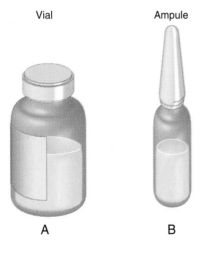

Vial   Ampule

A   B

Figure 4D–1
(A) Vial. (B) Ampule. (From Kee, J. L., and Marshall, S. M.: *Clinical Calculations*, 3rd ed. Philadelphia: WB Saunders, p. 124, 1996.)

SYRINGES

The syringe is composed of a barrel (outer shell), plunger (inner part), and the tip where the needle joins the syringe (Fig. 4D–2). Syringes are available in various types and sizes, the most common of which are the 3-mL and 5-mL sizes of tuberculin, insulin, and metal and plastic syringes for prefilled cartridges. Glass syringes may be used in the operating room and on special instrument trays. Selected injectable drugs are packaged in prefilled cartridges for Tubex and the Carpuject brand syringes. The tip of the syringe and inside of plunger should remain sterile.

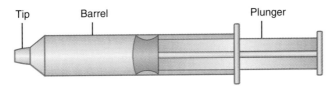

Tip   Barrel   Plunger

Figure 4D–2
Parts of a syringe. (From Kee, J. L., and Marshall, S. M.: *Clinical Calculations*, 3rd ed. Philadelphia: WB Saunders, p. 125, 1996.)

The 3-mL syringe is calibrated in tenths (0.1 mL) and minims. The amount of fluid in the syringe is determined by the black rubber end of the plunger (the inner end of the plunger) that is closest to the tip (Fig. 4D–3). *Remember:* Milliliter (mL) and cubic centimeter (cc) may be used interchangeably. An advance in safety needle technology is the "SafetyGlide shielding hypodermic needle" (Fig. 4D–4). The purpose of this type of needle is to reduce needle-stick injuries.

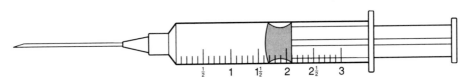

$\frac{1}{2}$ 1 $1\frac{1}{2}$ 2 $2\frac{1}{2}$ 3

Figure 4D–3
Three-milliliter syringe. (From Kee, J. L., and Marshall, S. M.: *Clinical Calculations*, 3rd ed. Philadelphia: WB Saunders, p. 124, 1996.)

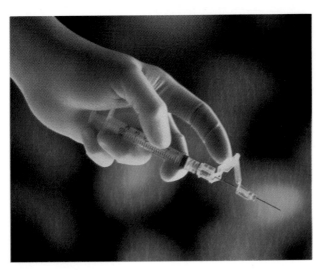

Figure 4D–4
Safety Glide needle. (Courtesy of Bectin-Dickinson Division, Franklin Lakes, NJ.)

The 5-mL syringe is calibrated in 0.2-mL marks. A 5-mL syringe is usually used when the fluid needed is more than 2.5 mL. It is frequently used when reconstituting the dry drug form with sterile bacteriostatic water or saline. Figure 4D–5 shows the 5-mL syringe and its markings.

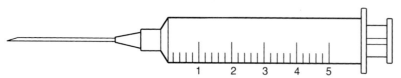

Figure 4D–5
Five-milliliter syringe. (From Kee, J. L., and Marshall, S. M.: *Clinical Calculations*, 3rd ed. Philadelphia: WB Saunders, p. 125, 1996.)

The **tuberculin syringe** is a 1-mL slender syringe with markings in tenths (0.1) and hundredths (0.01). It is also marked in minims (Fig. 4D–6). This syringe is used when the amount of drug solution to be administered is less than 1 mL and for pediatric and heparin dosages. Also the tuberculin syringe is available in a ½-milliliter syringe. Figure 4D–7 illustrates the 0.5 mL and the 1-mL tuberculin syringes.

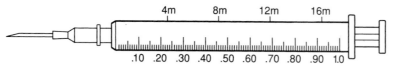

Figure 4D–6
Tuberculin syringe. (From Kee, J. L., and Marshall, S. M.: *Clinical Calculations*, 3rd ed. Philadelphia: WB Saunders, p. 126, 1996.)

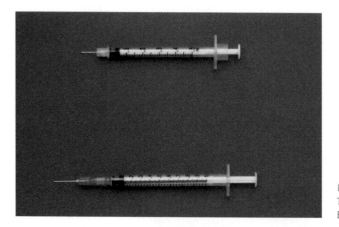

Figure 4D–7. Two types of tuberculin syringes. (Courtesy of Bectin-Dickinson Division, Franklin Lakes, NJ.)

The **insulin syringe** has the capacity of 1 mL; however, insulin is measured in units and insulin dosage *must not* be calculated in milliliters. Insulin syringes are calibrated as 2-U marks, and 100 U equal 1 mL (Fig. 4D–8). *Insulin syringes must be used for the administration of insulin.*

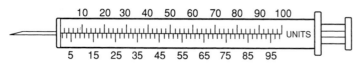

Figure 4D–8
Insulin syringe. (From Kee, J. L., and Marshall, S. M.: *Clinical Calculations*, 3rd ed. Philadelphia: WB Saunders, p. 126, 1996.)

Insulin syringes are available as low-dose insulin syringes. The 1-mL insulin syringe may be purchased with a permanent attached needle or a detachable needle (Fig. 4D–9).

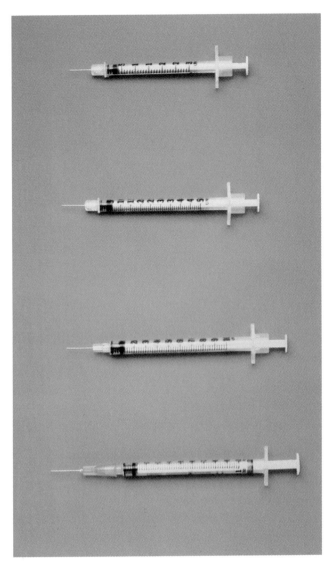

Figure 4D–9
Various types of insulin syringes. (Courtesy of Bectin-Dickinson Division, Franklin Lakes, NJ.)

Prefilled Drug Cartridges and Syringes

Many injectable drugs are packaged in prefilled, disposable cartridges. The disposable cartridge is placed into a Tubex injector or a reusable metal or plastic holder. Usually the prefilled cartridge contains 0.1 to 0.2 mL of excess drug solution. Based on the amount of drug to be administered, the excess solution must be expelled before administration. Figure 4D–10A illustrates the Tubex injector and cartridge; Figure 4D–10B shows the Hypak prefilled syringe.

Needles

Needle size has two components, gauge (diameter of the lumen) and length. The larger the **gauge,** the smaller the diameter of the **lumen,** and the smaller the gauge, the larger the diameter of the lumen. The more common gauge numbers of needles range from 18 to 26.

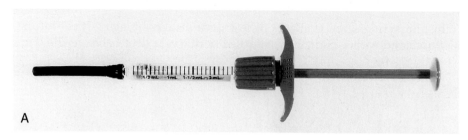

A

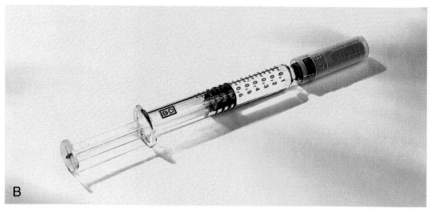

B

Figure 4D–10
(A) Prefilled cartridge and Tubex injector. (From Kee, J. L., and Marshall, S. M.: *Clinical Calculations*, 3rd ed. Philadelphia: WB Saunders, p. 126, 1996. Courtesy of Wyeth-Ayerst Laboratories, Philadelphia.) (B) Hypak Prefilled syringe. (Courtesy of Bectin-Dickinson Division, Franklin Lakes, NJ.)

Needle length varies from ⅜ to 2 in. Table 4D–1 lists the needle gauges and lengths for use in subcutaneous and intramuscular injections.

When choosing the needle length for an intramuscular injection, the size of the client and the amount of fatty tissue must be considered. A client with minimal fatty (subcutaneous) tissue may need a needle length of 1 inch. For an obese client, the length of the needle for an intramuscular injection would be 1.5 to 2 inches.

Many of the insulin syringes and prefilled cartridges have permanently attached needles. With other syringes, the needle can be changed to the desired needle size. Needle gauge and length are indicated on the syringe package or on the top cover of the syringe. It appears as gauge/length; for example, 20 g/1½.

Figure 4D–11 illustrates the parts of a needle.

Table 4D–1
Needle Size and Length

TYPE OF INJECTION	NEEDLE GAUGE	NEEDLE LENGTHS (INCHES)
Intradermal	25, 26	$\frac{3}{8}, \frac{1}{2}, \frac{5}{8}$
Subcutaneous	23, 25, 26	$\frac{3}{8}, \frac{1}{2}, \frac{5}{8}$
Intramuscular	19, 20, 21, 22	$1, 1\frac{1}{2}, 2$

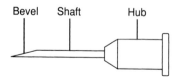

Bevel   Shaft   Hub

Figure 4D–11
Parts of a needle. (From Kee, J. L., and Marshall, S. M.: *Clinical Calculations*, 3rd ed. Philadelphia: WB Saunders, p. 126, 1996.)

ANGLES FOR INJECTIONS

For injections, the needle enters the skin at different angles. Intradermal injections are given at a 10- to 15-degree angle, subcutaneous injections at a 45- to 90-degree angle, and intramuscular injections at a 90-degree angle. Figure 3–19 in Chapter 3 illustrates the angles for intradermal, subcutaneous, and intramuscular injections.

PRACTICE PROBLEMS

I. Syringes and Needles

Think through and answer each question. Correct answers are given at the end of the section.

1. To mix 4 mL of bacteriostatic water in a vial with a powdered drug, which size syringe should be used?
2. To give 0.4 mL of drug solution subcutaneously, what type of syringe would you use?
3. Meperidine (Demerol) is available in a prefilled cartridge. Half of the drug solution is used. Should the remaining solution in the cartridge be saved for future use?
4. Which has the larger needle lumen, a 21-gauge needle or a 26-gauge needle?
5. Which needle has a length of ⅝ inch, a 21-gauge needle or a 25-gauge needle?
6. Which needle is used for an intramuscular injection, a 20-gauge needle with a 1.5-inch length or a 25-gauge needle with a ⅝-inch length?

INTERPRETING INJECTABLE DRUG LABEL

Drugs for injections are stored in liquid and powder form in vials and ampules. If the drug is in liquid form, the drug dose with its equivalent in milliliters is printed on the drug label. However, drugs in powder form have to be reconstituted (liquid form for use). Usually the instructions for reconstitution are given on the drug label and drug circular. If this is not the case, consult a pharmacist.

Example

Nafcillin sodium is the generic name; there is no brand (trade) name. The drug is for IM or IV administration. Instructions on the drug label read: "Add 6.6 mL of diluent; each vial contains 8 mL of drug solution."

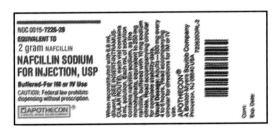

Another drug used as an example for interpreting injectable drug labels is Compazine. Prochlorperazine is the generic name and Compazine is the brand (trade) name. This drug comes in a 10-mL multidose vial. It can be administered deep IM or IV. The drug in the vial is in liquid form.

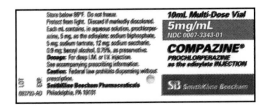

INTRADERMAL INJECTIONS

An **intradermal** injection is usually used for skin testing to diagnose the cause of an allergy or to determine the presence of a microorganism. The choice of syringe for intradermal testing is the tuberculin syringe with a 25-gauge needle.

The inner aspect of the forearm is frequently used for diagnostic testing because there is less hair in the area and the test results are more visible. The upper back may also be a testing site. The needle is inserted with the **bevel** upward at a 10- to 15-degree angle. Do not aspirate. Test results are read 48 to 72 h after the intradermal injection. A reddened or raised area is a positive reaction.

SUBCUTANEOUS INJECTIONS

Drugs injected into the **subcutaneous** (fatty) tissue are absorbed slowly because there are fewer blood vessels in the fatty tissue. The amount of drug solution administered subcutaneously is generally 0.5 to 1 mL at a 45-, 60-, or 90-degree angle. Drug solutions that are irritating to the fatty tissues are given intramuscularly because they can cause sloughing of the subcutaneous tissue.

The two types of syringes used for subcutaneous injections are the tuberculin syringe (1 mL), calibrated in 0.1 mL and 0.01 mL, and the 3-mL syringe, calibrated in 0.1 mL. The needle gauge commonly used is 25 or 26, and the length is ⅜ to ⅝ inch. Insulin is also administered subcutaneously and is discussed later in this section.

Calculations: Subcutaneous Injections

To calculate dosages for subcutaneous injections, use the basic formula of $D/H \times V$ or the ratio-and-proportion method (see Section 4B). Heparin is a drug frequently administered subcutaneously. It can be given at a 60- to 90-degree angle, depending on the amount of fatty tissue. The skin is lifted, and the heparin solution is injected into the subcutaneous tissue. Do not aspirate, and do not massage the injected site, because massage could cause small-vessel damage and bleeding.

Units (U) should be written out as a word and not as U only. When U is written, it may appear as O and thus the client could receive a higher dose of the drug.

Example

Order: heparin 2500 Units SC
Available: heparin 10,000 Units/mL in multiple-dose vial (10 mL)

Basic Formula:

$$\frac{D}{H} \times V = \frac{250\emptyset \text{ Units}}{1000\emptyset \text{ Units}} \times 1 \text{ mL} = \frac{25}{100} = 0.25 \text{ mL}$$

Ratio-and-Proportion Method:

$$\begin{array}{ccccccc} H & : & V & :: & D & : & x \\ 10{,}000 \text{ Units} & : & 1 \text{ mL} & :: & 2500 \text{ Units} & : & x \text{ mL} \end{array}$$

$$10{,}000x = 2500$$
$$x = \frac{25}{100} = 0.25 \text{ mL}$$

Answer: Heparin 2500 Units = 0.25 mL

II. Subcutaneous Injections

Use the formula you have chosen for calculating drug dosages from Section 4B. The same formula should be used when calculating oral, subcutaneous, intramuscular, insulin, and intravenous dosages. Refer to the conversion Table 4A–4 or 4B–1 as needed.

1. Order: heparin 4000 Units SC
   Available:

   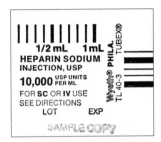

   How many mL should the client receive? _____

2. Order: heparin 7500 Units SC
   Available:

   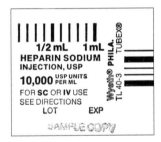

   How many mL should the client receive? _____

3. Order: atropine sulfate 0.5 mg SC
   Available:

   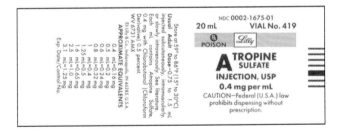

   How many mL should the client receive? _____

4. Order: epinephrine (Adrenalin) 0.2 mg, SC, STAT
   Available: epinephrine 1 mg/mL (1:1000) in ampule.
   What type of syringe would you use? _____

INSULIN INJECTIONS

Insulin is prescribed and measured in USP units. Most insulins are produced in concentrations of 100 Units/mL. Insulin should be administered with an insulin syringe, which is calibrated to correspond with the 100 Units of insulin. Insulin concentration is also available in 40 Units but is rarely used in the United States.

Insulin bottles and syringes are color-coded to avoid error. The 100 Units/mL (or U-100) insulin bottle and the 100 Units/mL syringe are coded orange. The 40 Units/mL (or U-40) insulin bottle and the 40 Units/mL syringe are coded red. *Always* match the insulin strength with the calibrated insulin syringe; the units of the insulin bottle and syringe should match. Administering insulin with a tuberculin syringe *should be avoided.*

Administration of medication requires attention to detail, and insulin is no exception. Insulin is ordered in units. For example, if the prescribed insulin dosage is 30 Units, withdraw 30 Units from a bottle of 100 Units of insulin using a 100-Unit calibrated insulin syringe (Fig. 4D–12).

Insulin is administered subcutaneously at a 45-, 60-, or 90-degree angle into the subcutaneous tissue. The subcutaneous absorption rate of insulin is slower because there are fewer blood vessels in the fatty tissue than in muscular tissue. The angle for administering insulin depends on the amount of fatty tissue. For an obese person, the angle may be 90 degrees; for a very thin person, the angle may be 45 to 60 degrees.

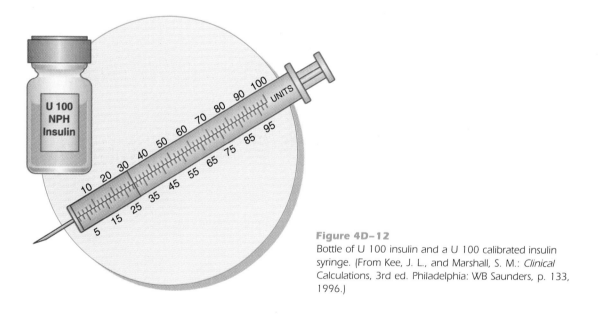

Figure 4D–12

Bottle of U 100 insulin and a U 100 calibrated insulin syringe. (From Kee, J. L., and Marshall, S. M.: *Clinical Calculations,* 3rd ed. Philadelphia: WB Saunders, p. 133, 1996.)

Types of Insulins

Insulins are clear (regular or crystalline insulin) and cloudy (NPH, lente) because of the substances protamine and zinc, which are used to prolong the action of insulin in the body. Only clear (regular) insulin can be given intravenously as well as subcutaneously. The source of insulin is beef, pork, beef-pork, and human (Humulin). Some individuals are allergic to beef insulin, so pork insulin is used because it has biologic properties similar to those of human insulin.

Insulin is categorized as fast-acting, intermediate-acting, and long-acting. The drug labels in the following example are arranged according to insulin action. Chapter 46 gives the peaks and durations of action of insulins.

A: Fast-Acting Insulin.

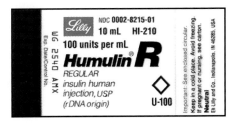

B: Intermediate-Acting Insulins.

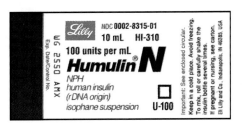
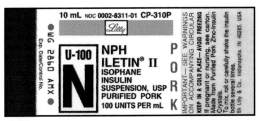

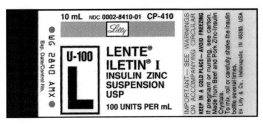

C: Long-Acting Insulin.

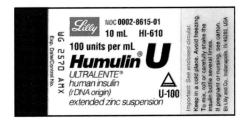

Mixing Insulins

Regular insulin is frequently mixed with insulin containing protamine (NPH) and zinc (lente). The following is an example of a method for mixing insulin:

Example

Order: Regular insulin 10 Units and NPH insulin 35 Units SC q 7 AM
Available: Regular insulin 100 U/mL and NPH insulin 100 U/mL. Insulin syringe: 100 U/mL.

Method

Step 1. Clean the rubber tops of the insulin bottles.
Step 2. Draw up 35 Units of air and inject into the NPH insulin bottle. Avoid letting the needle contact the NPH insulin solution. Withdraw the needle.

Step 3. Draw up 10 Units of air and inject into the regular insulin bottle.

Step 4. First, withdraw 10 Units of regular insulin. Regular insulin is always drawn up first.

Step 5. Insert needle into NPH bottle and withdraw 35 Units of NPH insulin. The total is 45 Units.

Step 6. Administer the two insulins immediately after mixing. Do *not* allow the insulin mixture to stand, because unpredicted physical changes may occur. Unpredicted changes are more common with protamine insulins, such as NPH, than with lente insulin.

PRACTICE PROBLEMS

III. Insulins

Indicate on the insulin syringe the amount of insulin that should be withdrawn for each type of insulin.

1. Order: lente insulin 30 Units SC
   Available: lente insulin 100 U/mL and insulin syringe 100 U/mL

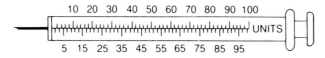

2. Order: NPH insulin 45 Units SC
   Available: NPH insulin 100 U/mL and insulin syringe 100 U/mL

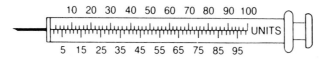

3. Order: regular insulin 15 Units and NPH insulin 25 Units SC
   Available: regular insulin 100 U/mL and NPH insulin 100 U/mL, and insulin syringe 100 U/mL

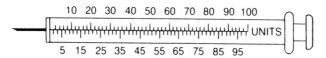

4. Order: regular insulin 6 Units and lente insulin 40 Units
   Available: regular insulin 100 U/mL and lente insulin 100 U/mL, and insulin syringe 100 U/mL

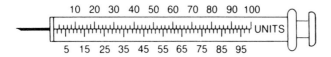

INTRAMUSCULAR INJECTIONS

Muscle has more blood vessels than the fatty tissue, so medications given by **intramuscular** (IM) injections are absorbed more rapidly than subcutaneous injections. The volume of solution for an IM injection is 0.5 to 3.0 mL, with the average being 1 to 2 mL. A volume of drug solution greater than 3 mL causes increased muscle tissue displacement and possible tissue damage. Occasionally, 5 mL of selected drugs, such as magnesium sulfate, may be injected into a large muscle, such as the dorsogluteal. A dose greater than 3 mL is usually divided and given at two different sites.

The needle gauges for intramuscular injections that contain thick solutions are 19 and 20, and for thin solutions are 20 and 21. Intramuscular injections are administered at a 90-degree angle. The needle length depends upon the amount of adipose (fat) and muscle tissues; the average needle length is 1.5 inches.

This section on intramuscular injections is divided into three subsections: (1) drug solutions for injection, (2) powdered drug reconstitution, and (3) mixing injectable drugs. An example is given for each subsection, and practice problems follow.

Sites of intramuscular injections are shown in Chapter 3.

Drug Solutions for Injection

Commercially premixed drug solutions are stored in vials and ampules for ready use. The drug label on the container gives the drug dose by weight and its equivalent in milliliters.

Example

Order: gentamicin (Garamycin) 50 mg IM
Available: gentamicin 80 mg/2 mL in a vial.

a. $\dfrac{D}{H} \times V = \dfrac{50}{80} \times 2 = \dfrac{100}{80} = 1.25$ mL

b.

H	:	V	::	D	:	x
80 mg	:	2 mL	::	50 mg	:	x mL

$$80x = 100$$
$$x = \frac{100}{80} = 1.25 \text{ mL}$$

Powdered Drug Reconstitution

Certain drugs lose their potency in liquid form; therefore, manufacturers package these drugs in powdered form. They are reconstituted using a **diluent** (bacteriostatic water or saline) before administration. The drug label or the instructional insert (accompanying pamphlet) frequently gives the type and amount of diluent to use. If the type and amount of diluent are not on the drug label or in the instructional insert, contact the pharmacist.

Usually, manufacturers determine the amount of diluent to mix with the drug powder to yield 1 to 2 mL/dose. The powdered drug occupies space; therefore, the volume of the drug solution is increased. Once the powdered drug has been reconstituted, the unused drug solution should be dated and initialed on the drug label. Unused drug solutions in vials are refrigerated and may be used for 48 h to 1 week according to the manufacturer's recommendation. Unused drug solutions in ampules are discarded.

Example

Solve the drug problem using the information on the drug label.
Order: aqueous penicillin 250,000 Units IM q4h

Available: aqueous penicillin 5,000,000 Units (5 million units).
The drug is in powdered form in a vial. The drug label states:

Diluent Added

(mL)	Units/mL
18	250,000
8	500,000
3	1,000,000

Add 18 mL of diluent. The drug powder is equivalent to 2 mL. Each 250,000 Units equals 1 mL. When working the problem, add 18 mL and 2 mL (powdered drug) = 20 mL.

a. $\dfrac{D}{H} \times V = \dfrac{250,000}{5,000,000} \times 20 = \dfrac{50}{50} = 1 \text{ mL}$

b.

H	:	V	::	D	:	x
5,000,000 Units	:	20 mL	::	250,000 Units	:	x mL

$$5,000,000x = 5,000,000$$

$$x = 1 \text{ mL}$$

Mixing Injectable Drugs

Drugs mixed together in the same syringe must be compatible to prevent precipitation. To determine drug compatibility, check drug reference texts or with a pharmacist. When in doubt about compatibility, do *not* mix drugs.

The three methods used for mixing drugs are (1) mixing two drugs in the same syringe from two vials, (2) mixing two drugs in the same syringe from one vial and one ampule, and (3) mixing two drugs in a prefilled cartridge from a vial.

METHOD 1: MIXING TWO DRUGS IN THE SAME SYRINGE FROM TWO VIALS

1. Draw air into the syringe to equal the amount of solution to be withdrawn from the first vial, and inject the air into the first vial. Do *not* allow the needle to come into contact with the solution. Remove the needle.
2. Draw air into the syringe to equal the amount of solution to be withdrawn from the second vial. Invert the second vial and inject the air. Withdraw the desired amount of solution from the second vial.
3. Change the needle, unless you will be using the entire volume in the first vial.
4. Invert the first vial, and withdraw the desired amount of solution.

METHOD 2: MIXING TWO DRUGS IN THE SAME SYRINGE FROM ONE VIAL AND ONE AMPULE

1. Inject air into the vial.
2. Remove the desired amount of solution from the vial.
3. Withdraw the desired amount of solution from the ampule.

METHOD 3: MIXING TWO DRUGS IN A PREFILLED CARTRIDGE FROM A VIAL

1. Check the drug dose and the amount of solution in the prefilled cartridge. If a smaller dose is needed, expel the excess solution.
2. Draw air into the cartridge to equal the amount of solution to be withdrawn from the vial. Invert the vial and inject the air.
3. Withdraw desired amount of solution from the vial. Be sure that the needle remains in the fluid, and do *not* take more solution than needed.

Mixing Drugs in the Same Syringe

Order: meperidine (Demerol) 25 mg and atropine sulfate 0.4 mg IM
Available: meperidine in a Tubex cartridge labeled 50 mg/mL
      Atropine sulfate in a multidose vial labeled 0.4 mg/mL
How many milliliters of each drug would you give and how are they mixed?

1. Meperidine dose

   a. $\dfrac{D}{H} \times V = \dfrac{25}{50} \times 1 = \dfrac{25}{50} = 0.5$ mL

   b.

H	:	V	::	D	:	x
50 mg	:	1 mL	::	25 mg	:	x mL

$$50x = 25$$
$$x = \frac{1}{2} = 0.5 \text{ mL}$$

2. Atropine dose:
   The label indicates 0.4 mg = 1 mL

Answer: Give meperidine 0.5 mL and atropine 1 mL.

PROCEDURE. Mix two drugs in the cartridge with one drug from a vial and the other drug in the prefilled cartridge.

1. Check the drug dose and volume on the prefilled cartridge.
2. Expel 0.5 mL and any excess drug solution (meperidine) from the cartridge (0.5 mL remains in the cartridge). Have another nurse witness the waste of a narcotic.
3. Draw 1 mL of air into the cartridge, and inject the air into the vial that contains the atropine.
4. Withdraw 1 mL of atropine from the vial into the meperidine solution in the cartridge.

PRACTICE PROBLEMS

IV. Intramuscular Injections

1. Order: cefazolin (Ancef) 500 mg IM q6h
   Available:

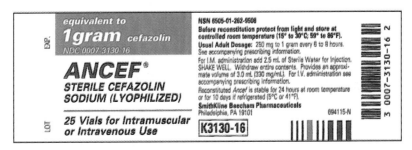

   How many milliliters (mL) would you give? _____

2. Order: procaine penicillin 400,000 Units IM q8h
   Available: procaine penicillin 300,000 Units/mL in a multiple-dose vial
   How many milliliters (mL) of procaine penicillin would you give?

SECTION D

3. Order: atropine sulfate 0.3 mg IM STAT
   Available: atropine sulfate

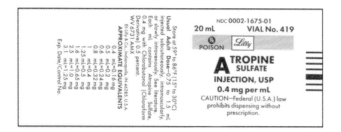

How many milliliters (mL) of atropine would you give? _____

4. Order: oxacillin 250 mg IM q6h
   Available:

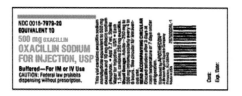

How many milliliters (mL) would you give? After the drug is reconstituted, how long can it be refrigerated?

5. Order: digoxin 0.25 mg IM q.d.
   Available: digoxin 0.5 mg/2 mL

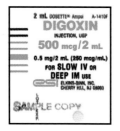

How many milliliters (mL) would you give? What should be done with the excess digoxin solution? (Usually parenteral digoxin is administered intravenously.)

6. Order: chlorpromazine (Thorazine) 50 mg IM STAT
   Available:

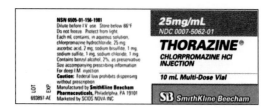

How many milliliters (mL) would you give? Can the vial be used again?

7. Order: meperidine 60 mg and hydroxyzine (Vistaril) 25 mg IM. These two drugs are compatible.
   Available: Hydroxyzine 100 mg/2 mL in vial

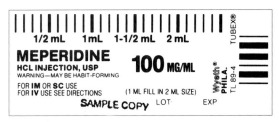

How many milliliters (mL) of meperidine and how many of hydroxyzine would you give? _____

Explain how the two drugs would be mixed in the cartridge.

8. Order: naloxone (Narcan) 0.5 mg IM and repeat in 3 min if needed
   Available:

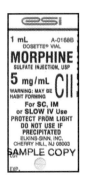

How many milliliters (mL) would you give per dose? _____

9. Order: morphine SO$_4$ 6 mg IM q4h PRN
   Available:

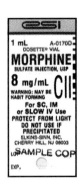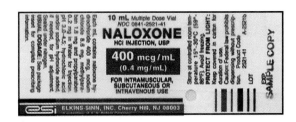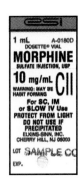

   a. Which morphine vial would you select? _____
      Explain _____
   b. How many milliliters (mL) of morphine would you administer per dose? _____
      Explain _____

10. Order: ampicillin 250 mg q6h IM
    Available:

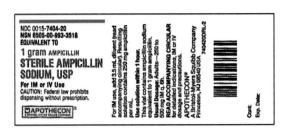

    a. How many milliliters (mL) of diluent would you add to the ampicillin vial? _____
    b. How many milliliters (mL) of ampicillin should the client receive per dose? _____
    c. How many milligrams (mg) should the client receive per day? _____

I. Syringes and Needles

1. 5-mL syringe
2. Tuberculin syringe (1 mL)
3. No, it should be discarded in the sink or toilet and witnessed by another RN or LPN, according to policy.
4. 21-gauge needle
5. 25-gauge needle
6. 20-gauge needle 1.5 (1½) inches in length

II. Subcutaneous Injections

1. a. $\dfrac{D}{H} \times V = \dfrac{4000}{10,000} \times 1 = \dfrac{4}{10} = 0.4 \text{ mL}$

   b.
H	:	V	::	D	:	x
10,000 Units	:	1 mL	::	4000 Units	:	x mL

   $$10,000x = 4000$$
   $$x = \dfrac{4000}{10,000} = 0.4 \text{ mL}$$

   Answer: heparin 4000 Units = 0.4 mL

2. 0.75 mL
3. The drug label reads: 1.25 mL = 0.5 mg of atropine. Also, under the word *atropine*, it reads 0.4 mg/mL

   a. $\dfrac{D}{H} \times V = \dfrac{0.5}{0.4} \times 1 = 1.25 \text{ mL}$

   b.
H	:	V	::	D	:	x
0.4 mg	:	1 mL	::	0.5 mg	:	x mL

   $$0.4x = 0.5$$
   $$x = \dfrac{0.5}{0.4} = 1.25 \text{ mL}$$

   Answer: atropine sulfate 0.5 mg = 1.25 mL

4. A tuberculin syringe should be used.

   a. $\dfrac{D}{H} \times V = \dfrac{0.2}{1.0} \times 1 = 1.0\sqrt{0.20} = 0.2 \text{ mL}$

   b.
H	:	V	::	D	:	x
1.0 mg	:	1 mL	::	0.2 mg	:	x mL

   $$1.0x = 0.2$$
   $$x = \dfrac{0.2}{1.0} = 0.2 \text{ mL}$$

   Answer: epinephrine 0.2 mg = 0.2 mL

III. Insulins

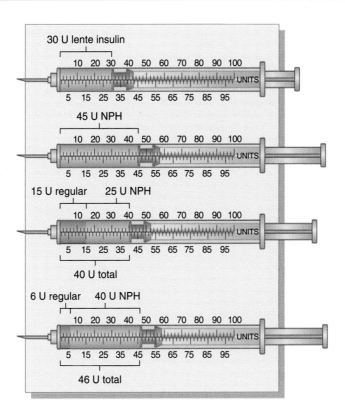

IV. Intramuscular Injections

1. Instructions on the drug label read: add 2.5 mL of sterile water. The drug solution equals 3.0 mL (drug powder is equal to 0.5 mL).
   Change 1 g to mg. 1 g = 1000 mg *or*

$$\text{Change 500 mg to g. } 500 \text{ mg} = 0.500 \text{ g } (0.5 \text{ g})$$

   a. $\dfrac{D}{H} \times V = \dfrac{0.5}{1 \text{ g}} \times 3 \text{ mL} = 1.5 \text{ mL}$

   b.
H	:	V	::	D	:	x
1000 mg	:	3 mL	::	500 mg	:	x mL

   $$1000x = 1500$$
   $$x = 1.5 \text{ mL}$$

   Answer: cefazolin 500 mg = 1.5 mL

2. 1.3 mL of procaine penicillin
3. The atropine drug label is marked as 0.4 mg/mL. The approximate equivalent of 0.3 mg is 0.8 mL as marked on the label. If the 0.3 mg = 0.8 mL is unknown, the problem may be calculated using 0.4 mg = 1 mL.

   a. $\dfrac{D}{H} \times V = \dfrac{0.3}{0.4} \times 1 = \dfrac{0.3}{0.4} = 0.75$, or 0.8 mL

   b.
H	:	V	::	D	:	x
0.4 mg	:	1 mL	::	0.3 mg	:	x mL

   $$0.4x = 0.3$$
   $$x = \dfrac{0.3}{0.4} = 0.75, \text{ or } 0.8 \text{ mL}$$

4. For oxacillin sodium, the drug label indicates that 2.7 mL of sterile water should be added to the vial containing 500 mg of drug. The total volume would be 3.0 mL.

a. $\dfrac{D}{H} \times V = \dfrac{250}{500} \times 3.0 = \dfrac{750}{500} = 1.5$ mL

b.
H	:	V	::	D	:	x
500 mg	:	3.0 mL	::	250 mg	:	x mL

$$500x = 750 = \dfrac{750}{500} = 1.5 \text{ mL}$$

Answer: Oxacillin 250 mg = 1.5 mL. It can be refrigerated for 96 h after it has been reconstituted.

5. a. $\dfrac{D}{H} \times V = \dfrac{0.25}{0.50} \times 2 = \dfrac{0.50}{0.50} = 1$ mL

b.
H	:	V	::	D	:	x
0.5 mg	:	2 mL	::	0.25 mg	:	x mL

$$0.5x = 0.5$$
$$x = 1 \text{ mL}$$

Expel 1 mL of digoxin solution from the Tubex cartridge before administering 1 mL.

6. Thorazine 50 mg = 2 mL. Yes, the vial can be used for multiple doses.
7. Meperidine 60 mg = 0.6 mL; hydroxyzine 25 mg = 0.5 mL
   Meperidine

a. $\dfrac{D}{H} \times V = \dfrac{60}{100} \times 1 = \dfrac{60}{100} = 0.6$ mL

b.
H	:	V	::	D	:	x
100 mg	:	1 mL	::	60 mg	:	x mL

$$100x = 60$$
$$x = 0.6 \text{ mL}$$

Hydroxyzine

a. $\dfrac{D}{H} \times V = \dfrac{25}{100} \times 2 = \dfrac{50}{100} = 0.5$ mL

b.
H	:	V	::	D	:	x
100 mg	:	2 mL	::	25 mg	:	x mL

$$100x = 50$$
$$x = 0.5 \text{ mL}$$

PROCEDURE

1. Check the meperidine dose and volume in the prefilled cartridge.
2. Expel any excess solution from the prefilled cartridge; 0.6 mL of solution should remain.
3. Draw 0.5 mL of air into cartridge and inject into the vial.
4. Withdraw 0.5 mL of hydroxyzine from the vial into the cartridge.
5. Total volume for the injection: meperidine and hydroxyzine = 1.1 mL

8. Naloxone (Narcan) 0.5 mg = 1.25 mL

   This is a multiple-dose vial containing 10 mL according to the label. Dose could be repeated in 3 minutes if needed.

9. a. Morphine vials 8 mg/mL and 10 mg/mL. Morphine 5 mg/mL vial could not be used because it is a single-vial dose.

   b. Morphine 8 mg/mL

   $$(1)\ \frac{D}{H} \times V = \frac{6\ mg}{8\ m} \times 1\ mL = \frac{6}{8} = 0.75\ mL$$

   Morphine 10 mg/mL

   $$(2)\ \frac{D}{H} \times V = \frac{6\ mg}{10\ mg} \times 1\ mL = \frac{6}{10} = 0.6\ mL$$

10. a. 3.5 mL of diluent (3.5 mL diluent + 0.5 mL of powdered drug = 4 mL of 1 g of ampicillin)

    b. 1 mL = 250 mg (1 g or 1000 mg = 4 mL)

    c. 250 mg × 4 (q6h) = 1000 mg or 1 g/d

SECTION 4E

Calculations of Intravenous Fluids

Outline

Objectives

- Describe the differences between continuous IV infusion and intermittent IV infusion.
- Define macrodrip and microdrip sets, KVO, and TKO.
- Calculate IV flow rate by using one of the given formulas.
- Explain how IV drug solutions administered by secondary set are calculated.
- Differentiate between volumetric and nonvolumetric IV regulators, and controllers and pump electronic regulators.

Terms

bolus

drop factor

electronic IV regulators

IVPB

KVO

macrodrip set

microdrip set

nonvolumetric regulator

PCA

primary IV sets

SASH procedure

secondary IV sets

TKO

volumetric regulator

INTRODUCTION

Intravenous (IV) fluid therapy is used for administering fluids containing water, dextrose, vitamins, electrolytes, and drugs. Today there are an increasing number of drugs administered by the intravenous route for direct absorption and fast action. Some drugs are given by IV push **(bolus).** Many of the drugs administered intravenously are irritating to the veins, so these drugs are diluted in 50 to 100 mL of fluid. Other drugs are delivered in a large volume of fluid over a period, such as 4 to 8 h.

There are two methods used to administer IV fluids and drugs: continuous IV infusion and intermittent IV infusion. Continuous IV administration replaces fluid loss, maintains fluid balance, and is a vehicle for drug administration. Intermittent IV administration is primarily used for giving IV drugs.

Nurses have an important role in the preparation and administration of intravenous solutions and IV drugs. The nursing functions and responsibilities during drug preparation include

- Knowledge of intravenous sets and their drop factors
- Calculating IV flow rates
- Mixing and diluting drugs in IV fluids
- Gathering equipment
- Knowledge of the drugs and the expected and untoward reactions

Nursing responsibilities continue with assessment of the client for effectiveness and untoward effects of the therapy and assessment of the IV site.

CONTINUOUS INTRAVENOUS ADMINISTRATION

When IV solutions are required, the health care provider orders the type and amount of IV solution in liters over a 24-h period or in milliliters per hour. The nurse calculates the IV flow rate according to the drop factor, the amount of fluids to be administered, and the time period.

Intravenous Sets

There are various IV infusion sets marketed by Abbott, Cutter, McGaw, and Travenol. The **drop factor,** the number of drops per milliliter, is normally printed on the packaging cover of the IV set. Sets that deliver large drops per milliliter (10 to 20 gtt/mL) are referred to as **macrodrip sets,** and those with small drops per milliliter (60 gtt/mL) are called **microdrip,** or **minidrip, sets.** Examples of drop factors, macrodrip sets, and microdrip sets are listed in Table 4E−1.

In most instances, the nurse has the choice of using either the macrodrip or microdrip set. If the IV rate is to infuse at 100 mL/h or more, the macrodrip set is usually used. If the infusion rate is less than (<) 100 mL/h or with pediatric client, the microdrip set is preferred. Slow drip rates of <100 mL/h make macrodrip adjustment difficult.

Table 4E−1
Intravenous Sets

MANUFACTURER	DROPS (GTT/ML)
MACRODRIP SETS	
Abbott	15
Cutter	20
McGaw	15
Travenol	10
MICRODRIP SETS	
Travenol	60
Minidrip sets	

At times, intravenous fluids are given at a slow rate to **keep vein open (KVO),** also called **to keep open (TKO).** The reasons for ordering KVO include a suspected or potential emergency situation for rapid administration of fluids and drugs and the need for an open line to give IV drugs at specified hours. For KVO, a microdrip set (60 gtt/mL) and a 250-mL IV bag may be used. KVO is usually regulated to deliver 10 mL/h.

Calculating Intravenous Flow Rate

Three different methods may be used to calculate IV flow rate (drops per minute, gtt/min). The nurse should select one method, memorize it, and consistently use it to calculate IV flow rate.

METHOD I: THREE-STEP

1. $\dfrac{\text{Amount of solution}}{\text{Hours to administer}} = \text{milliliters/hour (mL/h)}$

2. $\dfrac{\text{Milliliters per hour}}{60 \text{ minutes}} = \text{milliliters/minute (mL/min)}$

3. Milliliters per minute $\times$ drops per milliliter of IV set $=$ drops/minute (gtt/min)

METHOD II: TWO-STEP*

1. $\dfrac{\text{Amount of fluid}}{\text{Hours to administer}} = \text{milliliters/hour (mL/h)}$

2. $\dfrac{\text{Milliliters per hour} \times \text{Drops per milliliter (IV set)}}{60 \text{ minutes}} = \text{drops/minute (gtt/min)}$

If the milliliters per hour is known, then use step 2 to determine the drops per minute.

METHOD III: ONE-STEP

$$\dfrac{\text{Amount of fluid} \times \text{Drops per milliliter (IV set)}}{\text{Hours to administer} \times \text{Minutes per hour (60)}} = \text{drops/minute (gtt/min)}$$

Mixing Drugs for Continuous Intravenous Administration

Drugs such as potassium chloride and vitamins are frequently added to the IV solution bag for continuous IV infusion. Drugs should be added to the bag or bottle immediately before administering the intravenous fluid. Inject the drug into the rubber stopper on the IV bag or bottle and rotate the bag several times to ensure that the drug is dispersed throughout the solution (Fig. 4E–1). *Do not add the drug while the infusion is running unless the bag is rotated.* A drug solution injected into an upright infusing IV solution concentrates the drug into the lower portion of the IV bag, preventing it from being evenly dispersed. The client receives a concentrated drug solution, which may be harmful, for example, if the drug is potassium chloride. If drugs are injected into the IV bag prior to use, the bag should be refrigerated to maintain drug potency.

---

*The two-step method is the most popular method for IV calculation of the flow rate.

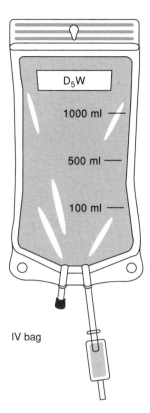

IV bag

SECTION E

There are various nutrients (e.g., dextrose) and electrolytes in commercially prepared intravenous solutions. The commonly used solutions are 5% dextrose in water (D_5W), normal saline (NSS), one-half normal saline (½ NSS), and lactated Ringer's. These types of solutions are abbreviated as listed in Table 4E–2.

Table 4E–2
Abbreviations of Solutions

INTRAVENOUS SOLUTIONS	ABBREVIATIONS
5% Dextrose in water	D_5W, 5% D/W
10% Dextrose in water	$D_{10}W$, 10% D/W
0.9% Sodium chloride, normal saline solution	0.9% NaCl, NSS
0.45% Sodium chloride, $\frac{1}{2}$ normal saline solution	0.45% NaCl, $\frac{1}{2}$ NSS
5% Dextrose in 0.9% sodium chloride	D_5NSS, 5% D/NSS, 5% D/0.9% NaCl
5% Dextrose in 0.45% sodium chloride	$D_5/\frac{1}{2}$ NSS, 5% D/$\frac{1}{2}$ NSS
	5% Dextrose in $\frac{1}{2}$ normal saline solution
Lactated Ringer's solution	LR

Example

Order: 1000 mL of 5% dextrose in water (D_5W) with potassium chloride (KCl) 20 mEq in 8h
Available: 1000 mL of 5% dextrose in water
 Potassium chloride 40 mEq/20 mL ampule
 IV set labeled 10 gtt/mL
Drug calculation: Using the basic formula and the ratio-and-proportion method

a. $\dfrac{D}{H} \times V = \dfrac{20}{40} \times 20 = \dfrac{400}{40} = 10$ mL of KCl

b.
H	:	V	::	D	:	x
40 mEq	:	20 mL	::	20 mEq	:	x mL

$$40x = 400$$
$$x = 10 \text{ mL of KCl}$$

The calculation of IV flow rate is described using the three methods outlined previously. However, it is strongly recommended that you select one method for determining IV flow rate.

Method I

1. $\dfrac{1000 \text{ mL}}{8 \text{ h}} = 125$ mL/h

2. $\dfrac{125 \text{ mL}}{60 \text{ min}} = 2.0\text{–}2.1$ mL/min

3. $2.1 \times 10 = 21$ gtt/min

Method II

1. $1000 \div 8 = 125$ mL/h

2. $\dfrac{125 \text{ mL/h} \times \overset{1}{\cancel{10}} \text{ gtt/mL}}{\underset{6}{\cancel{60}} \text{ min}} = \dfrac{125}{6} = 20\text{–}21$ gtt/min

Method III

$$\dfrac{1000 \text{ mL} \times \overset{1}{\cancel{10}} \text{ gtt/mL}}{8 \text{ h} \times \underset{6}{\cancel{60}} \text{ min}} = \dfrac{1000}{48} = 21 \text{ gtt/min}$$

PRACTICE PROBLEMS

I. Continuous Intravenous Flow Rates

Select one of the three methods for calculating IV flow rate.

1. Order: 1000 mL of $D_5/\frac{1}{2}$ NSS to infuse over 12 h
   Available: macrodrip set with 10 gtt/mL and a microdrip set with 60 gtt/mL
   a. Would you use a macrodrip or microdrip IV set?
   b. Calculate the IV flow rate in drops per minute according to the IV set that you selected.

2. Order: 3 L of IV solutions to infuse over 24 h
   1 L of D_5W and 2 L of $D_5/\frac{1}{2}$ NSS
   a. One liter is equal to how many milliliters?
   b. Each liter should infuse for how many hours?
   c. The institution uses a set with a drop factor of 15 gtt/mL. How many drops per minute should the client receive?

3. Order: 250 mL of D_5W to keep vein open (KVO)
   a. What type of IV set would you use?
      Why?
   b. Determine how many drops per minute the client should receive.

4. Order: 1000 mL of $D_5/\frac{1}{2}$ NSS, 1 vial of MVI (multiple vitamin), and 10 mEq of KCL (potassium chloride) in 10 h
   Available: 1000 mL of $D_5/\frac{1}{2}$ NSS
   Macrodrip set: 15 gtt/mL; microdrip set: 60 gtt/mL
   MVI: 5 mL vial
   KCl: 20 mEq/20 mL vial
   a. How many milliliters of KCl should be injected into the IV bag?
   b. How many drops per minute should the client receive using the macrodrip set and microdrip set?

5. A liter (1000 mL) of IV fluid was started at 9 AM and was to infuse for 8 h. The IV set delivers 10 gtt/mL. Four hours later only 400 mL were absorbed.
   a. How much IV fluid is left?
   b. Recalculate the flow rate for the remaining IV fluids.

INTERMITTENT INTRAVENOUS ADMINISTRATION

Some IV drugs are prescribed to be administered three to six times a day in a small volume of IV fluid (50 to 100 mL of D_5W or normal saline solution [NSS: 0.9% sodium chloride]). The drug solution is usually infused over a period of 15 min to 1 h. Separate tubing for IV drugs, the secondary line, is inserted into a port (rubber stopper) of the IV connector on the continuous, or **primary, IV line.** This type of IV administration is called intermittent IV therapy.

SECONDARY INTRAVENOUS SETS WITHOUT CONTROLLERS

Two IV sets available for administering IV drugs are (1) the calibrated cylinder (chamber) with tubing, such as the Buretrol, Volutrol, and Soluset, and (2) the secondary set, which is similar to a regular IV set except that the tubing is shorter (Fig. 4E–2). The **secondary set** is used mostly for infusing small volumes—50, 100, 250 mL and in pediatric for children's IV solution. The chamber of the Buretrol, Volutrol, and Soluset holds 150 mL of solution. Medication is injected into the chamber, then diluted with solution. These methods of administering IV drugs are referred to as **IV piggyback (IVPB).**

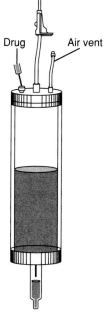

Drug   Air vent

Calibrated cylinder
(Buretrol)

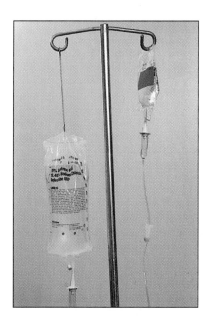

Secondary line B

Figure 4E–2
(A) The calibrated cylinder (Buretrol) is an example of a secondary intravenous (IV) device. (B) An example of a secondary line containing medication. The primary IV bag is 6 inches below the secondary IV bag. (A: From Kee, J. L., and Marshall, S. M.: *Clinical Calculations,* 3rd ed. Philadelphia: WB Saunders, p. 172, 1996. B: From Leahy, J. M., and Kizilay, P. E.: *Foundations of Nursing Practice: A Nursing Process Approach.* Philadelphia: WB Saunders, 1998.)

Drugs for IV infusion are diluted before infusion. Clinical agencies frequently have their own protocols for dilutions; the pharmacist and the drug circular are also resources for infusion guidelines. Guidelines and protocols help in preventing drug and fluid incompatibility.

When using the Buretrol, 15 to 30 mL of IV solution should be added to flush the drug out of the IV line once the infusion is completed.

When continuous IV fluid infusion is to be discontinued and intermittent drug therapy is to begin, an adapter is attached to the IV catheter or needle where the IV tubing was disconnected. Adapters have ports (stoppers) where needles, needleless, or IV tubing can be inserted as needed to continue drug therapy. The use of adapters increases the client's mobility by not having an IV line "tagging along," and is cost-effective because less IV tubing, solution, and equipment are needed.

The adapter may have short tubing, which is called the heparin lock. IV catheters and needles with adapters are kept free of blood clots by administering low doses of heparin after each drug infusion. In some institutions, this is known as the **SASH procedure.** SASH stands for:

S = Solution (saline) flush (2 mL)
A = Administer drug into rubber stopper
S = Solution (saline) flush (2 mL)
H = Heparin 1 : 100 solution (1 mL)

Before any drug is given, the IV tubing and adapter are flushed with 2 mL of saline solution for the purpose of clearing the line of heparin solution and assessing for IV patency. After the drug is administered, a 2-mL saline flush is given, followed by a low dose of heparin. In Figure 4E–3, the nurse is using the SASH procedure.

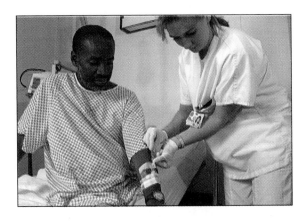

Figure 4E–3
To clear the line, the nurse performs the SASH procedure. (From Leahy J. M., and Kizilay, P. E.: *Foundations of Nursing Practice: A Nursing Process Approach.* Philadelphia: WB Saunders, 1998.)

ELECTRONIC INTRAVENOUS REGULATORS

Controllers and pumps are the two basic types of **electronic intravenous regulators** used in hospitals and some community settings. The electronic IV regulators are set to deliver a prescribed rate of intravenous solution. If the flow rate is obstructed, an alarm sounds.

Controllers operate by the pressure that gravity exerts on the fluid in the IV bag. A drop sensor is attached to the drip chamber to monitor the flow rate. The controller is the metal box through which the IV tubing is fed. It is set by the nurse for a flow rate in milliliters per hour, and the rate is displayed on the front panel of the controller. Since the controllers work by gravity, the IV solution bag should be at least 36 inches above the controller. Controllers are sensitive to any restrictions, such as infiltration or obstruction when a client is lying on the tubing. An alarm sounds when the set rate cannot be maintained.

IV pumps look like controllers, but they deliver intravenous solution against resistance. The flow rate is set in milliliters per hour. Pumps do not recognize infiltration. The alarm does not sound until the pump has exerted its maximum pressure to overcome resistance.

IV pumps are recommended for use with all central lines, such as femoral and subclavian sites. Controllers are used for peripheral lines, especially if fluid overload is a concern. Ongoing nursing assessment is essential whatever type of electronic IV regulator is used.

There are two types of flow control for electronic regulators, the volumetric and nonvolumetric regulators. The **volumetric regulators** deliver a specific volume of fluid at a specific rate, in milliliters per hour. The **nonvolumetric regulators** are designed to infuse at a drop rate in drops per minute. To determine whether the machine is volumetric or nonvolumetric, check to see whether the panel display is calibrated for mL/hr or gtt/min. Figure 4E–4 shows a combination IV controller and pump regulator. There are various electronic IV regulators for administering IV fluids and drugs (Fig. 4E–5).

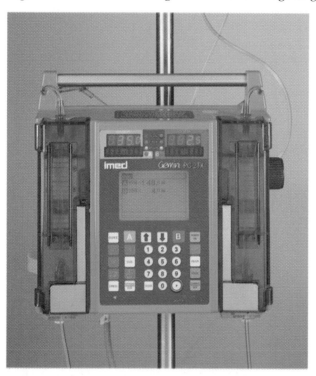

Figure 4E–4

IV pump and controller. (From Kee, J. L., and Marshall, S. M.: *Clinical Calculations*, 3rd ed. Philadelphia: WB Saunders, p. 174, 1996; Courtesy of IMED Corporation, San Diego, CA.)

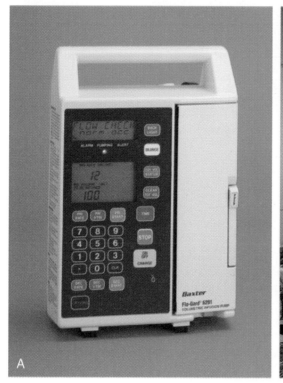
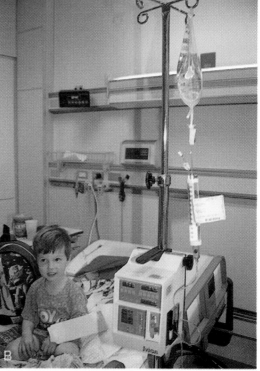

Figure 4E–5

(*A*) Flo-Gard volumetric infusion pump. (Courtesy of Baxter Healthcare Corp., Deerfield, IL.)
(*B*) Buretrol with an electronic regulator for IV drug administration. (From Bowden, V. R., Dickey, S. B., and Greenberg, C. S.: *Children and Their Families: A Continuum of Care*. Philadelphia: WB Saunders, 1998.)

Patient controlled analgesia (PCA) is another method of administering drugs intravenously. The objective of PCA is to provide a uniform serum concentration of drug(s), thus avoiding drug peaks and valleys. This method is designed to meet the needs of those clients who require at least 24 to 48 h of regular intramuscular narcotic injections.

Several reasons for the use of PCA include (1) effective pain control without the client feeling over-sedated, (2) considerable reduction in the amount of narcotic used (approximately one-half that of intramuscular delivery), and (3) clients' feelings of greater control over their pain.

There are choices available in the delivery of PCA. The pump is programmed to administer the prescribed medication (1) at client demand, (2) continuously, and (3) continuously and supplemented by client demand. Figure 4E–6 shows examples of PCA infusion pumps.

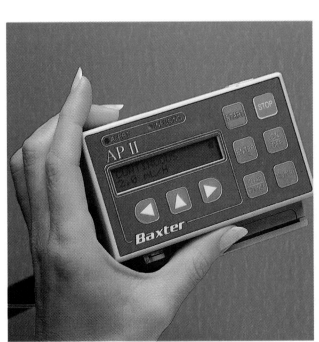
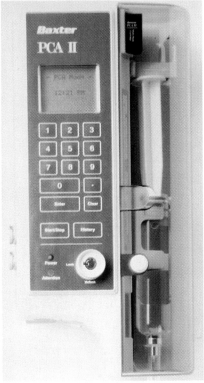

Figure 4E–6
Two examples of patient-controlled analgesic (PCA) infusion pumps. (From Monahan, F. D., and Neighbors, M.: *Medical-Surgical Nursing*, 2nd ed. Philadelphia: WB Saunders, p. 152, 1998. Courtesy of Baxter Healthcare Corp., Deerfield, IL.)

The health care provider's order must include:

- Drug ordered
- Loading dose: administered by the health care provider to obtain baseline serum concentration of analgesic
- PCA dose: amount to be administered each time client activates the button
- Lockout interval: time during which PCA cannot be administered
- Dose limit: the maximum amount the client can receive during a specified time

Client Teaching

- Inform the client that the pain should be tolerable, not necessarily absent.
- Advise the client of the pump's safety features, including the alarms.
- Instruct the client in use of control button (medication administered when button is *released*).
- Instruct the client to report any side effects or adverse reactions to the medication.
- Have naloxone (Narcan) easily accessible.

CALCULATING FLOW RATES FOR INTRAVENOUS DRUGS

Intravenous drug infusion rates depend on the drug dosing instructions, which indicate the amount of solution for dilution, and the length of infusion time. The nurse must first calculate the drug dose from the health care provider's order, then calculate the flow rate.

1. *Secondary Sets:* To find drops per minute for IV drugs, use calibrated cylinders (Buretrol, Volutrol), 50- to 250-mL bag (Add-A-Line), or any nonvolumetric regulator.

$$\frac{\text{Amount of solution} \times \text{Drops per milliliter of the set}}{\text{Minutes to administer}} = \text{Drops/minute (gtt/min)}$$

2. *Volumetric Regulators:* To find milliliters per hour

$$\text{Amount of solution} \div \frac{\text{Minutes to administer}}{\text{60 minutes/hour}} = \text{Milliliters/hour (mL/h)}$$

Problems for calculating IV drug dosage and IV flow rate in drops per minute and in milliliters per hour are given below.

Example

Order: ceftazidime (Fortaz) 1.5 g IV q6h
Available:

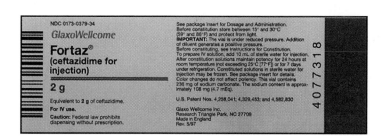

Set and solution: Cylinder set with drop factor of 60 gtt/mL; 500 mL of D$_5$W.
Instruction: Dilute ceftazidime 1.5 g in 100 mL of D$_5$W and infuse over 30 min.

1. Calculate drug dosage according to drug label.
2. Calculate drops per minute for drug solution.
3. Calculate milliliters per hour using volumetric pump rate.

Answer

1. Drug Calculation
   Drug label states to add 10 mL of sterile water (2 g = 10 mL)
   a. $\frac{D}{H} \times V = \frac{1.5\ \text{g}}{2.0\ \text{g}} \times 10\ \text{mL} = \frac{15}{2} = 7.5\ \text{mL of ceftazidime}$

   b. $\quad H \quad\quad : \quad\quad V \quad\quad :: \quad\quad D \quad\quad : \quad\quad x$
   $\quad\quad 2\ \text{g} \quad\quad : \quad\quad 10\ \text{mL} \quad\quad :: \quad\quad 1.5\ \text{g} \quad\quad : \quad\quad x\ \text{mL}$

   $$2x = 15$$
   $$x = 7.5\ \text{mL of ceftazidime}$$

2. IV Flow Calculation (Secondary Set)

$$\frac{\text{Amount of Solution} = \text{Drops per milliliter (set)}}{\text{Minutes to administer}} = \frac{100\ \text{mL} \times \overset{2}{\cancel{60}}\ \text{gtt}}{\underset{1}{\cancel{30}}\ \text{min}} = 200\ \text{gtt/min}$$

Inject 7.5 mL of ceftazidime in 100 mL of D₅W in the cylinder chamber.

Regulate IV flow rate to 200 gtt/min. It may be impossible to count 200 gtt/min. Instead of using the cylinder chamber, the nurse may use a secondary set that has a larger drop factor or a regulator. If the cylinder set is the only available secondary IV set, then the 200 gtt/min may be approximated.

3. Volumetric Pump Rate

$$\text{Amount of Solution} \div \frac{\text{Minutes to administer}}{60 \text{ minutes per hour}} = 100 \text{ mL} + 7.5 \text{ mL (drug)} \div \frac{30 \text{ min}}{60 \text{ min}}$$

$$= 107.5 \text{ mL} \times \frac{\overset{2}{\cancel{60}}}{\underset{1}{\cancel{30}}} = 215 \text{ mL/h}$$

Set volumetric rate at 215 mL/h to deliver drug in 30 min.

PRACTICE PROBLEMS

II. Intermittent Intravenous Set

Solve the IV drug problems by (1) calculating the drug dosage according to the drug label or information given and (2) calculating drops per minute for the drug solution.

1. Order: kanamycin 15 mg/kg/d in three divided doses (q8h) IV. Client weighs 50 kg. Available:

How many milliliters (mL) of kanamycin should the client receive per dose?
Set and solution: Cylinder set with a drop factor of 60 gtt/mL; 500 mL D₅W
Instruction: Dilute the drug in 75 mL of D₅W and infuse over 30 min.

2. Order: cefamandole (Mandol) 500 mg IV q6h
Available: cefamandole (Mandol) is in powdered form in a vial.

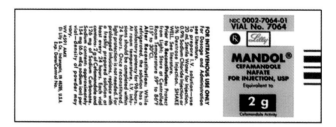

For reconstitution: Add 6.6 mL of diluent = 8 mL of drug solution (2 g = 8 mL)
Set and solution: Secondary set with 100 mL D₅W. Drop factor is 15 gtt/mL.
Instruction: Dilute in 100 mL of D₅W and infuse over 30 min.

3. Order: tobramycin (Nebcin) 50 mg IV q8h
Drug parameters: 3 mg/kg/day in three divided doses. Client weighs 65 kg.
Available:

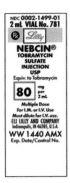

Set and solution: Cylinder IV set with drop factor of 60 gtt/mL; 500 mL D₅W

Set and solution: Cylinder IV set with drop factor of 60 gtt/mL; 500 mL D_5W
Instruction: Dilute tobramycin in 100 mL of ₅W and infuse over 40 min.
Is the tobramycin dose within safe parameters? Explain.

4. Order: piperacillin (Pipracil) 2.0 g IV q6h
   Available: piperacillin 4 g vial in powdered form. Add 7.8 mL of diluent to yield 10 mL of drug solution (4 g = 10 mL).
   Set and solution: Cylinder IV set with drop factor of 60 gtt/mL; 500 mL D_5W
   Instruction: Dilute piperacillin in 100 mL of D_5W and infuse over 45 min.
   Determine the volumetric pump rate for this problem in addition to the drug and IV flow calculations.

5. Order: ampicillin 500 mg IVq6h
   Available: Add 4.5 mL of diluent = 5 mL (2 g = 5 mL)

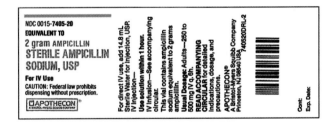

   Convert grams to milligrams.
   Set and solution: Cylinder set with drop factor of 60 gtt/mL; 500 mL of D_5W
   Instruction: Dilute ampicillin in 50 mL of D_5W and infuse over 15 min.
   Determine the volumetric pump rate for this problem in addition to the drug and IV flow calculations.

6. Order: ticarcillin (Ticar) 750 mg IV g6h
   Available:

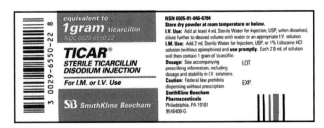

   How many mL should be given per dose?
   Set and solution: Cylinder IV set with drop factor of 60 gtt/mL; 500 mL D_5W
   Instruction: Dilute Ticar in 20 mL of D_5W and infuse over 30 min.

7. Order: digoxin 400 μg (0.40 mg) IV b.i.d. $\times$ 1 day
   Drug parameter: 10 to 15 μg/kg/day (1 mg) in divided doses
   Client's weight: 75 kg
   Available:

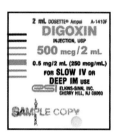

Instruction: Administer digoxin diluted in 4 mL of D_5W or 0.9% saline solution (NaCl) by direct intravenous injection over 5 or more min.
   a. Is the drug dose within safe parameter?
   b. How many milliliters (mL) of drug should the client receive per dose?

8. Order: diltiazem (Cardizem) 0.25 mg/kg IV bolus (direct intravenous) over 2 min.
   Client's weight: 178 pounds
   Available:

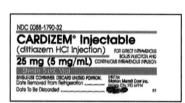 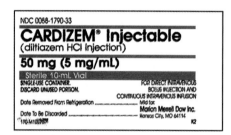

   a. Which Cardizem vial would you choose?
      Why? _____
   b. How many milligrams (mg) should the client receive?
   c. How many milliliters (mL) should be given direct IV?

9. Order: ranitidine HCl (Zantac) 50 mg IV q8h
   Available:

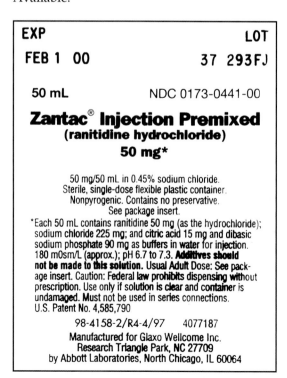

How many drops per minute should the client receive?
Set and solution: Secondary set with 50 mL of 1/2 NSS (0.45% NaCl). Drop factor of 15 gtt/mL.
Instruction: Infuse over 30 min.

10. Order: eptoposide (VePesid) 75 mg/m²/d for 5 consecutive days q 3–4 wk
Client weight: 134 lb; height: 66 inches
Use the nomogram to determine m² (BSA) (Fig. 4E–7).
Available:

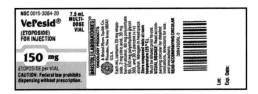

a. What is the client's BSA? _____
b. How many milligrams (mg) should the client receive?
c. How many milliliters (mL) of drug solution should the client receive?
   Set and solution: Secondary set with 250 mL of D₅W to run for 60 min. Drop factor is 15 gtt/mL.
   Determine the volumetric pump for this problem in addition to the drug and IV flow calculations.

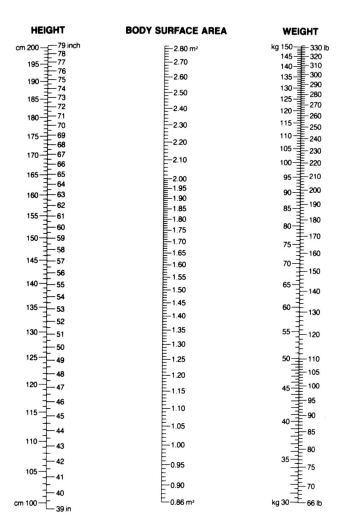

Figure 4E–7

Nomogram of body surface area for adults. *Directions:* (1) Find height. (2) Find weight. (3) Draw a straight line connecting the height and weight. (4) Where the line intersects on the Body Surface Area column is the body surface area (m²). (Sources: Deglin, Vallerand, and Russin: *Davis's Drug Guide for Nurses*, 2nd ed. Philadelphia: F. A. Davis, 1991; Lentner, C. (ed.): Geigy Scientific Tables, 8/E. Vol. 1. Basle, Switzerland: Ciba-Geigy, pp. 226–227, 1981.)

I. Continuous Intravenous Flow Rate

1. a. Microdrip set since the client is to receive 83 mL/h
   b. Two-step method: for continuous IV flow rate

   Step 1. $\dfrac{1000}{12} = 83$ mL/h

   Step 2. $\dfrac{83 \text{ mL/h} \times 1 \, \overset{1}{\cancel{60}} \text{ drops}}{\underset{1}{\cancel{60}} \text{ minutes}} = 83$ gtt/min

2. a. 1000 mL
   b. 8 h

   c. Step 1. $\dfrac{1000}{8} = 125$ mL/h

   Step 2. $\dfrac{125 \text{ mL/h} \times \overset{1}{\cancel{15}} \text{ gtt}}{\underset{4}{\cancel{60}} \text{ minutes}} = \dfrac{125}{4} = 31$ gtt/min

3. a. Microdrip set

   b. Step 1. $\dfrac{250}{24} = 10$ mL/h

   Step 2. $\dfrac{10 \text{ mL/h} \times \overset{1}{\cancel{60}} \text{ gtt}}{\underset{1}{\cancel{60}} \text{ minutes}} = 10$ gtt/min

4. a. $\dfrac{D}{H} \times V = \dfrac{10}{20} \times 20 = \dfrac{200}{20} = 10$ mL KCl

   b. $\dfrac{1000}{10} = 100$ mL

   Macrodrip set $\qquad \dfrac{100 \times \overset{1}{\cancel{15}}}{\underset{4}{\cancel{60}} \text{ min}} = 25$ gtt/min

   Microdrip set $\qquad \dfrac{100 \times \overset{1}{\cancel{60}}}{\underset{1}{\cancel{60}} \text{ min}} = 100$ gtt/min

5. a. 600 mL

   b. Step 1. $\dfrac{600}{4} = 150$ mL/h

   Step 2. $\dfrac{150 \text{ mL/h} \times \overset{1}{\cancel{10}}}{\underset{6}{\cancel{60}} \text{ minutes}} = 25$ gtt/min

II. Intermittent Intravenous Set

1. Use the One-Step for Intermittent IV Flow Rate Drug calculation:

   $\dfrac{D}{H} \times V = \dfrac{250 \text{ mg}}{500 \text{ mg}} \times 2 = \dfrac{500}{500} = 1$ mL of kanamycin

   Flow calculation: $\dfrac{75 \text{ mL} \times 60 \text{ (set)}}{30 \text{ minutes}} = \dfrac{4500}{30} = 150$ gtt/min

2. Drug calculation: Change 2 g to milligrams.

$$2\ g = 2.000\ mg \qquad \frac{D}{H} \times V = \frac{500}{2000} \times 8\ mL = \frac{4000}{2000} = 2\ mL\ Mandol$$

Flow calculation: $\dfrac{100\ mL \times \overset{1}{\cancel{15}}\ gtt\ (set)}{\underset{2}{\cancel{30}}\ minutes} = \dfrac{100}{2} = 50\ gtt/min$

3. Drug calculation: $\dfrac{D}{H} \times V = \dfrac{50}{80} \times 2 = \dfrac{100}{80} = 1.25\ mL$ of tobramycin

Flow calculation: $\dfrac{100\ mL \times \overset{3}{\cancel{60}}\ gtt\ (set)}{\underset{2}{\cancel{40}}\ minutes} = \dfrac{300}{2} = 150\ gtt/min$

Drug parameter: It is within safe parameters (3 kg × 65 = 195 mg/day). Client is receiving 50 mg × 3 = 150 mg/day.

4. Drug calculation: $\dfrac{D}{H} \times V = \dfrac{2}{4} \times 10 = \dfrac{20}{4} = 5mL$ of piperacillin

Flow calculation: 5 mL + 100 mL = 105 mL $\quad \dfrac{105\ mL \times \overset{4}{\cancel{60}}\ gtt\ (set)}{\underset{3}{\cancel{45}}\ minutes} = \dfrac{420}{3} =$

140 gtt/min

Volumetric pump rate:

$$\text{Amount of solution} \div \frac{\text{minutes to administer}}{60\ min} = \text{Milliliters/hour (mL/h)}$$

$$100\ mL + 5\ mL\ (drug) \div \frac{45\ min}{60\ min} = \quad 105\ mL \times \frac{\overset{4}{\cancel{60}}}{\underset{3}{\cancel{45}}} = \frac{420}{3} = 140\ mL/h$$

5. Drug calculation: Convert to milligrams.

$$2\ g = 2.000\ mg$$

$$\frac{D}{H} \times V = \frac{500}{2000} \times 5 = \frac{5}{4} = 1.25\ mL\ of\ ampicillin$$

Flow calculation: $\dfrac{50\ mL \times \overset{4}{\cancel{60}}\ gtt\ (set)}{\underset{1}{\cancel{15}}\ minutes} = \dfrac{200}{1} = 200\ gtt/min$

Volumetric pump rate: $50\ mL + 1.25\ mL \div \dfrac{15}{60} = \quad 51.25\ mL \times \dfrac{\overset{4}{\cancel{60}}}{\underset{1}{\cancel{15}}} = 205\ mL/h$

6. $\dfrac{D}{H} \times V = \dfrac{750\ mg}{1000\ mg} \times 4\ mL = \dfrac{3000}{1000} = 3\ mL$ of amikacin

H	:	V	::	D	:	x
1 g	:	4 mL	::	0.75 g	:	x mL

$$1\,x = 3 = \frac{3}{1}$$

$$x = 3\ mL\ of\ ticarcillin$$

Flow calculation: $\dfrac{20 \text{ mL} \times \overset{2}{\cancel{60}} \text{ gtt (set)}}{\underset{1}{\cancel{30}} \text{ minutes}} = \dfrac{40}{1} = 40 \text{ gtt/min}$

Volumetric pump rate:

$20 \text{ mL} + 3 \text{ mL} \div \dfrac{30}{60} = \quad 23 \text{ mL} \times \dfrac{\overset{2}{\cancel{60}}}{\underset{1}{\cancel{30}}} = 46 \text{ mL/h}$ (Increase in D_5W solution may be desired)

7. a. Drug dose is within safe parameters; 800 µg/d

   10 µg × 75 kg = 750 µg/d

   15 µg × 75 kg = 1125 µg/d

   b. $\dfrac{D}{H} \times V = \dfrac{400 \text{ µg}}{500 \text{ µg}} \times 2 \text{ mL} = \dfrac{800}{500} = 1.6 \text{ mL of digoxin}$

H	:	V	::	D	:	x
500 µg	:	2 mL	::	400 µg	:	x

   $500x = 800$

   $x = 1.6 \text{ mL of digoxin per dose}$

   Answer: Mix 1.6 mL of digoxin with 4 mL of diluent and administer the 5.6 mL by direct intravenous injection.

8. Client's weight: 178 lbs ÷ 2.2 = 81 kg
   a. Either Cardizem vial could be used. The Cardizem 25-mg vial is preferred because the dose is less than 25 mg and the balance of the solution would need to be discarded.
   b. 0.25 mg × 81 kg = 20.25 mg or 20 mg

   c. $\dfrac{D}{H} \times V = \dfrac{20 \text{ mg}}{25 \text{ mg}} \times 5 \text{ mL} = \dfrac{100}{25} = 4 \text{ mL of Cardizem}$

9. Flow calculation: $\dfrac{50 \text{ mL} \times \text{ gtt (set)}}{\underset{2}{\cancel{30}} \text{ minutes}} = \dfrac{50}{2} = 25 \text{ gtt/min}$

10. a. Client's BSA is 1.75.
    b. 75 mg × 1.75 (BSA) = 131.25 or 131 mg

    c. $\dfrac{D}{H} \times V = \dfrac{131}{150} \times 7.5 \text{ mL} = \dfrac{982.5}{150} = 6.55 \text{ or } 6.6 \text{ mL}$

    Flow calculation with secondary set: $\dfrac{250 \text{ mL} \times 15 \text{ gtt (set)}}{60 \text{ minutes}} = \dfrac{3750}{60} = 62.5 \text{ gtt/min}$

    Volumetric pump rate:

    $250 \text{ mL} + 6.6 \text{ mL} (256.6 \text{ or } 257 \text{ mL}) \div \dfrac{60}{60} = \quad 257 \text{ mL} \times \dfrac{\overset{1}{\cancel{60}}}{\underset{1}{\cancel{60}}} = 257 \text{ mL/h}$

Pediatric Drug Calculations

4

Outline

Objectives

- Utilize one of the two primary methods in determining pediatric drug dosage.
- Describe the dosage inaccuracies that may occur with pediatric drug formulas.
- Identify the steps in determining body surface area from a pediatric nomogram.
- Calculate the drug dosages correctly in the practice problems.

Terms

body surface area (BSA)   parameters

body weight

INTRODUCTION

Children drug dosages differ greatly from those for adults because of the physiologic differences between the two. Neonates and infants have immature kidney and liver function, which delays metabolism and elimination of many drugs. In neonates, drug absorption is different as a result of slow gastric emptying time. Decreased gastric acid secretion in children younger than 3 years old contributes to altered drug absorption. Neonates and infants have a lower concentration of plasma proteins, which can cause toxicity with drugs that are highly bound to proteins. Young children have less total body fat and more body water; therefore, lipid-soluble drugs require smaller doses when less than normal fat is present. Water-soluble drugs can require large doses because of a greater percentage of body water. It is the nurse's responsibility to ensure that a safe drug dosage is given and to closely monitor signs and symptoms of side effects and adverse drug reactions.

The purpose of learning how to calculate pediatric drug dosages is to ensure that children receive the correct dose within the approved therapeutic range. The two methods that are considered safe in administering drugs to children are the **body weight** (kg) and **body surface area** (BSA, or m^2) methods. Many manufacturers supply information in their literature concerning drug doses for children according to body weight. Also, manufacturers frequently give **parameters** for safe dose ranges. It is the nurse's responsibility to check the dose ranges given by the pharmaceutical manufacturers to be certain that the prescribed dose is within the parameters. Children's dosage can be determined from the adult dose using the body surface area rule. Older methods used in calculating children's dosages are Fried's rule and Young's rule, which are based on the child's age, and Clark's rule, which is based on the weight of the child. These older methods are mostly obsolete.

ORAL

Oral pediatric drug delivery usually requires the use of a calibrated measuring device because most drugs for small children are in liquid form. The measuring device can be a small plastic cup, an oral dropper, a measuring spoon, or an oral syringe (Fig. 4F–1). Some liquid medications come with their own calibrated droppers. The type of measuring device chosen depends on the age or the developmental level of the child. For infants and toddlers, the oral syringe and dropper can provide better drug delivery than a small cup can. A young child who is cooperative is able to use a small cup or measuring spoon. The cup or spoon may be rinsed with water or juice to ensure that the child has received all of the drug. Avoid giving oral medications to a crying child or infant because the drug could be easily aspirated or the child could "spit out" the drug. For the older child, some drugs are available in chewable form. Children should be told not to chew drugs that are enteric-coated or in timed-release form.

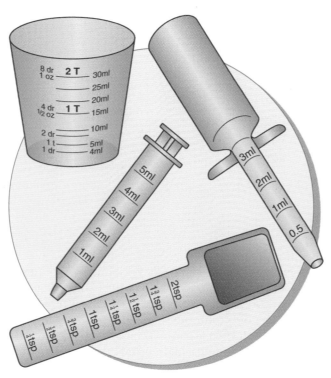

Figure 4F–1
Calibrated measuring devices. (From Kee, J. L., and Marshall, S. M.: *Clinical Calculations*, 3rd ed. Philadelphia: WB Saunders, p. 192, 1996.)

INTRAMUSCULAR

Intramuscular sites for drug administration are chosen on the basis of the age and muscle development of the child (Table 4F–1). All injections should be given in a manner that minimizes physical and psychosocial trauma. Explanations of injection administration should be given to children who can comprehend. With the very young child, distraction or brief restraint may be necessary. Comfort measures should immediately follow the injection.

Table 4F–1
Pediatric Guidelines for Intramuscular Injections*

	MUSCLE GROUP				
AGE	Rectus	Vastus Lateralis	Gluteus Maximus	Ventrogluteal	Deltoid
Birth to 2 yr	0.5–1 mL	0.5–1 mL	Not safe	Not safe	Not safe
2 to 3 yr	1 mL	1 mL	1 mL	1 mL	0.5 mL
3 to 7 yr	1.5 mL	1.5 mL	1.5 mL	1.5 mL	0.5 mL
7 to 16 yr	1.5–2 mL	1.5–2 mL	1.5–2 mL	1.5–2 mL	0.5–1 mL
16 yr to adult	2–2.5 mL	2–2.5 mL	2–3 mL	2–3 mL	1–2 mL

The safe use of all sites is based on normal muscle development and size of the child. Kee, J. L., and Marshall, S. M.: Clinical Calculations, 3rd ed. Philadelphia: WB Saunders, p. 193, 1996.

PEDIATRIC DOSAGE PER BODY WEIGHT

Example

Order: cefaclor (Ceclor) 50 mg q.i.d.
   Child weighs 15 lb or 6.8 kg (15 ÷ 2.2 = 6.8)
   Child's drug dosage: 20–40 mg/kg/day in three divided doses
   Available:

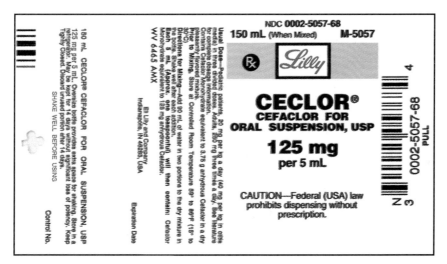

   Is the prescribed dose safe?
Answer:
Drug parameters: 20 mg × 6.8 kg = 136 mg/day
                          40 mg × 6.8 kg = 272 mg/day
Dosage order: 50 mg × 4 = 200 mg/day

Dosage is within safe parameters.

a. $\dfrac{D}{H} \times V = \dfrac{50}{125} \times 5 = \dfrac{250}{125} = 2$ mL

b. H : V :: D : x
   125 mg   :   5 mL   ::   50 mg   : x mL

$$125x = 250$$
$$x = 2 \text{ mL (cc)}$$

Cefaclor 50 mg = 2 mL. Give 2 mL four times a day.

PEDIATRIC DOSAGE PER BODY SURFACE AREA

To calculate pediatric dose by BSA, the child's height and weight are needed. Figure 4F–2 is the nomogram used to determine the BSA for infants and children.

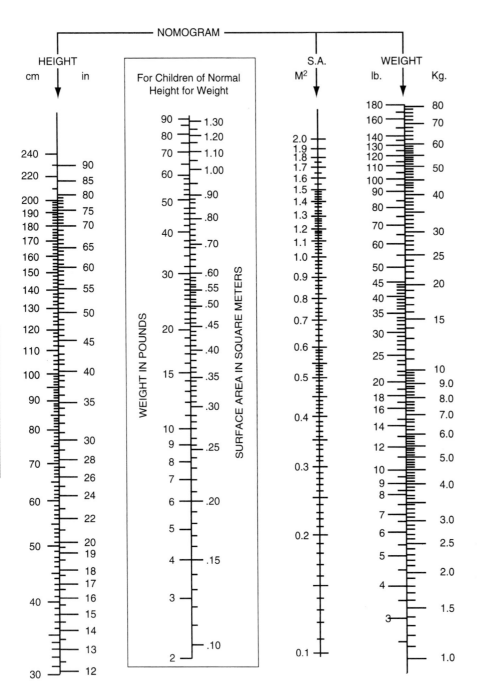

Figure 4F–2
Nomogram of body surface area for adults. *Directions:* (1) Find height. (2) Find weight (3) Draw a straight line connecting the height and weight. (4) Where the line intersects on the Body Surface Area column is the body surface area (m²). (Sources: Deglin, Vallerand, and Russin: *Davis's Drug Guide for Nurses*, 2nd ed. Philadelphia: F. A. Davis, 1991; Lentner, C. [ed.]: *Geigy Scientific Tables*, 8th ed. Vol. 1. Basle, Switzerland: Ciba-Geigy, pp. 226–227, 1981.)

Example

Order: methotrexate (Mexate) 50 mg weekly
  Child's height: 54 inches; weight: 90 lb (41 kg)
  Child's drug dosage: 25–75 mg/m²/week
  Child's height and weight intersect at 1.3 m² (BSA).
  Is the prescribed dose safe?

Answer:

Multiply the BSA, 1.3 m², by the minimum and maximum doses.

$$25 \text{ mg} \times 1.3 \text{ m}^2 = 32.5 \text{ mg}$$

$$75 \text{ mg} \times 1.3 \text{ m}^2 = 97.5 \text{ mg}$$

Dosage is considered safe within the parameters according to the child's body surface area (BSA).

PEDIATRIC DOSAGE FROM ADULT DOSAGE

To calculate the pediatric dosage from the adult dosage, determine the child's height and weight, and where they intersect on the nomogram is the body surface area in square meters. The formula for calculation is:

$$\frac{\text{Surface area (m}^2)}{1.73 \text{ m}^2} \times \text{Adult dose} = \text{Pediatric dose}$$

Example

Order: erythromycin (E-Mycin) 125 mg PO q.i.d.
  Child's height is 42 inches; weight is 60 lb
  Child's height and weight intersect at 0.9 m²
  The adult dose is 1000 mg/day.

$$\frac{0.9 \text{ m}^2}{1.73 \text{ m}^2} \times 1000 = \frac{900}{1.73} = 520 \text{ mg/day}$$

Drug dosage: 520 mg ÷ 4 times a day = 130 mg/dose
Dosage is within safe range.

PRACTICE PROBLEMS

I. Pediatric Dosing (Oral)

Solve the following problems using one of these three methods: body weight, body surface area, or pediatric dosage from adult dosage. The safe dosage is given in drug reference books.

1. Order: phenytoin (Dilantin) 50 mg b.i.d.
   Child weighs 44 lb (20 kg)
   Child's drug dosage: 4–8 mg/kg/day in two to three divided doses
   Available: Dilantin 30 mg/5 mL
   Is the prescribed dose safe? How many milliliters should the child receive for each dose?

2. Order: ethosuximide (Zarontin) 500 mg/d PO.
   Child weighs 26 kg
   Child's drug dosage: 20 mg/kg/day
   Available: ethosuximide syrup 250 mg/5 mL
   How many milligrams and milliliters should the child receive each day?

3. Order: dicloxacillin sodium (Dynapen) 100 mg q6h
   Child weighs 55 lb (_____ kg)
   Child's drug dosage range: < 40 kg, 12.5–25 mg/kg q6h
   Available:

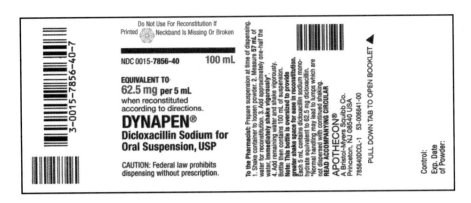

Is the prescribed dose safe? How many milliliters should be given for each dose?

4. Order: digoxin (Lanoxin), 35 μg/kg/loading dose (μg = mcg) PO
   Child weighs 10 kg
   Available: Lanoxin 50 μg/mL (0.05 mg/mL)
   a. How many micrograms or milligrams should the child receive?
   b. How many milliliters (mL) should be given for the loading dose?

5. Order: amoxicillin 200 mg PO q8h
   Child weighs 26 lb (12 kg)
   Child's drug dosage: 20–40 mg/kg/day in three divided doses
   Available:

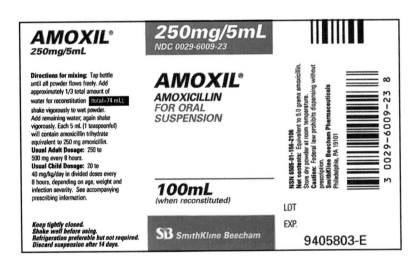

Is the prescribed dose safe? How many milliliters should be given every 8 h?

6. Order: theophylline sodium glycinate (Asbron G) 200 mg PO q6h
   Child is 12 years old and weighs 74 lb (34 kg)
   Child's drug dosage: 9–16 years old: 6 mg/kg/q6h
   Is the prescribed dose safe? _____

7. Order: amoxicillin and clavulanate potassium (Augmentin) 100 mg PO q8h
   Child's weight: 28 lb
   Child's drug dosage: 20–40 mg/kg/day
   Available:

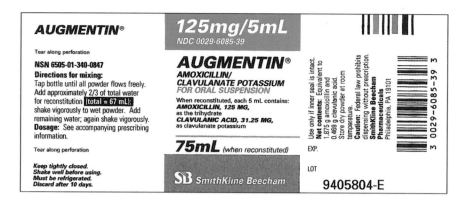

a. Is the prescribed drug dose within safe parameters? _____
b. How many mL should the child receive per dose?

8. Order: cefadroxil (Duricef) 75 mg PO q12h
   Child's weight: 20 lb
   Child's drug dosage: 30 mg/kg/day
   Available:

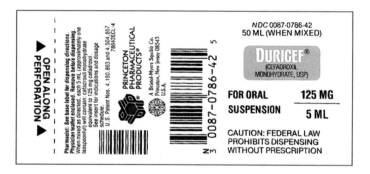

a. Is the prescribed drug dose within safe parameters? _____
b. How many mL should the child receive per dose?

9. Order: ampicillin 200 mg PO q6h
   Child weighs 27 kg
   Child's drug dosage: 25–50 mg/kg/day
   Available:

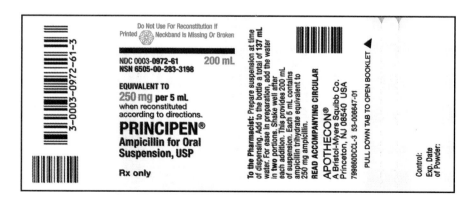

Is the prescribed dose safe? How many milligrams per dose?

10. Order: vinblastine (Velsar)
    Child's body surface area (BSA) is 1.2 m²
    Child's drug dosage: 2.5 mg/m²
    How many milligrams should the child receive?

PEDIATRIC CALCULATIONS FOR INJECTABLES

The same three methods used for calculating oral dosages for children are used for calculating injectable dosages. They are calculated from (1) body weight (kg), (2) body surface area (BSA, m²), and (3) the adult dose. Use the nomogram for BSA.

PRACTICE PROBLEMS

II. Pediatric Injectables

Solve the following drug problems and indicate whether the drug dose is within the safe parameters.

1. Order: tobramycin (Nebcin) 10 mg IM q8h
   Child's weight: 10 kg
   Child's drug dosage: 3 mg/kg/day in three divided doses
   Available:

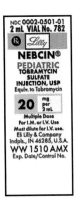

   a. Is dose within safe parameters? _____
   b. How many milliliters (mL) should the child receive per dose?

2. Order: promethazine (Phenergan) 20 mg IM q6h
   Child's weight: 45 kg
   Child's drug dosage: 0.25–0.5 mg/kg/dose; repeat every 4 to 6 h
   Available: Phenergan 25 mg/mL
   a. Is dose within safe parameters? _____
   b. How many milliliters (mL) should the child receive per dose?

3. Order: cefamandole (Mandol) 250 mg IM q6h
   Child's weight: 15 kg
   Child's drug dosage: 50–100 mg/kg/day in three to six divided doses
   Available:

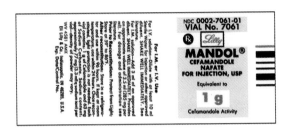

   a. Is the dose within safe parameters? _____
   b. How many milliliters (mL) should the child receive per dose?

4. Order: oxacillin sodium 250 mg IM q6h
   Child's weight: 15 kg
   Child's drug dosage: 50–100 mg/kg/day in divided doses
   Available:

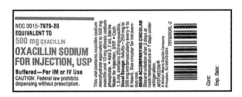

   a. How many milligrams (mg) should the child receive per day?
   b. How much diluent should be added?
   c. How many milliliters (mL) should the child receive per dose?
   d. Is dose within safe parameters? _____

5. Order: ampicillin sodium 75 mg q6h IM
   Child's weight: 17½ lb
   Child's drug dosage: 25–50 mg/kg/day
   Available:

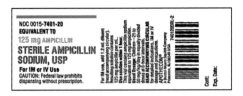

   a. How much diluent should be added?
   b. How many milligrams (mg) should the child receive per day?
   c. Is drug dosage per day within safe parameters? _____
      Explain _____

6. Order: nafcillin sodium 200 mg q6h IM
   Child's weight: 10 kg
   Child's drug dosage: 100–300 mg/kg/day in divided doses
   Available:

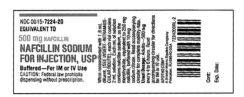

   a. How many milligrams (mg) will the child receive per day?
   b. Is the drug dosage per day within safe parameters? _____
   c. How many milliliters (mL) should the child receive per dose?

7. Order: The newborn is to receive AquaMEPHYTON (vitamin K) 0.5 mg immediately after delivery.
   Available:

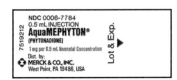 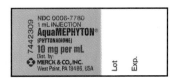

   a. Which AquaMEPHYTON container would you select?
   b. How many milliliters (mL) should the newborn receive?

8. Order: cefazolin (Ancef) 125 mg IM q6h
   Child's weight: 22 kg
   Child's drug dosage: 25–50 mg/kg/day in three to four divided doses (up to 100 mg/kg/day)
   Available:

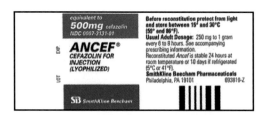

   a. How many milligrams (mg) should the child receive per day?
   b. Is the dose within safe parameters? _____
   c. The drug label does not give the amount of diluent to add to the Ancef powder. Check the pamphlet insert. With 3.4 mL of diluent added, is equivalent to 4 mL of drug solution.
   d. How many mL of cefazolin should the child receive per dose?

9. Order: hydroxyzine (Vistaril) 50 mg IM
   Child's height and weight: 47 inches, 45 lb
   Child's drug dosage: 30 mg/m²
   Available: Vistaril 25 mg/mL
   Is dose within safe parameters? _____

10. Order: methotrexate (Mexate) 50 mg IM weekly
    Child's height and weight: 56 inches, 100 lb
    Child's drug dosage: 25–75 mg/m²/week
    Available: methotrexate 2.5 mg/mL; 25 mg/mL; 100 mg/mL
    Is dose within safe parameters? _____

ANSWERS TO PRACTICE PROBLEMS

I. Pediatric Dosing (Oral)

1. Drug parameters:

   4 mg × 20 kg = 80 mg/day

   8 mg × 20 kg = 160 mg/day

   Dosage order: 50 mg × 2 (b.i.d.) = 100 mg/day
   Dosage is within safe parameters.

   a. $\dfrac{D}{H} \times V = \dfrac{50}{30} \times 5 = \dfrac{250}{30} = 8.3$ mL, or 8 mL

   b.
   $$H \quad : \quad V \quad :: \quad D \quad : \quad x$$
   $$30\ \text{mg} \quad : \quad 5\ \text{mL} \quad :: \quad 50\ \text{mg} \quad : \quad x\ \text{mL}$$

   $$30x = 250$$

   $$x = \frac{250}{30} = 8.3 \text{ mL}$$

   Administer 8 mL of phenytoin per dose.

2. Child's drug dosage: 20 mg × 26 kg = 520 mg, or 500 mg

   a. $\dfrac{D}{H} \times V = \dfrac{500}{250} \times 5 = \dfrac{2500}{250} = 10$ mL

b. $\begin{array}{ccccc} H & : & V & :: & D & : & x \\ 250 \text{ mg} & : & 5 \text{ mL} & :: & 500 \text{ mg} & : & x \text{ mL} \end{array}$

$$250x = 2500$$

$$x = 10 \text{mL}$$

Administer ethosuximide 10 mL/day.

3. a. Child weighs 25 kg (55 lb ÷ 2.2 = 25 kg)
   b. Drug parameters:

   $$12.5 \text{ mg} \times 25 \text{ kg} = 312.5 \text{ mg/day}$$

   $$25 \text{ mg} \times 25 \text{ kg} = 625 \text{ mg/day}$$

   Dosage order: 100 mg × 4 times a day (q6h) = 400 mg/day
   Dosage is within safe parameters.

   a. $\dfrac{D}{H} \times V = \dfrac{100}{62.5} \times 5 = \dfrac{500}{62.5} = 8$ mL of dicloxacillin

   b. $\begin{array}{ccccc} H & : & V & :: & D & : & x \\ 62.5 \text{ mg} & : & 5 \text{ mL} & :: & 100 \text{ mg} & : & x \text{ mL} \end{array}$

   $$62.5x = 500$$

   $$x = 8 \text{ mL of dicloxacillin}$$

4. Child's drug dosage:

   a. $35 \ \mu g \times 10 \text{ kg} = 350 \ \mu g$, or 0.35 mg

   $$350 \ \mu g = 0.350 \text{ mg}$$

   b. $\dfrac{D}{H} \times V = \dfrac{350 \ \mu g}{50 \ \mu g} \times 1 \text{ mL} = 7$ mL loading dose

   or

   $\dfrac{0.35 \text{ mg}}{0.05 \text{ mg}} \times 1 \text{ mL} = 7$ mL loading dose

5. Drug parameters:

   $$20 \text{ mg} \times 12 \text{ kg} = 240 \text{ mg/day}$$

   $$40 \text{ mg} \times 12 \text{ kg} = 480 \text{ mg /day}$$

   Dosage order: 200 mg × 3 (q8h) = 600 mg/day
   Dosage is *not* within safe parameters. Dose exceeds the drug parameters.
   Health care provider must be contacted.

6. Drug dosage: 6 mg × 34 kg = 204 mg, or 200 mg
   Dosage of 200 mg is within safe parameters.

7. a. Drug parameters: (28 lb ÷ 2.2 = 12.7 kg)

   $$20 \text{ mg} \times 12.7 \text{ kg} = 254 \text{ mg/day}$$

   $$40 \text{ mg} \times 12.7 \text{ kg} = 508 \text{ mg/day}$$

   Dosage order: 100 mg × 4 (q8h) = 400 mg/d
   Dosage is within safe parameters.
   b. 4 mL of Augmentin

8. 20 lb ÷ 2.2 = 9kg
   a. Drug parameters: 30 mg × 9 kg = 270 mg/day
   Drug dosage order: 75 mg × 2 (q12h) = 150 mg/day
   Drug dose is safe; it is below the drug parameter.
   b. 3 mL of Duricef

9. Drug parameters:

$$25 \text{ mg} \times 27 \text{ kg} = 675 \text{ mg/day}$$

$$50 \text{ mg} \times 27 \text{ kg} = 1350 \text{ mg/day}$$

Dosage order: 200 mg × 4 (q6h) = 800 mg/day
Dosage is within safe parameters.

a. $\dfrac{D}{H} \times V = \dfrac{200}{250} \times 5 = \dfrac{1000}{250} = 4$ mL of ampicillin

b.

H	:	V	::	D	:	x
250 mg	:	5 mL	::	200 mg	:	x mL

$$250x = 1000$$

$$x = 4 \text{ mL of ampicillin}$$

10. Drug dosage: 2.5 mg × 1.2 m² = 3 mg
Administer 3 mg vinblastine.

II. Pediatric Injectables

1. a. Tobramycin parameter: 3 mg/kg/day × 10 kg = 30 mg/day in three divided doses.
   Drug order: 10 mg × 3 (q8h) = 30 mg/day
   Dosage is within safe parameters.
   b. 10 mg = 1 mL/dose
   Child should receive 1 mL per dose.
2. a. Phenergan parameters: 0.25 mg/kg/dose × 45 kg = 11.25 mg/dose
                            0.50 mg/kg/dose × 45 kg = 22.5 mg/dose
   Drug order: Phenergan 20 mg IM per dose
   Dosage is within safe parameters.
   b. Phenergan 20 mg = 0.8 mL
3. a. Cefamandole parameters: 50 mg/kg/day × 15 kg = 750 mg/day
                              100 mg/kg/day × 15 kg = 1500 mg/day
   Drug order: cefamandole 250 mg × 4 doses = 1000 mg/day
   Dosage is within safe parameters.
   b. 0.89, or 0.9 mL
   The drug label states to add 3.0 mL of diluent, equaling 3.5 mL.
   Convert 1 g to 1000 mg.
4. a. 250 mg × 4 (q6h) = 1000 mg/day
   b. Add 2.7 mL of diluent = 3 mL of drug solution
   c. 1.5 mL
   d. Dosage is within safe parameters.
5. Child weighs 8 kg (17.5 lb ÷ 2.2 = 8 kg)
   a. 1.2 mL of diluent (see label)
   b. 75 mg × 4 (q6h) = 300 mg/day
   c. Dose per day is within safe parameters
      25 mg × 8 kg = 200 mg
      50 mg × 8 kg = 400 mg (200–400 mg/day)
6. a. 200 mg × 4 (q6h) = 800 mg/day
   b. Dose per day is safe but not in therapeutic range. Notify health care provider.
      100 mg × 10 kg = 1000 mg
      300 mg × 10 kg = 3000 mg
   c. Add 1.8 ml diluent = 2 mL (500 mg = 2 mL)
      Nafcillin 200 mg = 0.8 mL

7. a. Preferred selection is AquaMEPHYTON 1 mg = 0.5 mL
   b. *AquaMEPHYTON 1 mg = 0.5 mL*

$$\frac{D}{H} \times V = \frac{0.5 \text{ mg}}{1.0 \text{ mg}} \times 0.5 \text{ mL} = \frac{0.25}{1.0} = 0.25 \text{ mL}$$

   AquaMEPHYTON 10 mg = 1 mL

$$\frac{D}{H} \times V = \frac{0.5 \text{ mg}}{10 \text{ mg}} \times 1.0 \text{ mL} = \frac{0.5}{10} = 0.05 \text{ mL}$$

   For AquaMEPHYTON 1 mg = 0.5 mL. Give 0.25 mL. (Use a tuberculin syringe.)
   For AquaMEPHYTON 10 mg = 1 mL. Give 0.05 mL. (Use a tuberculin syringe; however, it would be difficult to give this small amount.)

8. a. 125 mg × 4 (q6h) = 500 mg
   b. 22 kg × 25 mg/kg/day = 550 mg
   22 kg × 50 mg/kg/day = 1100 mg
   22 kg × 100 mg/kg/day = 2200 mg (Range: 550–2200 mg)
   Drug dose per day is below the suggested child's drug dose range. The nurse should contact the health care provider. The daily drug dose may need to be increased because of the child's weight.
   c. Add 3.4 mL of diluent yielding 4 mL of drug solution.
   d. Give 1 mL of cefazolin (Ancef) per dose.

9. Height and weight intersect at 0.82 m².
   Hydroxyzine parameter: 30 mg/m² × 0.82 m² = 24.6 mg, or 25 mg
   Drug order: hydroxyzine 50 mg IM
   Dosage ordered is *not* within safe parameters. Dosage exceeds the drug parameters. *Do not* give the medication. Notify the health care provider.

10. Height and weight intersect at 1.38 m².
   Methotrexate parameters: 25 mg/m²/week × 1.38 m² = 34.5 mg/week
                          75 mg/m²/week × 1.38 m² = 103.5 mg/week
   Drug order: methotrexate 59 mg/week IM
   Dosage is within safe parameters.
   (1) If methotrexate 25 mg/mL is used, give 2 mL (50 mg) or
   (2) If methotrexate 100 mg/mL is used, give 0.5 mL. Because of the amount of solution, it may be more desirable to give 0.5 mL of the 100 mg/mL solution.

Unit II

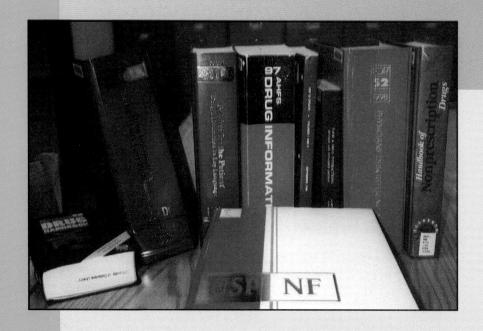

Contemporary Issues in Pharmacology

This unit comprises seven chapters covering a range of issues affecting drug therapy and nursing. Chapter 5, The Drug Approval Process (U.S. and Canadian), Resources, and Ethical Issues, covers drug standards and federal legislation on both American and Canadian drugs, which establish safety guidelines for drug use, drug names, and drug resources. Ethical considerations in the pharmacotherapeutic regimen are also addressed.

Chapter 6, Transcultural Considerations, helps the nurse understand and respond to unique cultural factors that may influence drug therapy for a particular client. Factors such as communication styles, family organization, spirituality and religion, health beliefs and practices, and traditional and folk medicine are discussed.

Chapter 7 covers drug interactions and drug abuse, two areas of special interest to nurses. Assessing drug interaction has always been and remains an ongoing function of the nurse. Because drug abuse is a national problem from which no portion of the population is immune, including health professionals, it is a topic of great concern to nurses.

Chapter 8, Herbal Therapy and Nursing Implications, explores the increasingly popular herbal-based preparations available over-the-counter. It covers the most commonly used herbs, discussing their indications, preparation, dosages, potential hazards, and tips for safe and effective use.

Drug therapy in children and elderly adults warrants special nursing considerations. Understanding the pharmacokinetic and pharmacodynamic effects specific to these age groups is especially important for identifying safe drug dosing and preventing adverse reactions. Chapter 9, Drug Therapy: Considerations Across the Lifespan, identifies aspects that require special attention when administering drugs to clients in these age groups.

With the increasing movement of health care into the community, nurses, above all other health care providers, are gaining more responsibilities and opportunities to guide clients in safe medication administration. Chapter 10, Medication Administration in Community Settings, focuses on aspects of drug therapy unique to the home, school, work place, and other alternative care settings.

The nurse's role in drug research, discussed in Chapter 11, is challenging. The nurse in general practice identifies specific needs that may be met by medications. As part of clinical drug trials, the nurse needs to be ever aware of informed consent and the client's response to drugs.

5
The Drug Approval Process (U.S. and Canadian), Resources, and Ethical Considerations

Outline

Objectives

- Explain the Food, Drug, and Cosmetic Act of 1938 and the two amendments to it.
- Explain the three Canadian schedules for drugs sold in Canada.
- Describe the function of nurse practice acts.
- Differentiate between chemical, generic, and brand names of drugs.
- List two drug resources (reference) books.
- Explain various ethical values that the nurse should consider in relation to health care.

Terms

American Hospital Formulary	*Drug Facts & Comparison*	nonfeasance
brand name	FDA	*PDR*
chemical name	generic name	pharmacology
controlled substance	malfeasance	*USP-DI*
DEA	misfeasance	*USP-NF*

INTRODUCTION

Pharmacology is the study of the effects of chemical substances on living tissues. Early drugs were derived from plants, animals, and minerals. Records of drug use date back to 2700 B.C. in the Middle East and China. The drugs most commonly used then were laxatives and emetics to induce vomiting.

In 1550 B.C., the Egyptians wrote their empirical observations of drug therapy on what has come to be known as the Ebers Medical Papyrus. They suggested castor oil as a laxative and opium for pain. They also suggested that moldy bread be applied to wounds and bruises 3500 years before Alexander Fleming's discovery of penicillin.

The Roman physician and writer Galen (131–201 A.D.) was considered an authority in medicine and pharmacy for hundreds of years. He initiated the common use of prescriptions and used several ingredients to treat a specific illness.

After the fall of the Roman Empire, medicine and pharmacy returned to the realms of folklore and tradition. During this time, however, Christian monks kept information on medicine and pharmacy in their monasteries and tended the sick and needy. The medicines used by the monks were derived from plants and herbs grown in the monastery gardens.

Around 1240 A.D., Arab doctors formulated the first set of drug standards and measurements (grains, drams, minims), known as the apothecary system. (Currently, the units of the metric system are used internationally to measure drugs; the apothecary system is being phased out.) In fifteenth-century England, apothecary shops were owned by barber-surgeons, physicians, and independent merchants dispensing herbal and chemical remedies.

In the eighteenth century, the following breakthrough drugs were introduced: the vaccine for smallpox, digitalis from the foxglove plant for strengthening and slowing the heart beat, and vitamin C from citrus fruit. In the nineteenth century, morphine and codeine were extracted from opium; atropine, bromides, and iodine were introduced; amyl nitrite was used to relieve the pain of angina; and the anesthetics ether and nitrous oxide were discovered.

In the early twentieth century, aspirin was derived from salicylic acid, and phenobarbital, insulin, and the sulfonamides were introduced. A vast majority of modern drugs date back to the early 1940s. Antibiotics (penicillin, tetracycline, streptomycin), antihistamines, and cortisone were marketed in the 1940s. In the 1950s, antipsychotic drugs, antihypertensives, oral contraceptives, and the polio vaccine were introduced.

DRUG STANDARDS AND LEGISLATION
Drug Standards

The set of drug standards used in the United States is the *United States Pharmacopeia* of 1820. The **U.S. Pharmacopeia National Formulary (USP-NF),** the current authoritative source for drug standards, is revised every 5 years by a group of experts in nursing, pharmaceutics, pharmacology, chemistry, and microbiology. Drugs included in the *USP-NF* have met high standards for therapeutic use, client safety, quality, purity, strength, packaging safety, and dosage form. Drugs that meet these standards have the initials USP following their official name.

The *International Pharmacopeia*, first published in 1951 by the World Health Organization (WHO), provides a basis for standards in strength and composition of drugs for use throughout the world. The book is published in English, Spanish, and French and, like the *USP-NF,* is revised every 5 years.

Federal Legislation

Through federal legislation, the public is protected from drugs that are impure, toxic, ineffective, or not tested before public sale. The primary purpose of this federal legislation is to ensure safety. America's first law to regulate drugs was the Federal Pure Food and Drug Act of 1906, which did not include drug effectiveness and drug safety.

1938: FOOD, DRUG, AND COSMETIC ACT

The Food, Drug, and Cosmetic Act of 1938 empowered a governing body, the **Food and Drug Administration (FDA),** to monitor and regulate the manufacture and marketing of drugs. It is the FDA'S responsibility to ensure that all drugs are tested for harmful effects and have labels with accurate information, and that detailed literature explaining adverse effects is enclosed with the drug packaging. The FDA can prevent the marketing of any drug that it judges to be incompletely tested or dangerous. Only those drugs that are considered safe by FDA are approved for marketing.

1952: DURHAM-HUMPHREY AMENDMENT OF THE 1938 ACT

The Durham-Humphrey amendment to the Food, Drug, and Cosmetic Act of 1938 distinguished between drugs that can be sold with or without prescription and those that should not be refilled without a new prescription. Those drugs that should not be refilled without a new prescription, such as narcotics, hypnotics, or tranquilizers, must be so labeled.

1962: KEFAUVER-HARRIS AMENDMENT OF THE 1938 ACT

The Kefauver-Harris amendment to the Food, Drug, and Cosmetic Act of 1938 resulted from the widely publicized thalidomide tragedy of the 1950s, in which pregnant European women who took the sedative-hypnotic thalidomide during the first trimester of pregnancy gave birth to babies with extreme limb deformities. The Kefauver-Harris amendment tightened controls on drug safety, especially experimental drugs, and required that adverse reactions and contraindications must be labeled and included in the literature. Also included in the amendment were provisions for the evaluation of testing methods used by manufacturers, the process for withdrawal of approved drugs when safety and effectiveness were in doubt, and the establishment of the effectiveness of new drugs before marketing.

1970: THE CONTROLLED SUBSTANCES ACT

In 1970, the Controlled Substances Act (CSA) of the Comprehensive Drug Abuse Prevention and Control Act, Title II, was passed by Congress. This act, designed to remedy the escalating problem of drug abuse, included several provisions: the promotion of drug education and research into the prevention and treatment of drug dependence; the strengthening of enforcement authority; the establishment of treatment and rehabilitation facilities; and the designation of schedules, or categories, for controlled substances according to abuse liability.

Controlled substances are described in five sched-ules, or categories, listed in Table 5–1. Schedule I drugs are *not* approved for medical use; schedule II through V drugs have accepted medical use. In addition, the abuse potential and extent of physical and psychological dependence are greatest with schedule I drugs. This dependency decreases as one moves through the schedule, with schedule V drugs having only very limited abuse potential. Some drugs might be listed in more than one schedule category. Codeine is a schedule II drug, but when codeine is added to acetaminophen, it becomes a schedule III drug, and when it is used in combination as a cough preparation, it becomes a schedule V drug.

NURSING INTERVENTIONS: CONTROLLED SUBSTANCES

- Account for all controlled drugs.
- Keep special controlled substance record for required information.
- Countersign all discarded or wasted medication.
- Ensure that records and drugs on hand match.
- Keep all controlled drugs locked up; narcotics must be kept under double lock.
- Be certain that only authorized persons have access to the keys.

In 1983, the **Drug Enforcement Administration (DEA)** of the Department of Justice was charged with the role of being the nation's sole legal drug enforcement agency. The Bureau of Narcotics and Dangerous Drugs, which preceded the DEA, is defunct.

Table 5–1
Schedule Categories of Controlled Substances

SCHEDULE	EXAMPLES OF SUBSTANCES	DESCRIPTION
I	Heroin, hallucinogenics (LSD, marijuana, mescaline, peyote, psilocybine)	Drugs with high abuse potential. No accepted medical use. Labeled C-I
II	Meperidine (Demerol), morphine, hydrocodone, hydromorphone, methadone, oxycodone, codeine, amphetamines, secobarbital, pentobarbital	High potential for drug abuse. Accepted medical use. Can lead to strong physical and psychological dependency. Labeled C-II
III	Codeine preparations, paregoric, nonnarcotic drugs (pentazocine, propoxyphene)	Medically accepted drugs. Potential abuse is less than that for schedules I and II. May cause dependence. Labeled C-III
IV	Phenobarbital, benzodiazepines (diazepam, oxazepam, lorazepam, chlordiazepoxide), chloral hydrate, meprobamate	Medically accepted drugs. May cause dependence. Labeled C-IV
V	Opioid controlled substances for cough and diarrhea, such as codeine in cough preparations	Medically accepted drugs. Very limited potential for dependence. Labeled C-V

Key: C, control.

NURSE PRACTICE ACTS

Every state has its own laws regarding drug administration by nurses. Generally, nurses cannot prescribe or administer drugs without a health care provider's order, but state laws vary. A practicing nurse should request a copy of the nurse practice act in the state in which she or he is licensed. In some states, a nurse who administers a drug without a physician's order is in violation of the nurse practice act and could have her or his license revoked.

In a civil court, the nurse can be prosecuted for giving the wrong drug or dosage, omitting a drug dose, or giving the drug by the wrong route. The legal terms for these offenses are

Misfeasance: negligence; giving the wrong drug or drug dose that results in the client's death

Nonfeasance: omission; omitting a drug dose that results in the client's death

Malfeasance: giving the correct drug but by the wrong route that results in the client's death

Canadian Drug Regulation

In Canada, the Health Protection Branch, Department of National Health and Welfare, is responsible for administering the two acts that are the foundation of the national drug laws. The manufacture, distribution, and sale of drugs (except narcotics) are controlled by the Canadian Food and Drug Act, amended in 1953. The manufacture, distribution, and sale of narcotic drugs are controlled by the 1961 Narcotics Control Act. Like the U.S. Controlled Substances Act, the Canadian act requires prescriptions and strict record keeping for all narcotics.

Drugs sold in Canada are assigned to one of the following schedules:

1. Schedule F. All prescription drugs (approximately 350) are available only with a prescription (written or verbal); thus, these drugs have essentially no potential for abuse.

2. Schedule G. Fourteen drugs in this group require written or verbal prescription and refills require a written prescription. These drugs have a moderate potential for abuse and must have a "C" on the label, similar to schedule III drugs in the United States.

3. Schedule H. These drugs have no recognized medical use and are potentially dangerous, similar to schedule I drugs in the United States. Their use is primarily limited to specialized medical research.

4. Narcotics. These drugs are dispensed only with written prescription and an "N" must appear on all advertisements and labels. Low-dose codeine (20 mg/30 mL and 8-mg tablets) is an exception and can be sold only by a pharmacist. Two additional medicinal ingredients, caffeine and acetylsalicylic acid, must be part of this codeine preparation.

Nonprescription drugs (over-the-counter preparations) are administered by the Pharmacy Acts of the respective Canadian provinces, which identify the place and conditions of sale. These drugs are assigned to one of three categories:

1. General proprietary. These drugs are for treatment of self-limiting minor illness, injury, or discomfort. The packaging information is considered adequate and the drug can be administered without consultation with a health care provider. These drugs can be purchased at any store.

2. Availability only through pharmacies. After consultation and approval by a health care provider, drugs designed to treat minor, self-limiting conditions are available through a pharmacy. Examples are cold remedies and laxatives.

3. Recommendation of a health care provider. This category requires recommendation by a health care provider. Examples include nitroglycerin, insulin, and muscle relaxants.

To address the proliferation of a variety of provincial schedules and regulations, the Health Protection Branch has proposed to "harmonize" regulations nationwide by creating a three-schedule system:

Schedule I: All prescription drugs (schedules F and G and narcotics)

Schedule II: Nonprescription, pharmacist-monitored drugs

Schedule III: Nonprescription drugs with no restrictions placed on location of sale

The initial harmonizing work is the development of specific criteria to identify the amount of professional involvement required for the sale and use of drug preparations. The initiation of schedule II presents special challenges.

In Canada, the therapeutic and toxic levels are monitored according to International System (SI) of units; this is also true in many European countries. The mole (mol) was adopted to express drug concentration in body fluid in molar units, such as millimoles per liter (mmol/L) instead of the traditional expression of mass units, milligrams per liter (mg/L). Some institutions in the United States use the International System of unit; however, the traditional use of mass units in the United States is still in use.

DRUG NAMES

Each drug may have several names. The **chemical name** describes the drug's chemical structure. The **generic name** is the official or nonproprietary name for the drug. This name is not owned by any pharmaceutical (drug) company and is universally accepted. Most drugs are ordered by their generic name. The **brand** or **trade name,** also known as the proprietary name, is chosen by the drug company and is usually a registered trade mark owned by that specific manufacturer. Drug companies market a compound using their given name (brand name). For example, Cardizem is the brand (proprietary) name registered with the manufacturer, and diltiazem HCl is the generic name recognized by the USP.

There are pros and cons to using generic drugs (Fig. 5–1). Generic drugs are usually cheaper and have the same active ingredients as in brand-name, or trade-name, drugs. However, some generic drugs have inert fillers and binders that may result in variations of drug effectiveness. The FDA publishes a list of approved generic drugs that are bioequivalents to brand-name drugs. Generic drugs are less expensive because manufacturers do not have to do extensive testing, because these drugs had been clinically tested for safety and efficacy by the pharmaceutical company that first formulated the drug. The health care provider and client must exercise care in choosing generic drugs because there may be some variation in the action of or response to them. Brand-name drugs are preferred when ordering anticonvulsants for seizures, anticoagulants (such as Coumadin), medication for congestive heart failure (Lanoxin), and aspirin when giving large doses for rheumatoid arthritis. A study showed that 23 seizure-free epileptic clients who switched to the generic drug experienced renewed seizure activity. The nurse should check with the health care provider or pharmacist when generic drugs are prescribed.

Throughout this text, both generic and brand names are given for drugs. Because many brand names may exist for a single generic name, the generic name is given *first* in lower case letters, followed by the most commonly used brand name in parentheses. With generic drugs, the name may be long and difficult to pronounce. Brand names always begin with a capital letter. An example of a generic and brand-name drug listing is "furosemide (Lasix)."

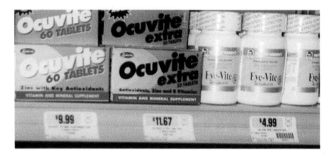

Figure 5–1
There is a $5.00 difference between the brand name and generic name vitamins.

DRUG RESOURCES

There are many resource reference books on drugs, including nursing texts that identify related nursing interventions and areas for health teaching.

The American Hospital Formulary Services (AHFS), Physicians' Desk Reference (PDR), Drug Facts and Comparisons (F & C), and the *United States Pharmacopeic—Drug Information (USP-DI)* are resources that provide valuable information of approved drugs. The method for presentation of the drugs varies.

American Hospital Formulary Service (AHFS) Drug Information is published yearly by the American Society of Health-System Pharmacists, Bethesda, Maryland. It is an excellent reference that provides accurate and complete drug information on nearly all prescription drugs marketed in the United States. This reference text contains drugs listed according to therapeutic drug classification. The information given for each drug includes chemistry and stability, pharmacologic actions, pharmacokinetics, uses, cautions per body system, precautions, contraindications, acute toxicity, drug interactions, dosage and administration, and preparations.

This reference book is updated yearly and updated regularly with monthly supplements. The supplementary editions contain new marketed drugs, their dosage forms and strengths, uses, and cautions. This text is unbiased in that it does not contain information about the drug from only a pharmaceutical company. Additionally, many drug handbooks are available as quick drug references. Most of these include nursing implications. When more information is needed about a drug, the *PDR* or the *American Hospital Formulary* frequently is suggested.

The ***Physicians' Desk Reference (PDR)*** lists several thousand drugs with complete drug information given by pharmaceutical companies. The *PDR* is published yearly. It contains seven sections, two of which are the most useful to nurses: the second (pink) section, which is the drug name index, and the sixth (white) section, which gives information about the drugs. The *PDR* is a useful drug resource, but it does not provide complete pharmacologic and therapeutic information and does not include nursing interventions. The drug information is reprinted drug package inserts supplied by the pharmaceutical company, which pays to have its drug listed in the *PDR*.

Drug Facts and Comparisons contains information on almost all drugs marketed in the United States. The reference consists of drug actions, indications, warnings and precautions, dosage and route for administration, adverse reactions, client information, overdosage, drug interactions, contraindications, and comparison charts and tables.

The ***United States Pharmacopeic—Drug Information (USP-DI)*** is a three-volume set that is available in most hospitals and pharmacies. Monthly supplements are available. Volumes IA and IB provide drug information for the health care provider. The sections in these volumes include pharmacology, precautions to consider, side and adverse effects, client consultation, general dosing information, and dosage forms. Volume II gives drug information for the client. It is a client-oriented volume that explains information in an understandable way for the client. The sections included in volume II are administration of drug, drug effects, indications, adverse reactions, dosage guidelines, and what to do for missed doses.

The Medical Letter on drugs and therapeutics is published biweekly by the Medical Letter, Inc., New Rochelle, New York. This is a nonprofit publication for physicians, nurse practitioners, and other health professionals. These biweekly issues cover one of two themes: (1) drugs for the treatment of disease entities such as HIV, peptic ulcers, or (2) two to four new drugs that have been approved by the FDA. The information included with each new drug is pharmacokinetics, clinical studies, dosage, adverse effects, interactions, and conclusion.

The *Handbook on Injectable Drugs* by Lawrence A. Trissel is published by the American Society of Hospital Pharmacists. It is an excellent reference for injectable medications, listing drug compatibility with other drugs, base fluids, and drugs available in large-volume parenterals. Also, it includes the pH of each drug and gives some dosing administration guidelines.

The **Internet** is a source for drug information. Drug-related Internet sites are given in Appendix I. Drug information can be posted by anyone, so the information may not always be accurate.

FOOD AND DRUG ADMINISTRATION PREGNANCY CATEGORIES

The FDA developed a classification system related to the effects of drugs on the unborn child (fetus). In the drug literature and drug reference books, a pregnancy category is indicated for most drugs. Categories A and B are considered to be within safe limits for drug use in pregnancy, especially in the first trimester. Table 5–2 lists the FDA pregnancy categories and describes each category's effect on the fetus.

POISON CONTROL CENTERS

Poison Control Centers (PCCs) are present in almost all cities. Telephone numbers for PCCs are listed in the front pages of most telephone books. The centers

Table 5–2
FDA Pregnancy Categories

CATEGORY	DESCRIPTION
A	No risk to fetus. Studies have not shown evidence of fetal harm.
B	No risk in animal studies, and well-controlled studies in pregnant women are not available. It is assumed there is little to no risk in pregnant women.
C	Animal studies indicate a risk to the fetus. Controlled studies on pregnant women are not available. Risk versus benefit of the drug must be determined.
D	A risk to the human fetus has been proved. Risk versus benefit of the drug must be determined. It could be used in life-threatening conditions.
X	A risk to the human fetus has been proved. Risk outweighs the benefit, and drug should be avoided during pregnancy.

provide information about the drug or toxic chemical compounds and the immediate action that should be taken to prevent injury or death. Client education about PCCs is a function of the nurse.

Each year, PCCs respond to more than 1.5 million cases related to a possible ingested drug or chemical toxic compound. About 90% of these cases are in children younger than 3 years and occur at home. Iron tablets, chocolate-covered laxatives, flavored acetaminophen, and flavored liquid medicines are common drugs that children ingest; in large doses they can be toxic to the child. Also, the consumption of most household cleaning chemicals and insecticides is extremely toxic to children.

The mortality rate from poisoning in the United States is about 12,000 deaths per year, of which 50% are from accidental causes and 50% are due to suicides. Immediate reporting of an excess drug or chemical ingestion followed by a proper action may prevent a death or more serious injury from the toxic agent.

ETHICAL CONSIDERATIONS

Ethical values related to drug administration and client care are an ongoing consideration for nurses. Nurses should be morally and ethically responsible

Table 5–3
American Nurses Association: Code of Ethics

1. The nurse provides services with respect for human dignity and the uniqueness of the client, unrestricted by considerations of social or economic status, personal attributes, or the nature of health problems.

2. The nurse safeguards the client's right to privacy by judiciously protecting information of a confidential nature.

3. The nurse acts to safeguard the client and the public when health care and safety are affected by the incompetent, unethical, or illegal practice of any person.

4. The nurse assumes responsibility and accountability for individual nursing judgments and actions.

5. The nurse maintains competence in nursing.

6. The nurse exercises informed judgment and uses individual competence and qualifications as criteria in seeking consultation, accepting responsibilities, and delegating nursing activities to others.

7. The nurse participates in activities that contribute to the ongoing development of the profession's body of knowledge.

8. The nurse participates in the profession's efforts to implement and improve standards of nursing.

9. The nurse participates in the profession's efforts to establish and maintain conditions of employment conducive to high-quality nursing.

10. The nurse participates in the profession's effort to protect the public from misinformation and misrepresentation and to maintain the integrity of nursing.

11. The nurse collaborates with members of the health professions and other citizens in promoting community and national efforts to meet the health needs of the public.

Source: American Nurses Association, 600 Maryland Ave, SW, Suite 100W, Washington, DC, 20024, A-03-30M 10/96 (1985—copyright).

for the client's total care. Drug administration should be correctly prepared and administered.

The American Nurses Association (ANA) and the Canadian Nurses Association (CNA) have a "Code of Ethics for Nurses." The ANA is in the process of updating its code. Both the ANA and CNA have developed similar standards for ethical practice in nursing. Table 5–3 lists the 11 standards of the ANA codes of ethics for nurses.

Nurses need to respect the rights, dignity, and wishes of clients. Clients have the right to know about their drugs, drug actions, and any side effects. They have the right to refuse drugs even after a thorough explanation of the drugs and desired effects are given. According to the ANA code of ethics, the nurse safeguards client's rights, safety, dignity, and health care. The nurse seeks consultation, accepts responsibility, and demonstrates competency in nursing care. The nurse's primary obligation is to the client.

SUMMARY

The nurse should be aware of the various federal acts and amendments related to the use and administration of drugs. The FDA sends out quarterly reports on new drugs, drugs that have been recalled, and other information regarding drug administration. Controlled substances should be checked according to the scheduled drug category of the Controlled Substances Act of 1970. There are many drug resource (reference) books on the market, and these books should be available to nurses in the practice setting. When the client is pregnant, the nurse is also responsible for checking the pregnancy category of the drug in a drug reference book before administering it.

Nurses should be cognizant of their ethical responsibilities toward clients in regards to health care and drug administration. The nurse should respect the rights, dignity, and safety of their clients.

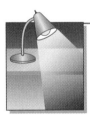

Study Questions

1. What are the provisions in the Food, Drug, and Cosmetic Act of 1938? What additional safeguards are included in the Durham-Humphrey amendment of 1952 and the Kefauver-Harris amendment of 1962?

2. Which controlled substance has the higher potential for drug abuse, controlled substance schedule II or schedule IV? Explain.

3. The Canadian Food and Drug Act of 1953 has identified three schedules for drug regulation. How does schedule F differ from schedule G?

4. What are the characteristics of the chemical name, generic name, and brand or trade name of a drug?

5. What are the titles of two drug resource books that are helpful in nursing practice?

6. Your client is taking a drug that is in pregnancy category B. Would this drug be safe? Explain.

7. Ethical values toward clients is a nursing responsibility. Give examples of nursing considerations related to ethical responsibilities of the nurse according to the ANA Code of Ethics.

6 Transcultural Considerations

LARRY D. PURNELL AND HELENE S. DEHAAN

Outline

Objectives

- Recognize verbal and nonverbal communication practices used by different ethnocultural individuals and groups.
- Assess clients in the context of biocultural ecology.
- Collaborate with traditional and folk practitioners.
- Assess clients for use of traditional and folk therapies.
- Increase the client's compliance with prescriptive therapies.

Terms

African-American	racial	biocultural ecology
Hispanic	spatial distancing	genetic
Jewish-American	European-American	hereditary
Amish	Asian/Pacific Islander	temporality
ethnocultural	American Indian	

INTRODUCTION

Racial, hereditary, and genetic influences have a profound effect on the way clients metabolize drugs and experience and tolerate side effects of medications (Matthews, 1995). Differences in the pharmacokinetics of drugs support processes, which are biologically or chemically mediated. These processes are related to the bioavailability of drugs, protein-binding, volume distribution, hepatic metabolism, and renal tubular absorption (Johnson, 1997). Factors affecting the efficacy and compliance with drug therapy include environment and culture (Finn, 1994). **Ethnocultural** perceptions and beliefs of illness and disease play an important role in the patient's compliance with and understanding of medical treatment and drug therapy (Levy, 1993).

Additionally, age, diurnal rhythms, gender, dietary practices, living conditions, and high-risk behaviors affect drug metabolism, efficacy, and patient compliance. To meet the needs of diverse ethnic and cultural groups, health care professionals need to have an understanding of the variables that influence compliance with medications, differences in physiologic responses to medications, and the patient's beliefs regarding medication (Purnell, 1998a).

Understanding clients' beliefs related to their desire and willingness to take medications can improve the health care provider's cultural competence in designing strategies to increase compliance among diverse ethnocultural populations (Levy, 1995). This is especially important when the cultural beliefs of the nurse are different from or in conflict with the cultural beliefs of the client, family, or group.

This chapter provides a brief overview of the cultural characteristics of the following groups: **African-Americans, American Indians, Amish, Asian/Pacific Islanders, Hispanics, Jewish-Americans,** and **European-Americans.**

THE PURNELL MODEL FOR CULTURAL COMPETENCE

This chapter uses selected domains and concepts from the Purnell Model for Cultural Competence to provide essential information in the context of ethnic, racial, and cultural responses to medication administration and compliance. The Purnell Model for Cultural Competence (Fig. 6–1) is a circle, with an outlying rim representing global society, a second rim representing community, a third rim representing family, and an inner rim representing the person; these are the macro aspects of the model.

The interior of the circle is divided into 12 pie-shaped wedges depicting cultural domains and their concepts. The domains have bidirectional arrows indicating that each domain relates to and is affected by all other domains; these are the micro aspects of the model.

The center of the model is empty and represents unknown aspects about the cultural group. Along the bottom of the model is an erose (jagged) line representing the nonlinear concept of cultural competence. This nonlinear line represents the degree of cultural competence attained by the health care provider or organization. Culturally competent nursing care requires that providers understand their culture and the client's culture and negotiate and integrate folk systems with allopathic care.

THE DOMAINS OF CULTURE

Overview/Heritage

Overview/heritage includes concepts related to origins, topography, economics, and education. Racial origin affects responses to some drugs; for example, Asian-Americans have increased sensitivity to beta-blockers, whereas African-Americans respond better to monotherapy for hypertension than do their European-American cohort groups (Levy, 1993). Topography, the landscape and surface configuration of terrain, may affect clients physiologically. For example, clients coming from high-altitude mountainous climates normally have increased red blood cell counts because of the lowered oxygen tension in the high-altitude climate. Clients coming from low-lying, swampy terrain are at an increased risk for dengue fever, malaria, and sickle cell anemia. The client's socioeconomic status has an impact on his or her ability to afford expensive prescription drugs. In some cases, the nurse can recommend a generic equivalent or other acceptable drug that is more affordable. The educational status of clients may determine how the nurse provides information to the client. For clients who are unable to read or do not have English language skills, the nurse may need to devise pictures to teach medication schedules. Directions should be provided to clients in their preferred language and at a level they can understand.

Communication

Communication includes concepts related to language, dialect, contextual use of the language, volume, and tone. Spatial distancing, touch, use of eye contact, preferred greetings, temporality, time, and format for names are also key concepts to understand for the nurse who wishes to be effective with assessing and counseling clients.

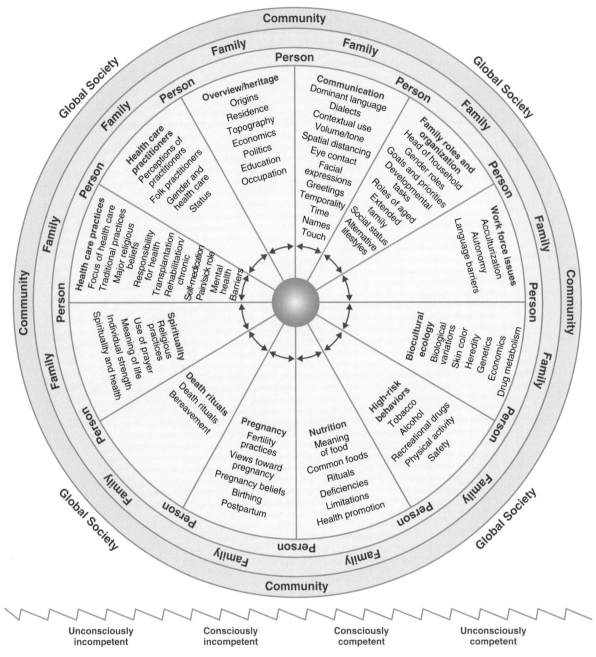

Figure 6–1
The Purnell Model for Cultural Competence. (Courtesy of Larry Purnell, Newark, DE.)

LANGUAGE

Given that 34.3% of the U.S. population prefers speaking a language other than English at home (Brunner, 1998), there are increased challenges for nurses to teach clients about their medication schedules and the side effects of medications. Because dialects may differ significantly, the nurse should attempt to identify a dialect-specific interpreter. Because clients may be able to read English but not speak or understand it, detailed written instructions are helpful.

The nurse needs to be aware of the contextual use of languages to better understand and communicate with culturally diverse clients. English and the Romance languages—Italian, Spanish, French, Portuguese, and Romanian—are low contexted languages with the majority of the message in the explicit verbal mode. In low contextual languages, many words are used to express a thought, and verbal skills are considered important. People may be uncomfortable with silence. However, in highly contexted languages such as Native American dialects, Chinese, and Vietnamese, the majority of the message is in the nonverbal mode. Few words are used to convey thoughts. Silence is considered important. In highly contexted languages, to interrupt someone or give a hasty response may be considered rude.

Not all languages have the numerous verb tenses that the English language has. For example, Finnish and Chinese only have the present tense; one must interpret the statement within its context. For example, the person may say "I go to store today, I go to store tomorrow, or I go to store yesterday." The nurse must give very precise instructions, such as "take one pill at bedtime." Because there is no future tense, the nurse should not say "you will/should take one pill at bedtime." Because the English language is the only language that uses contractions such as "don't" or "can't," the nurse must say "do not" or "can not" to prevent confusion and improve understanding among culturally diverse clients.

PARALANGUAGE

Some cultural groups such as African-Americans, European-Americans, and Arabs speak in a voice volume that may carry to those nearby. Asians and Native Americans usually speak in a lower volume voice. Because clients speak in a loud voice volume does not mean that they are angry, nor does speaking in a soft voice tone indicate that the person is reticent or not interested in the discussion. Likewise, the use of eye contact may vary among cultural groups and individuals. In general, European-Americans maintain eye contact without staring when conversing, which signals that the person is listening. Arabs and Greeks usually maintain intense eye contact in conversations, which should not be taken as aggression. Because many Asians and Pacific Islanders do not maintain eye contact with people in a perceived higher social status, this does not mean that they are not interested or listening to the conversation. They are demonstrating respect for the person's status.

Spatial distancing, the physical proximity between conversants, varies between and among cultural groups. Most European-Americans maintain approximately 18 to 24 inches when engaged in conversation with the health care provider. However, traditional Germans may see this as a violation of personal space, preferring to stand at a distance greater than 2 feet (Steckler, 1998). Traditional Arabs and some Hispanics may stand very close to each other with less than 18 inches between them. Even though the nurse may be uncomfortable with this close personal space, he or she should not take offense, but should accept it as a cultural variation.

TEMPORALITY

Temporality, whether the client stresses a past, present, or future orientation, needs to be considered when the nurse is caring for clients from diverse cultures. For example, many Portuguese, Haitians, and Hispanics are primarily present oriented; whatever is occurring at the moment is more important than what may occur later. With present-oriented clients, the nurse may need to take extra time and stress the importance of taking the medication. Future-oriented individuals are more likely to comply with prescription regimens.

Client orientation to clock time may also affect how the nurse perceives them. Mexican-Americans (Purnell, 1998b) and Brazilians (Coler, 1998) have a more relaxed perception of time than do European-Americans and the dominant U.S. health care system. For Mexican-Americans and Native Americans (Still & Hodgins, 1998), appointments are flexible, adherence to medication schedules is more fluid, and clients expect to be seen regardless of how late they arrive. If the provider does not see them, it may be interpreted as a noncaring behavior. However, in the dominant European-American health care system, a client with an appointment for 10:00 AM is expected to arrive before that time to ensure that he or she is ready for the appointment. For a client with a present-orientation that stresses flexibility, the nurse may need to adjust medication schedules to be congruent with the client's lifestyle.

GREETINGS

Culturally appropriate greetings demonstrate respect and enhance the therapeutic relationship between the nurse and client. The more informal style practiced by many Americans may not be acceptable with all cultural groups. Many traditional Asians, Hispanics, and Germans prefer to be addressed formally, using Mr., Mrs., Miss, or their title. To address them informally may be perceived as insolence or disrespectful behavior. Therefore, the nurse should always greet the client formally until told otherwise.

The format for names may cause confusion for nurses unfamiliar with diverse cultures. Among Hispanics, extended family names are common and may include a woman's married name and the last names of both parents. For example, Rosa Nunez y Arosemina would indicate a single woman whose father's last name is Nunez and whose mother's maiden name is Arosemina. If Rosa marries Jorge Sanchez, her complete name becomes Senora (depicting a married woman) Rosa Sanchez de Nunez y Arosemina. She would be called Mrs. Sanchez in a formal setting, and Rosa by her family and close friends. The traditional Korean woman does not take her husband's last name when she marries. However, because many Koreans know this causes confusion for health care providers in the United States, many are beginning to take their husband's name (Sabet, 1998). Thus, the nurse needs to specifically ask the client his or her family name and given name.

Family Organization

Family organization with the concepts of head of household and gender roles must be considered when the nurse is assessing and intervening with clients. The nurse must recognize that not all individuals adhere to the U.S. value of egalitarian decision making between men and women. Among traditional Central American Indian groups, men are expected to provide for their families in terms of outside resources and protect them from harm. When a family travels from their village, the procession looks something like this: The husband (or other adult male) leads the way, followed by the children who are old enough to walk. An older child may carry a smaller child. Bringing up the rear is the wife, who may be pregnant or breastfeeding an infant. In this order, the man is in a better position to protect the family from harm.

Women take care of the home and provide the majority of child care. Men work at a distance from the house or sometimes in another village, mixing more with the outside world. Therefore, they have a greater sphere of knowledge from which to make decisions. In cultures in which men are expected to make most decisions, the nurse is expected to direct questions to the man, even though the woman may provide the answers with the man being the spokesperson. When traditional women must work outside the home, family dynamics change. Men feel guilt for not being able to provide for their families, and women feel they are abandoning their children because they are working.

Biocultural Ecology

Biocultural ecology includes concepts related to biologic variations, heredity, genetics, endemics, and drug metabolism. To assess for oxygenation and cyanosis in dark-skinned people, the nurse must examine the sclera, conjunctiva, buccal mucosa, tongue, lips, nailbeds, palms, and soles of the feet rather than relying on skin tone. Jaundice can be determined in dark-skinned people by examining the sclera for a yellow pigmentation.

Genetic background can affect a client's response to drugs. For example, African-Americans have high rates of hypertension and respond better to monotherapy because their hypertension is usually related to volume expansion, decreased renin, and increased intracellular concentration of sodium and calcium (Levy, 1993). For Greeks and Greek-Americans with glucose-6-phosphate dehydrogenase deficiency, life-threatening hemolytic crises may occur if oxidating drugs such as quinine and chloramphenicol are prescribed (Tripp-Reimer & Sorofman, 1998). Many Asians and Pacific Islanders experience increased side effects of alcohol with facial flushing, tachycardia, and palpitations.

High-Risk Behaviors

The domain high-risk behaviors includes the use of tobacco, alcohol, and recreational drugs. Tobacco use causes more rapid elimination of medicines from the body; thus, the drug does not have its full therapeutic effect. Alcohol interferes with some psychotropic medications and enhances the effects of analgesics. Recreational use of drugs such as marijuana, antihistamine combinations, and cocaine may potentiate the effects of medications, resulting in increased side effects, an enhanced therapeutic response, or an overdose.

Nutrition

The domain nutrition includes concepts related to common foods and food rituals, limitations in obtaining nutritious foods, enzyme deficiencies, and how foods are used for health promotion and wellness. Each ethnocultural group has preferred foods and rituals that are passed on through the generations. Traditional Appalachian people frequently use extra lard to prepare fried foods. The diets of many Asian and Pacific Islanders are high in sodium. Some African-Americans use fatback to add extra flavor to vegetables. The proportion of fats, carbohydrates, and proteins may have an effect on how some drugs are absorbed or metabolized. Dietary consideration must be taken into account when prescriptions are given. Newer immigrants may have difficulty finding preferred native foods and not be aware of which foods to substitute to provide a nutritious diet. Asians, Pacific Islanders, Hispanics, and African-Americans have high incidences of lactose intolerance, resulting in maldigestion and bloating, although the condition is rare among children.

All societies have "prescriptions" for what is considered a healthy diet, although these prescriptions have great variability within each ethnocultural group. Among conservative Jews, milk and meat should not be eaten at the same meal. Among Haitians (Paperwalla & Colin, 1998), some Hispanics (Purnell, 1998b; Purnell, 1998e), Vietnamese (Nowak, 1998), Greeks (Tripp-Reimer & Sorofman, 1998), and Iranians (Lipson & Haifizi, 1998), foods are classified as "hot" or "cold" and a balance of these foods must be consumed at each meal or illness may result. Drugs are also classified as hot or cold. Antibiotics are considered hot and therefore should not be taken with cold water because their effect would be negated; use room temperature or tap water instead. Because hot and cold foods and conditions vary within each group, the nurse must specifically ask clients their food preferences and determine whether the diet interferes with drug absorption or interactions.

Spirituality

Spirituality includes concepts related to religious preference, meaning of life, and individual sources of strength. Clients' religious practices may prescribe what is acceptable in terms of diet (Islamic and orthodox Jewish), acceptability for genetic counseling, and use and choice of contraceptive methods. Muslims who celebrate the holiday Ramadan fast from sunup to sundown. Fasting also includes not taking medications. However, in times of illness, clients are permitted to take their prescribed medications, although the more devout may be reluctant to do so. The nurse can improve medication compliance by working with the client to determine an acceptable medication schedule during the holiday. Because clients do not eat on a normal daytime schedule, insulin administration must be adjusted accordingly.

MEANING OF LIFE

Among Mexican-Americans and Panamanian-Americans, family is usually the most important thing in their lives and gives meaning to life (Purnell, 1998). Thus, it can be especially important to include the family in teaching strategies. Illness is a family affair and should be treated accordingly.

Health Care Practices

Health care practices include the focus of health care, traditional medical practices, self-medication practices, barriers to accessing health care, the sick role, and perceptions of mental illness. The current focus of health care in the United States is undergoing a paradigm shift from acute care to one of wellness with health promotion and maintenance and disease and illness prevention. Whereas this concept is congruent with many ethnocultural groups, for some, prevention activities are unknown. For example, unacculturated Egyptian-Americans may refuse to have pap smears and mammograms because in Egypt these preventive measures are just beginning to be recognized and promoted (Meleis & Meleis, 1998).

COMPLEMENTARY, ALTERNATIVE, AND TRADITIONAL MEDICINE

Many people prefer their traditional medical practices either as complementary to or as an alternative to allopathic medicine (Fig. 6–2). Traditional Chinese medicine, Ayurvedic medicine, herbal and naturopathic medicine, and a host of other therapies may be preferred by some or used in conjunction with other

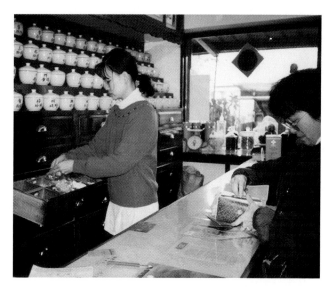

Figure 6–2
In some cultures, people may rely on traditional, nonprescription remedies.

therapies. Many ethnic people, accustomed to taking medications for only 2 or 3 days in their home countries, may believe that Western medicine is too strong, is supposed to only relieve symptoms, or has too many side effects. Thus, they may stop taking the medication when symptoms disappear.

SELF-MEDICATING PRACTICES

All clients self-medicate to some degree. Many use over-the-counter medications or folk remedies for the initial symptoms of an illness. Additionally, some ethnic groups may have family or friends bring medication that may not be available in the United States from their home country. For example, in Panama and throughout Central America, clients can purchase a wide variety of antibiotics, injectable vitamins, and even intravenous fluids without a prescription. To prevent contraindications in medication administration, the nurse must ask clients in a nonjudgmental manner whether they are taking any prescription medications, nonprescription medications, or herbal therapies (Fig. 6–3).

SICK ROLE

In some Hispanic and Arabic cultures, clients can enter the sick role without feelings of guilt or attached stigma. Any reason is acceptable for being ill and the person is relieved of normal responsibilities (Abu-Gharbieh, 1998; Purnell, 1998). However, among Germans and Polish people, clients may be expected to carry out their obligations unless they are severely ill (From, 1998; Steckler, 1998). This is one area in which the nurse can hasten the client's recovery with culturally appropriate counseling.

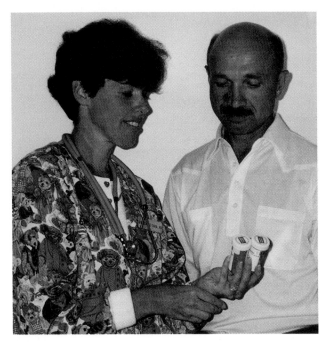

Figure 6–3
The nurse needs to ask the client about all medications and remedies he or she is taking, to be able to identify potential interactions with the prescribed medication regimen.

PAIN

Pain—the primary reason most people see a health professional—is expressed differently among ethnocultural groups. For example, among some Asians and Pacific Islanders, clients are reluctant to express pain because they believe it is God's will or a punishment for past sins (Miranda, Spangler, & McBride, 1998; Nowak, 1998; Sharts-Hopko, 1998). Among Arabs, clients are expected to openly express their pain and expect immediate relief, preferably through injectable or intravenous medication (Meleis & Meleis, 1998).

MENTAL ILLNESS

Mental illness is a culture-bound phenomenon. What is perceived as a mental illness in one culture may be seen as normal in another; for example, having visions and hallucinations about God is an expected behavior among some Hispanic groups (Dossey, 1998). Even though the "evil eye" occurs in numerous

cultures, someone from a culture who does not believe in the evil eye may see those who do believe in it as having a mental health problem. Thus, nurses must interpret a client's behavior within cultural boundaries.

Health Care Practitioners

The domain health care practitioners includes concepts related to the status of health care providers, folk practitioners, and gender and health care. For Arabs and Arab-Americans, the most respected health care provider is an experienced middle-aged to elderly male physician with several degrees (Lipson & Haifizi, 1998). Among Appalachian people, foreign-educated physicians may have difficulty being accepted because they are outsiders, not because of their ethnocultural background (Purnell & Counts, 1998). In many Arab countries, nursing is not seen as a desirable profession because it requires contact between the sexes (AbuGharbieh, 1998).

FOLK PRACTITIONERS

Many times, folk practitioners are preferred over allopathic educated physicians because treatments are less invasive. Folk practitioners are known to the client. Usually, they do not treat the symptoms of an illness; they remove the cause of the illness. Allopathic physicians can only treat the symptoms.

GENDER AND HEALTH CARE

Islamic women prefer health care providers of the same gender and may refuse treatment from male health care providers. However, the nurse should remind them that the *Koran* sanctions the use of male health care providers if female providers are not available. If only a male is available, physical examination should be performed through the clothes. Most European-American and African-American males and females generally accept care from either gender. More traditional and younger clients may prefer a same gender provider for intimate care. This should be accommodated whenever possible. Table 6–1 lists characteristics of selected domains for the major cultural groups in the United States.

Table 6–1
Health Care Practices and Compliance in Various Cultural Groups

CULTURAL GROUP	HEALTH CARE PRACTICES	NUTRITION	PROMOTING STRATEGIES FOR COMPLIANCE
African-Americans	Many delay seeking health care because of financial limitations and distrust in the formal medical establishment because of past inequities. Health care may be sought from family members and older community female leaders before professional health care providers.	Food, a symbol of health and wealth, is used to celebrate special events. Obesity usually is seen as positive. Food is also important for building blood. Diets are high in fat and low in fiber, fruits, and vegetables.	Develop a sound, trusting relationship. Identify conflicts in values and beliefs. Listen attentively. Respect cultural beliefs and values. The strengths of the family ties, church, and community organization are important resources for promoting adherence to medication regimens. Grandmothers have a significant voice in health care concerns.
Native Americans	Spirituality is central in their health care practice. Maintaining harmony with one's environment is stressed. Health promotion and maintenance may be difficult based on past acute care survival practices.	Food has a major significance in celebrations with numerous food rituals. Corn is an important staple and is used in ceremonial dances and healing practices. Generally, food is not associated with health promotion or illness. High-fat diet predominates and a lack of fruits and vegetables exists on many reservations.	Increase access to health care. Community involvement and culturally sensitive client education are important. Do not ask questions in public. If wrong answer is given, embarrassment may occur. Involve traditional healers and community leaders, including Native American church, in health promotion programs.
Amish	Very health conscious. Obtain medical care from physicians they know in nearby villages. Traditional home remedies are commonly used. Obligation is to care for oneself first before seeing a health care provider. Most do not participate in immunization practices. Do not like a lot of pills and strong medicine. Health foods are increasing among denominations.	Food has a major nutritional and social significance. Meals are large, high in fat, carbohydrates, and calories. High incidence of obesity.	Develop a trusting relationship. Use culturally consistent communication practices. Respect their cultural beliefs and practices. Allow time to make decisions. Must involve the family in all decisions. Incorporate traditional medicines with Western practices. Expect that a telephone call from the Amish for a health-related problem is a true emergency.
Asian/Pacific Islanders Chinese, Filipino, Japanese, Korean, Vietnamese, and other Indochinese.	Younger generations generally practice Western medicine. The elderly try traditional methods before seeking Western medicine. Self-medication and self-diagnosis are common. Traditional therapies include the following: acupuncture, acupressure, acumassage, moxibustion therapy, coining, and Chinese herbal therapies.	Food habits are important with balancing yin and yang qualities of foods. Many rituals revolve around food. Foods at meals have a specific order. Many diets are high in sodium.	Include family members in the plan of care. Encourage client to continue treatment after the initial response; many tend to stop treatment after the initial response. Address cultural issues directly. Incorporate traditional practices into Western practices. Include physical components of mental health illnesses and concerns to improve compliance. Ask the individual what he or she thinks caused the illness/problem. Address the individual formally until requested otherwise. Confidentiality is extremely important.

Table continued on following page

Table 6–1 Continued
Health Care Practices and Compliance in Various Cultural Groups

CULTURAL GROUP	HEALTH CARE PRACTICES	NUTRITION	PROMOTING STRATEGIES FOR COMPLIANCE
Hispanics Mexican-Americans, Cuban-Americans, Puerto Ricans, Latin Americans, Spanish-Americans	Strong valuing of the extended family. Use of home remedies, consultations with folk healers, herbalists, and masseuses influence their use of Western medicine. Fatalistic in their thinking; a higher power influences illness and health.	Many food rituals, depending on one's origin. Diet varies by country and region within the country. Hot and cold theory of balancing foods is common with most groups.	Identify conflicts in values and beliefs. Address cultural issues directly. Accommodate family values. Have instructions available in the language the client speaks or reads most easily. Demonstrate respect by addressing client formally until told otherwise. Incorporate folk and traditional practices with Western medicine. Ask about family matters first if condition is not life-threatening. Stress individual health care provider rather than the organization.
Jewish-Americans	Jewish-Americans are health conscious and practice preventive medicine. A well-immunized population. No folk healers in this group, but there are several home remedies, chicken soup being the most known.	Meals are used to satisfy hunger and teach discipline, and are the center of many religious celebrations. Food rituals are common and the laws of kashrut dictate which foods are permissible. Among the religious, all meat must be Kosher, which requires a ritual slaughtering of animals wherein the animal is killed as quickly as possible and all blood is drained from the animal as quickly as possible. Avoid pork and shellfish. Religious do not mix dairy and meat at the same meal.	Health promotion and disease prevention are important. Practitioners are held in high regard.
European-Americans and white ethnic groups	Most minimize or ignore symptoms until they interfere with work and activities of daily living. Sick role is not entered into easily. Use of traditional medicine varies but is common. Many are stoic with pain but there are broad variations, although Italians are more expressive than most other white ethnic groups. Expect health care providers to give explanations for all treatments and procedures.	British and French influence on US diet: high cholesterol and fat, low in fiber and complex carbohydrates. Descendants of southern Europeans have higher incidence of lactose intolerance.	Develop a sound, trusting relationship. Value the strengths of family ties and religious groups. Provide explanations for all prescriptions, treatments, and procedures.

NURSING PROCESS
TRANSCULTURAL CONSIDERATIONS

Assessment

- Assess ethnocultural and racial background.
- Assess length of time away from country of origin.
- Assess travel history, both within the country and outside the country.
- Assess language ability and preferred language for instruction.
- Assess nonverbal communication practices such as spatial distancing, temporality, and use of touch and eye contact.
- Assess high-risk health behaviors.
- Assess preferred foods, preparation practices, and eating patterns.
- Assess for illness and disease patterns commonly found in the client's family and cultural group.
- Assess use of traditional and folk practices.
- Assess use of traditional health care practitioners.

Planning

- Collaborate with client to reduce high-risk health behaviors.
- Develop a culturally congruent dietary plan that helps the client understand his or her dietary practices in relation to drug interactions.

Interventions

- Incorporate nonharmful traditional and folk practices with biomedical prescriptions.
- Collaborate with traditional and folk practitioners.
- Maintain culturally congruent communication practices to develop a trusting relationship with the client and family.
- Conduct a nutritional assessment to determine potential for drug-food interactions.
- Incorporate cultural beliefs and practices into the plan of care.

Client Teaching

- Involve family in teaching about prescriptive therapies.
- Provide explanation for all prescriptions, treatments, and procedures.
- Provide written instruction in the client's preferred language.

Evaluation

- Client correctly demonstrates understanding of prescriptive therapies and treatments.
- Client is compliant with prescriptive therapies of biomedical health care practitioners.
- Family members are involved in client's overall health plan.
- Client eliminates or decreases high-risk health behaviors.
- Client selects food choices congruent with prescriptive therapies.

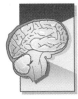

Critical Thinking in Action

Ana Maria de Navarro, age 63 years, picks vegetables along with several of her male relatives on a large farm. She has been recently diagnosed with hypertension and is 45 pounds overweight. She speaks minimal English, eats a traditional Mexican diet, and is the primary cook for the family. She is taking furosemide, 40 mg daily. Twice within the last month, she fainted while picking vegetables. Each time, her family took her to a shaded area where she regained consciousness within a few minutes. She admits to feeling dizzy when she awakes each morning but is glad that she no longer has headaches since she started taking her medicine. Her skin is dry and has decreased turgor. You are the public health nurse responsible for the employees in the migrant worker camp. You want her to keep a diary of her blood pressure and pulse four times a day for the next week. You speak minimal Spanish.

1. What type of medicine is furosemide?
2. Is the dose within therapeutic range?
3. Why is Ana Maria having dizziness?
4. Why did Ana Maria faint two times in the last month?
5. How might you teach her family to take and record Ana Maria's blood pressure and pulse?
6. At what times each day will you recommend her vital signs to be taken?
7. How will you communicate this with her and with her family?
8. What recommendation do you have for Ana Maria to combat her morning dizziness?
9. What recommendations do you have for her medication regimen?
10. If Ana Maria wanted to see a traditional healer, which one(s) might you recommend?
11. What culturally congruent goals might you collaborate on with Ana Maria?
12. What evaluation measures would you include in terms of nutrition and hydration?

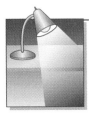

Study Questions

1. How does racial origin affect metabolism of pharmacologic agents?
2. How does the topography physiologically affect clients and what effect does it have on drug dosages?
3. What is meant by the contextual use of languages? Give an example of a highly contexted language. Give an example of a low contexted language.
4. Describe differences and similarities in nonverbal communications among Hispanics, American Indians, and European-Americans.
5. Identify strategies for improving medication compliance with each of the following ethnocultural groups: African-American, Native American, Amish, Asian/Pacific Islander, Hispanic, Jewish-American, and European-American.
6. Describe the format for names for Hispanics.
7. Why do most African-Americans respond better to monotherapy than do European-Americans?
8. List several reasons why most Asian/Pacific Islanders respond differently to pharmacologic agents than European-Americans and African-Americans.

9. What may occur if a client with glucose-6-dehydrogenase deficiency is prescribed an oxidating agent?

10. Explain what is meant by the "hot and cold" theory that is commonly practiced by Asian-Americans, Hispanic-Americans, and Greek-Americans.

11. How might you alter insulin administration for a client who celebrates Ramadan?

12. List three reasons some clients prefer traditional or folk practitioners instead of allopathic practitioners.

13. Discuss strategies for getting stoic individuals to accept medication for pain.

14. With what clients may therapeutic touch not be acceptable?

7

Drug Interaction, Over-the-Counter Drugs, and Drug Abuse

Outline

Objectives

* Define the term *drug interaction*.
* Explain the four pharmacokinetic processes related to drug interaction.
* Explain the three effects associated with pharmacodynamic interactions.
* Explain the effects of drug–food interactions.
* Explain the meaning of drug-induced photosensitiviy.
* Define the terms *drug abuse, drug misuse, addiction, physical dependence,* and *psychological dependence.*
* Identify the drugs associated with drug abuse.

Terms

addiction
additive effect
adverse drug reaction
antagonistic effect
drug abuse

drug incompatibility
drug interaction
habituation
over-the-counter drugs
photosensitivity

psychological dependence
synergistic effect
withdrawal

INTRODUCTION

Drug therapy has become complex because of the number of drugs. Drug–drug, drug–food, and drug–laboratory interactions have also become an increasing problem. Because of the possibility of numerous interactions, the nurse should be knowledgeable about drug interactions and should closely monitor client responses. Communication among members of the health team is essential.

DRUG INTERACTION

A **drug interaction** can be defined as an altered or modified action or effect of a drug as a result of interaction with one or more other drugs. It should not be confused with adverse drug reaction or drug incompatibility. An **adverse drug reaction** is an undesirable drug effect ranging from mild untoward effects to severe toxic effects, including hypersensitivity reaction and anaphylaxis. **Drug incompatibility** is a chemical or physical reaction that occurs among two or more drugs in vitro (outside the body).

Drug interactions can be divided into two categories: (1) pharmacokinetic interactions and (2) pharmacodynamic interactions. These two categories of drug interaction are discussed individually.

Pharmacokinetic Interaction

The pharmacokinetic interaction is a change that occurs in the absorption, distribution, metabolism or biotransformation, or excretion of one or both drugs.

ABSORPTION

When a person takes two drugs at the same time, the rate of absorption of one or both drugs can change. One drug can block, decrease, or increase the absorption rate of another drug. It can do this in one of three ways:

• By decreasing or increasing gastric emptying time
• By changing the gastric pH
• By forming drug complexes

Drugs that increase the speed of gastric emptying, such as laxatives, increase gastric and intestinal motility and cause a decrease in drug absorption. Most drugs are absorbed primarily in the small intestines; exceptions include barbiturates, salicylates, and theophylline. Narcotics and anticholinergic drugs (atropine-like drugs) decrease gastric emptying time and decrease gastrointestinal (GI) motility, thus causing an increase in absorption rate. The longer the drug remains in the stomach or intestine, the greater the amount of drug absorption (only for those drugs absorbed in the stomach).

When the gastric pH is decreased, a weak acid drug, such as aspirin, is less ionized and is more rapidly absorbed. Drugs that increase the pH of gastric juices decrease absorption of weak acid drugs. Antacids, such as Maalox and Amphojel, raise the gastric pH and block or slow absorption. Some drugs may react chemically. For example, tetracycline and the heavy-metal ions (calcium, magnesium, aluminum, iron) found in antacids form a complex, and the tetracycline is not absorbed. Tetracycline also can form complexes with dairy products. Milk products and antacids should be avoided for 1 h before and 2 h after consuming tetracycline.

Other drugs that can cause complexes with drugs besides antacids are kaolin-pectin, certain hypocholesterol drugs such as cholestyramine and colestipol, and activated charcoal. Because of the formed complexes, the drugs are less soluble, which results in less drug absorption.

Certain broad-spectrum antibacterials (antibiotics) such as erythromycin affect the GI flora, thereby causing an increase in absorption of digoxin, which depends on the flora in the intestine to metabolize digoxin.

DISTRIBUTION

Drug distribution to tissues can be affected by its binding to plasma/serum protein. Only drugs unbound to protein are free, active agents and can enter body tissues. Two drugs that are highly protein-bound and administered simultaneously can result in drug displacements. Factors that influence displacement of drugs are (1) the drug concentration in the blood, (2) protein-binding power of the drugs, and (3) volume of distribution (V_d).

Two drugs that are highly bound to protein or albumin compete for protein or albumin sites in the plasma. The result is a decrease in protein binding of one or both drugs; therefore, more free drug circulates in the plasma and is available for drug action. This effect can lead to drug toxicity. Drugs that are unbound to protein are free, active drugs and can cause a pharmacologic response. When two highly protein-bound drugs need to be taken concurrently, drug dosage of one or both drugs may need to be decreased to avoid drug toxicity.

Examples of drugs that are highly protein-bound include warfarin (anticoagulant); certain anticonvulsants, such as phenytoin and valproic acid; clofibrate; most nonsteroidal antiinflammatory drugs (NSAIDs); sulfonamides; tolbutamide; and quinidine. Warfarin is 99% protein-bound, thus allowing only 1% to be free drug. If 2% to 3% of warfarin is displaced in the albumin, the amount of free warfarin would be 3% to 4% instead of 1%. This increases the anticoagulant effect, and thus excess bleeding may result.

METABOLISM OR BIOTRANSFORMATION

Many drug interactions of metabolism occur with the induction (stimulation) or inhibition of the hepatic microsomal system. A drug can increase the metabolism of another drug by stimulating (inducing) liver enzymes. Drugs that promote induction of enzymes are called enzyme inducers. An example of an enzyme inducer is the barbiturates (e.g., phenobarbital). Phenobarbital increases the metabolism of beta blockers (propranolol [Inderal]), most antipsychotics, and theophylline. Increased metabolism promotes drug elimination and decreases plasma concentration of the drug. The result is a decrease in drug action. Sometimes, liver enzymes convert drugs to active or passive metabolites. The drug metabolites may be excreted or may produce an active pharmacologic response. Also, there are some drugs that are enzyme inhibitors.

The anticonvulsant drugs phenytoin and carbamazepine, alcohol, and rifampin are hepatic enzyme inducers that can increase drug metabolism, for example, for the anticoagulant drug warfarin. A larger dose of warfarin is usually needed while the client is taking a hepatic inducer. The metabolism aids in decreasing the amount of drug. If the drug inducer is withdrawn, warfarin dosages need to be decreased because less drug is being eliminated by hepatic metabolism. Usually, interaction occurs after 1 week of drug therapy and can continue for 1 week after the drug inducer is discontinued. Drugs with narrow therapeutic ranges should be closely monitored.

Cigarette smoking increases hepatic enzyme activity and can increase theophylline clearance. For smokers who are taking theophylline, the theophylline dose should be increased. With chronic alcohol use, hepatic enzyme activities are increased, whereas with acute alcohol use, metabolism is inhibited.

The antiulcer drug cimetidine is an enzyme inhibitor that decreases the metabolism of certain drugs, such as theophylline (antiasthmatic). As the result of decreasing theophylline metabolism, there is an increase in the plasma concentration of theophylline. The theophylline dose needs to be decreased to avoid toxicity. If cimetidine or any enzyme drug inhibitor is discontinued, the theophylline dosage should be adjusted. Certain drugs alter hepatic blood flow, causing a decrease in liver metabolism. Table 7–1 describes the effects of drug enzyme inducers and inhibitors.

EXCRETION

Most drugs are excreted in the urine and are filtered through the glomeruli. With some drugs, the excretion occurs in the bile, which passes into the intestinal tract. Drugs can increase or decrease renal excretion and have an effect on the excretion of other drugs. Drugs that decrease cardiac output, decrease blood flow to the kidneys, and decrease glomerular filtration can also decrease or delay drug excretion. The antidysrhythmic drug quinidine decreases the excretion of digoxin (a digitalis preparation); therefore, the plasma concentration of digoxin is increased and digitalis toxicity can occur. Furosemide (Lasix) decreases the glomerular filtration rate (GFR), which reduces clearance of drugs such as digoxin. A decrease in digoxin excretion could lead to an increase in serum digoxin levels. With a decrease in serum potassium level and a decrease in digoxin excretion, digoxin toxicity could occur (see Drug–Laboratory Interactions).

Probenecid (Benemid), a drug for gout, decreases penicillin excretion by competing for tubular reabsorption of penicillin in the kidneys. In some cases, this may be desirable to increase or maintain the plasma concentration of penicillin, which has a short half-life, for a longer time.

Changing urine pH affects drug excretion. The antacid sodium bicarbonate causes the urine to be alkaline. Alkaline urine promotes the excretion of drugs

Table 7–1
Drugs: Enzyme Inducer or Enzyme Inhibitor

DRUG CATEGORY	DRUG EFFECT
Drug enzyme inducer	Onset and termination of drug effect is slow, approximately 1 wk. Drug dosage may need to be increased with use of drug inducer. Drug dosage should be adjusted after termination of drug inducer. Monitor serum drug levels, especially if the drug has a narrow therapeutic drug range.
Drug enzyme inhibitor	Onset of drug effect usually occurs rapidly. Half-life (t½) of the second drug may be increased, causing a prolonged drug effect. Interaction may occur related to the dosage prescribed. Disease entities affect drug dosing. Monitor serum drug levels, especially if the drug has a narrow therapeutic range.

that are weak acids, such as aspirin and barbiturates. Alkaline urine also promotes reabsorption of weak base drugs. Acid urine promotes the excretion of drugs that are weak bases, such as quinidine.

With clients who have decreased renal or hepatic function, there is usually an increase in free drug concentration. It is essential to closely monitor such a client for drug toxicity when he or she is taking multiple drugs. Checking serum drug levels (therapeutic drug monitoring [TDM]) is especially important for drugs that have a narrow therapeutic range and are highly protein-bound, such as digoxin and phenytoin. Table 7–2 summarizes the drug interactions that affect pharmacokinetics.

Pharmacodynamic Interactions

Pharmacodynamic interactions are those that result in additive, synergistic (potentiation), or antagonistic drug effects. When two drugs are given that may or may not have similar actions, the combined effect may be additive (twice the effect), synergistic (greater than twice the effect), or antagonistic (the effect of either or both drugs is decreased).

ADDITIVE DRUG EFFECT

When two drugs with similar action are administered, the drug interaction is called an **additive effect** and is the sum of the effects of the two drugs. Addi-

Table 7–2
Pharmacokinetic Interactions of Drugs

PROCESS	DRUG	EFFECT
Absorption	Laxatives	Speeds gastric emptying time
		Increases gastric motility
		Decreases drug absorption
	Narcotics	Slows gastric emptying time
	Anticholinergics	Decreases gastric motility
		Increases drug absorption or decreases absorption depending on where the drug is delayed (gastric vs. intestinal)
	Aspirin	Decreases gastric pH
		Increases drug absorption
	Antacids	Increases gastric pH
		Slows absorption of acid drugs
	Antacids and tetracycline	Forms drug complexes
		Blocks drug absorption
Distribution	Anticoagulant and antiinflammatory (sulindac)	Competes for protein-binding sites
		Increases free drug; e.g., increases anticoagulant
Metabolism or biotransformation	Barbiturates	Promotes induction of liver enzymes
		Increases drug metabolism
		Decreases drug plasma concentration of the second drug
	Antiulcer (cimetidine)	Inhibits liver enzymes release
		Decreases drug metabolism of diazepam (Valium), phenytoin (Dilantin), morphine, etc.
		Increases drug plasma concentration of the second drug
Excretion	Antidysrhythmic (quinidine)	Decreases renal excretion of second drug; e.g., digoxin
		Increases digoxin concentration
	Antigout (probenecid)	Decreases excretion of penicillin by competing for tubular reabsorption
		Increases penicillin concentration
	Antacid (sodium bicarbonate)	Promotes excretion of weak acid drug; e.g., aspirin, barbiturates, sulfonamides
	Aspirin, ammonium chloride	Promotes excretion of weak base drugs; e.g., quinidine, theophylline
Other: Decrease cardiac output and renal blood flow	Most drug categories	Decreases drug excretion
		Increases drug plasma concentration

tive effects can be desirable or undesirable. For example, a desirable additive drug effect occurs when a diuretic and a beta blocker are given for hypertension: used in combination, these drugs lower the blood pressure and act as antihypertensive drugs. As another example, two analgesics, aspirin and codeine, can be given together for increased pain relief.

An example of an undesirable additive effect is that from two vasodilators: hydralazine (Apresoline) given for hypertension and nitroglycerin prescribed for angina. The result could be a severe hypotensive response. Another example is the interaction of aspirin and alcohol taken together, from which gastric bleeding can result. Both aspirin and alcohol can prolong bleeding time.

SYNERGISTIC DRUG EFFECT OR POTENTIATION

When two or more drugs are given together, one drug can potentiate or have a **synergistic effect** on the other drug, meaning that sometimes the effect is greater than the combined effect of two drugs from the same category. An example is the combination of meperidine (Demerol, a narcotic analgesic) and promethazine (Phenergan, an antihistamine). Phenergan enhances or potentiates the effect of Demerol. Actually, less Demerol is required when it is combined with Phenergan, which can be a desirable effect. An example of an undesirable effect occurs when two drugs, alcohol and a sedative-hypnotic drug such as chlordiazepoxide (Librium) or diazepam (Valium), are

Table 7–3
Drug Interaction with Anticoagulants and Prescription Drugs

PRESCRIPTION DRUGS	ANTICOAGULANT EFFECTS
Selected antilipids	
Fibrate group	Increased effect; may cause increase in bleeding
Statin group	
Lovastatin	Increased effect
Pravastatin	No known effects
Angiotensin-converting enzyme inhibitors	No known effects
Aminoglycoside	No known effects
Aspirin	Strong effects; can cause bleeding
Antineoplastic drugs	
Cytoxan, 5-fluorouracil, methotrexate, doxorubicin, vincristine	Increased effects; can cause bleeding
Cytoxan, mercaptopurine, mitotane	Decreased effects; Cytoxan may cause increased or decreased effects
Barbiturates	Reduced effect of anticoagulants
Benzodiazepine	No known effects
Beta blockers	No known effects
Selected cephalosporins	
Cefamandole	Increased effects; may cause bleeding
Nonsteroidal antiinflammatory drugs (NSAIDs)	
Ibuprofen	Normal doses; no effects
Diclofenac, ketoprofen, tolmetin	May increase effects
Quinolone antibiotics	Usually no effects
Ciprofloxacin, norfloxacin, ofloxacin, perfloxacin	Increased effects in isolated cases
Sulfonamides	
Bactrim-cotrimoxazole	Increased effects in 35% of persons
Tricyclic antidepressants	No known effects
Vitamin K	Decreased effects of anticoagulants
Food	
Aspartame (artifical sweetener)	Increased effects
Green vegetables (spinach, broccoli, Brussels sprouts)	Decreased effects; vegetables are rich in vitamin K
Alcohol	
Mild to moderate drinking	No effects unless heavy drinking
Heavy drinking	Increased effects if liver function is impaired

Table 7–4	
Pharmacodynamic Interactions of Drugs	
INTERACTIONS	EFFECT
Additive	In the same drug category, the drug effect is the sum of both drug effects.
Synergistic or potentiation	One drug potentiates or enhances the effect of the other drug (greater than effect of each alone).
Antagonistic	Two drugs in opposing drug categories cancel drug effects of both drugs.

combined, increasing central nervous system depression.

Some antibacterials (antibiotics) have an enzyme inhibitor added to the drug to potentiate the therapeutic effect of the drug. Examples are ampicillin with sulbactam, and amoxicillin with clavulanate potassium. Ampicillin and amoxicillin can be given without these inhibitors; however, the desired therapeutic effect may not occur because of the bacterial enzyme activity (e.g., beta-lactamase enzyme) causing bacteria resistance. The combination of the antibiotic with an added enzyme inhibitor (sulbactam or clavulanate potassium) inhibits bacterial enzyme activity, thus prolonging the effect of the antibacterial agent.

The use of two prescription drugs can have an additive and/or synergistic effect. An example is an anticoagulant such as warfarin with another drug. The effects of the second drug can increase, decrease, or have no effects on the anticoagulant. Table 7–3 lists the drugs that may be taken with an anticoagulant and the effects that the second drug has on the anticoagulant.

ANTAGONISTIC DRUG EFFECT

When two drugs are combined that have opposite, or **antagonistic effects,** the drugs cancel each other's drug effect. The actions of both drugs are nullified. An example of an antagonistic effect occurs when the adrenergic beta stimulant isoproterenol (Isuprel) and the adrenergic beta blocker propranolol (Inderal) are given together. The action of each drug is cancelled. Neither delivers the expected therapeutic effect.

With morphine overdose, naloxone is given as an antagonist (antidote) to block the narcotic response. This is a beneficial drug interaction of an antagonist. Table 7–4 summarizes the drug responses associated with pharmacodynamic interaction.

DRUG–FOOD INTERACTIONS

Food is known to increase, decrease, or delay drug absorption. Food can bind with drugs, causing less or slower drug absorption. An example of food binding with a drug is the interaction of tetracycline and dairy products. The result is a decrease in the plasma concentration of tetracycline. Because of the binding effect, tetracycline should be taken 1 h before or 2 h after meals and *should not* be taken with dairy products. There are a few drugs in which food increases drug absorption; examples include the antiinfective agent nitrofurantoin (Macrodantin), the beta blocker metoprolol (Lopressor), and the antilipemic lovastatin (Mevacor). These drugs should be taken at mealtime or with food.

The classic drug–food interaction occurs when an antidepressant of the monoamine oxidase (MAO) inhibitor type, e.g., Marplan, is taken with tyramine-rich foods such as cheese, wine, organ meats, beer, yogurt, sour cream, or bananas. More norepinephrine is released and the result could be a hypertensive crisis. These foods must be avoided when taking MAO inhibitors.

DRUG–LABORATORY INTERACTIONS

Abnormal plasma or serum electrolyte concentrations can affect certain drug therapies. If the client is taking digoxin (a digitalis preparation) and there are decreased serum potassium and serum magnesium levels or an increased serum calcium level, digitalis toxicity may result. Certain drugs, such as those from the thiazide diuretic group, can cause abnormal electrolyte concentrations. An example is hydrochlorothiazide (HydroDIURIL), which can decrease serum potassium, magnesium, and sodium levels, and can increase the serum calcium level. Because HydroDIURIL promotes potassium loss, the low serum potassium increases the plasma concentration of digoxin, thereby increasing the action. The result is digitalis toxicity (intoxication). When digoxin and HydroDIURIL are taken together, the nurse should observe the client for digitalis toxicity (nausea, vomiting, bradycardia [pulse less than 60 beats per minute], and stated visual problems).

DRUG-INDUCED PHOTOSENSITIVITY

Photosensitivity is a skin reaction caused by exposure to sunlight. It is caused by the interaction of a drug and exposure to ultraviolet A (UVA) light,

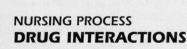

NURSING PROCESS
DRUG INTERACTIONS

Assessment

- Obtain a drug history of the over-the-counter (OTC) drugs the client is currently taking. There could be a drug interaction with the prescribed drug.
- Review all literature provided by drug companies and pharmacy.
- Assess for drug reaction when two highly protein-bound drugs are taken together daily. For example, the anticoagulant warfarin (Coumadin) and the antiinflammatory sulindac (Clinoril) have a high affinity to protein. Warfarin is displaced from the plasma protein, causing more free warfarin and a possible increase in bleeding.
- Assess the client for potential drug interaction problems related to an increased or decreased absorption rate of two drugs. Drug enzyme inducers that increase drug metabolism may result in a decrease in drug effect (increased drug metabolism leads to increased drug excretion).
- Assess the client for drug toxicity (overdose) when a drug enzyme inducer has been discontinued or when a drug enzyme inhibitor is taken concurrently with other drugs.
- Determine whether the client is a cigarette smoker. Tobacco is an enzyme inducer and can increase the metabolic rate of drugs. If a client is taking a drug such as theophylline to control asthma and also smokes, the drug dosage needs to be increased. For non-smokers, the theophylline dosage should be less or within the suggested drug range.
- Assess renal function by checking for adequate urine output; it should be greater than 600 mL/d. The guideline is 25 mL (cc)/h for adults.

Potential Nursing Diagnosis

- Risk of tissue injury related to the adverse reaction to drug interaction.

Planning

- The client will be aware of drug interactions and avoid drugs that may cause a severe drug reaction.
- The client will not take any OTC drugs without consultation with health care provider.

Nursing Interventions

- Notify the health care provider if a drug dose adjustment has not been ordered when a drug enzyme inducer has been discontinued.
- Recognize drugs of the same category that might have an additive effect. The additive drug effect might be undesirable and could cause a severe physiologic response.
- Notify the health care provider of drugs ordered that have antagonistic or opposite effects, such as beta stimulants and beta blockers.
- Consult a pharmacist about processing through a drug interaction computer program.

Client Teaching

- Advise clients not to take OTC drugs with prescribed drugs without first notifying the health care provider.

Evaluation

- Evaluate the effectiveness of the drugs and determine that the client is free of side effects.

Table 7-5
Drug-Induced Photosensitivity

DRUG INDUCED	OCCURRENCE
Amantadine	Was confirmed by positive photopatch testing
Amiodarone	Frequency may be 10% to 75%. Sunscreen lotion with UVA can inhibit photosensitivity
Benzodiazepines	Has been reported with drugs alprazolam and chlordiazepoxide
Carbamazepine	Frequency is less than 1%; however, photocopy machines can trigger photosensitivity
Corticosteroids	Was reported with positive photopatch testing and with use of hydrocortisone
Diphenhydramine	Was reported with positive photopatch testing with topical and oral use
Fluorouracil	Avoid sunlight with topical or IV use; erythema and hyperpigmentation could occur
NSAIDs	Aspirin, ibuprofen, and indomethacin have been reported to have low phototoxin effect; however, there is possibility for photosensitive effect with ibuprofen (dose related)
Methotrexate	Avoid sunlight to prevent severe photosensitive reaction (sunburn)
Calcium blockers	Diltiazem: possible phototoxic reaction Nifedipine: may cause phototoxicity with high drug doses
Phenothiazines	Reported cases of phototoxic reaction with chlorpromazine and other phenothiazines at high drug doses
Piroxicam	Was confirmed with positive photopatch testing; photosensitive reaction occurs after a few days of piroxicam and exposure to sunlight
Pyrazinamide	Skin color may change to reddish-brown; usually occurrence is dose-related
Quinolones (fluoroquin-olones)	Phototoxicity occurs with lomefloxacin, enoxacin, ofloxacin, and nalidixic acid; ciprofloxacin causes less photosensitivity
Sulfonamides	Photosensitive reaction has been reported
Sulfonylureas	Photosensitive reaction has been reported
Tetracyclines	Highly photosensitive; demeclocycline and doxycycline have a higher degree of photosensitive reaction than minocycline
Thiazines	Thiazide-induced photosensitivity has been reported; hydrochlorothiazide has a greater photosensitivity than bendroflumethiazide
Triamterene	Was confirmed by positive photopatch testing
Trimethoprim	Photosensitivity has been reported
Vinblastine	Photosensitivity of drug has been reported

KEY: NSAIDs: nonsteroidal antiinflammatory drugs.

which can cause cellular damage. Usually, the skin area that is exposed is affected.

Phototoxicity and *photoallergy* from drug-induced photosensitivity reactions are terms that are used interchangeably. Both are the result of light exposure but differ according to the wavelength of light and the photosensitive drug. Photosensitivity may be the result of the drug dose. The onset of phototoxicity with erythema can be rapid, occurring in 2 to 6 h of sunlight exposure. Examples of drugs that can induce photosensitivity are listed in Table 7-5.

Most photosensitive reactions can be avoided with the use of sunscreen block (UVA protection) ≥15 and by avoiding excessive sunlight. The higher the drug doses, the more likely that drug-induced photosensitivity will occur. Decreasing drug dose may decrease photosensitivity, if treatment is necessary; discontinuing the drug may be necessary.

OVER-THE-COUNTER DRUGS

Over-the-counter (OTC) drugs, drugs available without a prescription, are found in most households. (Fig. 7-1). Nurses need to be aware of these products and the implications of their use for their clients' drug therapy. OTC drugs provide both advantages and potential serious complications for the consumer.

The Durham-Humphrey amendment (1952) to the Food, Drug and Cosmetic Act of 1938 approved drugs that are safe for consumption and may be sold

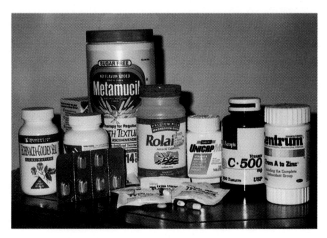

Figure 7–1
Commonly used over-the-counter preparations.

as nonprescription or over-the-counter (OTC) drugs. In 1962, the Kefauver-Harris amendment required proof of efficacy and safety of the drug. OTC drugs came under the scrutiny of the Food and Drug Administration (FDA) in 1970.

The FDA has the responsibility of monitoring the safety of drug therapy. This group of professionals is charged with (1) identifying standards for known active ingredients and (2) establishing mandatory labeling to assist the consumer in the proper use of the drug. The FDA OTC drug categories are listed in Table 7–6.

As a result of the review by the FDA panel, drugs are placed in one of three categories:

Category I: Drugs judged to be both safe and effective
Category II: Drugs judged to be either unsafe or ineffective, and which should not be included in nonprescription products
Category III: Drugs for which there are insufficient data to judge safety or efficacy

The FDA has recommended that drugs in category II be reformulated to be included in category I or removed from the market. (Note: Manufacturers can maintain the brand name after changing the components of an OTC product.) The FDA also has recommended that selected prescription drugs be reclassified so that they can be sold over the counter. As a result, it is vitally important that nurses be aware of current drug information, any changes in FDA recommendations, and the implications of this information for an informed client population.

It is important that both consumers and health care providers be knowledgeable about OTC products. The following cautions may be of assistance when OTC preparations are considered:

- Delay in professional diagnosis and treatment of serious or potentially serious conditions may occur if the client self-prescribes OTC drugs.
- Symptoms may be masked, thereby making diagnosis more complicated.
- Labels and instructions should be followed carefully.
- The client's health care provider or pharmacist should be consulted before OTC preparations are taken.
- Ingredients in OTC products may interact with medications that are prescribed by the health care provider or are self-prescribed by the client.
- Inactive ingredients (e.g., alcohol, dyes, and preservatives) may result in adverse reactions.
- A placebo effect could occur that fosters needless use of a potentially dangerous substance.
- Potential for overdose exists because of the use of several preparations with similar active ingredients. A double dose does not equal quicker recovery.

Table 7–6
FDA Over-the-Counter Drug Categories

Allergy treatment products (internal)
Analgesics—antipyretics (internal)
Antacids and antiflatulents
Antidiarrheal products
Antimicrobials
Antiperspirants
Antirheumatic products
Antitussives
Bronchodilators and antiasthmatic products
Cold remedies, decongestants
Contraceptive products
Dandruff products
Dentifrices and other dental products
Dermatologic products
Emetics and antiemetics
Hematinics
Hemorrhoidal products
Laxatives and cathartics
Ophthalmic products
Oral hygiene drug products
Sedatives and sleep aids
Stimulants
Sunburn prevention and treatment products
Vitamin–mineral supplements
Weight-loss aids
Miscellaneous products (OTC products not covered in above categories)

- Multiple medication users, whether prescription or OTC, are at increased risk as more medications are added to a therapy regimen.
- Interactions of selected prescription medications and OTC preparations are potentially dangerous. Many individuals routinely reach for aspirin, acetaminophen, and ibuprofen to relieve a discomfort or pain without being aware of these interactions. For example, an individual taking digoxin should avoid taking ibuprofen because it may increase the serum digoxin level, thereby resulting in digoxin toxicity; ibuprofen increases fluid retention, which could worsen the condition of a client with congestive heart failure; use of ibuprofen on a long-term basis may decrease the effectiveness of antihypertensive drugs.

Some of the OTC drugs had previously been prescription drugs, such as ibuprofen. The prescription drug Motrin became available as an OTC drug, ibuprofen, in 1984. Tagamet, another prescription drug, was made available as an OTC drug several years ago.

Several OTC drugs, such as cough medicines are composed of two to four compounds. One of the compounds may interact with a prescription drug that the client is taking.

Clients with asthma need to be aware that aspirin can trigger an acute asthma episode. Furthermore, aspirin is not recommended for children with flu symptoms or chickenpox because it has been associated with Reye's syndrome.

Clients with impaired renal function should avoid aspirin, acetaminophen, and ibuprofen because each can further decrease renal function, especially with long-term use. Aspirin and ibuprofen increase the effects of oral anticoagulants, so clients taking these medications may be at increased risk for bleeding.

The aforementioned examples are not inclusive. Caution is advised before using any OTC preparations, including antacids, decongestants, laxatives, and cough syrup (Fig. 7–2). Clients should check with their health care providers and read the drug labels before taking OTC medications in order to be aware of possible contraindications and adverse reactions.

Cold and Cough Remedies

Most OTC cold and cough remedies are for the purpose of relieving coughs, and nasal and sinus congestion. The majority of these OTC agents are sympathomimetic (stimulating the sympathetic nervous system) and contain ingredients such as phenylpropanolamine, pseudoephedrine, analgesic, and an antihistamine. These drugs are primarily safe for children older than 6 years (ages 2 to 6 years old with health

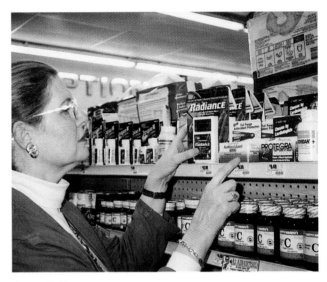

Figure 7–2

Consumers often have questions when choosing an over-the-counter preparation.

care provider's advice). Clients with heart disease, hypertension, or thyroid disease should not take these OTC preparations except with prior approval from their health care provider. Side effects of cold and cough OTC drugs that contain a sympathomimetic include headache, nervousness, increased blood pressure, and insomnia. The most common side effect of the antihistamine is drowsiness.

Health professionals should discuss the pros and cons of taking cold and cough remedies with their client and read the labels carefully. The recommended dose should not be exceeded for either adults or children.

Sleep Aids

Before 1979, most of the OTC sleep aids contained bromides, scopolamine, and/or a combination of antihistamines. The FDA has restricted the number of OTC sleep aids. Most OTC sleep aids currently contain an antihistamine with or without an analgesic such as aspirin or acetaminophen. The side effect of an antihistamine is drowsiness, which is useful as a sleep aid. If the client is having night pain that causes the sleeplessness, the analgesic with the antihistamine is helpful. In small children or elderly clients, these sleep aids may cause central nervous system (CNS) stimulation instead of sedation. These drugs should not be taken with a depressant drug because they can have an additive depressive effect on the CNS.

Weight-Control Drugs

For years, most weight-control drugs contained amphetamines. The amphetamines were prescription drugs prescribed to suppress the appetite. The effectiveness of the amphetamines was short-term because they were effective only so long as the blood level of the drug was present. Drug dependence was a problem associated with amphetamines. Side effects included nervousness, heart palpitations, increased blood pressure, and insomnia.

Currently, there are many OTC weight-control drugs on the market. The major ingredient in most OTC weight-control drugs is phenylpropranolamine, which is related to amphetamine and ephedrine. These drugs are less potent than amphetamine; however, they produce amphetamine-like side effects. The weight-control drugs are contraindicated for clients with heart disease, hypertension, diabetes mellitus, and thyroid disease.

Nonpharmacologic measures of consuming fewer calories and exercising more are the foundation of any weight loss program. If the client continues to eat large meals and snacks while taking weight-control drugs, little to no weight loss occurs.

Good information sources for OTC drugs include *The Handbook of Nonprescription Drugs*, American Pharmaceutical Association, Washington, DC (phone # 1-800-237-2742), and *Drug Facts and Comparisons* (updated monthly), JB Lippincott, Philadelphia. Both provide comprehensive comparisons on nonprescription drug products written for use by health care providers.

DRUG ABUSE

The definition of drug (or substance) abuse can differ among socioeconomic, ethnic, and cultural groups. It is not the misuse of drugs such as self-medicating with OTC drugs or taking prescription drugs other than as prescribed; sometimes, however, drug misuse could result in drug abuse. A broad definition of **drug abuse** is excessive self-administration of a drug that could result in **addiction** (physical dependence) and that could be detrimental to the individual's health. Some health professionals might find exceptions even with this broad definition.

A terminally ill cancer client who takes large doses of opiates to control pain is not considered to be abusing drugs; however, an otherwise healthy person self-administering large doses of opiates is. Two major substance abuse problems are the use of alcohol and nicotine (cigarette smoking). Ingesting an ounce or two of alcohol daily or weekly may not be considered a drug abuse problem by some, but in certain cultures and religions it could be.

Some of the categories of abused drugs include (1) central nervous system (CNS) depressants (such as alcohol, marijuana, narcotics [opiates]), analgesics (such as pentazocine [Talwin]), sedatives and hypnot-

ics, antipsychotics, and antianxiety drugs; (2) CNS stimulants (such as cocaine, amphetamines, caffeine); and (3) mind-altering or "psychedelic" drugs (such as lysergic acid diethylamide [LSD] and mescaline). Prescribed large doses of an antipsychotic drug to maintain well-being is not considered drug abuse. The Controlled Substances Act of 1970 set regulations for use of narcotics, such as establishing a requirement for record keeping. This act has been a help in reducing and detecting drug abuse.

With drug abuse, addiction frequently occurs and is a serious physical and behavioral problem. Characteristics of **addiction** include compulsive drug use, drug craving, and drug seeking. Addiction is physical dependence. **Withdrawal** is the physical effects, such as nausea and convulsions, that result when the drug is discontinued.

Psychological dependence, or **habituation,** is an intense desire or craving for the drug when it is not available. The person does not experience any physical or withdrawal effects. If the drug has been stopped and the psychological need is strong, the use of the drug could be reactivated by the abuser, initiating the cycle of drug abuse.

Chemical Impairment in Nurses

Of the 2.4 million nurses in the United States, it is estimated that 40,000 to 80,000 are chemically impaired; 20% may be chemically dependent. This problem frequently carries a stigma and is characterized by denial by the nurse.

The impaired nurse (1) is usually an adult at the onset of addiction, (2) most commonly initiates the behavior as an escape from life's problems, (3) is seldom "mainlining" the drug, and (4) continues to work. Indeed, chemically impaired nurses are considered to be capable and respected by their colleagues. Risk factors for drug abuse among nurses include overwork, chronic fatigue, physical illness, marital problems, insomnia, pending retirement, professional dissatisfaction, and the availability of drugs.

Evidence of impaired practice may involve behaviors related to the effects of the drug while under its influence and while in a state of withdrawal. Signs and symptoms depend on the particular drug being abused. Drug diversion (deliberate redirecting of a drug from a client or facility to the employee for his or her own or other use) is frequently a behavior of chemically impaired nurses. The most commonly abused chemicals include alcohol, meperidine (Demerol), oxycodone (Percodan), diazepam (Valium), alprazolam (Xanax), and flurazepam (Dalmane).

As a rule, coworkers and employers ignore or miss cues for some time about the abuse behaviors. Managers often fail to address the problem, and when they do, it is in a detrimental way.

NURSING PROCESS
DRUG ABUSE

Assessment

- Assess behavioral changes, such as lethargy or combativeness, that may suggest drug abuse.

Potential Nursing Diagnosis

- Situational low self-esteem related to personal problems.

Planning

- Person will become aware of drug habit and seek professional help.

Nursing Interventions

- Notify the charge nurse or health care provider if client has been receiving drugs, such as narcotics or hypnotics, over a long period of time, possibly resulting in drug abuse.
- Observe the client for physical withdrawal symptoms when a drug that creates physical dependence is discontinued. A mild symptom may be nausea, and severe symptoms include hallucination and convulsions.

Client Teaching

- Encourage the client to seek professional help in alleviating the drug habit.
- Encourage the family to be supportive of the client at all times.
- Encourage any health professional to seek help if a drug problem is suspected. Protecting a fellow employee or health professional suspected of drug abuse or drug diversion may result in serious complications for the individual and the nurse.
- Remind the client that professionals have a responsibility to protect public safety and health.

Evaluation

- Evaluate the effectiveness of identifying individuals who need professional help for their substance abuse and make appropriate reports and referrals.

Society generally and the health professions specifically are shifting their perspective on the chemical impairment of nurses from one of being a moral weakness to that of being a disease. This shift has facilitated the development of prevention and treatment programs. Education intervention can take many formats or directions; for example, incorporation of content on chemical impairment in the curricula of all nursing and staff development programs and the preparation of nurse specialists in addiction nursing.

Abbott (1987) outlines three approaches taken in the workplace when a chemically impaired nurse is identified: (1) administrative—involving dismissal, (2) enforcement—involving referral to narcotics divi-

sion and being treated like a criminal, and (3) co-operative—involving support and treatment. There is no agreement about how to deal with chemical abuse that is acceptable both personally and institutionally.

The tragedy of allowing a treatable disease to go untreated is costly in both human and economic terms. La Godna and Hendrix (1989) noted that the partial approximate cost of identifying an impaired nurse and filing a complaint to a board of nursing was $55,000, and it was a $32,000 economic loss to the identified nurse. Currently the costs are higher. Human costs may include a lowered self-esteem for both the impaired nurse and the informant, shame, and guilt. There may also be a loss of life. Boards of nursing have developed nondisciplinary programs to assist the impaired nurse and to protect the public safety. Some state nurses' associations offer support services.

The following questions pose many ethical dilemmas: What is the role of the regulatory board? Should the impaired nurse be reported? Whose responsibility is it to report the nurse? Should licenses be suspended or revoked when there is impaired practice?

It is incumbent on each nurse to know the rules and regulations of the state nurse practice act and its abuse component. Forty-eight state nurses' associations have peer assistance programs (PAPs) that provide one or all of the following services: information, referral, consultation, support groups, reentry, and monitoring. PAPs advocate that colleagues are more apt to report an impaired nurse if they know that help, rather than discipline, is the result.

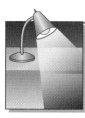

Study Questions

1. What is the meaning and importance of drug interaction?

2. What are the four pharmacokinetic processes related to drug interaction? Describe each process.

3. What are the three main effects associated with pharmacodynamic interaction?

4. What are the effects of drugs in food interactions? What are the implications for your nursing practice?

5. Define drug-induced photosensitivity. What are five drugs or drug groups that are attributed to photosensitivity?

6. List at least five potential disadvantages to the use of OTC preparations.

7. Define the following: drug abuse, drug misuse, addiction, physical dependence, and psychological dependence. What is the potential effect of each on your practice?

8. Which drugs are frequently associated with drug abuse? For what reasons?

9. List factors that contribute to chemical impairment in nurses.

10. Cite resources available to assist chemically impaired nurses. What rights do they have under most nurse practice acts?

11. What would you do if you discovered a peer taking drugs that he or she obtained illegally from the institution?

Herbal Therapy with Nursing Implications

Outline

Objectives

- Identify the herbal monographs associated with current therapy.
- Discuss at least four important points associated with consumer and health care provider education.
- Identify at least four common herbs and their associated toxicity.
- Identify at least eight of the most common herbal therapies and at least one situation in which they seem to be helpful.
- Describe the recommendations for labels on herbal therapy.

Terms

Dietary Supplement Health and Education Act of 1994

dried herbs

extracts

fresh herbs

herb

herbal monographs

oils

phytomedicine

salves

syrups

teas

tinctures

INTRODUCTION

Herbal therapy has surged in popularity in recent years. Marketing and the media have fueled the hype. Magazines, newspapers, local billboards, product displays in the grocery and drug stores are ablaze with products and ads. Herbal therapy has grown into a multimillion-dollar business as a result of the "back to nature" movement of the 1970s and the more health-conscious modern citizenry. In addition, herbal therapy is addressed in the professional literature with seeming increasing frequency and seriousness. Health care providers and consumers are both asking questions about herbal therapy such as "How effective is it?" "Are herbs toxic?" "In what ways do herbs mix with current medications?" What do these questions mean for the consumer and the health of the consumer?

An **herb,** according to Webster's New Collegiate Dictionary, is a "plant or plant part valued for its medicinal, savory, or aromatic qualities." Herbs have strong roots in Judeo-Christianity (tree of life). Also, herbs have long been and continue to be sources of both old and new drugs, such as foxglove (source of digitalis), snakeroot (source of reserpine), willow bark (source of salicin/aspirin), and Pacific yew tree (source of taxol). The therapeutic value of phytomedicine relates to several factors including dosage, potency, and purity.

This chapter describes selected aspects of herbal therapy including (1) herbal monographs, (2) Dietary Supplement Health and Education Act of 1994, (3) variety of preparations of herbs, (4) the most commonly used herbs, (5) herbs to treat selected common ailments, (6) potential hazards of herbs, (7) tips for consumers and health care providers, and (8) herbal resources.

HERBAL MONOGRAPHS

Therapeutic and qualitative are the two primary types of **herbal monographs.** Information on use, dosage, side effects, and contraindications are included in therapeutic monographs. Qualitative monographs have information on areas such as compliance with compounding guidelines and standards of purity. Integrating herbs into the American health care system requires both types of monographs, which the United States currently does not have.

Work is in progress on the development of these monographs by several organizations including United States Pharmacopeia (USP), World Organization (WHO), American Herbal Pharmacopeia (AHP), German Commission E, and European Scientific Cooperative of Phytomedicines (ESCOP):

- *United States Pharmacopeia (USP)*: The first edition was published in 1820 and since the early 1900s this work has been the authoritative source for therapeutic substances. Many originally botanical preparations have been replaced by synthetic analogues. Recently, USP undertook development of 15 to 20 monographs on herbs of high economic interest, such as garlic, ginger root, and valerian. Monographs have not yet been released.
- World Health Organization (WHO): WHO has compiled a list of 40 botanicals for which to develop qualitative and therapeutic monographs. This work was seen as supportive of the 1976 resolution to achieve adequate health care for the world's population by the year 2000.
- American Herbal Pharmacopeia (AHP): This group was founded in 1995 with a goal of developing 300 monographs. St. John's Wort, *Hypericum perforatum,* was the first monograph; 11 more are in the development process. It is anticipated that these monographs will be the most accurate and comprehensive in the English language.
- European Scientific Cooperative of Phytomedicines (ESCOP): This is an international cooperative of organizations working to develop botanical monographs. **Phytomedicines** are plant-based remedies. Fifty therapeutic monographs have already been developed.
- German Commission E: This group developed 330 therapeutic monographs between 1978 and 1993, when it was disbanded. About 77 of these monographs supported therapeutic recommendations. Lack of citations was a major limitation of these monographs. Monographs reported "reasonable certainty" of the efficacy of the specific herbal remedy.

The American Botanical Council is translating the Commission E monographs into English as an effort to bring more information to the American public. Much work remains to be done related to effects of preparations and the improvement of manufacturing and marketing processes.

Herbs were the original medicines. It has been estimated that phytomedicines are prescribed by the majority of physicians in Germany. This practice is promoted because the government's health insurance pays for botanical remedies. Americans have long used botanicals, but outside the mainstream. The United States exports significant quantities of herbs to Europe. Few pharmacy schools offer courses in botanical remedies.

It is reasonable to expect an associated expense of $350 million to bring a new drug to market. A botanical remedy cannot be patented; thus the manufacturer generally cannot justify the expense in the booming conventional medicine economy.

In 1992 Congress instructed the National Institutes of Health to develop an Office of Alternative Medicine to support studies of alternative therapies.

DIETARY SUPPLEMENT HEALTH AND EDUCATION ACT OF 1994

The **Dietary Supplement Health and Education Act of 1994** clarified marketing regulations for herbal remedies. Furthermore, it reclassified them as "dietary supplements," distinct from food or drugs. Herbal supplements can be marketed with suggested dosages. Consumers are reminded that premarket testing for safety and efficacy is not required, and manufacturing is not standardized. The physiologic effects of the product can be noted but no claims can be made about prevention or curing of specific conditions. For example, a claim cannot say the agent "prevents heart disease," but it can say that the agent "helps to increase blood flow to the heart." In addition, there is need for a disclaimer that the herb is not Food and Drug Administration (FDA) approved and that it is not meant to be used as a drug.

HERBAL PREPARATIONS

Herbal remedies take a variety of preparations and form. Examples include fresh aloe, dried ginger, peppermint oil, elderberry syrup, and chamomile tea. Following is a description of selected preparations and forms of herbs including: dried extracts, fresh oils, salves, teas, tinctures, syrups, capsules, and tablets.

Dried herbs are fresh herbs that have had the moisture removed by sun or heat. They can be stored for about 6 months. **Extracts** are made by isolating certain components, resulting in more reliable dosing. Dissolving the herb in a solvent such as alcohol or water is a common way to prepare an extract, which may or may not be standardized. **Fresh herbs** may decay after a few days because of enzyme activity; hence, they have a short life. Drying is a means of preservation. **Oils** are made by soaking dried herb in olive or vegetable oil and heating for an extended time. The vegetable oil promotes the concentration of some of the active components, and it may last for months if stored correctly. These infused oils are *not* essential oils. **Salves,** semisolid fatty preparations, are made by melting a wax in oil and having it cool and harden. Stored correctly, they last for several months as balms, creams, and ointments. **Teas** are made by soaking fresh or dried herbs in boiling water. It is recommended that only a 2- to 3-day supply be prepared at one time and that it be stored in the refrigerator. Teas may be used as a drink, added to baths, and applied topically in a compress. **Tinctures** are commonly made by soaking fresh or dried herbs in solvent such as water or alcohol. Both water- and fat-soluble components are concentrated in the final form. Alcohol promotes preservation, yielding a shelf-life of 1 year. Alcohol-free glycerin-based tinctures are available for people who do not consume alcohol.

Capsules are commonly a powdered form of dried supplement, but they may hold juices or oils. They have a slower effect than liquids because of decreased absorption. They store and travel well. Tablets are similar to capsules; they are a powder compressed with stabilizers and binders. **Syrups** are made by adding a sweetener, usually honey or sugar, to the herb and then cooking it. Syrups are used to treat colds, cough, and sore throat.

COMMONLY USED HERBAL REMEDIES

Most herbal therapies are used for chronic conditions, they are unlikely to cause harm, and they may provide some relief in selected situations (Fig. 8–1). This section discusses some of the more commonly used herbs.

ALOE VERA (Aloe barbadensis)
The juice is used externally for treatment of minor burns, insect bites, and sunburn. There has been some success with the treatment of dandruff, oily skin, and psoriasis. Taken internally, aloe vera is a powerful laxative. Menstrual flow is increased with small doses.

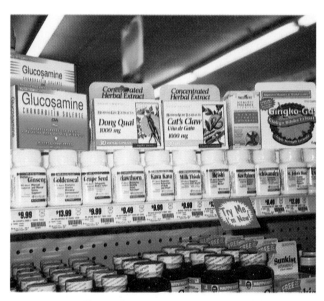

Figure 8–1
Commonly used herbal preparations.

CALENDULA (Calendula officinalis)

This popular herb is derived from marigold. It is used as a common topical remedy for skin irritations, bites and stings, strains and sprains, minor burns, and hemorrhoids. Mucilage is thought to have the ability to reduce inflammation and enhance wound healing. It is considered nontoxic.

CHAMOMILE (Matricaria recutita)

Dried flower heads of *Matricaria recutita* are ingredients of a popular tea for relief of digestive and gastrointestinal (GI) complaints. The tea is used for relief of irritable bowel syndrome and infant colic through antispasmodic and antiinflammatory effects on the GI tract. In addition, chamomile may have sedative effects.

Chamomile tea is prepared by steeping one teaspoon of flower heads for 10 to 15 minutes in boiling water drunk 3 to 4 times per day. An extremely rare allergic reaction of urticaria and bronchoconstriction may occur in an individual allergic to daisy or ragweed-type plants.

DONG QUAI (Angelica sinensis)

Dong quai, an all-purpose woman's tonic herb, has long been popular in China and Japan for treatment of menstrual cramps and to regulate the menstrual cycle. This herb has not been well studied and preparations are frequently mixed with fillers. It contains vitamin B_{12}, which may promote manufacture of blood cells. Rare side effects include fever and excessive menstrual bleeding. Herb experts tend to avoid its use.

ECHINACEA (Echinacea angustifolia)

Echinacea, a popular supplement, is used as an immune enhancer; it acts by furthering phagocytosis by means of increasing leukocytes and spleen cells and activating granulocytes. In addition, echinacea inhibits hyaluronidase activity and increases the release of tumor necrosis factor. The leaf preparation is given for respiratory and urinary tract infections. The root extract is used to treat flulike symptoms. Commission E recommends that echinacea preparations be avoided by persons with autoimmune diseases and those with abnormal T-cell functioning (e.g., human immunodeficiency virus [HIV], acquired immunodeficiency virus [AIDS], tuberculosis). Echinacea is used by native Americans to treat snakebite.

Echinacea should be purchased only from reliable sources; there are many reports of fraudulent substitution with other plants and varying potency. There is inconsistent recommendation of duration of treatment. Commission E recommends use of up to 8 weeks; others recommend a week's "drug holiday" (not taking the preparation for a specific time period) before continuing the therapy.

ELDERBERRY (Sambucus nigra)

Elderberry has a reputation of being a "one-plant medicine chest." Most popular uses include relief of cold and sore throat, and reduction of fever and flu-like symptoms. Elderberry is also credited with limited cough suppressant and laxative effects. Plant nutrients include vitamins, tannins, and flavonoids; recent studies suggest that elderberry prevents virus from attacking cells by binding to it. Bark and leaf products are not to be taken internally.

FEVERFEW (Chrysanthemum parthenium)

The plant compound parthenolide is believed to act as a serotonin antagonist, a mediator of vascular headaches from platelets. Feverfew is popular for relief of migraine headaches and relief of the accompanying nausea and vomiting.

Only standardized extracts should be used. Wide variation in the amount of active compound in plants and commercial capsules is a potential dosing problem. About 10% of users experience ulceration of the oral mucosa from chewing the fresh or dried leaves of *C. parthenium*, which requires refrigeration.

GARLIC (Allium sativum)

Garlic, which is the herb of endurance, is reported to lower cholesterol and triglyceride levels, decrease blood pressure, and reduce clotting capability of blood. It also acts as an antibiotic to treat infections and wounds both internally and externally. Warm garlic oil is used in the ear for treatment of earache.

GINGER (Zingiber officinale)

Ginger boosts the immune system. It is used to treat stomach and digestive disorders, including motion sickness. Long-time use as relief from nausea is validated by modern research. In addition, it may provide relief from pain, swelling, and stiffness of both osteoarthritis and rheumatoid arthritis (500–4000 mg/d).

GINKGO (Ginkgo biloba)

Ginkgo biloba, extract of one of the oldest plant species, is the most commonly prescribed herbal remedy worldwide. Crossing the blood–brain barrier, ginkgo has central nervous system (CNS) effects, increasing cerebral arterial dilation and increasing oxygen and glucose uptake. It assists cells during periods of hypoxia (e.g., during transient ischemic attacks) and decreases free-radical damage to neurons. In addition, there is inhibition of platelet adhesion and degranulation. Commission E monograph #55 lists the use of ginkgo for dementia syndromes, intermittent claudication, vertigo, and tinnitus. In addition, there is some evidence that it improves cognition and may be helpful in Alzheimer's disease, early stroke, and Raynaud's phenomenon.

Ginkgo biloba is generally given as 120 to 240 mg daily in two to three divided doses for up to 90 days. Rare side effects include headache and GI disturbances.

GINSENG (Panax ginseng)

Preparations of ginseng are taken for short-term relief of stress, to boost energy, and to give digestive support. Ginseng tends to support the immune system and assist in preventing chronic infections. Red Korean or Chinese ginseng may be overstimulating in chronic inflammatory conditions such as arthritis.

GOLDENSEAL (Hydrastis canadensis)

Goldenseal is frequently used with echinacea to ward off infection and promote wound healing. It is used to treat congestion associated with the common cold. In addition, it is used as a tonic and astringent. Active ingredients are deactivated in the stomach. Goldenseal is expensive and scarce; thus, it is frequently adulterated with fillers. Its ability to stimulate the immune system has been questioned, and it can be toxic if overused.

KAVA KAVA (Piper methysticum)

Kava kava has practical and ceremonial roles in the Pacific Island cultures. The root promotes sleep and muscle relaxation. Tea can help with urinary tract infections. Kava kava may be used in combination with other herbs such as valerian and St. John's wort for relaxation.

LICORICE (Glycyrrhiza glabra)

Licorice may have physiologic effects similar to aldosterone and corticosteroids related to glycyrrhizin, a major ingredient. Licorice may help with chronic fatigue syndrome. It relieves heartburn and indigestion by decreasing stomach acid. Side effects from excessive use of licorice include increased blood pressure, headache, lethargy, water retention, increased potassium excretion, and, rarely, heart failure. Licorice root (5–15 mg) is considered a safe dose when taken as tea; recommended use is limited to 6 weeks.

MILK THISTLE (Silybum marianum)

This herbal extract has the remarkable ability to prevent damage to liver cells and stimulate regeneration of liver cells. These findings have been validated by research. Milk thistle is widely used in Europe to treat hepatitis, cirrhosis, and fatty liver associated with drugs and alcohol.

PEPPERMINT (Mentha piperita)

Peppermint stimulates appetite and aids in digestion when taken internally. The digestive tract is protected by the tannins, and peppermint is used in treatment of bowel disorders. Hot peppermint tea stimulates circulation, reduces fever, clears congestion, and helps restore energy. Peppermint oil is an effective treatment for tension headache when rubbed on the forehead. Peppermint has been shown to be comparable to extra-strength Tylenol in relieving headache in research in Germany.

PSYLLIUM (Plantago)

The psyllium seed is widely used as a laxative. It is used in the treatment of hemorrhoids, colitis, Crohn's disease, and irritable bowel syndrome. A full dose is 1/2 teaspoon of seed soaked in water for 15 to 60 minutes taken at bedtime with at least 8 ounces of water.

SAGE (Salvia officinalis)

Sage is the herb of longevity. Sage in a poultice of dry leaves has wound-healing effects and is used as gargle tea for a sore throat. This tea also helps to dry up mother's milk and reduce hot flashes. Sage contains antibacterial, antioxidant, estrogenic compounds, and tannins, so it is recommended that this remedy be taken for only 1 to 2 weeks to avoid toxic effects.

ST. JOHN'S WORT (Hypericum perforatum)

The *British Medical Journal* (1996) reported a meta-analysis of 23 randomized trials comparing St. John's wort with another antidepressant or placebo. Results were that 55% of patients taking the active drug said it was helpful compared with 22% taking the placebo. Difficulties with analysis included lack of standardized preparation and wide range of doses. In addition, St. John's wort has at least 10 pharmacologically active components. The compound used for standardization is hypericin. Researchers recommend that further prospective trials be conducted to compare St. John's wort with standard antidepressant medication and to identify dosages, effectiveness in different stages of depression, and implications of long-term use. St. John's wort has been nicknamed "herbal Prozac" because of its great popularity in the United States and its use as a "tonic" for the nervous system. St. John's wort is used in combination with yarrow to treat enuresis.

The 1984 Commission E monograph on hypericin indicated the agent was an experimental monoamine oxidase (MAO) inhibitor for use in depression, anxiety, and psychogenic disturbances. The mechanism of action is unknown. Studies of reported antiviral effects are in progress.

The usual dose of St. John's Wort is 300 mg t.i.d. of extract (standardized to 0.3% hypericin). A tea can be prepared from 1 to 2 teaspoonsful of herb steeped for 10 minutes. One to two cups of tea per day for 4 to 6 weeks is recommended. Users need to apply sun screen freely when outdoors, although phototoxicity has not been reported in humans. Users of St. John's wort do not need to avoid tyramine-rich foods. It is considered a dietary supplement in the United States and has not been FDA approved; it is licensed in Germany for relief of anxiety, depression, and insomnia.

SAW PALMETTO (Serenoa repens)

Double-blind studies indicate that the herb saw palmetto relieves symptoms of benign prostatic hypertrophy and urinary conditions. Saw palmetto has earned the name "plant catheter." Other indications for this herb include use as an expectorant and treatment for colds, asthma, bronchitis, and thyroid deficiency. Recommended dose is 160 mg of standardized extract twice a day. Upset stomach is a rare side effect.

VALERIAN (Valeriana officinalis)

Valerian, a mild sedative and sleep-inducing agent, has the effect similar to benzodiazepines. It is popularly known as "herbal Valium." Most researchers report no hangover effect. A "dirty socks" odor is related to the dried plant, resulting in no risk of overdose. Preparations from fresh root are reported to be better relaxants and have a sweet aroma. There have been no reports of habituation and addiction. Drowsiness may occur, as with any relaxant. The dosage depends on the symptoms, such as insomnia and anxiety. To treat insomnia, 400 mg of tincture extract is recommended: 2.5 to 5.0 mg of solid extract at bedtime. For anxiety, a tea steeped with 1 teaspoon of dried herb is taken several times a day. About 5% to 10% of users report a stimulant effect.

YARROW (Achillea millefolium)

Yarrow, a wound-healing herb, stops wound bleeding. Yarrow has been used for more than a decade in healing lotions and ointments. Its antiinflammatory effects have been reported on skin and mucous membranes. Also, it is used to induce sweating (sudorific).

Yarrow is used for menstrual irregularities to reduce pain and heavy bleeding and to regulate the cycle. Furthermore, it enhances circulation and lowers blood pressure and has shown antispasmodic and antimicrobial activity. The most frequently reported side effect is contact dermatitis. Yarrow is not recommended in epileptic individuals or during pregnancy.

Summary

A summary of herbs and their properties is given in Table 8–1. Vitamins and elements commonly used in conjunction with herbal therapy are presented in Table 8–2.

USING HERBS TO TREAT SELECTED COMMON AILMENTS

Herbs also seem to be helpful in such conditions as cough, sore throat, cuts, and cholesterol chasers. For example, oil of eucalyptus is found in many cough medicines. Breathing and respiratory ailments are frequently eased with eucalyptus tea. The effectiveness of the aloe vera plant is known to many; gel from a broken leaf of the aloe potted house plant is spread directly on minor cuts. The fresh plant, easy to grow in pots or garden, is superior to commercial preparations. Lowering of cholesterol levels may be the most documented values of garlic and onions.

POTENTIAL HAZARDS OF HERBS

No preparations are safe in all situations and herbs are no exception. Consumers and health care providers need to be alert to potential hazards with herbal therapy.

Contamination is one area of concern, most likely resulting from lack of standards in manufacture and regulation of herbs. It is consumers' responsibility to educate themselves about herbs before use and to purchase products only from reputable dealers. Determination of the purity and concentration of a particular product can be determined only by assays, a costly process. Thus, most products have not had appropriate human toxicologic analysis.

Interaction with conventional drugs is another area requiring alertness. For example, an additive effect of digoxin can result from the use of cascara and senna. Also, elevation in the blood level of lithium may result from juniper and dandelion and other herbs with diuretic properties.

All compounds are not safe via all routes. For example, comfrey (symphytum officinale) has both internal and external preparations. Internal use is discouraged because hepatic damage may be fatal. For external use, comfrey is used as an ointment for relief of swelling associated with abrasions and sprains.

In 1997, the FDA proposed controls on dietary supplements containing ephedra, also known as ma huang, for weight loss and as an energy booster. Use of this supplement has markedly declined since reports of adverse effects came to light (e.g., palpitations, stroke). Ephedrine and pseudoephedrine, components of ephedra, have stimulant and bronchodilation effects.

The FDA proposed that the dosage not exceed 24 mg ephedrine per day as a dietary supplement. The

Text continued on page 183

Table 8–1
Summary of Herbs and Their Properties

COMMON NAME (SCIENTIFIC NAME) PART OF PLANT USED	OTHER NAMES	POPULAR LAYPRESS CLAIMS	SCIENTIFIC INFORMATION		ADVERSE EFFECTS/WARNINGS	ADDITIONAL COMMENTS/CONTRAINDICATIONS
			Scientific Properties/FDA Approval	German Commission E Recommendations		
Agrimony (*Agrimonia eupatoria*) leaves	Common agrimony	Astringent, inflammation of the throat, cystitis, gastroenteritis, gallbladder disorders, incontinence, hemostatic agent, analgesic, antiviral and antiinflammatory agent	Astringent	**Internally:** mild, acute diarrhea; inflammation of mouth and throat **Externally:** mild, superficial inflammation of the skin	No known adverse effects	
Aloe (*Aloe barbadensis*) fresh gel, dried juice	Barbados aloe, Curacao aloe	Emollient, laxative, minor burns, insect bites, skin irritations, minor cuts, wrinkles, regulates liver function, premenstrual syndrome (PMS), emmenagogue	FDA approved as a laxative	Acute constipation	May bring about abortion or premature birth; loss of electrolytes with chronic use	Avoid use if ileus present; do not use if pregnant or lactating
Angelica (*Angelica archangelica*) root, fruit, leaves	Garden angelica, European angelica	Emmenagogue, flavoring agent, abortifacient, carminative, stomachic, expectorant, relieves menstrual cramps and nervous insomnia, diuretic, diaphoretic	Conflicting evidence: possible spasmolytic properties and effects on secretion of gastric juice; others stating there is no scientific evidence to support claims	Approved for lack of appetite; dyspepsia	Photosensitiviy, dermatitis May be carcinogenic	Used as a flavoring in alcoholic beverages such as gin
Anise (*Pimpinella anisum*) fruits (commonly called seeds)	Anise plant, aniseed, common anise	Antispasmodic, aromatic, expectorant, tonic, carminative, aphrodisiac, emmenagogue, galactagogue	Expectorant, weakly spasmolytic, antibacterial	**Internally:** dyspeptic complaints **Internally and Externally:** catarrh of the respiratory tract	Allergic reactions of the skin, respiratory and GI tracts	Contraindication: allergy to aniseed or anethole
Bayberry Bark (*Myrica pensylvanica* and *M. cerifera*) root bark, berries		Astringent, circulatory stimulant, diaphoretic, colds, hemorrhoids, diarrhea	Mineralocorticoid activity, choleretic	No information		Potential carcinogen, therefore its use cannot be recommended
Balm (*Melissa officinalis*) leaves	Balm mint, bee balm, blue balm, cure-all, dropsy plant, garden balm, lemon balm	Antispasmodic, calmative, carminative, diaphoretic, hypotensive, stomachic, emmenagogue, insomnia, depression, relief of menstrual cramps, asthma, migraine, relief of toothache and cold sores	Sedative, carminative	Useful for nervous disorders that cause problems with sleep and for gastrointestinal disorders	No known adverse effects	

Table continued on following page

173

Table 8–1 Continued

Summary of Herbs and Their Properties

COMMON NAME (SCIENTIFIC NAME) PART OF PLANT USED	OTHER NAMES	POPULAR LAYPRESS CLAIMS	SCIENTIFIC INFORMATION		ADVERSE EFFECTS/WARNINGS	ADDITIONAL COMMENTS/CONTRAINDICATIONS
			Scientific Properties/FDA Approval	German Commission E Recommendations		
Black Cohosh (*Cimicifuga racemosa*) rhizome, root	Black snakeroot, rattleweed, rattleroot, squawroot, cimicifuga	Dysmenorrhea, antispasmodic, astringent, diuretic, expectorant, promotes labor, sedative, rheumatism, PMS, menopausal symptoms	May reduce secretion of luteinizing hormone	Premenstrual discomfort, dysmenorrhea, and climacteric symptoms	Stomach upset; no other information on toxicity	Long-term safety requires verification
Blessed Thistle (*Cnicus benedictus*) leaves, seeds	Holy thistle	Bitter tonic, astringent, diaphoretic, antibacterial, expectorant	Promotes secretion of saliva and gastric juice	Lack of appetite, dyspeptic complaints	Allergic reactions possible	
Boneset (*Eupatorium perfoliatum*) leaves, tops	Agueweed, crosswort, feverwort, Indian sage, sweating plant, wood boneset	Diaphoretic, cathartic, emetic, tonic, febrifuge, useful in "breaking up" mucus associated with the common cold and flu	Contains no compounds known to have therapeutic value, though this herb does appear to increase sweating	No information	Causes nausea	Caution in consumption of this herb is advised due to the possible presence of toxic alkaloids
Borage (*Borago officinalis*) leaves, tops	Bugloss, common bugloss, burage	Diuretic, astringent, febrifuge, tonic, galactagogue, antipyretic, pleurisy, peritonitis, diaphoretic, expectorant, laxative, antinflammatory	Astringent properties due to presence of tannin and mild expectorant action but no truly therapeutic effect has been found with this herb	No information	Slight constipating effects	Contains low levels of pyrrolizidine alkaloids which are potentially hepatotoxic and carcinogenic therefore consumption of this herb should only be done under medical supervision
Capsicum or Cayenne Pepper (*Capsicum* spp.) fruits	Chile pepper, red pepper	Stimulant, carminative, tonic, antiseptic, rubefacient, sialogogue, reduces symptoms of common cold, stomachic	FDA approved as a topical analgesic. It is marketed as a cream that may be effective when used topically for herpes zoster, diabetic neuropathy	No information	Avoid touching eyes or mucus membranes after applying product	
Cascara (*Rhamnus purshiana*) dried bark	Sacred bark, bitter bark	Laxative, bitter tonic, gallstones, liver ailments	FDA approved as a laxative; stimulates peristalsis	Constipation	Chronic use: increased loss of electrolytes	Contraindicated if ileus present; avoid use during pregnancy or lactation

Herb	Other names	Claimed/reported uses	Scientific evidence	Probable efficacy	Adverse effects/toxicity	Comments
Catnip (*Nepeta cataria*) leaves, tops	Catnep, catmint	Bronchitis, antidiarrheal agent, antiflatulent, digestive aid, astringent, antispasmodic, sedative, diaphoretic, mind-altering effects (smoked)	No scientific evidence to support claims	No information	No adverse effects reported	Patients may be able to drink the tea safely, although the safety of smoking this herb is not known
Chamomiles *Matricaria recutia, Chamaemelum nobile* flowering heads	German chamomile, Hungarian chamomile	Carminative, antiinflammatory, antispasmodic, antiinfective, antianxiety, diaphoretic, analgesic, local healing	Antiinflammatory and antispasmodic effects	Useful as antispasmodic, antiflatulent agents; inflammation of the mouth and throat	Contact dermatitis, anaphylaxis, hypersensitivity reactions	Persons allergic to ragweed, asters or chrysanthemums should use this herb with caution
Chaste Tree Berry (*Vitex agnuscastus*) fruit	Monk's pepper	PMS, dysmenorrhea menopause symptoms	Inhibits secretion of prolactin by the pituitary gland	Useful for a variety of menstrual disorders	Very limited toxicity data; may cause an itchy rash	
Comfrey (*Symphytum officinale*)	Blackwort, bruisewort, gum plant, healing herb, slippery root	Astringent, demulcent, emollient, expectorant, hemostatic, refrigerant, hoarseness, intestinal problems, bronchitis, pleurisy, rheumatism	Antiinflammatory action, promotes callus formation; contains pyrrolizidine alkaloids that may be hepatotoxic and carcinogenic	**Externally:** contusions, sprains, dislocations	Hepatotoxicity	The drug should only be applied to intact skin and used for no longer than 4 to 6 weeks in a year; internal use of comfrey should be avoided and comfrey should not be used in young children or pregnant or lactating women
Damiana (*Turnera aphrodisiaca*) leaves, stems	Blowball, cankerwort, lion's tooth, priest's crown, puffball, swine snout, white endive, wild endive	Aphrodisiac, laxative, antianxiety, urinary antisepetic, antidepressant	No scientific evidence to support claims	No information	No information available	Considered an "herbal hoax"
Dandelion (*Taraxacum officinale*) rhizome, roots, leaves	Tank kuei, dang qui	Digestive aid, laxative, diuretic, liver and gallbladder protectant, prevents iron-deficiency anemia, PMS, breast tenderness	According to Wichtl, this herb has choleretic and diuretic actions along with appetite-stimulating properties; Tyler states roots may aid digestion and have a slight laxative effect but there is no evidence to support a significant therapeutic benefit	Useful in biliary disorders, as a carminative, and to stimulate diuresis	Skin rash, no other significant side effects of toxicities noted	Preparations of dandelion may be taken for a period of up to 4 to 6 weeks
Dong quai (*Angelica sinensis*) root		Antispasmodic, dysmenorrhea, laxative, PMS, amenorrhea, hot flashes, insomnia, high blood pressure, prevents anemia, vaginal lubricant	No scientific evidence to support claims	No information	Photosensitization, contains coumarin derivatives	It is recommended to avoid all unnecessary exposure to this drug

Table continued on following page

Table 8-1 *Continued*
Summary of Herbs and Their Properties

COMMON NAME (SCIENTIFIC NAME) PART OF PLANT USED	OTHER NAMES	POPULAR LAYPRESS CLAIMS	SCIENTIFIC INFORMATION		ADVERSE EFFECTS/WARNINGS	ADDITIONAL COMMENTS/CONTRAINDICATIONS
			Scientific Properties/FDA Approval	German Commission E Recommendations		
Echinacea (*Echinacea augustifolia*, *E. pallida*, *E. purpurea*) rhizome, roots, leaves, tops	Sampson root, purple coneflower	Antiseptic, digestive, eczema, acne, migraine, antipyretic, antiflatulent, wound healing, immune stimulant to help fight colds, influenza	Immune-stimulant effect	Used to enhance resistance to infectious conditions in the upper respiratory tract	Allergies (infrequent)	Use of Echinacea root does not exclude concomitant administration of antibiotics; this herb should not be used by persons with conditions such as tuberculosis, AIDS, collagen diseases, multiple sclerosis
Ephedra (*Ephedra* spp.) stems	Ma huang	Antiasthmatic, nasal decongestant, vasodilator, antiallergic, hypertensive, circulatory stimulant, anorexiant	Effective nasal decongestant	No information	Increases blood pressure and heart rate, may cause insomnia, palpitations, dizziness, headaches, nervousness	Persons with heart disease, thyroid disease, hypertension and diabetes should use this herb with caution; FDA advisory in 1995 issued warning against products containing this herb
Eucalyptus (*Eucalyptus globulus*) leaves	Blue gum	Antiseptic, deodorant, expectorant, stimulant, indigestion, respiratory ailments	Secretomotor, expectorant, weakly spasmolytic	Catarrhal disorders of the respiratory passages	Nausea, vomiting, diarrhea	
Evening Primrose (*Oenothera biennis*) seed oil	Fever plant, field primrose, night willow-herb, king's cureall	Astringent, demulcent, depression, stimulating effect on liver, spleen and GI tract, skin rashes, PMS, weight loss	Conflicting evidence on efficacy of this herb; no data to support safety of prolonged consumption	No information		
Fennel (*Foeniculum vulgare*) root, fruit (commonly called seed)	Large fennel, sweet fennel, wild fennel	Demulcent, stomachic, antispasmotic, aromatic, carminative, diuretic, expectorant, stimulant, galactagogue, aromatic, rubefacient	Spasmolytic, increases gastrointestinal motility, secretolytic action in the respiratory tract; antiflatulent	Dyspeptic complaints, such as feelings of distention, flatulence; catarrh of the upper respiratory tract	*Fennel fruit:* allergic reaction of the skin and respiratory tract; *fennel volatile oil:* skin irritation, vomiting, seizures, respiratory problems, thus self-medication with oil is not recommended	Do not use in pregnancy

Herb	Common Names	Claims	Comments	Appropriate Uses	Adverse Effects	Precautions
Fenugreek (*Trigonella foenum-graecum*) seeds	Trigonella, Greek hay seed	Aphrodisiac, antidiabetic, expectorant, gout, demulcent, restorative, neuralgias, skin irritations, menstrual cycle stabilizer	Studies in small animals point to a number of potential applications but no data available in humans to support claims	**Internally:** anorexia **Externally:** local inflammation	Adverse skin reactions with repeated local applications	
Garlic (*Allium sativum*) bulb	Clove garlic	Antihelmintic, antispasmodic, diuretic, carminative, digestive, expectorant, treatment of atherosclerosis and high blood pressure, blood clotting disorders	Garlic appears to provide some protection against atherosclerosis and stroke and may reduce blood cholesterol and blood pressure	No information	Allergic reactions; reduction of clotting time; consumption of ≥5 cloves/day may cause heartburn, flatulence	Avoid large amounts in persons taking aspirin or other anticoagulant drugs
Ginger (*Zingiber officinale*) rhizome	Jamaica ginger, African ginger, black ginger, race ginger	Appetizer, carminative, diaphoretic, stimulant, prevention of motion sickness, rubefacient	Antiemetic, promotes salivary and gastric secretion; increases intestinal peristalsis	Dyspeptic complaints; prevention of symptoms of motion sickness	No known adverse effects	In patients with a history of gallstones, use only after consultation with a health care professional
Gingko (*Ginkgo biloba*) leaf extract	Maidenhair tree	Enhanced cerebral blood flow, tinnitus, vertigo, Alzheimer's, hemorrhoids, slows aging process, prevents cancer, antidepressant, improves memory	Ginkgo promotes vasodilation and improved blood flow in arteries and capillaries; acts as a free radical scavenger	Effective in treatment of circulatory disturbances and treating symptoms such as vertigo, weakened memory, mood swings	GI disturbances, headache, allergic skin reactions, restlessness	May interact with anticoagulants
Ginseng (*Panax ginseng*—Oriental) (*Panax quinque-folius*—American) Siberian ginseng (*Eleutherococcus senticosus*) roots	American ginseng; five-fingers, five-leafed ginseng	Adaptogen, demulcent, cure-all, antistress agents, aphrodisiac, menopausal symptoms, reduces cholesterol, increases energy, inhibits tumors	Solid clinical data supporting claims are lacking, although some studies have shown some beneficial pharmacologic effects	Useful for conditions manifested by lack of energy or poor concentration and during periods of convalescence	Insomnia, diarrhea, skin eruptions; menopausal bleeding	Concern exists over lack of standardized products, differences between Oriental and American plants. Recommended for use for only 3 months (Commission E)
Goldenseal (*Hydrastis canadensis*) rhizome, roots	Eye balm, eye root, ground raspberry, Indian plant, yellowroot, jaundice root, yellow puccoon	Bitter tonic, digestive aid, genitourinary conditions, menorrhagia, upper respiratory ills, irritated gums, canker sores, ringworm treatment, atrophic vaginitis	This herb may have some astringent and weak antiseptic properties but there is no scientific evidence to support claims	No information	No safety or efficacy data available when this herb is used internally	
Gotu Kola (*Centella asiatica*) leaves	Indian pennywort, hyrocotyle	Promote longevity, aphrodisiac, phlebitis, episiotomy healing, expectorant, leprosy, hypertension, ulcers, rheumatism, hot flashes, improves memory, antidepressant	May have some anti-inflammatory effects and may promote wound healing; no other claims have been substantiated	No information	Data not available	Do not confuse with kola which contains caffeine

Table continued on following page

Table 8–1 *Continued*
Summary of Herbs and Their Properties

COMMON NAME (SCIENTIFIC NAME) PART OF PLANT USED	OTHER NAMES	POPULAR LAYPRESS CLAIMS	SCIENTIFIC INFORMATION		ADVERSE EFFECTS/WARNINGS	ADDITIONAL COMMENTS/CONTRAINDICATIONS
			Scientific Properties/FDA Approval	German Commission E Recommendations		
Hawthorn (*Crataegus monogyna, C. laevigata*) fruits, leaves, flowers	May bush, May tree, thorn-apple tree, whitehorn	Antispasmodic, sedative, vasodilator, myocarditis, atherosclerosis, antihypertensive	Positive inotrope and chronotrope; increased coronary and myocardial circulation	Cardiac insufficiency corresponding to NYHA stages I and II; a feeling of pressure and tightness in the chest, mild bradycardia	Not known	Self-medication with this herb is not recommended
Hops (*Humulus lupulus*) strobile (floral part)	Hop vine	Sedative, mind-altering action, appetite, stimulant, antiflatulent agent, antiseptic, astringent	Studies have failed to confirm any of the claims	No information	Data not available	
Iceland Moss (*Cetraria islandica*) whole plant	Cetrari	Antiemetic, demulcent, galactogogue, tonic catarrh, gastroenteritis, anemia	Demulcent, weakly antibacterial	Irritation of mucous membranes of mouth and throat; lack of appetite	None known	Use of this herb in large quantities over extended periods of time is not recommended due to possible lead content
Juniper (*Juniperus communis*) fruit	Juniper berries	Diuretic, antiseptic, carminative, stomachic, tonic, rubefacient, antirheumatic, gastrointestinal infections	In animals, an increase in urinary output has been observed as well as smooth muscle contractions	Dyspeptic complaints (belching, heartburn, distension)	Renal damage may occur with prolonged use	Do not take during pregnancy or if renal disease present; do not take for longer than 4 weeks without consulting health care professional
Lady's-Mantle (*Alchemilla xanthochlora*) leaves, flowering shoot		Astringent, anorexia, diuretic, rheumatism, diarrhea, enteritis, menstrual problems, decreases menstrual flow, leucorrhea	Astringent	Useful for mild, nonspecific diarrhea and gastrointestinal complaints	May cause liver damage in rare cases	
Licorice (*Glycyrrhiza glabra*) rhizome, roots	Licorice root, sweet licorice, sweet wood	Expectorant, demulcent, flavoring agent, rheumatism, prevents cavities, prevents growth of certain cancerous tumors, stabilizes menstrual cycle, antiinflammatory effects	Has expectorant, antitussive, antiinflammatory, and antiallergic properties	Treatment of peptic ulcers, as a cough suppressant and expectorant	Headache, lethargy, sodium/water retention, heart failure, hypertension, cardiac arrest	Avoid in elderly and those with history of cardiovascular disease, kidney or liver problems Do not take longer than 4 to 6 weeks without consulting a health-care professional

178

Herb	Common names	Actions/Uses	Description	Indications	Hepatotoxicity	Comments
Life Root (*Senecio aureus*) entire plan	Ragwort, golden senecio, false valerian, squaw weed, cocash weed, grundy swallow	Emmenagogue, uterine diseases, diaphoretic, diuretic, abortifacient, urinary tract problems, various menstrual problems, expectorant	This drug is not safe to use due to presence of a toxic alkaloid	No information		
Marshmallow root (*Althaea officinalis*) root		Diarrhea, cystitis, demulcent, diuretic, emollient	Inhibits mucociliary activity, stimulates phagocytosis	Inflammation of mucous membranes of mouth and throat, upper respiratory tract and gastrointestinal tract	No known side effects	May delay the absorption of other drugs taken at the same time
Milk Thistle (*Silybum marianum*) fruit (commonly called seeds)	St. Mary's thistle, blessed thistle	Liver protectant, galactogogue, demulcent	Contains silymarin, which exerts a protectant effect on the liver	**Crude drug:** dyspeptic conditions **Preparations:** used as supportive treatment for chronic inflammatory conditions of the liver and liver cirrhosis	No known side effects	
Myrrh (*Commiphora* spp.) oleo-gum resin	Gum myrrh	Astringent, fragrance, antiseptic, carminative, stomachic, asthma, antimicrobial, anticatarrhal, emmenagogue	Mild astringent and antiseptic properties	Inflammation of the gums and mucus membranes of the mouth (gingivitis and stomatitis); pressure spots from prosthesis	No known side effects	Used in commercial mouthwashes, as a fragrance in soaps, cosmetics, perfumes and as a flavoring in food products
Nettle (*Urtica diocia*) above the ground plant, root	Common nettle, stinging nettle, great stinging nettle	Relief of heavy bleeding, endometriosis, cystitis, diuretic, astringent, antiasthmatic, tonic, antirheumatic, hair growth stimulator, treatment of benign prostatic hypertrophy (BPH) (root)	Nettle herb and root have well-established diuretic properties and there is some clinical evidence to support use of the root in the treatment of BPH	Urinary difficulties due to BPH	Local irritation and rash	
Passion flower (*Passiflora incarnata*) flower, fruit top	Maypops, passion vine, purple passion flower	Sedative, hypnotic, decreases muscle tension, relieves headaches, Parkinson's epilepsy, neuralgias, shingles, antispasmodic	Conflicting data exist; plant constituents may have both stimulant and sedative effects	Nervous conditions, mild sleeping problems, gastrointestinal complaints of nervous origin	No information available	
Peppermint (*Mentha piperita*) leaves, flowering tops	Lamb mint, American mint	Stomachic, carminative, flavoring agent, antispasmodic, diaphoretic, antiseptic, analgesic	Direct spasmolytic action on the smooth muscles of digestive tract, carminative, choleretic	Gastrointestinal and biliary complaints	No known side effects	If gallstones present, consult a health care professional prior to use [24]; caution in giving peppermint tea to infants or small children due to possible choking sensation from the menthol [11,20]

Table continued on following page

Table 8–1 *Continued*
Summary of Herbs and Their Properties

COMMON NAME (SCIENTIFIC NAME) PART OF PLANT USED	OTHER NAMES	POPULAR LAYPRESS CLAIMS	SCIENTIFIC INFORMATION			ADDITIONAL COMMENTS/CONTRAINDICATIONS
			Scientific Properties/FDA Approval	German Commission E Recommendations	ADVERSE EFFECTS/WARNINGS	
Psyllium (*Plantago psyllium, P. ovata, Plantago spp.*) seed	Plantago seed	Laxative, decreases blood cholesterol	FDA approved as a laxative; increases intestinal peristalsis	Constipation	Allergic reactions (rare)	Contraindications: intestinal obstruction
Red Raspberry (*Rubus idaeus* or *R. strigosus*) leaves	Wild red raspberry, garden raspberry	Astringent, uterine stimulant, menstrual cramps, antiemetic, laxative, controls frequent and excessive menstrual bleeding	May be effective as an antidiarrheal agent or for use in sore throats but claims have not been substantiated	Therapeutic use of this herb is not advocated due to lack of clinical trials	Avoid in pregnancy—no data on teratogenicity	
Sage (*Salvia officinalis*) leaves	Garden sage	Astringent, antihydrotic, flavoring agent, antispasmodic, relief of hot flashes, dries up mother's milk, epilepsy, insomnia, measles, seasickness, venereal disease, rheumatism	Antiseptic and local antiinflammatory due to the presence of tannins	Mouth wash or gargle for inflammations of mouth and throat; internally for use for digestive complaints and excessive perspiration	Mental and physical deterioration when used for a long period of time in small doses; convulsions and loss of consciousness in larger doses	Despite Commission E recommendations, others question whether sage should be used internally due to possible adverse effects; use as a spice in cooked foods it is likely safe
Sarsaparilla (*Smilax spp.*) roots	Honduras sarsap., Spanish sarsap., Mexican sarsap., Ecuadorian sarsap.	Anabolic steroid, diuretic expectorant, flavoring agent, menstrual stabilizer, carminative, diaphoretic, tonic, rhuematism, colds, fevers	Some evidence to support diuretic, expectorant and laxative effects	No information		Best use of this herb is as a flavoring agent in soft drinks; no anabolic steroid activity
Saw Palmetto (*Serenoa repens*) ripe fruits		Diuretic, BPH, urinary antiseptic, aphrodisiac, gastrointestinal infections, increase breast size, increase sperm production, reverse atrophy of testes and mammary glands	Has antiandrogenic properties and may have antiinflammatory actions; banned as a drug in the United States by the FDA	Treatment of BPH		
Scullcap (*Scutellaria lateriflora*) above the ground plant (may be spelled "skullkap" in the popular press)	Blue skullcap, blue pimpernel, helmet flower, hoodwort, mad-dog weed, sideside-flowering skullcap	Tonic, tranquilizer, antispasmodic, diuretic, rheumatism, neuralgia, delirium tremens, menstrual promoter, effective against rabies, relieves menstrual cramps, epilepsy	No scientific evidence to support claims	No information	Possible hepatotoxicity; hepatotoxicity may be due to adulteration or substitution	Ingestion of this drug should be avoided

Herb	Common names	Actions	FDA status	Uses	Adverse effects	Comments
Senna (*Cassia* spp.) leaflets		Cathartic	FDA approved as a laxative	No information	Diarrhea, nausea	Chronic and/or excessive use of this herb should be avoided
Shepherd's Purse (*Capsella bursa-pastoris*) aerial parts	Cocowort, pickpocket, St. Jame's weed, shepherd's heart	Diuretic, vasoconstrictor, blood pressure stabilizer, excessive menstruation uterine stimulant, astringent	Current information lacking	**Internally:** for treatment of excessive menstruation **Topically:** nose bleeds and bleeding injuries to skin	No known adverse effects	
Slippery Elm (*Ulmus rubra*) inner bark	Red elm	Demulcent, emollient, nutrient, astringent	Declared a safe and effective oral demulcent by the FDA	No information		Available in some commercial throat lozenges
St. John's Wort (*Hypericum perforatum*) leaves, tops	Amber, goatweed, Johnswort, Klamath weed	Antidepressant, antiinflammatory, antidiarrheal, astringent, rheumatism, gout, diuretic, gastritis	Astringent, mild antidepressant effect; possible anti-viral action	**Internally:** depression, anxiety, nervous conditions, dyspepsia complaints **Externally:** contusions, myalgias, first-degree burns	Photosensitization dermatitis	
Valerian (*Valeriana officinalis*) rhizome, roots	Wild valerian, garden heliotrope	Tranquilizer, carminative, antidepressant, hypotensive	Calming and sleep-inducing effects	Effective for treatment of insomnia and restlessness and gastrointestinal cramps		
Witch hazel (*Hamamelis virginiana*) leaves, bark	Snapping hazel, striped alder, tobacco wood, winterbloom	Astringent, hemostatic, sedative, tonic, vaginitis, hemorrhoids, menorrhagia, loss of uterine tone, analgesic astringent, antiinflammatory agent	FDA approved as an astringent	Useful as supportive therapy for acute, nonspecific diarrhea, and inflammation of mouth and gums	Stomach irritation, liver damage (rare)	Astringent activity of hamamelis water due to added alcohol

Used with permission from E.Q. Younghin and D.S. Israel: "A Review and Critique of Common Herbal Alternative Therapies," The Nurse Practitioner 21(10):39–62, 1996. © Springhouse Corporation.

NURSING PROCESS
HERBAL PREPARATION

Assessment

- Obtain baseline information about the client's use of nonconventional therapeutic agents.
- Identify product name, dosage, frequency, side effects, and client's perception of effectiveness.
- Identify all prescription and over-the-counter (OTC) medications taken by client; include dosage, frequency, side effects, and perceived effectiveness.

Potential Nursing Diagnoses

- Knowledge deficit
- Altered nutrition: less than body requirement
- Fatigue

Planning

- Client/family will verbalize an understanding of herbal therapy.
- Client/family will verbalize understanding of prescription and OTC medications.
- Client/family will identify strategies for optimal participation in their therapeutic regimen.
- Client/family will verbalize understanding of interaction between herbal therapy and prescription and OTC medications.

Nursing Interventions

- Monitor the client's response to herbal therapy.
- Monitor client's response to prescription and OTC medications.
- Consult dietitian and other specialists as necessary.
- Continue with same brand of herbal therapy; notify health care provider if considering changing brands/preparations.

Client Teaching

General
- Explain rationale for herbal therapy.
- Instruct client to first notify health care provider before substituting herbal product for prescription or OTC medication.
- Instruct client on need to read labels and heed the recommended information to be displayed on the label.
- Advise client of portion of plant used in preparation (e.g., flower or root).
- Advise client about optimal storage conditions of the herbal remedy.

Diet
- Instruct client about foods that enhance or diminish the action of the specific herbs.
- Instruct client about foods to avoid, if any, while taking herbs.

Side Effects
- Advise client of potential side effects of herbal therapy.
- Advise client of symptoms that require prompt reporting to the health care provider.

Self-Administration
- Instruct client on preparation of special remedies (e.g., steeping of specific teas).

Cultural Considerations

- Assess personal beliefs of clients from different cultures.
- Modify communication to meet client/family cultural needs.
- Communicate respect for client/family culture.
- Evaluate effectiveness of cultural competence in interactions.

Evaluation

- Evaluate the effectiveness of herbal remedies for alleviating symptoms.
- Evaluate client's use of resources.

Table 8-2
Vitamins and Elements Commonly Used with Herbal Therapy

Vitamin B$_6$
Antioxidants
  Vitamin A
  Vitamin C
  Vitamin E
Selenium
Zinc

label would warn against use for more than 7 days and that it is contraindicated at all times in persons with diseases such as diabetes mellitus, glaucoma, and hypertension. Common herbs and toxic effects are listed in Table 8-3.

TIPS FOR CONSUMERS AND HEALTH CARE PROVIDERS

The following are guidelines about prudent use of herbs:

- Do not take herbs if pregnant or attempting to become pregnant.
- Do not take herbs if nursing.
- Do not give herbs to babies or young children.
- Do not take a large quantity of any one herbal preparation.
- Buy only preparations that have the plant and their quantities listed on the packet; there is no guarantee of safety.
- Contact a health care provider *before* stopping a prescription medication.
- Store herbal remedy in a cool, dry, dark place; dark glass containers are preferred.
- Use only herbs that are bought currently and are fresh.

Table 8-3
Common Herbs and Toxic Effects

HERB	POTENTIAL TOXICITY
Adonis vernalis (pheasant's eye)	Sudden heart paralysis
Anemone pulsatilla (pasque flower)	Heart and nervous system damage
Arnica montana (arnica)	Damage to stomach and muscles (safe for external use)
Atropa belladonna (deadly nightshade)	Nervous system depression; respiratory depression
Bryonia dioica (bryony)	Damage to stomach and lungs
Cephaelis ipecacuanha (ipecac)	Violent vomiting
Convallaria majalis (lily-of-the-valley)	Heart and nervous system damage
Datura stramonium (thorn apple)	Nervous system damage; liver damage
Digitalis purpurea (foxglove)	Heart and central nervous system (CNS) damage; potentially lethal
Dryopteris filixmas (male fern)	CNS, eye, and heart damage
Gelsemium sempervirens (yellow jasmine)	Impaired breathing and heart function; loss of consciousness
Hedeoma pulegioides (pennyroyal)	Hepatotoxicity; stomach bleeding; shock; fetal toxicity
Hyoscyamus niger (henbane)	CNS depression, respiratory depression
Pausinystalia yohimbe (yohimbe)	Hypertension; heart damage; CNS damage
Podophyllum peltatum (American mandrake or mayapple)	Stomach damage; immune system damage; teratogenic
Rauwolfia serpentina (Indian snakeroot, rauwolfia)	Depression; sedation; stomach damage; CNS damage
Urginea maritime (squill)	Stomach and kidney damage; CNS damage
Veratrum viride (false hellebore)	Impaired heart and lung function; CNS damage
Viscum album (European mistletoe)	Gastrointestinal bleeding; CNS and heart damage

From Alschuler, L., Benjamin, S., Duke, J., D'Epiro, N. (1997). Herbal medicine: What works, what's safe. Patient Care, 31, 16, p. 49.

• Do *not* delay in seeking care from the health care provider for persisting or severe symptoms.
• Advise against belief in unsubstantiated claims of "miracle cures."

It is essential that both consumers and health care providers become aware of several crucial factors before trying the herbal therapy approach. Alschuler et al. has identified these to include the following:

• Consumers need to think of herbs as medicines; more is not necessarily better.
• Herbs are not placebos.
• Most herbal remedies are less potent than conventional drugs. However, when prescription and OTC drugs with similar actions are combined, there is an increased risk of adverse reactions.
• Results from conventional medicine may come faster.
• Safety, efficacy, and dosage are important; thus, multiple reliable sources should be consulted.

Labeling of the herbal products is an important aspect. The following recommended information should be on the label of herbal products:

• The scientific name of the product and the parts of the plant used in the preparation
• Manufacturer's name and address
• Batch and lot number
• Dates of manufacture and expiration; many products have short half-life

HERBAL RESOURCES

American Herbal Pharmacopeia
  P. O. Box 5159
  Santa Cruz, CA 95061
  (408) 461-6317
  E-mail: Herbal@got.net
United States Pharmacopeia
  12601 Twinbrook Parkway
  Rockville, MD 20852
  (301) 816-8250
American Botanical Council
  P. O. Box 201660
  Austin, TX 78720
  amebotcncl@aol.com
  http://www.herbalgram.org
Natural Health Village (legislative issues)
  http://www.netvillage.com/
The Alternative Medicine Home Page
  http://www.pitt.edu/~cbw/atlm.html
The U. S. Department of Agriculture
Agricultural Genome Information System
  http://probe.nalusda.gov

SUMMARY

Herbal medicine is the most widely used and oldest medicine throughout the world. Currently, there is no pressure from the U.S. government for quality control of herbal products. Hence, the buyer needs to be informed before purchasing the products and needs to deal only with reputable dealers. It is important that the client/family/consumer share with the health care provider use of herbal products in order that the optimal therapeutic plan can be implemented.

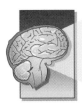

Critical Thinking in Action

A. B., a 49-year-old female accountant, reports periods of feeling tired that are increasing in frequency and intensity. On her health history she lists "no medications on a regular basis." During the nursing history you learn that she takes ginseng, ginkgo biloba 300 mg b.i.d., and licorice root 2 mg b.i.d. for the past 6 months. Occasionally she takes St. John's wort extract 300 mg t.i.d.

1. Is A. B. taking the recommended dose of ginseng and gingko biloba? If not, what modifications would you suggest that she consider?
2. A. B. tells you that she has arthritis. What modifications would be appropriate based on this new information?
3. What specific client teaching is appropriate for A. B. at this time?

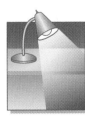

Study Questions

1. What is the most authoritative source for therapeutic substances?

2. What group was responsible for more than 300 therapeutic monographs between 1978 and 1993 and disbanded because of a lack of citations?

3. The Dietary Supplement Heath and Education Act of 1994 classified herbal remedies as what?

4. Can herbal remedies make claims about prevention or curing specific conditions?

Identify a common herb that best matches each of the following descriptions:

5. Serotonin antagonist for relief of migraine headache. Requires refrigeration.

6. Most commonly prescribed herbal remedy used in the treatment of dementia syndromes, vertigo, and tinnitus for up to 90 days.

7. Has at least 10 pharmacologically active components for the relief of depression and anxiety. Users do/do not need to avoid tyramine-rich foods?

8. Ephedra, ma huang, may be used as an energy booster or for weight loss. What are two reported adverse effects.?

9. List at least three recommended pieces of information for labels on herbal products.

10. What are five important areas of client teaching related to herbal therapy. Describe at least one specific suggestion for each area.

9

Drug Therapy Considerations Throughout the Life Span

Objectives

- Apply principles of pharmacokinetics of children to drug dosage and dosing interval.
- Explain drug dosage parameters for children and where dose ranges can be found.
- Explain the pharmacokinetics of the older adult (elderly) related to drug dosage.
- List reasons for noncompliance to drug regimen in the older adult.
- Give nursing implications related to drug therapy in children and the older adult.

Terms

compliance
noncompliance

older adult
pharmacodynamics

pharmacokinetics

GENERAL INTRODUCTION

Drug dosages are adjusted according to the client's age, weight, serum protein, and adipose tissue. Change in drug therapy is needed for low-birth-weight infants, newborns, infants, and older adults. A client's body water, fat, and protein are factors that need to be considered when determining drug dosage for the young and the old. Because of immature organs (infants) and declining organ functions (older adult), the effect of drug therapy should be closely monitored to prevent the risk of adverse reactions to drugs and possible drug toxicity.

Drug therapy changes throughout the life span, beginning with the infant and continuing through to the frail older adult. Traditionally, drug therapy focused on the middle-aged adult, but emphasis needs to be placed on the growing population of older adults. This chapter describes the physiologic changes, pharmacokinetics, and pharmacodynamics for drug therapy, bearing in mind these two ends of the continuum.

PEDIATRIC PHARMACOLOGY

Introduction

The majority of drugs administered to adults are also useful for children; however, the dosages are different. Drug doses for children may be adjusted according to the adult drug dose formula. Usually, a child's dose is calculated according to body weight or body surface area. Children's dosages are based on the maturation of the functions of the body's organs, body weight, and body surface area. Neonates (<1 month old) and infants (1 month to 1 year old) have alkaline gastric juices and immature liver and kidneys, which cause a decrease in the metabolism and excretion of drugs. The liver and kidneys mature by the age of 1 year, and the pH of gastric juices decreases to that of the normal adult level of pH 1 to 2.5 by the age of 3 years.

For some drugs used for children, the drug dosage is based on age. Fluoroquinolones or quinolones are potent antibacterials and should be avoided for children younger than 17 years of age because of their effect on skeletal bone growth. Verapamil, a calcium channel blocker or antagonist, should not be administered to children younger than 1 year of age because acute cardiorespiratory failure may occur. Adenosine is considered a safer drug for infants and children than verapamil. Valproic acid, an anticonvulsant, should not be given to a child 2 years of age or younger. Hepatic toxicity is a serious adverse reaction of valproic acid (Table 9–1).

Table 9–1
Selected Drugs to Avoid in Children Based on Age

DRUG	AGE TO AVOID DRUGS	POSSIBLE EFFECTS
Fluoroquinolones	<17 y	Less skeletal bone growth
Verapamil	<1 y	Acute cardiorespiratory failure
Valproic acid	<2 y	Hepatic toxicity

Pharmacokinetics

Pharmacokinetics in children differs from that of adults. Selection of drug dose and dosing interval is based on the effects of absorption, blood volume distribution, protein binding, drug metabolism, and drug elimination in children. Table 9–2 identifies the pharmacokinetics in infants and children. In infants (<1 year old), drug effects can be increased because of their immature renal and liver function. Drug response can be prolonged for the same reason. Drug levels decline more slowly in infants than adults; this is especially true for drugs given intravenously. In infants, drugs remain above the minimum effective concentration (MEC) levels longer than in adults. Also, drug effects and responses are more increased in low-birthweight infants than in average birthweight infants. As the child develops, the response to the medication is more similar to that of the adult; however, drug dosages differ from those of adults and need to be closely calculated and monitored.

Pediatric dose ranges (parameters) have been established for many drugs, and the ranges are reported in drug references such as the *Physicians' Desk Reference (PDR), American Hospital Formulary,* and drug handbooks. The nurse should check the dose ranges and specifically question those doses that are outside the range. Body weight and body surface area are the two most commonly used methods for calculating infants' and children's dosages (see Chapter 4F for drug calculations).

Pharmacodynamics

The immaturity of the organs in newborns and infants affects drug action, and drug dosage frequently needs to be adjusted accordingly. Receptor site sensitivity differs with the neonate, infant, and young child, so drug dosing may need to be decreased or increased.

Table 9–2
Pharmacokinetics in Infants and Children

PHASES	BODY EFFECTS AND POSSIBLE DRUG RESPONSES
Absorption	Reduced gastric acid production; gastric pH is higher than in adults. Drugs such as penicillin are absorbed poorly in a low gastric pH. Smaller drug dose may be required.
	Slow gastric emptying time due to a slow or irregular peristalsis may slow drug absorption. Drugs given orally usually take longer to reach peak plasma levels. Adults and older children have a faster absorption rate.
	First-pass elimination by the liver is reduced. More drug is available for distribution; thus, a smaller drug dose is required for those drugs with an extensive hepatic first-pass. Topical drugs may be absorbed faster than in adults because infants have a proportionally greater body surface area. In addition, their skin is thin and drugs pass through more readily. The increased systemic absorption could result in adverse effects. Steroid creams for dermatitis should be used sparingly.
Distribution	Infants and children have lower blood pressure, which affects blood flow to tissues. The liver and brain are proportionally larger and receive more blood flow; the kidneys receive less.
	Infants are composed of 65% to 75% water; premature infants are 85% water. Water-soluble drugs are diluted in the large volume of their body fluid. Because of drug dilution from the large volume of water, a larger drug dose is needed to achieve the desired plasma drug level.
	Since infants have decreased plasma protein-binding sites, lower doses are needed. With fewer available binding sites, there is more free drug. The serum albumin level is lower in infants. Protein-binding capacity usually is not the same as the adult until age 1. Drug doses should be decreased with most antibiotics, including cephalosporins and sulfonamides, as well as with phenobarbital and theophylline. All drugs should be checked for recommended pediatric dose range.
	The blood–brain barrier is not completely developed in the infant, so more drug passes into the cerebral cells.
Metabolism or biotransformation	There is a decreased activity of liver enzymes due to the immaturity of the infant liver; thus, the hepatic metabolism of drugs in infants is low until the age of 1. The half-life of drug may be more prolonged than it would be in an older child or adult; therefore, drug accumulation can occur. Drug dosage and dosing intervals should be considered when drug dosing for infants.
	Drug half-life in the older child can be shorter due to the increased metabolic rate. Higher doses for the older child might be needed to offset the increased metabolic rate.
Excretion	Drug elimination via the kidneys is decreased until after the first year of life. Blood flow volume through the kidneys is less than in adults, and the glomerular filtration rate is approximately 30% to 40% of the adult rate. A decrease in drug excretion leads to a longer half-life of the drug and possible drug toxicity. Many of the antibiotics and analgesics are slowly excreted. Children have a decreased ability to concentrate urine. Renal excretion of a drug is the net effect of glomerular filtration, active tubular secretion, and passive tubular reabsorption. In the presence of renal disease, a child may be unable to excrete a drug, leading to drug accumulation and possible toxicity.
	In childhood, the serum creatinine is less than the adult, <0.081 mg/dL. This is because of a lower muscle mass in children. Creatinine clearance test (estimated if necessary) is a better indicator of renal function.

Some drugs, such as aspirin, morphine, and phenobarbital, are more toxic to children than to adults. Likewise, other drugs have either the same effect or are less toxic than in adults. These include atropine, codeine, digoxin, meperidine (Demerol), and phenylephrine.

The rapidly developing tissues of infants and small children can be more sensitive to certain drugs. Tetracycline given during the last trimester of pregnancy and through early childhood (to age 8 years), can cause permanent discoloration of the teeth. Corticosteroid therapy given to the young child can result in suppression of growth. The child's height should be measured and his or her weight monitored. A dehydrated child runs the risk of development of toxic accumulations of drugs.

Figure 9–1 shows two 7-year-olds playing "dress up."

NURSING PROCESS
PEDIATRICS

Assessment

- Record the height, weight, and age of the child. Drug calculations are based on these three factors.

Potential Nursing Diagnoses

- Altered growth and development
- Altered (possible) tissue perfusion
- Altered patterns of urinary elimination
- Knowledge deficit

Planning

- The child receives drug dosage based on age, weight, and height. Most drug calculations for children are related to weight in kilograms or body surface area (BSA) (see Chapter 4F).

Nursing Interventions

- Use appropriate drug references to obtain the drug parameters or ranges, side effects, and contraindications for use of the drug when administering drugs to children.
- Monitor infants closely for side effects of drugs because of their immature liver and kidneys. Because infants and young children have limited communication skills, changes in their usual behavior pattern may be indicative of side effects.
- Communicate with the health care provider about drug dosages that are questionable for infants because of the drug's prolonged half-life and the infant's decreased drug excretion.
- Calculate the child's drug dose according to weight in kilograms or body surface area.

Client Teaching

- Instruct the responsible family member not to give over-the-counter (OTC) drugs to children without asking the health care provider.
- Instruct the family member to report side effects of the medication immediately to the health care provider.
- Advise mothers who are breastfeeding their newborn or infant to avoid taking OTC drugs or another person's medication because a portion of most drugs is excreted in breast milk.
- Advise the family member to keep medications out of reach of children.
- Instruct the family member to use child-resistant medication containers.

Evaluation

- Evaluate the family member's knowledge concerning the drug, drug dosage, schedule for drug administration, and side effects.
- Evaluate the child's physiologic and psychological response to the drug regimen.

GERIATRIC PHARMACOLOGY

Introduction

Twelve percent of the population is represented by persons older than 65 years of age, but this age group consumes approximately 25% of all medications. It is projected that, by the year 2005 older adults will con- stitute 18% of the population and will consume 40% of all medications.

Approximately 70% of clients older than 65 years of age take at least one prescribed drug yearly. **Older adults** take over-the-counter (OTC) drugs more frequently than the general population. About 15% of clients older than age 65, at the time of hospital admission, are not taking any medications. During hos-

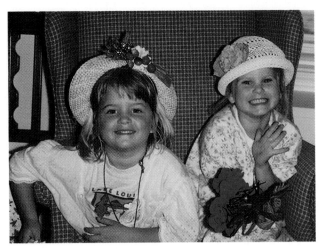

Figure 9–1
What special concerns related to medications may a caregiver of these two 7-year-olds playing "dress up" need to consider?

Table 9–3 Physiologic Changes in the Older Adult	
SYSTEM	**PHYSIOLOGIC CHANGE**
Gastrointestinal	↑ pH (alkaline) gastric secretions ↓ peristalsis with delayed intestinal emptying time
Cardiac and circulatory	↓ cardiac output ↓ blood flow
Hepatic	↓ enzyme function ↓ blood flow
Renal	↓ blood flow ↓ functioning nephrons (kidney cells) ↓ glomerular filtration rate

KEY: ↓ : *decrease,* ↑ : *increase*

pitalization, older adults take an average of three to five drugs. At the time of discharge from the hospital, approximately 30% of older adults are given three to five drug prescriptions. One-third of clients in nursing homes receive six to 12 drugs daily. Figure 9–2 shows a client with a "handful" of drugs.

The adverse reactions and drug interactions that occur in the older adult are three to seven times greater than those for middle-aged and young adults. Older adults consume numerous drugs because of chronic and multiple illnesses; they are, therefore, susceptible to adverse reactions and interactions. Additional problems that can cause adverse reactions from drugs include self-medication with OTC drugs, taking drugs that were prescribed for other health problems, consuming drugs ordered by several different health care providers, overdosing when symptoms do not subside, using drugs that were pre-

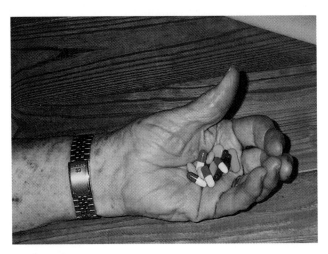

Figure 9–2
Does the client know what the medications are for and are they all necessary?

scribed for another person and, of course, the ongoing physiologic aging process.

Drug toxicity may develop in the older adult for drug doses that are within therapeutic range for the average adult. These therapeutic drug ranges are usually safe for young and middle-aged adults but are not always within safe range for older adults. It has been suggested for the elderly that the drug dose should initially be at a low to low average therapeutic range and then be gradually increased according to tolerance and lack of adverse reactions. This allows the older adult to avoid having a toxic reaction to the drug.

Physiologic Changes

The physiologic changes associated with the aging process have a major effect on drug therapy. Table 9–3 describes the physiologic changes occurring in the gastrointestinal (GI), cardiac and circulatory, hepatic (liver), and renal (kidney) systems of the older adult and how these changes can affect pharmacologic response to drug therapy.

Pharmacokinetics

Pharmacokinetic parameters for the older adult are described in Table 9–4.

ABSORPTION

Drug absorption from the GI tract is slowed in the older adult because of a decrease in blood flow and decrease in GI motility. In the older adult, acidic drugs are poorly absorbed because of their alkaline gastric secretions. Drugs remain in the GI tract because there is a decrease in gastric motility. However,

Table 9–4
Pharmacokinetics in Geriatrics

PHASES	BODY EFFECTS AND POSSIBLE DRUG RESPONSES
Absorption	A decrease in gastric acidity (increased gastric pH) alters absorption of weak acid drugs, such as aspirin.
	A decrease in blood flow to the gastrointestinal tract (40%–50% less) is due to a decrease in cardiac output. Because of the reduction of blood flow, absorption is slowed but not decreased.
	A reduction in gastrointestinal motility rate (peristalsis) may delay onset of action.
	A reduction in gastric emptying time.
Distribution	Due to a decrease in body water in the older adult, water-soluble drugs are more concentrated. There is an increase in fat-to-water ratio in the older adult; fat-soluble drugs are stored and are likely to accumulate.
	Older adults have a decrease in circulating serum protein. The two most common proteins are albumin and alpha$_1$ acid glycoprotein. Acidic drugs (e.g., nonsteroidal antiinflammatory drugs [NSAIDs] including aspirin, benzodiazepines, phenytoin, and warfarin) bind to albumin, and the basic drugs (e.g., beta-adrenergic blockers, tricyclic antidepressants, lidocaine) bind to alpha$_1$ acid glycoprotein. With fewer protein-binding sites, there is more free drug. It is the free, unbound drug that is available to body tissue at receptor sites.
	Drugs with a high affinity for protein, >90%, compete for protein-binding sites with other drugs. Drug interactions result due to a lack of protein sites and an increase in free drugs.
Metabolism	In the older adult, there is a decrease in hepatic enzyme production, hepatic blood flow, and total liver function. These decreases cause a reduction in drug metabolism.
	With a reduction in metabolic rate, the half-life (t½) of drugs increases, and drug accumulation can result. Metabolism of a drug inactivates the drug and drug metabolite and prepares it for elimination via the kidneys.
	When drug clearance by the liver is decreased, the drug half-life (t½) is prolonged, and when drug clearance is increased, the drug half-life is shortened. With prolonged t½, drug accumulation can result and drug toxicity could occur.
Excretion	The older adult has a decrease in renal blood flow and a decrease in glomerular filtration rate of 40%–50%. With a decrease in renal function, there is a decrease in drug excretion, and drug accumulation results. Drug toxicity should be assessed continually while the client is on the drug.

the absorption amount of an oral dose is not affected by age.

DISTRIBUTION

The elderly have a loss of protein-binding sites for drugs, which causes increased circulation of free drug and increased chance for adverse drug reaction. During the aging process, there is a loss of body water, thus, water-soluble drugs become more concentrated in the body. Because of an increase in body fat in the elderly, the lipid-soluble drugs are absorbed into the fat, causing a decrease in desired drug effects.

METABOLISM OR BIOTRANSFORMATION

Hepatic blood flow in the older adult may be decreased by 40% to 45%. Also, there is a decrease in liver size with age. Drug clearance by hepatic metabolism is affected more in older male adults than in female adults.

Liver dysfunction caused by the aging process de-

creases enzyme function, which decreases the liver's ability to metabolize and detoxify drugs, increasing the risk of drug toxicity.

The liver, as well as the kidneys, is a major organ responsible for drug clearance from the body. *Biotransformation* refers to drug metabolism that occurs in the liver (hepatic cells) and contributes to the clearance of drugs. Biotransformation can occur either in phase I by oxidation reaction or in phase II by conjugation reaction. The hepatic microsomal enzymes are responsible for phase I, oxidation reaction. The hepatic microsomal oxidation can be impaired by the aging process, liver diseases (cirrhosis, hepatitis), and drugs that reduce oxidation capability. Drug clearance by the liver is then reduced. An example of a drug that undergoes a phase I biotransformation oxidation reaction is diazepam (Valium). Diazepam is biotransformed to its active metabolites, desmethyldiazepam. In the elderly, the plasma–serum diazepam level would remain high because of an impaired phase I oxidation reaction. Other drugs that are biotransformed by phase I include barbiturates, codeine, ibuprofen, phenytoin, meperidine, lidocaine, certain benzodiazepines (alprazolam, flurazepam, midazolam, prazepam), and warfarin (Coumadin).

Phase II of biotransformation involves the conjugation or attachment of the drug to an inactive state. The hepatic conjugation is usually *not* influenced by older age, liver diseases, or drug interaction, so the drug is inactivated and excreted in the urine. Examples of drugs that are biotransformed or metabolized by phase II are aspirin, acetaminophen, certain benzodiazepines (lorazepam, oxazepam, temazepam), procainamide, and sulfanilamide. The benzodiazepines lorazepam, oxazepam, and temazepam that undergo conjugation reaction do not have active metabolites. The drug metabolic process, phase I or II, for drug clearance for the elderly client is an important consideration with drug selection.

To assess liver function, the liver enzymes need to be checked. Elevated levels indicate possible liver dysfunction. However, normal liver enzyme results may not indicate normal drug metabolism. The elderly could have normal liver function test results and still have impaired hepatic microsomal enzyme–drug oxidation reactions.

EXCRETION

Cardiac output and blood flow throughout the circulatory system is decreased, affecting blood flow to the liver and kidneys. After the age of 65 years, nephron function may be decreased by 35%, and after the age of 70 years, blood flow to the kidneys may be decreased by 40%.

Kidney function is assessed by monitoring urine output, laboratory values of blood urea nitrogen (BUN) and serum creatinine (Cr), and the creatinine clearance (Cl_{cr} or CrCl) test (estimated). Creatinine clearance is an indicator of glomerular filtration rate (GFR). To evaluate renal function based on serum creatinine alone may not be accurate for the elderly because of the decrease in the older adult's muscle mass. Creatinine is a byproduct of muscle catabolism; however, creatinine is primarily excreted by the kidneys. A decrease in muscle mass can cause a decrease in serum creatinine. With elderly clients, serum creatinine may be within normal values because of lack of muscle mass, but still there could be a decrease in renal function. With the young or middle-aged adult, serum creatinine would be increased with a decrease in renal function.

The 24-hour creatinine clearance test and the serum creatinine level should be used to evaluate renal function. If a 24-hour creatinine clearance (Cl_{cr}, CrCl) test is not feasible, there are formulas that can be used to estimate Cl_{cr} result such as:

$$Cl_{cr}(\text{males}) = \frac{(140 - \text{age}) \times \text{kg}}{72 \times \text{serum Cr level}} = \text{mL/min}$$

$$Cl_{cr}(\text{females}) = \text{value of males} \times 0.85 = \text{mL/min}$$

The normal creatinine clearance value for an adult is 80 to 130 mL/min.

With liver and kidney dysfunction, the efficacy of a drug dose is usually reduced. Multiple drug use may intensify drug effect in the older adult. When the efficiency of the hepatic and renal systems is reduced, the half-life of the drug is prolonged and drug toxicity is probable.

Factors contributing to adverse reactions in the older adult include a loss of protein-binding sites, which increases the amount of free circulating drug; a decline in hepatic first-pass metabolism; and a prolonged half-life of the drug because of decreased liver and kidney function. The time interval between doses of a drug may need to be increased for the older client.

Pharmacodynamics

Pharmacodynamics refers to how a drug interacts at the receptor site or at the target organ. Because there is a lack of affinity to receptor sites throughout the body in the older adult, the pharmacodynamic response may be altered. The older adult could be more or less sensitive to drug action because of age-related changes in the central nervous system, changes in the number of drug receptors, and changes in the affinity of receptors to drugs. Frequently, the drug dose needs to be lowered. Changes in organ functions are important to consider in drug dosing.

With the older adult, the compensatory response to physiologic changes is decreased. When a drug with vasodilator properties is administered and the sympathetic feedback does not occur quickly, orthostatic hypotension (rapid decrease in blood pressure when standing up quickly) could result. In the younger adult, the sympathetic response of vasoconstriction "kicks in" to avert a severe hypotensive effect.

Effects of Selected Drugs on Older Adults

Hypnotics, diuretics and antihypertensives, cardiac glycosides, anticoagulants, antibacterials (antibiotics), GI drugs (antiulcer, laxatives), antidepressants, and narcotic analgesics are drug categories for which drug effects on the elderly are possible. The number of drugs taken, drug interactions (see Chapter 7), and physical health of the elderly (cardiac, renal, and hepatic function) are factors associated with drug effects in the elderly population. Drug selection is extremely important. Drugs with a shorter half-life are less likely to cause problems as a result of drug accumulation than drugs with a long half-life. If severe side effects occur, the drug with a shorter half-life is eliminated more quickly than the drug with a longer half-life.

Drugs that are classified as phase II biotransformation are tolerated and eliminated more quickly than those that are from phase I (oxidation). If phase I drugs are used, the drug selection should be from those agents that have fewer active metabolites. Evaluation of hepatic and renal functions is imperative, especially if the older adult is taking multiple drugs. When side effects and adverse reactions occur, prescription and nonprescription drugs should be assessed.

HYPNOTICS

Insomnia is a frequently occurring problem for the older adult. Sedatives/hypnotics are the second most common group of drugs prescribed or taken OTC. Insomnia may be described as having difficulty in falling asleep, frequent awakenings during the night, or early morning awakenings with difficulty in falling back to sleep. Types of hypnotics differ according to the cause of insomnia. There are five benzodiazepine hypnotics (flurazepam, quazepam, temazepam, triazolam, and estazolam) that have been approved by the Food and Drug Administration (FDA) as hypnotics to control insomnia. For the elderly client, low doses of benzodiazepines with short or immediate action or half-lives usually are prescribed. Short-term therapy is suggested. Usually, benzodiazepines are prescribed at higher doses for sedative/hypnotic effects and at lower doses for the antianxiety effect. Approximately 35% of the older adult population takes a hypnotic.

Flurazepam HCl (Dalmane), the first benzodiazepine hypnotic, was introduced in 1970. It has three metabolites; thus, it is considered to be a short- and long-acting hypnotic. Its principal metabolite is desalkylflurazepam, which is long-acting, has a long half-life, and is slowly eliminated. This drug is not suggested for persons older than age 65. Drug hangover is a problem. Quazepam (Doral) has similar effects as flurazepam. It is a precursor of desalkylflurazepam and has a prolonged half-life.

Temazepam (Restoril) was introduced in 1981. It is biotransformed in the liver by conjugation and not by oxidation; thus, it is prescribed frequently for the elderly client. Its principal metabolite, glucuronide, is conjugated with no pharmacologic effects and is excreted in the urine. Temazepam is slowly absorbed, so it should be taken 1 to 2 h before bedtime. It is classified as an intermediate-acting benzodiazepine. Food delays its action. Temazepam is more effective for frequent awakenings during the night than for those who have a problem falling asleep.

Triazolam (Halcion) is an intermediate-acting benzodiazepine. It has a short half-life and is considered safe for the older adult at low doses (0.0625 to 0.125 mg). It is metabolized by hepatic microsomal oxidation, although the drug does differ from oxidized benzodiazepines. Triazolam helps with falling asleep and it also decreases frequent awakenings during the night. When stopping the drug, doses should be tapered rather than abruptly discontinued to avoid rebound insomnia. Estazolam is a new benzodiazepine. It is an intermediate- to long-acting drug. It is metabolized in the liver to two metabolites that are not highly potent.

Other benzodiazepines, lorazepam and oxazepam, can be used for insomnia. These agents have an intermediate half-life and should be taken 1 hour before bedtime. Other benzodiazepines are more effective as anxiolytics than as hypnotics.

DIURETICS AND ANTIHYPERTENSIVES

Diuretics are frequently prescribed for treatment of hypertension or congestive heart failure (CHF). For the older adult, the dose is usually reduced because of dose-related side effects. Hydrochlorothiazide (HydroDIURIL) is prescribed in low doses of 12.5 mg. Doses of 25 to 50 mg daily with chronic use can cause electrolyte imbalances (hypokalemia, hyponatremia, hypomagnesemia, hypercalcemia), hyperglycemia, hyperuricemia, and hypercholesterolemia.

Many older adults are hypertensive (blood pressure >140/90 mmHg). Nonpharmacologic methods are suggested (see Chapter 39), such as exercise, weight reduction if obese, reduction of salt intake and alcohol, and adequate rest. It could reduce the systolic and diastolic pressures by 8 to 10 mmHg. Drugs such as diuretics, beta-adrenergic blockers or antagonists, calcium channel blockers, angiotensin-converting (ACE) inhibitors, and centrally acting alpha₂ agonists are used as antihypertensive drugs. Calcium blockers and ACE inhibitors are frequently the agents of choice because of their low incidence of electrolyte imbalance and CNS side effects. Usually, antihypertensive dosing for the elderly begins with reduced doses that are gradually increased according to need, tolerance, and adverse reactions. Alpha₁ blockers or antagonists (prazosin, terazosin) and centrally acting alpha₂ agonists (methyldopa, clonidine, guanabenz, guanfacine) infrequently are prescribed for elderly clients because of their adverse reactions, such as orthostatic hypotension.

CARDIAC GLYCOSIDES

Digoxin is not always prescribed for long-term use because of its narrow therapeutic range (0.5 to 2 ng/mL) and the possibility of digitalis toxicity occurring. It is given for left ventricular failure, chronic atrial fibrillation, and for atrial tachycardia.

Its half-life is doubled (70 h) in clients who are older than 80 years of age. Most of the digoxin is eliminated by the kidneys, so a decline in kidney function (decreased GFR) could cause digoxin accumulation. With close monitoring of serum digoxin levels, creatinine clearance test, and vital signs (pulse should *not* be less than 60 bpm), digoxin is considered to be safe for the elderly.

ANTICOAGULANTS

Bleeding may occur with chronic use of anticoagulants for elderly clients. Warfarin (Coumadin) is 99% protein-bound; with a decrease in serum albumin, which is common among older adults, there is an increase in free, unbound circulating warfarin. There is a potential risk for bleeding. Elderly clients should have their prothrombin time (PT) or international normalized ratio (INR) checked periodically and the nurse should check for signs of bleeding.

ANTIBACTERIALS

Penicillins, cephalosporins, tetracyclines, and sulfonamides are considered to be safe for the elderly. If the elderly client has a decrease in renal drug clearance and the drug has a prolonged half-life, there should be a reduction of drug dose. Aminoglycosides, fluoroquinolones (quinolones), and vancomycin are excreted in the urine. These drug agents are not frequently prescribed for clients older than 75 years and, if they are prescribed, the drug dose is usually reduced.

GASTROINTESTINAL DRUGS

Histamine$_2$ (H$_2$) blockers and sucralfate are safer drugs than other antiulcer agents for the treatment of peptic ulcers. Cimetidine (Tagamet) was the first H$_2$ blocker or antagonist and is not suggested for the older adult because of its side effects and multiple potential drug interactions. Ranitidine, famotidine, and nizatidine may be prescribed for the elderly client instead of cimetidine.

Laxatives are frequently taken by the elderly. In long-term facilities such as nursing homes, 75% of the elderly clients take laxatives on a daily basis. Fluid and electrolyte imbalances may occur with excessive use. Increased GI motility with laxative use could decrease other drug absorptions. Nonpharmacologic measures should be encouraged, such as increasing fluid intake, consuming fiber foods such as prunes, and exercising.

ANTIDEPRESSANTS

The antidepressant drug dose for the older adult is normally 30% to 50% of the dose for the young and middle-aged adults. Drug dose should be gradually increased according to the client's tolerance and the desired therapeutic effect. There should be close monitoring for possible adverse reactions.

The tricyclic antidepressants are effective for the elderly client. They do have anticholinergic properties that can cause the following side effects: dry mouth, tachycardia, constipation, and urinary retention; they also can contribute to narrow-angle glaucoma. Fluoxetine, a bicyclic antidepressant, has fewer side effects than the tricyclics; the side effects are mostly dose-related. The monoamine oxidase (MAO) inhibitors are not often prescribed for the elderly because of their adverse reactions, such as drug–food interactions, which could result in hypertensive crisis and severe orthostatic hypotension (see Chapter 19).

NARCOTIC ANALGESICS

Narcotics when taken by the older adult can cause dose-related adverse reactions. Hypotension and respiratory depression may result from narcotic use.

Table 9–5
Noncompliance to Drug Regimen in the Older Adult

CAUSES	NURSING ACTIONS
Taking too many medications at different times (see Fig. 9–2)	Develop a chart indicating times to take drugs. Provide space to place a mark for each drug taken. Use an organizer device to mark with days and weeks.
Failure to understand the purpose or reason for drug	Explain the purpose, drug action, and importance of the medications. Provide time for questions and reinforcement. Reinforce with written information.
Impaired memory	Encourage family members or friends to monitor drug regimen.
Decreased mobility and dexterity	Advise family members or friends to have drugs and water or other fluid accessible. Assist older adult as needed.
Visual and hearing disturbances	Suggest eye and ear examinations (glasses or hearing aids).
Diminished finances	Contact the social services department of your institution.
Child-resistant drug bottles	Ensure that client has access to medications as appropriate.
Side effects or adverse reactions from the drug	Educate client and family about side effects to report to health care provider.

Close monitoring of vital signs is important while the elderly client is taking narcotic analgesics.

Noncompliance

Noncompliance with a drug regimen is a problem in all client categories, but especially with the older adult. Frequently, the older adult fails to ask questions during interactions with health care providers. Noncompliance can cause underdosing or overdosing that could be harmful to the elderly client's health. Some of the reasons for noncompliance are listed in Table 9–5.

Working with the older adult is an ongoing nursing responsibility. The nurse should plan strategies with the older adult and family or friends to encourage **compliance.** Daily contact with the client may be necessary at first. Mere ordering of medication does not mean that the client is able to get the drugs or is taking them correctly. Figure 9–3 shows the different medications to be taken by a client at different times; this complicated array of drugs can result in confusion and noncompliance. Older adults many times do not have the insurance to pay for medications and choose buying food instead of medications. Some older adults delay purchasing or never purchase the drugs. The older adult is more apt to experience serious side effects from drug administration than the

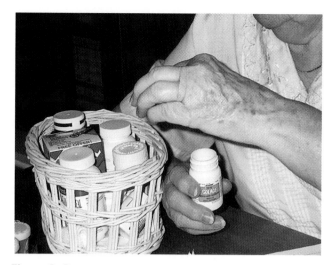

Figure 9–3
A possible cause of noncompliance in an elderly client is the need to take many different medications at different times.

young or middle-aged adult. If a drug such as ibuprofen (Motrin) is irritating to the GI tract, the older adult frequently will *not* take the drug. However, another drug, such as magnesium hydroxide (Maalox), may be given before the ibuprofen dose to decrease the side effects. Food can also decrease gastric irritation from ibuprofen.

NURSING PROCESS
GERIATRICS

Assessment

- Assess the older adult's sensorium or mental awareness. Is the person confused or disoriented? Is this state transitory?
- Obtain a history of kidney, liver, or GI disorder, and determine whether eyesight is failing. Kidney or liver disorders can cause a decrease in the function of these organs and can increase the half-life of drugs. Longer drug half-life and frequent drug dosing can result in drug toxicity. Assess the older adult's use of eyeglasses and check the date of the last eye examination.
- Determine whether the older person is taking OTC drugs, how often, and for what length of time. Specifically ask about laxatives and antacids, which can affect gastric pH, electrolyte balance, and GI motility; many people do not think of these agents as drugs. Remind the older adult or the family to tell the pharmacist about prescribed drugs when contemplating the purchase of OTC preparations.
- Assess for compliance of taking drugs correctly and reasons for noncompliance.

Potential Nursing Diagnoses

- Perceived constipation
- Urinary retention related to drug therapy
- Nutrition, altered: less than body requirements
- Altered health maintenance
- Knowledge deficit
- Noncompliance

Nursing Process continued on following page

Planning

- The older adult will take the prescribed medications as ordered.
- The drug therapy will be effective with no or few side effects.

Nursing Interventions

- Monitor the older adult's laboratory results in relationship to kidney and liver function. Are the BUN and serum creatinine levels within normal range (reference values)? Are the liver enzymes within normal range? Discuss the findings with the health care provider.
- Check the older adult's serum drug levels as ordered and report abnormal findings to the charge nurse or health care provider. Because of their reduced body water, elderly persons taking water-soluble drugs such as digoxin are likely to have higher blood levels.
- Communicate with the pharmacist or health care provider when the drug dose is in question. Check drug reference books for recommended drug doses for older adults.
- Observe the client for adverse reactions when multiple drugs are being taken. An older adult with hypertension and a failing heart (CHF) might be taking a diuretic (hydrochlorothiazide [HydroDIURIL]) and digoxin. The diuretic may cause potassium loss and, if potassium replacement is not ordered, digitalis toxicity may occur. Hypokalemia (low serum potassium) enhances the action of digoxin, causing the toxicity. The symptoms of digitalis toxicity may be a slow or irregular pulse rate (bradycardia, <60 bpm), nausea and vomiting, and blurred vision.
- Recognize a change in usual behavior or an increase in confusion associated with the drug regimen. Report these changes to the nurse or health care provider. In the elderly, who have possible decreases in cognitive ability, drug reactions and side effects may be difficult to detect. Communication skills may be poor.

Client Teaching

- Review the medications with the older adult and the family, including the reason for the medication, its route of administration, how often it is to be taken, common side effects, and when to notify the health care provider. Figures 9–4 and 9–5 show a client being instructed on drug use and how to keep a drug record.
- Explain to the older adult or the family the importance of compliance with the drug regimen. Emphasize taking the drug as prescribed, discarding unused or old drugs, and keeping a record of medication taken for reference. REMEMBER: the drugs are the property of the client and may not be disposed of without his or her permission.
- Be available to answer the client's questions. Be supportive of the older adult and the family. Discuss problems related to the medications.

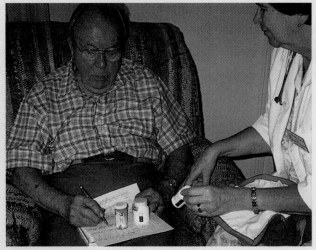

Figure 9–4
An older adult being instructed as to when medications should be taken.

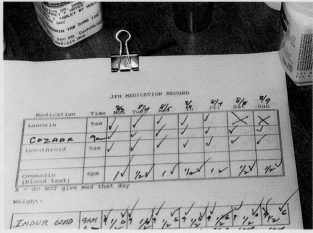

Figure 9–5
Keeping a medication record of drugs and when they are taken increases drug compliance.

Nursing Process continued on following page

Evaluation

- Evaluate the older adult's compliance to the drug regimen, and answer any questions the older adult may have.
- Evaluate the drug effect and the lack of side effects or adverse reactions.

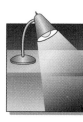

Study Questions

1. Are infants and children small adults? Explain. What are drug dose parameters for children and where can that information be obtained?

2. If a water-soluble drug is given to an infant, should the drug dose be increased or decreased? Explain.

3. Do infants have an increased or decreased number of protein-binding sites? When giving a drug that is highly protein-bound, would there be less or more free drug available? Explain.

4. Growing tissue in infants and small children can be more sensitive to certain drugs. With that in mind,

    a. What effect do corticosteroids have on infants?

    b. What effect does tetracycline have on children younger than 8 years old?

5. Explain the following pharmacokinetics related to children and drug therapy:

    a. Gastric emptying time

    b. Protein-binding sites

    c. Liver function

    d. Kidney function

6. Explain the following pharmacokinetics related to older adults and drug therapy:

    a. GI absorption

    b. Body water and water-soluble drugs

    c. Fat-soluble drugs

    d. Effect of liver function and metabolism on half-life

    e. Renal function

7. Noncompliance to the drug regimen is common in the older adult. Give reasons for the noncompliance. What are some nursing measures that might help to improve drug regimen compliance?

8. Cite major differences between children and adults that affect drug therapy.

9. Cite major factors that influence the effect of drugs on older adults.

10 Medication Administration in Community Settings

Objectives

- Describe common elements of client teaching about medication administration in community settings.
- Describe specific points related to administration of medications in the home.
- Identify specific points related to administration of medications in the school.
- Identify specific points related to administration of medications in the work site.
- Explain the application of the nursing process to medication administration.

INTRODUCTION

There has been a significant shift of health and illness care to community settings from the traditional institutions. The faces of a community are many, varied, and ever-changing (Fig. 10–1). With the movement of health care into the community, nurses, more than any other health care provider, have the opportunity to shape the health care of society. This chapter describes selected aspects of medication administration within each of the major community settings: home, school, and work sites. In all settings, client safety is of primary concern.

The process of medication administration in the home, school, and work site must be consistent with professional, legal, and regulatory requirements. In each setting, what will be taught about medications by the nursing personnel and the routes by which the medications may be administered must be identified. Once these decisions have been made, criteria for administration, instruction/client teaching, and ongoing supervision need to be developed, implemented, and subjected to evaluation. Mechanisms for communication and paper tracking must be in place to promote efficacy of the medication and avoidance of untoward responses and medication errors.

The backbone of health promotion and disease prevention is the client knowledge base. The role of the nurse in establishing this base is very important. (Refer to Chapter 2 for a comprehensive discussion of client teaching.) Assessment of learning needs and styles is an essential component of achieving the identified teaching goal (Fig. 10–2).

Regardless of the state and agency regulations related to medication administration in this environment, the following are suggested hints for client teaching associated with medication administration grouped into five categories: (1) general, (2) diet, (3) self-administration, (4) side effects, and (5) cultural considerations.

Within the general area, client safety is of primary concern. Thus, a client's physical abilities require on-

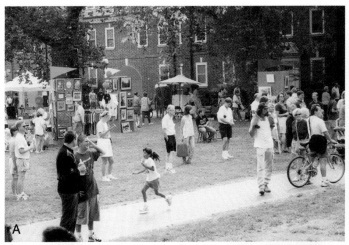

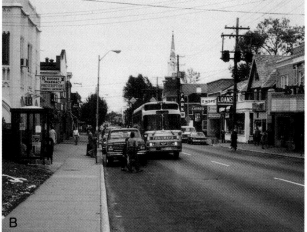

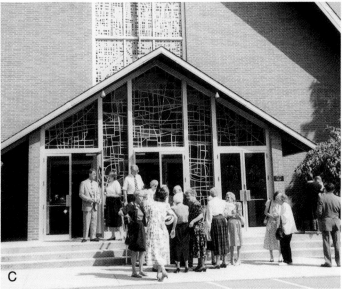

Figure 10–1
A-C, A community has many different faces.

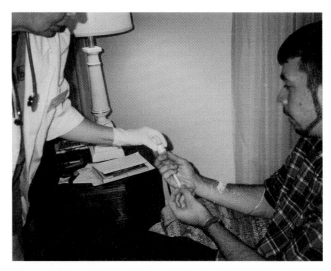

Figure 10–2
Effective client teaching is based on the individual client's learning needs.

going assessment. Capabilities of the client may be temporarily impaired with the use of certain drugs (e.g., narcotics, selected eye medications, and psychotropics). It is essential that clients be advised not to operate hazardous machinery during such times and to use caution at all other times. It is appropriate to discuss with clients or families what situations in the daily routine require full alertness and cannot be influenced by medication for the sake of safety.

There are safety concerns associated with the storage of medications. It is recommended that medications be kept in their original labeled containers with child-safe caps when needed. The client or family should be provided with written instructions (audio instructions if client is sight impaired) about the drug regimen. Large print may be helpful or very necessary. An important, yet frequently misunderstood, component of the instructions is the expected therapeutic effect and length of time to achieve a therapeutic response from the medication. There is wide variation (e.g., narcotics within 30 minutes; many antibiotics within 24 hours; and some psychotropics within 6 weeks). Having the client understand the expected time frame for results can markedly diminish his or her concerns and promote adherence to the therapeutic plan. Another part of the teaching plan is to advise the client or family about any necessary laboratory test monitoring of blood level of the medication and any possible drug-laboratory test interaction.

The client or family must be aware of the need to have adequate supply of necessary medications available at all times—at home, school, work, and while traveling. It is best to order prescription refills in advance; at least a week if the pharmacy is local. Allow several weeks if drugs are mail ordered. It is a good idea to pack extra medication when going on trips, both short and extended. This is preferred at all times, and essential for foreign travel.

Impress on the client or family to *first* contact the health care provider before using over-the-counter (OTC) preparations. Common OTC preparations that may cause problems are laxatives, diet aids, cold and cough preparations, and overdose of fat-soluble vitamins. Reinforce with the client or family the importance of follow-up appointments with health care providers. Encourage wellness check-ups, including preventive and restorative dental care because the presence of other conditions may impact on the current therapeutic regimen. In addition, advise them of the need to complete laboratory studies in a timely manner. Encourage clients to wear Medic-alert bands with medications and/or allergies indicated.

Reinforcement of the availability of community resources is important. Availability does not always equate with accessibility, so the client or family needs to be alert as to how to mobilize them according to individual needs. Matching community resources and client needs is a prerequisite. While acknowledging the variability of each, the following are offered as examples. The telephone book is a frequently overlooked resource that can direct clients and families to contacts and addresses of associations of relevant health conditions (e.g. American Heart Association and the American Cancer Society). Most agencies and associations have or direct the caller to a wealth of health education resources available in a variety of media (written, audiotapes, video, and occasionally in braille).

In addition, churches may have outreach groups in which volunteers pick up prescriptions and deliver them to the homebound client. Also, a call to the pharmacist frequently clarifies a client or family concern. Meals on Wheels enable clients to remain at home and implement compliance to taking medications with food. In a college town, students of the health professions may be motivated caregivers to assist clients or families in the community. Clients or families need to be encouraged to have a contact person for their concerns and questions, frequently a nurse. Use of appropriate resources is likely to increase compliance with and effectiveness of the therapeutic regimen.

Diet is the second area that requires the nurse's attention. There is an overall need to advise clients or families about possible drug-food interactions, detailing which foods are to be avoided and which foods are encouraged for specific nutrient value. For example, tyramine-rich foods are contraindicated with monoamine oxidase inhibitors (MAOIs), and potassium-rich foods are recommended for clients taking potassium-wasting diuretics. Alcohol may be contraindicated with selected medications. Lists of foods—

and pictures when appropriate—may be helpful to clients and others involved with the client's diet.

The third area of concern is self-administration of medications. Based on the client or family knowledge level, instructions should be given on all skills related to the drug regimen, for example, how to take pulse for clients taking digitalis preparations, correct use and cleaning of inhalers, and techniques for successful administration of parenteral medications. The nurse should allow time for instruction and questions, including demonstration of the skill and return demonstration. Clients should be given graphic illustrations for future reference, as appropriate. It is essential that the nurse provide the client or family with the name of a contact person and telephone number for questions and concerns. It is not uncommon for a client or family member to return demonstrate a skill with relative ease and then forget information or become confused when trying self-administration of the drug when alone.

Side effects are the fourth area for client teaching. The client or family should be advised about general side effects of the medications. This is not done to scare the clients, but rather to have them informed about the more commonly occurring side effects. The clients need to know when to notify their health care provider if they experience an adverse reaction.

Cultural considerations are the fifth general area of concern. Initially the nurse assesses the client's personal beliefs (Fig. 10–3). Based on these beliefs, the nurse then modifies communications to meet client or family cultural practices. The nurse needs to communicate respect for the client or family culture at all times. It is incumbent on the nurse to assess his or her own beliefs and biases related to cultural competence and diversity. Then one needs to evaluate the effectiveness of interactions and their acceptability within the cultural realm. (Refer to Chapter 6 for a comprehensive presentation of cultural considerations.)

Culturally sensitive and competent health care promotes client or family compliance with the therapeutic regimen. Respect for cultural diversity may be demonstrated by inclusion of traditional and folk practices into the plans for improved communication, health promotion, and disease prevention. Although applicable to multiple settings, some common cultural concerns are presented as examples for illustrative purposes (Purnell, 1998):

Home care: Hispanics and Asian/Pacific Islanders frequently say they agree with the plan out of respect for health care providers even though they may not intend to follow the plan. This practice may have dangerous or life-threatening outcomes. Egyptians are used to the oral tradition of communication and thus may not keep reliable written records for medication schedules and glucose monitoring results. A call from an Amish family is probably a true emergency because of their religious and cultural obligations to care for themselves first before seeking outside resources. Food rituals are important to the Appalachian, Jewish, Muslim, and Asian/Pacific Island people and must be incorporated into the plan of care if a prescription is to be followed. Self-medication and self-diagnosis are common among the Asians.

School: African-American grandmothers play a significant role in dealing with health care concerns and must be included in the plans for care. Because being overweight is seen as positive to many African-Americans, the health care provider may need to frequently reeducate clients in this cultural group and carefully explain the health risks associated with obesity.

Work site: African-Americans have increased risk for development of hypertension and prefer to be addressed formally. For Asian/Pacific Islanders, confidentiality is important, and they may not provide needed information if they perceive that the information may be shared and other community members may obtain knowledge about their health problems. It may be difficult for outsiders to develop rapport with Appalachian people because of past inequities from government agencies.

A summary of these guidelines is presented in Table 10–1.

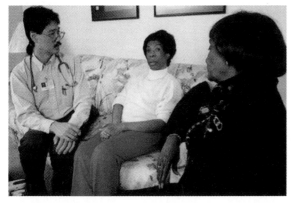

Figure 10–3
Providing culturally sensitive care starts with an assessment of the client's and family's particular beliefs, customs, and preferences. (From Swanson, J.M., Nies, M.A.: Community Health Nursing Promoting the Health of Aggregates, 2/E. Philadelphia: W.B. Saunders, 1997.)

HOME SETTING

The home setting provides the registered nurse with many challenges related to medication administration. A major question that quickly presents itself is "Who

Table 10–1
Summary of Hints for the Client Teaching About Medication Use/Administration in the Community

GENERAL

Client safety is of primary concern.
Client's physical abilities require ongoing assessment.
Keep or store medications in original labeled containers with child-safe caps when needed.
Provide client or family with written instructions (audio instructions if sight impaired) about the drug regimen.
Advise client or family about the expected therapeutic effect and length of time to achieve a therapeutic response from the medication; also the expected duration of treatment.
Advise client or family about possible drug-laboratory test interaction.
Advise client of nonpharmacologic measures to promote therapeutic response.
Advise client or family to have adequate supply of necessary medications available.
Caution against the use of over-the-counter (OTC) preparations without *first* contacting the health care provider.
Reinforce the importance of follow-up appointments with health care providers.
Encourage clients to wear Medic-alert band with medications and allergies indicated.
Reinforce that community resources are available and need to be mobilized according to the client or family needs.

DIET

Advise client/family/student/employee about possible drug-food interactions.
Advise client/family/student/employee what foods are contraindicated.
Advise client/family/student/employee regarding alcohol use.

SELF-ADMINISTRATION

Instruct client/family/student/employee regarding drug dose and dosing schedule.
Instruct client/family/student/employee on all psychomotor skills related to the drug regimen.
Provide client/family/student/employee with contact person and telephone number for questions and concerns.

SIDE EFFECTS

Advise client/family/student/employee about general side effects and adverse reactions of the medications.
Advise client/family/student/employee when to notify health care provider.

CULTURAL CONSIDERATIONS

Assess personal beliefs of client/family/student/employee.
Modify communications to meet cultural needs of client/family/student/employee.
Communicate respect for client/family/student/employee culture.

can administer medications in the home setting?" The response does not develop as quickly.

In general, medications are administered by licensed nurses in the home setting according to the order of the health care provider. Drugs that are administered by nursing personnel in the home must be approved by the Food and Drug Administration (FDA). The nurse also initiates instructions about the medication to the client or family (Fig. 10–4). The licensed nurse may also administer the medication on a short-term basis for a disease-related condition if a caregiver with an order from the health care provider is unable to do so.

The order from the health care provider must be current and complete (drug, dosage, frequency, route of administration, and signature). The medication must be labeled by the pharmacist or health care provider. The nurse should not administer any medica-

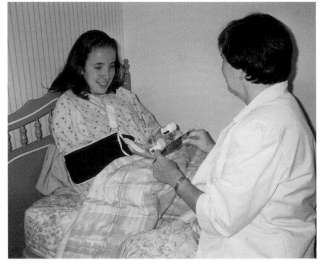

Figure 10–4
A vital aspect of home care is teaching clients about medications.

tion that is not properly labeled. It is the nurse's responsibility to contact the health care provider, pharmacist, or other group identified by the agency with any concerns about the medication for the specific client. The expiration date must be checked at the time of each administration. Storage and deterioration of the medication is also evaluated. Significant side effects, allergies, and adverse reactions are reported promptly to the health care provider; each client is assessed for allergies *before* starting the drug.

The establishment of policy and procedures for medication administration does promote safety and consistency; however, errors do occur. When a medication error occurs, it is reported to health care provider and nursing supervisor. The client and family are instructed when to notify the nurse or health care provider about adverse drug reactions; the health care provider is notified of all adverse drug reactions.

An agency policy for medication administration generally addresses guidelines for specific medications. Examples of these specific agents include allergy vaccines, chemotherapy, gamma-globulin, gold, experimental drugs, and narcotics. The guidelines are agency specific and may include that the first dose of allergy vaccine be given by the health care provider in a controlled environment or that family members be taught to administer narcotics to the client by the parenteral route if the order is so written by the health care provider. When the order is discontinued, the health care provider needs to be notified if any unused narcotics are in the home. Licensed practical nurses may not administer gamma-globulin intravenously, and family members may not be taught to administer selected drugs (e.g., Imferon). Chemotherapy for cancer commonly presents a special challenge. The client's blood work must be current before the administration of the chemotherapeutic drugs, the client must be under regular and ongoing care of a physician, and safety requirements may be identified (e.g., gloves and goggles may be used).

Certified home health aides work under the supervision of the registered nurse. The home health aides are commonly asked to administer medications to the clients by the client, family, or friends. In the current health care environment, the home health aide may receive pressure to administer medications. However, the home health aide may only have involvement of any kind with medications that the client customarily self-administers and then, only, in the capacity of assistance.

There are additional challenges related to medication administration in the home setting. One of these is compliance with the therapeutic regimen, especially the right drug, right dose, and right time. Some clients need and do not have a primary caregiver to oversee follow-up with medications and other aspects of care. The quality and preparation of meals may

also be a factor related to medication administration, such as what foods to avoid with certain medications and what foods complement a medication. In addition, it may be problematic for clients to get their medications and to get them in a timely manner. Furthermore, coordinated skill is required by the client or family as with the use of an inhaler or administration of insulin. In all of these situations, the nurse is frequently the person who coordinates the resources.

SCHOOL SETTING

Health and education are natural partners. The ability to learn is influenced by health factors.

Administration of medications in the school setting is of special concern. School health services are not immune from the phenomenon of downsizing of personnel. Thus, many school systems are dealing with questions such as "Where are the nurses?" and "Who is responsible for the administration of medication?"

In the absence of federal and state law, some school districts have elected not to employ school nurses. The average national caseload for a school nurse is 3098 students! This is a reality despite the long-standing recommendation of having one registered nurse for every 750 students. Coupled with this is the impact of a federal law that entitles children with handicaps to attend public schools in their residential areas. Hence, it is reasonable to assume that these children have special needs that require professional nursing services (Fig. 10–5).

In 1990, the Office of School Health Policy of the University of Colorado Health Sciences Center recognized that medication administration was a serious policy issue. The Massachusetts experience with de-

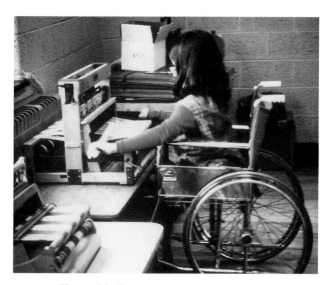

Figure 10–5
Many schoolchildren have special health needs.

Table 10-2
Standards for School Nursing Practice

1. The school nurse uses a clinical knowledge base in practice.
2. The school nurse uses a systematic approach to problem solving.
3. The school nurse contributes to the education of clients with special needs through use of the nursing process.
4. The school nurse uses effective communication skills.
5. The school nurse establishes and maintains a comprehensive school health program.
6. The school nurse collaborates with other school personnel and caregivers to meet students' needs.
7. The school nurse assists clients (students, families, and communities) to achieve optimal wellness via health education.
8. The school nurse contributes to nursing and school health through research and innovative practice.
9. The school nurse defines the nursing role, promotes quality care and professional growth, and demonstrates professional conduct.

---

velopment of its model had a goal "to develop regulations that provided minimum standards for the safe and proper administration of prescription medications in the Commonwealth schools" (Sheetz & Blum, 1998). The development of this model has many strengths, including representation of professional associations, community groups, and regulatory bodies. Consistent consent forms were designed and adopted and there were orientation and training programs for all personnel in school health positions. The established regulations apply to both public and nonpublic schools. This model appears to have applicability to other states that are grappling with the important child health issue of medication administration in the schools.

It is essential that the nurse be aware of the policies and procedures on medication administration for the specific state, county, or schools. The standards of practice for school nurses are presented in Table 10-2.

The policy for medication administration is necessary and should promote self-management programs of students with chronic conditions, such as asthma and diabetes. Nurses must be actively involved in the development of this policy and in ensuring that the needs of the individual students are met.

In some states or school systems, non-nurses may be responsible for medication administration. This presents additional concerns that need to be addressed such as adherence to instructions and adherence to the principle that medication administration is a process, more than "giving the student a pill." A major component of medication administration is assessment of the need for the medication and its effectiveness of action. The effectiveness of action includes being alert to side effects and adverse reactions that the client may experience.

While recognizing the variability between policies on medication administration, Igoe and Speer (1996) have identified the following basic requirements for administration of medications in schools:

1. Medications are given only with parents' written permission.
2. Medications requiring a prescription are given only on the written authorization of a health care provider.
3. For medications requiring a prescription, there must be an individual, pharmacy-labeled bottle for each student.
4. Medications must be recorded by the school personnel who administer them. This record states the student's name, medication, dosage, time, and the name of the person administering the medication.
5. Medications must be stored in a secure, locked, clean container or cabinet.

Child care and adult day services have similar rules for the administration of medications. In general, these facilities administer medications or supervise self-administration within the Nurse Practice Act of the specific state. In addition, most facilities require labeling of medications in accordance with the Pharmacy Rules and Regulations of the specific state. Guidelines for safe storage of medications must be followed, including being only accessible to personnel responsible for distribution of self-administration or administration of medications. Some states require that internal and external medications be stored separately. Care must be taken to ensure that prescription medications only be used for whom the medication was prescribed.

The National Association of School Nurses is a fine resource for information on the many faceted aspects of school nursing. They may be contacted at Lamplighter Lane, P. O. Box 1300, Scarboro, Maine, 14070; telephone: (207) 883-2217.

WORK SITE SETTING

Most adult Americans and many youth are employed and spend a significant amount of time at the work

Table 10-3
Standards for Occupational Health Nursing

1. The nurse collaborates with management in developing objectives for employee health services.
2. The nurse administers the employee health service.
3. The nurse defines nursing authority and responsibility and collaborates with management in determining the nurse's position in the organization.
4. The nurse administers nursing care and develops procedures and protocols with specific goals and interventions related to employee health needs.
5. The nurse coordinates responsibilities in health assessment and promotes health maintenance and prevention of illness and injury.
6. The nurse collaborates with other on-site members of the occupational health team to evaluate the work environment and uses outside resources as needed.
7. The nurse establishes and promotes working relationships with appropriate community agencies.

site on a regular basis. Thus, the work site is an ideal setting to promote personal health behaviors and decrease environmental hazards.

Healthy employees are more productive than unhealthy employees. This fact, coupled with the escalating costs of health care and insurance, has inspired many businesses to offer some type of health care at the work site. This care ranges from emergency first aid and work-related health and safety problems to the provision of primary care and referral services.

The American Association of Occupational Health Nurses (AAOHN) defines occupational health nursing as "the application of nursing principles to conserve the health of workers in all organizations." It emphasizes prevention, recognition, and treatment of illness and injury, and requires special skills and knowledge in the fields of health education and counseling, environmental health, rehabilitation, and human relations (AAOHN, 1988). The standards for practice developed by the AAOHN are presented in Table 10-3.

The nurse needs to be aware of the policies and procedures for administration of medication at the specific work site. There is great diversity in policy and procedure between settings. For example, the following are two of many current practices at work sites. At one setting, the registered nurse essentially follows protocols for selected employee complaints (e.g., back injuries, acute and chronic; burns, thermal, chemical, and electrical; eye emergencies; herpes; and adult immunizations). Each protocol includes the following areas with relevant information for the specific complaint: assessment, treatment/medications, patient education, referral, and follow-up. Medications are identified as appropriate, under treatment/medications section with the stated drug, dosage, frequency, and route.

Another site has established self-care stations for minor illnesses and injuries (Fig. 10-6). Each station has designated criteria for use. Examples of stations include "colds," superficial cuts, and menstrual cramps. Employees are oriented to this service as part of the orientation process. Upon arrival at the stations, the employee notes date, time, and signature on the sign-in sheet posted at each station. He or she indicates the chief complaint or reason for seeking medication and the specific OTC medications they have taken from the OTC preparations supplied at each station.

An excellent resource for care of clients in the work setting is the American Association of Occupational Health Nurses, 50 Lennox Pointe, Atlanta, Georgia, 30324; telephone: (404) 262-1162.

SUMMARY

This chapter discusses only a minute, but significant, portion of the nurse's role in a variety of community settings. Specifically, the focus is on selected concerns associated with the administration of medications and the need to practice in accordance with the Nurse Practice Act of a specific state. The role of the nurse in drug administration is growing in complexity. The nurse in the twenty-first century must have a strong knowledge base.

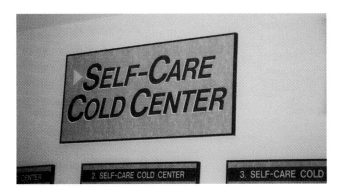

Figure 10-6
Some workplaces have "self-care" centers where employees can obtain over-the-counter preparations for such ailments as colds.

NURSING PROCESS
OVERVIEW OF MEDICATION ADMINISTRATION

Assessment

- Obtain appropriate vital signs and relevant laboratory test results for future comparisons and evaluation of the therapeutic response.
- Obtain drug history, including drug allergies.
- Identify high-risk clients/students/employees for reactions.
- Assess client's/student's/employee's capability to follow therapeutic regimen.
- Assess client/student/employee learning needs.

Potential Nursing Diagnoses

- Risk for injury related to possible adverse reaction
- Risk for ineffective management of therapeutic regimen
- Risk for impaired home maintenance management
- Knowledge deficit

Planning

- Identify goals.
- Promote therapeutic response and prevent or minimize adverse reactions.
- Identify strategies to promote adherence.
- Identify interventions.

Nursing Interventions

- Prepare equipment and environment; wash hands.
- Check for allergies and other assessment data.
- Check drug label three times; check expiration date.
- Be certain of drug calculation; verify dose with another registered nurse, as necessary.
- Pour liquids at eye level.
- Keep all drugs stored properly, especially related to temperature, light, and moisture.
- Avoid contact with topical and inhalation preparations.
- Verify client/student/employee identification.
- Administer only drugs you have prepared.
- Assist client to desired position.
- Discard needles and syringes in "sharps" container.
- Follow policy related to discarding drugs and controlled substances.
- Report drug errors immediately.
- Record all appropriate information in a timely manner.
- Record effectiveness of drugs administered and reason for any drugs refused.

Evaluation

- Evaluate effectiveness of medication(s) administered.
- Identify expected time frame of desired drug response; consider modification of therapy as needed.
- Determine client/student/employee satisfaction with regimen.
- Determine client/student/employee knowledge of medication regimen.

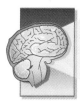

Critical Thinking in Action

The Rivera family: José age 30, wife Maria age 29 and 7 months pregnant, and children José Jr. age 10, Angel age 8, and Tony age 7 have recently moved into a new community. José is employed full time by a large credit card corporation and Maria is full-time "mom" and part-time cashier.

1. Give examples of culturally sensitive and competent care for the Rivera children in the school setting.
2. Identify culturally sensitive and competent care for the parents at the work sites.
3. What modifications would you suggest for a family of African-American heritage?

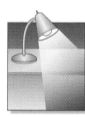

Study Questions

1. When teaching a client/student/employee about OTC preparations, what information does the nurse need to include?
2. What is the role of the certified home health aide in administration of medication in the home?
3. Describe the importance of advising the client/student/employee of the expected length of time for therapeutic effects of the medication.
4. What are the cultural considerations applicable to administration of medication?
5. What are the five basic requirements for administration of medication in the school according to Igoe and Speer?
6. What special skills and knowledge are necessary according to the AAOHN's definition of occupational health nursing?
7. What are the major points in the application of the nursing process to the administration of medications?

11 The Role of the Nurse in Drug Research

Outline

Objectives

- Identify basic ethical principles
- Relate three basic ethical principles governing informed consent and risk-to-benefit ratio
- Describe the objectives of each phase of human clinical experimentation
- Describe the role of the nurse in clinical drug trials using the nursing process

Terms

beneficence	experimental group	placebo
control group	informed consent	single-blind
double-blind	open-label study	triple-blind

INTRODUCTION

We often hear news broadcasts or read headlines announcing the release of a new drug for the treatment of acquired immunodeficiency syndrome (AIDS) or multiple sclerosis, an increase in a drug company's research and development budget, Food and Drug Administration (FDA) approval granted for promising drugs, or similar pharmacology-related news. Such news items signal increasing awareness of the importance of drug research.

Drug research and development is a complex process and one of interest and importance to professional nursing practice. The nursing process facilitates the integration of cutting-edge research.

This chapter is devoted to a description of basic ethical principles governing informed consent and risk-to-benefit ratio; preclinical testing and human clinical experimentation; and the role of the nurse in clinical drug trials using the nursing process.

BASIC ETHICAL PRINCIPLES

Three basic ethical principles are relevant to research involving human subjects: (1) respect for persons, (2) beneficence, and (3) justice.

Respect for Person

Individuals undergoing treatment in any health care system should be treated as independent persons who are capable of making decisions in their own interest. Individuals whose decision-making capability is diminished are entitled to protection. The nurse can determine this with consistent reassessment of the client's cognitive state. Clients should be made aware of the alternatives available to them in their health care, as well as the consequences that stem from those alternatives. Furthermore, the client's choice should be honored whenever possible. It is imperative that the nurse recognize when the client is not capable of rational decision making and is therefore entitled to protection.

Beneficence

Beneficence is the duty to not harm others, to maximize possible benefits, and to minimize possible harm that might occur in research. It is often not possible to know if something is beneficial unless it is tested and individuals have been exposed to the risks. A central question to this issue is "Who makes this decision—the client or those caring for the client?"

Justice

The principle of justice in the context of clinical drug trials means that social benefits and burdens can be allocated objectively and that those with equivalent circumstances should be treated equally.

The principles of respect for person, beneficence, and justice are integral to the issues of informed consent and risk-to-benefit ratio in research involving human subjects.

Informed Consent

Informed consent has dimensions beyond protection of the individual client's choice and includes

1. Promotion of individual autonomy
2. Protection of clients and subjects from harm
3. Avoidance of fraud and duress in health care
4. Encouragement for professionals to scrutinize their efforts in communicating information
5. Promotion of rational decision making among clients
6. Promotion of self-determination as a general social value.

Risk-to-Benefit Ratio

The risk-to-benefit ratio is one of the most complex problems faced by the researcher. All possible consequences of a clinical study must be analyzed and balanced with the inherent risks and the anticipated benefits. Physical, psychological, and social risks must be identified and weighed against the benefits. A requirement of the Department of Health and Human Services (DHHS) is that institutional review boards (IRBs) determine that "risks to subjects are reasonable in relation to anticipated benefits, if any, to subjects" (DHHS, 1981). No matter how noble the intentions, the calculation of risks and benefits by the researcher cannot be totally accurate or comprehensive.

Varying amounts of time are required for the process of identifying a potentially useful chemical and having it become available to the general population;

Table 11–1
Basic Sequence of the Development of a New Drug

Identification of potentially clinically useful chemical
Preclinical testing
Study designs
Human clinical experimentation
    Phase I
    Phase II
    Phases III and IV

in many cases, 10 years may elapse. Only 1 in 10,000 potential drugs endures the research and development process and is used in the clinical situation. Table 11–1 lists the basic sequence of the development of a new drug.

OBJECTIVES AND PHASES OF HUMAN CLINICAL EXPERIMENTATION

Preclinical Testing

Preclinical testing consists of in vitro and in vivo systems. In vitro experimentation is generally conducted in a test tube or other laboratory equipment, and in vivo testing is conducted using living organisms. This testing is followed by toxicity screening for the purposes of identifying (1) abnormal changes in animal organs related to drug administration and (2) the parameters of the safe therapeutic dose. Control and experimental groups of animals are compared. Participants in the **experimental group** receive the experimental intervention or treatment. Those in the **control group** do not receive the experimental intervention or treatment and provide a baseline against which to measure the effects of the treatment. Before initiating human studies, an assessment is made of the seriousness of the disease to be treated using this drug in relation to the drug's toxicity.

Human Clinical Experimentation

Clinical experimentation in drug research and development encompasses four phases, each with its own objectives. A brief description of each phase follows.

PHASE I

The objectives of phase I are to determine the human dosage range based on response in healthy human subjects and to identify the pharmacokinetics (absorption, distribution, metabolism/biotransformation, excretion/elimination) of the drug. Progression to the next phase occurs if there are no serious adverse effects demonstrated, the drug is eliminated in a reasonable amount of time, and the dose range is below that known to induce pathology in animals.

PHASE II

The objective of phase II is to demonstrate the safety and efficacy of the drug in subjects ($N = 100$) who have the disease that the drug is designed to treat. A multidisciplinary team approach (nurses, physicians, pharmacologists, statisticians, and research associates) is required to ensure that the data collected will answer the clinical questions. Phase III is initiated only

when acceptable efficacy and safety data are generated and clearly documented.

PHASES III AND IV

The objectives of phases III and IV are to demonstrate the safety and efficacy of the drug for a wide client population and to include long-term data if a chronic regimen is under consideration. The sponsor submits all relevant and analyzed data in a new drug application (NDA) to the FDA. In time, the FDA decides to approve, reject, or recommend withdrawal or resubmission. After the NDA research has been approved, phase IV addresses the long-term use of the drug.

Study Designs

An experimental design is required to determine cause and effect questions about the safety and efficacy of a drug. The experimental design must demonstrate that the researcher controls the method of treatment, uses different groups of subjects—some that receive treatment and control groups that receive no treatment or an alternative method of treatment—and assigns subjects randomly to treatment or control groups.

The following examples illustrate selected research designs.

A *descriptive* design would be a chart review of all clients hospitalized at University Hospital in a given year who received digoxin. In this situation, there is no control group, random assignment, or researcher manipulation of the treatment.

A *quasi-experimental* design would be comparison of intermittent intravenous (IV) device patency of those hospitalized clients who received heparin flushes and those who received saline flushes. This study has a nonmatched comparison group, but had no random assignment to treatment group. Such quasi-experimental designs may contribute valuable information but lack the power to ascribe cause because the variables are uncontrolled and potentially influential. Ethical decisions do not permit the use of the experimental design in all situations. For example, an experimental study to determine whether nicotine causes cancer would be unethical because individuals would have to be exposed to a carcinogenic substance.

The researcher designs the study to show the effect of the independent variable (the drug) on the dependent variables (clinical responses or reactions). Intervening variables are specific to the research question and may include age, sex, weight, disease and its state of severity, diet, and the subject's social environment. Controlled treatment groups in drug research trials can receive no drug, a different drug, a **placebo** (pharmacologically inert substance), or the same drug with a different dose, route, or frequency of administration.

A *crossover* design uses each subject in several different situations. In the first instance, the experimental group receives the drug and the control group receives an alternative form of treatment or no treatment. Then both groups receive no therapy. Finally, the experimental group receives the control form of therapy and the control group receives the drug. In this design, the subject serves as his or her own control.

The researcher wants to be able to generalize the findings from the sample of subjects to the larger target population, such as all women with breast cancer. A statistical method called probability sampling (subjects are randomly selected from the entire population) is recommended to provide relative confidence in the generalization of findings.

Various designs and techniques assist the researcher in reaching valid and generalizable conclusions. In a *matched-pair* design, the researcher identifies several variables that may influence the outcome, such as age, weight, or family history, then the subjects are matched for these variables. One of the pair is randomly assigned to the experimental group and the other to the control group. A less effective technique is nonrandom assignment to treatment group.

The **double-blind** technique is a powerful tool wherein neither the health care provider nor subject knows whether the subject is receiving the experimental or control form of therapy. In **triple-blind** studies, a researcher other than the prescribing health care provider collects data and is also unaware of the subject's treatment group. In a **single-blind** study, only the subject is unaware of which group he or she is assigned to. An **open-label study** indicates that all parties—data collectors, prescribing health care provider, and subject—know the treatment group assignment. The double-blind and triple-blind techniques are preferred for drug research because those involved in the study are not aware of the subject's treatment group, thereby removing a source of bias.

Nurses' Role

The nurse has a pivotal role in drug clinical trials. The research and development process for drug research requires the multifaceted roles of professional nursing practice. The nurse is both the client/family advocate and liaison between the client, health care provider, and research nurse responsible for the specific protocol. Nursing involvement is essential to the successful completion of clinical trials.

Asking relevant questions about informed consent and risk-to-benefit ratio is a major role of the nurse. Awareness of initial indicators of change in the client

and prediction of increased risk for adverse drug reaction are also dimensions of professional nursing practice.

RECENT DEVELOPMENTS: NEW FDA-APPROVED PRODUCTS AND THOSE WITH NEW INDICATIONS

Recent drug research and development has yielded few amazing cures for disease but has contributed new uses for some old medicines. For example, aspirin was reported to reduce the risk of colon cancer by almost 50%, and low doses of aspirin were found to be as effective as higher doses in preventing strokes. Ticlopidine (Ticlid), a platelet inhibitor, is available for individuals who cannot tolerate aspirin. Specific dosages of once prescription medications are available over-the-counter, such as Pepcid AC and Axid AR.

Examples of new products include naratriptan (Amerge), a selective 5-HT $1\beta/1\delta$ receptor agonist for treatment of acute migraines; tolterodine tartrate (Detrol), an antimuscarinic agent for treating symptomatic overreactive bladder; Lustra, for skin discoloration; sibutramine HCl (Meridia), in the management of obesity as adjunct to diet; clopidogrel (Plavix), to decrease atherosclerotic events via platelet aggregation inhibition; Prandin, a meglitinide analogue for diabetes; Singulair, a leukotriene receptor antagonist for treatment and prophylaxis of asthma; Teczem, calcium channel blocker plus angiotensin converting enzyme (ACE) inhibitor for treatment of hypertension; TriCor, a micronized fenofibrate for selective hyperlipidemias; Trovan, a broad-spectrum quinolone antibiotic; and sildenafil citrate (Viagra), for treating erectile dysfunction. Butenafine is the first in a new class of antifungals. A boon to pediatric medicine is Acel-Imune, a vaccine developed to protect against diphtheria, pertussis, and tetanus (DPT), which is expected to have fewer adverse reactions than the traditional DPT immunization. In addition, NovoPen 3 is an insulin delivery device.

Existing medications have received approval for expanded indications. Examples of these drugs include Pravachol to reduce risk of stroke or transient ischemic attack (TIA); Prevacid for gastroesophageal reflux disorder (GERD) treatment; DDAVP tablets for nocturnal enuresis; Zocor for reducing risk of stroke; Cipro oral suspension formula for adults; Atrovent nasal 0.03% for use in young children; Floxin Otic ear drop formulation; Tiazac for angina; Estratab for prevention of osteoporosis; and Flagyl ER, an oral, daily formulation for bacterial vaginosis. Midazolam HCl (Versed) was approved for use in newborns, infants, and children in the critical care settings and for painful procedures and preoperative sedation. Ofloxacin

(Floxin) is the first oral medication to be used as monotherapy in the treatment of acute pelvic inflammatory disease (PID) caused by *Chlamydia trachomatis* and/or *Neisseria gonorrhoeae*. In addition, monitoring recommendations for Clozaril have been eased to weekly for the first 6 months of therapy then bi-weekly for clients with acceptable white blood cell counts. Transdermal scopolamine has returned to the market as a patch to deliver 1 mg of drug over 3 days. Thalidomide has returned to the market as an FDA-approved drug for the treatment of leprosy.

NURSING PROCESS
CLINICAL DRUG TRIALS

Assessment

- Explore own beliefs about clinical trials.
- Recruit subjects.
- Assess subjects.
- Assess protocol.
- Demonstrate thorough knowledge of all inclusion/exclusion criteria for subjects (Table 11–2).
- Articulate observations and concerns to health care providers, sponsors, and pharmaceutical company.
- Communicate need for drug to address a specific need with the appropriate individuals.

Planning

- Develop fact sheet of protocol guidelines.
- Educate involved staff about protocol requirements.
- Provide input into budget negotiations.
- Coordinate personnel and budget, including office visits, special tests, and laboratory work.
- Ensure that subject consent is informed (Table 11–3, Fig. 11–1).
- Respond to subject's questions.

Nursing Interventions

- Screen subjects accurately and thoroughly based on established protocol.
- Adhere to protocol guidelines, including administration of drug.
- Monitor selected parameters. Observe and report toxicities promptly.
- Collect all data required by the sponsor (e.g., drug company).
- Communicate information in a complete, concise, accurate, and timely manner to the principal investigator and sponsor.
- Document data in a clear and timely manner.
- Record subjects' own evaluation; *seemingly unrelated responses may be significant*. At times, a drug is actually marketed for a different indication than the original testing.
- Report *all* deaths to physician, sponsor, Institutional Review Board, and FDA, whether or not the cause of death is drug-related.

Evaluation

- Consider the clarity of the research statement.
- Determine whether the research design is appropriate to answer research questions.
- Evaluate subject selection; for example, in an experimental design, were subjects randomly selected and randomly assigned? Were intervening variables identified and used when a matched-pair design was used?
- Determine the validity and reliability of measurement instruments.
- Are the actual sample and the target population comparable?
- Are the conclusions valid and based on data?
- Are the clinical findings significant?

Memorial Hospital
PERMISSION FOR CLINICAL INVESTIGATION

Completed by Client:

1. I hereby authorize Dr. _____ and/or such assistants as may be selected by him/her to conduct studies upon _____ for the following: _____

2. I further authorize Dr. _____ and/or such assistants as may be selected by him/her, to prescribe drugs or to perform certain procedures in connection with the diagnosis and treatment of my condition including the following drugs and/or extraordinary procedures: _____ _____

3. I have (have not) been made aware of certain risks, possible consequences and discomfort associated with these drugs or extraordinary procedures which are: _____ _____

4. I understand that no guarantee or assurance has been made as to the results that may be obtained although I have (have not) been advised of the possibility that certain benefits may be expected such as: _____

5. I have (have not) had explained to me alternative procedures/treatments/drugs that may be advantageous and they include the following: _____ _____

6. I have (have not) received an offer to answer any inquiries concerning the procedures involved _____

7. I have (have not) had explained to me all medical terminology in connection with this study _____

8. I understand that it is in the intent of the principal investigator to maintain the confidentiality of records identifying subjects in this study. The Food and Drug Administration, however, may possibly inspect the records to monitor compliance with published federal regulations.

9. I understand that I may withdraw this consent and discontinue participation in this study at any time, without prejudice to my care, by informing Dr. _____ of my desire to withdraw. _____ Yes, I understand _____ No, I do not understand

10. I understand that Department of Health and Human Services regulations require the Memorial Hospital to inform me of any provisions to provide for medical treatment for any physical injury which may occur as a result of this study. In this connection, I understand that the Memorial Hospital does not have a formal plan or program to provide for the cost of medical treatment or compensation for any physical injury which occurs as a result of this study and for which they do not have legal liability. However, in the unlikely event that I am injured as a result of my participation, I understand that I should promptly inform Dr. _____

SIGNED _____

RELATIONSHIP _____

ADDRESS _____ _____

DATED _____

Completed by witness:

I, the undersigned, hereby acknowledge that I was present during the explanation of the above consent for clinical investigation given by Dr. _____ to _____ during which the nature, purpose, risks, complications and consequences thereof were fully set forth and all questions answered and I was present while _____ signed the above consent.

Dated _____

_____
(witness)

_____
(address)

Figure 11–1
Example of informed consent.

Table 11-2
Inclusion/Exclusion Criteria for a Hypothetical Protocol for an Experimental Diuretic Medication

Inclusion

Males and females between the ages of 18 and 65 years

Weight between 50 and 100 kg

Subjects receiving cardiac medications only if dose has been stable for past 3 months

Subjects on sodium-restricted diet

Exclusion

Pregnant or nursing females

All females in childbearing years not responsibly using oral contraceptives

Severe damage or disease of cardiac, hepatic, renal, neurologic, or musculo-skeletal system

Clinically significant laboratory values

Table 11-3
Informed Consent Checklist

Participates voluntarily

Identifies related drugs, treatments, and techniques

Describes benefits and risks

Describes laboratory tests to monitor client's reactions

Identifies extent of confidentiality of results

Describes availability of emergency treatment for illness/injury, if any

States compensation for study-related injury, if any

States compensation for participation, if any

Writes consent clearly and understands easily at the 10th grade reading level

Provides name and telephone number of contact person for client questions and concerns

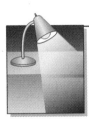

Study Questions

1. In what ways are informed consent and risk-to-benefit ratio related to drug research?
2. What are the objectives of the four phases of human experimentation?
3. What are the advantages and disadvantages of the various research designs?
4. What are the implications of clinical drug research for your nursing practice? Apply the nursing process.

Unit III

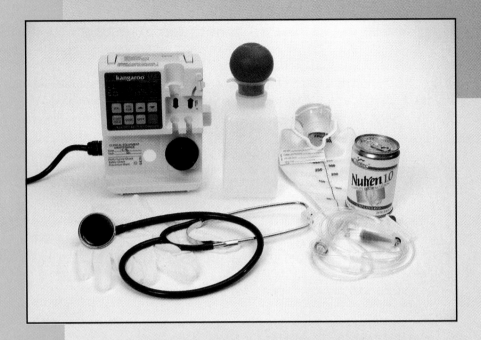

Nutrition and Electrolytes

The body requires vitamins, minerals, and electrolytes for cellular function. When there is a lack of these chemical components, replacement drug therapy is necessary. With regular nutritional dietary intake, vitamin, mineral, and electrolyte replacements are not needed.

Multiple vitamins have the highest sales volume of any over-the-counter (OTC) drugs. Usually, vitamin replacements are *not* necessary, especially for those who maintain a nutritionally balanced daily diet.

The vitamins discussed in Chapter 12 include the fat-soluble vitamins (vitamins A, D, E, and K) and the water-soluble vitamins (vitamin B complex—B_1, B_2, B_3, B_6, and B_{12}—and C). Iron is the primary mineral described. Other minerals discussed are copper, zinc, chromium, and selenium.

Body electrolytes are plentiful in extracellular fluid, intracellular fluid, and in the gastrointestinal mucosa. The cations (positively charged ions or electrolytes)—potassium (K), sodium (Na), calcium (Ca), and magnesium (Mg)—promote transmission and conduction of nerve impulses, and contractibility of muscles. Inadequate dietary intake and many disease entities contribute to electrolyte imbalances.

Drug replacements for potassium, sodium, calcium, and magnesium are discussed in Chapter 13. Implications for the nursing process are detailed for each of these electrolytes.

Nutritional support is discussed in Chapter 14.

Vitamin and Mineral Replacement 12

Outline

Objectives

- List the four groups into which vitamin supplements are divided.
- Differentiate between water- and fat-soluble vitamins.
- Identify food sources and deficiency conditions associated with each vitamin.
- Define the term *recommended dietary allowance* (RDA).
- Explain the need for iron and foods that are high in iron content.
- Explain the uses for iron, copper, zinc, chromium, and selenium.
- Describe the nursing interventions including client teaching related to vitamin and mineral uses.

Terms

fat-soluble vitamins   megavitamin   RDA
iron   minerals   water-soluble vitamins

INTRODUCTION

This chapter discusses two topics: vitamins and minerals. These substances are needed in correct portions for normal body function. Overuse of vitamins and minerals, particularly fat-soluble vitamins and iron, may lead to vitamin or iron toxicity.

VITAMINS

Vitamins are organic chemicals that are necessary for normal metabolic functions and for tissue growth and healing. The body only needs a small amount of vitamins daily, which can be easily obtained through one's diet. A well-balanced diet has all the vitamins and minerals needed for body functioning. The intake of vitamins should be increased during periods of rapid body growth, by those who are pregnant or are breastfeeding, by those with a debilitating illness, and by those with inadequate diets, for example, alcoholics and some geriatric clients. Children who have poor nutrient intake or are malnourished may need vitamin replacement. Persons on fad or restrictive diets frequently have vitamin deficiencies.

The sale of vitamins in the United States is a multibillion dollar business (Fig. 12–1). Some people take vitamins to relieve tiredness or to improve general overall health, both of which are inappropriate indications for vitamin therapy. Vitamins are *not* necessary if the individual consumes a well-balanced daily diet. Vitamin deficiencies can cause cellular and organ dysfunction that may result in a slow recovery from illness. Vitamin supplements are necessary for the vi-

Table 12–1
Justification for Vitamin Supplements

CATEGORIES	DEFICIENCIES
Inadequate absorption	Malabsorption, diarrhea, infectious and inflammatory diseases
Inability to utilize vitamins	Liver disease (cirrhosis, hepatitis), renal disease, certain hereditary deficiencies
Increased vitamin losses	Fever from infectious process, hyperthyroidism, hemodialysis, cancer, starvation, crash diets
Increased vitamin requirements	Early childhood, pregnancy, debilitating disease (cancer, alcoholism), gastrointestinal surgery, special diets

tamin deficiencies described in Table 12–1, but vitamins frequently are taken prophylactically rather than for therapeutic purposes.

The United States Department of Agriculture (USDA) Food Guide Pyramid (Fig. 12–2) provides a guide to daily food choices. Eating a variety of foods and getting the appropriate number of calories and grams of fat for a healthy weight are recommended.

The pyramid recommends the following:

- Bread, cereal, rice, and pasta group—6 to 11 servings
- Vegetable group—3 to 5 servings
- Fruit group—2 to 4 servings
- Milk, yogurt, and cheese group—2 to 3 servings
- Meat, poultry, fish, dry beans, eggs, and nut group—2 to 3 servings
- Fats, oils, and sweets—use sparingly; limit fat to 30% of calories

The National Academy of Sciences Food and Nutrition Board publishes the United States **recommended dietary allowance (RDA)** for daily dose requirements of each vitamin. The Food and Drug Administration (FDA) requires that all vitamin products be labeled according to the amount of vitamin content and the proportion of the RDA the vitamin product provides. Individuals should be encouraged to check the RDA listed on a vitamin container to determine whether the product provides the RDA dose requirements (Fig. 12–3). The recommended allowances may need to be modified for clients who are ill.

Fat-Soluble Vitamins

Vitamins fall into two general categories: fat-soluble and water-soluble. The **fat-soluble vitamins** are A, D,

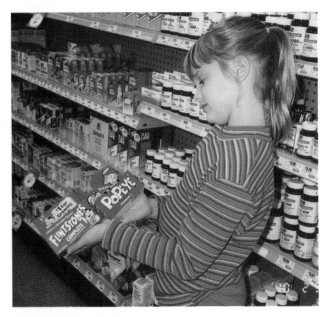

Figure 12–1
Would a less-expensive generic children's vitamin be just as good?

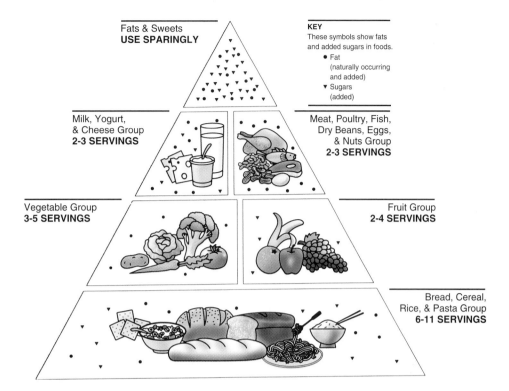

Figure 12–2
The U.S. Department of Agriculture Food Guide Pyramid.

E, and K. They are metabolized slowly, can be stored in fatty tissue, liver, and muscle in significant amounts, and are excreted in the urine at a slow rate. Vitamins A and D are toxic if taken in excess amounts over time. Vitamin A can be stored in the liver for up to 2 years. Vitamins E and K are less toxic than vitamins A and D. Foods rich in vitamin A are fruits, yellow and green vegetables, fish, and dairy products; foods rich in vitamin D are milk, dairy products, and margarine; foods rich in vitamin E are oils, margarine, milk, grains, and meats; and foods rich in vitamin K are green leafy vegetables, meats, eggs, cheese, and milk.

VITAMIN A

Vitamin A is essential for the maintenance of epithelial tissues, skin, eyes, hair, and bone growth. It has been used for the treatment of skin disorders such as acne; however, excess doses can be toxic. During pregnancy, excess amounts of vitamin A (>6000 international units [IU]) might have a teratogenic effect (birth defect) on the fetus. Chart 12–1 describes the effects of vitamin A. The nursing process can be applied as the drug data are obtained and the drug is administered.

Pharmacokinetics

When a person is deficient in vitamin A, the vitamin is absorbed faster than if there is no deficiency or intestinal obstruction. A portion of vitamin A is stored in the liver and with liver disease, this function can be inhibited. Massive doses of vitamin A may cause hypervitaminosis A, symptoms of which are loss of hair and peeling skin.

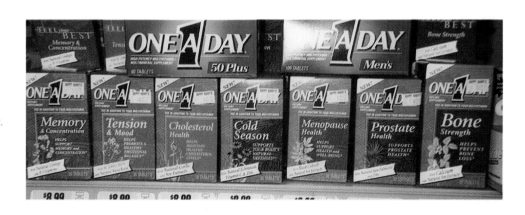

Figure 12–3
Drug companies offer vitamin supplements for specialized needs.

Chart 12–1.   Fat-Soluble Vitamin: Vitamin A

VITAMIN A

Drug Name

Vitamin A
  (Acon, Aquasol A)
Fat-soluble vitamin
Pregnancy Category: A

Dosage

A & C >8 y: PO: 100,000–500,000 IU
daily × 3 d; then 50,000 daily × 14 d
Maintenance: 10,000–20,000 IU q.d. × 60 d
C 1–8 y: IM: 17,000–35,000 IU daily × 10 d
Maintenance:
4–8 y: 15,000 IU daily × 60 d
1–<4 y: 10,000 IU daily × 60 d

Contraindications

Hypervitaminosis A, pregnancy (massive doses)

Drug-Lab-Food Interactions

Decrease absorption of mineral oil, cholestyramine, oral contraceptives, corticosteroids

Pharmacokinetics

Absorption: PO: 1h
Distribution: PB: UK
Metabolism: t½: weeks–months
Excretion: Urine and feces

Pharmacodynamics

PO: Onset: 1–2 h
        Peak: 4–5 h
        Duration: UK

Therapeutic Effects/Uses

To treat vitamin A deficiency, prevent night blindness, treat skin disorders, promote bone development

Mode of Action: Essential for growth, bone and teeth development, vision, integrity of skin and
mucous membranes, and reproduction

Side Effects

Headache, fatigue, drowsiness, irritability, anorexia, vomiting, diarrhea, dry skin, visual
changes

Adverse Reactions

Evident only with toxicity: leukopenia, aplastic
anemia, papilledema, increased intracranial
pressure, hypervitaminosis A

Assessment and Planning

Interventions

Evaluation

NURSING PROCESS

KEY: A: adult; C: child; <: less than; UK: unknown; PO: by mouth; PB: protein-binding; t½: half-life.

The RDA for vitamin A supplement is 5000 IU. Excess use of vitamin A should be avoided because this vitamin is stored in the liver, kidneys, and fat and is slowly excreted from the body. Excess vitamin A is stored in the liver for up to 2 years. Vitamin A toxicity affects multiple organs, especially the liver. The dose for healthy clients should not be greater than 7500 IU in order to prevent the occurrence of vitamin A toxicity.

Mineral oil, cholestyramine, alcohol, and antili-
pemic drugs decrease the absorption of vitamin A. Vitamin A is excreted through the kidneys and feces.

Pharmacodynamics

Vitamin A is necessary for many biochemical pro-
cesses. It aids in the formation of the visual pigment needed for night vision, it is needed in bone growth and development, and it promotes the integrity of the mucosal and epithelial tissues. An early sign of vitamin A deficiency (hypovitaminosis A) is night blind-

ness. This may progress to dryness and ulceration of the cornea and to blindness.

Vitamin A taken orally begins to take effect in 1 to 2 h and peaks in 4 to 5 h. Its duration of action is unknown. Because vitamin A is stored in the liver, the vitamin may be available to the body for days, weeks, or months.

VITAMIN D

Vitamin D has a major role in regulating calcium and phosphorus metabolism and is needed for calcium absorption from the intestines. Dietary vitamin D is absorbed in the small intestine and requires bile salts for absorption. There are two compounds of vitamin D: vitamin D_2, ergocalciferol, a synthetic fortified vitamin D; and vitamin D_3, cholecalciferol, a natural form of vitamin D influenced by ultraviolet sunlight through the skin. Once absorbed, vitamin D is converted to calcifediol in the liver. Calcifediol is then converted to an active form, calcitriol, in the kidneys.

Calcitriol, the active form of vitamin D, functions as a hormone and, with parathyroid hormone (PTH) and calcitonin, regulates calcium and phosphorus metabolism. Calcitriol and PTH stimulate bone reabsorption of calcium and phosphorus. Excretion of vitamin D is primarily in bile; only a small amount is excreted in the urine. If serum calcium levels are low, more vitamin D is activated; when serum calcium levels are normal, activation of vitamin D is decreased.

Excess vitamin D ingestion (>40,000 IU) results in hypervitaminosis D and may cause hypercalcemia (an elevated serum calcium level). Anorexia, nausea, and vomiting are early symptoms of vitamin D toxicity.

VITAMIN E

Vitamin E has antioxidant properties that protect cellular components from being oxidized and red blood cells from hemolysis. Vitamin E depends on bile salts, pancreatic secretion, and fat for its absorption. Vitamin E is stored in all tissues, especially the liver, muscle, and fatty tissue. About 75% is excreted in the bile.

Taking 400 to 800 IU of vitamin E per day is considered useful in reducing the numbers of nonfatal myocardial infarctions (MIs). It has been reported that a person taking 200 IU a day for several years can reduce the risk of coronary artery disease (CAD). This vitamin protects the heart and arteries because of its antioxidant effects (inhibits the oxidation of other compounds by blocking a group of harmful chemicals called free radicals).

Side effects of large doses of vitamin E may include fatigue, weakness, nausea, gastrointestinal upset, headache, and breast tenderness. Vitamin E may prolong the prothrombin time (PT). Those persons taking warfarin should have their PT monitored closely. Iron and vitamin E should not be taken to-gether, because iron can interfere with the body's absorption and use of vitamin E.

VITAMIN K

Vitamin K occurs in four forms: vitamin K_1 (phytonadione) is the most active form; vitamin K_2 (menaquinone) is synthesized by intestinal flora; and vitamin K_3 (menadione) and vitamin K_4 (menadiol) have been produced synthetically. Vitamin K_2 is not commercially available. Vitamin K_1 and K_2 are absorbed in the presence of bile salts. Vitamin K_3 and K_4 do not need bile salts for absorption. After vitamin K is absorbed, it is stored primarily in the liver and in other tissues. One-half of vitamin K comes from the intestinal flora and the remaining portion comes from one's diet.

Vitamin K is needed for synthesis of prothrombin and the clotting factors VII, IX, and X. For oral anticoagulant overdose, vitamin K_1 (phytonadione) is the vitamin that is most effective in preventing hemorrhage. The commercial drugs for vitamin K_1 are Mephyton, AquaMEPHYTON, and Konakion, and the commercial drug for vitamin K_4 is Synkayvite.

Water-Soluble Vitamins

Water-soluble vitamins are the B-complex vitamins and vitamin C. This group of vitamins is not usually toxic unless taken in extremely excessive amounts. Water-soluble vitamins are not stored by the body and are readily excreted in the urine. Protein-binding of water-soluble vitamins is minimal. Foods that are high in vitamin B are grains, cereal, bread, and meats. Citrus fruits and green vegetables are high in vitamin C. If the fruits and vegetables are cut, washed, or cooked, a large amount of vitamin C is lost.

VITAMIN C

Vitamin C (ascorbic acid) is absorbed from the small intestine. Vitamin C aids in the absorption of iron and in the conversion of folic acid. Vitamin C is not stored in the body and is excreted readily in the urine. A high serum vitamin C level that results from excessive dosing of vitamin C is excreted by the kidneys unchanged.

The average dose of vitamin C for an adult per day is 50 to 100 mg. Some individuals take as much as 500 mg to 6000 mg a day for purposes such as treatment of upper respiratory infections, cancer, or hypercholesterolemia. Massive doses of vitamin C can cause diarrhea and GI upset. Chart 12–2 gives drug information on vitamin C.

Pharmacokinetics

Vitamin C is absorbed readily through the GI tract and is distributed throughout the body fluids. The

Chart 12–2. Water-Soluble Vitamin: Vitamin C

VITAMIN C

Drug Names

Vitamin C, Ascorbic Acid
　　Ascorbicap, Cecon, Cevalin, Solucap C)
　　🍁 Apo-C, Ce-Vi-Sol, Redoxon
Pregnancy Category: C

Dosage

Prophylactic:
A: PO: 45–60 mg/d
C: PO: 20–50 mg/d
Severe deficit: Scurvy
A: PO: IM: IV: 150–500 mg/d in 1 to 2 divided
　　doses
C: PO: IM: IV: 100–300 mg/d in 1 to 2 divided
　　doses
Pregnancy and Lactation:
A: PO: 60–80 mg/d

Contraindications

Caution: Renal calculi, gout, anemia: sickle cell, sideroblastic, thalassemia

Drug-Lab-Food Interactions

Decrease ascorbic acid uptake taken with salicylates; may decrease effect of oral anticoagulants; may decrease elimination of aspirins

Pharmacokinetics

Absorption: PO: quickly
Distribution: PB: UK
Metabolism: t½: UK
Excretion: In the urine; unchanged with high doses

Pharmacodynamics

PO: Onset:>2 d
　　Peak: UK
　　Duration: UK

Therapeutic Effects/Uses

To prevent and treat vitamin C deficiency (scurvy); increase wound healing; for burns

Mode of Action: A water-soluble vitamin, essential for collagen formation and tissue repair (bones, skin, blood vessels)

Side Effects

Headaches, fatigue, drowsiness, nausea, heartburn, vomiting, diarrhea

Adverse Reactions

Kidney stones, crystalluria, hyperuricemia
Life-threatening: Sickle cell crisis, deep vein thrombosis

Assessment and Planning
Interventions
Evaluation
NURSING PROCESS

KEY: A: adult; C: child; PO: by mouth; PB: protein-binding; t½: half-life; UK: unknown; >: greater than; 🍁: Canadian drug names.

kidneys completely excrete vitamin C, mostly unchanged.

Pharmacodynamics

Vitamin C is needed for carbohydrate metabolism and protein and lipid synthesis. Collagen synthesis also requires vitamin C for capillary endothelium, connective tissue and tissue repair, and osteoid tissue of the bone.

Large doses of vitamin C may decrease the effect of oral anticoagulants. Oral contraceptives can decrease vitamin C concentration in the body. Smoking decreases serum vitamin C levels.

The use of **megavitamin therapy,** massive doses of vitamins, is questionable at best. Megadoses of vitamins can cause toxicity and might result in minimal desired effect. Most authorities believe that vitamin C does not cure or prevent the common cold; rather, they believe that vitamin C has a placebo effect. Moreover, megadoses of vitamin C taken with aspirin or sulfonamides may cause crystal formation in the urine (crystalluria). Excessive doses of vitamin C can cause a false-negative occult (blood) stool result and false-positive sugar result in the urine when tested by the Clinitest method. If large doses of megavitamins are to be discontinued, a gradual reduction of dosage is necessary to avoid vitamin deficiency.

VITAMIN B COMPLEX

Vitamin B_1 (thiamine), vitamin B_2 (riboflavin), vitamin B_3 (nicotinic acid, or niacin), and vitamin B_6 (pyridoxine) are four of the vitamin B complex members. This B-complex group is water-soluble. Thiamine is used to treat peripheral neuritis, which may occur from alcoholism or beriberi. Riboflavin may be given to manage dermatologic problems, such as scaly dermatitis, cracked corners of the mouth, and inflammation of the skin and tongue. Niacin is given to alleviate pellagra and hyperlipidemia, for which large doses are required. However, large doses may cause GI irritation and vasodilation, resulting in a flushing sensation. Pyridoxine is administered to correct vitamin B_6 deficiency. It may also help alleviate the symptoms of neuritis caused by isoniazid (INH) therapy for tuberculosis.

FOLIC ACID (FOLATE)

Folic acid is absorbed from the small intestine and the active form of folic acid (folate) is circulated to all tissues. One-third of folate is stored in the liver and the rest is stored in tissues. Four-fifths of folate is excreted in the bile and one-fifth in the urine.

Folic acid is essential for body growth. It is needed for DNA synthesis, and without folic acid there is a disruption in cellular division. Chronic alcoholism, poor nutritional intake, malabsorption syndromes, pregnancy, and drugs that cause inadequate absorption (phenytoin, barbiturates) or folic acid antagonists (methotrexate, triamterene, trimethoprim) are causes of folic acid deficiencies. Symptoms of folic acid deficiencies include anorexia, nausea, stomatitis, diarrhea, fatigue, alopecia, and blood dyscrasias (megaloblastic anemia, leukopenia, and thrombocytopenia). These symptoms are usually not noted for 2 to 4 months after folic acid storage is depleted.

Folic acid deficiency during the first trimester of pregnancy can affect the development of the central nervous system (CNS) of the fetus. This may cause neural tube defects (NTDs) such as spina bifida, which is a defective closure of the bony structure of the spinal cord, or anencephaly, lack of brain mass formation. It is imperative that the pregnant woman take adequate folic acid supplements, 400 μg/day, starting with the first trimester of pregnancy in order to prevent the development of CNS anomalies.

There is some evidence that 400 to 800 μg (0.4 to 0.8 mg) of folic acid per day can decrease the incidence of coronary artery disease. It is thought that folic acid decreases the amino acid homocysteine in the blood, which may contribute to heart disease.

Too-high doses of folic acid may mask signs of vitamin B_{12} deficiency—a risk in the elderly. Clients taking phenytoin (Dilantin) to control seizures should be cautious about taking folic acid. This vitamin can lower the serum phenytoin level, which could increase the risk of seizures. The phenytoin dose would need to be adjusted in such clients.

VITAMIN B_{12}

Vitamin B_{12}, like folic acid, is essential for DNA synthesis. Vitamin B_{12} aids in the conversion of folic acid to its active form. With active folic acid, vitamin B_{12} promotes cellular division. It is also needed for normal hematopoiesis (development of red blood cells in bone marrow) and to maintain nervous system integrity, especially the myelin.

The gastric parietal cells produce an intrinsic factor that is necessary for the absorption of vitamin B_{12} through the intestinal wall. Without the intrinsic factor, little or no vitamin B_{12} is absorbed. After absorption, vitamin B_{12} binds to the protein transcobalamin II and is transferred to the tissues. Most vitamin B_{12} is stored in the liver. Vitamin B_{12} is slowly excreted, and it can take 2 to 3 years for stored vitamin B_{12} to be depleted and a deficit noticed.

Vitamin B_{12} deficiency is uncommon unless there is a disturbance of the intrinsic factor and intestinal absorption. Pernicious anemia (lack of the intrinsic factor) is the major cause of vitamin B_{12} deficiency. Vitamin B_{12} deficiency can develop in strict vegetarians who do not consume meat, fish, or dairy products. Other possible causes of vitamin B_{12} deficiency include malabsorption syndromes (cancer, celiac disease, certain drugs), gastrectomy, Crohn's disease, and liver and kidney diseases. Symptoms may include numbness and tingling in the lower extremities, weakness, fatigue, anorexia, loss of taste, diarrhea, memory loss, mood changes, dementia, psychosis, and megaloblastic anemia with macrocytes (overenlarged erythrocytes [RBC]) in blood, and megaloblasts (overenlarged erythroblasts) in the bone marrow.

To correct vitamin B_{12} deficiency, cyanocobalamin in crystalline form can be given for severe deficits intramuscularly. It cannot be given intravenously because of possible hypersensitive reactions. It also can be given orally and is found in multiple vitamin preparations.

Table 12–2 lists both the fat-soluble and water-soluble vitamins with their functions, suggested food sources, and selected deficiency conditions. Table 12–3 lists fat- and water-soluble vitamins, their RDA

Table 12–2
Vitamins: Functions, Suggested Food Sources, and Selected Deficiency Conditions

VITAMIN	FUNCTION	FOOD SOURCES	DEFICIENCY CONDITIONS
A	Required for development and maintenance of healthy eyes, gums, teeth, skin, hair, and selected glands. Needed for fat metabolism.	Whole milk, butter, eggs, leafy green and yellow vegetables and fruits,* liver	Dry skin, poor tooth development, night blindness
B_1 (thiamine)	Promotes use of sugars (energy). Required for good function of nervous system and heart.	Enriched breads and cereals, yeast, liver, pork, fish, milk	Sensory disturbances, retarded growth, fatigue, anorexia
B_2 (riboflavin)	Promotes body's use of carbohydrates, proteins, and fats by releasing energy to cells. Required for tissue integrity.	Milk, enriched breads and cereals, liver, lean meat, eggs, leafy green vegetables†	Visual defects, such as blurred vision and photophobia; cheilosis; rash on nose; numbness of extremities
B_6 (pyridoxine)	Important in metabolism, synthesis of proteins, and formation of red blood cells.	Lean meat, leafy green vegetables, whole-grain cereals, yeast, bananas	Neuritis, convulsions, dermatitis, anemia, lymphopenia
B_{12} (cobalamin)	Functions as a building block of nucleic acids and to form red blood cells. Facilitates functioning of nervous system.	Liver, kidney, fish, milk	Gastrointestinal disorders, poor growth, anemias
Folic acid	Helps in formation of genetic materials and proteins for the cell nucleus. Assists with intestinal functioning and prevents selected anemias.	Leafy green vegetables, yellow fruits and vegetables, yeast, meats	Decreased WBC count and clotting factors, anemias, intestinal disturbances, depression
Pantothenic acid	Promotes body's use of carbohydrates, fats, and proteins. Essential for formation of specific hormones and nerve-regulating substances.	Eggs, leafy green vegetables, nuts, liver, kidney, skimmed milk	Natural deficiency unknown in man
Niacin	In all body tissues. Necessary for energy-producing reactions. Assists nervous system.	Eggs, meat, liver, beans, peas, enriched bread, and cereals	Retarded growth, pellagra, headache, memory loss, anorexia, insomnia
Biotin	Synthesis of fatty acids and energy production from glucose. Required by body chemical systems.	Eggs, milk, leafy green vegetables, liver, kidney	Natural deficiency unknown in man
C (ascorbic acid)	Helps tissue repair and growth. Required in formation of collagen.	Citrus fruits, tomatoes, leafy green vegetables, potatoes	Poor wound healing, bleeding gums, scurvy, predisposition to infection
D (calciferol)	Promotes use of phosphorus and calcium. Important for strong teeth and bones.	Vitamin D–fortified milk, egg yolk, tuna, salmon	Rickets, deficit of phosphorus and calcium in blood
E	Protects fatty acids and promotes the formation and functioning of red blood cells, muscle, and other tissues.	Whole-grain cereals, wheat germ, vegetable oils, lettuce, sunflower seeds	Breakdown of red blood cells
K	Essential for blood clotting.	Leafy green vegetables, liver, cheese, egg yolk	Increased clotting time, leading to increased bleeding and hemorrhage

*Yellow fruits and vegetables include apricots, cantaloupe, carrots, rutabaga, pumpkin, squash, and sweet potatoes.
†Leafy green vegetables include Brussels sprouts, chard, broccoli, kale, spinach, and turnip and mustard greens.

Table 12–3
Fat- and Water-Soluble Vitamins: RDA, Dosages for Vitamin Deficiencies, and Therapeutic Ranges

VITAMIN	RDA	DOSAGES FOR VITAMIN DEFICIENCIES	THERAPEUTIC RANGES
FAT-SOLUBLE			
Vitamin A	Male: 1000 μg or 5000 IU Female: 800 μg or 4000 IU Preg: 1000 μg, 5000 IU Lact: 1200 μg, 6000 IU	10,000–20,000 IU or 3000–6000 μg/dL	30–70 μg/dL Deficit: < 20 μg/dL
Vitamin D	Male and Female: 40–80 μg; 200–400 IU	Mild: 50–125 μg/dL Moderate to severe: 2.5–7.5 mg/d; 2500–7500 μg	Unknown
Vitamin E	Male: 10 mg/d; 15 IU Female: 8 mg/d; 12 IU Preg: 10–12 mg/d	Malabsorption: 30–100 mg/d Severe deficit: 1–2 mg/kg/d or 50–200 IU/kg/d	0.5–0.7 mg/dL Deficit: < 0.5 mg/dL
Vitamin K	Male: 70–80 μg/d Female: 60–65 μg/d Taking broad-spectrum antibiotic: 140 μg/d Preg: 65 μg/d	5–15 mg/d	Based on prothrombin time (PT) results
WATER-SOLUBLE			
Vitamin C	Male and female: 60 mg/d Preg: 70 mg/dL Lact: 95 mg/dL	150–300 mg *Burns: 500–2000 mg/d*	Serum: > 1.30 mg/dL WBC: > 15 mg/dL *Deficit:* Serum < 0.2 mg/dL WBC; < 7 mg/dL
Vitamin B₁ (thiamine)	Male: 1.5 mg Female: 1.1 mg Preg: 1.5 mg Lact: 1.6 mg	30–60 mg/d	Urine: < 50 μg/d
Vitamin B₂ (riboflavin)	Male: 1.4–1.7 mg Female: 1.2–1.3 mg Preg: 1.6 mg Lact: 1.8 mg	5–25 mg/d Prophylactic: 3 mg/d	Urine: < 50 μg/d
Vitamin B₃ (nicotinic acid or niacin)	Male: 15–19 mg/d Female: 13–15 mg/d Preg: 18 mg/d Lact: 20 mg/d	Prevention: 5–20 mg/d Deficit: 50–100 mg/d Pellagra: 300–500 mg in 3 divided doses Hyperlipidemia: 1–2 g/d in 3 divided doses	Unknown
Vitamin B₆ (pyridoxine)	Male: 2.0 mg/d Female: 1.6 mg/d Preg: 2.1 mg/d Lact: 2.2 mg/d	25–100 mg/d *Isoniazid therapy prophylaxis* 25–50 mg/d *Peripheral neuritis* 50–200 mg/d	Serum: > 50 ng/mL Urine: < 1.0 mg/d
Folic acid (folate)	Male and female: 400 μg/d Preg: 600–800 μg/d Lact: 600–800 μg/d	1–2 mg/d	Serum folate: 6–20 ng/mL RBC: 160–600 ng/mL *Deficit:* Serum: < 3–4 ng/mL RBC: <140 ng/mL
Vitamin B₁₂	Male and female: 3 μg/d Preg: 4 μg/d	100 mg/dL 14 d *Pernicious anemia:* 50–100 μg/d or 1000 μg/wk × 3 wk	150–900 pg/mL *Deficit:* <100 pg/mL *Schilling test* >30% normal

KEY: *Preg: pregnancy; Lact: lactation; d: day; wk: week; >: greater than; <: less than.*

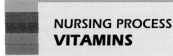

NURSING PROCESS
VITAMINS

Assessment

- Assess the client for vitamin deficiency before start of and regularly throughout therapy. Explore such areas as inadequate nutrient intake, debilitating disease, and GI disorders.
- Assess 24- and 48-h diet history.

Potential Nursing Diagnoses

- Altered nutrition; less than body requirements

Planning

- Client will eat a well-balanced diet that includes the foods and servings recommended in the food pyramid.
- Client with vitamin deficiency will take vitamin supplements as prescribed.

Nursing Interventions

- Administer vitamins with food to promote absorption.
- Store drug in light-resistant container.
- When administering vitamins in drop form, use the supplied calibrated dropper for accurate dosing. Solution may be administered mixed with food or dropped into the mouth.
- Administer IM primarily for clients unable to take by PO route (e.g., GI malabsorption syndrome).
- Recognize need for vitamin E supplements for infants receiving vitamin A to avoid hemolytic anemia.

Client Teaching

General
- Instruct client to take the prescribed amount of drug.
- Inform clients (adults and children) to read vitamin labels in determining which vitamin would be appropriate for them (Fig. 12–4).
- Discourage the client from taking megavitamins over a long period unless these are prescribed for a specific purpose by the health care provider. To discontinue long-term megavitamin therapy, a gradual decrease in vitamin intake is advised to avoid a vitamin deficiency. Megadoses of vitamins can be toxic.
- Inform the client that missing vitamins for 1 or 2 days is not a cause for concern because deficiencies do not occur for some time.
- Advise the client to check the expiration dates on vitamin containers before purchasing and taking them. Potency of the vitamin is reduced after the expiration date.
- Instruct the client to avoid taking mineral oil with vitamin A on a regular basis because it interferes with the absorption of the vitamin. If needed, take mineral oil at bedtime.
- Explain to the client that there is no scientific evidence that megadoses of vitamin C (ascorbic acid) will cure a cold.
- Alert the client not to take megadoses of vitamin C with aspirin or sulfonamides because crystals may form in the kidneys and urine.
- Instruct the client to avoid excessive intake of alcoholic beverages. Alcohol can cause vitamin B-complex deficiencies.

Diet
- Advise the client to eat a well-balanced diet that includes the recommended amounts and types of food detailed in the food pyramid. Vitamin supplements are not necessary if the person is healthy and receives proper nutrition on a regular basis.
- Instruct the client about foods rich in vitamin A, including whole milk, butter, eggs, leafy green and yellow vegetables, fruits, and liver. Foods rich in other vitamins are listed in Table 12–2.

Nursing Process continued on following page

Side Effects
- Instruct the client that nausea, vomiting, headache, loss of hair, and cracked lips (symptoms of hypervitaminosis A) should be reported to the health care provider. Early symptoms of hypervitaminosis D are anorexia, nausea, and vomiting.

Evaluation

- Evaluate the effectiveness of the client's diet for the inclusion of the appropriate amounts and types of food from the food pyramid. Have the client keep a periodic diet chart for a complete week.
- Determine whether the client with malnutrition is receiving appropriate vitamin therapy.

values, dosages for vitamin deficiencies, and therapeutic serum blood or urine ranges.

MINERALS

Various **minerals,** such as iron, copper, zinc, chromium, and selenium, are needed for body function.

Iron

Iron (ferrous sulfate, gluconate, or fumarate) is vital for hemoglobin regeneration. Sixty percent of the iron in the body is found in hemoglobin. One of the

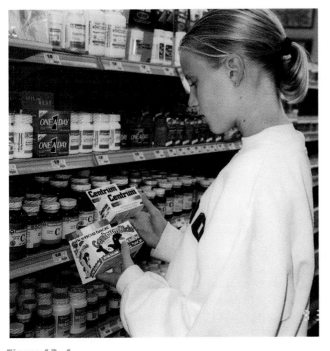

Figure 12–4
This 12-year-old is trying to decide whether an adult or a children's vitamin would be more appropriate for her needs.

causes of anemia is iron deficiency. A normal diet contains 5 to 20 mg of iron per day. Foods rich in iron include liver, lean meats, egg yolks, dried beans, green vegetables (such as spinach), and fruit. Food and antacids slow the absorption of iron, and vitamin C increases iron absorption.

During pregnancy, an increased amount of iron is needed, but during the first trimester of pregnancy, megadoses of iron are contraindicated because of its possible teratogenic effect on the fetus. Larger doses of iron are required during the second and third trimesters of pregnancy.

The infant and child dose of iron, ages 6 months to 2 years old, is 1.5 mg/kg. For the adult, 50 mg/day is needed for hemoglobin regeneration. The ferrous sulfate tablet is 325 mg, of which 65 mg is elemental iron. Therefore, one tablet of ferrous sulfate is sufficient as a daily iron dose when indicated. Chart 12–3 describes the effects of iron preparations.

PHARMACOKINETICS

Iron is absorbed by the intestines and goes into the plasma as heme, or it may be stored as ferritin. Although food decreases absorption by 25% to 50%, it may be necessary to take iron preparations with food to avoid GI discomfort. Vitamin C may slightly increase iron absorption, whereas tetracycline and antacids can decrease absorption.

PHARMACODYNAMICS

Iron replacement primarily is given to correct or control iron-deficiency anemia, which is diagnosed by a laboratory blood smear. Positive findings for this anemia are microcytic (small), hypochromic (pale) erythrocytes (red blood cells [RBC]). Clinical signs and symptoms include fatigue, weakness, shortness of breath, pallor, and, in cases of severe anemia, increased GI bleeding. The dosage of ferrous sulfate for prophylactic use is 300 to 325 mg/day; for therapeu-

Chart 12–3. Antianemia, Mineral: Iron

IRON

Drug Name

IRON
Ferrous sulfate (Feosol, Fer-Iron)
Ferrous gluconate (Fergon, Fetinic)
Ferrous fumarate (Feostat, Fumerin)
Mineral
Pregnancy Category: A

Dosage

A: PO: 300–325 mg q.i.d.: increase to 650 mg q.i.d. as needed and/or tolerated
Pregnancy: PO: 300–600 mg/d
C ≥ 2 y: PO 8 mg/kg q.d. in divided doses

Contraindications

Hemolytic anemia, peptic ulcer, ulcerative colitis

Drug-Lab-Food Interactions

Increased effect of iron with vitamin C; decreased effect of tetracycline, antacids, penicillamine

Pharmacokinetics

Absorption: PO: 5–30% intestines
Distribution: PB: UK
Metabolism: $t_{\frac{1}{2}}$: UK
Excretion: Urine, feces, bile

Pharmacodynamics

PO: Onset: 4 d
Peak: 7–14 d
Duration: 3–4 mo

Therapeutic Effects/Uses

To prevent and treat iron deficiency anemia

Mode of Action: Enables RBC development and oxygen transport via hemoglobin

Side Effects

Nausea, vomiting, diarrhea, constipation, epigastric pain; elixir may stain teeth

Adverse Reactions

Pallor, drowsiness
Life-threatening: Cardiovascular collapse, metabolic acidosis

Assessment and Planning — Interventions — Evaluation — NURSING PROCESS

KEY: A: adult; C: child; PO: by mouth; PB: protein-binding; $t_{\frac{1}{2}}$: half-life; UK: unknown; ≥: equal to or greater than.

tic use, the dosage is 600 to 1200 mg/day in divided doses.

The onset of action for iron therapy takes days, and its peak action does not occur for days or weeks; therefore, the client's symptoms are slow to improve. Increased hemoglobin and hematocrit levels occur within 3 to 7 days.

Iron toxicity is a serious cause of poisoning in children. As few as 10 tablets of ferrous sulfate (3 g) taken at one time can be fatal within 12 to 48 h. The child can hemorrhage because of the ulcerogenic effects of unbound iron, causing shock. Parents should be cautioned against leaving iron tablets that look like candy (M & M's) within a child's reach; most iron products are distributed in bubble packs.

Copper

Copper is needed for the formation of red blood cells and connective tissues. Copper is a cofactor of many enzymes and its function is in the production of norepinephrine and dopamine (neurotransmitters). Excess serum copper levels may be associated with Wilson's disease, which is an inborn error of metabolism that allows for large amounts of copper to accumulate in the liver, brain, cornea (brown or green Kayser-Fleischer rings), or kidney.

A prolonged copper deficiency may result in anemia, which is not corrected by taking iron supplements. Abnormal blood and skin changes caused by a copper deficiency include a decrease in white blood cell count, glucose intolerance, and a decrease in skin and hair pigmentation. Mental retardation might also occur in the young.

The RDA for copper is 1.5 to 3 mg per day. Most adults consume about 1 mg per day. Foods rich in copper are shellfish (crabs and oysters), liver, nuts, seeds (sunflower, sesame), legumes, and cocoa.

Zinc

The use of zinc has greatly increased in the past few years (Fig. 12–5). It is thought by some that zinc can alleviate the common cold. Some individuals take as much as 200 mg/day. The adult RDA is 12 to 19 mg. Foods rich in zinc include beef, lamb, eggs, and leafy and root vegetables.

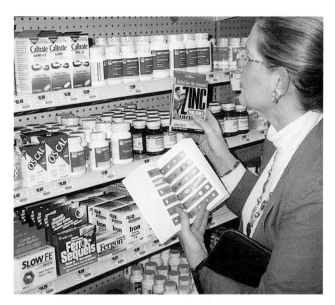

Figure 12–5
The use of zinc and other mineral supplements, such as iron and selenium, is on the rise.

Large doses, more than 150 mg, may cause a copper deficiency, a decrease in high-density lipoprotein (HDL) cholesterol (friendly cholesterol), and a weakened immune response. Zinc can inhibit tetracycline absorption. Clients taking zinc and an antibiotic should not take them together; zinc should be taken at least 2 hours after taking an antibiotic.

Chromium

Chromium is said to be helpful in the control of non–insulin-dependent diabetes. It is thought that this mineral helps to normalize blood glucose by increasing the effects of insulin on the cells. If a client is taking large doses of chromium and an oral hypoglycemic agent or insulin, the glucose level should be monitored closely for a hypoglycemic reaction. The dose of an oral hypoglycemic drug or insulin may need to be decreased. Some clients with an impaired glucose tolerance or prediabetic clients may benefit by taking chromium.

There is no RDA for chromium; however, 50 to 200 μg/day is considered within the normal range for children older than 6 years old and adults. Foods rich in chromium include meats, whole-grain cereals, and brewer's yeast.

Selenium

Selenium acts as a cofactor for an antioxidant enzyme that protects protein and nucleic acids from oxidative damage. Selenium works with vitamin E. It is thought that selenium has an anticarcinogenic effect, and doses greater than 200 μg may reduce the risk of lung, prostate, and colorectal cancer. Excess doses of more than 200 μg might cause weakness, a loss of hair, dermatitis, nausea, diarrhea, and abdominal pain. Also, there may be a garlic-like odor from the skin and breath.

The RDA for selenium is 40 to 75 μg (higher dose for men and a lower dose for women). Foods rich in selenium include meats (especially liver), seafood, eggs, and dairy products.

NURSING PROCESS
ANTIANEMIA, MINERAL: IRON

Assessment

- Obtain a history of anemia or health problems that may lead to anemia.
- Assess the client for signs and symptoms of iron deficiency anemia, such as fatigue, malaise, pallor, shortness of breath, tachycardia, and cardiac dysrhythmia.
- Assess the client's RBC count, hemoglobin, hematocrit, iron level, and reticulocyte count before start of and throughout drug therapy.

Potential Nursing Diagnoses

- Fatigue
- Altered nutrition; less than body requirements

Planning

- Client will consume foods rich in iron.
- Client with iron deficiency anemia or with low hemoglobin will take iron replacement as recommended by the health care provider, resulting in laboratory results within the desired range.

Nursing Interventions

- Encourage the client to eat a nutritious diet to obtain sufficient iron. Iron supplements are not needed unless the person is malnourished, pregnant, or has abnormal menses.
- Store drug in light-resistant container.
- Administer IM injection of iron by the Z-track method to avoid leakage of iron into the subcutaneous tissue and skin, because it irritates and stains the skin.

Client Teaching

General
- Instruct the client to take the tablet or capsule between meals with at least 8 oz of juice or water to promote absorption. If gastric irritation occurs, instruct the client to take with food.
- Advise client to swallow whole the tablet or capsule.
- Instruct client to maintain sitting upright position for 30 min to prevent esophageal corrosion from reflux.
- Do not administer the iron tablet within 1 h of ingesting antacid, milk, ice cream, or other milk products like pudding.
- Advise client to increase fluids, activity, and dietary bulk to avoid or relieve constipation. Slow-release iron capsules decrease constipation and gastric irritation.
- Instruct adults not to leave iron tablets within reach of children. If a child swallows many tablets, induce vomiting and immediately call the local poison control center; the telephone number is in the front of most telephone books (include this number on emergency reference list). Keep ipecac available; it is an over-the-counter drug.
- Instruct client to take prescribed amount of drug to avoid iron poisoning.
- Be alert that iron content varies among iron salts; therefore, do not substitute one for another.
- Advise client that drug treatment for anemia is generally less than 6 months.

Diet
- Counsel the client to include iron-rich foods in diet, such as liver, lean meats, egg yolk, dried beans, green vegetables, and fruit.

Side Effects
- Instruct the client taking the liquid iron preparation to use a straw to prevent discoloration of teeth enamel.
- Alert the client that the drug turns stools a harmless black or dark green.

Nursing Process continued on following page

• Instruct client about signs and symptoms of toxicity, including nausea, vomiting, diarrhea, pallor, hematemesis, shock, and coma, and report occurrence to health care provider.

Evaluation

• Evaluate the effectiveness of the drug therapy by determining that the client is not fatigued or short of breath and that the hemoglobin is within the desired range.

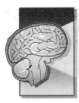

Critical Thinking in Action

A. P. is pregnant and is taking two tablets of 325 mg of ferrous sulfate. She has a 2-year-old daughter.

1. What precautions should A. P. take in regard to the container of ferrous sulfate? Explain.
2. If A. P. asks whether she should take more than two tablets of iron a day, what would your response be?
3. A. P. states that she is constipated and wonders if the iron is the cause. How can this problem be alleviated? What would be an appropriate response?

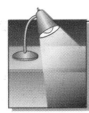

Study Questions

1. Vitamin A is classified in what vitamin category? What foods are high in vitamin A? How does vitamin A differ from vitamin C?
2. What are the nursing interventions when megadoses of vitamins are discontinued?
3. Why is vitamin D important? Which is the most active form of vitamin K? Where is this vitamin stored in the body?
4. What is the approved use of vitamin C (ascorbic acid)? What is the nonapproved use of the drug?
5. What are the common names of vitamins B_1, B_2, B_3, and B_6? What are the uses of these vitamin B-complex drugs?
6. How are folic acid and vitamin B_{12} similar? Why is folic acid important during the first trimester of pregnancy?
7. What is the most common cause of vitamin B_{12} deficiency? Explain.
8. List three nursing interventions and client teaching guides for clients receiving iron preparations. High doses of ferrous sulfate can result in what condition?

13 Fluid and Electrolyte Replacement

Outline

Objectives

- Define osmolality and tonicity.
- Give the iso-osmolality range for serum and intravenous solutions.
- Describe the four classifications of intravenous fluids.
- Differentiate between cations and anions of electrolytes.
- List the major functions of cations.
- List examples of potassium, calcium, and magnesium supplements.
- Explain the methods for correcting potassium, calcium, and magnesium excess.
- Describe several signs and symptoms of hypokalemia, hyperkalemia, hyponatremia, hypernatremia, hypocalcemia, and hypercalcemia.
- Explain the pharmacokinetics and pharmacodynamics of oral and intravenous potassium chloride and calcium salts.
- Describe the assessments, nursing interventions, and client teaching for fluid, potassium, sodium, calcium, and magnesium imbalances.

Terms

anion

cation

electrolytes

hypercalcemia

hyperkalemia

hypermagnesemia

hypernatremia

hyperosmolar

hypocalcemia

hypokalemia

hypomagnesemia

hyponatremia

hypo-osmolar

iso-osmolar

osmolality

tonicity

INTRODUCTION

Fluid replacement is based on body fluid needs. The adult body is approximately 60% water, the human embryo is 97% water, and the newborn infant is 77% water. Of the 60% adult body water (fluid), 40% of the body fluid is the intracellular fluid (cells) and 20% of the body fluid is the extracellular fluid, of which 15% is interstitial (tissue) fluid and 5% is intravascular or vascular fluid (Table 13–1).

Electrolytes in the body are substances that carry either a positive charge **(cation)** or a negative charge **(anion).** Cations and anions are described in Table 13–2. The functions of cations are the transmission of nerve impulses to muscles and the contraction of skeletal and smooth muscles.

The cations of the electrolytes are most plentiful in the cells (potassium, magnesium, and some calcium), in the extracellular fluid (ECF) that is within the blood vessels and tissue spaces (sodium and some calcium), and in the gastrointestinal (GI) tract. Anions are attached to cations. Figure 13–1 illustrates those electrolytes that are plentiful in the stomach and in the intestines.

Fluid and electrolyte replacements based on fluid and specific electrolyte deficits and excesses are described in this chapter.

BODY FLUIDS

The concentration of body fluid is described as **osmolality** and osmolarity; these terms are frequently used interchangeably. Osmolality is the osmotic pull exerted by all particles (solutes) per unit of water, expressed as osmoles or milliosmoles per kilogram (mOsm/kg) of water. There are three types of fluid concentration based on the osmolality of body fluids:

1. **Iso-osmolar** fluid, which has the same proportion of weight of particles (e.g., sodium, glucose, urea, protein) and water
2. **Hypo-osmolar** fluid, which has fewer particles than water

Table 13–1
Body Fluid Volume

FLUID COMPARTMENT		PERCENT
Intracellular (cellular) fluid (ICF)		40
Extracellular fluid (ECF)		20
Interstitial fluid (tissue spaces)	15%	
Intravascular fluid (vascular fluid)	5%	—
Total body fluid		60

Table 13–2
Cations and Anions

CATIONS	ANIONS
Potassium (K$^+$)	Chloride (Cl$^-$)
Sodium (Na$^+$)	Bicarbonate (HCO$_3^{--}$)
Calcium (Ca^{++})	Phosphate (PO$_4^{--}$)
Magnesium (Mg^{++})	Sulfate (SO$_4^{--}$)

3. **Hyperosmolar** fluid, which has more particles than water. The plasma/serum osmolality (concentration of circulating body fluids) can be calculated if the serum sodium level is known or the sodium, glucose, and blood urea nitrogen (BUN) levels are known. Sodium is the main extracellular electrolyte and its major function is to regulate body fluids. The two formulas used for estimating serum osmolality are

1. Double the serum sodium (Na) = serum osmolality

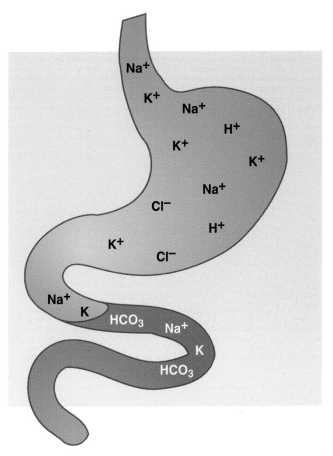

Figure 13–1
Plentiful electrolytes in the gastrointestinal tract include potassium (K), sodium (Na), hydrogen (H), bicarbonate (HCO$_3$), and chloride (Cl).

2. $2 \times \text{serum Na} + \dfrac{\text{BUN}}{3} + \dfrac{\text{Glucose}}{18} = \begin{array}{l}\text{serum}\\ \text{osmolality}\end{array}$

The second formula is more accurate in estimating the correct serum osmolality.

Normal serum osmolality is 275 to 295 mOsm/kg. If the serum osmolality is less than 275 mOsm/kg, the body fluid is hypo-osmolar (fewer particles than water); if the serum osmolality is greater than 295 mOsm/kg, the body fluid is hyperosmolar (more particles and less water). Hypo-osmolality of body fluid may be the result of excess water intake or fluid overload (edema) caused by an inability to excrete excess water. Hyperosmolality of body fluid could be caused by severe diarrhea, increased salt and solutes (protein) intake, inadequate water intake, diabetes, ketoacidosis, or sweating.

The terms osmolality and **tonicity** have been used interchangeably, and although they are similar, they are different. Osmolality is the concentration of body fluids, and tonicity is the effect of fluid on cellular volume. Increased osmolality (hyperosmolality) can result from impermeant solutes such as sodium and permeant solutes such as urea (BUN). Hypertonicity results from an increase of impermeant solutes such as sodium but *not* of permeant solutes such as urea (BUN). Hyperosmolality of body fluid occurs with increased serum sodium and BUN levels; however, it may also cause isotonicity because BUN does not affect tonicity. Serum osmolality is a better indicator of the concentration of solutes in body fluids than tonicity. Tonicity is primarily used as a measurement of the concentration of intravenous solutions.

FLUID REPLACEMENT

Intravenous Solutions

With fluid volume deficit from the extracellular body compartment, there is a loss of fluid from the interstitial (tissue) spaces and from the vascular (blood vessel) spaces. Intravenous (IV) fluids in various concentrations are available for replacing body fluid loss. The osmolalities of many IV fluids are similar to serum osmolality, with the exception that the osmolality of solutions is wider. The average serum osmolality is 290 mOsm/kg H_2O. For an IV solution, the iso-osmolar range is 240 to 340 mOsm/L. This is determined by using a factor of 50: subtract 50 from 290 mOsm to equal 240 and add 50 to 290 to equal 340. If the osmolality of the IV solution is <240 mOsm, it is a hypotonic solution; if it is >340 mOsm, it is a hypertonic solution. Isotonic solutions include dextrose 5% in water (D_5W), which has 250 mOsm; normal saline solution or 0.9% NaCl (sodium chloride), which has 310 mOsm; lactated Ringer's solution, which has 275 mOsm; and Ringer's solution, which has 310 mOsm. These isotonic solutions have osmolalities similar to the extracellular and intracellular fluids. With fluid volume loss, isotonic IV solutions are usually indicated.

Dextrose in water, when used continuously or administered rapidly, becomes a hypotonic solution instead of being isotonic. The dextrose is rapidly metabolized to water and carbon dioxide (CO_2). Five percent dextrose in water (D_5W) should only be given intravenously and never subcutaneously. Normal saline solution or an isotonic solution of dextrose and saline may be administered subcutaneously.

There are four classifications of IV solutions used for fluid replacements:

• Crystalloids
• Colloids
• Lipids
• Blood and blood products

Crystalloids include dextrose, saline, and lactated Ringer's solutions. This group of solutions is used for replacement and maintenance fluid therapy. Colloids are volume expanders that include dextran solutions, amino acids, hetastarch, and plasmanate. Dextran is not a substitute for whole blood, because it does not have any products that can carry oxygen. Dextran 40 tends to interfere with platelet function and can prolong bleeding time. Hetastarch is a nonantigenic volume expander and lasts for more than 24 h, but it may persist for weeks in the body. Hetastarch is an isotonic solution (310 mOsm/L) that can decrease platelet and hematocrit counts, and is contraindicated for clients with bleeding disorders, congestive heart failure (CHF), and renal dysfunction. Plasmanate is a commercially prepared protein product that is used instead of plasma or albumin to replace body protein.

Blood and blood products are whole blood, packed red blood cells, plasma, and albumin. A unit of packed red blood cells contains whole blood without plasma. The advantages for using packed cells instead of whole blood are that there is a decreased chance for causing circulatory overload, a smaller risk of a reaction to plasma antigens, and a possible reduction in the risk of transmitting serum hepatitis. Whole blood should not be used to correct anemia unless the anemia is severe. A unit of whole blood elevates the hemoglobin by 0.5 to 1.0 g, and a unit of packed red blood cells elevates the hematocrit by three points. Lipids are administered as fat emulsion solution and are usually indicated when IV therapy lasts longer than 5 days. Lipids add to balancing the client's nutritional needs. Total parenteral nutrition (TPN) or hyperalimentation is normally implemented for cli-

Table 13–3
Intravenous Solutions

SOLUTIONS	OSMOLALITY (TONICITY)	TOTAL mOsm	DEXTROSE mOsm	Na⁺	K⁺	Ca⁺⁺	Cl⁻	LACTATE	COMMENTS
CRYSTALLOIDS									
NaCl 0.45% (sodium chloride)	Hypo	154	—	77	—	—	77	—	Helpful to establish renal function. Not to be used constantly. Could cause water intoxication.
NaCl 0.9%	Iso	310	—	154	—	—	154	—	Normal saline solution. Restores extracellular fluid volume and replaces sodium chloride deficit.
Dextrose 2.5% in 0.45% NaCl	Iso	279	125	77	—	—	77	—	Helpful in establishing renal function–urine output.
Dextrose 5% in 0.2% saline	Iso	326	250	38	—	—	38	—	Useful for daily maintenance of body fluids and when less Na and Cl are required.
Dextrose 5% in 0.33% saline	Hyper/iso	352	250	51	—	—	51	—	Same as above. May be isotonic because dextrose is rapidly metabolized.
Dextrose 5% in 0.45% saline	Hyper	404	250	77	—	—	77	—	Useful for daily maintenance of body fluids and nutrition and for treating fluid volume deficits.
Dextrose 5% in saline 0.9%	Hyper	560	250	154	—	—	154	—	Replacement of fluid, sodium, chloride, and calories.
Dextrose 10% in saline 0.9%	Hyper	810	500	154	—	—	154	—	Replacement of fluid, sodium, chloride, and calories.
Dextrose 5% in water (50 g) (dextrose 10% is occasionally used)	Iso/hypo	250	250	—	—	—	—	—	Helpful in rehydration and elimination. May cause urinary sodium loss. Good vehicle for IV potassium. May be hypotonic because dextrose is rapidly metabolized.
Lactated Ringer's solution	Iso	274	—	130	4	3	109	28	This solution resembles the electrolyte composition of normal blood serum and plasma. The amount of potassium available is not sufficient for the body's daily potassium requirement.

Table continued on following page

Table 13–3 *Continued*
Intravenous Solutions

SOLUTIONS	OSMOLALITY (TONICITY)	TOTAL mOsm	DEXTROSE mOsm	Na+	K+	Ca++	Cl−	LACTATE	COMMENTS
Dextrose 5% in lactated Ringer's solution	Hyper	524	250	130	4	3	109	28	Same contents as lactated Ringer's plus calories.
Ringer's solution	Iso	312	—	147	4	5	156	—	Does not contain lactate, which can be harmful to people who cannot metabolize lactic acid.
Dextrose 5% in Ringer's solution	Hyper	562	250	147	4	4	156	—	Same contents as Ringer's solution plus calories.
M/6 sodium lactate	Iso	334	—	167	—	—	—	167	Supplies sodium without chloride. Lactate has some caloric value and is metabolized to CO_2 for excretion or increases bicarbonate in alkalosis.
Hyperosmolar saline 3% NaCl	Hyper	990	—	495	—	—	495	—	Helpful for severe hyponatremia by raising Na osmolality of the blood. Helpful in eliminating intracellular fluid excess.
Ionosol B with dextrose 5%	Hyper	—	250	57	25	—	49	25 (also Mg 5 and P 7)	Useful in treating clients requiring polyionic parenteral replacement, e.g., alkalosis due to vomiting, diabetic acidosis, fluid losses from burns, and postoperative fluid volume deficit.
Ionosol D-CM with dextrose 5%	Hyper	—	250	138	12	5	108	50 (also Mg 3)	Useful for electrolyte replacement of duodenal fluid losses because of intestinal suction or biliary or pancreatic drainage and to correct mild acidosis.

SOLUTIONS	OSMOLALITY	TOTAL mOsm	DEXTROSE mOsm	Na+	K+	Ca++	Mg++	Cl−	HCO3	COMMENTS
Isolyte R with 5% dextrose (McGraw)	Hyper	378	250	40	16	5	3	40	24 (acetate)	For maintenance therapy: Contains multiple electrolytes. May be isotonic because dextrose is rapidly metabolized.
Normosol M (Abbott)	Hypo	112	—	40	13	—	3	40	16 (acetate)	For maintenance therapy.

Table continued on following page

Table 13–3 *Continued*
Intravenous Solutions

SOLUTIONS	OSMOLALITY (TONICITY)	TOTAL mOsm	DEXTROSE mOsm	Na$^+$	K$^+$	Ca^{++}	Mg^{++}	Cl$^-$	HCO$_3$	COMMENTS
Normosol M with 5% dextrose (Abbott)	Hyper	362	250	40	13	—	3	40	16 (acetate)	For maintenance therapy. May be isotonic because dextrose is rapidly metabolized.
Normosol R (Abbott)	Iso	296	—	140	5	—	3	98	50	For replacement therapy. Contains multiple electrolytes.
Normosol R with 5% dextrose (Abbott)	Hyper	546	250	140	5	—	3	98	50	Same as above with calories.
Isolyte E	Hyper	568	250	140	10	5	3	103	57	For replacement therapy. Is isotonic without the 5% dextrose.

SOLUTIONS	OSMOLALITY	CALORIC VALUE	mEq/L (mOsm)			MISCELLANEOUS	COMMENTS
			Na$^+$	K$^+$	Cl$^-$		
COLLOIDS							
Protein Solutions Aminosol 5%	Iso	175	<10	17	—	Amino acids	Provides protein and fluid for body. Prevents shock and promotes wound healing.
Aminosol 5% with dextrose 5%	Hyper	345	<10	17	—	Amino acids	Provides protein, calories, and fluid for body; especially helpful for clients who are old and malnourished and for those with hypoproteinemia resulting from other causes. Not to be used in severe liver damage.
Plasma Expander Dextran 40 10% in normal saline (0.9%) or 5% dextrose in water (500 mL bottle)	Hyper						Dextran is a colloidal solution used to increase plasma volume. Dextran 40 is a short-lived plasma volume expander (4–6 h). Useful in early shock by correcting hypovolemia, and increasing arterial pressure, pulse pressure, and cardiac output. It improves microcirculatory flow by reducing red blood cell aggregation in the capillaries (increases small vessel perfusion). *Caution:* It should not be used for clients who are severely dehydrated, have renal disease, have thrombocytopenia, or are actively hemorrhaging.

Table continued on following page

Table 13–3 *Continued*
Intravenous Solutions

SOLUTIONS	OSMOLALITY	CALORIC VALUE	Na⁺	K⁺	Cl⁻	MISCELLANEOUS	COMMENTS
			mEq/L (mOsm)				
Dextran 70 6% in normal saline (0.9%) or 5% dextrose in water	Hyper						Dextran 70 is a long-lived plasma volume expander (20 h). Useful for shock or impending shock caused by hemorrhage, surgery, or burns. It can interfere with platelet function, thus causing prolonged bleeding. Blood for type and cross-match should be drawn before starting Dextran; it tends to coat RBC. Dextran 70 is seldom administered.

SOLUTIONS	VOLUME (mL)	Na⁺	K⁺	Cl⁻	COMMENTS
BLOOD PRODUCTS					
Whole blood	500–1000	142	5	103	Replacement for blood loss that is greater than 1 L (2 pints or units). One unit of blood elevates the hemoglobin by 0.5–0.75 g/dL.
Packed red blood cells	250	5	20	13	Replacement of blood loss for clients who do not require excess fluid. Prevents overload of fluid for clients with CHF. It minimizes potential risks of viral transmission.
Plasma	250	38	1	25	Volume expander. It does not require type and cross-match.
Albumin (5%–25%)	100	16	0	2	Volume expander. Helps to increase plasma oncotic (osmotic) pressure caused by malnutrition, liver disease.
LIPIDS					
Fat emulsions (10% & 20%)					Contains soybean or safflower oil and egg phosphatides. Used for prolonged parenteral nutrition to provide essential fatty acids. Avoid for clients with high hyperlipemia. Use cautiously for clients with severe liver or pulmonary disease.

Solution chart reviewed by Abbott Laboratories Clinical Research Associate and Baxter Laboratories Clinical Information Manager. Selected portions from Abbott Laboratories: Wall Chart, Intravenous and Other Solutions, North Chicago, October 1968; Traveenol Laboratories, Inc.: Guide to Fluid Therapy, Deerfield, IN, 1981: Kee, J. L., Paulanka, B. J.: Fluids and Electrolytes with Clinical Applications, 6/E. New York: Delmar Publishers, 1999; Brensilver, J. M., Goldberger, E: A Primer of Water, Electrolyte, and Acid–Base Syndromes, 8/E. Philadelphia: F. A. Davis, 1996; Methany N.: Fluid and Electrolyte Balance: Nursing Considerations, 3/E. Philadelphia: J. B. Lippincott, 1996.

ents who require long-term IV therapy. TPN is discussed in Chapter 14.

Table 13–3 lists various IV solutions in the four classifications according to their osmolality, caloric and electrolyte compositions, and general comments.

Daily water requirements differ according to age and medical problems. The approximate daily water need for a client weighing 70 kg is 30 mL per kg of

NURSING PROCESS
FLUID REPLACEMENT

Assessment

- Assess vital signs and use for future baseline values. Report abnormal findings.
- Check the client's laboratory findings, especially the hematocrit and BUN. If both values are elevated, this may be due to fluid volume deficit (dehydration). If the BUN is >60 mg/dL, renal impairment is most likely the cause.
- Check urine output. Report if the urine output is <25 mL/h or 600 mL/day. Normal urine output should be >35 mL/h or 1000 to 1200 mL/day.
- Check urine specific gravity (SG). Normal range is 1.005 to 1.030. If the urine specific gravity is greater than 1.030, hypovolemia or dehydration may be the cause.
- Check the types of intravenous fluid ordered per day. Report to the health care provider if there is continuous use of one type of IV fluid such as 5% dextrose in water (D_5W). This could cause hypo-osmolality of body fluid.
- Check client's weight and record for a baseline level.

Nursing Diagnoses

- Risk for fluid volume excess related to excess volume infused, rapidly infused IV fluids, or volume infused too great for client's physical size or condition
- Risk for fluid volume deficit related to inadequate fluid intake
- Altered tissue perfusion (vascular) related to decreased blood circulation or inadequate fluid replacement

Planning

- Client will not develop fluid volume deficit or excess as the result of intravenous fluid replacement.
- Client will be hydrated; vital signs and urine output will be within the normal ranges.

Nursing Interventions

- Monitor vital signs and report abnormal findings. Rapid pulse rate could be indicative of hypovolemia (decrease in body fluids). Blood pressure changes should be reported. Decrease in blood pressure occurs when hypovolemia is severe and shock is occurring.

Nursing Process continued on following page

body weight, or 2000 mL per day. In pounds, the calculation is 15 mL per pound. A client weighing 150 pounds should receive 2250 mL of water daily. If the client has a fever, water needs increase by 15%. A client loses water daily: 400 to 500 mL through skin by normal evaporation, 400 to 500 mL from breathing, 100 to 200 mL in feces, and 1000 to 1200 mL in urine.

When IV fluids are prescribed for 24 hours, the total amount of IV fluid ordered is usually 2000 to 3000 mL. Normally, there is more than one type of solution used. Three liters of dextrose 5% in water per day causes a hypo-osmolar body fluid state, and water intoxication (intracellular fluid volume excess) can occur. If hypertonic IV solutions such as dextrose in normal saline solution only are used, dehydration can occur as a result of hyperosmolality, which pulls fluid from the cells and promotes fluid excretion. Usually there are one or two isotonic solutions (this could include D_5W) and one or two hypertonic solutions administered per day.

ELECTROLYTES

Potassium

Potassium (K^+), an important cellular cation, is 20 times more prevalent in the cells (intracellular fluids [ICF]) than in the vessels (intravascular fluid, or plasma). The normal plasma or serum level (these terms are frequently used interchangeably) for potassium is 3.5 to 5.3 milliequivalents per liter (mEq/L). A serum potassium level less than 3.5 mEq/L is called **hypokalemia,** and a serum potassium level greater than 5.3 mEq/L is called **hyperkalemia.** Potassium has a narrow normal range. Too little potassium (hypokalemia), less than 2.5 mEq/L, or too much potassium (hyperkalemia), more than 7.0 mEq/L, may lead to cardiac arrest.

Potassium is poorly stored in the body, so daily potassium intake is necessary. The recommended potassium intake is approximately 40 to 60 mEq daily,

- Monitor urine output. Report if the urine output is less than 600 mL/day. This could be due to fluid volume deficit or CHF from fluid overload.
- Monitor weight daily. A gain of 2.2 to 2.5 pounds is equivalent to 1 L of fluid. If the client gained 5 pounds in one day, it may indicate that the client is retaining 2 L of fluid. This could be a sign of fluid overload.
- Check for signs and symptoms of fluid volume deficit (dehydration) such as excess thirst (mild dehydration). Marked thirst, dry mucous membranes, poor skin turgor, decrease in urine output, tachycardia, and slight decrease in systolic blood pressure are indicators of marked dehydration.
- Check for signs and symptoms of fluid volume excess (fluid overload) such as constant, irritated cough; dyspnea; neck vein engorgement; hand vein engorgement; and moist rales in the lung.
- Monitor laboratory results daily, especially BUN, hemoglobin, and hematocrit. Elevated values can indicate dehydration.
- Monitor the types of fluids the client is receiving. Report if only one type of IV fluid is being prescribed daily. This can cause fluid imbalance (hypo-osmolality or hyperosmolality).
- Monitor IV injection site for infiltration or phlebitis.

Client Teaching

- Instruct the client that thirst means there is a mild fluid deficit. Increasing fluid intake is important. Elderly clients' thirst mechanisms are frequently decreased. The nurse should offer fluids as needed to the elderly.
- Inform the client to report frequent vomiting or diarrhea. When vomiting and diarrhea occur constantly or over several days, severe fluid volume imbalance can result.
- Encourage the client to monitor fluid intake and output. Inform the client to report abnormal findings such as diuresis, weight gain or loss, peripheral edema, or tight shoes and rings to the health care provider.

Evaluation

- Evaluate that the intravenous therapy has replaced the client's body fluids.
- Evaluate that the IV therapy has not caused a deficit or an excess of the client's body fluids.

consumed in such foods as fruits, fruit juices, and vegetables, or in the form of potassium supplements. Bananas and dried fruits are higher in potassium content than oranges and fruit juices.

FUNCTIONS

Potassium is necessary for the transmission and conduction of nerve impulses, and for the contraction of skeletal, cardiac, and smooth muscles. It is also needed for the enzyme action needed to change carbohydrates to energy (glycolysis) and amino acids to protein. Potassium promotes glycogen (energy) storage in hepatic (liver) cells. It also regulates the osmolality (solute concentration) of cellular fluids.

HYPOKALEMIA

Whenever cells are damaged from trauma, injury, surgery, or shock, potassium leaks from the cells into the intravascular fluid and is excreted by the kidneys. With cellular loss of potassium, potassium shifts from the blood plasma into the cell to restore the cellular potassium balance. Thus, hypokalemia usually results. Vomiting and diarrhea also decrease serum potas-

sium levels. Between 80% and 90% of potassium in the body is excreted in the urine; 8% is excreted in the feces. If the kidneys shut down or are diseased, potassium accumulates in the intravascular fluid and hyperkalemia results.

When the serum potassium level is between 3.0 and 3.5 mEq/L, 100 to 200 mEq of potassium chloride (KCl) is needed to increase the serum potassium level 1 mEq (e.g., 3.0 to 4.0 mEq). If the serum potassium level is less than 3.0 mEq/L, then 200 to 400 mEq of KCl is needed to increase the serum potassium level 1 mEq. Potassium chloride cannot rapidly correct a severe potassium deficit.

Potassium can be given orally or intravenously and is combined with an anion, such as chloride or bicarbonate. Oral potassium can be given as a liquid, powder, or tablet. Potassium is extremely irritating to the gastric and intestinal mucosa, so *it must be given with at least a half glass of fluid* (juice or water) or, preferably, a full glass of fluid. Because cardiac arrest (standstill) results from excessive potassium, intravenous potassium must be diluted in IV fluids—it cannot be given as an IV push or IV bolus. Nurses must re-

Table 13–4	
Potassium Supplements	
PREPARATION	**DRUG**
Oral liquid	Potassium chloride: 10% = 20 mEq/15 mL, 20% = 40 mEq/15 mL
	Kay Ciel (potassium chloride)
	Kaochlor 10% (potassium chloride)
	Kaon-Cl 20% (potassium chloride)
	Potassium Triplex (potassium acetate, bicarbonate, citrate). Rarely used.
Oral tablet or capsule	Potassium chloride (enteric-coated tablet)
	Kaon (potassium gluconate)
	Kaon-Cl (potassium chloride)
	Slow-K (potassium chloride, 8 mEq)
	Kaochlor (potassium chloride)
	K-Lyte (potassium bicarbonate-effervescent tablet)
	K-Lyte/Cl (potassium chloride)
	K-Dur (potassium chloride)
	Micro-K (potassium chloride)
	Ten-K (potassium chloride)
	K-Tab (potassium chloride)
Intravenous potassium	Potassium chloride in clear liquid in multidose vial or ampule (2 mEq/mL)

member that, when administering any type of potassium, *it must be diluted.* Table 13–4 lists the potassium preparations used to treat hypokalemia.

Signs and symptoms of hypokalemia include nausea and vomiting, dysrhythmias, abdominal distention, and soft, flabby muscles. If the serum potassium level is a low normal, foods high in potassium should be suggested, such as fruit juices, citrus fruits, dried fruits, bananas, nuts (peanut butter), some sodas and tea, and vegetables such as potatoes, broccoli, and green leafy vegetables.

Certain drugs promote potassium loss, such as potassium-wasting diuretics (hydrochlorothiazide [HydroDIURIL], furosemide [Lasix], ethacrynic acid [Edecrin]) and cortisone preparations. Clients receiving these drugs should increase their potassium intake by consuming foods rich in potassium or by taking potassium supplements. Their serum potassium levels should be monitored for abnormal serum potassium levels. Potassium must be used cautiously in clients with renal insufficiency. If the urine output

is less than 600 mL/day, the health care provider should be notified, especially if a potassium supplement is ordered.

Chart 13–1 compares the pharmacokinetics and pharmacodynamics of oral and intravenous potassium preparations. The nursing process is based on the drug data.

Pharmacokinetics

Oral liquid potassium is absorbed faster than tablets or capsules; the pharmaceutic phase is decreased. Sustained-release capsules such as Micro-K, Slow-K, and K-Tab release the potassium over a period of time. Plenty of water, no less than 4 oz, must be taken with oral potassium preparations. The capsule may be taken with a meal or immediately after eating.

Intravenous potassium is immediately absorbed in the vascular fluids. Intravenous potassium must be diluted in IV solutions anal *never* given as a bolus or an IV push. Between 80% and 90% of the potassium in body fluids is excreted in the urine; 8% is excreted in feces.

Pharmacodynamics

Potassium maintains neuromuscular activity; therefore, serum potassium levels should be closely monitored. Onset of action of oral potassium may be within 30 min; for intravenous potassium, it is immediate. Duration of action of potassium is not known; however, it may vary according to the dose taken. An electrocardiogram (ECG) should be closely monitored when large doses are administered.

HYPERKALEMIA

Hyperkalemia usually results from renal insufficiency or from the administration of large doses of potassium over time. For a mildly elevated serum potassium level, such as 5.3 to 5.5 mEq/L, restricting foods rich in potassium may correct the excess potassium level. If renal insufficiency or failure is present, additional measures must be taken.

Drugs that might be ordered for hyperkalemia (serum potassium >5.3 mEq/L) are listed in Table 13–5. To immediately decrease a temporary potassium excess in the serum potassium level, sodium bicarbonate, calcium gluconate, or insulin and glucose may be prescribed. Sodium polystyrene sulfonate (Kayexalate) with sorbitol is ordered for severe hyperkalemia. This drug therapy exchanges a sodium ion for a potassium ion in the body and is a more permanent means of correcting hyperkalemia.

Signs and symptoms of hyperkalemia include nausea, abdominal cramps, oliguria (decreased urine output), tachycardia and later bradycardia, weakness, and numbness or tingling in the extremities. For mild hyperkalemia, foods rich in potassium are usually restricted.

Chart 13–1.   Electrolyte: Potassium

POTASSIUM

Assessment and Planning

Drug Name

Potassium chloride
   (Kaochlor, Kaon-Cl, Kay Ciel, Micro-K,
K-Dur)
Potassium replacement
Pregnancy Category: A

Dosage

A: *Hypokalemia (maintenance):*
PO: 20 mEq in 1–2 divided doses
Hypokalemia (correction):
PO: 40–80 mEq in 3–4 divided doses
IV: 20–40 mEq diluted in 1 L of IV solution

Contraindications

Renal insufficiency or failure, Addison's disease,
hyperkalemia, severe dehydration, acidosis, potassium-sparing diuretics
Caution:
Cardiac disorders, burns

Drug-Lab-Food Interactions

Increase serum potassium level with ACE inhibitors, potassium-sparing diuretics
Lab: May *increase* serum potassium level
(>5.5 mEq/L)

Interventions

Pharmacokinetics

Absorption: PO: rapidly absorbed, 95% in body
fluids
Distribution: PB: UK
Metabolism: t½: UK
Excretion: 80%–90% in urine; 10% in feces

Pharmacodynamics

PO: Onset: 30 min
     Peak: 1–2 h
     Duration: UK
IV: Onset: Rapid
     Peak: 1–1.5 h
     Duration: UK

NURSING PROCESS

Therapeutic Effects/Uses

To correct potassium deficit; strengthen cardiac and muscular activities.

Mode of Action: Transmits and conducts nerve impulses; contracts skeletal, smooth, and cardiac
muscles.

Evaluation

Side Effects

Nausea, vomiting, diarrhea, abdominal cramps,
irritability, rash (rare)

Adverse Reactions

Oliguria, ECG changes (peaked T waves, wid-
ened QRS complex, prolonged PR interval), GI
ulceration
Life-threatening: Cardiac dysrhythmias, respiratory distress, cardiac arrest

KEY: A: adult; PO: by mouth; IV: intravenous; UK: unknown; PB: protein-binding; t½: half-life; >: greater than; ACE: angiotensin-
converting enzyme; ECG: electrocardiogram.

EFFECT OF DRUGS ON POTASSIUM BALANCE

Potassium-wasting diuretics are a major cause of hypokalemia. Diuretics are divided into two categories:
potassium-wasting and potassium-sparing drugs. Potassium-wasting diuretics excrete potassium and other
electrolytes such as sodium and chloride in the urine.
Potassium-sparing diuretics retain potassium but excrete sodium and chloride in the urine. Table 13–6
lists the trade and generic names of potassium-
wasting, potassium-sparing diuretics, and combined
potassium-wasting/potassium-sparing diuretics.

Laxatives, corticosteroids, antibiotics, and potassium-wasting diuretics are the major drug groups
that can cause hypokalemia. The drug groups that
may cause hyperkalemia include oral and intravenous
potassium salts, central nervous system (CNS) agents,
and potassium-sparing diuretics. Table 13–7 lists the
drugs that affect potassium balance.

Table 13–5
Correction of Potassium Excess (Hyperkalemia)

DRUG THERAPY	RATIONALE
IV Sodium bicarbonate (HCO_3)	By elevating the pH level, potassium moves back into the cells, thus lowering the serum level.
10% Calcium gluconate	Calcium decreases the irritability of myocardium resulting from hyperkalemia. It does not promote potassium loss.
Insulin and glucose	The combination of insulin and glucose moves potassium back into the cells. This lasts about 6 h. Repeating these agents is not always as effective.
Sodium polystyrene sulfonate (Kayexalate) and sorbitol 70%	Kayexalate is used as a cation exchange for severe hyperkalemia. It can be given orally or rectally. *Orally:* Kayexalate: 15 g, 1–4 × 1 day. Sorbitol 70%: 20 mL with each dose. *Rectally:* Kayexalate: 30–50 g. Sorbitol 70%: 50 mL. Mix with 100–150 mL of water. (Retention enema for 20–30 min)

Sodium

Sodium is the major cation in the extracellular fluid (vessels and tissue spaces). The normal serum or plasma sodium level is 135 to 145 mEq/L. A serum sodium level less than 135 mEq/L is called **hyponatremia,** and a serum sodium level greater than 145 mEq/L is called **hypernatremia.**

FUNCTIONS

Sodium is the major electrolyte that regulates body fluids. It promotes the transmission and conduction of nerve impulses. It is part of the sodium/potassium pump that causes cellular activity. Sodium shifts into cells as potassium shifts out of the cells, repeatedly, to maintain water balance and neuromuscular activity. When sodium shifts into the cell, depolarization occurs; when sodium shifts out of the cell, potassium shifts back into the cell and repolarization occurs. Sodium combines readily with chloride (Cl) or bicarbonate (HCO_3) to promote acid–base balance.

HYPONATREMIA

Sodium loss can result from vomiting, diarrhea, surgery, and potent diuretics. Signs and symptoms of hyponatremia include muscular weakness, headaches, abdominal cramps, nausea, and vomiting. The serum sodium level should be monitored as necessary.

For a serum sodium level between 125 and 135 mEq/L, normal saline (0.9% sodium chloride) may increase the sodium content in the vascular fluid. If the serum sodium level is 115 mEq/L, a hypertonic, 3% saline solution may be necessary.

HYPERNATREMIA

When the serum sodium level is elevated above 145 mEq/L, sodium restriction is indicated. Signs and symptoms of hypernatremia are flushed skin, elevated body temperature and blood pressure, and rough, dry tongue. An increase in serum sodium can

Table 13–6
Potassium-Wasting and Potassium-Sparing Diuretics

POTASSIUM-WASTING DIURETICS	POTASSIUM-SPARING DIURETICS	COMBINATION DIURETICS

Thiazides
  Chlorothiazide (Diuril)
  Hydrochlorothiazide (Hydro-DIURIL)
Loop diuretics
  Furosemide (Lasix)
  Ethacrynic acid (Edecrin)
Carbonic anhydrase inhibitors
  Acetazolamide (Diamox)
Osmotic diuretic
  Mannitol
	Aldosterone antagonist
	  Spironolactone (Aldactone)
	  Triamterene (Dyrenium)
	  Amiloride (Midamor)
		Aldactazide
		Spironazide
		Dyazide
		Moduretic

From Kee, J. L., Paulanka, B. J.: Fluids and Electrolytes with Clinical Applications, *6/E. New York: Delmar Publishers, 1999.*

Table 13–7
Drugs Affecting Potassium Balance

POTASSIUM IMBALANCE	DRUGS	RATIONALE
Hypokalemia (serum potassium deficit)	Laxatives Enemas (hyperosmolar)	Laxative abuse can cause potassium depletion.
	Corticosteroids	
	Cortisone	Ion exchange agent.
	Prednisone	Steroids promote potassium loss and sodium retention.
	Kayexalate	Exchange potassium ion for a sodium ion.
	Licorice	Licorice action is similar to aldosterone, promoting K loss and Na retention.
	Levodopa / L-Dopa Lithium	Increases potassium loss via urine.

	Antibiotic I
	  Amphotericin B
	  Polymyxin B
	  Tetracycline (outdated)
	  Gentamicin
	  Neomycin
	  Amikacin
	  Tobramycin
	  Cisplatin
		Toxic effect on renal tubules, thus decreasing potassium reabsorption.

	Antibiotic II
	  Penicillin
	  Ampicillin
	  Carbenicillin
	  Ticarcillin
	  Nafcillin
	  Piperacillin
	  Aziocillin
		Potassium excretion is enhanced by the presence of nonreabsorbable anions.

	Alpha-adrenergic blockers Insulin and glucose	These agents promote movement of potassium into cells, thus lowering the serum potassium level.

	Beta$_2$ agonists
	  Terbutaline
	  Albuterol
	Estrogen
	Potassium-wasting diuretics
		See Table 13–6.

Hyperkalemia (serum potassium excess)	Potassium choice (oral or IV) Potassium salt (no salt) K penicillin	Excess ingestion or infusion of these agents can cause a potassium excess.
	KPO$_4$ enema Indomethacin Captopril (Capoten) Heparin	Decreases renal excretion of potassium.

	CNS agents
	  Barbiturates
	  Sedatives
	  Narcotics
	  Heroin
	  Amphetamines
		These CNS agents are usually characterized by muscle necrosis and cellular shift of potassium from cells to serum.

	Nonsteroidal anti-inflammatory drugs (NSAIDS); ibuprofen	Blocks cellular potassium uptake.
	Alpha agonists Beta blockers	
	Succinylcholine Cyclophosphamide	Loss of potassium from cells.
	Potassium-sparing diuretics	See Table 13–6.

From Kee, J. L., Paulanka, B. J.: Fluids and Electrolytes with Clinical Applications, *6/E. New York: Delmar Publishers, 1999.*

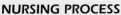

NURSING PROCESS
ELECTROLYTE: POTASSIUM

Assessment

- Assess for signs and symptoms of hypokalemia (decreased serum potassium) and hyperkalemia (elevated serum potassium). Symptoms of hypokalemia include nausea, vomiting, cardiac dysrhythmias, abdominal distention, and soft flabby muscles. Symptoms of hyperkalemia include oliguria, nausea, abdominal cramps, and tachycardia and, later, bradycardia, weakness, and numbness or tingling in the extremities.
- Assess serum potassium level; normal serum potassium level is 3.5 to 5.3 mEq/L. Report serum potassium deficit or excess to the health care provider.
- Obtain baseline vital sign (VS) and ECG readings. Report abnormal findings. The VS and ECG results can be compared with future VS and ECG readings.
- Assess the client for signs and symptoms of digitalis toxicity when receiving a digitalis preparation (digoxin) and a potassium-wasting diuretic (hydrochlorothiazide, furosemide) or a cortisone preparation (prednisone). A decreased serum potassium level enhances the action of digitalis. Signs and symptoms of digitalis toxicity are nausea, vomiting, anorexia, bradycardia (pulse rate <60 or markedly decreased), cardiac dysrhythmias, and visual disturbances.

Potential Nursing Diagnoses

- Altered nutrition, less than body requirements
- Impaired tissue integrity

Planning

- Client's serum potassium level will be within normal range in 2 to 4 d.
- Client with hypokalemia will eat foods rich in potassium, such as fruits, fruit juices, and vegetables. Client with hyperkalemia will avoid potassium-rich foods.

Nursing Interventions

- Give oral potassium with a sufficient amount of water or juice (at least 6 to 8 oz) or at mealtime. Potassium is extremely irritating to the gastric mucosa.
- Dilute IV potassium chloride in the IV bag and invert the bag several times to promote thorough mixing of potassium with IV fluids. Potassium *cannot* be given IM. *Potassium should never be given as an IV bolus or push.* Giving IV potassium directly into the vein causes cardiac dysrhythmias and cardiac arrest.
- Monitor the amount of urine output. If the client is receiving potassium and the urine output is <25 mL/h or <600 mL/d, potassium accumulation occurs. Remember, 80% to 90% of potassium is excreted in the urine. Report results to the health care provider.
- Monitor the serum potassium level. Hypokalemia occurs if the serum potassium value is <3.5 mEq/L; hyperkalemia occurs when the serum potassium value is >5.3 mEq/L.
- Monitor the ECG. With hypokalemia, the T wave is flat or inverted, the ST segment is depressed, and the QT interval is prolonged. With hyperkalemia, the T wave is narrow and peaked, the QRS complex is spread, and the PR interval is prolonged.
- Check the IV site for infiltration if the client is receiving potassium in the IV fluids. Potassium can cause tissue necrosis if it infiltrates into the fatty tissue (subcutaneous tissue). The IV fluid with potassium should be discontinued when infiltration occurs.
- Monitor clients receiving various medications for hyperkalemia, such as sodium bicarbonate, calcium gluconate, insulin and glucose, and Kayexalate and sorbitol, for signs and symptoms of continuing hyperkalemia or of developing hypokalemia.
- Prepare and administer Kayexalate orally or by retention enema, according to the drug circular. The client should have a cleansing enema before the retention enema. A

Nursing Process continued on following page

suggested method for preparation and administration of Kayexalate retention enema is as follows:

1. Use warm fluid to prepare (do not heat).
2. Mix with 20% dextrose in water or sorbitol.
3. Keep particles in suspension by stirring periodically and administer at body temperature by gravity.
4. Encourage the client to retain the enema for 30 to 60 min minimum.
5. Flush tubing with 50 to 100 mL of fluid before clamping for retention.
6. After completion, irrigate the colon with 2 quarts of flushing liquid and drain the fluid contents.

Client Teaching

General

- Advise the client to have the serum potassium level checked at regular intervals when taking drugs that are potassium supplements or that decrease potassium levels.
- Instruct the client to drink a full glass of water or juice when taking oral potassium supplements. Potassium preparations can be taken during or after a meal. Explain to the client that potassium is very irritating to the stomach.
- Instruct the client to comply with the prescribed potassium dose, regular laboratory tests, and medical follow-up related to the health problem and drug regimen.

Diet

- Instruct the client who is taking a potassium-wasting diuretic or a cortisone preparation to eat potassium-rich foods, including citrus fruit juice, fruits (bananas, plums, oranges, cantaloupes, raisins), vegetables, and nuts.

Side Effects

- Instruct the client to report signs and symptoms of hypokalemia and hyperkalemia. See Assessment for the list. When taking large amounts of potassium supplements, hyperkalemia could result.

Evaluation

- Evaluate the client's serum potassium level and ECG. Report to the health care provider if the level remains abnormal. Potassium replacements and diet may need modification.

result from consuming certain drugs, such as cortisone preparations, cough medications, and selected antibiotics.

Calcium

Calcium is found in approximately equal proportion in the ICF and ECF. The serum calcium range is 4.5 to 5.5 mEq/L, or 9 to 11 mg/dL. A calcium deficit, less than 4.5 mEq/L, is called **hypocalcemia,** and a calcium excess, greater than 5.5 mEq/L, is called **hypercalcemia.** About half of the calcium in the body fluid is bound to protein. Calcium that is unbound to protein is free, ionized calcium and can cause a physiologic response. If the serum protein (albumin) levels are decreased, there is more free circulating calcium even when the serum calcium level is decreased.

Modern blood analyzers allow the ionized calcium (iCa) level to be measured. The normal serum ionized calcium range is 2.2 to 2.5 mEq/L, or 4.25 to 5.25 mg/dL. Certain changes in the blood composition can either increase or decrease the serum iCa level. When an individual is acidotic, calcium is released from the serum protein and increases the serum iCa level. During alkalosis, calcium is bound to protein and there is less iCa.

FUNCTIONS

Calcium promotes normal nerve and muscle activity. It increases contraction of the heart muscle (myocardium). This cation also maintains normal cellular permeability and promotes blood clotting by converting prothrombin into thrombin. In addition, calcium is needed for the formation of bone and teeth.

Vitamin D is needed for calcium absorption from the GI tract. Aspirin and anticonvulsants can alter vitamin D, affecting calcium absorption. Loop or high-ceiling diuretics (furosemide [Lasix]; see Chapter 38), steroids (cortisone), magnesium preparations, and phosphate preparations promote calcium loss. Conversely, thiazide diuretics (hydrochlorothiazide

NURSING PROCESS
ELECTROLYTE: SODIUM

Assessment

- Assess the client for signs and symptoms of hyponatremia and hypernatremia. See signs and symptoms in this chapter.
- Check the serum sodium level. Report abnormally low sodium levels (<125 mEq/L), because prompt medical care is required.
- Obtain history of health problems that may lead to sodium loss or excess.

Potential Nursing Diagnosis

- Risk for fluid volume excess related to water retention

Planning

- Client's serum sodium level will be within normal range in 3 to 5 days.
- Edema will be decreased in client with sodium retention.

Nursing Interventions

- Monitor the medical regimen for correction of hyponatremia, such as water restriction, intravenous normal saline (0.9% sodium chloride), and 3% saline solution to correct a serum sodium level of <115 mEq/L.
- Monitor serum sodium levels. Report abnormal level.

Client Teaching

- Instruct the client with hypernatremia to avoid foods rich in sodium, such as canned foods, lunch meats, ham, pork, pickles, potato chips, and pretzels. Instruct the client to avoid using salt when cooking or adding salt to food at the table.
- Emphasize the importance of reading labels on food products.

Evaluation

- Evaluate the client's serum sodium level. Report if sodium imbalance continues.

[HydroDIURIL]) increase the serum calcium level.

HYPOCALCEMIA

Inadequate calcium intake causes calcium to leave the bone to maintain a normal serum calcium level. Fractures may occur if calcium deficit persists because of calcium loss from the bones (bone demineralization). Hypoparathyroidism, vitamin D deficiency, and receiving multiple blood transfusions are causes of hypocalcemia.

Signs and symptoms of hypocalcemia include anxiety, irritability, and tetany (twitching around the mouth, tingling and numbness of fingers, carpopedal spasm, spasmodic contractions, laryngeal spasm, and convulsions). If metabolic acidosis is present with hy-

pocalcemia, tetany symptoms are absent because calcium leaves protein sites during an acidotic state; thus, more ionized calcium is available. During an alkalotic state, more calcium binds with protein. There is less ionized calcium, and tetany symptoms usually occur.

Many calcium preparations can be administered orally or intravenously. For treatment of calcium deficit, oral calcium tablets, capsules, or powder and IV calcium solutions may be given. Calcium preparations are combined with various salts, such as chloride, carbonate, gluconate, glucceptate, and lactate. Calcium for IV use should be mixed with 5% dextrose in water and *not mixed* in a saline solution. Sodium encourages calcium loss. Chart 13–2 compares the pharmacokinetics and pharmacodynamics of calcium preparations.

Chart 13–2. Calcium

CALCIUM

Drug Name

Calcium chloride (IV)
Calcium carbonate
    (Os-cal, Tums, Caltrate, Megacal)
Calcium gluconate (Kalcinate)
Calcium lactate
Calcium replacement
Pregnancy Category: C
Drug Forms: Tab, cap, liq, inj

Dosage

Antacid use:
A; PO: 0.5–1 g q4–6h (dose varies according to the calcium salt)
Osteoporosis:
A: PO: 1–2 g b.i.d.
    IV: 0.5–1 g q.d., q.o.d.
Tetany:
A: IV 4–16 mEq
C: IV: 0.5–0.7 mEq/kg t.i.d., q.i.d.
Hypocalcemia:
C: PO: 500 mg/d in divided doses

Contraindications

Hypercalcemia, renal calculi, digitalis toxicity, ventricular fibrillation
Caution:
Renal or respiratory disorders, GI hypomotility

Drug-Lab-Food Interactions

Increase digitalis toxicity: digoxin;
Decrease calcium effect: saline solution; *decrease* effect of calcium channel blockers, verapamil; *decrease* absorption of tetracycline; *increase* serum calcium level: thiazide diuretics

Pharmacokinetics

Absorption: PO: 35% absorbed, requires vitamin D
Distribution: PB: UK
Metabolism: $t\frac{1}{2}$ UK
Excretion: 20% in urine; 70% in feces, some in saliva

Pharmacodynamics

PO: Onset: UK
    Peak: UK
    Duration: 2–4 h
IV: Onset: Rapid
    Peak: UK
    Duration: 2–3 h

Therapeutic Effects/Uses

To correct calcium deficit or tetany symptoms, prevent osteoporosis.

Mode of Action: Transmits nerve impulses, contracts skeletal and cardiac muscles, maintains cellular permeability; promotes strong bone and teeth growth.

Side Effects

Nausea, vomiting, constipation, pain, drowsiness, headache, muscle weakness

Adverse Reactions

Hypercalcemia, ECG changes (shortened QT interval), metabolic alkalosis, heart block, rebound hyperacidity
Life-threatening: Renal failure, cardiac dysrhythmias, cardiac arrest

(Side margin labels: Assessment and Planning; Interventions; Evaluation; NURSING PROCESS)

KEY: A: adult; C: child; PO: by mouth; IV: intravenous; UK: unknown; PB: protein-binding; $t\frac{1}{2}$ half-life.

Pharmacokinetics

Vitamin D promotes calcium absorption from the GI tract; phosphorus inhibits calcium absorption. The pH affects the amount of circulating, free ionized calcium. When pH is decreased (acidic), there is more free calcium because it has been released from protein-binding sites. With an increased pH, more calcium is bound to protein.

Pharmacodynamics

A calcium deficit causes tetany symptoms and, if severe, can be life-threatening. Rapid administration of intravenous calcium may cause tingling and warm sensations and a metallic taste. Calcium needs to be administered at a moderate rate, and infiltration should be avoided. Calcium can be given undiluted IV in emergency situations.

HYPERCALCEMIA

Elevated serum calcium may be due to hyperparathyroidism, hypophosphatemia, tumors of the bone, prolonged immobilization, multiple fractures, and drugs such as the thiazide diuretics. Pathologic fractures might occur because of thinning of the bone resulting from calcium loss from the bony structure. Calcium leaves the bone and accumulates in the vascular fluid. Signs and symptoms of hypercalcemia are flabby muscles, pain over bony areas, and kidney stones of calcium composition.

EFFECT OF DRUGS ON CALCIUM BALANCE

Phosphate preparations, corticosteroids, loop diuretics, aspirin, anticonvulsants, magnesium sulfate, and mithramycin are some of the groups of drugs that can lower the serum calcium level. Excess calcium

---

Table 13–8
Drugs Affecting Calcium Balance

CALCIUM IMBALANCE	DRUGS	RATIONALE
Hypocalcemia (serum calcium deficit)	Magnesium sulfate Propylthiouracil (Propacil) Colchicine Plicamythin (Mithramycin) Neomycin Excessive sodium citrate	These agents inhibit parathyroid hormone (PTH) secretion and decrease the serum calcium level.

	Acetazolamide
	Aspirin
	Anticonvulsants
	Glutethimide (Doriden)
	Estrogens
	Aminoglycosides
	   Gentamicin
	   Amikacin
	   Tobramycin
		These agents can alter the vitamin D metabolism that is needed for calcium absorption.

	Phosphate preparations: oral, enema, and intravenous
	   Sodium phosphate
	   Potassium phosphate
		Phosphates can increase the serum phosphorus level and decrease the serum calcium level.

	Corticosteroids
	   Cortisone
	   Prednisone
		Steroids decrease calcium mobilization and inhibit the absorption of calcium.

	Loop diuretics Furosemide (Lasix)	Loop diuretics reduce calcium absorption from the renal tubules.
Hypercalcemia (serum calcium excess)	Calcium salts Vitamin D	Excess ingestion of calcium and vitamin D and infusion of calcium can increase the serum Ca level.
	IV lipids	Lipids can increase the calcium level.

	Kayexalate androgens
	Diuretics
	   Thiazides
	   Chlorthalidone (Hygroten)
		These agents can induce hypercalcemia.

From Kee, J. L., Paulanka, B. J.: Fluids and Electrolytes with Clinical Applications, 6/E. New York: Delmar Publishers, 1999.

Table 13–9
Calcium Preparations

CALCIUM NAME	DRUG FORM	DRUG DOSE
ORALS		
Calcium carbonate	650–1500 mg tablets	400 mg/g*
Calcium citrate	950 mg tablet	211 mg/g*
Calcium lactate	325–650 mg tablets	130 mg/g*
Calcium gluconate	500–1000 mg tablets	90 mg/g*
INTRAVENOUS		
Calcium chloride	10 mL size	272 mg/g*; 13.5 mEq
Calcium gluceptate	5 mL size	90 mg/g*; 4.5 mEq
Calcium gluconate	10 mL size	90 mg/g*; 4.5 mEq

Elementary calcium is 1 gram (1 g).
From Kee, J. L., Paulanka, B. J.: Fluids and Electrolytes with Clinical Applications, 6/E. New York: Delmar Publishers, 1999.

salt ingestion and infusion, and thiazide and chlorthalidone diuretics are conditions that can increase the serum calcium level. Table 13–8 lists the drugs that affect calcium balance.

CLINICAL MANAGEMENT OF CALCIUM IMBALANCE

Clinical management of hypocalcemia consists of oral supplements and intravenous calcium diluted in 5% dextrose in water (D_5W). Calcium should *not* be diluted in a normal saline solution (0.9% NaCl) because the sodium promotes calcium loss. Table 13–9 lists the oral and intravenous preparations of calcium salts, their dosages, and drug form. Calcium carbonate can cause GI upset because it produces carbon dioxide. For better calcium absorption, calcium supplements should contain vitamin D and oral calcium should be taken 30 minutes before meals. Table 13–10 gives guidelines for the suggested clinical management for hypocalcemia.

The goal for managing hypercalcemia is to correct the underlying cause of the serum calcium excess. Drugs such as calcitonin or IV saline solution administered rapidly and followed by a loop diuretic can be used to promote rapid urinary excretion of calcium.

Magnesium

Magnesium, a sister cation to potassium, is most plentiful in the intracellular fluid (ICF). When there is a loss of potassium, there is also a loss of magnesium. The normal serum magnesium level is 1.5 to 2.5 mEq/L or 1.8 to 3.0 mg/dL. A magnesium deficit is called **hypomagnesemia**, and a magnesium excess

is called **hypermagnesemia**. Daily magnesium requirement is 8 to 20 mEq.

FUNCTIONS

Magnesium promotes the transmission of neuromuscular activity; it is an important mediator of neural transmission in the central nervous system (CNS). Like potassium, it promotes contraction of the myocardium. It activates many enzymes for the metabolism of carbohydrates and protein. It is responsible for the transportation of sodium and potassium across cell membranes.

Table 13–10
Suggested Clinical Management for Hypocalcemia

CALCIUM DEFICIT	SUGGESTED CLINICAL MANAGEMENT
Mild	Oral calcium salts with vitamin D; take twice a day.
	10% IV calcium gluconate (10 mL) in D_5W solution; administer slowly, 1 to 3 mL per minute.
Moderate	10% IV calcium gluconate (10 to 20 mL) in D_5W solution; administer slowly, 1 to 3 mL per minute.
Severe	10% IV calcium gluconate (100 mL) in 1 liter of D_5W; administer over 4 hours.

From Kee, J. L., Paulanka, B. J.: Fluids and Electrolytes with Clinical Applications, 6/E. New York: Delmar Publishers, 1999.

ELECTROLYTE: CALCIUM

Assessment

- Assess the client for signs and symptoms of hypocalcemia (decreased serum calcium), such as tetany (twitching of the mouth, tingling and numbness of the fingers, facial spasms, spasms of the larynx, and carpopedal spasm), muscle cramps, bleeding tendencies, and weak cardiac contractions.
- Check the serum calcium levels (normal, 4.5–5.5 mEq/L, or 8.5–10.5 mg/dL) for hypocalcemia and hypercalcemia. Report abnormal test results. Serum ionized calcium (iCa) (normal, 2.2–2.5 mEq/L, or 4.25–5.25 mg/dL) indicates free circulating calcium and is more accurate for determining calcium imbalance.
- Obtain VS and ECG readings. Report abnormal findings. VS and ECG results can be compared with future VS and ECG readings.
- Obtain a current drug history for the client. Calcium enhances the effect of digoxin. An elevated serum calcium level, when taken with digoxin, can cause digitalis toxicity. Signs and symptoms of digitalis toxicity include nausea, vomiting, anorexia, bradycardia (pulse rate <60 or markedly decreased), cardiac dysrhythmias, and visual disturbances. Thiazide diuretics can increase the serum calcium level. Drugs that decrease the effect of calcium are calcium channel blockers, tetracycline, and sodium chloride.

Potential Nursing Diagnoses

- Altered nutrition, less than body requirements
- Impaired tissue integrity

Planning

- Client's serum calcium level will be within normal range by 3 to 7 days.
- Tetany symptoms will cease. Client will eat foods rich in calcium or take calcium supplements as ordered.
- Client with hypercalcemia will avoid foods rich in calcium, such as milk products.

Nursing Interventions

- Monitor VS. Report abnormal findings. Compare with baseline VS. Monitor pulse rate if the client is taking digoxin. Bradycardia is a sign of digitalis toxicity.
- Administer IV fluids slowly with 10% calcium gluconate or chloride. Calcium should be administered with D₅W and not saline solution because sodium promotes calcium loss. Calcium should not be added to solutions containing bicarbonate because rapid precipitation occurs.
- Check IV site for infiltration if the client is receiving calcium in IV fluids. Calcium can cause tissue necrosis (sloughing of the tissue) if it infiltrates into the subcutaneous tissue. Calcium gluceptate is the only calcium preparation that can be given IM.
- Monitor the serum calcium and iCa levels. Hypocalcemia occurs if the serum calcium value is <4.5 mEq/L, or <8.5 mg/dL, or if iCa is <2.2 mEq/L. Hypercalcemia occurs if the serum calcium value is >5.5 mEq/L, or >10.5 mg/dL, or if iCa is >2.5 mEq/L.
- Monitor ECGs. With hypocalcemia, the ST segment is lengthened and the QT interval is prolonged. With hypercalcemia, the ST segment is decreased and the QT interval is shortened.

Client Teaching

General

- Instruct the client to avoid overuse of antacids and to prevent the habit of chronic use of laxatives. Excessive use of certain antacids may cause alkalosis, decreasing calcium ionization. Chronic use of laxatives decreases calcium absorption from the GI tract. Suggest fruits and foods rich in fiber for improving bowel elimination.
- Instruct the client taking calcium supplements to check that the calcium tablet is absorbable. To do this, put 1 tablet into 1 oz of white vinegar. Stir every 3 min. The tablet should break up or dissolve within 30 min.
- Take oral calcium supplements with meals or after meals to increase absorption.

Nursing Process continued on following page

Diet
• Suggest that the client consume foods high in calcium, such as milk, milk products, and protein-rich foods. Protein and vitamin D are needed to enhance calcium absorption.

Side Effects
• Instruct the client to report symptoms related to calcium excess or hypercalcemia, including flabby muscles, pain over bony areas, ECG changes, and kidney (calcium form) stones.

Evaluation

• Evaluate the client's serum calcium level. Report if calcium imbalance continues.
• Determine whether side effects caused by previous untreated hypocalcemia are absent.

When there is a magnesium deficit, there frequently is a potassium or calcium deficit. A serum magnesium deficit increases the release of acetylcholine from the presynaptic membrane of the nerve fiber. This increases neuromuscular excitability. A serum magnesium excess has a sedative effect on the neuromuscular system, which can result in a loss of deep tendon reflexes. Cardiac (ventricular) dysrhythmias can occur as a result of hypomagnesemia. Hypotension and heart block may result from hypermagnesemia.

Hypomagnesemia is probably the most undiagnosed electrolyte deficiency. This is most likely because hypomagnesemia is asymptomatic until the se-

Table 13–11
Drugs Affecting Magnesium Balance

MAGNESIUM IMBALANCE	DRUGS	RATIONALE

Hypomagnesemia (serum magnesium deficit)	Diuretics
	  Furosemide (Lasix)
	  Ethacrynic acid (Edecrin)
	  Mannitol
		Diuretics promote urinary loss of magnesium.

	Antibiotics
	  Gentamicin
	  Tobramycin
	  Carbenicillin
	  Capreomycin
	  Neomycin
	  Polymyxin B
	  Amphotericin B
	Digitalis
	Calcium gluconate
	Insulin
		These agents can cause magnesium loss via kidney.

	Laxatives Cisplatin	Laxative abuse causes magnesium loss via the gastrointestinal tract.

	Corticosteroids
	  Cortisone
	  Prednisone
		Steroids can decrease serum magnesium level.

Hypermagnesemia (serum magnesium excess)	Magnesium salts:
	Oral and enema
	  Magnesium hydroxide (MOM)
	  Magnesium sulfate (Epsom) salt
	  Magnesium citrate
	  Magnesium sulfate (maternity)
		Excess use of magnesium salts could increase serum magnesium level.
		
		Use of excess $MgSO_4$ in treatment of toxemia could cause hypermagnesemia.

	Lithium	Hypermagnesemia is associated with lithium.

From Kee, J. L., Paulanka, B. J.: Fluids and Electrolytes with Clinical Applications, 6/E. New York: Delmar Publishers, 1999.

NURSING PROCESS
ELECTROLYTE: MAGNESIUM

Assessment

- Assess the client for signs and symptoms of magnesium deficit or excess. Hypomagnesemia includes tetany-like symptoms caused by hyperexcitability (tremors, twitching of the face) and ventricular tachycardia that leads to ventricular fibrillation and hypertension. Hypermagnesemia includes lethargy, drowsiness, weakness, paralysis, loss of deep tendon reflexes, hypotension, and heart block.
- Check serum magnesium levels for magnesium imbalance. Symptoms of magnesium deficit may or may not be seen until the serum level is below 1.0 mEq/L.
- Check clients receiving digitalis preparations for digitalis toxicity. A magnesium deficit, as with a potassium deficit, enhances the action of digitalis, causing digitalis toxicity.

Potential Nursing Diagnosis

- Altered nutrition: less than body requirements related to insufficient intake of foods that are rich in magnesium
- Decreased cardiac output related to hypomagnesemia or hypermagnesemia.

Planning

- Client's serum magnesium level will be within normal range in 2 to 5 days.

Nursing Interventions

- Report to the health care provider if the client is NPO (nothing by mouth) and receiving IV fluids without magnesium salts for weeks. Administer IV magnesium sulfate in solution slowly to prevent a hot or flushed feeling. Monitor vital signs.
- Monitor urinary output. Most of the body's magnesium is excreted by the kidneys. Report if the urine output is less than 600 mL/day.
- Check hypomagnesemia clients who are taking digoxin for digitalis toxicity; e.g., nausea and vomiting, bradycardia. Magnesium deficit enhances the action of digoxin (digitalis preparations).
- Monitor vital signs. Report abnormal findings to the health care provider.
- Monitor serum electrolyte results. Report a low serum potassium or calcium level. Low serum magnesium levels may be attributed to hypokalemia or hypocalcemia. When correcting a potassium deficit, potassium is not replaced in the cells until magnesium is replaced. A serum magnesium level of 1.0 mEq/L or less can cause cardiac arrest.
- Check for Trousseau's and Chvostek's signs of severe hypomagnesemia. Tetany symptoms occur in both magnesium and calcium deficits.
- Have IV calcium gluconate available for emergency reversal of hypermagnesemia from overcorrection of a magnesium deficit.

Client Teaching

- Instruct the client to eat foods rich in magnesium (green vegetables, fruits, fish and seafood, grains, nuts, and peanut butter).
- Instruct the client with hypermagnesemia to avoid routine use of laxatives and antacids that contain magnesium. Suggest that the client check drug labels.

Evaluation

- Evaluate the client's serum magnesium level. Report if the serum level remains abnormal.
- Observe for signs and symptoms of hypomagnesemia and hypermagnesemia.

rum magnesium level approaches 1.0 mEq/L. The total serum magnesium concentration is not representative of the cellular magnesium levels.

To correct severe hypomagnesemia, intravenous magnesium sulfate ($MgSO_4$) may be given. For hypermagnesemia, calcium gluconate may be given to decrease the serum magnesium level.

EFFECT OF DRUGS ON MAGNESIUM BALANCE

Sodium inhibits tubular absorption of magnesium and calcium. Long-term administration of saline infusions may result in losses of magnesium and calcium.

Diuretics, certain antibiotics, laxatives, and steroids are drug groups that promote magnesium loss. Hypomagnesemia, like hypokalemia, enhances the action of digitalis and causes digitalis toxicity. Magnesium sulfate corrects hypomagnesemia and symptoms of digitalis toxicity.

An excess intake of magnesium salts is the major cause of serum magnesium excess. Two drug groups that contain magnesium and could cause hypermagnesemia are laxatives such as magnesium sulfate, milk of magnesia, and magnesium citrate; and antacids such as Maalox, Mylanta, and DiGel. Table 13–11 lists the drugs that affect magnesium balance.

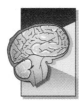

Critical Thinking in Action

J. S., 72 years old, has been vomiting and has had diarrhea for 2 days. J. S. takes digoxin 0.25 mg/day and HydroDIURIL 50 mg/day. His serum potassium level is 3.2 mEq/L. He complains of being dizzy. His blood pressure is slightly lower than usual. The nurse assesses his physiologic status and notes that his muscles are weak and flabby, his abdomen is distended, and peristalsis is diminished.

1. What contributing factors causes J. S.'s potassium imbalance?
2. What signs and symptoms indicate that J. S. is in potassium imbalance?
3. What interventions should be taken for alleviating this potassium imbalance?
4. How much potassium chloride would be needed to elevate J. S.'s serum potassium by 1 mEq?

J. S. was ordered intravenously 1 liter of 5% dextrose in water (D_5W) with 30 mEq of potassium chloride (KCl), and 1 liter of 5% dextrose in 0.45% NaCl (1/2 of normal saline). He was also prescribed oral KCl 15 mEq, t.i.d. × 2 days. Oral KCl is available in 15 mEq/10 mL.

5. Explain the method for diluting KCl in IV fluids. Can KCl be given intramuscularly, subcutaneously or as an IV bolus (push)? Explain.
6. What instructions would you give J. S. for taking oral potassium supplements?
7. What happens if J. S.'s urine output decreases while he is receiving intravenous and oral potassium? What would be your responsibility?
8. Because J. S. is taking a diuretic and digoxin, what should the nurse include with client teaching? Give examples.

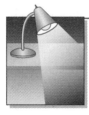

Study Questions

1. What is the average range of the osmolality of body fluids? If your client's serum sodium is 140 mEq/L, BUN is 12 mg/dL and glucose is 100 mg/dL, what is your client's serum osmolality?
2. The client is receiving 1000 mL of D_5/0.9% NaCl (5% dextrose in normal saline solution). What is the osmolality of this intravenous solution? Explain.

3. What is the difference between crystalloids and colloids? Give examples of each.

4. Your client gained 15 pounds in 2 days. It is determined that the weight gain is due to body fluid retention. The weight gain could be equivalent to how many liters of fluid (water)?

5. What is the normal serum potassium range? Your client has been vomiting and has weak, flabby muscles. The client's pulse is irregular. What type of potassium imbalance would you suspect?

6. What are the nursing implications of giving oral potassium supplements and for giving IV potassium chloride? Name the groups of foods that are rich in potassium.

7. What are the drugs used to correct severe hyperkalemia? How are they administered?

8. What drugs may cause an elevated serum sodium level? What health problem may result?

9. In hypocalcemia, the serum calcium level is less than what level? What are the symptoms of hypocalcemia?

10. Why are clients with hypocalcemia and hypercalcemia at high risk of having fractures?

11. What are the functions of magnesium? Describe specific client teaching for clients with hypomagnesemia or hypermagnesemia.

14 Nutritional Support

Outline

Objectives

- Explain the differences between enteral nutrition and parenteral nutrition.
- Describe the routes for enteral feedings.
- Give examples of enteral solutions and explain the differences.
- Explain the advantages and differences of the methods used for delivery of enteral nutrition.
- Describe the complications that may occur with use of enteral nutrition and parenteral nutrition.
- List the nursing interventions for clients receiving enteral nutrition and parenteral nutrition.

Terms

bolus

continuous feedings

cyclic method

enteral nutrition

intermittent enteral feedings

intermittent infusion

nasogastric tube

nutritional support

parenteral nutrition

total parenteral nutrition

Valsalva maneuver

INTRODUCTION

Nutrients are needed for cell growth, cellular function, enzyme activity, carbohydrate-fat-protein synthesis, muscular contraction, wound healing, immune competence, and gastrointestinal (GI) integrity. Inadequate nutrient intake can result from surgery, trauma, malignancy, and other catabolic illnesses. Without adequate nutritional support, protein catabolism (breakdown), malnutrition, and diminished organ functioning affect the GI, liver, renal, cardiac, and respiratory systems. The functioning of the immune system also is decreased.

Clients who are well nourished can usually tolerate a lack of nutrients for 14 days without major health problems. However, clients who are critically ill may only tolerate a lack of nutrient support for a short period of time (a few days to a week) before signs of impaired organ function, infection, or morbidity result. If nutritional support is started within hours of an injury, as in the cases of severe trauma or burns, recovery is more rapid. When the injury is due to minor surgery, there is no severe bodily harm caused by lack of nutritional support for days. Early nutritional support improves intestinal and liver blood flow and function, enhances wound healing, decreases the occurrence of infection, and improves the general outcome of the health situation for the critically ill as well as for the client with a minor injury. "Early fed" injured clients have a positive nitrogen balance and less chance for bacterial infections; thus, they also have a decrease in institutional length of stay.

Dextrose 5% in water (D_5W), normal saline, and lactated Ringer's solution are not forms of nutritional support, although these solutions do provide fluids and some electrolytes. A client requires 2000 calories per day; critically ill clients may require 3000 to 5000 calories per day. In cases of burns, the caloric need could be greater. Clients who remain NPO (nothing by mouth) for an extended period of time become malnourished. Delayed nutritional support by even 5 days for the trauma or neurologic (cervical fracture) client could hamper wound healing and increase the risk of developing an infection.

There are two routes for administering **nutritional support,** enteral and parenteral. **Enteral nutrition,** which involves the GI tract, can be given orally or by feeding tubes (tube feeding). If the client can swallow, the nutrient preparations can be taken by mouth; if the client is unable to swallow, a tube is inserted into the stomach or small intestine. **Parenteral nutrition** involves administering high caloric nutrients through large veins, for example, the subclavian vein. This method is called **total parenteral nutrition (TPN)** or hyperalimentation. Parenteral nutrition is more costly (approximately three times more expensive) than en-

teral nutrition, and the benefits are not significant. In fact, with TPN there is a higher infection rate. The use of TPN does not promote effective GI integrity, liver function, or body weight gain, as does enteral nutrition. Enteral feedings require a functioning small intestine. TPN is necessary when the GI tract is incapacitated; if there is intestinal obstruction, uncontrolled vomiting, or high risk for aspiration; or to supplement inadequate oral intake.

This chapter is divided into enteral nutrition and parenteral nutrition. Routes for nutritional administration, nutritional preparations, methods for delivery, complications, and the nursing process are discussed for each.

ENTERAL NUTRITION

When enteral nutrition is prescribed, there should be adequate small bowel function with digestion, absorption, and GI motility. To determine whether there is a lack of GI motility, the nurse assesses for abdominal distention and a decrease or absence of bowel sounds. In critically ill clients, frequently there is a decrease or absence in gastric emptying time; then TPN may be necessary. The preferred method for nutritional support is enteral feedings for clients with intact gastric emptying and with a decreased risk of aspiration.

Routes for Enteral Feedings

Oral, gastric by **nasogastric tube** or gastrostomy, and small intestinal by nasoduodenal, or nasojejunal, or by jejunostomy tube are the routes used for enteral feedings. Use of nasogastric tube through oral (mouth) or nasal cavities is the most common route for short-term enteral feedings. The gastrostomy, nasoduodenal/jejunal, and jejunostomy tubes are used for long-term enteral feedings. Figure 14–1 displays the four types of GI tubes used for enteral feedings. If aspiration is a concern, the small intestinal route is suggested.

Enteral Solutions

Several types of liquid formulas are commercially available for enteral feedings. These solutions differ according to their various nutrients, caloric values, and osmolality. There are three groups of solutions for enteral nutrition: blenderized; polymeric, which includes milk-based and lactose-free; and elemental or monomeric. The commercial preparations are listed according to their groups in Table 14–1. Components of the enteral solutions include (1) carbohydrates in the form of dextrose, sucrose, lactose, starch or dextrin (the first three are simple sugars that can be

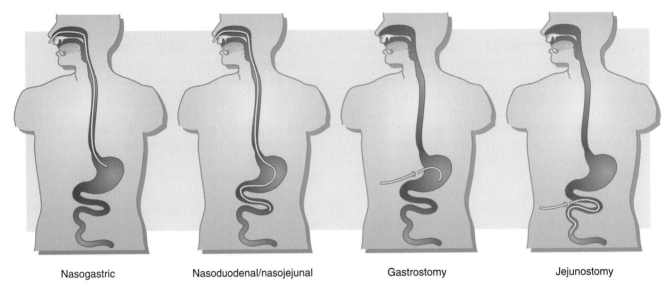

Nasogastric   Nasoduodenal/nasojejunal   Gastrostomy   Jejunostomy

Figure 14–1
Types of gastrointestinal tubes for enteral feedings. A *nasogastric* tube is passed from the nose into the stomach. A weighted *nasoduodenal/nasojejunal* tube is passed through the nose into the duodenum/jejunum. A *gastrostomy* tube is introduced through a temporary or permanent opening on the abdominal wall (stoma) into the stomach. A *jejunostomy* tube is passed through a stoma directly into the jejunum.

absorbed quickly); (2) protein in the form of intact proteins, hydrolyzed proteins, or free amino acids; and (3) fat in the form of corn oil, soybean oil, or safflower oil (some have a higher oil content than others). With all enteral nutrition, sufficient water to maintain hydration is essential.

Blended formulas for enteral solutions are liquid in consistency to pass through the tube. These are indi-

Table 14–1
Commercial Preparations for Enteral Feeding

TYPE	COMMERCIAL PREPARATIONS (MANUFACTURER)	COMMENTS
I. Blenderized	Compleat B (Sandoz) Formula 2 (Cutter) Vitaneed (Sherwood)	Blended natural foods; ready to use
II. Polymeric Milk-based	Meritene (Sandoz) Instant Breakfast (Carnation) Sustacal Powder (Mead Johnson)	Pleasant tasting oral supplements; provide intact nutrients
Lactose-free	Ensure, Jevity, Osmolite (Ross) Sustacal Liquid, Isocal, Ultracal (Mead Johnson) Fibersource, Resource (Sandoz) Entrition, Nutren (Clintec) Attain, Comply (Sherwood)	May be used as tube feeding, meal replacement, or oral supplement; made with intact protein isolates, oligosaccharides and starches, and fats; provide 1 kcal/mL (others available providing up to 2 kcal). Adequate quantities meet reference daily intakes for vitamins and minerals; ready to use; isotonic (except Ensure and Sustacal)
III. Elemental or monomeric formulas	Vital HN (Ross) Vivonex T.E.N. (Sandoz) Criticare HN (Mead Johnson) Travasorb (Clintec) Peptamen (Clintec) Reabilan (O'Brian)	Partially digested nutrients for feeding; hypertonic (except for Reabilan and Peptamen); require reconstitution (except for Peptamen, Reabilan, and Criticare)

From Davis, J. R., and Sherer, K.: Applied Nutrition and Diet Therapy for Nurses, 2/E. Philadelphia: WB Saunders, p. 349, 1994.

vidually prepared based on the client's nutritional need. Frequently, baby food is used with liquid added. If the food particles are too large, the tube can become clogged.

There are two groups of polymeric solutions, milk-based and lactose-free. Most of the milk-based polymeric preparations come in powdered form to be mixed with milk or water. Many of these milk-based polymeric solutions do not provide complete nutritional requirements unless given in large amounts. Frequently, they are used as a supplement to meet nutritional needs. The lactose-free polymeric solutions are commercially prepared in liquid form for replacement feedings. Many of these solutions are isotonic (300 to 340 mOsm/kg H_2O), and the breakdown of nutrients includes 50% carbohydrates, 15% protein, 15% fat, and 20% other nutrients. Examples of these include Ensure, Isocal, and Osmolite (Fig. 14–2). These polymeric solutions provide 1 calorie per milliliter of feeding.

The elemental or monomeric solutions are useful for partial GI tract dysfunction. They are available in powdered and liquid forms. The nutrients from these solutions are rapidly absorbed in the small intestine. They are more expensive than the other enteral solutions.

Methods for Delivery

Enteral feedings may be given by bolus, intermittent drip or infusion, continuous drip, or cyclic infusion. The bolus method was the first method used to deliver enteral feedings. With the **bolus** method, 250 to 400 mL of solution is rapidly administered through a syringe or funnel into the tube four to six times a day. This method takes about 10 minutes and many times is not tolerated well because a massive volume of solution is given in a short period of time. This method can cause nausea, vomiting, aspiration, abdominal cramping, and diarrhea. A healthy client can tolerate the rapidly infused solution. This method is seldom used unless the client is ambulatory.

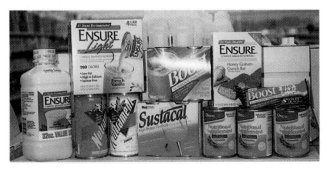

Figure 14–2
A typical selection of over-the-counter supplemental feeding products.

Intermittent enteral feedings are administered every 3 to 6 hours over 30 to 60 minutes by gravity drip or pump infusion. Three hundred to 400 mL of solution is usually given at each feeding. A feeding bag is commonly used. **Intermittent infusion** is considered an inexpensive method for administering enteral nutrition.

Continuous feedings are prescribed for the critically ill or for those receiving feedings into the small intestine. The enteral feedings are given by an infusion pump, such as the Kangaroo set, at a slow rate over 24 hours. Approximately 50 to 125 mL of solution is infused per hour (Fig. 14–3).

The **cyclic method** is another type of continuous feeding that is infused over 8 to 16 hours daily (day or night). The daytime hours are suggested for clients who are restless or for those who have a greater risk for aspiration. The nighttime schedule allows more freedom during the day for the clients who are ambulatory.

Complications

Dehydration can occur if an insufficient amount of water is given with the feedings or between feedings. Some of the enteral solutions are hyperosmolar and can draw water out of the cells to maintain serum iso-osmolality.

Aspiration may occur if the client is fed while he or she is lying down or is unconscious. The head of the bed should be elevated at least 30 degrees. The nurse should check for gastric residual by gently aspirating the stomach contents before administering the next enteral feeding.

One of the major problems of enteral feeding is diarrhea. This could be due to rapid administration of feeding, high caloric solutions, malnutrition, GI bacteria (Clostridium difficile), and drugs. Antibacterials (antibiotics) and drugs that contain magnesium such as antacids (Maalox) and sorbitol (used as a filler for certain drugs) are associated with the occurrence of diarrhea. Many oral liquid drugs are hyperosmolar, which tends to pull water into the GI tract and cause diarrhea.

Diarrhea usually can be managed or corrected by decreasing the rate of infusion of the solution, diluting the solution, changing the enteral solution, discontinuing the drug, or increasing the client's daily water intake.

Enteral Medications

Most drugs that can be administered orally can also be given via enteral tube. The drug must be in liquid form or dissolved into a liquid. Drugs that cannot be

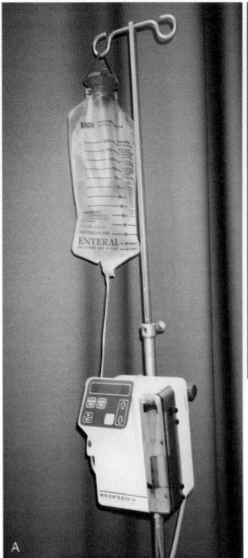

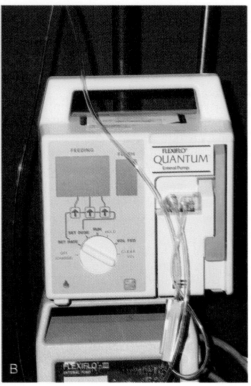

Figure 14–3
Examples of enteral infusion pumps for intermittent, continuous, and cyclic enteral feedings.

dissolved are time-release forms, enteric-coated forms, sublingual forms, and bulk-forming laxatives.

The liquid medication must be properly diluted when administered through the feeding tube. The drug dose is usually given as a bolus and then followed with water. Most liquid medications are hyperosmolar (>1000 mOsm/kg H_2O) when compared with the osmolality of the secretions of the GI tract (130 to 350 mOsm/kg H_2O). Although the hyperosmolality of liquid medication was once thought to be well tolerated by the GI tract, abdominal distention and cramping, vomiting, and diarrhea can result from the administration of undiluted hyperosmolar liquid medications and electrolyte solutions. Liquid medication should be diluted with water to reduce the osmolality to 500 mOsm/kg H_2O (mildly hypertonic) in order to decrease GI intolerance. Table 14–2 lists the osmolalities of various commercial drug suspensions and solutions.

CALCULATION FOR DILUTION OF ENTERAL MEDICATIONS

Three steps should be followed to determine the amount of water needed for diluting liquid medications:

Step 1. Calculate the drug order to find the volume of the drug:

$$\frac{D}{H} \times V \quad \text{or} \quad H : V :: D : x$$

D: Desired dose: drug dose ordered by health care provider.
H: On-hand dose: drug dose on label of container (bottle, vial, or ampule).
V: Vehicle: form and amount in which the drug is available (tablet, capsule, liquid).

NURSING PROCESS
ENTERAL NUTRITION

Assessment

- Assess that the tape around the tube is secured.
- Assess the client's tolerance to the enteral feeding, including possible GI disturbance (nausea, cramping, diarrhea). These are common complications of enteral feeding.
- Assess urine output. Record result for future comparison.
- Obtain client's weight, which can be used for future comparisons.
- Assess for bowel sounds. Diminished or absent bowel sounds should be reported immediately to the health care provider.
- Assess baseline laboratory values. Compare with future laboratory results.

Nursing Diagnoses

- Risk for fluid volume deficit related to inadequate fluid intake or excess fluid loss
- Risk for diarrhea related to enteral feedings
- Risk for aspiration related to enteral feedings via nasogastric tube

Planning

- The client will receive adequate nutritional support through enteral feedings.
- Complication, diarrhea, related to enteral feedings will be managed.

Nursing Interventions

- Check tube placement by aspirating gastric secretion or injecting air into the tube to listen by stethoscope for air movement in the stomach. However, injecting air to check for placement may be misleading because the tube may be in the base of the lung and air flow there produces similar sounds as when the tube is placed in the stomach. For placement of the tube for small intestine route, an X-ray confirmation may be needed.
- Check for gastric residual before enteral feeding. A residual of more than 50% of previous feeding indicates delayed gastric emptying. Notify the health care provider. Usually the residual is 0 to 100 mL.
- Check continuous route for gastric residual every 2 to 4 hours. If residual is more than 50 mL, stop infusion for 30 min to 1 hour and then recheck.
- Before feeding, raise the head of the bed to a 30-degree angle. If elevating the head of the bed is not advisable, then position the client on his or her right side.
- Deliver the enteral feeding according to the method ordered: bolus, gastric, or small intestine.
- Flush feeding tube accordingly: intermittent feeding, 30 mL before and after; continuous feeding, every 4 hours; medications, 30 mL before and after. If tube obstruction occurs, flush with warm water or cola.
- Monitor adverse effects of enteral feedings such as diarrhea. To manage or correct diarrhea, decrease flow rate for the enteral feedings and, as diarrhea lessens, gradually increase the feeding rate. Enteral solution may be diluted and then gradually increased to full strength. However, diluted solution can decrease the nutrient intake. Determine whether the drugs could be causing the diarrhea.
- Dilute the drug solution's osmolality to 500 mOsm when giving liquid medication through the tube. Use the formula in the text. Consult with the health care provider.
- Monitor vital signs. Report abnormal findings.
- Give additional water during the day to prevent dehydration. Consult with the health care provider.
- Weigh the client to determine weight gain or loss. Compare with the baseline weight. The client should be weighed at the same time each day, with the same scale and the same amount of clothing.
- Change feeding bag daily. Do not add new solution to old solution in the feeding bag. The nutritional solution should not be ice cold, but at room temperature.

Nursing Process continued on following page

Client Teaching

• Instruct the client to report any problems related to enteral feedings such as diarrhea, sore throat, and abdominal cramping.

Cultural Considerations

• Respect cultural beliefs concerning refusal to receive enteral or TPN nutrition. Explain the reason for adequate nutrition and find ways that nutritional needs can be met.
• Communicate, verbally or in writing, how enteral nutrition is used by various cultural groups such as in third-world countries.

Evaluation

• Determine that the client is receiving prescribed nutrients daily and is free of complications associated with enteral feedings.

Step 2. Find the osmolality of the drug (check drug literature or with pharmacist) and liquid dilution. Use 500 mOsm as a constant for the desired osmolality.

$$\frac{\text{known mOsm}}{\text{desired mOsm}} \times \text{volume of drug} =$$
$$\text{total volume of liquid}$$

Step 3. Determine the volume of water for dilution:

total volume of liquid − volume of drug =
volume of water for dilution

Order: acetaminophen 650 mg, q6h, PRN for pain

Table 14–2
Osmolality of Selected Drugs

DRUG	AVERAGE mOsm
Acetaminophen elixir, 65 mg/mL	5400
Amoxicillin suspension, 50 mg/mL	2250
Cephalexin (Keflex) suspension, 50 mg/mL	1950
Cimetidine (Tagamet) solution, 60 mg/mL	5500
Digoxin elixir, 50 μg/mL	1350
Docusate sodium (Colace) syrup, 3.3 mg/mL	3900
Furosemide (Lasix) solution, 10 mg/mL	2050
Lithium citrate syrup, 1.6 mEq/mL	6850
Milk of magnesia suspension	1250
Potassium chloride liquid, 10%	3550
Prochlorperazine syrup, 1 mg/mL	3250
Theophylline solution, 5.33 mg/mL	800

Drug Available: Acetaminophen elixir 65 mg/mL Average mOsm/kg = 5400 (see Table 14–2)

Step 1. Calculate the volume of drug:

$$\frac{D}{H} \times V = \frac{650 \text{ mg}}{65 \text{ mg}} \times 1 \text{ mL} = 10 \text{ mL}$$
or

$$\begin{array}{cccc} H & : V & D & :x \\ 65 \text{ mg}:1 \text{ mL} & :: & 650 \text{ mg}:x \text{ mL} \\ & 65x = 650 \\ & x = 10 \text{ ml of drug} \end{array}$$

Step 2. Find the osmolality of drug and total liquid dilution:

$$\frac{\text{known mOsm (5400)}}{\text{desired mOsm (500)}} \times \text{volume of drug (10)} =$$
$$\frac{5400}{500} \times 10 = 108 \text{ mL of liquid}$$

Step 3. Determine the volume of water for dilution:

total volume of liquid (108 mL)
− volume of drug (10 mL)
= 98 mL of water for dilution

PARENTERAL NUTRITION

Total Parenteral Nutrition

Total parenteral nutrition (TPN), also called hyperalimentation or intravenous hyperalimentation (IVH), is the primary method for providing complete nutrients by the parenteral or intravenous route. TPN is an infusion of hyperosmolar glucose, amino acids, vitamins, electrolytes, minerals, and trace elements; it can meet a client's total nutritional needs. TPN is indicated for clients with severe burns who are in negative nitrogen balance; clients with GI disorders, when the GI tract needs a complete rest; and clients with debilitating diseases such as metastatic cancer or acquired immunodeficiency syndrome (AIDS).

The average percent of dextrose in TPN is 25%. This high glucose concentration is mixed with commercially prepared protein and lipid sources. Fat emulsion supplement therapy provides an increased number of calories and is a carrier of fat-soluble vitamins. Vitamins and electrolytes are added before administration. Electrolytes are frequently added immediately before the infusion according to the client's serum electrolyte levels. High glucose concentrations are irritating to peripheral veins, so TPN is administered through central venous lines such as the subclavian or internal jugular.

Enteral feedings should be considered before TPN. Enteral feeding is less costly, poses less risk of sepsis, and maintains GI integrity. When enteral nutrition cannot be used because of severe GI disorders, TPN should be prescribed. TPN does enhance wound healing and provides the necessary nutrients to prevent cellular catabolism.

Complications

Complications associated with TPN can result from catheter insertion and TPN infusion. Table 14–3 lists the complications associated with TPN.

Complications include pneumothorax, hemothorax, hydrothorax, air embolism, infection, hyperglycemia, hypoglycemia, and fluid overload (hypervolemia). For the prevention of an air embolism, the client should be taught the **Valsalva maneuver,** which is to take a breath, hold it, and bear down while the nurse is changing infusion bags or bottles and changing tubing. Strict asepsis is necessary when changing IV tubing and dressings at the insertion site. Gloves, masks, and antibacterial ointment usually are necessary. TPN is an excellent medium for organism growth. Hypertonic dextrose in a protein hydrolysate solution promotes yeast and bacteria growth. It has been reported that these organisms do not grow as rapidly in the preferred crystalline amino acid solution as they do in a protein hydrolysate solution. Most TPN solutions are prepared by the pharmacist with the use of a laminar air flow hood.

Hyperglycemia occurs primarily as the result of the hypertonic dextrose solution when TPN is initiated.

Table 14–3
Complications of Total Parenteral Nutrition

COMPLICATION	CAUSES	SYMPTOMS
CATHETER INSERTION		
Pneumothorax	Accidental puncture of the pleural cavity.	Sharp chest pain. Decreased breath sounds.
Hemothorax	Catheter damages the large vein.	Same as pneumothorax.
Hydrothorax	Catheter perforates the vein, releasing solution into the chest.	Same as pneumothorax.
TOTAL PARENTERAL NUTRITION INFUSION		
Air embolism	Intravenous (IV) tubing disconnected. Catheter not clamped. Injection port fell off. Improper changing of IV tubing (no Valsalva maneuver).	Coughing, shortness of breath, chest pain, cyanosis.
Infection	Poor aseptic technique when catheter inserted. Contamination when changing tubing. Contamination when solution is mixed. Contamination when dressing is changed.	Temperature >100°F or 37.7°C. Tachycardia; chills; sweating; redness; swelling; drainage at insertion site; pain in the neck, arm, or shoulder; lethargy.
Hyperglycemia	Fluid infused too rapidly. Insufficient insulin coverage. Infection.	Nausea, headache, weakness, thirst, elevated blood glucose.
Hypoglycemia	Fluids stopped abruptly. Too much insulin infused.	Pallor, cold, clammy skin. Increased pulse rate, "shaky feeling," headache, blurred vision.
Fluid overload hypervolemia	Increased IV rate. Fluids shift from cellular to vascular spaces due to hypertonic solutions.	Cough, dyspnea, neck vein engorgement, chest rales, weight gain.

NURSING PROCESS
TOTAL PARENTERAL NUTRITION

Assessment

- Obtain baseline vital signs for future comparison.
- Obtain baseline weight.
- Check laboratory results. Electrolytes, glucose, and protein levels frequently change during TPN therapy. Early laboratory results are useful for future comparison.
- Check urine output. Report abnormal findings.
- Check the label on the TPN solution. Compare the solution with the order.

Potential Nursing Diagnoses

- Risk for fluid volume excess related to excess fluid infusion or renal dysfunction
- Risk for fluid volume deficit related to osmotic diuresis resulting from hyperosmolar TPN solution
- Risk for infection related to TPN solution that has a high glucose concentration.
- Ineffective breathing pattern related to complication from the insertion of subclavian line

Planning

- The client's nutrient needs will be met via TPN.
- The common complication from TPN therapy, infection, will be avoided.

Nursing Interventions

- Monitor vital signs. Report changes.
- Monitor body weight and compare with baseline weight.
- Monitor laboratory results and report abnormal findings, especially electrolytes, protein, glucose. Compare laboratory changes with the baseline findings.
- Monitor intake and output. Fluid volume deficit or excess could occur. Because the TPN solution is hyperosmolar, fluid shift occurs, which can cause osmotic diuresis.
- Monitor temperature changes for possible infection or febrile state. Use aseptic technique when changing dressings and solution bottles or bags.
- Check blood glucose level periodically. When TPN therapy is started, there may be a transient elevated glucose level until the beta cells adjust to the secretion of insulin. If this occurs, the flow rate for TPN should be started slowly and gradually increased as the blood glucose level decreases. Regular insulin may be added to the TPN fluids to correct elevated glucose levels.
- Refrigerate TPN solution that is not in use. High glucose concentration is an excellent medium for bacterial growth.
- Monitor the flow rate of TPN. Start with 60 to 80 mL/h and increase the rate slowly to the ordered level to avoid hyperglycemia.
- Have the client perform the Valsalva maneuver to avoid air embolism by taking a breath, holding it, and bearing down. If the line is opened to air when changing the solution bag or bottle and IV tubing, an air embolus could occur.
- Observe cardiac status because the Valsalva maneuver can cause cardiac dysrhythmias.
- Check for signs and symptoms of overhydration, including coughing, dyspnea, neck vein engorgement, or chest rales. Report findings.
- Follow the institution's procedure for changing dressing and tubing. Usually, tubing is changed daily and the dressing is changed every 24 hours for the first 10 days and then every 48 hours thereafter.
- Do not draw blood, give medications, or check central venous pressure via the TPN line. Results could be invalid.

Client Teaching

- Provide emotional support to the client and family before and during TPN therapy.
- Be available to discuss the client's concerns or refer the client to the appropriate health care provider.

Nursing Process continued on following page

Instruct the client to notify the health care provider immediately with any discomforts or reactions.
• Keep the client informed of progress and effectiveness of TPN.

Evaluation

• Evaluate the client's positive and negative response to the TPN therapy.
• Determine periodically whether the client's serum electrolytes, protein, and glucose levels are within desired ranges.
• Evaluate nutritional status by weight changes, energy level, feeling of well-being, symptom control, or healing.

This occurs until the pancreas adjusts to the hyperglycemic load and therefore may be transient. It also occurs when the infusion rate for TPN is too rapid. In some cases, insulin is added to the TPN solution, which tends to be more effective than administering the insulin subcutaneously. Usually 1 liter of solution is ordered for the first 24 hours when initiating TPN therapy. This allows the pancreas to accommodate to the increased glucose concentration of the solution. Additional daily increases of 500 to 1000 mL are ordered until the desired daily volume of 2½ to 3 liters is reached.

Sudden interruption of TPN therapy can cause hypoglycemia. After the glucose level is decreased, the insulin level remains, causing a hypoglycemic state. It is suggested that an isotonic dextrose solution be administered for 12 to 24 hours after TPN therapy is discontinued. A gradual decrease in the hourly infusion rate of TPN may also be used to discontinue TPN therapy. This process decreases the possibility of a hypoglycemic reaction.

TPN solutions and tubing should be changed every 24 hours. Dressing changes are required every 48 to 72 hours, according to the hospital policy. In some institutions, the dressing is changed every 24 hours for the first 7 to 10 days.

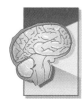

Critical Thinking in Action

M. M. had abdominal surgery and received D₅W and D₅ 0.45% NaCl for 4 days. A nasogastric tube was inserted for enteral nutrition. It was determined that the function of M. M.'s GI tract was intact.

1. Why would M. M. receive enteral nutrition? For short-term or long-term therapy?
2. Differentiate between the Ensure solution that M. M. is receiving and other forms of enteral solutions.
3. What possible complications should be considered while M. M. is receiving enteral nutrition?
4. If diarrhea develops, how can it be managed or corrected?
5. M. M. was receiving enteral nutrition by a bolus method which was later switched to an intermittent method. Explain the advantages and disadvantages of both methods.

M. M. was ordered amoxicillin suspension 250 mg, q.i.d., and potassium chloride solution 10% (15 mEq/10 mL), q12h. These medications are to be given through the enteral tubing.

6. How many mL of amoxicillin should M. M. receive per dose? How much water dilution is needed to reduce the drug osmolality to 500 mOsm?
7. How many mL of potassium chloride should M. M. receive per dose? How much water dilution is needed to reduce the drug osmolality to 500 mOsm?

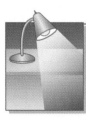

Study Questions

1. What are the differences between enteral nutrition and parenteral nutrition? Would D_5W, normal saline solution (0.9% NaCl), and lactated Ringer's solution be a form of nutritional support? Explain.

2. What are the four methods of delivery for enteral nutrition? How do these four methods differ from each other?

3. What are the three groups of solution used for enteral nutrition? Give an example from each group.

4. What complications can occur with the use of enteral feedings? Explain.

5. Your client is receiving cimetidine (Tagamet) solution 200 mg, t.i.d. How many mL should your client receive? How much water is needed to reduce the osmolality to 500 mOsm?

6. When is TPN therapy preferred over enteral therapy for nutritional support?

7. What is the composition of TPN solution? Normal dextrose percent is _____.

8. The osmolality of TPN solution is _____.

9. What are the major complications associated with TPN? Explain.

10. How is the Valsalva maneuver performed? What is its purpose?

11. If the blood glucose level is elevated, what are some interventions to reduce the glucose level?

Unit IV

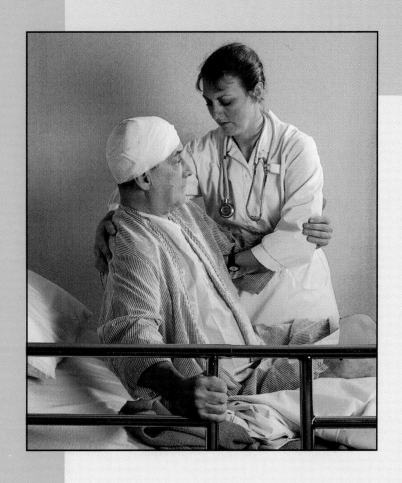

Neurologic and Neuromuscular Agents

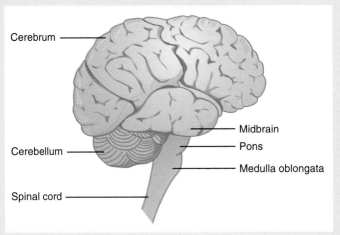

Figure IV–1
Brain and spinal cord.

The nervous system is composed of all nerve tissues: brain, spinal cord, nerves, and ganglia. The purpose of the nervous system is to receive stimuli and transmit information to nerve centers for an appropriate response. There are two types of nervous systems: the central nervous system and the peripheral nervous system.

The **central nervous system (CNS),** composed of the brain and spinal cord, regulates body functions (Fig. IV–1). The CNS interprets information sent by impulses from the **peripheral nervous system (PNS)** and returns the instruction through the PNS for appropriate cellular actions. Stimulation of the CNS may either increase nerve cell (neuron) activity or block nerve cell activity.

The PNS consists of two divisions: the **somatic nervous system (SNS)** and the **autonomic nervous system (ANS).** The SNS is voluntary and acts on skeletal muscles to produce locomotion and respiration. The ANS, also called the visceral system, is involuntary and controls and regulates the functioning of the heart, respiratory system, gastrointestinal system, and glands. The ANS, a large nervous system that functions without our conscious control, has two subdivisions: the sympathetic and the parasympathetic.

The sympathetic nervous system of the ANS is referred to as the **adrenergic system** because its neurotransmitter is *norepinephrine.* The parasympathetic nervous system is referred to as the **cholinergic system** because its neurotransmitter is *acetylcholine.* Because organs are innervated by both the sympathetic and the parasympathetic systems they can produce opposite responses. The sympathetic response is excitability, and the parasympathetic response is inhibition.

The sympathetic and the parasympathetic nerve pathways originate from different locations in the spinal cord. These nervous systems send information by two types of nerve fibers, the preganglionic and the postganglionic, and by the ganglion

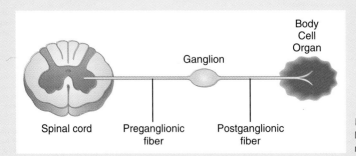

Figure IV–2
Preganglionic and postganglionic nerve fibers.

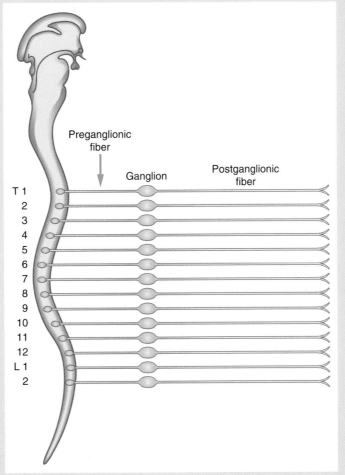

Figure IV-3
Sympathetic nerve fibers.

between these fibers (Fig. IV-2). The preganglionic nerve fiber carries messages from the CNS to the ganglion, and the postganglionic fiber transmits impulses from the ganglion to body tissues and organs.

The sympathetic nervous system is also referred to as the **thoracolumbar division** of the ANS because the preganglionic fibers originate from the thoracic (T1 to

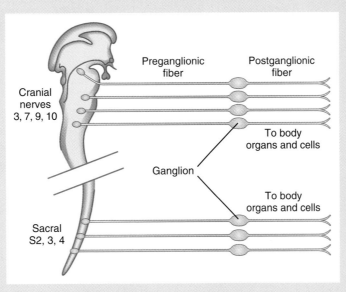

Figure IV-4
Parasympathetic nerve fibers.

T12) and the upper lumbar segments (L1 and L2) of the spinal cord. The sympathetic preganglionic fibers are short from the spinal cord to the ganglion, and the sympathetic postganglionic fibers are long from the ganglion to the body cells. Figure IV–3 illustrates the sympathetic preganglionic fibers from the spinal cord.

The parasympathetic nervous system is referred to as the **craniosacral division** of the ANS because the preganglionic fibers originate with the cranial nerves III, VII, IX, and X from the brain stem and the sacral segments S2, S3, and S4 from the spinal cord. The parasympathetic preganglionic fibers are long from the spinal cord to the ganglion, and the parasympathetic postganglionic fibers are short from the ganglion to the body cells. Figure IV–4 illustrates the parasympathetic preganglionic fibers from the spinal cord.

Drugs that affect the sympathetic and the parasympathetic nervous systems are discussed in Chapters 20, 21, and 22. Drugs that stimulate and depress the CNS are discussed in Chapters 15, 16, and 17. Amphetamines and amphetamine-like drugs, anorexiants, analeptics, and xanthines (caffeine) stimulate the CNS. Some of these drugs are used therapeutically for narcolepsy and attention deficit disorder (ADD). The group of drugs that depress the CNS are sedative-hypnotics, anesthetics, narcotics, and nonnarcotic agents. Drugs used to control convulsions (anticonvulsants, discussed in Chapter 18) are considered depressants of the CNS. The drug groups for controlling psychiatric disorders, discussed in Chapter 19, also affect CNS response. For neuromuscular disorders, such as parkinsonism, myasthenia gravis, multiple sclerosis, and Alzheimer's disease, the drugs have varying effect on the nervous system and muscles, and are discussed in Chapter 23.

Figure IV–5 is a schematic breakdown of the nervous systems in the body.

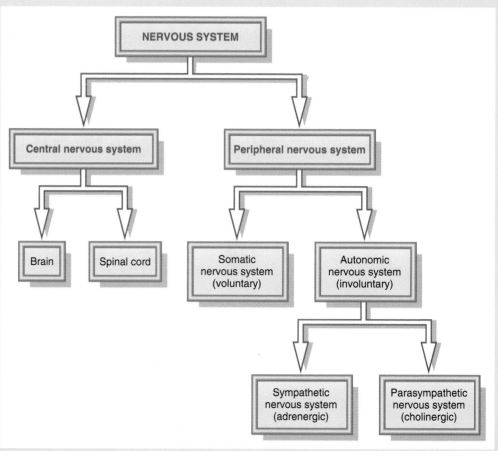

Figure IV–5
The body's nervous system.

Central Nervous System Stimulants

15

Outline

Objectives

- Explain the effects of stimulants on the central nervous system.
- Define narcolepsy and attention deficit disorder.
- List the drugs that are used for narcolepsy and attention deficit disorder.
- Identify the common side effects of amphetamines, anorexiants, analeptics, doxapram, and caffeine.
- Identify at least four nursing interventions when administering CNS stimulants.

Terms

amphetamines

analeptics

anorexiants

attention deficit disorder (ADD)

attention deficit hyperactivity disorder (ADHD)

autonomic nervous system (ANS)

axons

central nervous system (CNS)

dependence

hyperkinesis

narcolepsy

neurons

neurotransmitters

peripheral nervous system (PNS)

tolerance

INTRODUCTION

Numerous drugs can stimulate the **central nervous system (CNS),** but the medically approved use of these drugs is limited to the treatment of narcolepsy, attention deficit disorder (ADD) in children, obesity, and the reversal of respiratory distress. The major group of CNS stimulants includes amphetamines and caffeine, which stimulate the cerebral cortex of the brain; analeptics and caffeine, which act on the brain stem and medulla to stimulate respiration; and anorexiants, which act to some degree on the cerebral cortex and on the hypothalamus to suppress appetite. The amphetamines and related anorexiants have been greatly abused. Long-term use of amphetamines can produce psychological **dependence** and **tolerance,** a condition in which larger and larger doses of a drug are needed to reproduce the initial response. Gradually increasing a drug dose and then abruptly stopping the drug may result in depression and withdrawal symptoms.

AMPHETAMINES

Amphetamines stimulate the release of the **neurotransmitters,** norepinephrine and dopamine, from the brain and the sympathetic nervous system (peripheral nerve terminals). The amphetamines cause euphoria and alertness; however, they can also cause sleeplessness, restlessness, tremors, and irritability. Cardiovascular problems, such as increased heart rate, palpitations, cardiac dysrhythmias, and increased blood pressure, can result from continuous use of amphetamines.

The half-life of amphetamines varies from 4 to 30 h. Amphetamines are excreted faster in acid than in alkaline urine. When CNS toxicity or cardiac toxicity is suspected, decreasing the urine pH aids in the excretion of the drug. An acid urine decreases the half-life of the amphetamine. Table 15–1 lists the amphetamines and amphetamine-like drugs, their dosages, uses, and considerations.

Table 15–1
Amphetamines and Amphetamine-like Drugs

GENERIC/BRAND NAME	ROUTE AND DOSAGE	USES AND CONSIDERATIONS
AMPHETAMINES		
Amphetamine sulfate CSS II	*Narcolepsy* A: PO: 5–20 mg, q.d.–t.i.d.; *max:* 60 mg/d C > 6–12y: PO: 5 mg/d *ADD* C 3–5 y: PO: 2.5 mg/d C 6–12 y: PO: 5 mg/d, *max:* 40 mg/d	For narcolepsy, ADD. Dosage should be minimal to control symptoms in ADD. CNS and cardiac toxicity could occur. *Pregnancy category:* C; PB: UK; t½: 10–30 h.
Dextroamphetamine sulfate (Dexedrine) CSS II	*ADD* C 3–5 y: PO: 2.5 mg/d C 6–12 y: PO: 5 mg/d, *max:* 40 mg/d	Uses similar to those of amphetamines. Drug has been used for obesity and narcolepsy. *Pregnancy category:* C; PB: UK; t½: UK.
Methamphetamine HCl (Desoxyn) CSS II	C: PO: 2.5–5 mg daily; increase to 20 mg as needed in 2 divided doses	For ADD. Could cause CNS and cardiac toxicity. *Pregnancy category:* C; PB: UK; t½: UK.
AMPHETAMINE-LIKE DRUGS Methylphenidate HCl (Ritalin) CSS II	See Chart 15–1	For ADD and ADHD in children. Dose is increased weekly until symptoms are alleviated. Absorption is affected by food. For narcolepsy. *Pregnancy category:* C; PB: UK; t½: 1–3 h.
Pemoline (Cylert) CSS IV	C > 6 y: PO: 37.5 mg daily and increase weekly; average: 50–75 mg/d; *max:* 112.5 mg/d	For ADD and ADHD in children. Less potent and fewer side effects than Desoxyn and Ritalin. Insomnia may occur; reduce dose. *Pregnancy category:* B; PB: 50%; t½: 9–12 h.

KEY: A: adult; C: child; CSS: controlled substance schedule; PB: protein-binding; PO: by mouth; CNS: central nervous system; t½: half-life; UK: unknown; >: greater than.

Side Effects and Adverse Reactions

Amphetamines can cause adverse effects in the central nervous, cardiovascular, gastrointestinal (GI), and endocrine systems. The side effects and adverse reactions include restlessness, insomnia, tachycardia, hypertension, heart palpitations, dry mouth, anorexia, weight loss, diarrhea or constipation, and impotence.

AMPHETAMINE-LIKE DRUGS FOR NARCOLEPSY AND ADD

Amphetamine-like drugs are given for the treatment of narcolepsy and **attention deficit disorder (ADD)** or **attention deficit hyperactivity disorder (ADHD)**.

Narcolepsy is characterized by falling asleep during normal waking activity (e.g., while driving a car or talking with someone). Sleep paralysis, the condition of muscle paralysis that is normal during sleep, usually accompanies narcolepsy and affects the voluntary muscles. The person is unable to move and may collapse.

ADD or ADHD is the inability to learn and to interact socially because of hyperactivity (excessive and purposeless activity) and a decrease in attention span. This condition occurs most frequently in children. The incidence is three to seven times more common in boys than girls. This problem may continue through the teen-age years. Some professionals state that ADD is often incorrectly diagnosed and many children receive unnecessary treatment for months to years.

The child with ADD may display poor coordination, and there may be abnormal electroencephalographic (EEG) findings. Intelligence is usually not affected. This problem has also been called minimal brain dysfunction, hyperactivity in children, **hyperkinesis,** and hyperkinetic syndrome with learning disorder. Counseling or psychotherapy as well as drug and diet therapy may be needed to decrease or alleviate the hyperactive behavior.

Amphetamine and amphetamine-like stimulants are given to increase the child's attention span and improve daytime sleepiness. Sedatives are not indicated. Two amphetamine-like drugs, methylphenidate (Ritalin) and pemoline (Cylert), are usually prescribed for treating ADD and narcolepsy rather than the amphetamines owing to their lower incidence of side effects. However, dextroamphetamine (Dexedrine) may be prescribed for some ADD clients. Amphetamine and amphetamine-like drugs should not be taken in the evening or before bedtime because insomnia may result.

ADD and ADHD can persist or may be first identified in adulthood. Symptoms in the young adult with ADD/ADHD include stress intolerance, outbursts of anger, difficulty in concentration, and inability to complete tasks. Chart 15–1 compares the pharmacokinetics, pharmacodynamics, and therapeutic effects of methylphenidate and pemoline in treating ADD and narcolepsy.

Pharmacokinetics

Methylphenidate and pemoline are well absorbed from the GI mucosa. Although pemoline has a longer half-life than methylphenidate, the drugs are usually administered to children once a day before breakfast. However, methylphenidate may be given twice a day, before breakfast and lunch. Because food affects the absorption rate, the drug should be given 30 to 45 minutes before meals. These drugs should not be given 6 h before sleep because they may cause insomnia. Both drugs are excreted in the urine; 40% of methylphenidate is excreted unchanged.

Pharmacodynamics

Methylphenidate and pemoline help to correct ADD by decreasing hyperactivity and improving attention span. These amphetamine-like drugs are considered more effective in treating ADD than amphetamines. Amphetamines are generally avoided because they have a higher potential for abuse, habituation, and tolerance. Methylphenidate is slightly more effective than pemoline for ADD, but the side effects and adverse reactions of pemoline are less severe.

Sympathomimetic drugs, such as decongestants, enhance the actions of methylphenidate and pemoline. Antihypertensives and barbiturates can decrease the action of these drugs. Foods with caffeine content should be avoided because they increase drug action.

ANOREXIANTS

Obesity has been treated with prescribed amphetamines or over-the-counter (OTC) amphetamine-like drugs. Amphetamines have been recommended as **anorexiants** (appetite suppressants) for short-term use (4 to 12 weeks). Because of tolerance, psychological dependence, and abuse, amphetamines are *not* recommended currently for use as appetite suppressants. The OTC choice for short-term use of an appetite suppressant is phenylpropanolamine (Dexatrim) because it causes fewer systemic side effects and has less of a potential for abuse. Most of the anorexiants used to suppress appetite (Table 15–2) do not have the serious side effects associated with amphetamines. To lose weight, emphasis should be placed on proper

Chart 15–1. Amphetamine-like Drugs

AMPHETAMINE-LIKE DRUGS

Assessment and Planning — NURSING PROCESS

Drug Names

Methylphenidate HCl (M) (Ritalin, Ritalin SR)
Pregnancy Category: C
Pemoline (P) (Cylert)
Central Nervous System Stimulants
Pregnancy Category: B

Dosage

(M) *Attention deficit disorder:*
C >6 y: PO: 5 mg before breakfast and lunch; if necessary increase dosage weekly by 5–10 mg; max: 60 mg/d
SR: Not recommended for initial treatment
Narcolepsy:
A: PO: 10 mg, b.i.d.–t.i.d. 30 min before meals
(P) *Attention deficit disorder:*
C >6 y: PO: 37.5 mg daily and increase weekly; average dose: 50–75 mg/d; max: 112.5 mg/d

Contraindications

(M&P) Hypersensitivity
(M) Hyperthyroidism, anxiety, history of seizures, motor tics, Tourette's syndrome, glaucoma
Caution: (M) Hypertension, depression, alcoholism, pregnancy
(P) Impaired renal or hepatic function, psychosis
(M&P) not to be used for children <6 y

Drug-Lab-Food Interactions

(M) *Increase* hypertensive crisis with MAOIs
(M) *Increase* effects of oral anticoagulants, anticonvulsants, tricyclic antidepressants
(M&P) May *decrease* effects of decongestants, antihypertensives, barbiturates; may alter effects of insulin therapy
Food: Caffeine (coffee, tea, colas, chocolate) may *increase* effects
Lab: (P) May *increase* AST, ALT, LDH

Interventions

Pharmacokinetics

Absorption: (M&P) Well absorbed from GI tract
Distribution: PB: (M) UK, (P) 50%
Metabolism: $t\frac{1}{2}$: (M) 1–3 h, (P) 10–14 h
Excretion:
(M) 40% excreted unchanged in urine
(P) Excreted in the urine

Pharmacodynamics

(M) **PO:** Onset: 0.5–1 h
Peak: 1–3 h
Duration: 4–6 h
SR: 4–8 h
(P) **PO:** Onset: 0.5–1 h
Peak: 2–4 h
Duration: 8 h

Evaluation

Therapeutic Effects/Uses

(M&P) To correct hyperactivity caused by ADD, increase attention span, and treat fatigue
(M) To control narcolepsy

Mode of action: Acts primarily on the cerebral cortex, reticular activatory system

Side Effects

(M&P) Anorexia, vomiting, diarrhea, insomnia, dizziness, nervousness, restlessness, irritability

Adverse Reactions

(M&P) Tachycardia, growth suppression
(M) Palpitations, transient loss of weight in children, increased hyperactivity
(P) Dyskinetic movements (face, lips, tongue), hepatitis, jaundice
Life-threatening: (M) Exfoliative dermatitis, uremia, thrombocytopenia

KEY: PO: by mouth; PB: protein-binding; $t\frac{1}{2}$: half-life, UK: unknown, A: adult, C: child, SR: sustained release; MAOI: monoamine oxidase inhibitor; AST: aspartate aminotransferase; ALT: alanine aminotransferase; ADH: antidiuretic hormone.

Table 15–2
Anorexiants and Analeptics

DRUG	ROUTE AND DOSAGE	USES AND CONSIDERATIONS
ANOREXIANTS		
Benzphetamine HCl (Didrex) CSS III	A: PO: 25–50 mg q.d.–t.i.d.	Similar to amphetamines. Potential for abuse. Avoid taking drug during pregnancy. *Pregnancy category:* X; PB: UK, $t_{\frac{1}{2}}$: 6–12 h.
Dextroamphetamine sulfate (Dexedrine) CSS II	A: PO: 5–10 mg 1 to 3 × d 30–60 min a.c.	To treat obesity. Can cause restlessness and insomnia. For short-term use. *Pregnancy category:* C; PB: UK; $t_{\frac{1}{2}}$: 30–35 h.
Dexfenfluramine (Redux)	A: PO: 15 mg, b.i.d. with meals	It is used in the management of obesity. It does not produce CNS stimulation. Contraindications include pulmonary hypertension, taking MAOIs. *Pregnancy category:* PK: UK; $t_{\frac{1}{2}}$: 17–20 h.
Diethylpropion HCl (Dospan, Tenuate, Tepanil) CSS IV	A: PO: 25 mg t.i.d.; SR: 75 mg daily	For appetite suppression by stimulating the appetite control center in the hypothalamus. Take 1 h before meals. For short-term use. *Pregnancy category:* B; PB: UK; $t_{\frac{1}{2}}$: 2–3 h.
Fenfluramine HCl (Pondimin) CSS IV	A: PO: 20 mg t.i.d.; a.c.; max: 120 mg/d May increase weekly	To treat exogenous obesity. Should be taken 1 h before meals. Can depress mood and motor activity, and may increase blood pressure (BP). *Pregnancy category:* C; PB: UK: $t_{\frac{1}{2}}$: 20 h
Mazindol (Mazanor, Sanorex) CSS IV	A: PO: Initial: 2 mg/d A: PO: 1 mg t.i.d. a.c.; or 2 mg daily	To manage obesity. To be taken 1 h before meals or daily dose before lunch. May increase heart rate. BP usually unchanged. Is a potential abused drug. *Pregnancy category:* C; PB: UK; $t_{\frac{1}{2}}$: 2.5–9 h.
Phendimetrazine tartrate (Anorex, Adipost, Trimcaps, Prelu-2) CSS III	A: PO: 17.5–35 mg 1 h a.c. b.i.d.–t.i.d.; max: 70 mg t.i.d.	To manage obesity. Should be taken 1 h before meals. Usually no change in heart rate or blood pressure. CNS stimulation (mood and motor activity). *Pregnancy category:* C; PB: UK; $t_{\frac{1}{2}}$: 2–10 h.
Phenmetrazine HCl (Preludin) CSS II	A: PO: 25 mg b.i.d.–t.i.d.; SR: 75 mg daily; max: 75 mg daily	Short-term use to manage obesity. Should be taken 1 h before meals. Increases CNS, heart rate, and blood pressure. High abuse potential. *Pregnancy category:* C; PB: UK; $t_{\frac{1}{2}}$: UK.
Phentermine HCl (Adipex-P, Fastin, Ionamin) CSS IV	A: PO: 8 mg t.i.d. a.c.; or 15–37.5 mg/d	To control appetite. Should be taken before meals. Increases heart rate and blood pressure. Low abuse potential. *Pregnancy category:* C; PB: UK; $t_{\frac{1}{2}}$: 20 h.
Phenylpropanolamine HCl (Acutrim, Control, Dexatrim, Prolamine)	A: PO: 25 mg a.c. t.i.d.; or SR: 75 mg/d in morning	To control weight gain. Should be taken before meals. OTC drugs. May increase heart rate and blood pressure. Low abuse potential. *Pregnancy category:* C; PB: UK; $t_{\frac{1}{2}}$: 4–7 h.

Table continued on following page

Table 15–2 *Continued*
Anorexiants and Analeptics

DRUG	ROUTE AND DOSAGE	USES AND CONSIDERATIONS
ANALEPTICS: METHYLXANTHINES		
Caffeine	*Neonatal apnea:* Infant and C: PO-IM-IV. 5–10 mg/kg on day 1; then 2.5–5 mg/d *Therapeutic range:* 5–20 mg/mL	Used for newborns with apnea to stimulate respiration; increases heart rate and blood pressure. Given through a nasogastric tube, intramuscularly, or intravenously. *Pregnancy category:* C; PB: 25%–35%; $t_{\frac{1}{2}}$: A: 3–5 h, neonate: 40–144 h.
OTC drugs (Nō Dōz, Tirend), coffee	A: 100–200 mg q 3–4 h as needed	Restores mental alertness. Contains citrated caffeine. Brewed coffee contains 60–180 mg of caffeine per cup.
Theophylline	Infants: NGT; 5 mg/kg on day 1; then 2 mg in divided doses	Used for newborns with apnea to stimulate respiration. Given through a nasogastric tube.
CNS STIMULANT FOR MIGRAINE		
Sumatriptan succinate (Imitrex)	A: SC: 6 mg single dose; may repeat in 1 h; max: 12 mg/d	To treat acute migraine attacks. Promotes vasoconstriction of the carotid arteries. *Pregnancy category:* C; PB: 20%; $t_{\frac{1}{2}}$: 2 h.
RESPIRATORY STIMULANT		
Doxapram HCl (Dopram)	A: IV: 0.5–1 mg/kg; inf: 1–2 mg/min; max: 3 g/d *Neonatal apnea:* Initially: 0.5 mg/kg/h Maintenance: 0.5–2.5 mg/kg/h titrated to lowest effective rate	Used in adults only for chronic obstructive pulmonary disease (COPD). Used to treat sedative-hypnotic overdose to correct respiratory depression. It can increase blood pressure. *Pregnancy category:* B; PB: UK; $t_{\frac{1}{2}}$: A: 2.5–4 h, neonate: 7–10 h.

KEY: A: adult; a.c.: before meals; C: child; CSS: Controlled Substance Schedule; max: maximum; NGT: nasogastric tube; PB: protein-binding; PO: by mouth; SC: subcutaneous; SR: sustained-release; $t_{\frac{1}{2}}$: half-life; UK: unknown; MAOI: monoamine oxidase inhibitor.

diet, exercise, and behavioral modifications. Reliance on appetite suppressants should be discouraged. Those individuals who are taking anorexiants should be under a health care provider's supervision.

Side Effects and Adverse Reactions

Children younger than 12 years old should *not* take anorexiants, and self-medication with anorexiants should be discouraged. Long-term use of these drugs frequently results in such severe side effects as nervousness, restlessness, irritability, insomnia, heart palpitations, and hypertension.

ANALEPTICS

Analeptics, which are CNS stimulants, mostly affect the brain stem and spinal cord but also affect the cerebral cortex. The primary use of an analeptic is to stimulate respiration. One subgroup of analeptics is the xanthines (methylxanthines), of which caffeine and theophylline are the main drugs. Depending on the dose, caffeine stimulates the CNS, and large doses stimulate respiration. Table 15–3 lists the concentration of caffeine in various beverages. Newborns with respiratory distress might be given caffeine to increase respiration. Theophylline is used mostly to relax the bronchioles; however, it has also been used to

Table 15–3
Caffeine Content in Beverages

COFFEE, TEA, AND CHOCOLATE (5-oz cup)

Regular coffee	
Brewed	60 to 180 mg
Instant	30 to 120 mg
Decaffeinated coffee	
Brewed	2 to 5 mg
Instant	1 to 5 mg
Tea	
Brewed	20 to 100 mg
Instant	20 to 50 mg
Hot chocolate	2 to 50 mg
Chocolate milk	2 to 7 mg

SOFT DRINKS (12-oz cup)

Storm	58 mg
Mountain Dew	55 mg
Coca-Cola and Diet Coca-Cola	45 mg
Pepsi and Diet Pepsi	36 mg
Sprite, 7-Up, ginger ale	0 mg

increase respiration in newborns. Table 15–2 lists the analeptics, their dosages, uses, and considerations.

Side Effects and Adverse Reactions

The side effects from caffeine are similar to those from anorexiants: nervousness, restlessness, tremors, twitchings, palpitations, and insomnia. Other side effects include diuresis (increased urination), GI irritation (nausea, diarrhea), and, rarely, tinnitus (ringing in the ear). More than 500 mg of caffeine affects the CNS and heart. High doses of caffeine in coffee, chocolate, and cold-relief medications can cause a psychological dependence. The half-life of caffeine is 3½ hours; however, metabolism is slowed and the half-life is prolonged in liver disease and in pregnancy. Caffeine is contraindicated during pregnancy because the effect on the fetus is not known.

RESPIRATORY CNS STIMULANT

Doxapram (Dopram), a CNS and respiratory stimulant, is used to treat respiratory depression caused by drug overdose, postanesthetic respiratory depression, and chronic obstructive pulmonary disease (COPD). It is administered intravenously. The onset of action is within 20 to 40 seconds with a peak action within 2 minutes. Side effects are infrequent; however, with an overdose, hypertension, tachycardia, trembling, and convulsions may occur.

TREATMENT OF MIGRAINE HEADACHES

A unilateral throbbing head pain, accompanied by nausea, vomiting, and photophobia usually occurs with migraine headaches. Migraine attacks frequently occur in persons in their twenties and thirties, and in women symptoms are decreased or absent after menopause. The migraine headaches are caused by arterial dilation.

Drugs to treat migraines include (1) aspirin-like analgesics, (2) opioid analgesics, (3) ergot alkaloids, and (4) triptans. For mild migraine attacks, aspirin, ibuprofen, naproxen (Aleve), or acetaminophen may be prescribed. Aspirin may be used in combination with caffeine. Meperidine (Demerol) and butorphanol nasal spray (Stadol NS) are the opioid analgesics occasionally given.

Ergotamine tartrate, a nonspecific serotonin agonist and vasoconstrictor, has been prescribed for years to treat moderate to severe migraine headaches. It should be taken early during a migraine attack. Nausea and vomiting might occur; an antiemetic may be given to decrease these symptoms. Ergotamine is available in sublingual tablets or with caffeine in oral tablets and suppositories. Dihydroergotamine, ergot alkaloid, can be administered subcutaneously, intramuscularly, intravenously, and by means of a nasal spray.

The triptans (5-HT$_1$ receptor agonists) are the most recently developed group of drugs for the treatment of migraine headaches. Sumatriptan (Imitrex), a selective serotonin receptor agonist with a short duration of action, was the first triptan drug. It is considered to be more effective than ergotamine for treating acute migraine attacks. Sumatriptan is administered subcutaneously, by oral tablets, and by nasal spray. Three triptans in tablet form recently approved by the FDA are naratriptan (Amerge), rizatriptan (Maxalt), and zolmitriptan (Zomig).

NURSING PROCESS

CENTRAL NERVOUS SYSTEM STIMULANT: METHYLPHENIDATE HCI (RITALIN)

Assessment

- Determine whether there is a history of heart disease, hypertension, hyperthyroidism, parkinsonism, or glaucoma; in such cases, drug is usually contraindicated.
- Assess vital signs to be used for future comparisons. Pay close attention to clients with cardiac disease because drug may reverse effects of antihypertensives.
- Assess the client's mental status; e.g., mood, affect, aggressiveness.
- Assess height, growth, weight of children.
- Assess complete blood count (CBC), differential white blood cells (WBCs), and platelets before and during therapy.

Potential Nursing Diagnoses

- Behavior disorders (impulsiveness, short attention span, and distractibility) related to interference with peer relationships, learning, and discipline
- Potential for family crisis related to dysfunctional behavior

Planning

- Client will be free of hyperactivity.
- Client will not experience side effects or adverse reactions to therapy. Client will increase attention span.

Nursing Interventions

- Monitor vital signs. Report irregularities.
- Monitor height, weight, and growth of children.
- Monitor the client for withdrawal symptoms (e.g., nausea, vomiting, weakness, headache).
- Monitor the client for side effects (e.g., insomnia, restlessness, nervousness, tremors, irritability, tachycardia, or elevated blood pressure). Report findings.

Client Teaching

General
- Instruct the client to take drug before meals.
- Instruct the client to avoid alcohol consumption.
- Encourage the use of sugarless gum to relieve dry mouth.
- Instruct the client to monitor weight twice a week and to report weight loss.
- Instruct the client to avoid driving and using hazardous equipment when experiencing tremors, nervousness, or increased heart rate.
- Instruct the client not to abruptly discontinue the drug; the dose must be tapered off to avoid withdrawal symptoms. Consult the health care provider before modifying the dose.
- Encourage the client to read the labels on OTC products because many contain caffeine. A high caffeine plasma level could be fatal.
- Instruct the nursing mother to avoid taking all CNS stimulants. These drugs pass into the breast milk and can cause the infant to be hyperactive or restless.
- Encourage the family to seek counseling for children with attention deficit disorder or attention deficit hyperactivity disorder. Drug therapy alone is not an appropriate therapy program. Notify school nurse of drug therapy regimen.
- Explain to client or family that long-term use may lead to drug abuse.

Diet
- Instruct the client to avoid caffeine-containing foods.
- Instruct parents to provide children with a nutritional breakfast because drug may have anorexic effects.

Nursing Process continued on following page

Side Effects

• Instruct the client about drug side effects and the need to report tachycardia and palpitations. Monitor children for onset of Tourette's syndrome.

Evaluation

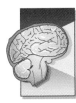

• Evaluate the effectiveness of drug therapy. The client is not hyperactive and does not have adverse effects from drug.
• Monitor weight, sleep patterns, and mental status.

Critical Thinking in Action

M. P., 67 years old, wants to lose 30 pounds. She wants to take an OTC diet pill but does not want to exercise or be on a diet.

1. Would you suggest a diet pill? Why or why not?
2. What does the nurse need to assess concerning this client's physical status before suggesting a "diet pill" or weight loss program?
3. What behavior modification may you suggest related to losing weight?
4. In what ways could diet control and exercise help this client? Explain.
5. Would you suggest a weight loss program such as Weight Watchers or Jenny Craig? How do these programs differ? Would one program benefit her more than the other? Explain.

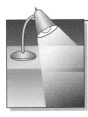

Study Questions

1. A 5-year-old boy was diagnosed as having attention deficit disorder (ADD). What is ADD? What drugs are effective in controlling this problem?
2. What are appetite suppressants called? Why are amphetamines not recommended for the treatment of obesity?
3. The client has hypertension. Why are amphetamines not recommended for hypertensive clients? List the side effects of amphetamines.
4. A mother is breastfeeding her infant daughter. She wants to lose 30 lb and plans to take an OTC anorexiant. What would your response be? Explain.

16 Central Nervous System Depressants Sedative-Hypnotics and Anesthetics

Outline

Objectives

- Identify the types and stages of sleep.
- Identify several nonpharmacologic ways to induce sleep.
- Define *hangover, dependence, tolerance, withdrawal symptoms,* and *REM rebound.*
- Explain which drugs might cause the above adverse effects.
- List examples of short-acting and intermediate-acting barbiturates used as sedative-hypnotics.
- List three benzodiazepines developed for hypnotic use.
- Give the nursing interventions related to barbiturates and benzodiazepine hypnotics.
- Describe the stages of anesthesia.
- Explain the uses for topical anesthetics.
- Identify examples of general and local anesthetics and their major side effects.

Terms

anesthetics
balanced anesthesia
barbiturates
caudal anesthesia
dependence
epidural anesthesia

hangover
hypnotic effect
infiltration anesthesia
insomnia
nerve block anesthesia
NREM sleep

saddle block
REM sleep
sedation
spinal anesthesia
tolerance
withdrawal symptoms

INTRODUCTION

Drugs that are central nervous system (CNS) depressants cause varying degrees of depression (reduction in functional activity) within the central nervous system. The degree of depression depends primarily on the drug and the amount of drug taken. The broad classification of CNS depressants includes sedative-hypnotics, general and local anesthetics, analgesics, narcotic analgesics, anticonvulsants, antipsychotics, and antidepressants. The last five groups of drugs are presented in separate chapters. Sedative-hypnotics and general and local anesthetics are covered in this chapter.

Sleep disorders, such as **insomnia** (inability to fall asleep), occur in 5% to 10% of healthy adults, 20% to 25% of hospitalized clients, and approximately 75% of psychiatric clients. Insomnia occurs more frequently in women and increases with age. Sedative-hypnotics are frequently ordered for sleep disorders.

Types and Stages of Sleep

People spend approximately one-third of their lives, or as much as 25 years, sleeping. Normal sleep is composed of two definite phases: **REM, or rapid eye movement,** and **NREM, or nonrapid eye movement.** Both REM and NREM occur cyclically during sleep at about 90-minute intervals (Fig. 16–1). The four successively deeper stages of NREM sleep end with an episode of REM sleep and the cycle begins again. If sleep is interrupted, the cycle begins again with stage 1 of NREM sleep.

It is during the REM sleep phase that individuals experience most of their recallable dreams. Individuals perform better during their waking hours if they experience all types and stages of sleep. Children have few REM sleep periods and have longer periods of stage 3 and 4 NREM sleep. Older adults (elderly) have a decrease in stage 3 and 4 of NREM sleep and have frequent waking periods.

It is difficult to arouse a person during REM sleep. The period of REM sleep episodes becomes longer during the sleep process. Frequently, if the person is aroused from REM sleep, he or she may recall a vivid, bizarre dream. If these dreams are unpleasant, they may be called *nightmares.* Sleep walking or *nightmares* that occur in children take place during NREM sleep.

Nonpharmacologic Methods

Various nonpharmacologic methods should be used for promoting sleep before using sedative-hypnotics or over-the-counter (OTC) sleep aids. Once the nurse discovers why the client cannot sleep, she or he may suggest the following ways for promoting sleep:

1. Arise at a specific hour in the morning.
2. Take few or no daytime naps.
3. Avoid drinks that contain caffeine 6 h before bedtime.
4. Avoid heavy meals or strenuous exercise before bedtime.
5. Take a warm bath, read, or listen to music before bedtime.
6. Decrease exposure to loud noises.
7. Avoid drinking copious amounts of fluids before sleep.
8. Drink warm milk before bedtime.

SEDATIVE-HYPNOTICS

The mildest form of CNS depression is **sedation,** which at lower dosages of certain CNS depressants diminishes physical and mental responses but does not affect consciousness. Sedatives are used mostly during the daytime. Increasing the drug dose can produce a **hypnotic effect**—not hypnosis, but a form of "natural" sleep. Sedative-hypnotic drugs are sometimes the same drug; however, certain drugs are used more often for their hypnotic effect. With very high doses of sedative-hypnotic drugs, anesthesia may be achieved. An example of an ultrashort-acting barbitu-

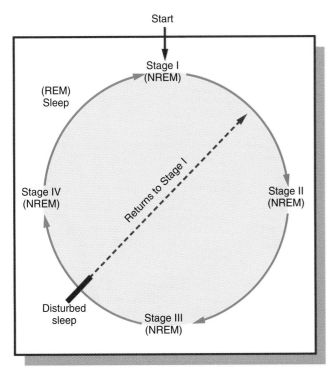

Figure 16–1
Types and stages of sleep. REM: rapid eye movement (dreaming); NREM: nonrapid eye movement (four stages).

rate used to produce anesthesia is thiopental sodium (Pentothal).

Sedatives were first prescribed for reducing tension and anxiety. Barbiturates were used first for their antianxiety effect, until the early 1960s when benzodiazepines were introduced. Because of the many side effects of barbiturates and their potential for physical and mental dependency, they are less frequently prescribed. Similarly, the chronic use of any sedative-hypnotic should be avoided.

Because of the high incidence of sleep disorders, hypnotic drugs are one of the most frequently prescribed drugs. More than $35 million is spent each year for OTC sleep aids, such as Nytol, Sominex, Sleep-Eze, Tylenol PM. The primary ingredient in OTC sleep aids is an antihistamine, such as diphenhydramine, and not barbiturates or benzodiazepines.

There are short-acting hypnotics and intermediate-acting hypnotics. Short-acting hypnotics are useful in achieving sleep because they allow the client to awaken early in the morning without experiencing lingering side effects. Intermediate-acting hypnotics are useful for sustaining sleep; however, after using one the client may experience residual drowsiness

(hangover) in the morning. This may be undesirable if the client is active and requires mental alertness. The ideal hypnotic promotes natural sleep without disrupting normal patterns of sleep and produces no hangover or undesirable effect. Table 16–1 lists the common side effects and adverse reactions associated with sedative-hypnotic use and abuse.

Hypnotic drug therapy should be short term to prevent drug **dependence** and drug **tolerance.** Interrupting hypnotic therapy can decrease drug tolerance. However, abruptly discontinuing a high dose of hypnotic that has been taken over a long period of time could cause **withdrawal symptoms.** At high doses, the dose should be tapered to avoid withdrawal symptoms. The lowest dose should be taken to obtain sleep. Clients with severe respiratory disorders should avoid hypnotics, which could cause an increase in respiratory distress. Normally, hypnotics are contraindicated during pregnancy.

The category of sedative-hypnotics includes barbiturates, benzodiazepines, and piperidinediones, among others. Each of these is discussed separately. Drug charts are included for barbiturates and benzodiazepines.

Table 16–1
Common Side Effects and Adverse Reactions of Sedative-Hypnotics

SIDE EFFECTS AND ADVERSE REACTIONS	EXPLANATION OF THE EFFECTS
Hangover	A hangover is residual drowsiness resulting in impaired reaction time. The intermediate and long-acting hypnotics are frequently the cause of drug hangover. The liver biotransforms these drugs into active metabolites that persist in the body, causing drowsiness.
REM Rebound	REM rebound, which results in vivid dreams and nightmares, frequently occurs after taking a hypnotic over a prolonged period and then abruptly stopping. However, it may occur after taking only one hypnotic dose.
Dependence	Dependence is the result of chronic use of hypnotics. Physical and psychological dependence can result. Physical dependence results in the appearance of specific withdrawal symptoms when a drug is discontinued after prolonged use. The severity of withdrawal symptoms depends on the drug and the dosage. Symptoms may include muscular twitching and tremors, dizziness, orthostatic hypotension, delusions, hallucinations, delirium, and seizures. The withdrawal symptoms start within 24 h and can last for several days.
Tolerance	Tolerance results when there is a need to increase the dosage over time to obtain the desired effect. It is mostly due to an increase in drug metabolism by liver enzymes. Barbiturates is one drug category that can cause tolerance after prolonged use. Tolerance is reversible when the drug is discontinued.
Excessive Depression	Long-term use of a hypnotic may result in depression, which is characterized by lethargy, sleepiness, lack of concentration, confusion, and psychologic depression.
Respiratory Depression	High doses of sedative-hypnotics can suppress the respiratory center in the medulla.
Hypersensitivity	Skin rashes and urticaria can result when taking barbituates. Such reactions are rare.

Table 16–2
Sedative-Hypnotics: Barbiturates and Others

GENERIC (BRAND)	ROUTE AND DOSAGE	USES AND CONSIDERATIONS
BARBITURATES: SHORT-ACTING		
Pentobarbital sodium (Nembutal Sodium)	See Chart 16–1.	For sedative or sleep. Can be used for induction to general anesthesia. *Pregnancy category:* D; PB: 35%–45%; t½: 4 h, 30–50 h (2nd phase) Methohexital sodium. See Table 16–5
Secobarbital sodium (Seconal Sodium) CSS II	*Preoperative sedative:* A: PO: 100–300 mg before surgery C: PO: 50–100 mg or 2–6 mg/kg max: 100 mg *Hypnotic:* A: PO/IM: 100–200 mg h.s. C: IM 3–5 mg/kg; max: 100 mg *Status epilepticus:* A: IV: 5.5 mg/kg; repeat in 3–4 h *With spinal anesthesia:* A: IV: 50–100 mg; infuse over 30 sec; max: 250 mg/dose	For sedation or sleep. Also preanesthetic sedation. *Pregnancy category:* D; PB: UK; t½: 15–40 h
BARBITURATES: IN-TERMEDIATE-ACTING		
Amobarbital sodium (Amytal Sodium)	*Sedative:* A: PO: 30–50 mg b.i.d.–t.i.d. C: PO: 2 mg/kg/d in 3–4 divided doses *Hypnotic:* A: PO/IM: 65–200 mg h.s. C: IM: 2–3 mg/kg A and C: IV: 65–200 mg	As a sedative and short-term hypnotic; to control acute convulsive episodes; and for insomnia. Take 0.5–1 h before bedtime. *Pregnancy category:* D; PB: 50%–60%; t½: 20–40 h
Aprobarbital (Alurate)	*Sedative:* A: PO: 40 mg t.i.d. *Hypnotic:* A: PO: 40–160 mg h.s.	As a sedative and short-term hypnotic; use no longer than 2 wk. *Pregnancy category:* D, PB: <50%; t½: 15–40 h
Butabarbital sodium (Butisol Sodium) CSS III	*Sedative:* A: PO: 15–30 mg t.i.d., q.i.d. *Hypnotic:* A: PO: 50–100 mg h.s. *Preoperative sedative:* A: PO: 50–100 mg, 1–1.5 h before surgery	To relieve anxiety and for short-term hypnotic for insomnia. Avoid alcohol with all barbiturates. *Pregnancy category:* D; PB: <50%; t½: 60–120 h
OTHER SEDATIVE-HYPNOTICS		
Chloral hydrate CSS IV	*Sedative:* A: PO: 250 mg t.i.d. pc C: PO: 8.3 mg/kg t.i.d. pc; max: 1000 mg/d or 500 mg/dose *Hypnotic:* A: PO: 500 mg–1g h.s. (15–30 min before sleep) C: PO: 50 mg/kg h.s.; max: 1000 mg	For sedative or sleep. Used in mid 1800s. No hangover and less respiratory depression. Give with meals or fluids to prevent gastric irritation. Give 15–30 min prior to sleep. *Pregnancy category:* C; PB: 70%–80%; t½: 8–10 h
Ethchlorvynol (Placidyl)	*Sedative:* A: PO: 100–200 mg, b.i.d., t.i.d. *Hypnotic:* A: PO: 0.5–1 g, h.s. for 1 wk only	A barbiturate-like drug. For sedation and sleep. Use no longer than 1 wk. Caution: renal or liver disease and drug abuse. Give with food or fluid to decrease nausea and vomiting. It has a short duration of action. *Pregnancy category:* C; PB: UK; t½: 20–100 h

Table continued on following page

Table 16–2 Continued
Sedative-Hypnotics: Barbiturates and Others

GENERIC (BRAND)	ROUTE AND DOSAGE	USES AND CONSIDERATIONS
Paraldehyde (Paral) CSS IV	*Sedative:* A: PO: 5–10 mL q4–6h PRN in water or juice: max: 30 mL C: PO: 0.3 mL/kg *Hypnotic:* A: PO: 10–30 mL h.s.	Exhaled via the lungs. Strong odor and disagreeable taste. Seldom used today; has been used to control delirium tremens (DTs) in alcoholics. Can be used for drug poisoning, status epilepticus, and tetanus to control convulsions. *Pregnancy category:* C; PB: UK; $t_{\frac{1}{2}}$: 7.5 h

KEY: *A: adult; C: child; PO: by mouth; IM: intramuscular; IV: intravenous; pc: after meals; UK: unknown; PB: protein-binding; $t_{\frac{1}{2}}$: half-life; h.s.: hour of sleep; max: maximum; <: less than; CSS: Controlled Substance Schedule; PRN: as needed.*

Barbiturates

Barbiturates were introduced as a sedative in the early 1900s. More than 2000 barbiturates have been developed, but only 12 are currently marketed. The barbiturates are classified as long-acting, intermediate-acting, short-acting, and ultrashort-acting. The long-acting group includes phenobarbital and mephobarbital and is used for controlling seizures in epilepsy. The ultrashort-acting barbiturate, thiopental sodium (Pentothal), is used as general anesthesia. Phenobarbital, introduced in 1912, is still in use.

The short-acting barbiturates secobarbital (Seconal) and pentobarbital (Nembutal) are used to induce sleep for those who have difficulty falling asleep. These drugs may cause the person to awaken early in the morning. The intermediate-acting barbiturates amobarbital (Amytal), aprobarbital (Alurate), and butabarbital (Butisol) are useful as sleep sustainers for maintaining long periods of sleep. Because these drugs take approximately 1 h for the onset of sleep, they are not prescribed for those who have trouble getting to sleep. Vital signs should be closely monitored in persons taking these two groups of barbiturates.

Barbiturates increase CNS depression in the elderly and should not be taken by the elderly for sleep. Nonpharmacologic approaches to sleep should first be promoted.

Barbiturates should be restricted to short-term use (2 weeks or less) because of their numerous side effects, including tolerance to the drug. In the United States, barbiturates are classified as class II in the schedule of the Controlled Substances Act. In Canada, barbiturates are classified as schedule G. The barbiturates are listed in Table 16–2 and described in more detail in Chart 16–1, with a focus on the short-acting barbiturate pentobarbital (Nembutal). Nursing process is based on the drug data.

PHARMACOKINETICS

Pentobarbital (Nembutal) has been available for nearly half a century and was the hypnotic of choice until the introduction of benzodiazepines in the 1960s. It has a slow absorption rate and is moderately protein-bound. The long half-life is mainly due to the formation of active metabolites resulting from liver metabolism.

PHARMACODYNAMICS

Pentobarbital is primarily used to induce sleep and for sedation needs. It has a rapid onset with a short duration of action; thus, it is considered a short-acting barbiturate. The onset of action is slower when administered intramuscularly than when administered orally.

There are many drug interactions associated with pentobarbital. Alcohol, narcotics, and other sedative-hypnotics used in combination with pentobarbital may further depress the central nervous system. Pentobarbital increases hepatic enzyme action, thus causing an increased metabolism and decreased effect of drugs, such as oral anticoagulants, glucocorticoids, tricyclic antidepressants, and quinidine. Pentobarbital may cause hepatotoxicity if taken with large doses of acetaminophen.

Benzodiazepines

Selected benzodiazepines (minor tranquilizer or anxiolytic), introduced with chlordiazepoxide (Librium) in the 1960s as antianxiety agents, are ordered as sedative-hypnotics for inducing sleep. Five benzodiazepines marketed as hypnotics are flurazepam (Dalmane), temazepam (Restoril), triazolam (Halcion), estazolam (ProSom), and quazepam (Doral) (see Table 16–2). Increased anxiety might be the cause of insom-

Chart 16-1. Sedative-Hypnotic: Barbiturate

PENTOBARBITAL SODIUM

Assessment and Planning

Drug Name

Pentobarbital sodium
(Nembutal Sodium), ❦ Novopentobarb
  Short-acting barbiturate
CSS II
Pregnancy Category: D

Dosage

Sedative:
A: PO: 20–30 mg t.i.d.
C: PO: 2–6 mg/kg/d in 3 divided doses
Hypnotic:
A: PO: 100–200 mg h.s.
C: PO: 30–120 mg h.s.
Also based on age and weight
Preoperative:
A: PO/IM/IV: 100 mg; repeat if needed

Contraindications

Respiratory depression, severe hepatic disease, pregnancy (fetal immaturity), nephrosis

Drug-Lab-Food Interactions

Decrease: respiration with alcohol, CNS depressants; incompatible in solution with numerous drugs such as codeine, insulin, penicillin G, hydrocortisone, phenytoin

NURSING PROCESS — **Interventions**

Pharmacokinetics

Absorption: PO: 90% absorbed slowly
Distribution: PB: 35%–45%
Metabolism: $t\frac{1}{2}$: 4 h (first phase); 30–50 h (second phase)
Excretion: In urine as metabolites

Pharmacodynamics

PO: Onset: 15–30 min
  Peak: 0.5–1 h
  Duration: 3–6 h
IM: Onset: 10–15 min
  Peak: 0.5–1 h
  Duration: 3–6 h
IV: Onset: Immediate
  Peak: 2–5 min
  Duration: 15–60 min

Evaluation

Therapeutic Effects/Uses

To treat insomnia; used for sedation, preoperative medication, barbiturate coma (for controlling increased intracranial pressure).

Mode of Action: Depression of the CNS, including the motor and sensory activities.

Side Effects

Nausea, vomiting, diarrhea, lethargy, drowsiness, hangover, dizziness, rash

Adverse Reactions

Drug dependence or tolerance, urticaria, hypotension (rapid IV)
Life threatening: Respiratory distress, laryngospasm

KEY: A: adult; C: child; PO: by mouth; PB: protein-binding; $t\frac{1}{2}$: half-life; IM: intramuscular; IV: intravenous; CNS: central nervous system; ❦: Canadian drug names.

NURSING PROCESS
SEDATIVE-HYPNOTIC: BARBITURATE

Assessment

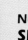

- Obtain baseline vital signs for future comparison.
- Determine whether there is a history of insomnia or sleep disorder.
- Assess renal function. Urine output should be >600 mL/day. Renal impairment could prolong drug action by increasing the half-life of the drug.
- Assess potential for fluid volume deficit, which would potentiate hypotensive effects.

Potential Nursing Diagnosis

- Sleep pattern disturbance

Planning

- Client will receive adequate sleep without hangover when taking the hypnotic.

Nursing Interventions

- Recognize that continuous use of a barbiturate might result in drug abuse.
- Monitor vital signs, especially respirations and blood pressure.
- Raise bedside rails of older adults and clients who are receiving a hypnotic for the first time. Confusion may occur, and injury may result.
- Observe the client, especially an older adult or a debilitated client, for adverse reactions to the pentobarbital; see Chart 16–1.
- Check the client's skin for rashes. Skin eruptions may occur in clients taking barbiturates.
- Observe the client for withdrawal symptoms when pentobarbital has been taken over a prolonged period of time and then discontinued.
- Administer intravenous (IV) pentobarbital at a rate of less than 50 mg/min. Do *not* mix pentobarbital with other medications. Intramuscular (IM) injection should be given deep in a large muscle such as the gluteus medius.

Client Teaching

General
- Instruct the client to use nonpharmacologic ways to induce sleep, such as enjoying a warm bath, listening to music, drinking warm fluids, and avoiding drinks with caffeine for 6 hours before bedtime.
- Instruct the client to avoid alcohol and antidepressant, antipsychotic, and narcotic drugs while taking the barbiturate. Respiratory distress may occur when these drugs are combined.
- Advise the client not to drive a motor vehicle or operate machinery. Caution is always encouraged.
- Instruct the client to take the hypnotic 30 min before bedtime. Short-acting hypnotics such as pentobarbital take effect within 15 to 30 min.
- Encourage the client to check with the health care provider about OTC sleeping aids. Drowsiness may result from taking these drugs, and therefore caution in driving is advised.

Side Effects
- Advise the client to report adverse reactions, such as hangover, to the health care provider. Drug selection or dosage might need to be changed.

Nursing Process continued on following page

• Instruct the client that hypnotics such as pentobarbital should be gradually withdrawn, especially if it has been taken for several weeks. Abrupt cessation of the hypnotic may result in withdrawal symptoms (tremors, muscle twitching).

Evaluation

• Evaluate the effectiveness of pentobarbital. Usually, this drug is given before surgery.
• Evaluate respiratory status to ensure that respiratory distress has not occurred.

Chart 16–2.   Sedative-Hypnotic: Benzodiazepine

FLURAZEPAM HCl

		NURSING PROCESS
Drug Name *Flurazepam HCl* (Dalmane), 🍁 Apo-Fluraze-pam, novoflupam Benzodiazepine hypnotic CSS IV *Pregnancy Category:* X	**Dosage** A: PO: 15–30 mg h.s. Elderly: PO: 15 mg h.s.	*Assessment and Planning*
Contraindications Hypersensitivity to benzodiazepine, pregnancy, lactation, intermittent porphyria **Caution:** Renal, liver, or mental disorders; elderly, debilitation	**Drug-Lab-Food Interactions** May *increase* effect with cimetidine *Decrease* effect with antacids, smoking *Decrease* CNS function with alcohol, CNS depressants, anticonvulsants **Lab:** Increase AST, ALT, ALP, bilirubin *False negatives:* Clinistix, Diastix	

Pharmacokinetics
 	
Absorption: PO: well absorbed
Distribution: PB: 97%
Metabolism: t½ 2–3 h; metabolites: 45–100 h
Excretion: In urine as active metabolites
	Pharmacodynamics
	
	PO: Onset: 15–45 min
	   Peak: 0.5–1 h
	   Duration: 7–10 h
		Interventions

Therapeutic Effects/Uses To treat insomnia. **Mode of Action:** Depression of the CNS, neurotransmitter inhibition.		
Side Effects Drowsiness, lethargy, hangover (residual sedation), dizziness, lightedheadedness, anxiety, nausea, vomiting, diarrhea, confusion, disorientation	**Adverse Reactions** Tolerance, psychological and/or physical dependence, hypotension, mental depression **Life-threatening:** Coma from overdose, leukopenia (rare)	*Evaluation*

KEY: A: adult; PO: by mouth; PB: protein-binding; t½: half-life; CNS: central nervous system; 🍁: Canadian drug names. ALP: alkaline phosphatase; ALT: alanine aminotransferase; AST: aspartate aminotransferase.

nia for some clients, so lorazepam (Ativan), alprazolam, or oxazepam can be used to alleviate the anxiety. These drugs are classified as schedule IV according to the Controlled Substances Act.

Benzodiazepines can suppress stage 4 of NREM sleep, which may result in vivid dreams or nightmares, and can delay REM sleep, except for temazepam. Benzodiazepines are effective for sleep disorders for several weeks longer than other sedative-hypnotics; however, they should not be used for longer than 3 to 4 weeks as a hypnotic to prevent REM rebound. Flurazepam (Dalmane) was the first benzodiazepine hypnotic introduced, and it is described in Chart 16–2. Triazolam (Halcion) is a short-acting hypnotic with a half-life of 2 to 5 h. It does not produce any active metabolites. Complaints of adverse reactions to prolonged use of triazolam, such as loss of memory, have led to its being taken off the market in Great Britain; it is being reviewed by the Food and Drug Administration (FDA). The advisory group in Great Britain is recommending that the legislative body reinstate triazolam. Currently, it is seldom prescribed.

The short-acting benzodiazepines are considered safer than the barbiturates. These benzodiazepines have short to intermediate half-lives and are frequently prescribed along with chloral hydrate for the elderly. In many cases, the client is encouraged to take the benzodiazepine no more than four times a week to avoid side effects and drug dependency.

It has been reported that older women have more difficulty in sleep patterns than older men. The main sleep problem with older adults is frequent awake periods. Disturbance in sleep may be due to discomfort and pain. The OTC drug Tylenol PM contains acetaminophen and diphenhydramine. Occasionally, a nonsteroidal antiinflammatory drug (NSAID) such as ibuprofen may alleviate the discomfort that was preventing sleep.

Small doses of benzodiazepine are recommended for clients with renal or hepatic dysfunction. For benzodiazepine overdose, the benzodiazepine antagonist flumazenil may be prescribed.

PHARMACOKINETICS

Flurazepam is well absorbed through the gastrointestinal (GI) mucosa. Flurazepam is rapidly metabolized in the liver to active metabolites and has a long half-life of 45 to 100 h. Flurazepam is highly protein-bound, and if it is taken with other highly protein-bound drugs, more free drug is available, which increases the risk of adverse effects.

PHARMACODYNAMICS

Flurazepam is used to treat insomnia by inducing and sustaining sleep. It has a rapid onset of action and intermediate- to long-acting effects. The normal

recommended dose of a benzodiazepine may be too much for the older adult, so half of the dose is recommended initially to prevent overdosing.

Alcohol or narcotics taken with a benzodiazepine may cause an additive depressive CNS response. Cimetidine (Tagamet) decreases metabolism of flurazepam, thus increasing its action. Barbiturates decrease the effectiveness of flurazepam by increasing the metabolism of the benzodiazepine. There are other drug interactions that should be carefully assessed when administering a benzodiazepine as a hypnotic.

Piperidinediones

The piperidinediones resemble barbiturates. These sedative-hypnotics were introduced in the mid-1950s and include glutethimide, which has similar effects as the short-acting barbiturates. These drugs were marketed to be nonaddictive; however, they can be addictive and can cause severe adverse reactions, such as vasomotor collapse, serious blood dyscrasias (aplastic anemia), and allergic reactions. Gastric irritation rarely occurs.

If glutethimide is used over several weeks, a gradual tapering of the dose is necessary to avoid severe withdrawal symptoms, including hallucination and convulsion. Over the past decade, there has been a declining use of the piperidinedione group.

Chloral Hydrate

Other sedative-hypnotic drugs are ethchlorvynol (Placidyl), chloral hydrate, and paraldehyde (Paral). Chloral hydrate was first introduced in the 1860s. It is used to induce sleep and to decrease nocturnal awakenings; it does not suppress REM sleep. There is less occurrence of hangover, respiratory depression, and tolerance with chloral hydrate than with other sedative-hypnotics. It has been used effectively with older adults and can be given with mild liver dysfunction, but it should be avoided if severe liver or renal disorder is present. Gastric irritation is a common complaint, so the drug should be taken with sufficient water. Drugs that interact with chloral hydrate include other CNS depressants, furosemide, and oral anticoagulants.

Table 16–3 describes the sedative-hypnotics, their dosages, uses, and considerations.

ANESTHETICS

Anesthetics are classified as general and local. General anesthetics depress the central nervous system, alleviate pain, and cause a great loss of consciousness. The first anesthetic, nitrous oxide (laughing gas), was used for surgery in the early 1800s. It is still an effec-

SEDATIVE-HYPNOTIC: BENZODIAZEPINE

Assessment

- Obtain baseline vital signs and laboratory tests (AST, ALT, bilirubin) for future comparisons.
- Obtain drug history. Taking CNS depressants with benzodiazepine hypnotics can depress respirations. Flurazepam is highly protein-bound. Report if the client is taking other highly protein-bound drugs such as warfarin (Coumadin). Drug displacement can occur with two highly protein-bound drugs, causing an increase in circulating drugs.
- Ascertain the client's problem with sleep disturbance.

Potential Nursing Diagnosis

- Sleep pattern disturbance

Planning

- Client will remain asleep for 6 to 8 h.

Nursing Interventions

- Monitor vital signs. Check for signs of respiratory distress, such as slow, irregular breathing patterns.
- Raise bedside rails of older adults or clients receiving flurazepam for the first time. Confusion may occur, and injury may result.
- Observe the client for side effects of flurazepam, such as hangover (residual sedation), lightheadedness, dizziness, or confusion. The metabolites of flurazepam have a long half-life, so cumulative effects of the drug can occur.

Client Teaching

General
- Instruct the client to use nonpharmacological ways to induce sleep, such as enjoying a warm bath, listening to music, drinking warm fluids such as milk, and avoiding drinks with caffeine after dinner.
- Instruct the client to avoid alcohol and antidepressant, antipsychotic, and narcotic drugs while taking sedative-hypnotics. Severe respiratory distress may occur when these drugs are combined.
- Advise the client to take flurazepam before bedtime. Flurazepam takes effect within 15 to 45 min.
- Suggest that the client urinate before taking flurazepam to prevent sleep disruption.
- Encourage the client to check with the health care provider about OTC sleeping aids. Drowsiness may result from taking these drugs; therefore, caution in driving is advised.

Side Effects
- Instruct the client to report adverse reactions, such as hangover, to the health care provider. Drug selection or dosage may need to be changed if hangover occurs.

Cultural Considerations

- Ask the transcultural person about methods that family members have used to promote sleep.
- Suggest nonpharmacologic alternatives that may be effective for inducing sleep for the person.

Evaluation

- Evaluate the effectiveness of flurazepam in promoting sleep.
- Determine whether side effects such as hangover occur after several days of taking flurazepam. Another hypnotic may be prescribed if side effects remain.

Table 16–3
Sedative-Hypnotics: Benzodiazepines-Nonbenzodiazepines

GENERIC (BRAND)	ROUTE AND DOSAGE	USES AND CONSIDERATIONS
BENZODIAZEPINES		
Alprazolam (Xanax) CSS IV	A: PO: 0.25–0.5 mg h.s.	For alleviating anxiety which may be the cause of sleeplessness. *Pregnancy category:* D; PB: UK; t½: 12–15 h
Estazolam (ProSom) CSS IV	A: PO: 1–2 mg h.s. Elderly: PO: 0.5 mg h.s.	New benzodiazepine hypnotic for treatment of insomnia. Should not be used for longer than 6 weeks. Decreases the frequency of nocturnal awakeness. *Pregnancy category:* X; PB: 93%; t½: 10–24 h
Flurazepam HCl (Dalmane)	See Chart 16–2	For insomnia. Should not be used for longer than 4 weeks. *Pregnancy category:* X; PB: 97%; t½: 2–3 h; metabolites: 45–100 h
Lorazepam (Ativan) CSS IV	*Insomnia:* A: PO: 2–4 mg h.s.	Used as a preoperative sedative and to reduce anxiety. *Pregnancy category:* D; PB: 85%; t½: 12–14 h
Oxazepam (Serax) CSS IV	A: PO: 10–30 mg h.s.	For alleviating anxiety, which may be the cause of sleeplessness. *Pregnancy category:* C; PB: UK; t½: 4–12 h
Quazepam (Doral) CSS IV	A: PO: 7.5–15 mg h.s.	To treat insomnia and to decrease nocturnal awakenings. Avoid alcohol with this drug and all benzodiazepines. *Pregnancy category:* X; PB: >95%; t½: 39 h
Temazepam (Restoril) CSS IV	*Hypnotic:* A: PO: 15–30 mg h.s.	To treat insomnia and to decrease nocturnal awakenings. Also has sedative effects. *Pregnancy category:* X; PB: 96%; t½: 10–20 h
Triazolam (Halcion) CSS IV	*Hypnotic:* A: PO: 0.125–0.5 mg h.s. (0.5 mg with caution) Elderly: PO: 0.125–0.25 mg h.s.	For management of insomnia. Should not be used for longer than 7–10 d at a time to avoid tolerance. Avoid alcohol and smoking when taking triazolam. *Pregnancy category:* X; PB: 89%; t½: 2–4 h
BENZODIAZEPINE ANTAGONIST		
Flumazenil (Romazicon)	A: IV: 0.2 mg over 30 sec; may repeat with 0.3 mg in 30 sec. *Max:* 3 mg total dose	Management of benzodiazepine overdose or reversal of sedative effects of benzodiazepine with general anesthesia. *Pregnancy category:* UK; PB: UK; t½: UK.
NONBENZODIAZEPINES		
Zolpidem tartrate (Ambien)	A: PO: Initially 5 mg; maint: 5–15 mg h.s.; average: 10 mg h.s.; use for 7–10 d	A benzodiazepine-like drug. For treatment of insomnia. *Pregnancy category:* B; PB: 79–92%; t½: 1.5–4 h
PIPERIDINEDIONES		
Glutethimide (Doriden) CSS III	*Hypnotic:* A: PO: 250–500 mg h.s.; repeat in 4 h if necessary	For insomnia. Resembles barbiturates. Caution in use: renal disease and mental depression. Withdraw drug gradually to prevent withdrawal symptoms (rebound insomnia). *Pregnancy category:* C; PB: 50%; t½: 10–20 h

KEY: A: adult; C: child; CSS: Controlled Substance Schedule; h.s.: hour of sleep; PB: protein-binding; PO: by mouth; t½: half-life.

tive anesthetic and is frequently used in dental surgery. In the mid-1800s, ether and chloroform were introduced. Ether, a highly flammable volatile liquid, has a pungent odor and can cause nausea and vomiting after it has been administered. It is seldom used, probably because of the hazard of possible explosion and its noxious odor. Chloroform is toxic to liver cells and is no longer used.

Balanced Anesthesia

Balanced anesthesia, a combination of drugs, is frequently used in general anesthesia. Balanced anesthesia generally includes

1. A hypnotic given the night before
2. Premedication, such as a narcotic analgesic or a benzodiazepine (e.g., midazolam [Versed]) and an anticholinergic (e.g., atropine) to decrease secretions given about 1 h before surgery
3. A short-acting barbiturate, such as thiopental sodium (Pentothal)
4. An inhaled gas, such as nitrous oxide and oxygen
5. A muscle relaxant as needed

Balanced anesthesia minimizes cardiovascular problems, decreases the amount of general anesthetic needed, reduces possible postanesthetic nausea and vomiting, minimizes the disturbance of organ function, and increases recovery from anesthesia. Because the client is not receiving large doses of general anesthetics, there are fewer adverse reactions.

Stages of Anesthesia

General anesthesia proceeds through four stages (Table 16–4), during the third stage of which the surgical procedure is usually performed. If an anesthetic agent is given immediately before the inhalation anesthesia, the third stage can occur without the early stages of anesthesia being observed. However, if the drug is given slowly, all stages of anesthesia are usually observed.

Assessment Before Surgery

The client's response to anesthesia may differ according to variables related to the health status of the individual. These variables include age (young and elderly), a current health disorder (renal or liver), pregnancy, history of heavy smoking, obesity, and frequent use of alcohol and drugs. These problems need to be identified before surgery because the type and amount of the anesthetic might need to be adjusted.

Inhalation Anesthetics

During stage 3 anesthesia, inhalation anesthetics (gas or volatile liquids administered as gas) are used to deliver general anesthesia. Certain gases, such as nitrous oxide and cyclopropane, are absorbed quickly, have a rapid action, and are eliminated rapidly. Cyclopropane was the popular inhalation anesthetic for 30 years (1930 to 1960), but because of its highly flammable state as ether, it is no longer used. In the late 1950s, halothane was introduced as a nonflammable alternative. Other inhalation drugs introduced as anesthetics include methoxyflurane in the 1960s, enflurane in the 1970s, isoflurane in the 1980s, desflurane in 1992, and the newest seroflurane in 1995.

Intravenous Anesthetics

Intravenous anesthetics may be used for general anesthesia or for the induction stage of anesthesia. For outpatient surgery of short duration, an intravenous anesthetic might be the chosen form of anesthesia. Previously, thiopental sodium (Pentothal), an ultrashort-acting barbiturate, was the general anesthetic for short-term surgery. It is still used for the rapid induction stage of anesthesia and in dental procedures. Presently, droperidol (Innovar), etomidate (Amidate), and ketamine hydrochloride (Ketalar) are used intravenously as general anesthetics. Intravenous anesthetics have rapid onsets and short durations of action. Table 16–5 describes the inhalation and intravenous anesthetics used for general anesthesia.

Table 16–4
Stages of Anesthesia

STAGE	NAME	DESCRIPTION
1	Analgesia	Begins with consciousness and ends with loss of consciousness. Speech is difficult; sensations of smell and pain are lost. Dreams and auditory and visual hallucinations may occur. This stage may be referred to as the induction stage.
2	Excitement or delirium	Produces a loss of consciousness due to depression of the cerebral cortex. Confusion, excitement, or delirium occur. Short induction time.
3	Surgical	Surgical procedure is performed during this stage. There are four phases. The surgery is usually performed in phase 2 and upper phase 3. As anesthesia deepens, respirations become more shallow and respiratory rate is increased.
4	Medullary paralysis	Toxic stage of anesthesia. Respirations are lost and circulatory collapse occurs. Ventilatory assistance is necessary.

Table 16–5
Inhalation and Intravenous Anesthetics

DRUG	INDUCTION TIME	CONSIDERATIONS
INHALATION: VOLATILE LIQUIDS		
Ether	Slow	Highly flammable. Has no severe effect on the cardiovascular system or liver.
Halothane (Fluothane)	Rapid	Introduced in the 1950s. Highly potent anesthetic. Rapid recovery. Could decrease blood pressure. Has a bronchodilator effect. Contraindicated in obstetrics.
Methoxyflurane	Slow	Introduced in the 1960s. Used during labor. Drug dose is usually less than other anesthetics and it does not suppress uterine contraction. Could cause hypotension. Contraindicated in renal disorders.
Enflurane (Ethrane)	Rapid	Introduced in 1970s. Similar to halothane. Can depress respiratory function; thus, ventilatory support may be necessary. Not to be used during labor because uterine contractions could be suppressed. Avoid with clients with seizure disorders.
Isoflurane (Forane)	Rapid	Introduced in 1980s. Frequently used in inhalation therapy. Has a smooth and rapid induction of anesthesia and rapid recovery. Could cause hypotension and respiratory depression. Not to be used during labor because it suppresses uterine contraction. Has minimal cardiovascular effect.
Desflurane	Rapid	The newest volatile liquid anesthetic. Similar to isoflurane. Rapid recovery after anesthetic administration has ceased. Could cause hypotension and respiratory depression.
Sevoflurane (Ultane)	Rapid	For induction and maintenance during surgery. It may be given alone or combined with nitrous oxide. Rate of elimination is similar to desflurane.
INHALATION: GAS		
Nitrous Oxide (laughing gas)	Very rapid	Rapid recovery. Has minimal cardiovascular effect. Should be given with oxygen. Low potency.
Cyclopropane	Very rapid	Highly flammable and explosive. Seldom used.
INTRAVENOUS (ULTRA-SHORT BARBITURATES)		
Thiopental Sodium (Pentothal)	Rapid	Has short duration of action. Used for rapid induction of general surgery. Keep client warm; shivering and tremors may occur. Can depress respiratory center and ventilatory assistance might be necessary.
Methohexital sodium (Brevital sodium)	Rapid	Has a short duration. Frequently used for induction and with other drugs as part of balanced anesthesia. An inhalation anesthesia usually follows.
Thiamylal Sodium (Surital)	Rapid	Used for induction of anesthesia and anesthesia for electroshock therapy.
BENZODIAZEPINES		
Diazepam	Moderate to rapid	For induction of anesthesia. No analgesic effect.
Midazolam	Moderate to rapid	For induction of anesthesia and for endoscopic procedures. IV drug can cause conscious sedation. Avoid if a cardiopulmonary disorder is present.

Table continued on following page

Table 16–5 *Continued*
Inhalation and Intravenous Anesthetics

DRUG	INDUCTION TIME	CONSIDERATIONS
OTHERS		
Droperidol and Fentanyl (Innovar)	Moderate to rapid	A neuroleptic analgesic when combined with fentanyl (potent opiate narcotic). Frequently used with a general anesthetic. Can also be used as a preanesthetic drug. Also used for diagnostic procedures. May cause hypotension and respiratory depression.
Etomidate (Amidate)	Rapid	Used for short-term surgery, or as induction of anesthesia, or with a general anesthetic to maintain the anesthetic state.
Ketamine Hydrochloride (Ketalar)	Rapid	Used for short-term surgery or for induction of anesthesia. It increases salivation, blood pressure, and heart rate. May be used for diagnostic procedures. Avoid with history of psychiatric disorders.
Propofol (Diprivan)	Rapid	For induction of anesthesia and may be used with general anesthesia. Short duration of action. May cause hypotension and respiratory depression. Pain can occur at the injection site; thus, may be mixed with a local anesthetic such as lidocaine to decrease pain.

Topical Anesthetics

Use of topical anesthetic agents is limited to mucous membranes, broken or unbroken skin surfaces, and burns. Topical anesthetics come in different forms, such as solution, liquid spray, ointment, creams and gel. The purpose is to decrease the sensitive nerve endings of the affected area.

Local Anesthetics

Local anesthetics block pain at the site where the drug is administered, allowing consciousness to be maintained. Uses for local anesthetics include dental procedures, suturing of skin lacerations, short-term (minor) surgery at a localized area, spinal anesthesia by blocking nerve impulses (nerve block) below the insertion of the anesthetic, and such diagnostic procedures as lumbar puncture and thoracentesis.

Most local anesthetics are divided into two groups, the esters and the amides, according to their basic structures. The amides have a very low incidence of causing an allergic reaction.

The first local anesthetic used was cocaine hydrochloride in the late 1800s. Procaine hydrochloride (Novocain), a synthetic of cocaine, was discovered in the early 1900s. Lidocaine hydrochloride (Xylocaine) was developed in the mid-1950s to replace procaine, except in dental procedures. Lidocaine has a rapid onset and a long duration of action, is more stable in solution, and causes fewer hypersensitivity reactions than procaine. Since the introduction of lidocaine, many local anesthetics have been marketed. Table 16–6 describes the various types of local anesthetics according to short-, moderate-, and long-acting effects.

Spinal Anesthesia

Spinal anesthesia requires a local anesthetic be injected in the subarachnoid space at the third or fourth lumbar space. If the local anesthetic is given too high in the spinal column, the respiratory muscles could be affected, and respiratory distress or failure could result. Headaches might result following spinal anesthesia (a "spinal"), possibly as a result of a decrease in cerebrospinal fluid pressure caused by a leak of fluid at the needle insertion. Encouraging the client to remain flat following surgery with spinal anesthesia and to take increased fluids usually decreases the likelihood of leaking spinal fluid. Hypotension also can result following spinal anesthesia.

Various sites of the spinal column can be used for a **nerve block** with a local anesthetic (Fig. 16–2). A **spinal block** is the penetration of the anesthetic into the subarachnoid membrane, the second layer of the spinal cord. An **epidural block** is the placement of the local anesthetic in the outer covering of the spinal cord, or the dura mater. A **caudal block** is placed near the sacrum. A **saddle block** is given at the lower end of the spinal column to block the perineal area. Blood pressure should be monitored during administration of these types of anesthesia, because a decrease in blood pressure resulting from the drug and

Table 16–6
Local Anesthetics

ANESTHETICS	TYPE	USES AND CONSIDERATIONS
SHORT-ACTING ($\frac{1}{2}$–1 h)		
Chloroprocaine (Nesacaine)	Ester	For infiltration, caudal and epidural anesthesia. Onset of action is 6–12 min.
Procaine HCl (Novocain)	Ester	Introduced in 1905. For nerve block, infiltration, epidural and spinal anesthesias. Useful in dentistry. Caution in use for clients allergic to ester-type anesthetics.
MODERATE-ACTING (1–3 h)		
Lidocaine (Xylocaine)	Amide	Introduced in 1948. For nerve block, infiltration, epidural and spinal anesthesias. Allergic reaction is rare. Used to treat cardiac dysrhythmias (see Chapter 37).
Mepivacaine HCl (Carbocaine HCl; Isocaine; Polocaine)	Amide	For nerve block, infiltration, caudal and epidural anesthesias. May be used in dentistry.
Prilocaine HCl (Citanest)	Amide	For peripheral nerve block, infiltration, caudal and epidural anesthesias. May be used in dentistry.
LONG-ACTING (3–10 h)		
Bupivacaine (Marcaine, Sensorcaine)	Amide	For peripheral nerve block, infiltration, caudal, and epidural anesthesias.
Dibucaine HCl (Nupercainal)	Amide	For topical use (creams and ointment) to affected areas.
Etidocaine (Duranest)	Amide	For peripheral nerve block, infiltration, caudal and epidural anesthesias.
Tetracaine HCl (Pontocaine)	Ester	For spinal anesthesia (high and low saddle block). Also for topical use to affected areas, such as the eye to anesthetize the cornea; nose and throat for bronchoscopy; to the skin for relief of pain, pruritis (itching).

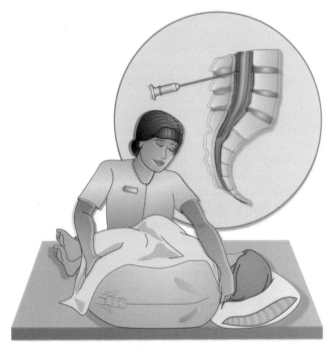

Figure 16–2
Positioning a client for spinal anesthetic.

procedure might occur. A saddle block is frequently used for clients in labor (see Chapter 47).

Nurses play an important role in client assessment before and after general and local anesthesia. Preparing the client for surgery by explaining the preparations and completing the preoperative orders, including premedications, are necessary to enhance the safety and effectiveness of the anesthesia and surgery.

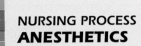

NURSING PROCESS
ANESTHETICS

Assessment

- Obtain baseline vital signs.
- Obtain a drug history, noting drugs that affect the cardiopulmonary systems.

Potential Nursing Diagnosis

- Pain

Planning

- Client will participate in preoperative preparation and understand postoperative care.
- Client's vital signs will remain stable following surgery.

Nursing Interventions

- Monitor the client's postoperative state of sensorium. Report if the client remains non-responsive or confused for a time.
- Check preoperative and postoperative urine output. Report deficit of hourly or 8-hour urine output.
- Monitor vital signs following general and local anesthesia; hypotension and respiratory distress may result.
- Administer an analgesic or a narcotic-analgesic with caution until the client fully recovers from the anesthetic. To prevent adverse reactions, dosage might need to be adjusted if the client is under the influence of the anesthetic.

Client Teaching

- Explain to the client the preoperative preparation and postoperative nursing assessment and interventions.

Evaluation

- Evaluate client's response to the anesthetics. Continue to monitor the client for adverse reactions.

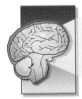

Critical Thinking in Action

J. Z., a 72-year-old woman, has difficulty staying asleep. She asks the nurse whether she should take Nytol or Sominex before bedtime.

1. Before J. Z. takes any sleep aid or hypnotic, what nursing assessments should be made?
2. Describe the nursing plan that should be presented to J. Z. that might help her sleep disturbance.
3. Would J. Z. be a candidate for taking a barbiturate or benzodiazepine? Explain.
4. What follow-up plan should the nurse have related to J. Z.'s sleep problem?

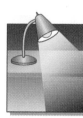

Study Questions

1. What are the advantages of using benzodiazepine hypnotics instead of barbiturates for sleep disorders?

2. Why should renal function be assessed by the nurse? What minimal daily urine output is considered adequate?

3. What is a hangover resulting from a hypnotic? What are the nursing interventions?

4. What is the meaning of withdrawal symptoms from hypnotic use? How can they be prevented? What are the symptoms and the nursing interventions for each?

5. Why should vital signs be closely monitored following general and local anesthesia?

6. What is balanced anesthesia? Give the rationale for its use.

7. What are the nursing interventions, including client teaching, of a client having spinal anesthesia?

Nonnarcotic and Narcotic Analgesics

17

Outline

Objectives

* Define the types of pain: acute, chronic, superficial, visceral, and somatic.
* Differentiate between nonnarcotic and narcotic analgesics. Explain when these drug groups are indicated.
* Identify the serum therapeutic ranges of acetaminophen and aspirin.
* Name the side effects of aspirin and narcotics.
* Explain the methadone treatment program.
* Give the nursing interventions, including client teaching, related to nonnarcotic analgesics and narcotic analgesics.

Terms

abstinence syndrome

analgesics

methadone treatment program

mixed narcotic agonist-antagonist

narcotic

narcotic agonist

narcotic antagonist

nonnarcotic

NSAIDs

orthostatic hypotension

prostaglandins

somatic

visceral

INTRODUCTION

Analgesics, both nonnarcotic and narcotic, are prescribed for the relief of pain; the choice of drug depends on the severity of the pain. Mild to moderate pain of the skeletal muscle and joints frequently is relieved with the use of nonnarcotic analgesics. Moderate to severe pain in the smooth muscles, organs, and bones usually requires a narcotic analgesic.

There are five classifications and types of pain:

- Acute pain, which could be mild, moderate, or severe
- Chronic pain
- Superficial pain
- **Somatic** (bones, skeletal muscles, and joints) pain
- **Visceral,** or deep, pain.

Table 17–1 lists the types of pain and the drug groups that may be effective in relieving each type of pain.

NONNARCOTIC ANALGESICS

Nonnarcotic analgesics—aspirin, acetaminophen, ibuprofen, and naproxen—are not addictive and are less potent than narcotic analgesics. They are used to treat mild to moderate pain and may be purchased over-the-counter (OTC). These drugs are effective for the dull, throbbing pain of headaches, dysmenorrhea (menstrual pain), pain from inflammation, minor abrasions, muscular aches and pain, and mild to moderate arthritis. Most of the analgesics lower an elevated body temperature, thus having an antipyretic effect. Some analgesics, such as aspirin, have antiinflammatory and anticoagulant effects as well.

Salicylates and Nonsteroidal Antiinflammatory Drugs

Aspirin (ASA), a salicylate, is the oldest nonnarcotic analgesic drug still in use. Adolf Bayer marketed the original formulation in 1899, and currently aspirin can be purchased under many names and with added ingredients. Examples are Bufferin, Ecotrin (enteric-coated tablet), Anacin (containing caffeine), and Alka-Seltzer. Aspirin's primary effect is as an analgesic for pain, but it also has an antipyretic effect. Aspirin should not be used and is contraindicated for any elevated temperature in a child younger than 12 years, regardless of the cause because of the danger of Reye's syndrome (neurologic problems associated with viral infection and treated with salicylates). Acetaminophen (Tylenol) is used instead of aspirin in these circumstances.

Aspirin is also classified as an antiinflammatory drug and is discussed with the nonsteroidal antiinflammatory drugs **(NSAIDs)** in depth in Chapter 24. Aspirin and the NSAIDs relieve pain by inhibiting the enzyme, cyclooxygenase, which is needed for the biosynthesis of prostaglandins. There are two enzyme forms of cyclooxygenase, symbolized as COX-1 and

Table 17–1 **Types of Pain**		
TYPE OF PAIN	**DEFINITION**	**DRUG TREATMENT**
Acute	Pain occurs suddenly and responds to treatment	Mild pain: Nonnarcotic (acetaminophen, NSAIDs [aspirin, Motrin, Advil]) Moderate pain: Combination of nonnarcotic and narcotic (codeine and acetaminophen) Severe pain: Narcotic
Chronic	Pain persists for greater than 6 months and is difficult to treat or control	Nonnarcotic drugs are suggested. Narcotics if used should: 1. be by oral route 2. have a long half-life 3. include adjunct therapy 4. not cause respiratory depression
Superficial	Pain from surface areas such as the skin and mucous membrane	Mild pain: Nonnarcotic Moderate pain: Combination of narcotic and nonnarcotic analgesic drug
Visceral (deep pain)	Pain from smooth muscles and organs	Narcotic drugs
Somatic	Pain of the skeletal muscle, ligaments, and joints	Nonnarcotics: NSAIDs (aspirin, Motrin, Advil). Also act as an antiinflammatory drug and muscle relaxant

COX-2. COX-1 protects the stomach lining and regulates blood platelets, thus promoting blood clotting. COX-2 triggers pain and inflammation at the injured site. Two groups of analgesics, salicylates (aspirin) and NSAIDs, inhibit or block both COX-1 and COX-2. By inhibition of COX-1, protection to the stomach lining is markedly decreased, fever and pain are reduced, and blood clotting is decreased. Stomach bleeding and ulcers may occur when COX-1 is blocked; thus, aspirin and NSAID agents can cause gastric discomfort and bleeding. When COX-2 is inhibited, pain is reduced and inflammation is suppressed. Many arthritic clients would benefit from a drug that blocks COX-2 but not COX-1 in order to maintain stomach lining protection (Fig. 17–1).

Pharmaceutical companies are developing new analgesics, especially for arthritic clients, which would block only COX-2 for decreasing pain and inflammation and not block COX-1. Therefore, the stomach lining would still be intact (no gastric bleeding and ulcers), and the pain and inflammation would be decreased. The two new COX-2 inhibitors that were expected to be approved by the Food and Drug Administration (FDA) in 1998–1999 are Celebra (Monsanto) and Vioxx (Merck). Clients at risk for stroke or heart attacks who take an aspirin to prevent blood clotting by decreasing platelet aggregation would not benefit from COX-2 inhibitors. If COX-1 enzyme were not blocked, increased blood clotting would remain even though there would be protection to the stomach lining.

Many researchers believe that COX-2 inhibitors may prevent some types of cancer such as cancer of the colon. Fruits and vegetables block COX-2 enzyme naturally; they protect the colon from malignant growths.

Prostaglandins accumulate at injured tissue sites, causing inflammation and pain. All NSAIDs have an analgesic effect, as well as an antipyretic and antiinflammatory action. Aspirin, ibuprofens (Motrin IB, Nuprin, Advil, Medipren), and naproxen (Aleve) can be purchased as OTC drugs. In addition to its analgesic, antipyretic, and antiinflammatory properties, aspirin decreases platelet aggregation (clotting). Some health care providers may therefore prescribe one 81-mg or 325-mg aspirin tablet every day or one 325-mg tablet every other day as a measure to prevent transient ischemic attacks (TIAs, or "small strokes"), heart attacks, or any thromboembolic episode.

SIDE EFFECTS AND ADVERSE REACTIONS

A common side effect of aspirin and NSAIDs is gastric irritation. These drugs should be taken with food, at mealtime, or with a full glass of fluid to help reduce this problem. If aspirin or an NSAID is taken for dysmenorrhea during the first 2 days of menstruation, excess bleeding might occur (more so with aspirin than with ibuprofen).

Some clients are hypersensitive to aspirin. Tinnitis, vertigo, bronchospasm, and urticaria are some of the symptoms indicating hypersensitivity or overdose of the salicylate product. Certain foods contain salicylates, such as prunes, raisins, paprika, and licorice. Those who have a hypersensitivity to aspirin and salicylate products may be sensitive to other NSAIDs. This hypersensitivity may be related to inhibition of the enzyme cyclooxygenase by the salicylate product.

Acetaminophen

The analgesic acetaminophen (*para*-aminophenol derivative) is a popular nonprescription drug taken by infants, children, adults, and older adults for pain, discomfort, and fever (Fig. 17–2). It constitutes 25% of all OTC drugs sold. Acetaminophen (Tylenol, Panadol, Tempra), first marketed in the mid-1950s, is a safe, effective analgesic and antipyretic drug used for muscular aches and pains and for fever caused by viral infections. It causes little to no gastric distress and does not interfere with platelet aggregation. There is no link between acetaminophen and Reye's syndrome, and it does not increase the potential for

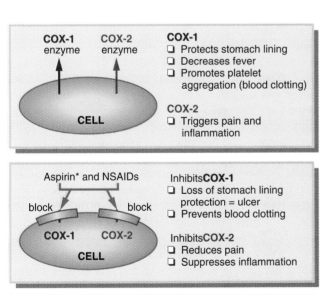

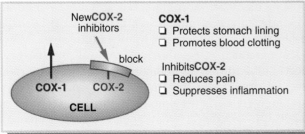

*Aspirin is only one of the NSAIDs

Figure 17–1
Uses of COX-1 and COX-2 inhibitors.

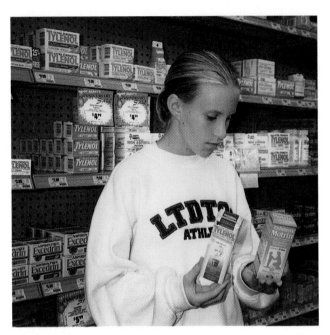

Figure 17–2

This 12-year-old girl injured her foot playing soccer. Which of these analgesics—acetaminophen (Tylenol) or ibuprofen (Motrin)—should she choose to relieve her pain and inflammation?

excessive bleeding if taken for dysmenorrhea, as do aspirin and NSAIDs. Acetaminophen does not have the antiinflammatory properties of aspirin, so it is not the drug of choice for any inflammatory process. See Chart 17–1.

PHARMACOKINETICS

Acetaminophen is well absorbed from the gastrointestinal (GI) tract. Rectal absorption may be erratic as a result of the presence of fecal material, or a decrease in blood flow to the colon. Because of acetaminophen's short half-life, it can be administered every 4 h as needed with a maximum dose of 4 g/day. Greater than 85% of acetaminophen is metabolized to drug metabolites by the liver.

Large doses or overdoses can be toxic to the hepatic cells; therefore, when large doses are administered over a long period, the level of acetaminophen in serum should be monitored. The therapeutic serum range is 5 to 20 μg/mL. Liver enzyme levels (aspartate aminotransferase [AST], alanine aminotransferase [ALT], alkaline phosphatase [ALP]), and serum bilirubin should be monitored.

PHARMACODYNAMICS

Acetaminophen weakly inhibits the prostaglandin synthesis, which decreases pain sensation. It is effective in eliminating mild to moderate pain and headaches, and is useful for its antipyretic effect. It does not possess antiinflammatory action. Its onset of action is rapid and the duration of action is 5 h or less.

Severe adverse reactions may occur with an overdose, so acetaminophen in liquid or chewable form should be out of a child's reach.

SIDE EFFECTS AND ADVERSE REACTIONS

An overdose of acetaminophen can be extremely toxic to the liver cells, causing hepatotoxicity. Death could occur in 1 to 4 days from hepatic necrosis. If a child or adult ingests excessive amounts of acetaminophen tablets or liquid, the poison control center should be contacted immediately, or the child or adult should be taken to the emergency department. Early symptoms of hepatic damage include nausea, vomiting, diarrhea, and abdominal pain.

Table 17–2 lists the commonly used nonnarcotic analgesics, their dosage, uses, and considerations.

NARCOTIC ANALGESICS

Narcotic analgesics, called **narcotic agonists,** are prescribed for moderate and severe pain. In the United States, the Harrison Narcotic Act of 1914 required that all forms of opium must be sold with a prescription and could no longer be a nonprescription drug. The Controlled Substances Act of 1970 classified addicting drugs in five schedule categories according to their potential for drug abuse (see Chapter 7).

In 1803, a German pharmacist isolated morphine from opium. Morphine, a prototype opioid, is obtained from the sap of seed pods of the opium poppy plant. This drug was used as early as 350 B.C. to relieve pain. Codeine is another drug obtained from opium. In the past 40 years, many synthetic and semisynthetic narcotics have been developed, with approximately 20 narcotics marketed for clinical use.

Narcotic analgesics **(narcotics)** act mostly on the central nervous system, whereas nonnarcotic analgesics (analgesics) act on the peripheral nervous system at the pain receptor sites. Narcotics not only suppress pain impulses but can suppress respiration and coughing by acting on the respiratory and cough centers in the medulla of the brain stem. One example of such a narcotic is morphine, which is a potent analgesic that can readily depress respirations. Codeine is not as potent as morphine, but it relieves mild to moderate pain and suppresses cough. It can also be classified as a cough suppressant (antitussive). Many of the narcotics possess antitussive and antidiarrheal effects, in addition to relieving pain. An important effect of opioids on the CNS is their suppression of the cough reflex. Most opioids, with the exception of meperidine (Demerol), have an antitussive (cough suppression) effect. The opioids have two isomers (levo and dextro). The levo-isomers of opioids produce an analgesic effect; however, both levo- and dextro-isomers possess an antitussive response. The

Chart 17–1.   Analgesic: Acetaminophen

ACETAMINOPHEN

Drug Name

Acetaminophen
   (Tylenol, Tempra, Panadol), 🍁 Robigesis,
   Atasol
Para-aminophenol analgesic
Pregnancy Category: B

Dosage

A: PO: 325–650 mg q4–6h PRN; max:
   4000 mg/d; rectal supp: 650 mg q.i.d.
C: 0–3 mo: PO: 40 mg 4–5×/d
   4 mo–1 y: PO: 8 mg 4–5×/d
   1–2 y: PO: 120 mg 4–5×/d
   2–3 y: PO: 160 mg 4–5×/d
   4–5 y: PO: 240 mg 4–5×/d
   6–8 y: PO: 320 mg 4–5×/d
   9–10 y: PO: 400 mg 4–5×/d
   >11 y: PO: 480 mg 4–5×/d
C: 2–5 y: Rectal: 120 mg 4–5×/d
   6–12 y: Rectal: 325 mg 4–5×/d

Contraindications

Severe hepatic or renal disease, alcoholism; hypersensitivity

Drug-Lab-Food Interactions

Increase effect with caffeine, diflunisal
Decrease effect with oral contraceptives, anticholinergics, cholestyramine, charcoal

Pharmacokinetics

Absorption: PO: rapidly absorbed; rectal: erractic
Distribution: PB: 20%–50%; crosses the placenta, in breast milk
Metabolism: t½: 1–3.5 h
Excretion: In urine as metabolites

Pharmacodynamics

PO: Onset: 10–30 min
        Peak: 1–2 h
        Duration: 3–5 h
Rectal: Onset: UK
        Peak: UK
        Duration: 4–6 h

Therapeutic Effects/Uses

To decrease pain and fever.

Mode of Action: Inhibition (weakly) or prostaglandin synthesis, inhibition of hypothalamic heat-regulator center.

Side Effects

Anorexia, nausea, vomiting, rash

Adverse Reactions

Severe hypoglycemia, oliguria, urticaria
Life-threatening: Hemorrhage, hepatotoxicity, hemolytic anemia, leukopenia, thrombocytopenia

Assessment and Planning

Interventions

NURSING PROCESS

Evaluation

KEY: A: adult; C: child; PO: by mouth; PB: protein-binding; t½: half-life; UK: unknown: >: greater than; 🍁: Canadian drug names; ALT: alanine aminotransferase; AST: asparate aminotransferase.

Table 17–2
Analgesics

GENERIC (BRAND)	ROUTE AND DOSAGE	USES AND CONSIDERATIONS
SALICYLATES		
Aspirin (Bayer, Ecotrin, Astrin)	*Analgesic:* A: PO: 325–650 mg, q4h, *max:* 4 g/d C: PO: 40–65 mg/kg/d in 4–6 divided doses; *max:* 3.6 g/d	Effective in relieving headaches, muscle pain, inflammation and pain from arthritis, and as mild anticoagulant. Serum therapeutic range: headache: 5 mg/dL; inflammation: 15–30 mg/dL. Can displace other highly protein-bound drugs. If taken with acetaminophen, GI bleeding could result. Side effects: gastric discomfort, tinnitus, vertigo, deafness (reversible), increased bleeding. Should be taken with foods or at mealtime. It should *not* be taken with alcohol. *Pregnancy category:* D; 55%–90%; $t\frac{1}{2}$: 2–20 h (high doses)
Diflunisal (Dolobid)	A: PO: Initially: 1000 mg; maint: 500 mg q8–12h	Used for mild to moderate pain. Considered to be less toxic than aspirin. *Pregnancy category:* C; PB: 99%, $t\frac{1}{2}$: 8–12 h
PARA-AMINOPHENOL		
Acetaminophen (Tylenol, Panadol, Tempra)	See Chart 17–1	Used for mild to moderate pain. Serum therapeutic range: 5–20 μm/mL. Safe to take if flu symptoms are present. Does *not* cause gastric distress or interfere with platelet aggregation. Overdose or prolonged, high dosage can cause liver toxicity. *Pregnancy category:* B; PB: 20%–50%; $t\frac{1}{2}$: 1–3.5 h
NSAIDs: PROPIONIC ACID		
Ibuprofen (Motrin, Advil, Nuprin, Medipren)	*Pain:* A: PO 200–800 mg q4–6h; *max:* 3200 mg/d *Fever:* A: PO 200–400 mg t.i.d–q.i.d C: 6 mo–12 y: PO: 5–10 mg/kg t.i.d–q.i.d.	For mild to moderate muscle aches and pains. Causes some gastric distress but less than aspirin. Should be taken with food, at mealtime, or with plenty of fluids. *Pregnancy category:* B; PB: 98%; $t\frac{1}{2}$: 2–4 h
MISCELLANEOUS		
Methotrimeprazine HCl (Levoprome)	*Sedative-analgesic:* A: C: >12 y: PO: 6–25 mg/d in divided doses with meals; IM: 10–12 mg q4–6h PRN (deep IM) Elderly: IM: 5–10 mg q4–6h *Postanalgesia:* A and C: >12 y: IM: 2.5–7.5 mg q4–6h PRN	Treatment of moderate to severe pain. May be used before and after surgery for pain and sedation. Has properties of phenothiazines, analgesia, and sedative/hypnotic. *Pregnancy category:* C; PB: UK; $t\frac{1}{2}$: 20 h
Tramadol (Ultram)	A: PO: 50–100 mg q4–6h, PRN, *max:* 400 mg/d Elderly >75 y: *max:* 300 mg/d *Hepatic dysfunction:* 50 mg q12h *Renal disorder:* Cl_{Cr} (CrCl) <30 mL/min: 50–100 mg q12h	Used for moderate to severe pain. Contraindicated in severe alcoholism or with use of narcotics. Nausea, vomiting, dizziness, constipation, headache, and anxiety may occur. *Pregnancy category:* C; PB: UK; $t\frac{1}{2}$: UK

KEY: A: adult; C: child; IM: intramuscular; PB: protein-binding; PO: by mouth; $t\frac{1}{2}$: half-life; UK: unknown; >: more than; PRN: as necessary; GI: gastrointestinal.

NURSING PROCESS
ANALGESIC: ACETAMINOPHEN

Assessment

- Obtain a medical history of liver dysfunction. Overdosing or extremely high doses of acetaminophen can cause hepatotoxicity.
- Ascertain the severity of the pain. Nonnarcotic NSAIDs such as ibuprofen or a narcotic may be necessary for relieving pain.

Potential Nursing Diagnoses

- Risk for injury
- Pain

Planning

- Client's pain will be relieved or controlled.

Nursing Interventions

- Check liver enzyme tests such as ALT, ALP, GGT (gamma-glutamyl transferase), 5-NT (5'nucleotidase), and bilirubin for elevations for clients taking high doses or overdoses of acetaminophen.

Client Teaching

General
- Instruct the client to keep acetaminophen out of children's reach. Acetaminophen for children is available in flavored tablets and liquid. High doses can cause hepatotoxicity. Self-medication of acetaminophen should not be used longer than 10 d for adults and 5 d for children without the health care provider's approval.
- Instruct the parent to call the poison control center immediately if a child has taken a large or unknown amount of acetaminophen. Ipecac should be available in the home.
- Check acetaminophen dosage on package level. Do *not* exceed the recommended dosage.

Side Effects
- Instruct the client to report side effects. Overdosing can cause severe liver damage and death.
- Check the serum acetaminophen level when toxicity is suspected. The normal serum level is 5 to 20 μg/mL; the toxic level is >50 μg/mL, and levels of >200 μg/mL could indicate hepatotoxicity. The antidote for acetaminophen is acetylcysteine (Mucomyst). The dosage is based on the serum acetaminophen level.

Evaluation

- Evaluate the effectiveness of acetaminophen in relieving pain. If pain persists, another analgesic may be needed.
- Determine whether the client is taking the dose as recommended and no side effects are observed or reported.

dextro-isomers do not cause physical dependence, whereas the levo-isomers of opioids produce a physical dependence to the drug.

Other synthetic cough suppressants on the market are discussed in Chapter 35.

Common side effects of most opioids include nausea and vomiting (particularly in ambulatory clients), constipation, moderate decrease of blood pressure, orthostatic hypotension with high doses, respiratory depression with high doses, urinary retention (usually in the elderly), and antitussive effects (except with meperidine).

Opioid Use in Children and Elderly Adults

CHILDREN

It is more difficult to determine pain in children; thus, pain management for the young becomes complex. Many children are fearful of injections, and when they are in severe pain, some children will not verbalize their discomfort. Communication skills are needed by the nurse in determining the child's need for relief of pain. Nurses find that the "ouch scale" presented in Figure 17–3 is helpful in determining the pain level in many children. Also, the parent may be of help in identifying the presence and degree of the child's pain. Crying and whining from the child may be an indicator for need of pain relief, or it may indicate other needs.

A child, like an adult, should be given medication *before* the pain becomes severe. The use of oral liquid medication for pain relief, if appropriate, is generally more acceptable to the child. The nurse, using drawings and pictures related to areas of pain in the body and pain relief with smiling faces, may alleviate the child's fear and help with drug compliance.

ELDERLY ADULTS

Usually, elderly adults require adjustment to drug doses to avoid severe side effects. Many elderly adults take many medications for health problems, thus increasing the possibility of drug interactions and drug side effects. As a person ages, the liver and renal functions decrease, causing the metabolism and excretion of the drug to be slowed. Drug accumulation can occur. In elderly adults, side effects from use of narcotics become more pronounced. Meperidine (Demerol), pentazocine (Talwin), and proproxyphene (Darvon) tend to be more toxic in elderly adults.

Small doses of narcotic analgesic is not always the answer for the elderly. The nurse needs to monitor the elderly adult taking narcotic analgesics closely for adverse reactions.

Morphine

Morphine, an extraction from opium, is a potent narcotic analgesic (Chart 17–2). Morphine is effective against acute pain resulting from acute myocardial infarction (AMI) or cancer and for dyspnea resulting from pulmonary edema. It may be used as a preoperative medication. Although it is effective in relieving severe pain, it can cause respiratory depression, orthostatic hypotension, miosis, urinary retention, constipation resulting from reduced bowel motility, and cough suppression. Table 17–3 lists the desirable and undesirable effects of morphine and other opioids. An antidote for morphine excess or overdose is the narcotic antagonist naxolone (Narcan).

PHARMACOKINETICS

Morphine may be taken orally, although gastrointestinal (GI) absorption can be somewhat erratic. For severe pain, such as with AMI, it is given intravenously. Morphine is 30% protein-bound. Oral morphine undergoes first hepatic pass; thus, the liver metabolizes the oral drug before use. Only a small amount of the morphine crosses the blood–brain barrier to produce an analgesic effect. Morphine crosses the placenta and is present in the mother's breast milk. It has a short half-life and 90% is excreted in the urine.

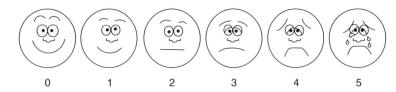

0   1   2   3   4   5

1. Explain to the child that each face is for a person who feels happy because he has no pain (hurt, or whatever word the child uses) or feels sad because he has some or a lot of pain.

2. Point to the appropriate face and state, "This face is . . ."
    0-"very happy because he doesn't hurt at all."
    1-"hurts just a little bit."
    2-"hurts a little more."
    3-"hurts even more."
    4-"hurts a whole lot."
    5-"hurts as much as you can imagine, although you don't have to be crying to feel this bad."

3. Ask the child to choose the face that best describes how he feels. Be specific about which pain (e.g., "shot" or incision) and what time (e.g., now? earlier? before lunch?).

Figure 17–3

A scale for rating the intensity of pain in children. (From Wong, D.: Nursing Care of Infants and Children, 6/E. St. Louis: Mosby, 1999.)

Chart 17–2.   Narcotic: Morphine

MORPHINE SULFATE

Assessment and Planning | **NURSING PROCESS**

Drug Name

Morphine sulfate
   (Duramorph, MS Contin, Roxanol SR),
      ❋ Epimorph, Statex
Narcotic opiate
CSS II
Pregnancy Category: B

Dosage

A: PO: 10–30 mg q4h PRN
SR: 30 mg, q8–12h
IM/SC: 5–15 mg PRN
IV: 4–10 mg q4h PRN: diluted; inject over 5 min
Epidural: 2–10 mg over 24 h
C: IM/SC: 0.1–0.2 mg/kg PRN; max: <15 mg/dose

Contraindications

Asthma with respiratory depression, increased intracranial pressure, shock
Caution: Respiratory, renal, or hepatic diseases; myocardial infarction; elderly; very young

Drug-Lab-Food Interactions

Increase effects of alcohol, sedatives-hypnotics, antipsychotic drugs, muscle relaxants
Lab: Increase AST, ALT

Pharmacokinetics

Absorption: PO: varies; IV: rapid
Distribution: PB: UK; crosses placenta, in breast milk
Metabolism: $t\frac{1}{2}$: 2.5–3 h
Excretion: 90% in urine

Pharmacodynamics

PO: Onset: variable
       Peak: 1–2 h
       Duration: 4–5 h; SR: 8–12 h
SC/IM: Onset: 15–30 min
       Peak: SC: 50–90 min
            IM: 0.5–1 h
       Duration: 3–5 h
IV: Onset: rapid
       Peak: 20 min
       Duration: 3–5 h

Interventions

Therapeutic Effects/Uses

To relieve severe pain.

Mode of Action: Depression of the CNS; depression of pain impulses by binding with the opiate receptor in the CNS.

Side Effects

Anorexia, nausea, vomiting, constipation, drowsiness, dizziness, sedation, confusion, urinary retention, rash, blurred vision, bradycardia, flushing, euphoria, pruritus

Adverse Reactions

Hypotension, urticaria, seizures
Life-threatening: Respiratory depression, increased intracranial pressure

Evaluation

KEY: A: adult; C: child; PO: by mouth; SR: sustained-release; IM: intramuscular; SC: subcutaneous; IV: intravenous; PB: protein-binding; $t\frac{1}{2}$: half-life; UK: unknown; <: less than; PRN: as necessary; ❋: Canadian drug name; ALT: alanine aminotransferase; AST: aspartate aminotransferase.

Table 17–3
Desirable and Undesirable Effects of Morphine and Other Opioids

DESIRABLE EFFECTS	UNDESIRABLE EFFECTS
Suppress pain	Drowsiness
Suppress cough	Decrease mental alertness
Decrease oxygen demand of the myocardium	Decrease respiration
Euphoria	Miosis
Slightly decrease body temperature	Increase intracranial pressure
Increase release of prolactin and antidiuretic hormone (ADH), which may be useful during large volume of fluid loss	Decrease peristalsis
	Decrease gastric acid secretion
	Stimulate chemoreceptor trigger zone (CTZ) that can cause vomiting

PHARMACODYNAMICS

Morphine binds with the opiate receptor in the CNS. Parenterally, the onset of action is rapid, especially intravenously. Onset of action is slower for subcutaneous and intramuscular injections. Duration of action with all types of drug administration is 3 to 5 h except with sustained-release products such as MS Contin, which has a duration of action of 8 to 12 h.

The opioid interacts with receptors in the brain and in the spinal cord to produce an analgesic effect. The patient-controlled analgesia (PCA) is an alternative route for morphine administration for relief of pain. Within predetermined limits, the client controls the narcotic analgesic according to pain need by pushing a button that releases a specific dose of analgesic into the intravenous line. The health care provider titrates the narcotic analgesic dose by regulating the time intervals (every several minutes) at which the drug can be received. There is a lockout mechanism on the PCA machine that prevents the client from constantly pushing the button and causing a drug overdose.

Meperidine

One of the first synthetic narcotics, meperidine (Demerol), became available in the mid-1950s. It is classified as a schedule II drug according to the Controlled Substances Act. Meperidine has a shorter duration of action than morphine, and its potency varies according to the dosage. Meperidine, which can be given orally, intramuscularly, and intravenously, is the most commonly used narcotic for alleviating postoperative pain. It does not have the antitussive property of opium preparations.

During pregnancy, meperidine is preferred to morphine because it does not diminish uterine contractions and causes less neonatal respiratory depression. Meperidine causes less constipation and urinary retention than morphine. Meperidine is not indicated for clients with chronic pain, severe liver dysfunction, severe coronary artery disease (CAD), and those with cardiac dysrhythmias. When elderly adults and clients with advanced cancer receive large doses of meperidine, neurotoxicity (nervousness, tremors, agitation, irritability, seizures) have been reported. Meperidine should not be prescribed for long-term use. Drug data related to meperidine are covered in Chart 17–3.

PHARMACOKINETICS

Meperidine is usually administered intramuscularly for postoperative pain because it is absorbed faster and more completely by this method than in an oral preparation. The oral meperidine dose may need to be increased to achieve the same effect as the intramuscular injection dose. It is considered to have a moderate half-life and can therefore be administered several times a day at specified intervals. Also, its protein-binding is not prolonged. Meperidine is metabolized in the liver to an active metabolite; therefore, the dose needs to be decreased for clients with hepatic or renal insufficiency. It is excreted in the urine, mostly as metabolites.

PHARMACODYNAMICS

Meperidine should not be taken with alcohol or sedative-hypnotics because the combination of these drugs causes an additive CNS depression. A major side effect of meperidine is a decrease in blood pressure, so blood pressure should be monitored while the client is taking meperidine, especially if the client is an older adult.

Table 17–4 lists the narcotics, their dosages, uses, and considerations.

NURSING PROCESS
NARCOTIC ANALGESIC I: MORPHINE SULFATE

Assessment

- Obtain a medical history. Contraindications to use of morphine include severe respiratory disorders, increased intracranial pressure (ICP), and severe renal disease. Morphine may increase ICP and seizures.
- Obtain a drug history. Report if a drug-drug interaction is probable. Morphine increases the effects of alcohol, sedatives or hypnotics, antipsychotic drugs, and muscle relaxants and might cause respiratory depression.
- Assess vital signs and urinary output. Note the depth and rate of respirations. Morphine can cause urinary retention.

Potential Nursing Diagnoses

- Pain related to surgery, injury
- Ineffective breathing patterns related to excess morphine dosage

Planning

- Client will be free of pain, or the intensity of pain will be lessened.

Nursing Interventions

- Administer the narcotic before pain reaches its peak to maximize the effectiveness of the drug.
- Monitor vital signs at frequent intervals to detect respiratory changes. Respirations of <10/min can indicate respiratory distress.
- Monitor the client's urine output; urine output should be at least 600 mL/d.
- Check bowel sounds for decreased peristalsis, a cause of constipation caused by morphine. Dietary change or mild laxative might be needed.
- Check for pupil changes and reaction. Pinpoint pupils can indicate morphine overdose.
- Have naloxone (Narcan) available as an antidote if morphine overdose occurs.
- Check child's dose of morphine before its administration; dose is 0.1 to 0.2 mg/kg/q4h, intramuscularly or subcutaneously; maximum dose 15 mg/dose.

Client Teaching

General
- Instruct the client not to take alcohol or CNS depressants with any narcotic analgesics such as morphine. Respiratory depression can result.
- Suggest nonpharmacological measures to relieve pain as client is recuperating from surgery. If necessary, a nonnarcotic analgesic may be prescribed.

Side Effects
- Alert the client that with continuous use, narcotics such as morphine can become addicting. If addiction occurs, inform the client about methadone treatment programs and other resources in the area.
- Instruct the client to report dizziness or difficulty in breathing while taking morphine. Dizziness could be due to orthostatic hypotension. Advise the client to ambulate with caution or only with assistance.

Evaluation

- Evaluate the effectiveness of morphine in lessening or alleviating the pain.
- Evaluate the stability of vital signs. Report any decrease in blood pressure.

Chart 17–3. Narcotic: Meperidine

MEPERIDINE HCl

Assessment and Planning

Drug Name

Meperidine HCl
(Demerol HCL), ♣ Pethadol, Pethidine HCl
Synthetic narcotic
CSS II
Pregnancy Category: B

Dosage

A: PO/SC/IM/IV: 50–150 mg q3–4h PRN
C: PO/IM/IV: 1 mg/kg q4–6h; max: <100 mg q4h

Contraindications

Alcoholism; head trauma; increased intracranial pressure; severe hepatic, renal, and pulmonary diseases; MAO inhibitors

Drug-Lab-Food Interactions

Increase CNS depression with alcohol, sedative-hypnotics, and other CNS depressants
Lab: Increase serum amylase, AST, ALT, bilirubin

NURSING PROCESS

Interventions

Pharmacokinetics

Absorption: PO: 50% absorbed; IM: well absorbed
Distribution: PB: 60%–70%
Metabolism: $t\frac{1}{2}$: 3–8 h
Excretion: In urine, mostly as metabolites

Pharmacodynamics

PO: Onset: 15 min
Peak: 1 h
Duration: 4 h
IM/SC: Onset: 10–15 min
Peak: 0.5–1 h
Duration: –4 h
IV: Onset: 1–5 min
Peak: 5–10 min
Duration: 2 h

Evaluation

Therapeutic Effects/Uses

To relieve moderate to severe pain.

Mode of Action: Synthetic morphine-like substances, depression of pain impulses by binding to the opiate receptor in the CNS.

Side Effects

Nausea, vomiting, constipation, headache, dizziness, drowsiness, hypotension, sedation, confusion, abdominal cramps, euphoria, blurred vision, rash, tinnitus, tremors

Adverse Reactions

Bradycardia, severe hypotension, convulsion, physical and/or psychologic dependence, seizures
Life-threatening: Respiratory depression, cardiovascular collapse, increased intracranial pressure

KEY: A: adult; C: child; PO: by mouth; SC: subcutaneous; IM: intramuscular; IV: intravenous; <: less than; PRN: as necessary; ♣: Canadian drug names; MAO: monoamine oxidase; CNS: central nervous system.

Table 17–4
Narcotics: Opium and Synthetics

GENERIC (BRAND)	ROUTE AND DOSAGE	USES AND CONSIDERATIONS
Codeine (sulfate, phosphate) CSS II	A: PO/SC/IM: 15–60 mg q4–6h PRN C: PO/SC/IM: 0.5 mg/kg dose q4–6h	Is effective for mild to moderate pain. Can be used with a nonnarcotic (acetaminophen) for pain relief. Has antitussive properties. Can decrease respiration, and cause physical dependence and constipation. *Pregnancy category:* C; PB: 70%, $t_{\frac{1}{2}}$: 2.5 h.
Hydromorphone HCl (Dilaudid) CSS II	A: PO: 1–6 mg q4–6h PRN SC/IM/IV: 1–4 mg q4–6h PRN Rectal: 3 mg q6–8h PRN	For severe pain. Potent narcotic, 5–10 times more potent than morphine. Can decrease respiration, may cause constipation. Effective in controlling pain in terminal cancer. *Pregnancy category:* C; PB: 62%; $t_{\frac{1}{2}}$: 1–3 h
Levorphanol tartrate (Levo-Dromoran) CSS II	A: PO/SC/IV: Initially: 2 mg PO/SC/IV: 2–3 mg q6–8 h PRN	For moderate to severe pain. Has similar side effects as morphine. *Pregnancy category:* B; PB: 50%–60%; $t_{\frac{1}{2}}$: 10–16 h
Meperidine (Demerol)	See Chart 17–3	For moderate pain. Can decrease blood pressure and cause dizziness. In head injury, can increase intracranial pressure. *Pregnancy category:* B; PB: 60%–70%; $t_{\frac{1}{2}}$: 3–8 h
Morphine sulfate	See Chart 17–2	Potent narcotic for severe pain. IV morphine is given to relieve cardiac pain due to a myocardial infarction. Can cause respiratory depression, physical dependence, orthostatic hypotension, and constipation. May cause nausea and vomiting due to increased vestibular sensitivity. *Pregnancy category:* B; PB: UK; $t_{\frac{1}{2}}$: 2.5–3 h
Oxycodone HCl with acetaminophen (Percocet) and oxycodone terephthalate with aspirin (Percodan) CSS II	A: PO: 5 mg q4–6h PRN or 5–10 mg q6h PRN C: 6–12 y: 1.25 mg q6h PRN 12–17 y: 2.5 mg q6h PRN	For moderate to severe pain. Percocet contains acetaminophen; Percodan contains aspirin and can cause gastric irritation, so it should be taken with food or plenty of liquids. *Pregnancy category:* B; PB: UK; $t_{\frac{1}{2}}$: 2–3 h
Propoxyphene HCl (Darvon) Propoxyphene napsylate (Darvon-N) CSS IV	A: PO: HCL: 65 mg q4h PRN; *max:* 390 mg/d A: PO: napsylate: 100 mg q4h PRN; *max:* 600 mg/d	For mild pain. Weak analgesic. Darvon-compound contains aspirin, and Darvocet-N contains acetaminophen. Is not a constipating drug; has little effect on physical dependence. *Pregnancy category:* C; PB: >90%; $t_{\frac{1}{2}}$: 12 h
Alfentanil (Alfenta)	A: IV: 8–40 μg/kg	An opioid analgesic with a rapid onset of action. It may be given for the induction of anesthesia or administered by continuous infusion with nitrous oxide and oxygen. *Pregnancy category:* C; PB: UK; $t_{\frac{1}{2}}$: UK.
Fentanyl (Duragesic, Sublimaze) CSS II	*Preoperative:* A: IM/IV: 50–100 μg q1–2h PRN (0.05–0.1 mg) C: 2–12 y: 1.7–3.3 μg/kg A: Transdermal patch: 72-h effect	Short-acting potent narcotic analgesic. It may be used with short-term surgery. Also, drug is available as a transdermal patch for controlling chronic pain. *Pregnancy category:* C; PB: 80%–89%; $t_{\frac{1}{2}}$: 3.6 h
Sufentanil citrate (Sufenta) CSS II	*Primary anesthetic:* A: IV: 8–30 μg/kg with 100% O_2 and muscle relaxant C: IV: 10–25 μg/kg with 100% O_2 and muscle relaxant *Adjunct to anesthesia:* IV: 1–8 μg/kg	It is a potent synthetic narcotic and is used as part of the balanced anesthesia group. Also may be used as a primary anesthetic. *Pregnancy category:* C; PB: 93%; $t_{\frac{1}{2}}$: 1–3 h
Remifentanil (Ultiva)	A: IV: Infusion rate: 0.05–2 μg/min IV: Postop: 0.025–0.2 μg/min	The newest opioid analgesic. Rapid onset of action; short-acting duration (5 to 10 min). Can cause respiratory depression, hypotension, and bradycardia. *Pregnancy category:* UK; PB: UK; $t_{\frac{1}{2}}$: UK

Table continued on following page

Table 17–4 *Continued*
Narcotics: Opium and Synthetics

GENERIC (BRAND)	ROUTE AND DOSAGE	USES AND CONSIDERATIONS
Methadone (Dolophine)	A: PO: IM: 2.5–10 mg q3–4h PRN Elderly: 2.5 mg q8–12h *Detoxification* A: PO/SC/IM:15–40 mg/d; *max:* 120 mg/d	Similar to morphine but has a longer duration of action. Used in drug abuse programs. Helps in alleviating the craving for opioids. Peak action occurs in 30 min to 1 hour. *Pregnancy category:* C; PB: UK; $t_{\frac{1}{2}}$: 15–25 h
FOR NARCOTIC ADDICTION		
Levomethadyl acetate HCl (Orlaam)	A: IM: Initially: 10–40 mg 3×/wk: maint: 60–90 mg 3×/wk; *max:* 140 mg 3×/wk (M, W, F regimen)	To manage narcotic addiction. *Pregnancy category:* UK; PB: UK; $t_{\frac{1}{2}}$: UK

KEY: A: adult; C: child; CSS: Controlled Substances Schedule; IM: intramuscular; IV: intravenous; PO: by mouth; PRN: as necessary; PB: protein-binding; SC: subcutaneous; $t_{\frac{1}{2}}$: half-life; UK: unknown.

SIDE EFFECTS AND ADVERSE REACTIONS

Many side effects are known to accompany the use of narcotics, and the nurse needs to be vigilant when administering these drugs. Of particular importance are signs of respiratory depression (respiration <10/ min). Other side effects include **orthostatic hypotension** (decrease in blood pressure when rising from sitting or lying position), tachycardia, drowsiness and mental clouding, constipation, and urinary retention. Also, pupillary constriction (a sign of toxicity), tolerance, and psychological and physical dependence may occur with prolonged use.

Increased metabolism of narcotics contributes to tolerance, which causes an increased need for higher doses of the narcotic. If chronic use of the narcotic is discontinued, withdrawal symptoms (called **abstinence syndrome**) usually occur within 24 to 48 h after the last narcotic dose. Abstinence syndrome is due to physical dependence. Irritability, diaphoresis (sweating), restlessness, muscle twitching, and increase in pulse rate and blood pressure are examples of withdrawal symptoms. Withdrawal symptoms from narcotics are most unpleasant but are not as severe or life-threatening as those that accompany withdrawal from sedative-hypnotics—a process that may lead to convulsions.

CONTRAINDICATIONS

Use of narcotic analgesics is contraindicated for clients with head injuries. Narcotics decrease respiration, thus causing an accumulation of carbon dioxide (CO_2). With an increase in CO_2 retention, blood vessels dilate (vasodilation), especially cerebral vessels, which causes increased intracranial pressure.

Narcotic analgesics given to a client with a respiratory disorder only intensify the respiratory distress. In the asthmatic, opiates decrease respiratory drive while simultaneously increasing airway resistance.

Narcotics may cause hypotension and are not indicated for clients in shock or those who have very low blood pressure. If a narcotic is necessary, the dosage needs to be adjusted; otherwise, the hypotensive state may worsen. For the older adult or a person who is debilitated, the narcotic dose usually needs to be decreased.

In treating moderate to severe pain, there are combination drugs of an analgesic and a narcotic analgesic. An example is hydrocodone and ibuprofen (Vicoprofen), which is a combination of an NSAID and an opioid. Another combination for treating mild to moderate pain is acetaminophen and codeine. Using a combination of drugs for pain helps to decrease drug dependency from a possible long-time use of a narcotic agent.

Transdermal opioid analgesics provide a continuous "around the clock" pain control that is helpful to clients who suffer from chronic pain. The transdermal method is not useful for acute or postoperative pain. An example of an opioid analgesic in a transdermal patch is fentanyl (Duragesic). This patch comes in various strengths—25, 50, 75, and 100 μg/h. Fentanyl is also available for intramuscular and intravenous use. Fentanyl is more potent than morphine. For the elderly adult, the use of a lower fentanyl transdermal dose is usually suggested. Caution should be taken for prescribing fentanyl for clients weighing less than 110 pounds. Maximum serum fentanyl levels occur within 24 hours when the patch is first applied.

NURSING PROCESS
NARCOTIC ANALGESIC II: MEPERIDINE (DEMEROL)

Assessment

- Obtain drug history from the client of drugs he or she is currently taking. Report if a drug-drug interaction is probable. CNS depressants enhance the action of meperidine; thus, respiratory depression can occur.
- Obtain baseline vital signs for future comparisons. Meperidine tends to decrease systolic blood pressure.
- Assess type of pain, location, and duration before giving meperidine.

Potential Nursing Diagnosis

- Pain related to surgery or injury

Planning

- Client's pain will be decreased or alleviated. Drug dosing may need to be repeated.

Nursing Interventions

- Administer meperidine before the pain reaches its peak to maximize the effectiveness of the drug.
- Monitor vital signs to compare blood pressure with baseline pressure. Hypotension is a side effect of meperidine. Note whether the client is having any breathing dysfunction.
- Have naloxone (Narcan) available, which can reverse respiratory depression resulting from narcotic overdose.
- Check urine output and bowel sounds. Urinary retention and constipation are side effects of meperidine.
- Check older adults for side effects of meperidine. Confusion may occur, so use of side rails and other precautions should be taken. Dosage may need to be decreased.

Client Teaching

General
- Instruct the client not to take alcohol or CNS depressants with meperidine because of increased depression of the CNS and of respirations.
- Inform the client that drug dependence could occur with continual use of meperidine. If severe pain is still present, another narcotic analgesic or analgesic may be prescribed.

Side Effects
- Instruct the client to report side effects such as dizziness resulting from orthostatic hypotension, headaches, constipation, blurred vision, or decreased urine output. Report findings to the health care provider.

Cultural Considerations
- Respect cultural and religious beliefs concerning refusal of narcotic analgesics.
- Accept Asian and other cultural groups' use of alternative measures in relief of pain.

Evaluation

- Evaluate the effectiveness of the narcotic analgesic in lessening or alleviating the pain. If pain persists after several days, the cause should be determined or the narcotic should be changed.
- Evaluate the stability of vital signs. Abnormal signs, such as decreased blood pressure, should be reported.

NARCOTIC AGONIST-ANTAGONISTS

In the past 20 years, **mixed narcotic agonist-antagonists,** medications in which a narcotic antagonist, such as naloxone (Narcan) is added to a narcotic agonist, were developed in hopes of decreasing narcotic abuse. Pentazocine (Talwin), the first mixed narcotic analgesic, can be given orally (tablet) and by injection (SC, IM, and IV). Pentazocine is classified as a schedule IV drug. Butorphanol tartrate (Stadol), buprenorphine (Buprenex), and nalbuphine hydrochloride (Nubain) are examples of other mixed narcotic agonist-antagonist analgesics. Reports are that pentazocine and butorphanol can cause dependence. These drug agents are considered safe during labor, but safety during early pregnancy has not been established.

Chart 17–4 details the pharmacologic behavior of pentazocine and Table 17–5 lists the various agonist-antagonist narcotics.

Pharmacokinetics

Pentazocine can be administered orally, intramuscularly, or intravenously. It is absorbed well from the GI tract and is rapidly absorbed parenterally. It has a short half-life and is moderately protein-bound. Pentazocine is metabolized in the liver and is excreted in the urine.

Pharmacodynamics

Pentazocine is effective in alleviating moderate pain. Onset of action is rapid, and peak time occurs within 15 min for intravenous administration and 1 to 2 h for oral and intramuscular administrations. Duration of action is the same for all routes of administration, which is approximately 3 h.

NARCOTIC ANTAGONISTS

Narcotic antagonists are antidotes for overdoses of narcotic analgesics. The narcotic antagonists have a higher affinity to the opiate receptor site than the narcotic being taken. The narcotic antagonist blocks the receptor and displaces any narcotic that would be at the receptor, thus inhibiting the narcotic action. Naloxone (Narcan), administered intramuscularly or intravenously, naltrexone hydrochloride (ReVia), administered orally by tablet or liquid, and nalmefene (Revex) are pure narcotic antagonists. Levallorphan tartrate (Lorfan), administered by injection, has some weak agonist properties; however, it has a strong narcotic antagonist effect. These drugs reverse the respiratory and CNS depression caused by the narcotics and are perfect examples of pharmacologic antagonists. Table 17–6 lists the narcotic antagonists.

TREATMENT FOR NARCOTIC-ADDICTED PERSONS

Throughout the country there are many **methadone treatment programs** to help the narcotic-addicted person to withdraw from heroin or similar narcotics without causing withdrawal symptoms. Methadone is a narcotic, but it causes less dependency than the narcotics it is replacing. The half-life of methadone is longer than most narcotics, so it needs to be given only once a day. The dosage is from 15 to 40 mg per day; maximum is 120 mg/d.

There are two types of methadone programs: weaning programs and maintenance programs. In a weaning program, the person receives a dose of methadone for the first 2 days that is approximately the same as the dose of the "street" drug to which she or he is addicted. After 2 days, the methadone dose may be decreased by 5 to 10 mg per day or as indicated until the person is completely weaned from methadone. In a maintenance program, the person is given the same methadone dose every day. The dose may be less than that of the street drug, but it remains the same dose every day.

Chart 17–4. Narcotic: Agonist-Antagonist

PENTAZOCINE LACTATE

Drug Name

Pentazocine lactate
  (Talwin)
Narcotic agonist-antagonist
CSS II
Pregnancy Category: C

Dosage

A: PO: 50–100 mg q3–4h PRN: max: 600 mg/d
IM/IV: 30 mg q3–4h PRN; max: 360 mg/d

Contraindications

Alcoholism; head trauma; severe respiratory, renal, and/or hepatic disease hypersensitivity to naloxone
Caution: Severe heart disease

Drug-Lab-Food Interactions

Increase CNS depression with alcohol, sedative-hypnotics, antipsychotics, muscle relaxants

Pharmacokinetics

Absorption: PO: well absorbed
Distribution: PB: 60%
Metabolism: $t_{\frac{1}{2}}$: 2–3 h
Excretion: In urine (small amount excreted unchanged); in feces (small amount)

Pharmacodynamics

PO: Onset: 15–30 min
    Peak: 1–2 h
    Duration: 2–4 h
IM: Onset: 15–20 min
    Peak: 1 h
    Duration: –4 h
IV: Onset: minutes
    Peak: 15 min
    Duration: 3 h

Therapeutic Effects/Uses

To relieve moderate to severe pain.

Mode of Action: Inhibition of pain impulses transmitted in the CNS by binding with the opiate receptor, pain threshold is increased.

Side Effects

Nausea, vomiting, constipation, dizziness, sedation, headaches, confusion, euphoria, rash, blurred vision, dysuria

Adverse Reactions

Hallucinations, urinary retention, urticaria, tachycardia
Life-threatening: Respiratory depression, shock

Assessment and Planning — **Interventions** — **Evaluation** — **NURSING PROCESS**

KEY: A: adult; C: child; PO: by mouth; IM: intramuscular; IV: intravenous; UK: unknown; PB: protein-binding; $t_{\frac{1}{2}}$: half-life; max: maximum; CSS: Controlled Substances Schedule.

Table 17–5
Narcotics: Agonist-Antagonists

GENERIC (BRAND)	ROUTE AND DOSAGE	USES AND CONSIDERATIONS
Buprenorphine HCl (Buprenex) CSS V	A: IM/IV: Initially: 0.3 mg q6h; may increase to 0.6 mg q6h PRN	For moderate to severe pain associated with surgery, cancer, ureteral calculi, myocardial infarction, and trauma. Avoid alcohol and CNS depressants. *Pregnancy category:* C; PB: 96%; t½: 2–3 h
Butorphanol tartrate (Stadol)	A: IM: 1–4 mg q3–4h PRN IV: 0.5–2 mg q3–4h PRN Nasal spray: 1 mg (1 spray) q3–4h	Management of moderate to severe pain for cancer, renal calculi, labor, musculoskeletal, and burns. *Pregnancy category:* C; PB: >90%; t½: 2.5–4 h
Dezocine (Dalgan)	A: IM: 5–20 mg q3–6h PRN: *max:* 120 mg/d IV: 2.5–10 mg q3–6h PRN	To control moderate to severe pain. *Pregnancy category:* C; PB: UK; t½: 2.2–2.6 h
Nalbuphine HCl (Nubain)	A: SC/IM/IV: 10–20 mg q3–4h PRN; *max:* 160 mg/d	To control moderate to severe pain. May be used as a supplement to surgical anesthesia. Use for clients with respiratory depression. *Pregnancy category:* B; PB: UK; t½: 5 h
Pentazocine lactate (Talwin)	See Chart 17–4	To control moderate to severe pain. May be used as a supplement with surgery. Use with caution if hepatic, renal, or respiratory dysfunction is present. *Pregnancy category:* C; PB: 60%; t½: 2–3 h

KEY: A: adult; C: child; CSS: Controlled Substances Schedule; IM: intramuscular; IV: intravenous; PB: protein-binding; SC: subcutaneous; t½: half-life; UK: unknown; CNS: central nervous system.

Table 17–6
Narcotic Antagonists

GENERIC (BRAND)	ROUTE AND DOSAGE	USES AND CONSIDERATIONS
Nalmefene (Revex)	A: IM/IV: 0.25 µg/kg initially; repeat 0.25 µg/kg at 2- to 5-min intervals PRN	Reverse opioid overdose and respiratory depression. Long half-life. Naloxone has a shorter half-life with shorter withdrawal effects. *Pregnancy category:* UK; PB: UK; t½: UK
Naloxone HCl (Narcan)	Opiate overdose; *Narcotic-induced respiratory distress:* A: IV: 0.4–2 mg; may repeat q2–3min; *max:* 10 mg C: IV: 0.01–0.1 mg/kg; may repeat q2–3min; *max:* 10 mg *Postoperative RD:* A: IV: 0.1–0.2 mg; may repeat q2–3min PRN C: IV/IM: 0.005–0.01 mg/kg; may repeat q2–3min PRN	To treat narcotic overdose. May be given rapidly IV in small amounts with repeats at 2- to 3-min intervals PRN. Approved for use in neonates to reverse respiratory depression induced by maternal opioid use. *Pregnancy category:* B; PB: UK; t½: 1–1.5 h
Naltrexone HCl (Trexan, ReVia)	A: PO: 25–50 mg/d	Treatment of opioid abuse and alcohol abuse. Three to five times more potent than naloxone. Long duration of action. Decreases but does not prevent the craving for opioids. Use after the client is off opioids for 7 or more days. Do not give if client is in opiate withdrawal; it can precipitate a withdrawal reaction. High doses can cause hepatotoxicity. *Pregnancy category:* C; PB: UK; t½: 4–13 h

KEY: A: adult; PO: by mouth; IV: intravenous; PB: protein-binding; UK: unknown; t½: half-life; PRN: as necessary.

NURSING PROCESS
MIXED NARCOTIC ANALGESIC: PENTAZOCINE (TALWIN)

Assessment

- Obtain a drug history from the client. Report if a drug-drug interaction is probable. When taken with pentazocine, CNS depressants can cause respiratory depression.
- Obtain baseline vital signs for future comparison.
- Assess the type of pain, duration, and location before giving the drug.

Potential Nursing Diagnosis

- Pain related to surgery or trauma

Planning

- Client will be free of pain, or the intensity of pain will be lessened.

Nursing Interventions

- Monitor vital signs. Note any changes in respirations.
- Check bowel sounds. Decreased peristalsis may result in constipation. A mild laxative may be necessary.
- Check urine output. Report if urine output is <30 mL/h or <600 mL/d.
- Administer IV pentazocine diluted in sterile water or undiluted. Do not mix with barbiturates.

Client Teaching

General
- Instruct the client not to consume alcohol or CNS depressants while taking pentazocine. Respiratory depression can occur.
- Suggest nonpharmacologic methods for lessening pain, such as changing position or ambulation.

Side Effects
- Instruct the client to report side effects to pentazocine such as dizziness, headaches, constipation, dysuria, rash, or blurred vision. Hallucinations, tachycardia, and respiratory depression are adverse reactions that might occur.

Cultural Considerations

- Accept various cultural groups' use of alternative methods in relief of pain.

Evaluation

- Evaluate the effectiveness of pentazocine in relieving pain. If ineffective, another narcotic analgesic may be ordered.
- Evaluate the stability of the vital signs. Note whether there is a change in respirations, pulse rate, or blood pressure. Report abnormal findings.

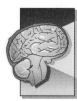

Critical Thinking in Action

R. J., 79 years old, had abdominal surgery for colon resection. The narcotic analgesic meperidine (Demerol), 75 mg, q 3 to 4 h, was prescribed following the surgery. R. J. did not ask for "pain medication" because he thought he might become addicted to the narcotic. The nurse noted that he was restless and grimacing when he moved in bed. He refused to breathe deeply and cough when instructed to do so. The nurse compared his vital signs to his baseline findings. His pulse rate had increased and his systolic blood pressure had decreased by 6 mmHg.

1. Should the nurse give the meperidine? Explain.
2. What would your reaction be to R. J. in regard to his restlessness, grimacing, and refusal to deep breathe and cough?
3. What is the significance of the changes in the vital signs?
4. What classic side effects of narcotic analgesics should the nurse assess?
5. What nonpharmacologic measures might be helpful to R. J. for decreasing his pain?

After the first day, R. J. asked for meperidine every 3 h. On the fifth day after surgery, the health care provider discontinued the meperidine and prescribed acetaminophen with codeine.

6. Why was the narcotic analgesic order changed?
7. R. J. does not want to ambulate. What is an appropriate nursing response?

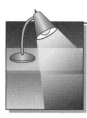

Study Questions

1. A client has had major surgery. What type of analgesic best meets the client's needs? Explain.
2. A client is complaining of flu symptoms and is taking aspirin for fever and to relieve the achiness associated with the flu. What is an appropriate intervention? Why?
3. Aspirin is a mild nonnarcotic analgesic. Name drug categories in which aspirin is used and explain each.
4. What is the most common side effect of nonnarcotics? What nursing measures can be used to decrease or alleviate this side effect?
5. What are the advantages and disadvantages of using acetaminophen?
6. A client is physically dependent on a "street" narcotic. What type of program could be of help in decreasing or eliminating the drug addiction? How would you explain the program to the client?
7. A child took approximately 20 acetaminophen tablets. What should the parent do? What is the serious toxic effect of acetaminophen?
8. What are the serious side effects of narcotic analgesics?
9. When do withdrawal symptoms occur? Describe the symptoms.

Anticonvulsants

18

Outline

Objective

- Describe the two international classifications of seizures and give examples of types of seizures.

- Differentiate between the types of seizures.

- Give the pharmacokinetics, side effects and adverse reactions, therapeutic plasma phenytoin level, contraindications for use, and drug interactions of the hydantoin, phenytoin (Dilantin).

- Describe the uses for hydantoins, long-acting barbiturates, succinimides, oxazolidones, benzodiazepines, carbamazepine, and valproate.

- Explain the nursing interventions, including client teaching, related to the use of hydantoins and other anticonvulsants.

Terms

anoxia

anticonvulsants

atonic seizures

clonic seizures

electroencephalogram (EEG)

hydantoins

hyperplasia

idiopathic

seizures: grand mal, petit mal, psychomotor

status epilepticus

teratogenic

tonic seizures

INTRODUCTION

Epilepsy, a seizure disorder, occurs in approximately 1% of the population. The **seizure** associated with epilepsy results from abnormal electric discharges from the cerebral neurons and is characterized by a loss or disturbance of consciousness and usually by a convulsion (abnormal motor reaction). The **electroencephalogram (EEG),** computerized tomography (CT), and magnetic resonance imaging (MRI) are useful in diagnosing epilepsy. The EEG records abnormal electric discharges of the cerebral cortex. Fifty percent of all epilepsy cases are considered to be primary, or **idiophatic** (of unknown cause), and 50% are considered secondary to trauma, brain anoxia, infection, or cerebrovascular disorders (CVA, or stroke).

Epilepsy is a chronic, usually life-long disorder. Approximately 75% of persons with seizures had their first seizure before 18 years of age. Isolated seizures could result from fever, hypoglycemic reaction, electrolyte imbalance (hyponatremia), acid–base imbalance (acidosis or alkalosis), and alcohol or drug withdrawal. When these conditions are corrected, the seizures cease. Recurrent seizures may result from birth and perinatal injuries, head trauma, congenital malformations, neoplasms (tumors), and idiopathic or unknown causes.

INTERNATIONAL CLASSIFICATION OF SEIZURES

There are various types of and names for seizures, such as grand mal (tonic-clonic), petit mal (absence), and psychomotor. The international classification of seizures (Table 18–1) describes two categories of seizure: generalized and partial seizure. A person may have more than one type of seizure.

Drugs used for epileptic seizures are called **anticonvulsants,** or antiepileptics. Anticonvulsant drugs suppress the abnormal electric impulses from the seizure focus to other cortical areas, thus preventing the seizure but *not* eliminating the cause of the seizure. Anticonvulsants are classified as central nervous system (CNS) depressants.

ANTICONVULSANTS

Before 1850, there were various remedies for control of seizures. In 1857, the use of potassium bromide was the first treatment successful in controlling seizures. Bromide was used for years even though the drug was habit-forming and caused side effects. Phenobarbital was introduced in 1918 and phenytoin (Dilantin) in 1938. Both phenobarbital and phenytoin are still used for seizure disorders. With the use of anticonvulsants, 75% of epileptics are free of seizures.

There are many types of anticonvulsants used in treating epilepsy, including the hydantoins (phenytoin, mephenytoin, ethotoin), long-acting barbiturates (phenobarbital, mephobarbital, primidone), succinimides (ethosuximide), oxazolidones (trimethadione), benzodiazepines (diazepam, clonazepam), carbamazepine, and valproate (valproic acid). Anticonvulsants are not used for all types of seizures; for example, the hydantoin phenytoin, is effective in treating **grand mal** (tonic-clonic) seizures and **psychomotor** seizures but is not effective in treating **petit mal** (absence) seizures. Anticonvulsants are usually taken throughout the person's lifetime. In some cases, the health care provider might discontinue the anticonvulsant if there has not been a seizure in the past 3 to 5 years.

Action of Anticonvulsants

The anticonvulsant drugs work in one of three ways: (1) suppressing sodium influx by the drug binding to the sodium channel when it is inactivated, thus prolonging the channel inactivation and thereby preventing neuron firing; (2) suppressing the calcium influx, thus preventing the electric current generated by the calcium ions to the T calcium channel; and (3) increasing the action of gamma-aminobutyric acid (GABA), which inhibits neurotransmitter throughout the brain; seizure activity is suppressed. The drugs that suppress sodium influx are phenytoin, carbamazepine, valproic acid, and lamotrigue. Valproic acid and ethosuximide are examples of drugs that suppress calcium influx. Examples of drug groups that enhance the action of GABA are barbiturates and benzodiazepines. Gabapentin promotes GABA release. A new anticonvulsant, vigabarin, inhibits the degradation of GABA from enzyme action.

Hydantoins

The first anticonvulsant used to treat seizures was phenytoin, a **hydantoin** discovered in 1938 that is still the most commonly used drug for controlling seizures. It has the least toxic effects, has a small effect on general sedation, and is nonaddicting. However, this drug should not be used during pregnancy because it can have a **teratogenic** effect on the fetus.

Drug dosage for phenytoin as well as for other anticonvulsants varies according to the age of the client. Newborns, persons with liver disease, and the older adult require a lower dosage because of a decrease in metabolism resulting in more available drug. Children and young and middle-aged adults have an increased metabolism rate. The drug dosage is adjusted according to the therapeutic plasma or serum level. Phenytoin has a narrow therapeutic

Table 18–1
International Classification of Seizures

CATEGORY	CHARACTERISTICS
GENERALIZED SEIZURES	Convulsive and nonconvulsive; involve both cerebral hemispheres of the brain.
Tonic-clonic seizure	Also called grand mal seizure; most common form of seizures. In the tonic phase, the skeletal muscles contract or tighten in a spasm, lasting 3 to 5 seconds. In the clonic phase, there is a dysrhythmic muscular contraction, or jerkiness, of the legs and arms, lasting 2 to 4 minutes.
Tonic seizure	Sustained muscle contraction.
Clonic seizure	Dysrhythmic muscle contraction.
Absence seizure	Also called petit mal seizure; brief loss of consciousness, lasting less than 10 seconds; fewer than three spike waves on the electroencephalogram (EEG) printout; usually occurs in children.
Myoclonic seizure	Isolated clonic contraction or jerks lasting 3 to 10 seconds; may be limited to one limb (focal myoclonic) or involve the entire body (massive myoclonic); may be secondary to a neurologic disorder, such as encephalitis or Tay-Sachs disease.
Atonic seizure	Head drop; loss of posture; sudden loss of muscle tone. If the lower limbs are involved, this could cause the client to collapse.
Infantile spasms	Muscle spasm.
PARTIAL SEIZURES	Involve one hemisphere of the brain. There is no loss of consciousness in simple partial seizures, but there is a loss of consciousness in complex partial seizures.
Simple seizure	Occurs in motor, sensory, autonomic, and psychic forms; no loss of consciousness.
Motor	Formally called the jacksonian seizure; involves spontaneous movement that spreads; can develop into a generalized seizure.
Sensory	Visual, auditory, or taste hallucinations.
Autonomic response	Paleness, flushing, sweating, or vomiting.
Psychologic	Personality changes.
Complex seizure	There is a loss of consciousness. Client does not recall behavior immediately before, during, and immediately after the seizure.
Psychomotor	Complex symptoms: automatisms (repetitive behavior such as chewing or swallowing motions), behavioral changes, and motor seizures.
Cognitive	Confusion or memory impairment.
Affective	Bizarre behavior.
Compound	May lead to generalized seizures such as tonic-clonic, tonic.

range of 10 to 20 μg/mL. The benefits of an anticonvulsant become apparent when the serum drug level is within the therapeutic range; if, however, the drug level is below the desired range, the client is not receiving the required drug dosage to prevent seizures. Also, if the drug level is above the desired range, drug toxicity may result. Monitoring the therapeutic serum drug range is of utmost importance to ensure drug effectiveness. Chart 18–1 lists the pharmacologic data associated with phenytoin.

PHARMACOKINETICS

Phenytoin is slowly absorbed from the small intestine. It is a highly protein-bound (85% to 95%) drug; a decrease in serum protein or albumin can increase the free phenytoin serum level. With a small to average drug dose, the half-life of phenytoin is approximately 22 h; however, the range can be from 6 to 45 h. Phenytoin is metabolized to inactive metabolites, and that portion is excreted in the urine.

PHARMACODYNAMICS

The pharmacodynamics of orally administered phenytoin include onset of action within 30 min to 2 h, peak serum concentration in 1.5 to 3 h, steady state of serum concentration in 7 to 10 days, and a duration of action dependent on the half-life. Oral phenytoin is most commonly ordered as a sustained-release capsule. The peak concentration time is 4 to 12 h (sustained-release).

Intravenous infusion of phenytoin should be administered by direct injection into a large vein. The

Chart 18–1.   Anticonvulsants

ANTICONVULSANT

Drug Name

Phenytoin
   (Dilantin)
Anticonvulsant, hydantoin
Pregnancy Category: D

Dosage

A: PO: 100 mg, t.i.d.
IV: LD: 10–15 mg/kg/d; infusion <50
   mg/min; *max:* 300 mg/d
C: 4–8 mg/kg/d in divided doses
Therapeutic serum range: 10–20 μg/mL
Toxic level: 30–50 μg/mL

Contraindications

Hypersensitivity, heart block, psychiatric disorders, pregnancy

Drug-Lab-Food Interactions

Increase effects with cimetidine, isoniazid, chloramphenicol; *decrease* effects with cisplatin, folic acid, and vinblastine
Decrease effects of anticoagulants, oral contraceptives, antihistamines, corticosteroids, theophylline, cyclosporin, quinidine, dopamine, rifampin
Food: Those rich in folic acid

Pharmacokinetics

Absorption: PO: slowly absorbed; IM: erratic rate of absorption
Distribution: PB: 85%–95%
Metabolism: t$\frac{1}{2}$: 6–45 h; average: 22 h
Excretion: In urine, small amount; in bile and feces, moderate amount

Pharmacodynamics

PO: Onset: 0.5–2 h
   Peak: 1.5–3 h
   Duration: 6–12 h
IV: Onset: minutes–1 h
   Peak: 2 h
   Duration: >12 h

Therapeutic Effects/Uses

To prevent grand mal and complex partial seizures.

Mode of Action: Reduces motor cortex activity by altering transport of ions.

Side Effects

Headache, diplopia, confusion, dizziness, sluggishness, decreased coordination, ataxia, slurred speech, rash, anorexia, nausea, vomiting, hypotension (IV), pink-red/brown discoloration of urine

Adverse Reactions

Leukopenia, hepatitis, depression, gingival hyperplasia, gingivitis, nystagmus, hirsutism
Life-threatening: Aplastic anemia, thrombocytopenia, agranulocytosis, Stevens-Johnson syndrome, hypotension, ventricular fibrillation

KEY: A: adult; C: child; PB: protein-binding; t$\frac{1}{2}$: half-life; PO: by mouth; IV: intravenous; >: greater than; <: less than.

drug may be diluted in saline solution; however, dextrose solution should be avoided because of drug precipitation. Continuous intravenous infusion should not be used. Infusion rates of more than 50 mg/min may cause hypotension or cardiac dysrhythmias, especially with elderly and debilitated clients. Local irritation at the injection site may be noted and sloughing may occur. Intramuscular injection of phenytoin is irritating to tissues and may cause damage. For this reason and its erratic absorption rate, intramuscular administration of phenytoin is discouraged.

Mephenytoin is a potent hydantoin and much more toxic than phenytoin. It is used for severe grand mal or psychomotor seizures that do not respond to phenytoin or other anticonvulsant therapy. The newest hydantoin, ethotoin, produces similar responses as phenytoin and has a shorter half-life of 3 to 6 h, therefore, decreasing the chance of cumulative drug effects.

SIDE EFFECTS AND ADVERSE REACTIONS

The severe side effects of hydantoins include gingival hyperplasia, or overgrowth of the gum tissues (reddened gums that bleed easily); neurologic and psychiatric effects, such as slurred speech, confusion, depression, and thrombocytopenia (low platelet count); and leukemia (low white blood cell count). Clients on hydantoins for long periods might have an elevated blood sugar (hyperglycemia), which results from the drug inhibiting the release of insulin. Less severe side effects include nausea, vomiting, constipation, headaches, alopecia, and hirsutism.

DRUG-DRUG INTERACTIONS

Drug-drug interaction is common with hydantoins because they are highly protein-bound. Hydantoins compete with other drugs, such as anticoagulants and aspirin, for plasma protein-binding sites. The hydantoins displace the anticoagulants and aspirin, causing more free drug and increasing their activity. Drugs, such as sulfonamides and cimetidine (Tagamet), can increase the action of hydantoins by inhibiting liver metabolism, which is necessary for drug excretion. Absorption of hydantoins can be decreased by antacids, calcium preparations, and antineoplastic drugs. Antipsychotics can lower the seizure threshold and can increase seizure activity. The client should be closely monitored for seizure occurrence.

Barbiturates

Phenobarbital, a long-acting barbiturate, is still prescribed for treating grand mal seizures and acute episode of **status epilepticus** seizures (rapid succession of epileptic seizures), meningitis, toxic reactions, and eclampsia. Possible teratogenic effects and other side effects related to phenytoin are less pronounced with phenobarbital. Problems associated with phenobarbital include its cause of general sedation and client tolerance to the drug. Discontinuance of phenobarbital should be gradual to avoid recurrence of seizures.

Succinimides

The succinimide drug group is used to treat absence or petit mal seizures, and it may be used in combination with other anticonvulsants to treat such seizures. Ethosuximide is the succinimide of choice; the other formulations, methsuximide and phensuximide, are used mainly for petit mal refractory seizures.

Oxazolidones/Oxazolidinedione

The oxazolidones, trimethadione and paramethadione, are also prescribed to treat petit mal seizures. Trimethadione was the first drug developed for petit mal and for that reason is prescribed more frequently than paramethadione. There are many severe side effects associated with this group of anticonvulsants. Trimethadione may be used in combination with other drugs or singly for treating refractory petit mal seizures.

Benzodiazepines

The three benzodiazepines that have anticonvulsant effects are clonazepam, clorazepate dipotassium, and diazepam. Clonazepam is effective in controlling petit mal (absence) seizures; however, tolerance may occur 6 months after drug therapy starts, and consequently, clonazepam dosage has to be adjusted. Clorazepate dipotassium is frequently administered in adjunctive therapy for treating partial seizures.

Diazepam is primarily prescribed for treating acute status epilepticus and must be administered intravenously to achieve the desired response. The drug has a short-term effect; thus other anticonvulsants, such as phenytoin or phenobarbital, need to be given during or immediately following diazepam.

Iminostilbenes

Carbamazepine, an iminostilbene, is effective in treating refractory seizure disorders that have not responded to other anticonvulsant therapies. It is used to control grand mal and partial seizures and a combination of these seizures.

Carbamazepine is also used for psychiatric disorders, such as bipolar disease, as an analgesic in trigeminal neuralgia, and for treating alcohol withdrawal. However, the drug has not been approved by the Food and Drug Administration (FDA) for treatment of the aforementioned disorders.

Valproate

Valproic acid has been prescribed for petit mal, grand mal, and mixed types of seizures. Care should be taken when giving this drug to very young children and clients with liver disorders because hepatotoxicity is one of the possible adverse reactions. Liver enzymes should be monitored.

Table 18-2 lists the various anticonvulsants, their dosages, uses, and considerations. Table 18-3 lists selected anticonvulsants that are frequently prescribed to treat seizure disorders. Anticonvulsant dosages usually start low and gradually increase over a period of weeks until the serum drug level is within therapeutic range or the seizures stop. Serum anticonvulsant drug levels should be closely monitored to prevent toxicity.

Table 18-2
Anticonvulsants

GENERIC (BRAND)	ROUTE AND DOSAGE	USES AND CONSIDERATIONS
BARBITURATES		
Amobarbital (Amytal) CSS II	*Status epilepticus:* A: IM/IV: 75–500 mg; *max:* IM: 500 mg; IV: 1,000 mg Therapeutic serum range: 1–5 μg/mL	For acute convulsive episode and to control status epilepticus. Infusion rate should not exceed 100 mg/min for adult and 60 mg/m^2/min for children. *Pregnancy category:* D; PB: 50%–60%; t$\frac{1}{2}$: 20–25 h
Mephobarbital (Mebaral) CSS II	A: PO: 400–600 mg/d C: PO: 6–12 mg/kg/d in divided doses or C >5 y: 32–64 mg t.i.d./q.i.d. C <5 y: 16–32 mg t.i.d./q.i.d. Therapeutic serum range: 15–40 μg/mL	For grand mal and petit mal (absence) seizures. May be used in combination with other anticonvulsants. Also used to manage delirium tremens. May cause drowsiness and dizziness. *Pregnancy category:* D; PB: UK; t$\frac{1}{2}$: 34 h
Phenobarbital (Luminal) CSS IV	*Status epilepticus:* Neonate: IV: LD: 15–20 mg/kg single or divided dose A & C: IV: 15–18 mg/kg; *max:* 30 mg/kg *Maintenance:* Neonate: PO/IV: 3–4 mg/kg/d in 1–2 divided doses Infant: 5–6 mg/kg/d in 1–2 divided doses C: PO: 1–5 y; 6–8 mg/kg/d in 1–2 divided doses; 6–12 y: 4–6 mg/kg/d in 1–2 divided doses A: PO: 1–3 mg/kg/d; 100–300 mg/d Therapeutic serum range: 15–40 μg/mL	Long-acting barbiturate. Used for grand mal (tonic-clonic), partial seizures, and to control status epilepticus. May be used in combination with phenytoin. High doses given to the elderly or children may cause confusion, depression, irritability. Long-term use with high doses could cause physical dependence. *Pregnancy category:* D; PB: 20%–40%; t$\frac{1}{2}$: A: 50–140 h; C: 35–75 h
Primidone (Mysoline)	A: PO: 125–250 mg b.i.d./q.i.d. C <8 y: PO: $\frac{1}{2}$ of adult dose Therapeutic serum range: 5–10 μg/mL	Barbiturate-like drug. Used to manage grand mal and psychomotor seizures. Take with food if the drug causes GI distress. *Pregnancy category:* D; PB: 99%; t$\frac{1}{2}$: 10–24 h
BENZODIAZEPINES (ANXIOLYTICS)		
Clonazepam (Klonopin)	A: PO: 0.5–1 mg t.i.d.; gradually increase dose q3d until seizures are controlled C: PO: 0.01–0.03 mg/kg/d; gradually increase Therapeutic serum range: 20–80 ng/mL	For petit mal, myoclonus, and status epilepticus. May be used when petit mal (absence) seizures are refractory to succinimides or valproic acid. *Pregnancy category:* C; PB: 85%; t$\frac{1}{2}$: A: 20–50 h; C: 24–36 h
Clorazepate (Tranxene) CSS IV	A: PO: 7.5 mg t.i.d. C >9 y: PO: 7.5 mg b.i.d.	May be used for partial seizures and as adjunctive therapy for seizures. *Pregnancy category:* D; PB: 97%; t$\frac{1}{2}$: 48 h
Diazepam (Valium)	*Status epilepticus:* A: IV: 5–10 mg, 2–5 mg/min C: IV: 1 mg over 3 min	For status epilepticus (drug of choice). Administer intravenously and repeat q10–15 min up to 30 mg PRN; then q2–4 h PRN. *Pregnancy category:* D; PB: 98%; t$\frac{1}{2}$: 20–50 h

Table continued on following page

Table 18-2 *Continued*
Anticonvulsants

GENERIC (BRAND)	ROUTE AND DOSAGE	USES AND CONSIDERATIONS
Lorazepam (Ativan) CSS IV	*Status epilepticus:* Neonate: IV: 0.05 mg/kg over 2–5 min Infants & C: 0.1 mg/kg over 25 min; *max:* 4 mg/single dose A: IV: 4 mg over 2–5 min; *max:* 8 mg; may repeat in 10–15 min for all ages Therapeutic serum range: 50–240 ng/mL	To control status epilepticus. Infusion rate should not exceed 2 mg/min. *Pregnancy category:* D; PB: 85%; t$\frac{1}{2}$: 10–16 h

HYDANTOINS

Ethotoin (Peganone)	A: PO: 1–3 g/d in divided doses C: PO: 0.5–1 g/d Therapeutic serum range: 15–50 μg/mL	For grand mal, psychomotor seizures. *Pregnancy category:* D; PB: UK; t$\frac{1}{2}$: 3–9 h
Mephenytoin (Mesantoin)	A: PO: Initially: 50–100 mg; 100–200 mg t.i.d. C: PO: Initially: 50–100 mg; 100–400 mg/d in divided doses Therapeutic serum range: 25–40 μg/mL	For grand mal, psychomotor, focal (simple) seizures. Severe adverse reaction may include blood dyscrasias. *Pregnancy category:* C; PB: UK; t$\frac{1}{2}$: 7 h; metabolite: 100–144 h
Phenytoin (Dilantin)	See Chart 18–1.	For tonic-clonic (grand mal) and psychomotor seizures. Phenytoin is not effective for petit mal (absence) seizures. Adverse reactions include gingival hyperplasia and CNS effects. Severe adverse reactions include aplastic anemia, agranulocytosis. *Pregnancy category:* D; PB: 85%–95%; t$\frac{1}{2}$: 22 h

IMINOSTILBENE

Carbamazepine (Tegretol)	A: PO: 200 mg b.i.d.; increasing doses as needed C: PO: 10–20 mg/kg/d in divided doses Therapeutic serum range: 5–12 μg/mL	For grand mal, psychomotor, mixed seizures. Used in treating seizures that do not respond to other anticonvulsants. *Pregnancy category:* C; PB: 75%–90%; t$\frac{1}{2}$: 15–30 h

OXAZOLIDONES

Paramethadione (Paradione)	A: PO: 300–600 mg t.i.d./q.i.d. C: PO: 13 mg/kg t.i.d. or 335 mg/m^2 t.i.d. or 300–900 mg/d in divided doses	For petit mal (absence) seizures. May be used when refractory to other anticonvulsants. *Pregnancy category:* D; PB: UK; t$\frac{1}{2}$: 1–4 h
Trimethadione (Tridione)	Same as paramethadione	For petit mal seizures. May be used when refractory to other anticonvulsants. It has many side effects. After prolonged use, drug should be withdrawn gradually. *Pregnancy category:* D; PB: <10%; t$\frac{1}{2}$: 6–12 d

SUCCINIMIDES

Ethosuximide (Zarontin)	A: PO: 250 mg b.i.d.; increase dose gradually C: 3–6 y: PO: 250 mg/d Therapeutic serum range: 40–100 μg/mL	For petit mal and myoclonic seizurs. Gastric irritation is common; may take with food. *Pregnancy category:* C; PB: UK; t$\frac{1}{2}$: A: 50–60 h, C: 25–30 h

Table continued on following page

Table 18–2 *Continued*
Anticonvulsants

GENERIC (BRAND)	ROUTE AND DOSAGE	USES AND CONSIDERATIONS
Methsuximide (Celontin)	A & C: PO: Initially: 300 mg/d for 1 wk; may increase at intervals	For petit mal (absence) seizures when refractory to other drugs. High occurrence of toxicity; more so than ethosuximide. *Pregnancy category:* C; PB: UK; $t\frac{1}{2}$: 2–4 h
Phensuximide (Milontin)	A: C: PO: 0.5–1 g, b.i.d., t.i.d.	Similar to methsuximide. *Pregnancy category:* C; PB: UK; $t\frac{1}{2}$: 5–12 h
VALPROATE		
Valproic acid (Depakene)	A & C: PO: 15 mg/kg; *max:* 60 mg/kg/d in divided doses Therapeutic serum range: 40–100 μg/mL	For grand mal, petit mal, psychomotor, and myoclonic seizures. Doses may be increased weekly by 5–10 mg/kg/d until seizures are controlled. Avoid during pregnancy. *Pregnancy category:* D; PB: 90%; $t\frac{1}{2}$: 6–16 h
MISCELLANEOUS		
Acetazolamide (Diamox)	Commonly used with other anticonvulsants: A: PO/IM/IV: 375 mg daily; *max:* 250 mg q.i.d. or PO SR: 250–500 mg daily or b.i.d. C: PO: 8–30 mg/kg in divided doses; *max:* 1.5 g/d	For grand mal, petit mal (absence), and focal seizures. Adequate fluid intake should be maintained to prevent kidney stones. *Pregnancy category:* D; PB: 90%; $t\frac{1}{2}$: 2.5–6 h
Gabapentin (Neurontin)	*Adjunctive therapy for partial seizures:* A: PO: 900–1800 mg/d in 3 divided doses; max time between doses: 12 h	Used as adjunctive therapy for partial seizures. It promotes GABA release. To avoid GI upset, give drug with food. If drug is discontinued, dose should be gradually reduced to avoid occurrence of seizures. *Pregnancy category:* C; PB: <3%; $t\frac{1}{2}$: 5–7 h
Felbamate (Felbatol)	A: PO: 1200 mg/d in divided doses C >2 y: PO: 45 mg/kg/d in divided doses	To treat partial and secondary generalized seizures. Also used in adjunctive therapy for the treatment of Lennox-Gastaut syndrome in children. Weak inhibitory effect on GABA-receptor binding. **Contraindications:** client with a blood disorder (reported incidences of aplastic anemia from use of the drug). *Pregnancy category:* C; PB: UK; $t\frac{1}{2}$: UK
Lamotrigine (Lamictal)	A: PO: Initially: 25 mg q.o.d. for 2 weeks; 25 mg/d for 2 weeks. *Maint:* 25–50 mg/d for 1–2 wk; up to 75–150 mg b.i.d.	Used for partial seizures and in adjunctive anticonvulsant therapy. Also to treat tonic-clonic, absence, atypical absence, myoclonic seizures, and for the treatment of Lennox-Gastaut syndrome in infants and children. It blocks the sodium influx. May be given with other anticonvulsants. *Pregnancy category:* C; PB: UK; $t\frac{1}{2}$: 12.5–25 h (half-life is increased when given with other anticonvulsants).
Vigabatrin (Sabril)	A: PO: 1–4 g/d in divided doses C: PO: 50–150 mg/d in divided doses	To treat complex partial seizures and used in adjunctive anticonvulsant therapy. It permits more GABA in the brain. Inhibits the enzyme that destroys GABA. New anticonvulsant drug. *Pregnancy category:* UK; PB: UK; $t\frac{1}{2}$: UK

Table continued on following page

Table 18–2 *Continued*
Anticonvulsants

GENERIC (BRAND)	ROUTE AND DOSAGE	USES AND CONSIDERATIONS
Magnesium sulfate	*Preeclampsia or eclampsia:* A: IV: Initially: 4 g in 250 mL D₅W; then 4 g IM: follow with 4 g IM q4h PRN or Inf: 1–4 g/h *Hypomagnesemic seizures:* A: IV: 1–2 g (19% sol) over 20 min; follow with 1 g IM q4–6h based on blood levels	To control seizures in toxemia of pregnancy due to eclampsia or preeclampsia. *Pregnancy category:* B; PB: UK; t½: UK

KEY: A: adult; C: child; CNS: central nervous system; CSS: Controlled Substances Schedule; GI: gastrointestinal; IM: intramuscular; inf: infusion; IV: intravenous; LD: loading dose; PB: protein-binding; PO: by mouth; t½: half-life; UK: unknown; >: greater than; <: less than; GABA: gamma aminobutyric acid.

Anticonvulsants and Pregnancy

During pregnancy, seizure episodes increase 25% in epileptic women. Hypoxia that may occur during seizures places the epileptic mother and the child (fetus) at risk.

Many of the anticonvulsant drugs have teratogenic properties that increase the risk for malformations;

Table 18–3
Selected Anticonvulsants to Treat Seizure Disorders

SEIZURE DISORDER	DRUG THERAPY
Tonic-clonic (grand mal)	Phenytoin Carbamazepine Valproic acid Lamotrigine Primidone Phenobarbital
Partial (complex-secondarily generalized)	Phenytoin Carbamazepine Primidone Phenobarbital
Absence (petit mal)	Ethosuximide Valproic acid Lamotrigine Clonazepam
Myoclonic, atonic, atypical absence	Valproic acid Lamotrigine Clonazepam
Status epilepticus	Diazepam Lorazepam Phenytoin

however, many epileptic women give birth to normal infants. Phenytoin and carbamazepine have been linked to fetal anomalies such as cardiac defects and cleft lip and palate. Trimethadione should not be given to women of childbearing age because of its strong teratogenic effect. It has been reported that valproic acid is known to cause neural tubal defects (spinal bifida) in 2% to 3% of pregnant women taking the drug. As expected, the highest incidence of birth defects occurs when the woman is taking combinations of anticonvulsant drugs.

Anticonvulsant drugs increase the loss of folate (folic acid) in the pregnant woman; thus, daily folate supplements should be taken. Anticonvulsants tend to act as inhibitors of vitamin K, which contributes to hemorrhaging in infants shortly after birth. Frequently, mothers taking anticonvulsants are given an oral vitamin K supplement during the last week or 10 days of the pregnancy, or vitamin K is administered to the infant soon after birth.

Anticonvulsants and Febrile Seizures

Seizures associated with fever usually occur in children between the ages of 3 months and 5 years old. Epilepsy develops in approximately 2.5% of children who have had one or more febrile seizures. Prophylactic anticonvulsant treatment such as phenobarbital or diazepam may be indicated for high-risk clients. Valproic acid should not be given to children because of the possible hepatotoxic effect.

NURSING PROCESS
ANTICONVULSANTS: PHENYTOIN

Assessment

- Obtain a medication history from the client, including current drugs. Report if a drug-drug interaction is probable.
- Check urinary output to determine if adequate (>600 mL/d).
- Check laboratory values related to renal and liver function. If both blood urea nitrogen (BUN) and creatinine levels are elevated, a renal disorder should be suspected. Elevated serum liver enzymes, such as alkaline phosphatase (ALP), alanine aminotransferase (ALT), μ-glutamyl transferase (GGT), and/or 5'-nucleotidase, indicate a hepatic disorder.

Potential Nursing Diagnoses

- Risk for injury
- Altered oral mucous membranes

Planning

- Client will be free of seizures and will adhere to anticonvulsant therapy.
- Side effects of phenytoin will be minimal and closely monitored.

Nursing Interventions

- Monitor serum drug levels of anticonvulsant to determine overdosing or underdosing of drug; promote compliance to regimen.
- Protect the client from hazards in the environment, such as sharp objects and table corners, during a seizure.
- Determine whether the client is receiving adequate nutrients. Phenytoin may cause anorexia, nausea, and vomiting.
- Women taking oral contraceptives and anticonvulsants may need to use an additional contraceptive method.

Client Teaching

General
- Instruct the client to shake the suspension form well before pouring.
- Instruct the client not to drive or perform other hazardous activity when beginning anticonvulsant therapy. Until the client adapts to drug dosage, drowsiness is apt to occur.
- Alert female clients contemplating pregnancy to consult with the health care provider because phenytoin and valproic acid may have a teratogenic effect.
- During pregnancy, seizures frequently increase because of increased metabolism rates, and serum phenytoin levels should be closely monitored. Most anticonvulsants are classified in the D pregnancy category.
- Inform the client that alcohol and other CNS depressants can cause an added depressive effect on the body and should be avoided.
- Advise the client to obtain an alert ID card and medic alert bracelet or tag that indicates the health problem and the drug taken.
- Instruct the client not to abruptly stop the drug therapy but rather to withdraw the prescribed drug gradually under medical supervision to prevent seizure rebound (reoccurrence of seizures).
- Instruct the client of the need for preventive dental check-ups.
- Instruct the client to take the prescribed anticonvulsant, get laboratory tests as ordered, and to keep follow-up visits with the health care provider.
- Teach the client not to self-medicate with over-the-counter (OTC) drugs without first consulting the health care provider.

Nursing Process continued on following page

- Instruct the diabetic client to monitor serum glucose levels more closely than usual because phenytoin may inhibit insulin release, thus causing an increase in glucose level.
- Inform the client of the existence of national, state, and local associations that provide resources, current information, and support.

Diet
- Instruct the client to take the anticonvulsant at the same time every day with food or milk. If liquid form is used, shake well before ingesting the drug.

Side Effects
- Advise the client that urine may be a harmless pinkish-red or reddish-brown.
- Instruct the client to maintain good oral hygiene; use a soft toothbrush to prevent gum irritation and bleeding.
- Teach the client to report symptoms of sore throat, bruising, and nosebleeds, which may indicate a blood dyscrasia.
- Instruct the client to inform the health care provider of adverse reactions such as gingivitis, nystagmus (involuntary movement of the eyeball), slurred speech, rash, and dizziness.

Cultural Considerations

- There may be a lack of understanding among certain cultural groups, such as Hispanics, Asians, and first-generation Europeans, related to the importance of taking anticonvulsants on a daily basis for life.
- A written drug schedule may be needed for members of cultural groups who do not understand the importance of the prescribed drug regimen.
- Follow-up by a community nurse may be needed to determine the client's compliance to the drug regimen.

Evaluation

- Evaluate the effectiveness of the drug in controlling seizures.
- Continue to monitor phenytoin serum levels to determine whether they are within the desired range. High serum levels of phenytoin are frequently indicators of phenytoin toxicity.

Table 18–4
Selected Anticonvulsants: Pharmacokinetics, Pharmacodynamics, and Therapeutic Ranges

| | PHARMACOKINETICS | | | PHARMACODYNAMICS | | | |
DRUG	Protein-Binding (%)	$t\frac{1}{2}$	Excretion	PO Onset	Peak Time (hr)	Duration of Action (hr)	THERAPEUTIC SERUM RANGE
Phenytoin (Dilantin)	85–95	6–45 h (average: 22 h)	Kidneys, bile, and GI	30 min–2 h	1.5–3	6–12	10–20 µg/mL
Phenobarbital	20–45	2–6 d	50%–75% in urine	30–60 min	8–12	6–24	15–40 µg/mL
Ethosuximide (Zarontin)	UK	60 h (adult) 30 h (child)	25% in urine unchanged	UK	>4	12–60	40–100 µg/mL
Clonazepam (Klonopin)	UK	20–50 h	Kidneys and feces	20–60 min	1–2	6–12	20–80 ng/mL
Carbamazepine (Tegretol)	75	25–65 h	75% in urine, 25% in feces	Varies	4–7	6–12	5–12 µg/mL
Valproic acid (Depakene)	90	6–16 h	kidneys	20–30 min	1–4	24	40–100 µg/mL

KEY: GI: gastrointestinal; UK: unknown; >: greater than.

Anticonvulsants and Status Epilepticus

Status epilepticus, a continuous seizure state, is considered a medical emergency. If treatment is not begun immediately, death could result. The choices of pharmacologic agents are intravenous diazepam or lorazepam followed by intravenous administration of phenytoin. These drugs should be administered slowly to avoid respiratory depression.

SUMMARY

The pharmacologic behavior of specified anticonvulsants is summarized in Table 18–4.

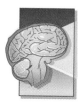

Critical Thinking in Action

S. S., age 26 years, is taking phenytoin (Dilantin) 100 mg, t.i.d. to control grand mal seizures. S. S. and her husband are contemplating starting a family.

1. For the nurse, what action should be taken in regard to client family planning?

S. S. complains of frequent "upset stomach" and "bleeding gums" when brushing her teeth.

2. To decrease GI distress, what can be suggested?
3. To alleviate bleeding gums, what client teaching for S. S. may be included?
4. The nurse checks S. S.'s serum phenytoin level. What are the indications of an abnormal serum level? What appropriate actions should be taken?

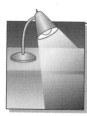

Study Questions

1. What are the differences between generalized and partial seizures according to the international classification of seizures?
2. What are the implications of liver disease or kidney disease for a person taking anticonvulsants? Explain.
3. What is the therapeutic serum range of phenytoin? Is it considered to have a narrow or a wide range? Why should it be closely monitored?
4. What is gingival hyperplasia? Name the drug that might cause this. Give the nursing interventions for decreasing this problem.
5. What are the drug-drug interactions between hydantoins and other drugs? Give examples.
6. What drugs are used to treat status epilepticus? By what route should these drugs be given?
7. What type of seizures are benzodiazepines effective in treating? What is another classification for benzodiazepines?

Antipsychotics, Anxiolytics, and Antidepressants

19

Outline

Objectives

- Differentiate between the three groups of drugs: antipsychotics, anxiolytics, and antidepressants.
- Name the general side effects associated with antipsychotics (typical and atypical), anxiolytics, and antidepressants.
- Give the nursing interventions, including client teaching, for antipsychotics, anxiolytics, and antidepressants.
- Explain the uses of lithium, the serum or plasma therapeutic range, side effects and adverse reactions, and nursing interventions.

Terms

affective disorder
akathisia
antidepressants
antiemetic
antipsychotics
anxiolytics
atypical antipsychotics
bipolar affective disorder
blood dyscrasias
dopamine
dyskinesia

dysphoria
dystonia
electroconvulsive therapy
extrapyramidal reactions
(symptoms/syndrome/EPS)
manic-depressive
monoamine oxidase (MAO)
inhibitors
neuroleptic
orthostatic hypotension
parkinsonism

phenothiazines
psychosis
reactive depression
schizophrenia
second-generation antide-
pressants
selective serotonin reuptake
inhibitors
tardive dyskinesia
tricyclic antidepressants
unipolar depression

INTRODUCTION

Chapters 16 to 18 discuss central nervous system (CNS) depressants: sedative-hypnotics, anesthetics, narcotic and nonnarcotic analgesics, and anticonvulsants. This chapter covers the last group of CNS depressants: antipsychotics, anxiolytics, and antidepressants, which are used to control symptoms of mental disorders. Antipsychotics are also known as neuroleptics and psychotropics. The preferred name for this group is either antipsychotics or neuroleptics. **Neuroleptic** refers to any drug that modifies psychotic behavior, thus exerting an antipsychotic effect. Anxiolytics are also called antianxiety drugs or sedative-hypnotics. Certain anxiolytics are used for sleep disorders and withdrawal symptoms from alcoholic intoxication. This group of drugs is used to treat anxiety. Antidepressants have been called mood elevators. They are used for depressive episodes with accompanying feelings of hopelessness and helplessness. Lithium, effective for bipolar affective disorder (manic-depressive illness), can be classified separately as a mood stabilizer.

ANTIPSYCHOTICS
Psychosis

Psychosis is symptomatic in a variety of mental or psychiatric disorders. Psychosis is usually characterized by more than one symptom, such as difficulty in processing information and coming to a conclusion, delusions, hallucinations, incoherence, catatonia, and aggressive or violent behavior. Schizophrenia, a chronic psychotic disorder, is the major category of psychosis in which many of these symptoms are manifested.

Schizophrenia usually occurs in adolescence or early adulthood. People with this psychotic disorder have been divided into two groups: those with positive symptoms and those with negative symptoms. The positive symptoms may be characterized by exaggeration of normal function (such as agitation), incoherent speech, hallucination, delusion, and paranoia. The negative symptoms are characterized by a decrease or loss in function and motivation. There is a poverty of speech content, poor self-care, and social withdrawal. The negative symptoms tend to be more chronic and persistent. The typical or traditional group of antipsychotics is more helpful for managing positive symptoms than the negative symptoms. Since 1984, a new group of antipsychotics, called atypical, have been found to be more useful in treating both the positive and negative symptoms of schizophrenia.

Antipsychotics comprise the largest group of drugs used to treat mental illness. Specifically, these drugs improve the thought processes and behavior of clients with psychotic symptoms, especially those with **schizophrenia** and other psychotic disorders. They are not used for treating anxiety or depression. The theory is that psychotic symptoms result from an imbalance in the neurotransmitter **dopamine** in the brain. Sometimes these antipsychotics are called dopamine antagonists. Antipsychotics block D_2 dopamine receptors in the brain, thereby reducing the psychotic symptoms. Many of the antipsychotics block the chemoreceptor trigger zone and vomiting (emetic) center in the brain, producing an **antiemetic** effect. By blocking dopamine, **extrapyramidal reactions,** or **symptoms** of parkinsonism, such as tremors, mask-like facies, rigidity, and shuffling gait, may occur. Many clients taking high-potency antipsychotic drugs may require long-term medication for parkinsonian symptoms.

Antipsychotic Agents

Antipsychotics are divided into two major categories: typical (or traditional) and atypical. The typical/traditional antipsychotics, introduced in 1952, are subdivided into phenothiazines and the nonphenothiazines, which include butyrophenones, dibenzoxazepines, dihydroindolones, and thioxanthenes.

The phenothiazines and thioxanthenes block norepinephrine, causing sedative and hypotensive effects early in treatment. The butyrophenones block only the neurotransmitter dopamine.

The second category of antipsychotics is the atypical agents. Clozapine, discovered in the 1960s and made available in Europe in 1971, was the first atypical antipsychotic agent. It was not marketed in the United States until 1990 because of adverse hematologic reactions. Atypical antipsychotics are effective for treating schizophrenia and other psychotic disorders for clients who do not respond to the typical/traditional antipsychotic agents.

MECHANISMS OF ACTION

Antipsychotics block the actions of dopamine and thus may be classified as dopaminergic antagonists. There are five subtypes of dopamine receptors, D_1 through D_5. All antipsychotics block the D_2 (dopaminergic) receptor, which in turn promotes the presence of extrapyramidal symptoms, resulting in pseudoparkinsonism. The atypical antipsychotics have a weak affinity for D_2 receptors, stronger affinity to D_4 receptors, and block the serotinin receptor. These agents cause fewer extrapyramidal symptoms than the typical (phenothiazines) antipsychotic agents, which have a strong affinity to the D_2 receptors.

ADVERSE EFFECTS

Pseudoparkinsonism that resembles symptoms of Parkinson's disease is a major side effect of typical antipsychotic drugs. Symptoms of pseudoparkinsonism or extrapyramidal symptoms (EPS) include stooped posture, mask-like facies, rigidity, tremors at rest, shuffling gait, pill-rolling motion of the hand, and bradykinesia. When clients take high-potency typical antipsychotic drugs, these symptoms are more pronounced. Clients taking low-strength antipsychotics, such as chlorpromazine (Thorazine), are not as likely to have symptoms of pseudoparkinsonism as those taking fluphenazine (Prolixin).

During early treatment with typical antipsychotic agents for schizophrenia and other psychotic disorders, two adverse extrapyramidal reactions that may occur are **acute dystonia** and **akathisia. Tardive dyskinesia** is a later phase of extrapyramidal reaction to antipsychotics. Use of anticholinergic drugs helps to decrease pseudoparkinsonism symptoms and the symptoms of acute dystonia and akathisia. They have little effect for alleviating tardive dyskinesia.

The symptoms of *acute dystonia* usually occur in 5% of clients taking typical antipsychotics within days of treatment. Characteristics of the reaction include muscle spasms of face, tongue, neck, and back; facial grimacing; abnormal or involuntary eye upward movement; and laryngeal spasms that can impair respiration. This condition is treated with anticholinergic/antiparkinsonism drugs, such as benztropine (Cogentin). The benzodiazepine lorazepam may also be prescribed.

Incidence of *akathisia* occurs in approximately 20%

of clients taking a typical antipsychotic drug. With this reaction, the client has trouble standing still. The client is restless, paces the floor, and is in constant motion (e.g., rocks back and forth). This condition is best treated with benzodiazepine (lorazepam) or beta blocker (propranolol).

Tardive dyskinesia is a serious adverse reaction occurring in clients who have taken a typical antipsychotic drug for longer than a year. The dose and duration of the antipsychotic factor into the prevalence for development of tardive dyskinesia. Characteristics of tardive dyskinesia include protrusion and rolling of the tongue, sucking and smacking movements of the lips, chewing motion, and involuntary movement of the body and extremities. In the elderly, these reactions are more frequent and severe. The drug should be stopped. Other benzodiazepines, calcium channel blocker, or beta blockers are helpful in some cases in decreasing this condition. No one agent is effective for all clients. High doses of vitamin E may be helpful and is currently under investigation. Clozapine has been effective for treating tardive dyskinesia. Figure 19–1 shows the characteristics of pseudoparkinsonism, acute dystonia, akathisia, and tardive dyskinesia.

PHENOTHIAZINES

In 1952, chlorpromazine hydrochloride (Thorazine) was the first phenothiazine introduced for treating

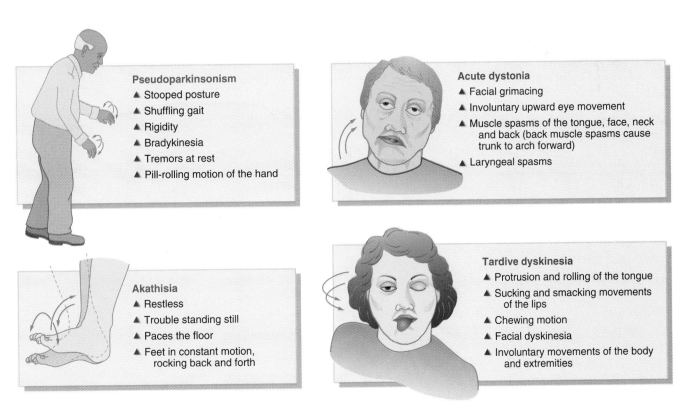

Figure 19–1

Characteristics of pseudoparkinsonism, acute dystonia, akathisia, and tardive dyskinesia.

psychotic behavior in clients in psychiatric hospitals. The phenothiazines are subdivided into three groups: aliphatic, piperazine, and piperidine, which differ mostly in their side effects. Chlorpromazine is in the aliphatic group. The aliphatic phenothiazines produce a strong sedative effect, decrease blood pressure, and may cause moderate extrapyramidal symptoms (EPS) (pseudoparkinsonism).

Triflupromazine (Vesprin) is administered intramuscularly; it has similar incidence of side effects as chlorpromazine (Thorazine). Orthostatic hypotension is not as pronounced with triflupromazine as it is with chlorpromazine.

The piperazine phenothiazines produce a low sedative and a strong antiemetic effect, and they have little effect on the blood pressure. They also cause more extrapyramidal symptoms (EPS) than the other phenothiazines. Examples of piperazine phenothiazines include prochlorperazine (Compazine), acetophenazine (Tindal), fluphenazine (Prolixin), perphenazine (Trilafon), and trifluoperazine (Stelazine).

The piperidine phenothiazines have a strong sedative effect, cause few EPS, have a low to moderate effect on the blood pressure, and have no antiemetic effect. Thioridazine (Mellaril) and mesoridazine (Serentil) are examples of piperidine phenothiazines. Mesoridazine is a metabolite of thioridazine. Table 19–1 summarizes the effects of the phenothiazines.

Most of the antipsychotics can be given orally (tablet or liquid), intramuscularly, or intravenously. For oral use, the liquid form might be preferred because some clients hide tablets to avoid taking them. Also, the absorption rate is faster with the liquid form. The peak serum drug level occurs in 2 to 3 h. The antipsychotics are highly protein-bound (>90%), and the excretion of the drug and its metabolites is very slow. The drug is metabolized by the liver enzymes to phenothiazine metabolites. The metabolites can be detected in the urine several months after the medication has been discontinued. Phenothiazine metabolites may cause a harmless pinkish to red-brown urine color. The *full* therapeutic effects of antipsychotics may not be evident for 3 to 6 weeks following initiation of therapy; however, an observable therapeutic response may be apparent after 7 to 10 days. The dosage for the antiemetic effect is lower than for the antipsychotic effect.

Chart 19–1 compares the aliphatic phenothiazine chlorpromazine hydrochloride (Thorazine) with the piperazine phenothiazine prochlorperazine maleate (Compazine). These two phenothiazines are the early antipsychotics, and although they were marketed for treatment of psychosis, each has a different primary use today. Chlorpromazine is used to manage psychotic disorders, and prochlorperazine is used mainly for treatment of nausea and vomiting.

Pharmacokinetics

The oral absorption of chlorpromazine and prochlorperazine is variable; the liquid form has a faster absorption rate. Both drugs are strongly protein-bound and have a long half-life; the drug may accumulate. Both chlorpromazine and prochlorperazine are metabolized by the liver and are excreted as metabolites in the urine. They cross the placenta readily and are excreted in breast milk. With hepatic dysfunction, the phenothiazine dose may need to be decreased because of lack of drug metabolism in the liver, thus causing an elevation in drug level.

Table 19–1
Effects of Phenothiazines (Varies within class)

GROUP	SEDATION	HYPOTENSION	EPS	ANTIEMETIC
Aliphatic	+++	+++	++	++
Chlorpromazine and triflupromazine				+++
Piperazine	++	+	+++	+++
Piperidine	+++	+++	+	—
Nonphenothiazines				
Haloperidol	+	+	+++	++
Loxapine	++	++	+++	—
Molindone	+/++	+	+++	—
Thiothixene	+	+	+++	—
Atypical antipsychotics				
Risperidone	+	+	+/0	—

KEY: —: no effect; +: mild effect; ++: moderate effect; +++: severe effect; EPS: extrapyramidal symptoms.

Chart 19-1. Antipsychotics (Neuroleptics)

Assessment and Planning

Drug Name

Aliphatic Phenothiazine
Chlorpromazine (C)
   (Thorazine), ♣ chlorpromanyl, Largactil
Pregnancy Category: C

Piperazine Phenothiazine
   Prochlorperazine (P) (Compazine),
♣ Stemetil
Pregnancy Category: C

Dosage

(C) *Psychoses*
A: PO: 10–25 mg, b.i.d.–q.i.d.; increase by 20–50 mg/d q3–4 d
Max: 800 mg/d in 4 divided doses (usual dose is 200 mg/d)
IM/IV: Initially: 25–50 mg; may repeat in 1 h; then q3–4h PRN
Max: 400 mg q4–6h
C: PO: 0.55 mg/kg, q4–6h
C: >6 mo: IM/IV: 0.55 mg/kg or 15 mg/m² q6–8h
Max: 6 mo–5 y: 40 mg/d; 5–12 y: 75 mg/d

(P) *Severe nausea and vomiting, psychoses*
A: PO: 5–10 mg, t.i.d.–q.i.d.
PO: SR: 10–15 mg, q12h

PR: 25 mg b.i.d.–t.i.d.
IM: 5–10 mg q3–4h
IV: 2.5–5 mg q6–8h
Max: all routes: 40 mg/d
C: PO: 2.5 mg t.i.d., 5 mg b.i.d.
Max: 15 mg/d
PR: 2.5 mg t.i.d.–q.i.d.
IM: 0.13 mg/kg q3–4h

Contraindications

(C & P): Coma, bone marrow depression
(C): Hepatic, renal, or coronary disease, cerebral insufficiency, severe hypotension, CNS depression
(P): Severe liver disease, cardiovascular disease, narrow angle glaucoma, seizures

Drug-Lab-Food Interactions

(C & P): Drug: *Increase* CNS depression with alcohol, CNS depressants, narcotics, sedative-hypnotics; tricyclic antidepressants *increase* hypotensive and anticholinergic effects; *decrease* absorption with antacids, antidiarrheals
Lab: *Increase* AST, ALT, and alkaline phosphatase; false pregnancy test, false PKU; *decrease* hemoglobin, hematocrit, leukocytes, platelets

Interventions — **NURSING PROCESS**

Pharmacokinetics

Absorption: (PO)
(C & P): varies
Distribution: PB:
(C): 95%
(P): >90%

Metabolism: t½:
(C): 8–30 h
(P): 23 h
Excretion: (C & P): in urine as metabolites

Pharmacodynamics

(C): PO: Onset: 30–60 min
   Peak: 2–4 h
   Duration: 4–6 h
PO: SR: Onset: 30–60 min
   Peak: 2–4 h
   Duration: 10–12 h
PR: Onset: 1–2 h
   Peak: 3 h
   Duration: 3–4 h
IM: Onset: 15–30 min
   Peak: 30 min
   Duration: 4–8 h

IV: Onset: 5–10 min
   Peak: 10 min
   Duration: UK
(P): PO: Onset: 30–40 min
   Peak: UK
   Duration: 3–4 h
PO: SR: Onset: 30–40 min
   Peak: UK
   Duration: 10–12 h

PR: Onset: 1 h
   Peak: UK
   Duration: 3–4 h
IM: Onset: 10–20 min
   Peak: UK
   Duration: 4–12 h
IV: Onset: 5 min
   Peak: UK
   Duration: UK

Evaluation

Therapeutic Effects/Uses

(C): To treat psychosis (schizophrenia), intractable hiccups, preoperative sedation, behavioral problems in children. Secondary use is to control nausea and vomiting. (P): To treat nausea and vomiting. Secondary use is to treat psychosis.

Mode of Action: Alteration in dopamine effect on CNS, depression of limbic system and cerebral cortex that controls aggression.

Side Effects

(C & P): Sedation, dizziness, headaches, dry mouth and eyes, urinary retention; extrapyramidal symptoms
(P): Blurred vision, restlessness, pink-reddish urine, euphoria or depression

Adverse Reactions

(C & P): Hypotension, tachycardia, leukopenia, tardive dyskinesia, ECG changes
(C): Seizures
Life-threatening: (C & P): Agranulocytosis, circulatory failure, respiratory depression, neuroleptic malignant syndrome

*Extrapyramidal symptoms/reactions include symptoms of pseudoparkinsonism.
KEY: A: adult; C: child; PO: by mouth; PB: protein-binding; t½: half-life; UK: unknown; ECG: electrocardiogram; CNS: central nervous system; SR: sustained-release capsules; IM: intramuscular; IV: intravenous; ♣: Canadian drug names. AST: aspartate aminotransferase; ALT: alanine aminotransferase; PKU: phenylketonuria.

Pharmacodynamics

Chlorpromazine is primarily prescribed for psychotic disorders and prochlorperazine for nausea and vomiting. Prochlorperazine has anticholinergic properties and should be cautiously administered to clients with glaucoma, especially narrow-angle glaucoma. Because hypotension is a side effect of these phenothiazines, any antihypertensives being administered at the same time can cause an additive hypotensive effect. Narcotics and sedative-hypnotics administered simultaneously with these phenothiazines can cause an additive CNS depression. Antacids decrease the absorption rate of both drugs and all phenothiazines. Give 1 h before or 2 h after giving a phenothiazine.

The onset of action of oral, intramuscular, and intravenous administration of chlorpromazine and prochlorperazine are similar. The sustained release preparations prolong the duration time of both drugs. These drugs should be administered rectally only if the oral method is not tolerated. Erratic absorption of the suppository frequently occurs. Intramuscularly, the drugs should be administered deeply in the dorsogluteal muscle. They are extremely irritating to the subcutaneous tissue.

NONPHENOTHIAZINES

The many groups of nonphenothiazine include butyrophenone, dibenzoxazepines, dihydroindolone, and thioxanthene.

Frequently prescribed nonphenothiazine is the butyrophenone haloperidol (Haldol), whose pharmacologic behavior is similar to that of the phenothiazines. Haloperidol is a potent antipsychotic drug in which the equivalent prescribed dose is smaller than drugs of lower potency; e.g., chlorpromazine. Drug dose for haloperidol is 0.5 to 5 mg, whereas the drug dose for chlorpromazine is 10 to 25 mg. Chart 19–2 provides the drug data related to haloperidol.

Pharmacokinetics

Haloperidol is absorbed well through the gastrointestinal (GI) mucosa. It has a long half-life and is highly protein-bound, so the drug may accumulate. Most of haloperidol is excreted in the urine.

Pharmacodynamics

Haloperidol alters the effects of dopamine by blocking the dopamine receptors; thus sedation and EPS may occur. The drug is used to control psychoses and decrease signs of agitation in adults as well as children. Dosages need to be decreased in the older adult due to decreased liver function and potential side effects. It may be prescribed for children with hyperactive behavior. Haloperidol has anticholinergic activity; thus, care should be taken in administering it to clients with a history of glaucoma.

Haloperidol has similar onset of action, peak time

of concentration, and duration of action to those of the phenothiazines. The nurse needs to observe the client for EPS. Skin protection is necessary when taking the drug for a period of time because of the possible side effect of photosensitivity.

From the dibenzoxazepine group, loxapine (Loxitane) is a moderate potent agent. It has moderate sedative and orthostatic hypotensive effects and a strong EPS effect. The typical antipsychotic, molindone hydrochloric acid (Moban) from the dihydroindolone group, is a moderate potent agent. It has low sedative and orthostatic hypotensive effects and a strong EPS effect.

In the last nonphenothiazine group, known as thioxanthene, is thiothixene (Navane), a highly potent typical antipsychotic drug. It has side effects similar to those of molindone with low sedative and orthostatic hypotensive effects and a strong EPS effect.

Side Effects and Adverse Reactions

There are several common side effects associated with antipsychotics. The most common side effect for all antipsychotics is drowsiness. Many of the antipsychotics have some anticholinergic effects, such as dry mouth, increased heart rate, urinary retention, and constipation. Blood pressure decreases with the use of antipsychotics; aliphatic and piperidine types cause a greater decrease in blood pressure than the others. EPS are most prevalent with the phenothiazines, butyrophenones, and thioxanthenes and include pseudoparkinsonism, akathisia, dystonia, and tardive dyskinesia. In 20% of clients taking antipsychotics for long-term therapy tardive dyskinesia may develop. Most antiparkinsonism anticholinergics are not always effective for treating tardive dyskinesia. These EPS can begin 5 to 30 days after initiation of antipsychotic therapy. Anticholinergic drugs may be given to control EPS. High dosing or long-term use of antipsychotics can cause **blood dyscrasias** (blood cell disorders), e.g., agranulocytosis. White blood cell (WBC) count should be closely monitored and reported if there is an extreme decrease in the WBCs.

Dermatologic side effects seen early in drug therapy are pruritus and marked photosensitivity. Use of sunscreen, hats, protective clothing, and staying out of the sun are suggested.

Drug Interactions

Because phenothiazine lowers the seizure threshold, dosage adjustment of an anticonvulsant may be necessary. If either aliphatic phenothiazine or the thioxanthene group is administered, a higher dose of anticonvulsant might be necessary to prevent seizures.

Antipsychotics interact with alcohol, hypnotics, sedatives, narcotics, and benzodiazepines to potentiate the sedative effects of antipsychotics. Atropine counteracts the EPS and potentiates antipsychotic ef-

Chart 19–2. Antipsychotic: Nonphenothiazine

HALOPERIDOL

Assessment and Planning

Drug Name

Haloperidol
   (Haldol), 🍁 Peridol
Antipsychotic, neuroleptic
   (nonphenothiazine)
Pregnancy Category: C

Dosage

A: PO: 0.5–5 mg b.i.d.–t.i.d.
IM: Decanoate: 50–100 mg q4wk
IM: 2–5 mg q4h PRN
C: PO: 0.15 mg/kg/d in divided doses (not for child <3 y)
Elderly: Decreased doses than for younger adult; PO: 0.5–2 mg b.i.d.–t.i.d.

Contraindications

Narrow-angle glaucoma; severe hepatic, renal, and cardiovascular diseases; bone marrow depression; Parkinson's disease; blood dyscrasias; CNS depression; subcortical brain damage

Drug-Lab-Food Interactions

Drug: *Increase* sedation with alcohol, CNS depressants; *increase* toxicity with anticholinergics, CNS depressants, lithium; *decrease* effects with phenobarbital, carbamazepine; *decrease* effects with caffeine

Interventions / NURSING PROCESS

Pharmacokinetics

Absorption: PO: 60% absorbed
Distribution: PB: 80%–90%
Metabolism: $t\frac{1}{2}$: 15–35 h
Excretion: In urine and feces

Pharmacodynamics

PO:	Onset: erratic
	Peak: 2–6 h
	Duration: 24–72 h
IM:	Onset: 15–30 min
	Peak: 30–45 min
	Duration: 4–8 h
IM: Decanoate:	Onset: UK
	Peak: 6–7 d
	Duration: 3–4 wk

Evaluation

Therapeutic Effects/Uses

To treat acute and chronic psychoses, for children with severe behavior problems who are combative, to suppress narcotic withdrawal symptoms, to treat schizophrenia resistant to other drugs, to treat Tourette's syndrome, to treat symptoms of dementia in elderly.

Mode of Action: Alteration of the effect of dopamine on CNS; mechanism for antipsychotic effects are unknown.

Side Effects

Sedation, extrapyramidal symptoms, orthostatic hypotension, headache, photosensitivity, dry mouth and eyes, blurred vision

Adverse Reactions

Tachycardia, seizures, urinary retention, tardive dyskinesia
Life-threatening: Laryngospasm, respiratory depression, cardiac dysrhythmias, neuromalignant syndrome (NMS)

KEY: A: adult; C: child; PO: by mouth; IM: intramuscular; PB: protein-binding; $t\frac{1}{2}$: half-life; CNS: central nervous system; UK: unknown; <: less than; 🍁: Canadian drug names.

fects. Use of antihypertensives can cause an additive hypotensive effect.

Antipsychotics should *not* be given with other antipsychotic or antidepressant drugs except to control psychotic behavior for selected individuals who are refractory to drug therapy. Usually if one antipsychotic drug is ineffective, then another one is prescribed. Individuals should *not* take alcohol or other CNS depressants (such as narcotic analgesics and barbiturates) with antipsychotics because additive depression is likely to occur. Geriatric clients may require a decreased dosage to reduce side effects.

Table 19-2

Phenothiazines and Nonphenothiazines

GENERIC (BRAND)	DRUG POTENCY	ROUTE AND DOSAGE	USES AND CONSIDERATIONS
PHENOTHIAZINES			
Aliphatics			
Chlorpromazine HCl (Thorazine)	Low	See Chart 19–1	Effective for acute psychosis; for decreasing agitation in the elderly without causing confusion; and for intractable hiccups. It has a strong sedative effect, and can cause orthostatic hypotension. *Pregnancy category:* C; PB: 95%; $t\frac{1}{2}$: 8–30 h
Promazine HCl (Sparine)	Uk	A: PO: 10–200 mg q4–6h IM: 50–150 mg; may repeat × 1 C >12 y: PO: 10–25 mg q4–6h	For psychotic disorders. Not effective for an acutely agitated psychotic client. Can cause orthostatic hypotension. *Pregnancy category:* C; PB: ≥90%; $t\frac{1}{2}$: ≥24 h
*Triflupromazine (Vesprin)	Moderate	A: PO: 10–50 mg b.i.d.–t.i.d. IM: 60–150 mg/d C >2 y: PO: 0.5–2 mg/kg/d in 3 divided doses	Similar to promazine HCl. Not to be used for client with psychosis and having depression. *Pregnancy category:* C; PB: ≥90%; $t\frac{1}{2}$: ≥24 h
Piperazines			
Fluphenazine HCl (Prolixin)	High	A: PO: 1–5 mg t.i.d.–q.i.d. Elderly: 1–2.5 mg/d; also long-acting weekly/biweekly dosages Therapeutic range: 5–20 ng/mL	For moderate to severe psychosis. Extrapyramidal symptoms (EPS) are likely. *Pregnancy category:* C; PB: ≥90%; $t\frac{1}{2}$: 5–15 h
Perphenazine (Trilafon)	Moderate	A: PO: 4–16 mg b.i.d., t.i.d., or q.i.d.	For psychotic disorders; control severe nausea and vomiting; and treat intractable hiccups. Used also prior to chemotherapy to prevent nausea. *Pregnancy category:* C; PB: ≥90%; $t\frac{1}{2}$: 9.5 h
Prochlorperazine maleate (Compazine)	Low	A: PO: 5–10 mg t.i.d.–q.i.d.; *max:* 40 mg/d (can be higher for psychotic behavior)	For mild psychotic behavior. Effective antiemetic, given either orally, deep IM, or rectally. Causes less sedation and hypotension. Marked EPS. *Pregnancy category:* C; PB: ≥90%; $t\frac{1}{2}$: 23 h
Acetophenazine maleate (Tindal)	Moderate	A: PO: 20 mg, b.i.d.–q.i.d.; *max:* 120 mg/d	For psychosis. Higher doses for schizophrenia. *Pregnancy category:* C; PB: ≥90%; $t\frac{1}{2}$: UK
*Trifluoperazine HCl (Stelazine)	High	A: PO: 1–5 mg b.i.d.; *max:* 40 mg/d C: PO: 1 mg q.i.d.–b.i.d.	Management of psychotic disorders. To control excessive tension and anxiety. Can cause EPS. Dilute liquid in 120 mL of water, milk, or juice. *Pregnancy category:* C; PB: ≥90%; $t\frac{1}{2}$: ≥24 h
Piperidines			
Mesoridazine besylate (Serentil)	Low-Moderate	A: PO: 50 mg t.i.d.; gradually increase Optimal response: 100–400 mg/d Elderly: $\frac{1}{3}$–$\frac{1}{2}$ adult dose	For psychosis and schizophrenia, severe anxiety, chronic brain syndrome (smaller doses). Few EPS. Can cause hypotensive effects. *Pregnancy category:* C; PB: 92%–99%; $t\frac{1}{2}$: 24–48 h
*Thioridazine HCl (Mellaril)	Low	A: PO: 50–100 mg t.i.d.; *max:* 800 mg/d Elderly: $\frac{1}{3}$–$\frac{1}{2}$ adult dose	For psychosis. Higher doses for severe psychosis. Lower doses (10–50 mg t.i.d.) for marked depression, alcohol withdrawal, intractable pain. Few EPS. Little antiemetic effect. Can cause orthostatic hypotension. *Pregnancy category:* C; PB: ≥90%; $t\frac{1}{2}$: 24–34 h

Table continued on following page

Table 19–2 *Continued*
Phenothiazines and Nonphenothiazines

GENERIC (BRAND)	DRUG POTENCY	ROUTE AND DOSAGE	USES AND CONSIDERATIONS
NONPHENOTHIAZINES			
Butyrophenone			
Droperidol (Inapsine)	Moderate-High	A: IM/IV: 2.5–10 mg 30–60 min before anesthesia C: IM/IV: 0.088–0.165 mg/kg	Primarily prescribed as a preoperative drug administered alone or in conjunction with a narcotic. Has antiemetic properties. May decrease blood pressure and increase heart rate. *Pregnancy category:* C; PB: UK; $t_{\frac{1}{2}}$: 2 h
Haloperidol (Haldol)	High	See Chart 19–2	For acute psychosis. Also for children with severe behavior problems who are combative. Used to suppress narcotic withdrawal symptoms and for schizophrenia that is resistive to drugs. Likely to cause EPS. Has minimal sedative, hypotensive, and anticholinergic effects. *Pregnancy category:* C; PB: 80%–90%; $t_{\frac{1}{2}}$: 15–35 h
Dibenzoxazepine			
Loxapine (Loxitane)	Moderate	A: PO: Initially: 10 mg b.i.d.; then may increase to 50–100 mg/d Elderly: $\frac{1}{3}$–$\frac{1}{2}$ regular adult dose	For acute psychosis and schizophrenia. Likely to cause EPS. Overdose can cause cardiac toxicity or neurotoxicity. *Pregnancy category:* C; PB: 95%; $t_{\frac{1}{2}}$: 5 h
Dihydroindolone			
Molindone HCl (Moban)	Moderate	A: PO: Initial: 50–75 mg in 3–4 divided doses A: PO: 5–50 mg t.i.d.–q.i.d. Elderly: $\frac{1}{3}$–$\frac{1}{2}$ adult dose	Management of schizophrenia. Can cause EPS. Has less sedative effect. *Pregnancy category:* C; PB: UK; $t_{\frac{1}{2}}$: 1.5 h
Thioxanthenes			
Chlorprothixene HCl (Taractan)		A: PO: 25–50 mg t.i.d.; gradually increase to 500–600 mg/d	For psychosis and schizophrenia. Sedative effect is common. Few incidences of EPS. Can cause orthostatic hypotension. Take with food to decrease GI distress. *Pregnancy category:* C; PB: UK; $t_{\frac{1}{2}}$: 3–34 h
Thiothixene HCl (Navane)	High	A: PO: 2 mg t.i.d.; *max:* 60 mg/d; IM: 4 mg b.i.d.–q.i.d.; *max:* 30 mg/d	Management of psychotic disorders, especially acute and chronic schizophrenia. Can cause EPS. *Pregnancy category:* C; PB: ≥90%; $t_{\frac{1}{2}}$: 24–34 h
Atypical Antipsychotics			
Clozapine (Clozaril)	Low	A: PO/IM: Initially: <50 mg/d; if tolerated, gradually increase to 300–450 mg/d in divided doses	For severely ill schizophrenic clients, especially those who do not respond to other antipsychotics. With long-term use, monitor white blood cell count. *Pregnancy category:* B; PB: 95%; $t_{\frac{1}{2}}$: 8–12 h
Olanzapine (Zyprexa)	Uk	A: PO: 5 mg/d initially, 5–10 mg/d thereafter	It is effective in treating positive and negative symptoms of schizophrenia. Does not cause EPS symptoms. May cause headaches, dizziness, agitation, insomnia, and somnolence. *Pregnancy category:* C; PB: UK; $t_{\frac{1}{2}}$: 27–30 h
Quetiapine (Seroquel)	Uk	A: PO: 25 mg/d initially, 25–50 mg b.i.d. first week; *max:* 400 mg/d	New drug, effective in treating positive and negative symptoms of schizophrenia. Is not likely to cause EPS. May cause dizziness, headache, insomnia. *Pregnancy category:* UK; PB: UK; $t_{\frac{1}{2}}$: UK

Table continued on following page

Table 19–2 *Continued*
Phenothiazines and Nonphenothiazines

GENERIC (BRAND)	DRUG POTENCY	ROUTE AND DOSAGE	USES AND CONSIDERATIONS
Sertindole (Serlect)	Uk	A: PO: 4 mg/d initially, then 20 mg/d	Newest atypical agent. Improves positive and negative symptoms of schizophrenia. May cause little EPS. May cause dizziness, headache, constipation, ejaculatory disturbances. *Pregnancy category:* UK; PB: UK; $t\frac{1}{2}$: UK
Risperidone (Risperdal)	Low	A: PO: 1–3 mg b.i.d. Elderly: $\frac{1}{3}$–$\frac{1}{2}$ adult dose	Management of psychotic disorders. Side effects include EPS, insomnia, anxiety, agitation. *Pregnancy category:* C; PB: 90%; $t\frac{1}{2}$: 24 h

*Avoid spilling liquid on skin. Contact dermatitis could result.
KEY: A: adult; C: child; PO: by mouth; IM: intramuscular; IV: intravenous; <: less than; ≥: equal to or greater than; PB: protein-binding; $t\frac{1}{2}$: half-life; EPS: extrapyramidal symptoms; UK: unknown.

When discontinuing antipsychotics, the drug dosage should be reduced gradually to avoid sudden recurrence of psychotic symptoms. Table 19–2 lists the antipsychotic drugs (phenothiazines and nonphenothiazines), their dosages, uses, and considerations.

ATYPICAL (SEROTONIN/DOPAMINE ANTAGONISTS) ANTIPSYCHOTICS

A new category for antipsychotics was marketed in the United States in the early 1990s. This group, **atypical antipsychotics,** differs from the typical or traditional antipsychotics because the atypical agents are effective in treating both positive and negative symptoms of schizophrenia. The typical antipsychotics have not been effective in the treatment of negative symptoms. Two advantages of the atypical agents is that they are effective in treating negative symptoms and are not likely to cause EPS or tardive dyskinesia. The four atypical drugs available include clozapine (Clozaril), risperidone (Risperdal), olanzapine (Zyprexa), and quetiapine (Seroquel). These agents have a greater affinity for blocking serotonin and dopaminergic D_4 receptors than primarily blocking the dopaminergic D_2 receptor that is responsible for mild and severe extrapyramidal symptoms.

Clozapine was the first atypical antipsychotic agent used to treat schizophrenia and other psychoses. It does not cause acute EPS, although tremors and occasional rigidity have been reported. The serious adverse reaction of clozapine is agranulocytosis, a decrease in the production of granulocytes, which results in a decrease in the body's defense mechanism, and seizures. Currently it is only indicated for the treatment of the severely ill schizophrenic client

who has not responded to the traditional antipsychotic drugs. If the WBC (leukocytes) level is less than 3000 mm³, clozapine should be discontinued. The white blood cell count needs to be closely monitored. Seizures have been reported in 3% of clients taking the drug. Dizziness, sedation, tachycardia, orthostatic hypotension, and constipation are common side effects.

Another atypical agent for treating positive and negative symptoms of schizophrenia is risperidone (Risperdal). Its action is similar to that of clozapine and the occurrence of EPS and tardive dyskinesia is very low. It does not cause agranulocytosis.

Another new atypical agent is olanzapine (Zyprexa). This drug, like clozapine and risperidone, is effective for treating positive and negative symptoms of schizophrenia. It does not cause agranulocytosis.

The latest atypical agent is quetiapine (Seroquel), which has recently been approved by the Food and Drug Administration (FDA). Like all the other atypical antipsychotics, it is less likely to cause EPS. Tardive dyskinesia for long-term use has not been determined.

ANXIOLYTICS

Anxiolytics or **antianxiety drugs** are primarily used for treating anxiety and insomnia. The major group of anxiolytics are the benzodiazepines (a minor tranquilizer group). Long before benzodiazepines were prescribed for anxiety and insomnia, barbiturates were used. Benzodiazepines are considered more effective than barbiturates because they enhance the action of gamma-aminobutyric acid (GABA), an inhibitory neu-

NURSING PROCESS
PHENOTHIAZINE AND NONPHENOTHIAZINE

Assessment

- Obtain baseline vital signs (VS) for use in future comparison.
- Obtain a history from the client of present drug therapy. If client is taking an anticonvulsant, drug dose might need to be increased because antipsychotics tend to lower seizure threshold.
- Assess mental status, cardiac, eye, and respiratory disorders before start of drug therapy and continue daily.

Potential Nursing Diagnoses

- Altered thought processes
- Activity intolerance
- Sensory-perceptual alteration

Planning

- Client's psychotic behavior will be controlled by drug(s) and psychotherapy.

Nursing Interventions

- Monitor vital signs. Orthostatic hypotension is likely to occur.
- Remain with client while he or she takes the medication. Some clients hide drugs.
- Avoid skin contact with liquid concentrates to prevent contact dermatitis. Liquid must be protected from light and should be diluted with fruit juice.
- Administer oral doses with food or milk to decrease gastric irritation.
- Administer by IM route deep into the muscle because the drug is irritating to the fatty tissue. Do *not* inject into subcutaneous tissue. Check blood pressure for marked decrease 30 min after drug is injected.
- Do not mix in same syringe with heparin, pentobarbital, cimetidine, or dimenhydrinate.
- Chill suppository in the refrigerator for 30 min before removing foil wrapper.
- Observe the client for extrapyramidal syndrome (EPS), especially clients taking typical/traditional antipsychotics: *acute dystonia* (spasms of the tongue, face, neck, and back), *akathisia* (restlessness, inability to sit still, foot-tapping), *pseudoparkinsonism* (muscle tremors, rigidity, shuffling gait), and *tardive dyskinesia* (lip smacking, protruding and darting tongue, and constant chewing movement). Report these promptly to the health care provider.
- Monitor for symptoms of neuroleptic malignant syndrome (NMS): increased fever, pulse, and blood pressure; muscle rigidity; increased creatine phosphokinase and WBC count; altered mental status; acute renal failure; varying levels of consciousness; pallor; diaphoresis; tachycardia; and dysrhythmias.
- Monitor urine output. Urinary retention may result.
- Monitor serum glucose level.

Client Teaching

General

- Instruct the client to take the drug exactly as ordered. In schizophrenia and other psychotic disorders, antipsychotics do not cure the mental illness but do prevent symptoms. Many clients on medication can function outside the institution setting. Compliance with drug regimen is extremely important.
- Advise the client that medication may take 6 wk or longer to achieve full clinical effect.

Nursing Process continued on following page

NURSING PROCESS *Continued*

PHENOTHIAZINE AND NONPHENOTHIAZINE

- Instruct the client not to consume alcohol or other CNS depressants such as narcotics; these drugs intensify the depressant effect on the body.
- Instruct the client not to abruptly discontinue the drug. Seek advice from the health care provider before making any changes in dosage.
- Encourage the client to read labels on over-the-counter (OTC) preparations. Some are contraindicated when taking antipsychotics.
- Adjust drug dose if client smokes, as necessary. Smoking increases the metabolism of some antipsychotics.
- Advise client to maintain good oral hygiene by frequent brushing and flossing.
- Encourage the client to talk with the health care provider regarding family planning. The effect of antipsychotics on the fetus is not fully known; however, there may be teratogenic effects on the fetus.
- Advise the client that phenothiazine passes into breast milk. This could cause drowsiness and unusual muscle movement in the baby.
- Instruct the client on the importance of routine follow-up examinations.
- Encourage the client to obtain laboratory tests on schedule. WBCs are monitored for 3 mo, especially during the start of drug therapy. Leukopenia, or decreased WBCs, may occur. Be alert to symptoms of malaise, fever, and sore throat, which may be an indication of agranulocytosis, a serious blood dyscrasia. Report this promptly to the health care provider, especially when taking clozapine.
- Encourage the client to wear an ID bracelet indicating the medication taken.
- Inform the client that tolerance to sedative effect develops over a period of days or weeks.

Side Effects

- Instruct the client to avoid potentially dangerous situations, such as driving, until drug dosing has been stabilized.
- Inform the client about EPS; instruct the client to promptly report symptoms to the health care provider.
- Photosensitivity may occur; instruct the client to avoid direct sunlight or to use a sun block and protective clothing. Sunbathing can cause a skin rash.
- Advise the client of orthostatic hypotension and possible dizziness.
- Advise the client who is taking aliphatic phenothiazines, such as chlorpromazine, that the urine might be pink or red-brown; this discoloration is harmless.
- Inform the client that changes may occur related to sexual functioning and menstruating. Women could have irregular menstrual periods or amenorrhea, and men might experience impotence and gynecomastia (enlargement of breast tissue).
- Suggest lozenges or hard candy if mouth dryness occurs. Advise the client to consult the health care provider if dry mouth persists for more than 2 wk.
- Advise the client to avoid extremes in temperatures and increased exercise.
- Advise the client to rise slowly from sitting or lying to standing to prevent a sudden decrease in blood pressure.

Cultural Consideration

- Recognize that various cultural groups may have difficulty in accepting the client's mental disorder.

Evaluation

- Evaluate the effectiveness of the drug; the client is free of psychotic symptoms at the *lowest* dose possible.
- The client can cope with everyday living situation and attend to activities of daily living.
- Determine if any side effects of or adverse reactions to the drug have occurred.

rotransmitter within the CNS. Benzodiazepines have fewer side effects and may be less dangerous in overdosing. Long-term use of barbiturates causes drug intolerance and dependence and may cause respiratory distress. Currently, barbiturates are not the choice of drug for anxiety. Table 19–3 lists the approved uses for benzodiazepines. Drugs used to treat insomnia, which includes the benzodiazepines, are discussed in Chapter 16. Antihistamines are discussed in Chapter 35. Beta blockers that may be given for anxiety are discussed in Chapter 39.

A limited degree of anxiety might be considered normal; however, when the anxiety is excessive and could be disabling, anxiolytics may be prescribed. The action of anxiolytics resembles that of the sedative-hypnotics, but not that of the antipsychotics.

There are two types of anxiety—primary and secondary. Primary anxiety is not caused by a medical condition or by drug use; secondary anxiety is related to selected drug use or medical or psychiatric disorders. The anxiolytics are not usually given for secondary anxiety unless the medical problem is untreatable, severe, and causing disability. In this case, the drug could be given for a short period to alleviate any acute anxiety attacks. These agents treat the symptoms but do not cure them. Long-term use of anxiolytics is discouraged because tolerance develops within weeks or months, depending on the drug agent. Drug tolerance can occur in less than 2 to 3 months for meprobamate and phenobarbital.

Some of the symptoms of a severe or panic attack of anxiety include dyspnea (difficulty in breathing), choking sensation, chest pain, heart palpitations, dizziness, faintness, sweating, trembling and shaking, and fear of losing control. *Nonpharmacologic measures should be used for decreasing anxiety before giving anxiolytics.* These measures might include using a relaxation technique, psychotherapy, or support groups.

Benzodiazepines

Benzodiazepines have multiple uses, such as anticonvulsants, antihypertensives, sedative-hypnotics, preoperative drugs, and anxiolytics. Most of the benzodiazepines are used mainly for severe or prolonged anxiety; examples include chlordiazepoxide (Librium), diazepam (Valium), chlorazepate dipotassium (Tranxene), oxazepam (Serax), lorazepam (Ativan), alprazolam (Xanax), prazepam (Centrax), and halazepam (Paxipam). The three most frequently prescribed benzodiazepines are diazepam (Valium), alprazolam (Xanax), and lorazepam (Ativan). Table 19–4 describes the various uses for benzodiazepines. Many of the benzodiazepines, such as diazepam (Valium), are used for more than one purpose.

Benzodiazepines are lipid-soluble and are absorbed readily from the GI tract. They are highly protein-bound (80% to 98%). They could displace other highly protein-bound drugs, so the drug dosage for clients with liver or renal disease should be lowered accordingly to avoid possible cumulative effects. Traces of benzodiazepine metabolites could be present in the urine for weeks or months after the person has stopped taking the drug. These are controlled substance schedule IV (CSS IV) drugs.

In 1962, the first benzodiazepine, chlordiazepoxide (Librium), became widely used for its sedative effect. Diazepam (Valium) was the most frequently prescribed drug in the early 1970s and was called a miracle drug by many. Diazepam is the prototype drug of benzodiazepine and is described in Chart 19–3.

Table 19–3
Approved Uses for Benzodiazepines

PRESCRIBED USES	DRUGS
Anxiety	Alprazolam (Xanax) Chlordiazepoxide (Librium) Chlorazepate (Tranxene) Diazepam (Valium) Halazepam (Paxipam) Ketazolam (Loftan) Lorazepam (Ativan) Oxazepam (Serax) Prazepam (Centrax)
Anxiety associated with depression	Alprazolam (Xanax) Clonazepam (Klonopin) Lorazepam (Ativan) Oxazepam (Serax)
Insomnia: Short-term use	Estazolam (Prosom) Flurazepam (Dalmane) Quazepam (Doral) Oxazepam (Serax) Temazepam (Restoril) Triazolam (Halcion)
Seizures and status epilepticus	Clonazepam (Klonopin) Clorazepate (Tranxene) Diazepam (Valium) status epilepticus Lorazepam (Ativan) status epilepticus
Alcohol withdrawal	Clorazepate (Tranxene) Chlordiazepoxide (Librium) Diazepam (Valium) Oxazepam (Serex)
Skeletal muscle spasms	Diazepam (Valium)
Preoperative medications	Chlordiazepoxide (Librium) Diazepam (Valium) Lorazepam (Ativan) Midazolam (Versed)

Table 19–4
Anxiolytics

GENERIC (BRAND)	ROUTE AND DOSAGE	USES AND CONSIDERATIONS
ANTIHISTAMINES		
Hydroxyzine HCl (Atarax, Vistaril)	A: PO: 50–100 mg t.i.d.–q.i.d. IM: 25–100 mg C <6 y: 25 mg b.i.d. C >6 y: 25 mg b.i.d.–q.i.d.	For anxiety and tension; control nausea and vomiting. May be used as a preoperative and postoperative drug to reduce narcotic dose. Side effects include drowsiness, dizziness, dry mouth, hypotension. *Pregnancy category:* C; PB: UK; $t\frac{1}{2}$: 3–7 h
BENZODIAZEPINES		
Alprazolam (Xanax) CSS IV	A: PO: 0.25–0.5 mg t.i.d. Elderly: 0.25 mg b.i.d.–t.i.d.; *max:* 4 mg/d	Management of anxiety and panic disorders and anxiety associated with depression. Side effects include drowsiness, dry mouth, and lightheadedness. *Pregnancy category:* D; PB: 80%; $t\frac{1}{2}$: 12–15 h
Chlordiazepoxide HCl (Librium) CSS IV	*Anxiety disorders:* A: PO: 5–25 mg t.i.d.–q.i.d. C: PO: 5 mg b.i.d.–q.i.d. *Acute alcohol withdrawal:* A: PO/IM/IV: 50–100 mg; *max:* 300 mg/d Elderly: $\frac{1}{2}$ adult dose	Effective for alcohol withdrawal syndrome (DTs), anxiety, and tension. Dose should be less for the older adult. *Pregnancy category:* D; PB: 90%–98%; $t\frac{1}{2}$: 6–30 h
Clorazepate dipotassium (Tranxene) CSS IV	A: PO: 15–60 mg/d in divided doses Elderly: 7.5 mg b.i.d.	For anxiety, alcohol withdrawal syndrome, and partial seizures. Avoid taking alcohol or CNS depressants with chorazepate. Drowsiness and dizziness may occur. *Pregnancy category:* C; PB: 80%–90%; $t\frac{1}{2}$: 0.5–1 h
Diazepam (Valium)	See Chart 19–3	For anxiety disorders, alcohol withdrawal syndrome, status epilepticus, muscle spasm, sedation. Avoid alcohol intake. *Pregnancy category:* D; PB: 98%; $t\frac{1}{2}$: 25–50 h
Halazepam (Paxipam)	A: PO: 20–40 mg t.i.d.–q.i.d. Elderly; 20 mg daily/b.i.d.	Management of anxiety disorders. Drowsiness, sedation, confusion, headaches and hypotension may occur. *Pregnancy category:* D; PB: 97%; $t\frac{1}{2}$: 14 h
Lorazepam (Ativan) CSS IV	A: PO: 2–6 mg/d in divided doses A: IM/IV: 2–4 mg Elderly: $\frac{1}{2}$ adult dose	For short-term relief of anxiety. Can be used as preoperative drug. Has been given prior to chemotherapy. Drowsiness and dizziness may occur. *Pregnancy category:* D; PB: 90%; $t\frac{1}{2}$: 10–20 h
Oxazepam (Serax)	A: PO: 10–30 mg t.i.d.–q.i.d. Elderly: 10–15 mg, t.i.d.–q.i.d.	For mild to moderate anxiety. To control alcohol syndrome. Drowsiness, dizziness may occur. *Pregnancy category:* C; PB: 85%–95%; $t\frac{1}{2}$: 3.5–21 h
Prazepam (Centrax) CSS IV	A: PO: 10 mg t.i.d.–q.i.d. Elderly: 10–15 mg/d in divided doses	To relieve anxiety disorders. *Pregnancy category:* D; PB: 97%; $t\frac{1}{2}$: 30–200 h
PROPANEDIOL		
Meprobamate (Equanil, Miltown) CSS IV	A: PO: 400 mg t.i.d.–q.i.d. C: PO: 100–200 mg b.i.d.–t.i.d.	An original anxiolytic drug. For short-term relief of anxiety. Promotes sleep in anxious clients. Avoid alcohol intake. *Pregnancy category:* D; PB: UK; $t\frac{1}{2}$: 6–16 h
AZAP'RONES		
Buspirone HCl (BuSpar)	A: PO: Initial: 5 mg, b.i.d.–t.i.d. A: PO: 15–30 mg/d in divided doses; *max:* 60 mg/d Elderly: *max:* 30 mg/d	For anxiety and anxiety-related depression. Takes several weeks before anxiolytic effects occur. Common side effects include drowsiness, dizziness, headache, nausea. *Pregnancy category:* B; PB: 95%; $t\frac{1}{2}$: 2–3 h
BENZODIAZEPINE ANTAGONIST		
Flumazenil (Romazicon)	A: IV: 0.2 mg over 30 sec; repeat 0.3–0.5 mg at 1 min intervals; *max:* 3 mg in an hour	Used to partially or completely reverse benzodiazepine dose due to sedation, anesthesia, and overdose. It should not be used with antipsychotics or antidepressants. *Pregnancy category:* C; PB: UK; $t\frac{1}{2}$: UK

KEY: A: adult; C: child; CSS: Controlled Substance Schedule; PB: protein-binding; PO: by mouth; $t\frac{1}{2}$: half-life; UK: unknown.

Chart 19–3. Anxiolytics

DIAZEPAM

Drug Name

Diazepam
(Valium), ✤ Apo-diazepam, Diazemuls, Novodipam
Benzodiazepine
CSS IV
Pregnancy Category: D

Dosage

Anxiety:
A: PO/IM/IV: 2–10 mg b.i.d.–q.i.d.
Elderly: 2.5 mg b.i.d.
C <6 mo: 1–2.5 mg t.i.d.–q.i.d.
Musculoskeletal spasm:
A: PO: 2–10 mg b.i.d.–q.i.d.
IM: 5–10 mg q3–4h
Preoperative sedation:
A: IV: 5–15 mg 15 min before event
Status epilepticus:
A: IV: 5–10 mg q10–20 min; *max:* 30 mg
C <6 y: 0.2–0.5 mg/kg q15–30 min; *max:* 5 mg total dose
C >6 y: 0.2–0.5 mg/kg q15–30 min; *max:* 10 mg total dose
IV: *max:* 5 mg/3 min

Contraindications

Hypersensitivity, CNS depression, shock, coma, narrow-angle glaucoma, pregnancy, lactation
Caution: Hepatic or renal dysfunction; epilepsy, elderly and infants; history of drug abuse; depression, addiction-prone, or suicidal tendency

Drug-Lab-Food Interactions

Drug: *Increase* effects of diazepam with alcohol, oral contraceptives, CNS depressants, cimetidine, disulfiram, fluoxetine, isoniazid, ketoconazole, levodopa, metoprolol, propoxyphene, propranolol, valproic acid; toxic effects with MAOIs; *decrease* effects with rifampin, cigarettes, theophylline; *increase* effects of digoxin, phenytoin
Do not mix or dilute with other drugs in syringe
Lab: *Increase* bilirubin

Pharmacokinetics

Absorption: Rapid from GI tract; erratic from IM administration; most rapid and complete from deltoid muscle
Distribution: Widely PB: 98%
Metabolism: $t\frac{1}{2}$: 25–50 h
Excretion: In urine

Pharmacodynamics

PO: Onset: 30–60 min
Peak: 1–2 h
Duration: 2–3 h (varies)
IM: Onset: 15–30 min
Peak: 1–2 h
Duration: $1–1\frac{1}{2}$ h (varies)
IV: Onset: 1–5 min
Peak: 15–30 min
Duration: 15–60 min

Therapeutic Effects/Uses

To control anxiety, preoperative sedation, skeletal muscle relaxant, to treat status epilepticus, alcohol withdrawal, convulsive disorders, anterograde amnesia.

Mode of Action: Depression of limbic and subcortical CNS and skeletal muscle relaxation, shortens stage 4 and REM sleep.

Side Effects

Drowsiness, dizziness, syncope, orthostatic hypotension, blurred vision, nausea, vomiting, fatigue, confusion

Adverse Reactions

ECG changes, tachycardia, psychological and physical dependence with long-term use
Life threatening: Laryngospasm

NURSING PROCESS: Assessment and Planning; Interventions; Evaluation

KEY: A: adult; C: child; PO: by mouth; IM: intramuscular; IV: intravenous; PB: protein-binding; CNS: central nervous system; MAOI: monoamine oxidase inhibitor; GI: gastrointestinal; $t\frac{1}{2}$: half-life; >: greater than; <: less than; ✤: Canadian drug names.

PHARMACOKINETICS

Diazepam is highly lipid-soluble and the drug is rapidly absorbed from the GI tract. The intravenous route of administration is used more frequently than the intramuscular (IM) route. IM administration results in slow, erratic absorption and lower peak plasma levels. IM administration into the deltoid muscle results in better absorption. The drug is highly protein-bound and the half-life is long (20 to 80 h). Cumulative effects may result. The drug is excreted primarily in the urine.

PHARMACODYNAMICS

Diazepam acts on the limbic and subcortical levels of the central nervous system. The onset of action is 0.5 to 1 h by mouth and 1 to 5 min intravenously. Most oral doses of benzodiazepines serum levels peak in 1 to 2 hours. Oxazepam levels peak in 3 hours and prazepam levels peak in 6 hours. Duration of action varies; by mouth the average is 2 to 3 h. The longest duration of action is 1 h intravenously.

It is recommended that benzodiazepines be prescribed for no longer than 3 to 4 months. Beyond the 4 months, the effectiveness of the drug lessens. Table 19–4 lists the anxiolytics, their dosages, uses, and considerations.

Before benzodiazepines, the propanediol drug meprobamate (Equanil, Miltown) was used to treat anxiety. Meprobamate was preferred over the use of barbiturates because of fewer side effects. Currently, meprobamate is occasionally prescribed for short-term relief of anxiety and for its muscle relaxant properties. Alcohol should be avoided when taking meprobamate or any of the benzodiazepines.

Hydroxyzine hydrochloride (Atarax, Vistaril) and diphenhydramine hydrochloride (Benadryl) are antihistamines. They cause drowsiness and have a sedative effect and are used for short-term relief of anxiety. Because they do not cause tolerance, these drugs could be used temporarily when other antianxiety drugs have been abused.

The newest anxiolytic is buspirone hydrochloride (BuSpar), developed for alleviating anxiety. It does not have many of the side effects associated with benzodiazepines, such as sedation and physical and psychological dependency. Buspirone might not become effective until 1 to 2 weeks after continuous use.

Flurazepam, temazepam, triazolam, estazolam, and quazepam are benzodiazepines used primarily for insomnia (see Chapter 16).

SIDE EFFECTS AND ADVERSE REACTIONS

The side effects associated with benzodiazepines are sedative effect, dizziness, headaches, dry mouth, blurred vision, rare urinary incontinence, and constipation. Adverse reactions include leukopenia (decreased white blood cell count) with symptoms of

Table 19–5
Suggested Treatment for Overdose of Benzodiazepines

1. Administer an emetic and follow with activated charcoal if the client is conscious; gastric lavage if the client is unconscious.
2. Administer the benzodiazepine antagonist flumazenil (Romazicon) intravenously if required.
3. Maintain an airway, give oxygen as needed for decreased respirations, and monitor vital signs.
4. Give intravenous vasopressors for severe hypotension.
5. Request for a mental health consultation.

NOTE: Dialysis has little value in removing benzodiazepine from the bloodstream.

fever, malaise, and sore throat; tolerance to the drug dosage with continuous use; and physical dependency. Table 19–5 lists guidelines for treating benzodiazepine overdose.

Benzodiazepines should not be abruptly discontinued because withdrawal symptoms are likely to occur. Withdrawal symptoms due to benzodiazepines are similar to those from the sedative-hypnotics (agitation, nervousness, tremor, anorexia, muscular cramps, sweating); however, they are slower to develop, taking 2 to 10 days and could last several weeks. It would depend on the half-life of the benzodiazepine. When discontinuing a benzodiazepine, the drug dosage should be gradually decreased over a period of days depending on dose or length of time on the drug. Alcohol and other CNS depressants should *not* be taken with benzodiazepines, because respiratory depression could result. Smoking, caffeine, and sympathomimetics decrease the effectiveness of benzodiazepines. Benzodiazepines are contraindicated during pregnancy because of the possible teratogenic effects on the fetus.

ANTIDEPRESSANTS
Depression

Depression is the most common psychiatric problem, affecting approximately 10% to 20% of the population. Only one-third of the depressed persons receive medical or psychiatric help. Depression is primarily characterized by mood changes and loss of interest in normal activities.

Contributing causes of depression include genetic predisposition, social and environmental factors, and biologic conditions. It is also thought that depression may be due to insufficient monoamine neurotransmit-

NURSING PROCESS
ANXIOLYTICS

Assessment

- Assess for suicidal ideation.
- Obtain a history of the client's anxiety reaction.
- Determine the client's support system (family, friends, groups), if any.
- Obtain the client's drug history. Report possible drug-drug interaction.

Potential Nursing Diagnoses

- Anxiety
- Mobility, impaired physical

Planning

- Client's anxiety and stress will be reduced through nonpharmacologic methods, anxiolytic drugs, or support/group therapy.

Nursing Interventions

- Administer by IM route in large muscle mass, and inject drug slowly.
- Observe the client for side effects of anxiolytics. Recognize that drug tolerance and physical and psychological dependency can result with most anxiolytics.
- Recognize that anxiolytic dosages should be less for the elderly, children, and debilitated persons than for middle-aged adults.
- Monitor vital signs, especially blood pressure and pulse; orthostatic hypotension may occur.
- Do not mix Valium with other drugs because precipitation will result.
- Give Vistaril by Z-track method.
- Encourage the family to be supportive of the client.

Client Teaching

General
- Advise the client not to drive a motor vehicle or operate dangerous equipment when taking anxiolytics because sedation is a common side effect.
- Instruct the client not to consume alcohol or CNS depressants such as narcotics while taking an anxiolytic.
- Instruct the client on ways to control excess stress and anxiety, such as relaxation techniques.
- Inform the client that effective response may take 1 to 2 wk.
- Encourage the client to follow drug regimen and not to abruptly stop taking the drug after prolonged use because withdrawal symptoms can occur. Drug dose is usually tapered when drug is discontinued.

Side Effects
- Instruct the client to arise slowly from the sitting to standing position to avoid dizziness from orthostatic hypotension.

Evaluation

- Evaluate the effectiveness of drug therapy by determining if the client is less anxious and more able to cope with stresses and anxieties.
- Determine if the client is taking the anxiolytic drug as prescribed and is adhering to client teaching instructions.

ters (norepinephrine and/or serotonin) in the brain. Some signs of major depression include loss of interest in most activities, depressed mood, weight loss or gain, insomnia or hypersomnia, loss of energy, fatigue, feeling of despair, inability to think or concentrate, and suicidal thoughts. About two-thirds of all suicides are related to depression. Antidepressants can mask suicidal tendencies.

The three types of depression are (1) reactive or exogenous, (2) major or unipolar, and (3) bipolar affective (previously referred to as manic-depressive) disorder. **Reactive** or **exogenous depression** usually has a sudden onset resulting from a precipitating event. The client knows why he or she is depressed such as a person's response to a loss (loss of a loved one). The person may refer to this as the "blues." Usually this type of depression lasts for months. A benzodiazepine agent may be prescribed. **Major, unipolar,** or **endogenous depression** is characterized by loss of interest in work and home, inability to complete tasks, and deep depression **(dysphoria).** Major depression can be either primary (not related to other health problems) or secondary to a health problem, such as physical or psychiatric disorder or drug use. Antidepressants have been effective in treating major depression. **Bipolar affective disorder** involves swings between two moods, the manic (euphoric) and the depressive (dysphoria). Lithium is the drug of choice for treating this type of disorder, although new drugs, such as depakote, will be offered within a few years.

Electroconvulsive therapy (ECT) was used to treat psychosis and depression before the introduction of antipsychotics and antidepressants. ECT is still used, although not as frequently as in the past, for clients who are extremely depressed, suicidal, or do not respond to antidepressant therapy. ECT is not as traumatic as it once was. The use of thiopental (short-acting anesthetic) and succinylcholine (short-acting neuromuscular blocking agent), which reduces the severe convulsive movements, has made ECT a more safe and desirable method for treating depression. The use of ECT does not affect the person's memory or intellectual function.

Antidepressant Agents

The antidepressants are divided into three groups: (1) tricyclic antidepressants (TCAs) or tricyclics, (2) second-generation antidepressants, which became available in the late 1980s and are subdivided as selective serotonin reuptake inhibitors (SSRIs) and atypical antidepressants, and (3) **monoamine oxidase (MAO) inhibitors.** The tricyclics and MAO inhibitors were marketed in the late 1950s. The SSRI agents are popular antidepressants because they do not cause sedation,

hypotension, anticholingeric effects, or cardiotoxicity as do many of the TCAs.

TRICYCLIC ANTIDEPRESSANTS

The tricyclic antidepressants (TCAs) are frequently prescribed drugs to treat major depression because they are effective and less expensive than the SSRIs and other drugs. Imipramine was the first TCA marketed in the last 1950s.

Tricyclic antidepressants block the uptake of the neurotransmitters norepinephrine and serotonin in the brain. The clinical response of TCAs follows 2 to 4 weeks of drug therapy. If there is no improvement after 2 to 4 weeks, the antidepressant is slowly withdrawn and another antidepressant is prescribed. Polydrug therapy, giving several antidepressants or antipsychotics together, is to be avoided because of possible serious side effects.

The tricyclics have been effective for treating major/unipolar depression. This group of drugs elevates mood, increases interest in daily living and activity, and decreases insomnia. For agitated depressed persons, amitriptyline (Elavil), doxepin (Sinequan), or trimipramine (Surmontil) may be prescribed because of their highly sedative effect. Frequently, TCAs are given at night to minimize the problems caused by their sedative action. When discontinuing TCAs, the drugs should gradually be decreased to avoid withdrawal symptoms, such as nausea, vomiting, anxiety, and akathisia. Imipramine hydrochloride (Tofranil) is used for the treatment of enuresis (involuntary discharge of urine during sleep in children).

The tricyclics have many side effects, such as orthostatic hypotension, sedation, anticholinergic effects, cardiac toxicity, and seizures. Rising from a sitting position too rapidly can cause dizziness and lightheadedness; thus, the client should be instructed to rise to an upright position slowly to avoid **orthostatic hypotension.** This group of antidepressants block the histamine receptors, thus sedation is likely to occur. The TCAs block the cholinergic receptors that can cause anticholinergic effects, such as tachycardia, urinary retention, constipation, dry mouth, and blurred vision. The most serious adverse reaction to tricyclics is cardiac toxicity, such as dysrhythmias that may result from high doses of the drug.

The TCA drugs are categorized as tertiary or secondary amines. The tertiary amines include amitriptyline, imipramine, trimipramine, and doxepin. The secondary amines include desipramine, nortriptyline, and protriptyline. Amoxapine (Ascendin) and maprotiline (Ludiomil) are atypical antidepressants; however, they are similar to the tricyclic secondary amines. Amoxapine and maprotiline are sometimes considered to be members of the TCAs because of their pharmacologic similarities. The TCA drugs desi-

Chart 19-4. Antidepressants

Drug Name

Tricyclic antidepressant
Amitriptyline HCl (E) (Elavil), 🍁 Apo-
Amitriptyline, Novotriptyn
Pregnancy Category: D

Selective Serotonin Reuptake Inhibitor

Fluoxetine (P) (Prozac)
Pregnancy Category: B

Dosage

(E)
A: PO: 25 mg b.i.d.–q.i.d.; increase to 150–200 mg/d; dose may be given as a single h.s. dose
IM: 20–30 mg q.i.d.
C >13 y: PO: 10 mg t.i.d. and 20 mg h.s.
Elderly: PO: 10 mg t.i.d. 20 mg h.s.
Therapeutic Serum Range: 100–200 ng/mL
(P)
A: PO: 20 mg in a.m.
max: 80 mg/d in divided doses
Elderly: 10 mg/d initially. May increase by 10–20 mg q2 wk
Therapeutic range: 90–300 ng/mL

Contraindications

(E & P) Recovery from acute myocardial infarction (AMI), taking MAOIs
Caution: (E & P): Severe depression with suicidal tendency, severe liver or kidney disease, (E) Narrow-angle glaucoma, seizures, prostatic disease

Drug-Lab-Food Interactions

(E & P):
Drug: *Increase* effects of CNS, respiratory depression, and hypotensive effect with alcohol and CNS depressants
(E) *Increase* sedation, anticholinergic effects with phenothiazines, and haloperidol; *increase* toxicity with cimetidine; *decrease* effect of clonidine, guanethidine
Hypertensive crisis and death may occur with MAOIs.
Lab: Altered ECG readings

Pharmacokinetics

Absorption: PO:
 (E & P): well absorbed
Distribution: PB:
 (E) 95%, (P) 95%
Metabolism: $t_{\frac{1}{2}}$:
 (E) 10–50 h; (P) 2–3 d
Excretion: (E & P) Excreted primarily in urine

Pharmacodynamics

Antidepressant Effect
(E):
PO: Onset: 1–3 wk
 Peak: 2–6 wk
 Duration: UK
(P):
PO: Onset: 2–4 wk
 Peak: 2–4 wk
 Duration: weeks

Therapeutic Effects/Uses

(E & A): To treat depression with or without melancholia, depressive phase of bipolar disorder, depression associated with organic disease, alcoholism, migraine headaches, mixed symptoms of anxiety and depression, or urinary incontinence.

Mode of Action: Serotonin and norepinephrine increased in nerve cells due to blockage from nerve fibers.

Side Effects

(E): Sedation, drowsiness, blurred vision, dry mouth and eyes, extrapyramidal syndrome (EPS), urinary retention, constipation, weight gain, dizziness, nervousness
(P): Headache, nervousness, restlessness, insomnia, tremors, GI distress

Adverse Reactions

(E): Orthostatic hypotension, cardiac dysrhythmias
Life threatening: (E): Agranulocytosis, thrombocytopenia, leukopenia.
(E & P): Seizures

Assessment and Planning

Interventions

Evaluation

NURSING PROCESS

KEY: A: adult; C: child; PO: by mouth; PB: protein-binding; MAOI: monoamine oxidase inhibitor; ECG: electrocardiogram; CNS: central nervous system; GI: gastrointestinal; $t_{\frac{1}{2}}$: half-life; UK: unknown; <: less than; >: greater than; 🍁: Canadian drug names.

pramine and nortriptyline are major metabolites of imipramine and amitriptyline.

SECOND-GENERATION ANTIDEPRESSANTS (SELECTIVE SEROTONIN REUPTAKE INHIBITORS AND ATYPICAL ANTIDEPRESSANTS)

In the late 1980s, a group of antidepressants that did not have TCA chemical structure were identified. This group was first classified as second-generation antidepressants. Today they have been reclassified as **selective serotonin reuptake inhibitors** (SSRIs) and atypical antidepressants. The action of the atypical antidepressants are not well defined. The SSRIs block the reuptake of serotonin into the nerve terminal of the CNS, thereby enhancing its transmission at the serotonergic synapse. SSRIs do not block the uptake of dopamine or norepinephrine, and they do not block cholinergic and alpha$_1$-adrenergic receptors. These two groups of drugs are more commonly used to treat depression than are the TCAs, even though they are more costly. There are fewer side effects with SSRIs and atypical antidepressants than with TCAs.

Four SSRIs have been marketed since 1988: fluoxetine (Prozac), fluvoxamine (Luvox), sertraline (Zoloft), and paroxetine (Paxil). Celexa and cipramil are new SSRIs. The primary use of SSRIs is for major (unipolar) depressive disorders. They are also effective for treating anxiety disorders such as obsessive-compulsiveness, panic, phobias, posttraumatic stress disorders, and other forms of anxiety. Fluvoxamine (Luvox) is useful for treating obsessive-compulsive disorders in children and adults. SSRIs have also been used for treating eating disorders and selected drug abuses. Miscellaneous uses for SSRIs include decreasing premenstrual tension syndrome, preventing migraine headaches, and preventing or minimizing aggressive behavior in clients with borderline personality disorder.

Fluoxetine (Prozac) has been effective in 50% to 60% of clients who fail to respond to TCA therapy (TCA-refractory depression). Of all the SSRIs, fluoxetine is the most commonly prescribed antidepressant. Chart 19–4 compares the tricyclic amitriptyline HCl (Elavil) with the SSRI fluoxetine (Prozac). Both drugs are antidepressants and represent different classifications. Table 19–6 lists the side effects of the various antidepressants.

Pharmacokinetics

Amitriptyline and fluoxetine are strongly protein-bound. The half-life of amitriptyline is shorter than it is for fluoxetine. The cumulative effect may therefore result from long-term use of fluoxetine. Both drugs are excreted by the kidneys.

Pharmacodynamics

Both amytriptyline and fluoxetine are well absorbed; however, their antidepressant effects develop slowly over several weeks. The onset of antidepressant effect of amitriptyline and fluoxetine is between 1 and 4 wk; however, the peak concentration times of amoxapine and fluoxetine are about the same. The durations of action for both drugs have not been determined but they are estimated to be several weeks. The drug dose for the elderly should be decreased to reduce side effects.

Side Effects and Adverse Reactions

Amitriptyline produces strong anticholinergic effects such as dry mouth and eyes, blurred vision, urinary retention, and constipation. Amitriptyline can cause EPS. The sedative and cardiotoxicity effects of amitriptyline are most pronounced; however, sedative effects decrease with continuous use of the drug. Care should be taken when administering these amitriptyline drugs to clients with a history of glaucoma. Fluoxetine has fewer side effects than amitriptyline. GI distress and insomnia are the major side effects of fluoxetine.

The general side effects of tricyclics are sedation, orthostatic hypotension, and anticholinergic symptoms, such as decreased salivation, urinary retention, constipation, and increased heart rate. If the client overdoses, fatal ventricular dysrhythmia may occur. Other side effects of TCAs include allergic reactions (skin rash, pruritus, petechiae), gastrointestinal symptoms (nausea, vomiting, anorexia, diarrhea, epigastric distress), sexual dysfunction (impotence, amenorrhea, gynecomastia), and blood cell disorders or blood dyscrasias (leukopenia, thrombocytopenia, and agranulocytosis). Table 19–6 lists the side effects of antidepressants. TCAs decrease seizure threshold; therefore, clients with seizure disorders may need to have the TCA dose increased and serum levels closely monitored. Table 19–7 lists the tricyclic, SSRIs, and atypical antidepressants.

Some clients may experience sexual dysfunction when taking SSRIs. Men have discontinued taking fluoxetine (Prozac) after experiencing a decrease in sexual arousal. Some women have become anorgasmic on paroxetine HCl (Paxil).

MONOAMINE OXIDASE INHIBITORS

The third group of antidepressants is the monoamine oxidase inhibitors (MAOIs). The enzyme monoamine oxidase inactivates norepinephrine, dopamine, epinephrine, and serotonin. By inhibiting monoamine oxidase, the levels of these neurotransmitters rise. In the body there are two forms of monoamine oxidase (MAO) enzyme: MAO-A and MAO-B. These enzymes are found primarily in the liver and brain. MAO-A inactivates dopamine in the brain, whereas MAO-B

Table 19–6
Side Effects of Antidepressants

ANTIDEPRESSANT CATEGORY	ANTICHOLINERGIC EFFECT	SEDATION	HYPOTENSION	GI DISTRESS	CARDIOTOXICITY	SEIZURES	INSOMNIA/ AGITATION
TRICYCLIC ANTIDEPRESSANTS							
Amitriptyline (Elavil)	++++	++++	+++	—	++++	+++	—
Clomipramine (Anafranil)	++++	++++	++	—	++++	++	—
Desipramine (Norpramin)	+	++	++	—	++	++	+
Doxepin (Sinequan)	+++	++++	++	—	++	++	—
Imipramine (Tofranil)	+++	+++	+++	+	++++	++	+
Nortriptyline (Aventyl)	+	+++	+	—	+++	++	—
Protriptyline (Vivactil)	+++	+	++	—	+++	++	+
Trimipramine (Surmontil)	+++	++++	+++	—	++++	++	
SELECTIVE SEROTONIN REUPTAKE INHIBITORS							
Fluoxetine (Prozac)	—	+	—	+++	—	0/+	++
Fluvoxamine (Luvox)	—	++	—	+++	—	—	++
Paroxetine (Paxil)	—	+	—	+++	—	—	++
Sertraline (Zoloft)	—	+	—	+++	—	—	++
ATYPICAL (HETEROCYCLIC) ANTIDEPRESSANTS							
Amoxapine (Asendin)	+++	++	+	—	+	+++	++
Bupropion (Wellbutrin)	++	—	0/+	+	+	++++	++
Nefazodone (Serzone)	+	++	+	+	0/+	—	—
Trazodone (Desyrel)	—	+++	++	+	+	+	
Maprotiline (Ludiomil)	+++	+++	+	—	++	+++	
Monoamine Oxidase Inhibitors (MAOIs)	—	+	++	+	—	—	++

KEY: —: no effect; +: mild effect; ++: moderate effect; +++: strong effect; ++++: severe effect.

inactivates norepinephrine and serotonin. The MAOIs are nonselective; thus, they inhibit both MAO-A and MAO-B. Inhibition of MAO by MAOIs is thought to relieve the symptoms of depression. Three MAOIs are currently prescribed: tranylcypromine sulfate (Par-nate), isocarboxazid (Marplan), and phenelzine sulfate (Nardil). These MAOIs are discussed in Table 19–7.

Monoamine oxidase inhibitors (MAOIs) are as effective as TCAs for treating depression but because of adverse reactions such as the risk of hypertensive cri-

Table 19–7

Antidepressants: Tricyclic Antidepressants, SSRIs and Atypical Antidepressants, and Mood Stabilizers (Antimanic)

GENERIC (BRAND)	ROUTE AND DOSAGE	USES AND CONSIDERATIONS
TRICYCLIC ANTIDEPRESSANTS		
Amitriptyline HCl (Elavil, Endep, Enovil)	See Chart 19–4 *Therapeutic serum range:* 100–200 ng/mL	For depression. Can be given at bedtime to avoid daytime drowsiness. May be used for intractable pain, eating disorders (anorexia and bulimia) associated with depression. *Pregnancy category:* D; PB: 95%; $t\frac{1}{2}$: 10–50 h
Clomipramine HCl (Anafranil)	A: 25–100 mg/d in divided doses; *max:* 250 mg/d; after titration; entire dose may be given h.s. Elderly: 20–30 mg/d	To treat obsessive-compulsive disorder. May be used for alleviating anxiety or panic disorder. Tremor, dizziness, weight gain, and dry mouth are common side effects. *Pregnancy category:* C; PB: 97%; $t\frac{1}{2}$: 20–30 h
Desipramine HCl (Norpramin, Pertofrane)	A: PO: 25 mg t.i.d. or 75 mg h.s.; increase to 200 mg/d; *max:* 300 mg/d Elderly: 25–50 mg/d in divided doses; *max:* 150 mg/d *Therapeutic serum range:* 150–250 ng/mL	For depression. Has been used for attention deficit disorder (ADD). Take with food if GI distress occurs. Common side effects include drowsiness, dry mouth, increased appetite, urinary retention, and postural hypotension. *Pregnancy category:* D; PB: 90%–95%; $t\frac{1}{2}$: 12–60 h
Doxepin HCl (Sinequan)	A: PO: 75–100 mg/d h.s. or in divided doses; *max:* 300 mg/d Elderly: 25–50 mg/d *Therapeutic serum range:* 30–50 ng/mL	For depression and anxiety related to involutional depression or manic-depressive disorder. Has less effect on cardiac status than other drugs in this group. *Pregnancy category:* C; PB: 80%–85%; $t\frac{1}{2}$: 6–8 h
Imipramine HCl (Tofranil)	A: PO: 75 mg/d (h.s. or 25 mg t.i.d.); *max:* 300 mg/d IM: Initially: *max:* 100 mg/d in divided doses Elderly: 25–100 mg in divided doses C <12 y: PO: 25–50 mg h.s. C >12 y: PO: 75 mg h.s. *Therapeutic serum range:* 150–250 ng/mL	For depression. Can be taken at bedtime to lessen dangers from sedative effect. Take with food if GI distress occurs. Avoid taking with alcohol or CNS depressants. Common side effects include drowsiness, dry mouth, hypotension, delayed micturition. *Pregnancy category:* D; PB: 90%–95%; $t\frac{1}{2}$: 8–15 h
Nortriptyline HCl (Aventyl)	A: PO: 25 mg t.i.d.–q.i.d.; *max:* 150 mg/d Elderly: 30–50 mg/d in divided doses *Therapeutic serum range:* 50–150 ng/mL	For depression. Similar to imipramine HCl. *Pregnancy category:* D; PB: 90%–95%; $t\frac{1}{2}$: 18–28 h
Protriptyline HCl (Vivactil)	A: PO: 15–40 mg/d in divided doses; increase gradually; *max:* 60 mg/d Elderly: 5 mg t.i.d.; *max:* 20 mg/d *Therapeutic serum range:* 70–250 ng/mL	For depression. Has little sedative effect. Effects are similar to imipramine HCl. *Pregnancy category:* C; PB: 92%; $t\frac{1}{2}$: 60–98 h
Trimipramine maleate (Surmontil)	A: 75–150 mg/d in divided doses or all h.s.; *max:* 200 mg/d Elderly: *max:* 100 mg/d	For depression. Similar to imipramine HCl. *Pregnancy category:* C; PB: 95%; $t\frac{1}{2}$: 20–26 h

Table continued on following page

Table 19–7 *Continued*
Antidepressants: Tricyclic Antidepressants, SSRIs and Atypical Antidepressants, and Mood Stabilizers (Antimanic)

GENERIC (BRAND)	ROUTE AND DOSAGE	USES AND CONSIDERATIONS
SECOND GENERATION ANTIDEPRESSANTS (ATYPICAL)		
Amoxapine (Asendin)	A: PO: 25 mg b.i.d.–q.i.d.; increase 150–200 mg/d; dose may be given as a single one	For depression with anxiety and reactive depression. Do not take with MAO inhibitors. Side effects include drowsiness, dizziness, EPS, postural hypotension, increased appetite, urinary retention. *Pregnancy category:* C; PB: >90%; $t_{\frac{1}{2}}$: 8 h
Bupropion HCl (Wellbutrin)	A: PO: Initially: 200 mg/d as b.i.d.; increase gradually to 300 mg/d in divided doses; *max:* 450 mg/d	For depression. May cause increased risk of seizures. Avoid with a history of seizures. Many side effects. *Pregnancy category:* B; PB: >80%; $t_{\frac{1}{2}}$: 50 h
Maprotiline HCl (Ludiomil)	A: PO: 75 mg h.s. or in divided doses; *max:* 150 mg/d Elderly: 25 mg/d; *max:* 75 mg/d	Same as amoxapine. Can be taken at bedtime. *Pregnancy category:* B; PB: 88%; $t_{\frac{1}{2}}$: 21–25 h
Nefazodone HCl (Serzone)	A: PO: Initial: 200 mg/d in 2 divided doses; *maint:* 300–600 mg/d in divided doses Elderly: PO: 50 mg b.i.d. to start	The newest antidepressant. For depression. It is effective for long-term use for longer than 6–8 wk. It should not be used with MAO inhibitors, and should not be used within 14 d after discontinuing MAO inhibitors. *Pregnancy category:* C; PB: UK; $t_{\frac{1}{2}}$: UK
Trazodone HCl (Desyrel)	A: PO: 75 mg h.s. or 50 mg t.i.d.–q.i.d.; *max:* 600 mg/d	For depression. Can be taken at bedtime to lessen dangers from sedative effect. Drowsiness, lightheadedness, orthostatic hypotension, and dry mouth might occur. Take with food to decrease GI distress. *Pregnancy category:* C; PB: 85%–95%; $t_{\frac{1}{2}}$: 5–10 h
SELECTIVE SEROTONIN REUPTAKE INHIBITORS		
Fluoxetine HCl (Prozac)	A: PO: 20 mg in a.m.; *max:* 80 mg/d in divided doses	For depression, anxiety, addictions, bulimia, and obsessive-compulsive disorder. Can cause insomnia and decrease appetite. Increase in suicide attempts have been reported; same as with other antidepressant drugs used. Usually takes 3 wk to become effective. *Pregnancy category:* B; PB: 95%; $t_{\frac{1}{2}}$: 7–9 d
Paroxetine HCl (Paxil)	A: PO: 20 mg/d in a.m.; *max:* 50 mg/d Elderly: PO: Initially: 10 mg/d; *max:* 40 mg/d	For depression and obsessive-compulsive disorders. Lower dose for the elderly and those with renal and hepatic disorders. Side effects include dizziness, insomnia, headache, nausea, dry mouth, tremors, postural hypotension. *Pregnancy category:* B; PB: 90%–95%; $t_{\frac{1}{2}}$: 21 h, elderly: 68 h
Sertraline HCl (Zoloft)	A: PO: 50 mg/d; *max:* 200 mg/d	Management of major depression disorders. Do *not* take with MAO inhibitors or tricyclics. Take with food if GI distress occurs. Urine may be pink-red-brown color. *Pregnancy category:* B; PB: 98%; $t_{\frac{1}{2}}$: 26 h
Fluvoxamine (Luvox)	A: PO: 50 mg h.s., increase by 50 mg in 5 to 7 d; *max:* 300 mg/d C 8–18 y: PO: 25 mg h.s., increase by 25 mg, *max:* 200 mg/d Elderly: decrease dose	To treat obsessive-compulsive disorder and depression. Caution: Do not use in renal or hepatic disorder. *Pregnancy category:* C; PB: UK; $t_{\frac{1}{2}}$: 13–15 h

Table continued on following page

Table 19–7 *Continued*

Antidepressants: Tricyclic Antidepressants, SSRIs and Atypical Antidepressants, and Mood Stabilizers (Antimanic)

GENERIC (BRAND)	ROUTE AND DOSAGE	USES AND CONSIDERATIONS
MONOAMINE OXIDASE INHIBITORS		
Isocarboxazid (Marplan)	A: PO: 10–20 mg/d; *max:* 60 mg/d	For depression that is refractory to tricyclics. Avoid certain foods such as cheese, beer, figs, shrimp, banana, and chocolate, and avoid drugs, e.g., tricyclic antidepressants. *Pregnancy category:* C; PB: UK; t½: UK
Phenelzine sulfate (Nardil)	A: PO: 50 mg t.i.d.; 1 mg/kg in divided doses; *max:* 90 mg/d Elderly: *max:* 45–60 mg/d	For depression. Avoid certain foods and drugs (see Isocarboxazid). *Pregnancy category:* C; PB: UK; t½: UK
Tranylcypromine sulfate (Parnate)	A: PO: 10 mg t.i.d.; *max:* 60 mg/d Elderly: *max:* 45 mg/d	Same as isocarboxazid and phenelzine sulfate.
MOOD STABILIZER		
Lithium carbonate: lithium citrate	See Chart 19–5	For bipolar affective disorder. Monitor serum lithium levels. Toxic: 2.0 mEq/L and greater. *Pregnancy category:* D; PB: UK; t½: 21–30 h

KEY: A: adult; C: child; PO: by mouth; IV: intravenous; UK: unknown; PB: protein-binding; t½: half-life; MAO: monoamine oxidase; EPS: extrapyramidal symptoms; maint: maintenance; GI: gastrointestinal; CNS: central nervous system.

sis resulting from food and drug interactions, only 1% of clients taking antidepressants are taking an MAOI. MAOIs are not the antidepressants of choice. Currently, MAOIs are usually prescribed when the client does not respond to tricyclic antidepressants or second generation antidepressants. However, MAO inhibitors are used for mild, reactive, and atypical depression (chronic anxiety, hypersomnia, and fear). MAO inhibitors and tricyclics should *not* be taken together for treating depression.

Drug and Food Interactions

Certain drugs and food interactions with MAOIs can be fatal. Any drugs that are CNS stimulants or sympathomimetics, such as vasoconstrictors, cold medications containing phenylephrine, pseudoephedrine, and phenylpropanolamine, can cause a hypertensive crisis when taken with an MAO inhibitor. Also foods that contain tyramine, such as cheese (cheddar, Swiss, bleu), cream, yogurt, coffee, chocolate, bananas, raisins, Italian green beans, liver, pickled herring, sausage, soy sauce, yeast, beer, and red wines, have sympathomimetic-like effects and can cause a hypertensive crisis (Table 19–8). These types of food and drugs *must be avoided.* Frequent blood pressure monitoring is essential when the client is taking MAO inhibitors. Client teaching regarding foods and OTC drugs to avoid is an important nursing responsibility.

Because of the danger associated with a hypertensive crisis, many psychiatrists will not prescribe MAO inhibitors for depression, unless they sense the client's

Table 19–8

Foods That Can Cause a Hypertensive Crisis When Taken with Monoamine Oxidase Inhibitors*

FOODS	EFFECTS
Cheese (cheddar, Swiss, bleu)	Sweating
	Tremors
Bananas, raisins	Bounding heart rate
Pickled foods	Increased blood pressure
Red wine, beer	Increased temperature
Cream, yogurt	
Chocolate, coffee	
Italian green beans	
Liver	
Yeast	
Soy sauce	

*Avoid taking barbiturates, tricyclic antidepressants, antihistamines, central nervous system depressants, and over-the-counter cold medications with monoamine oxidase inhibitors.

NURSING PROCESS
ANTIDEPRESSANTS

Assessment

- Assess the client's baseline vital signs (VS) and weight for future comparison.
- Check the client's liver and renal function by assessing urine output (>600 mL/d), BUN, and serum creatinine and liver enzyme levels.
- Obtain a history of episodes of depression; assess mental status and for suicidal tendencies.
- Obtain the client's drug history. CNS depressants can cause an additive effect. Antidepressants that cause anticholinergic-like symptoms are contraindicated if the client has glaucoma.
- Assess for tardive dyskinesia and neuroleptic malignant syndrome (NMS), including hyperpyrexia, muscle rigidity, tachycardia, cardiac dysrhythmias.

Potential Nursing Diagnoses

- Potential for violence and injury
- Anxiety
- Social isolation
- Ineffective coping

Planning

- Client's depression or manic-depressive behavior will be decreased.

Nursing Interventions

- Observe the client for signs and symptoms of depression: mood changes, insomnia, apathy, or lack of interest in activities.
- Check the client's vital signs. Orthostatic hypotension is common. Check for anticholinergic-like symptoms: dry mouth, increased heart rate, urinary retention, or constipation. Check weight two or three times per week.
- Monitor the client for suicidal tendencies when marked depression is present.
- If the client is taking an anticonvulsant, observe the client for seizures; antidepressants lower the seizure threshold. The anticonvulsant dose might need to be increased.
- Provide the client with a list of foods to avoid, especially with MAOIs. These include cheese, red wine, beer, liver, bananas, yogurt, sausage, and others.
- Check the client for extremely high blood pressure when taking MAO inhibitors. Sympathomimetic-like drugs and foods containing tyramine may cause a hypertensive crisis if taken with MAO inhibitors.

Nursing Process continued on following page

ability to comply with the drug and food regimen. However, this group of drugs is effective for treating depression if properly taken.

Side Effects and Adverse Reactions
Side effects of MAOIs include CNS stimulation (agitation, restlessness, insomnia), orthostatic hypotension, and anticholinergic effects.

MOOD STABILIZER: LITHIUM FOR BIPOLAR DISORDER
The last antidepressant drug to be discussed in this chapter is lithium, which is used to treat bipolar af-

fective disorder. Lithium was first used as a salt substitute in the 1940s, but because of lithium poisoning, it was banned from the market. Some refer to lithium as an antimania drug that is effective in controlling manic behavior that arises from underlying depression. It is most effective in controlling the manic phase. Lithium has a calming effect without impairing intellectual activity. It controls any evidence of flight of ideas and hyperactivity. If the person stops taking lithium, manic behavior may return.

Lithium is an inexpensive drug, but it has to be closely monitored. Lithium has a narrow therapeutic serum range, 0.8 to 1.5 mEq/L. Serum lithium levels

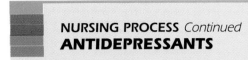

NURSING PROCESS *Continued*
ANTIDEPRESSANTS

Client Teaching

General

- Instruct the client to take the medication as prescribed. Compliance is important.
- Inform the client that the full effectiveness of the drug may not be evident until 1 to 2 wk after the start of therapy.
- Encourage the client to keep medical appointments.
- Instruct the client not to consume alcohol or any CNS depressants due to their addictive effect.
- Instruct the client not to drive or be involved in potentially dangerous mechanical activity until stabilization of drug dose has been established.
- Instruct the client not to abruptly stop taking the drug. Drug dose should be gradually decreased.
- Encourage the client who is planning pregnancy to consult with the health care provider about possible teratogenic effects of the drug on the fetus.
- Take with food if GI distress occurs.

Side Effects

- Advise the client that antidepressants may be taken at bedtime to decrease the dangers from the sedative effect. Have client check with the health care provider. Transient side effects include nausea, drowsiness, headaches, and nervousness.

Cultural Considerations

- If Asian client is taking an antipsychotic, such as TCA or lithium, the drug dose may need to be decreased. Explanation may be needed.
- Explain to the Hispanic client that the dose for the antidepressant drug may be lower than is required for other cultural groups.

Evaluation

- Evaluate the effectiveness of the drug therapy. The client's depression is controlled or has ceased.

---

greater than 1.5 to 2.0 mEq/L are toxic. The serum lithium level should be monitored biweekly until the therapeutic level has been obtained and then monitored monthly on the maintenance dose. Serum sodium levels also need to be monitored because lithium tends to deplete sodium. Use lithium with caution, if at all, in clients taking diuretics. Chart 19–5 lists the pharmacologic behavior of lithium.

Pharmacokinetics

More than 95% of the lithium is absorbed through the GI tract. The average half-life of lithium is 24 h; however, in the older adult, the half-life can be up to 36 h. Because of its long half-life, cumulative drug action may result. Lithium is metabolized by the liver and most of the drug is excreted unchanged in the urine.

Pharmacodynamics

Lithium is prescribed mostly for the manic phase of manic-depressive illness. The onset of action is fast, but the client may not receive the desired effect for 5 to 6 days. Increased sodium intake increases renal excretion, so the sodium intake needs to be closely monitored. Increased urine output can result in body fluid loss and dehydration.

Table 19–7 lists the mood stabilizer lithium—its dosage, uses, and considerations. Anticonvulsants such as tegretol and valproic acid have been used in place of lithium. A new agent, depakote, will be used to treat bipolar disorder.

Side Effects and Adverse Reactions

Many side effects from taking lithium can be annoying to the client, such as dry mouth, thirst, increased

Chart 19–5. Mood Stabilizer: Lithium

MOOD STABILIZER (ANTIMANIC)

Assessment and Planning

Drug Name

Lithium carbonate
  (Eskalith, Lithane, Lithonate, Lithobid), ✥
  Carbolith, Lithizine
Pregnancy Category: D

Dosage

A: PO: 300–600 mg t.i.d.; *maint:* 300 mg t.i.d.–
q.i.d.; *max:* 2.4 g/d
Elderly: lower dosage
TDR: 0.5–1.5 mEq/L

Contraindications

Liver and renal disease, pregnancy, lactation, severe cardiovascular disease, severe dehydration, brain tumor or damage, sodium depletion, children <12 y
Caution: Thyroid disease

Drug-Lab-Food Interactions

Drug: May *increase* lithium level with thiazide diuretics, methyldopa, haloperidol, NSAIDs, antidepressants, carbamazepine, theophylline, aminophylline, sodium bicarbonate, phenothiazines
Food: *Increase* sodium intake; lithium may cause sodium depletion
Lab: *Increase* urine and blood glucose, protein

Interventions

Pharmacokinetics

Absorption: PO: well absorbed
Distribution: PB: UK
Metabolism: t½: 21–30 h; >36 h with renal impairment or in elderly
Excretion: 98% in urine, mostly unchanged

Pharmacodynamics

Antimanic effects:
PO: Onset: 5–7 d
       Peak: 10–21 d
       Duration: days
PO SR: Peak: 5–7 d

Evaluation

Therapeutic Effects/Uses

To treat bipolar manic-depressive psychosis, manic episodes.

Mode of Action: Alteration of ion transport in muscle and nerve cells; increased receptor sensitivity to serotonin.

Side Effects

Headache, lethargy, drowsiness, dizziness, tremors, slurred speech, dry mouth, anorexia, vomiting, diarrhea, polyuria, hypotension, abdominal pain, muscle weakness, restlessness

Adverse Reactions

Urinary incontinence, clonic movements, stupor, azotemia, leukocytosis, nephrotoxicity
Life-threatening: Cardiac dysrhythmias, circulatory collapse

NURSING PROCESS

KEY: A: adult; C: child; PO: by mouth; PB: protein-binding; t½: half-life; UK: unknown; NSAID: nonsteroidal antiinflammatory drug; TDR: therapeutic drug range; ✥: Canadian drug names.

urination (loss of water and sodium), weight gain, bloated feeling, metallic taste, and edema of the hands and ankles. In pregnancy, lithium may have teratogenic effects in the unborn.

Lithium and NSAIDs should not be given together on a continuous basis and should not be prescribed for clients who have a cardiac sick sinus syndrome. If the client has been taking lithium for a long period of time, the laboratory tests to determine thyroid function should be closely monitored.

Table 19–9 lists some drugs and drug classes that may cause psychiatric symptoms.

Text continued on page 362

NURSING PROCESS
MOOD STABILIZER: LITHIUM

Assessment

- Assess for suicidal ideation.
- Assess the client's baseline vital signs (VS) for future comparison.
- Assess client's neurologic status, including gait, level of consciousness, reflexes, and tremors.
- Check the client's hepatic and renal function by assessing urine output (>600 mL/d), whether blood urea nitrogen (BUN), and serum creatinine and liver enzyme levels are within normal range. Assess for toxicity. Draw weekly blood levels initially and then every 1 to 2 mo. Therapeutic serum levels for acute mania are 1.0 to 1.5 mEq/L; for maintenance, levels are 0.6 to 1.2 mEq/L. Signs and symptoms of toxicity at serum levels of 1.5 to 2.0 mEq/L are persistent nausea and vomiting, severe diarrhea, ataxia, blurred vision, and tinnitus; at 2.0 to 3.5 mEq/L, signs and symptoms are excessive output of dilute urine, increasing tremors, muscular irritability, psychomotor retardation, mental confusion, and giddiness; and at >3.5 mEq/L, levels are life threatening and may result in impaired consciousness, nystagmus, seizures, coma, oliguria/anuria, cardiac dysrhythmias, myocardial infarction, and cardiovascular collapse. Withhold medications and notify health care provider immediately if any of these occur.
- Obtain a history of episodes of depression or manic-depressive behavior.
- Obtain the client's drug history. Diuretics, NSAIDs (e.g., ibuprofen), tetracyclines, methyldopa, and probenecid decrease renal clearance of lithium, thus causing lithium accumulation.

Potential Nursing Diagnoses

- Potential for injury or violence related to excessive hyperactivity
- Ineffective individual coping
- Noncompliance

Planning

- Client's manic-depressive behavior will be decreased.

Nursing Interventions

- Observe the client for signs and symptoms of depression: mood changes, insomnia, apathy, or lack of interest in activities.
- Check the client's vital signs. Orthostatic hypotension is common.
- When drawing blood to check for lithium levels, draw samples immediately before the next dose (8 to 12 h after the previous dose). Monitor for signs of lithium toxicity. Report high (>1.5 mEq/L) or toxic (>2.0 mEq/L) serum lithium levels immediately to the health care provider.
- Monitor client for suicidal tendencies when marked depression is present.
- Monitor the client's urine output and body weight. Fluid volume deficit may occur as a result of polyuria.
- Observe the client for fine and gross motor tremors and presence of slurred speech, which are signs of adverse reaction.
- Check the client's cardiac status. Loss of fluids and electrolytes may cause cardiac dysrhythmias.
- Monitor the client's serum electrolytes. Report abnormal findings.

Client Teaching

General

- Instruct the client to take lithium as prescribed. Emphasize the importance of adherence to the therapy, laboratory tests, and follow-up visits with the health care provider. If lithium is stopped, manic symptoms will reappear.

Nursing Process continued on following page

NURSING PROCESS *Continued*
MOOD STABILIZER: LITHIUM

- Encourage the client to keep medical appointments. Have client check with the health care provider before taking OTC preparations.
- Instruct the client not to drive a motor vehicle or be involved in potentially dangerous mechanical activity until stable lithium level is established.
- Advise the client to maintain adequate fluid intake: 2 to 3 L/d initially and 1 to 2 L/d maintenance. Fluid intake should increase in hot weather.
- Instruct the client to take the lithium with meals to decrease gastric irritation.
- Inform the client that the effectiveness of the drug may not be evident until 1 to 2 wk after the start of therapy. Compliance in taking the prescribed lithium doses on a daily basis is a major problem with bipolar clients. When the client has a period of emotional stability, he or she does not believe that the drug is needed; thus, the client stops taking the lithium.
- Encourage the client who is planning pregnancy to consult with the health care provider about possible teratogenic effects of the drug on the fetus, especially during the first 3 months.
- Encourage the client to wear or carry an ID tag or bracelet indicating the drug taken.

Diet
- Advise the client to avoid caffeine products (coffee, tea, or colas) because they can aggravate the manic phase of the bipolar disorder.
- Instruct the client to maintain adequate sodium intake and to avoid crash diets that affect physical and mental health.

Side Effects
- Instruct the client to contact the health care provider for early symptoms of toxicity: diarrhea, drowsiness, loss of appetite, muscle weakness, nausea, vomiting, slurred speech, trembling; and for late symptoms of toxicity: blurred vision, confusion, increased urination, convulsions, severe trembling, and unsteadiness.

Evaluation

- Evaluate the effectiveness of the drug therapy. The client is free of bipolar behavior.
- Client verbalizes understanding of symptoms of toxicity.
- Client demonstrates a subsiding or resolution of the symptoms.

Table 19–9
Drugs that Cause Psychiatric Symptoms

DRUG	REACTIONS	COMMENTS
Acyclovir (*Zovirax*)	Hallucinations, fearfulness, confusion, insomnia, hyperacusis, paranoia, depression	At high doses, particularly in patients with chronic renal failure
Alprazolam (*Xanax*)	See Benzodiazepines	
Amantadine (*Symmetrel**)	Illusions, visual hallucinations, delusions	Risk increases with duration of therapy; more common in elderly
Amitriptyline (*Elavil**)	See Antidepressants, tricyclic	
Amphetamine-like drugs	Bizarre behavior, hallucinations, paranoia, agitation, anxiety, manic symptoms Depression	Usually with overdose or abuse; can occur with inhaler abuse On withdrawal
Anabolic steroids	Psychosis, mania, depression, anxiety, aggressiveness, paranoia	Most reports based on abuse

Table continued on following page

Table 19–9 *Continued*
Drugs that Cause Psychiatric Symptoms

DRUG	REACTIONS	COMMENTS
Anticholinergics and atropine	Confusion, memory loss, disorientation, depersonalization, delirium, auditory and visual hallucinations, fear, paranoia, agitation, bizarre behavior	More frequent in elderly and children with high doses; has occurred with transdermal scopolamine
	Sudden incoherent speech, delirium with high fever, flushed dry skin, hallucinations, retrograde amnesia	From eye drops, particularly when mistaken for nose drops
Anticonvulsants	Agitation, confusion, delirium, depression psychosis, aggression, mania, toxic encephalopathy, nightmares	Usually with high doses or high plasma concentrations
Antidepressants, tricyclic	Mania or hypomania, delirium, hallucinations, paranoia	Patients with bipolar disorder at highest risk for mania; anticholinergic effects may cause delirium in elderly
Antihistamine H_1-blockers	Hallucinations	Especially with overdosage of sedating antihistamines
Asparaginase (*Elspar*)	Confusion, depression, paranoia	May occur frequently
Atropine	See Anticholinergics and atropine	
Baclofen (*Lioresal**)	Hallucinations, paranoia, nightmares, mania, depression, anxiety, confusion	Sometimes with high doses, but usually after sudden withdrawal
Barbiturates	Excitement, hyperactivity, visual hallucinations, depression, delirium-tremens-like syndrome	Especially in children and the elderly, or on withdrawal
Benzodiazepines	Rage, hostility, paranoia, hallucinations, delirium, depression, nightmares, anterograde amnesia, mania	During treatment or on withdrawal; may be more common in elderly
Beta-adrenergic blockers	Depression, psychosis, delirium, anxiety, nightmares, hallucinations	With oral or ophthalmic preparations; incidence of depression may be overestimated
Bromocriptine (*Parlodel*)	Mania, delusions, hallucinations, paranoia, aggressive behavior, schizophrenic relapse, depression, anxiety	Not dose-related; may persist weeks after stopping drug
Buprenorphine (*Buprenex*)	See Narcotics	
Bupropion (*Wellbutrin; Zyban*)	Psychosis, agitation, anxiety, nightmares, mania	Agitation, anxiety most common
Buspirone (*BuSpar*)	Vivid dreams, delirium, mania, panic attack	In a few patients
Caffeine	Anxiety, confusion, psychotic symptoms	With excessive doses
Calcium-channel blockers	Depression	Several reports
Captopril (*Capoten**)	Mania, anxiety, hallucinations	Several cases
Carbamazepine (*Tegretol**)	See Anticonvulsants	
Cephalosporins	Euphoria, delusions, depersonalization, illusions	Renal disease is a risk factor
Chlorambucil (*Leukeran*)	Hallucinations, lethargy, seizures, stupor, coma	In 5 of 6 patients at high dosage
Chloroquine (*Aralen**)	Confusion, delusions, hallucinations, mania	Several reports
Cimetidine (*Tagamet*)	See Histamine H_2-receptor antagonists	
Ciprofloxacin (*Cipro*)	See Fluoroquinolone antibiotics	
Clarithromycin (*Biaxin*)	Mania	Reported in two patients
Clomipramine (*Anafranil*)	See Antidepressants, tricyclic	
Clonazepam (*Klonopin*)	See Benzodiazepines	
Conidine (*Catapres**)	Depression, delirium, psychosis	May resolve with continued use
Clorazepate (*Tranxene**)	See Benzodiazepines	

Table 19–9 *Continued*
Drugs that Cause Psychiatric Symptoms

DRUG	REACTIONS	COMMENTS
Clozapine (*Clozaril*)	Delirium; psychosis following abrupt withdrawal	Less with slow dose titration
Cocaine	Anxiety, agitation, psychosis	Can occur with topical use
Codeine	See Narcotics	
Corticosteroids (prednisone, cortisone, ACTH, others)	Psychosis, mania, depression	1%–3% incidence, may be dose-related; can occur on withdrawal
Corticosteroids, inhaled	Hyperactivity, aggressiveness, disinhibition	Several cases
Cycloserine (*Seromycin**)	Agitation, depression, psychosis, anxiety	Multiple reports
Cytarabine (*Cytosar-U**)	Confusion	Especially with high doses
Dapsone	Insomnia, agitation, hallucinations, mania, depression	Several reports; may occur even with low doses
Deet (*Off**)	Mania, hallucinations	With excessive or prolonged use
Desipramine (*Norpramin**)	See Antidepressants, tricyclic	
Diazepam (*Valium**)	See Benzodiazepines	
Digitalis glycosides	Delirium, depression, decreased libido, psychosis, mania, visual hallucinations	Dose-dependent; elderly at higher risk
Diltiazem (*Cardizem**)	See Calcium-channel blockers	
Disopyramide (*Norpace**)	Hallucinations, paranoia, panic, depression	Within 24–48 hours after starting
Disulfiram (*Antabuse**)	Catatonia, delirium, depression, psychosis	Not related to alcohol reactions
Dronabinol (*Marinol*)	Anxiety, disorientation, psychosis	Most disturbing in the elderly
Erythropoietin (*Epogen; Procrit*)	Visual hallucinations	Reported in dialysis patients
Estrogens	Panic attacks, depression	Several reports
Famotidine (*Pepcid*)	See Histamine H_2-receptor antagonists	
Fenfluramine (*Pondimin*)	See Amphetamine-like drugs	
Fluoroquinolone antibiotics	Psychosis, agitation, depression, hallucinations, paranoia, Tourette-like syndrome	Most reports of psychosis with ciprofloxacin
Fluoxetine (*Prozac*)	See Selective serotonin reuptake inhibitors	
Fluvoxamine (*Luvox*)	See Selective serotonin reuptake inhibitors	
Ganciclovir (*Cytovene*)	Psychosis, delirium	Several cases
Histamine H_2-receptor antagonists	Delirium, confusion, psychosis, mania, aggressiveness, decreased libido, depression	Especially elderly and seriously ill
HMG-CoA reductase inhibitors ("statins")	Anxiety, depression, obsessions, delusions	Several case reports
Ibuprofen (*Motrin**)	See Nonsteroidal anti-inflammatory drugs	
Ifosfamide (*Ifex*)	Encephalopathy, hallucinations, emotional lability	Several cases
Indomethacin (*Indocin**)	See Nonsteroidal anti-inflammatory drugs	
Interferon alfa (*Roferon-A; Intron A*)	Irritability, emotional lability, depression, agitation, paranoia	Depression has been documented in clinical trials
Interleukin-2	Hallucinations, disorientation	In 2% of one series, but may have been related to brain metastases
Isoniazid (*INH**)	Psychosis, hallucinations	Several reports
Isotretinoin (*Accutane*)	Depression, suicidality	Several reports
Ketamine (*Ketalar**)	Nightmares, hallucinations, crying, delirium	Acute; frequent with usual doses
Levodopa (*Dopar**)	Hallucinations, delusions, mania, depression, anxiety, panic attacks, confusion	Dose-dependent; anxiety may occur in "off" phase
Lidocaine (*Xylocaine**)	See Procaine derivatives	

Table continued on following page

Table 19–9 *Continued*
Drugs that Cause Psychiatric Symptoms

DRUG	REACTIONS	COMMENTS
Lorazepam (*Ativan**)	See Benzodiazepines	
Lovastatin (*Mevacor*)	See HMG-CoA reductase inhibitors	
Maprotiline (*Ludiomil**)	Hallucinations, agitation, disorientation	Several reports
Mefloquine (*Lariam*)	Encephalopathy, depression, confusion, psychosis, hallucinations, aggression, agitation, anxiety	In 0.5% with treatment and 1/15,000 with prophylaxis
Meperidine (*Demerol**)	See Narcotics	
Methadone (*Dolophine**)	See Narcotics	
Methandrostenolone (*Dianabol*)	See Anabolic steroids	
Methyldopa (*Aldomet**)	Depression, amnesia, nightmares, psychosis	Incidence of depression may be overestimated
Methylphenidate (*Ritalin**)	Hallucinations, anxiety, encephalopathy	In children and adults
Methyltestosterone	See Anabolic steroids	
Methysergide (*Sansert*)	Depersonalization, hallucinations, agitation	Several reports
Metoclopramide (*Reglan**)	Depression, anxiety, mania	Several case reports
Metrizamide (*Amipaque*)	Confusion, hallucinations, depression, anxiety	May be prolonged
Metronidazole (*Flagyl**)	Depression, agitation, uncontrollable crying, disorientation, hallucinations	Two cases with oral use; hallucinations with high IV dose in one man
Monoamine oxidase inhibitors	Mania or hypomania	
Morphine	See Narcotics	
Nalorphine	See Narcotics	
Naproxen (*Anaprox; Naprosyn*)	See Nonsteroidal anti-inflammatory drugs	
Narcotics	Nightmares, anxiety, agitation, euphoria, dysphoria, depression, paranoia, hallucinations	Usually with high doses; also occurs with intrathecal morphine
Nifedipine (*Procardia**)	See Calcium-channel blockers	
Nizatidine (*Axid*)	See Antihistamine H_2-receptor antagonists	
Nonsteroidal anti-inflammatory drugs	Depression, paranoia, psychosis	Uncommon
Norfloxacin (*Noroxin*)	See Fluoroquinolone antibiotics	
Nortriptyline (*Aventyl**)	See Antidepressants, tricyclic	
Ofloxacin (*Floxin*)	See Fluoroquinolone antibiotics	
Ondansetron (*Zofran*)	Panic attack, dysphoria	Two cases
Oxandrolone (*Anavar*)	See Anabolic steroids	
Oxymetholone (*Anadrol*)	See Anabolic steroids	
Paroxetine (*Paxil*)	See Selective serotonin reuptake inhibitors	
Penicillin G procaine	See Procaine derivatives	
Pentazocine (*Talwin*)	See Narcotics	
Pergolide (*Permax*)	Hallucinations, paranoia, confusion, anxiety, depression	During treatment or on withdrawal
Phenelzine (*Nardil*)	See Monoamine oxidase inhibitors	
Phentermine (*Fastin**)	See Amphetamine-like drugs	
Phenylpropanolamine (*Dexatrim**)	Psychosis, mania, irritability, aggressiveness, hallucinations, confusion, anxiety, depression	Usually in combination products; children and adults with history of mood or psychotic disorders at higher risk

Table 19–9 *Continued*
Drugs that Cause Psychiatric Symptoms

DRUG	REACTIONS	COMMENTS
Phenytoin (*Dilantin**)	See Anticonvulsants	
Pilocarpine (*Pilocar**)	Confusion, agitation, memory loss	Topical ocular use especially in elderly and demented patients
Pravastatin (*Pravachol*)	See HMG-CoA reductase inhibitors	
Primidone (*Mysoline**)	See Anticonvulsants	
Procaine derivatives	Fear of imminent death, hallucinations, illusions, agitation, depersonalization	Probably due to procaine
Progestins, implanted (*Norplant*)	Major depression, panic disorder	Two cases
Propafenone (*Rythmol*)	Agitation, delusions, disorientation, mania, paranoia	Several reports
Propoxyphene (*Darvon**)	See Narcotics	
Propranolol (*Inderal**)	See Beta-adrenergic blockers	
Pseudoephedrine (in *Actifed**)	Hallucinations, paranoia, bipolar disorder	Reported with usual dosage in children and with overuse in one adult
Quinidine	Confusion, agitation, psychosis	Usually dose-related
Ranitidine (*Zantac*)	See Histamine H_2-receptor antagonists	
Salicylates	Agitation, confusion, hallucinations, paranoia	Chronic intoxication
Scopolamine	See Anticholinergics and atropine	
Selective serotonin reuptake inhibitors	Mania; hypomania, aggression or impulsivity on withdrawal	Incidence of mania estimated at 1% in depressed patients without bipolar disorder
Selegiline (*Eldepryl*)	Hallucinations, mania, nightmares, behavioral disturbance, confusion, hypersexuality, delusions	Several reports
Simvastatin (*Zocor*)	See HMG-CoA reductase inhibitors	
Sulfonamides	Confusion, disorientation, depression, euphoria, hallucinations	Several reports
Sulindac (*Clinoril**)	See Nonsteroidal anti-inflammatory drugs	
Sumatriptan (*Imitrex*)	Panic-like somatic symptoms	Especially with history of anxiety
Theophylline	Withdrawal, mutism, hyperactivity, anxiety, mania	With high serum concentrations
Thiabendazole (*Mintezol*)	Psychosis	Occasional
Thiazide diuretics	Depression, suicidal ideation	After weeks' to months' use
Tizanidine (*Zanaflex*)	Hallucinations	Visual hallucinations or delusions reported in 3% of patients
Tranylcypromine (*Parnate*)	See Monoamine oxidase inhibitors	
Trazodone (*Desyrel**)	Delirium, hallucinations, paranoia, mania	Several reports
Triazolam (*Halcion*)	See Benzodiazepines	
Trihexyphenidyl (*Artane**)	See Atropine and anticholinergics	
Trimethoprim-sulfamethoxazole (*Bactrim**)	Delirium, psychosis	Several reports
Valproic acid (*Depakene**)	See Anticonvulsants	
Verapamil (*Isoptin**)	See Calcium-channel blockers	
Vinblastine (*Velban**)	Depression, anxiety	May occur commonly
Vincristine (*Oncovin**)	Hallucinations	May be dose-related
Zolpidem (*Ambien*)	Psychosis, hallucinations, sensory distortions	Women may be at greater risk; higher doses may increase risk

Also available with other brand names or generically.
Adapted from The Medical Letter on Drugs and Therapeutics, 40 (1020), 1998.

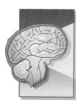

Critical Thinking in Action

F. S., 75 years old, is receiving risperidone, 3 mg b.i.d., to control a psychotic disorder. She has taken the drug for 6 months. She has become agitated and is complaining of insomnia.

1. What is the relation between F. S.'s drug dose and her complaints? Explain.
2. What further assessment should be made concerning F. S. and the drug regimen? How does the risperidone compare with other antipsychotics?

S. T., 37 years old, is receiving fluoxetine (Prozac) for depression.

1. What are the similarities and differences between fluoxetine and TCAs?
2. What needs to be included in teaching S. T. about fluoxetine?

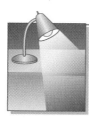

Study Questions

1. Your client is taking the phenothiazine promazine (Sparine). What side effects associated with phenothiazines are similar to the side effects from anticholinergics and pseudoparkinsonism? Why should the blood pressure be closely monitored? What do you tell the client about the color of the urine?

2. What group of drugs has antiemetic properties? What is the route of administration for a client who is vomiting?

3. Haloperidol (Haldol) is a drug frequently used in psychiatry. How is it different from other antipsychotics?

4. What is the major group of anxiolytics called? A client receiving a drug from this category should be observed for what side effects? Client teaching is important regarding the use of alcohol or OTC drugs and discontinuing the anxiolytic. Why?

5. The client is receiving imipramine hydrochloride (Tofranil). Imipramine is from what drug category? Why do some clients take the drug at bed-time?

6. The client is taking tranylcypromine sulfate (Parnate), an MAO inhibitor. What should the nurse teach the client regarding food and drugs? Why?

7. Lithium is effective for what type of psychiatric disorder? What is the therapeutic serum lithium level? Why should the urinary output and vital signs be closely monitored?

Autonomic Nervous System

20

Outline

Objectives

- Differentiate between the autonomic and the somatic nervous systems, and between the sympathetic and parasympathetic nervous systems.
- Explain how drugs that mimic and block the sympathetic and parasympathetic nervous systems have opposite effects and similar effects on organ tissue.
- List terms that identify sympathetic stimulants and depressants, and parasympathetic stimulants and depressants.

Terms

acetylcholine

adrenaline

adrenergic

autonomic nervous system (ANS)

central nervous system (CNS)

cholinergic

neurotransmitter

norepinephrine

parasympathetic nervous system

parasympatholytics

parasympathomimetics

peripheral nervous system (PNS)

sympathetic nervous system

sympatholytics

sympathomimetics

INTRODUCTION

The **central nervous system (CNS),** which consists of the brain and spinal cord and is the primary nervous system of the body, was previously discussed in Unit IV. The **peripheral nervous system (PNS),** located outside the brain and spinal cord, is made up of two divisions; the autonomic and the somatic. After interpretation by the CNS, the PNS receives stimuli and initiates responses to those stimuli.

The **autonomic nervous system (ANS),** also called the visceral system, acts on smooth muscles and glands. Its functions include control and regulation of the heart, respiratory system, gastrointestinal (GI) tract, bladder, eyes, and glands. The ANS innervates (acts on) smooth muscles, but it is an involuntary nervous system over which a person has little or no control. We breathe, our heart beats, and peristalsis occurs without our realizing it. However, unlike the autonomic nervous system, the somatic nervous system is a voluntary system that innervates skeletal muscles, over which we do have control.

The two sets of neurons in the autonomic component of the peripheral nervous system are (1) the afferent, or sensory, neurons, and (2) the efferent, or motor, neurons. The afferent neurons send impulses to the CNS, where they are interpreted. The efferent neurons receive the impulses (information) from the brain and transmit those impulses through the spinal cord to the effector organ cells. The efferent pathways in the autonomic nervous system are divided into two branches: the sympathetic and the parasympathetic nerves, which are collectively called the sympathetic nervous system, and the parasympathetic nervous system (Fig. 20–1).

The sympathetic nervous system and the parasympathetic nervous system act on the same organs but produce opposite responses in order to provide homeostasis (balance) (Fig. 20–2). Drugs act on the sympathetic and parasympathetic nervous systems by either stimulating or depressing responses.

SYMPATHETIC NERVOUS SYSTEM

The **sympathetic nervous system** is also referred to as the **adrenergic** system because, at one time, it was believed that **adrenaline** was the **neurotransmitter** that innervates the smooth muscle. The neurotransmitter is, however, **norepinephrine.** Drugs that mimic the effect of norepinephrine are called adrenergic drugs, **sympathomimetics,** or adrenomimetics. They are also known as **adrenergic agonists** because they *initiate* a response at the adrenergic receptor sites. Drugs that block the effect of norepinephrine are called **adrenergic blockers, sympatholytics,** or adrenolytics. These are known as adrenergic antagonists because they *prevent* a response at the receptor sites.

The adrenergic receptor organ cells are of four types: alpha$_1$, alpha$_2$, beta$_1$, and beta$_2$ (Fig. 20–3). Norepinephrine is released from the terminal nerve ending and stimulates the cell receptors to produce a response.

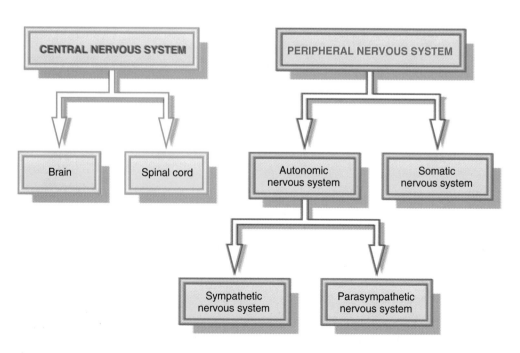

Figure 20–1

Subdivisions of the peripheral nervous system.

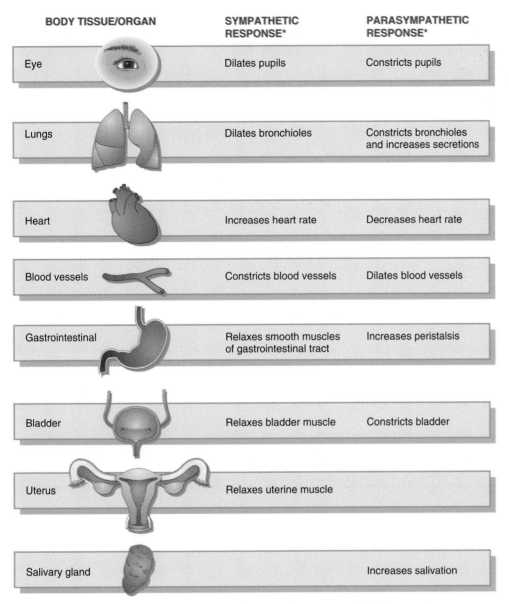

BODY TISSUE/ORGAN	SYMPATHETIC RESPONSE*	PARASYMPATHETIC RESPONSE*
Eye	Dilates pupils	Constricts pupils
Lungs	Dilates bronchioles	Constricts bronchioles and increases secretions
Heart	Increases heart rate	Decreases heart rate
Blood vessels	Constricts blood vessels	Dilates blood vessels
Gastrointestinal	Relaxes smooth muscles of gastrointestinal tract	Increases peristalsis
Bladder	Relaxes bladder muscle	Constricts bladder
Uterus	Relaxes uterine muscle	
Salivary gland		Increases salivation

Figure 20–2
Sympathetic and parasympathetic effects on body tissues.

*The sympathetic and parasympathetic nervous systems have opposite responses on body tissues and organs.

PARASYMPATHETIC NERVOUS SYSTEM

The **parasympathetic nervous system** is referred to as the **cholinergic** system because the neurotransmitter at the end of the neuron that innervates the muscle is **acetylcholine.** Drugs that mimic acetylcholine are called **cholinergic drugs,** or **parasympathomimetics.** They are **cholinergic agonists** because they *initiate* a cholinergic response; conversely, drugs that block the effect of acetylcholine are called **anticholinergic,** or **parasympatholytics.** They are also known as **cholinergic antagonists** because they *inhibit* the effect of acetylcholine on the organ.

The cholinergic receptors at organ cells are either nicotinic or muscarinic, meaning that they are stimulated by the alkaloids nicotine and muscarine, respectively (see Fig. 20–3). Acetylcholine stimulates the receptor cells to produce a response, but the enzyme, acetylcholinesterase, may inactivate acetylcholine before it reaches the receptor cell.

Drugs that mimic the neurotransmitters norepinephrine and acetylcholine produce responses opposite to each other in the same organ. For example, an adrenergic drug (sympathomimetic) increases the heart rate, whereas a cholinergic drug (parasympathomimetic) decreases the heart rate (see Fig. 20–2). However, a drug that mimics the sympathetic ner-

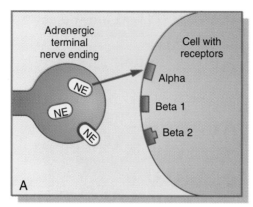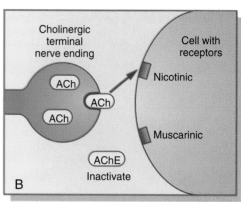

Figure 20–3
Sympathetic and parasympathetic transmitters and receptors. NE: norepinephrine; Ach: acetylcholine; AchE: acetylcholinesterase.

vous system and a drug that blocks the parasympathetic nervous system can cause similar responses in the organ; for instance, the sympathomimetic and the parasympatholytic drugs both increase the heart rate. The adrenergic blocker and the cholinergic drug both decrease heart rate.

Many name classifications are given to drugs that mimic or block both the sympathetic nervous system and the parasympathetic nervous system (Table 20–1). The nurse needs to become familiar with these names. Drug names and specific actions are discussed in Chapters 21 and 22.

Table 20–1
Autonomic Nervous Systems: Sympathetic and Parasympathetic

SYMPATHETIC STIMULANTS	PARASYMPATHETIC STIMULANTS
	DIRECT-ACTING
Sympathomimetics (adrenergics, adrenomimetics, or adrenergic agonists) *Action:* Increase blood pressure Increase pulse rate Relax bronchioles Dilate pupils of eyes Uterine relaxation Increase blood sugar	*Parasympathomimetics (cholinergics, or cholinergic agonists)* *Action:* Decrease blood pressure Decrease pulse rate Constrict bronchioles Constrict pupils of eyes Increase urinary contraction Increase peristalsis
	INDIRECT-ACTING
	Cholinesterase Inhibitors (anticholinesterase) *Action:* Increase muscle tone
SYMPATHETIC DEPRESSANTS	**PARASYMPATHETIC DEPRESSANTS**
Sympatholytics (adrenergic blockers, adrenolytics, or adrenergic antagonists) *Action:* Decrease blood pressure Decrease pulse rate Constrict bronchioles	*Parasympatholytics (anticholinergics, cholinergic antagonists, or antispasmodics)* *Action:* Increase pulse rate Decrease mucus secretions Decrease gastrointestinal motility Increase urinary retention Dilate pupils of eyes

Opposite responses on organ tissue are caused by sympathomimetics and parasympathomimetics, and by sympatholytics and parasympatholytics. Sympathomimetics and parasympatholytics cause similar organ responses as do sympatholytics and parasympathomimetics.

SUMMARY

There are two subdivisions of the autonomic nervous system: the sympathetic and the parasympathetic nervous systems. These nervous systems have opposite effects on organ tissues. Drugs can either stimulate or block both of these nervous systems through their receptors. Table 20–2 lists the organ responses from drugs that act on these systems.

Table 20–2
Sympathetic and Parasympathetic Responses to Drugs

SYMPATHETIC	PARA-SYMPATHETIC	RESPONSE
Sympathomimetic	Para-sympathomimetic	Opposite response
Sympatholytic	Para-sympatholytic	Opposite response
Sympathomimetic	Para-sympatholytic	Similar response
Sympatholytic	Para-sympathomimetic	Similar response

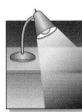

Study Questions

1. What are the divisions of the central nervous system and the peripheral nervous system? What is their interrelationship?

2. What does the autonomic nervous system control and regulate? What does the somatic nervous system control and regulate?

3. Drugs that mimic and block the sympathetic and parasympathetic nervous systems have opposite and similar effects on organ tissue. Explain this phenomenon.

4. What terms are used to classify sympathetic stimulants and depressants? What are their actions on the body?

5. What terms are used to classify parasympathetic stimulants and depressants? What are their actions on the body?

21 Adrenergics and Adrenergic Blockers

Outline

Objectives

- Name the adrenergic receptors and give examples of their major responses.
- Describe the difference between selective adrenergic drugs and nonselective drugs.
- Give drug names of selective and nonselective adrenergic drugs.
- List major side effects of adrenergic drugs.
- Explain nursing interventions, including client teaching, associated with adrenergic drugs.
- List examples of drugs that are selective and nonselective adrenergic blockers.
- Describe the uses of alpha blockers and beta blockers.
- List the general side effects of adrenergic blockers.
- Describe nursing interventions, including client teaching, associated with adrenergic blockers.

Terms

adrenergic blockers
adrenergic neuron blockers
adrenergic receptors
alpha blockers

beta blockers
catecholamines
nonselectivity

selectivity
sympathomimetics
sympatholytics

Table 21–1
Effects of Adrenergics at Receptors

RECEPTOR	PHYSIOLOGIC RESPONSES
Alpha$_1$	Increases force of contraction of heart. Vasoconstriction: increases blood pressure. Mydriasis: dilates pupils of the eyes. Glandular (salivary): decreases secretion. Bladder and prostate: capsule increases contraction and ejaculation.
Alpha$_2$	Inhibits the release of norepinephrine, dilates blood vessels, and produces hypotension; decreases gastrointestinal motility and tone.
Beta$_1$	Increases heart rate and force of contraction; increases renin secretion, which increases blood pressure.
Beta$_2$	Dilates the bronchioles; promotes gastrointestinal and uterine relaxation; promotes increase in blood sugar through glycogenolysis in the liver; increases blood flow in the skeletal muscles.

INTRODUCTION

Two groups of drugs that affect the sympathetic nervous system, the adrenergics (**sympathomimetics** or **adrenomimetics**) and the adrenergic blockers (**sympatholytics** or **adrenolytics**) are discussed in this chapter. Lists of adrenergic drugs and adrenergic blockers, their dosages, and uses are also included. For explanation of the autonomic nervous system (adrenergic and cholinergic), see Chapter 20.

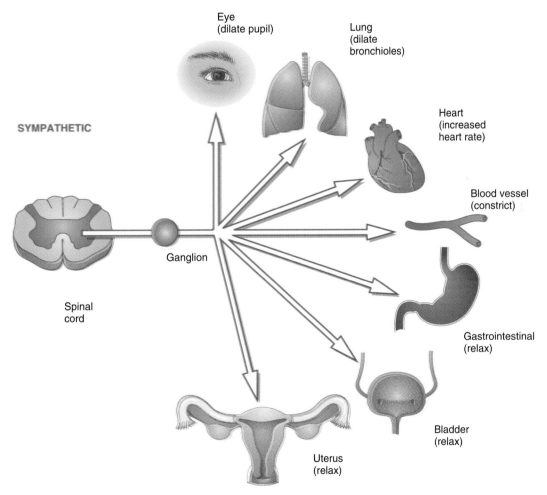

Figure 21–1

Sympathetic responses. Stimulation of the sympathetic nervous system or use of sympathomimetic (adrenergic) drugs can cause the pupils and bronchioles to dilate, the heart rate to increase, blood vessels to constrict, and the muscles of the gastrointestinal tract, bladder, and uterus to relax, decreasing contractions.

ADRENERGICS

Drugs that stimulate the sympathetic nervous system are called adrenergics, adrenergic agonists, sympathomimetics, or adrenomimetics because they mimic the sympathetic neurotransmitters (norepinephrine and epinephrine). They act on one or more **adrenergic receptor** sites located on the cells of smooth muscles, such as the heart, walls of the bronchioles, gastrointestinal (GI) tract, urinary bladder, and ciliary muscle of the eye. There are many adrenergic recep-

tors. The four main receptors are alpha$_1$, alpha$_2$, beta$_1$, and beta$_2$, which mediate the major responses described in Table 21–1 and illustrated in Figure 21–1.

The alpha-adrenergic receptors are located in the vascular tissues (vessels) of smooth muscles. When the **alpha$_1$-receptor** is stimulated, the arterioles and venules are constricted, thereby increasing peripheral resistance and blood return to the heart. Circulation is improved and blood pressure is increased. When there is too much stimulation, the blood flow is decreased to the vital organs. The **alpha$_2$-receptor** is

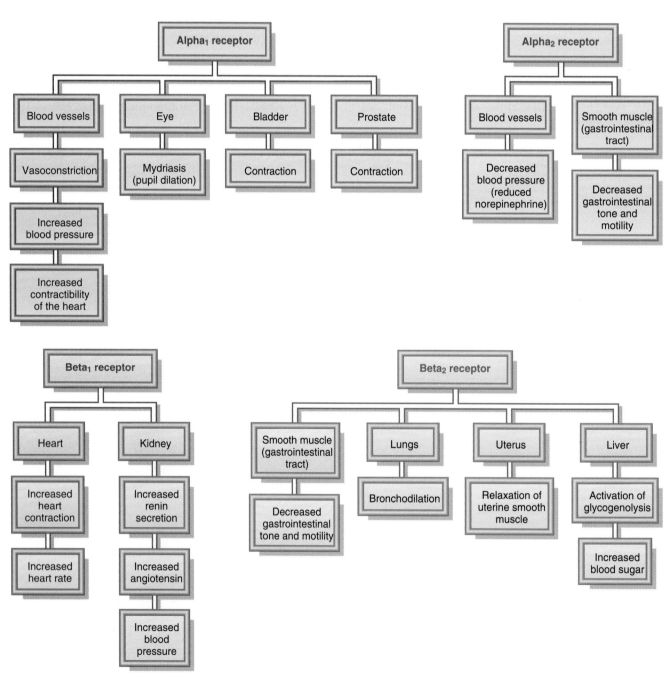

Figure 21–2

Effects of activation of alpha$_1$, alpha$_2$, beta$_1$, and beta$_2$ receptors.

located in the postganglionic sympathetic nerve endings, and when stimulated, it inhibits the release of norepinephrine, thus leading to a decrease in vasoconstriction. This results in a decrease in blood pressure.

The **beta$_1$-adrenergic receptors** are located primarily in the heart. Stimulation of the beta$_1$ receptor increases myocardial contractility and heart rate. The **beta$_2$-receptors** are found mostly in the smooth muscles of the lung, the arterioles of skeletal muscles, and the uterine muscle. Stimulation of the beta$_2$-receptor causes (1) relaxation of the smooth muscles of the lungs, resulting in bronchodilatation, (2) increase in blood flow to the skeletal muscles, and (3) relaxation of the uterine muscle, resulting in a decrease in uterine contraction (see Table 21–1 and Fig. 21–2).

Another adrenergic receptor is dopaminergic and is located in the renal, mesenteric, coronary, and cerebral arteries. When this receptor is stimulated, the vessels dilate and blood flow increases. Only dopamine can activate this receptor.

Inactivation of Neurotransmitters

After the transmitter, such as norepinephrine, has performed its function, the action must be stopped to prevent prolonging the effect. The three ways transmitters are inactivated are by (1) promoting reuptake of the transmitter back into the neuron (nerve cell terminal), (2) enzymatic transformation or degradation, and (3) diffusion away from the receptor. The mechanism of norepinephrine reuptake plays a more important role in inactivation than the enzymatic action. Following the reuptake of the transmitter in the neuron, the transmitter may be degraded or reused. The two enzymes that inactivate the metabolism of

norepinephrine are (1) monoamine oxidase (MAO), which is inside the neuron, and (2) catechol-*o*-methyl-transferase (COMT), which is outside the neuron.

Drugs can stop the termination of the neurotransmitter such as norepinephrine by two methods: (1) inhibiting the norepinephrine reuptake, which prolongs the action of the transmitter, and (2) inhibiting the degradation of norepinephrine by enzyme action.

Classification of Sympathomimetics/ Adrenomimetics

The sympathomimetic drugs that stimulate adrenergic receptors are classified into three categories according to their effects on organ cells: (1) direct-acting sympathomimetics, which directly stimulate the adrenergic receptor (e.g., epinephrine or norepinephrine); (2) indirect-acting sympathomimetics, which stimulate the release of norepinephrine from the terminal nerve endings (e.g., amphetamine); and (3) mixed-acting (both direct and indirect acting) sympathomimetics, which stimulate the adrenergic receptor sites and stimulate the release of norepinephrine from the terminal nerve endings (Fig. 21–3).

Ephedrine is an example of mixed-acting sympathomimetic. This drug acts indirectly by stimulating the release of norephinephrine from the nerve terminals, and acts directly on the alpha$_1$- and beta$_1$- and beta$_2$-receptors. Ephedrine-like epinephrine increases heart rate and blood pressure, but it is not as potent a vasoconstrictor as epinephrine. It is helpful to treat idiopathic orthostatic hypotension and hypotension resulting from spinal anesthesia. It also stimulates beta$_2$-receptors, which dilate bronchial tubes, and is useful in treating mild forms of bronchial asthma.

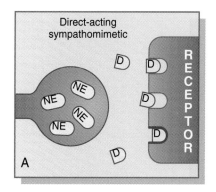
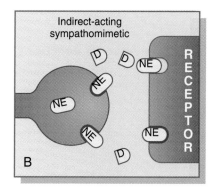
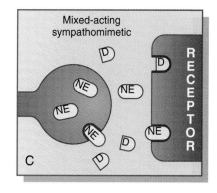

Figure 21–3
(A) Direct-acting, (B) indirect-acting, and (C) mixed-acting sympathomimetics.

Chart 21-1. Adrenergic Agonist: Epinephrine

SYMPATHOMIMETIC

Drug Name

Epinephrine
  (Adrenalin)
Pregnancy Category: C

Dosage

Asthma anaphylaxis:
A: SC: 0.1–0.5 mL of 1:1000 PRN
  IV: 0.1–0.25 mL of 1:1000 with additional
  dilution. IV: 0.1–0.25 mg or 1–2.5 mL of
  1:10,000 infused over 5–10 min
C: SC: 0.01 mL/kg of 1:1000
  IV: 0.01 mL/kg of 1:1000 with additional dilution. IV: 0.1 mg or 10 mL 1:100,000 infused
  over 5–10 min

Contraindications

Cardiac dysrhythmias, cerebral arteriosclerosis,
pregnancy, narrow-angle glaucoma, cardiogenic
shock
Caution: Hypertension, prostatic hypertrophy,
hyperthyroidism, pregnancy, diabetes mellitus
(hyperglycemia could result)

Drug-Lab-Food Interactions

Decrease epinephrine effect with methyldopa,
beta blockers, and alpha-adrenergic blockers
(e.g., phentolamine)
Lab: *Increase* blood glucose, serum lactic acid

Pharmacokinetics

Absorption: SC/IM/IV: Rapidly
Distribution: PB: UK; in breast milk
Metabolism: t½: UK
Excretion: In urine unchanged

Pharmacodynamics

SC/IM: Onset: 3–10 min
    Peak: 20 min
    Duration: 20–30 min
IV: Onset: Immediate
    Peak: 2–5 min
    Duration: 5–10 min
Inhal: Onset: 1 min
    Peak: 3–5 min
    Duration: 1–3 min

Therapeutic Effects/Uses

To treat allergic reaction, anaphylaxis, bronchospasm, cardiac arrest.

Mode of Action: Action on one or more adrenergic sites; promotion of CNS and cardiac stimulation,
and bronchodilation.

Side Effects

Anorexia, nausea, vomiting, nervousness, tremors, agitation, headache, pallor, insomnia, syncope, dizziness

Adverse Reactions

Palpitations, tachycardia, dyspnea
Life-threatening: Ventricular fibrillation, pulmonary edema

Assessment and Planning

Interventions

Evaluation

NURSING PROCESS

KEY: A: adult; C: child; SC: subcutaneous; IV: intravenous; UK: unknown; PB: protein-binding; t½: half-life; IM: intramuscular; CNS: central
nervous system; PRN: as needed.

Catecholamines are the chemical structures of a
substance (either endogenous or synthetic) that can
produce a sympathomimetic response. Examples of
endogenous catecholamines are epinephrine, norepinephrine, and dopamine. The synthetic catecholamines are isoproterenol and dobutamine. There are
also noncatecholamines (e.g., phenylephrine, metapro-

terenol, and albuterol) that stimulate the adrenergic
receptors. Most noncatecholamines have a longer duration of action than the endogenous or synthetic catecholamines.

Many of the adrenergic drugs stimulate more than
one of the adrenergic receptor sites. An example is
epinephrine (Adrenalin), which acts on alpha$_1$-, beta$_1$-,

Chart 21–2. Beta-Adrenergic: Albuterol

BETA$_2$-AGONIST

Drug Name

Albuterol
   (Proventil, salbutamol, Ventolin), 🍁 Novo-
   salmol
Pregnancy Category: C

Dosage

A: PO: 2–4 mg, t.i.d., q.i.d.
   SR: 4–8 mg, q12h
   Inhal: 1–2 puffs q4–6h PRN
   Nebulizer: 0.5 mL of 0.5% sol in
      3 mL of 0.9% NaCl in 5–15 min
C: (2–6 y): PO: 0.1 mg/kg/t.i.d.
   (6–12 y): PO: 2 mg, t.i.d., q.i.d.
   (6–12 y): Inhal: same as adult

Contraindications

Caution: Severe cardiac disease, hypertension, hyperthyroidism, diabetes mellitus, pregnancy

Drug-Lab-Food Interactions

Increase effect with other sympathomimetics; may *increase* effect with MAO inhibitors and tricyclic antidepressants
Antagonize effect with beta-adrenergic blockers (beta-blockers)
Lab: May *increase* glucose level slightly; may *decrease* serum potassium level

Pharmacokinetics

Absorption: well absorbed from the GI tract
Distribution: PB: UK
Metabolism: t$\frac{1}{2}$: PO: 2.5–6 h; Inhal: 3.5–5 h
Excretion: 75% excreted in the urine

Pharmacodynamics

PO: Onset: 30 min
         Peak: 2–3 h
         Duration: 4–6 h
Inhal: Onset: 5–15 min
         Peak: 0.5–2 h
         Duration: 3–6 h

Therapeutic Effects/Uses

To treat bronchospasm, asthma, bronchitis, and other COPD

Mode of Action: It stimulates the beta$_2$ adrenergic receptors in the lungs, which relaxes the bronchial smooth muscles.

Side Effects

Tremor, dizziness, nervousness, restlessness

Adverse Reactions

Palpitations, reflex tachycardia, hallucinations
Life-threatening: Cardiac dysrhythmias

Assessment and Planning

Interventions

Evaluation

NURSING PROCESS

KEY: A: adult; C: child; PO: by mouth; inhal: inhalation; PB: protein-binding; t$\frac{1}{2}$: half-life; UK: unknown; MAO: monoamine oxidase; PRN: as needed; GI: gastrointestinal; 🍁: Canadian drug names.

and beta$_2$-adrenergic receptor sites. The responses from these receptor sites include an increase in blood pressure, pupil dilation, increase in heart rate (tachycardia), and bronchodilatation. In certain types of shock (i.e., cardiogenic, anaphylactic), epinephrine is a useful drug because it increases blood pressure, heart rate, and air flow through the lungs through bronchodilatation. Because epinephrine affects three different adrenergic receptors, it lacks **selectivity;** in other words, it is considered **nonselective** to one receptor. Side effects result when more responses occur than are desired. Chart 21–1 lists the pharmacologic behavior of epinephrine.

Epinephrine

PHARMACOKINETICS

Epinephrine can be administered by parenteral routes, inhalation, or topically. It should not be given orally because it is rapidly metabolized in the gastrointestinal (GI) tract and liver; thus, inadequate serum levels occur. The percentage by which the drug is protein-bound and its half-life are unknown. Epinephrine is metabolized by the liver and excreted in the urine.

PHARMACODYNAMICS

Epinephrine is frequently used in emergencies to combat anaphylaxis, which is a life-threatening allergic response. It is a potent inotropic (force of muscular contraction) drug, causing the blood vessels to constrict, thus increasing the blood pressure, and causing the heart rate to increase and the bronchial tubes to dilate. High doses can result in cardiac dysrhythmias; therefore, the electrocardiogram (ECG) should be monitored. Epinephrine can also cause renal vasoconstriction, thereby decreasing renal perfusion and urinary output.

Epinephrine is usually prescribed subcutaneously or intravenously. The drug can also be administered by inhalation.

The onset of action and peak concentration times are rapid. The use of decongestants with epinephrine has an additive effect. When epinephrine is administered with digoxin, cardiac dysrhythmias may occur. Beta blockers can cause a decrease in action of epinephrine. Epinephrine is also discussed with the emergency drugs in Chapter 52.

Isoproterenol hydrochloride (Isuprel), an adrenergic drug, activates beta$_1$- and beta$_2$-receptors. It is more specific than epinephrine, because it acts on two different adrenergic receptors but is not completely selective. The response to beta$_1$- and beta$_2$-stimulation is an increase in heart rate and bronchodilation. When a client takes isoproterenol to control asthma by dilating the bronchi, an increase in heart rate also occurs as a result of beta$_1$-stimulation. When isoproterenol is used in excess, severe tachycardia can result.

Albuterol

Albuterol sulfate (Proventil) is selective for beta$_2$-adrenergic receptors, so the response is purely bronchodilation. An asthmatic client may therefore respond better by taking albuterol than isoproterenol because its primary action is on the beta$_2$-receptor. By using selective sympathomimetics, there are fewer undesired responses (side effects). However, high dosages of albuterol may affect the beta$_1$ receptors, causing an increase in heart rate. Chart 21–2 lists the drug data related to albuterol.

PHARMACOKINETICS

Albuterol sulfate (Proventil, Ventolin) is well absorbed from the GI tract and is extensively metabolized by the liver. The half-life of the drug differs slightly according to the route of administration (oral route is 2.5 h and inhalation is 3.5 h).

PHARMACODYNAMICS

The primary use of albuterol is to prevent and treat bronchospasms. With inhalation, the onset of action of albuterol is faster than with oral administration, although the duration of action is the same for both oral and inhalation preparations.

Tremors, restlessness, and nervousness may occur when high doses of the drug are taken—side effects that are most likely due to the reflex effect of beta$_1$. If albuterol is taken with a monoamine oxidase (MAO) inhibitor, a hypertensive crisis can result. Beta blockers may inhibit the action of albuterol. Albuterol and the beta$_2$ drugs are also discussed in Chapter 36.

Clonidine (Catapres) and methyldopa (Aldomet) are selective alpha$_2$-adrenergic drugs that are used primarily to treat hypertension. The accepted theory for the action of alpha$_2$ drugs is that they regulate the release of norepinephrine by inhibiting its release. Alpha$_2$ drugs are also believed to produce a cardiovascular depression by stimulating alpha$_2$-receptors in the central nervous system (CNS), leading to a decrease in blood pressure (discussed in Chapter 39).

Names of adrenergic drugs, the receptors they activate, dosage information, and common uses are listed in Table 21–2.

SIDE EFFECTS AND ADVERSE REACTIONS

Side effects frequently result when the drug dosage is increased or the drug is nonselective (acting on several receptors). Side effects that are commonly associated with adrenergic drugs include hypertension, tachycardia, palpitations, dysrhythmias, tremors, dizziness, urinary difficulty, nausea, and vomiting.

ADRENERGIC BLOCKERS (ANTAGONISTS)

Drugs that block the effects of the adrenergic neurotransmitter are called **adrenergic blockers,** adrenergic antagonists, or sympatholytics. They are antagonists to the adrenergic agonists by blocking the alpha- and beta-receptor sites. Most adrenergic blockers block either the alpha- or the beta-receptor. They block the effects of the neurotransmitter either directly by occupying the alpha- or the beta-receptors, or indirectly by inhibiting the release of the neurotransmitters norepinephrine and epinephrine. The three sympatholytic

Table 21–2

Adrenergic Drugs (Alpha, Beta₁, and Beta₂)

GENERIC (BRAND)	ROUTE AND DOSAGE	USES AND CONSIDERATIONS
Epinephrine (Adrenalin) Alpha₁, beta₁, and beta₂	See Chart 21–1	For nonhypovolemic shock, cardiac arrest, acute anaphylaxis, acute asthmatic attack. Pulse rate and blood pressure will greatly increase. Bronchial tubes will dilate. *Pregnancy category:* C; PB: UK; t½: UK
Ephedrine HCl Ephedrine sulfate (Ephedsol, Ectasule) Alpha₁, beta₁, and beta₂	A: PO: 25–50 mg t.i.d./q.i.d. SC/IM: 25–50 mg; IV: 10–25 mg PRN; *max:* 150 mg/24 h C > 2 y: PO: 2–3 mg/kg/d or 25–100 mg/m²/d in 4–6 divided doses	To treat hypotensive states, bronchospasm, nasal congestion, orthostatic hypotension. Effective for relief of symptoms of hay fever, sinusitis, and allergic rhinitis. Also may be used for treating mild cases of asthma. Drug resistance may occur with prolonged use of ephedrine. If this occurs, stop drug for 3–5 d and then resume. *Pregnancy category:* C; PB: UK; t½: 3–6 h
Norepinephrine bitartrate (levarterenol, Levophed) Alpha₁ and beta₁	A: IV: 4 mg in 250–500 mL of D₅W or NSS infused initially 8–12 μg/min, then 4 μg/min; monitor blood pressure	For shock. It is a potent vasoconstrictor. It increases blood pressure and cardiac output. The blood pressure should be closely monitored every 2–5 min during infusion. IV flow is titrated according to blood pressure. *Pregnancy category:* D; PB: UK; t½: UK
Metaraminol bitartrate (Aramine) Alpha₁ and beta₁	A: IV/Inf: 15–100 mg in 500 mL of D₅W C: IV/Inf: 0.04 mg/kg (each 1 mg diluted in 25 mL of D₅W)	Treatment of acute hypotension. Infusion rate should be adjusted according to blood pressure. *Pregnancy category:* C; PB: UK; t½: UK
Dopamine HCl (Intropin) Alpha₁ and beta₁	A: IV/INF: 1–5 μg/kg/min initially; gradually increase 5–10 μg/kg/min; *max:* 50 μg/kg/min C: IV: usually the same	To correct hypotension. It does not decrease renal function in doses <5 μg/kg/min. *Pregnancy category:* C; PB: UK; t½: 2 min
Midodrine (ProAmatin) Alpha₁	A: PO: 10 mg t.i.d.	To treat symptomatic orthostatic hypotension. Blood pressure may increase by 15 to 30 mmHg in 1 hour with one 10-mg dose. *Pregnancy category:* C; PB: UK; t½: 3–4 h
Phenylephrine HCl 12-hour spray (oxymetazoline HCl) (Neo-Synephrine) Alpha	*Nasal decongestant:* A: Instill: 2–3 sprays or gtt of 0.25%–0.5% sol C <6 y: Instill: 2–3 gtt of 0.125% sol C 6–12 y: Instill: 2–3 gtt of 0.25% sol Also available IM, IV	To treat nasal congestion; acts as a decongestant. Used for clients with common cold, sinusitis, and with allergic rhinitis. Have client blow nose before drug is administered. *Pregnancy category:* C; PB: UK; t½: 2.5 h
Pseudoephedrine HCl (Sudafed, Actifed, Co-Tylenol, PediaCare) Alpha and beta₁	*Nasal decongestant:* A: PO: 60 mg q.i.d./q6h PO/SR: 120 mg q12h; *max:* 240 mg/d C 2–6 y: PO: 15 mg q6h; *max:* 60 mg/d C 6–12 y: PO: 30 mg q6h; *max:* 120 mg/d	To treat nasal congestion. OTC drug. Check label for contraindications. Avoid taking with a history of hypertension, cardiac disease, diabetes mellitus, etc. *Pregnancy category:* C; PB: UK; t½: 9–16 h
Phenylpropanolamine HCl Decongestant (Dimetapp, Dristan, Contac 12 hour, Triaminicol, Triaminic)	*Nasal decongestant:* A: PO: 25 mg q4h PRN PO/SR: 75 mg q12h PRN C 2–6 y: PO: 6.25 mg q4h PRN C 6–12 y: 12.5 mg q4h PRN	To treat nasal congestion; acts as OTC drugs
Anorexiant (Dexatrim, Dietac, Control) Alpha and beta₁	*Appetite suppressant:* A: PO/SR: 75 mg q.d. (before breakfast); PO: 25 mg t.i.d. a.c.	To control weight gain. OTC drug. Client should check with health care provider before taking an appetite suppressant. *Pregnancy category:* C; PB: UK; t½: 3–4 h

Table continued on following page

Table 21–2 *Continued*
Adrenergic Drugs (Alpha, Beta₁, and Beta₂)

GENERIC (BRAND)	ROUTE AND DOSAGE	USES AND CONSIDERATIONS
Isoproterenol HCl (Isuprel) Beta₁ and beta₂	A: SL: 10–20 mg t.i.d. *max:* 60 mg/d; Inhal: 1–2 puffs q4–6 h PRN; IV: 0.01–0.02 mg OR 2–20 μg/min via infusion C: SL: 5–10 mg t.i.d. Inhal: Same as adult; IV: 2.5 μg/min OR 0.1 μg/kg/min via infusion	To treat cardiac decompensation, congestive heart failure (increases myocardial blood flow and cardiac output), and asthmatic attack. This drug increases heart rate and dilates bronchial tubes. *Pregnancy category:* C; PB: UK; $t_{\frac{1}{2}}$: 2.5–5 min
Metaproterenol sulfate (Alupent, Metaprel) Beta₁ (some) and beta₂	A&C: >9 y: PO: 10–20 mg t.i.d./q.i.d. C <6y: PO: 1–2.6 mg/kg/d in 3–4 divided doses C 6–9 y: PO: 10 mg t.i.d./q.i.d. A&C: >12 y: inhal: 2–3 puffs q3–4h; *max:* 12 puffs/d	Treatment for bronchospasm, acute heart block (only used in atropine-refractory bradycardia). By stimulating beta₁, the heart rate is increased but not as strongly as with isoproterenol HCl. The drug dilates the bronchial tubes. *Pregnancy category:* C; PB: UK; $t_{\frac{1}{2}}$: UK
Albuterol (Proventil, Ventolin) Beta₂	A: PO: 2–4 mg t.i.d./q.i.d. PO/SR: 4–8 mg q12h; Inhal: 1–2 puffs q4–6h PRN; Nebulizer: 0.5 mL of 0.5% sol in 3 mL of 0.9% NaCl in 5–15 min C: 2–6 y: PO: 0.1 mg/kg t.i.d. 6–12 y: PO: 2 mg t.i.d./q.i.d. C: 6–12 y: Inhal: Same as adult	To relieve bronchospasm, due to acute and chronic obstructive airway disease such as asthma, bronchitis, emphysema. It stimulates the beta₂ receptors of the bronchi, thus promoting bronchodilation. *Pregnancy category:* C; PB: UK; $t_{\frac{1}{2}}$: 2.5–5 h
Dobutamine HCl (Dobutrex) Beta₁	A or C: IV: 2.5–20 μg/kg/min initially; increase dose gradually; *max:* 40 μ/kg/min	To treat cardiac decompensation due to depressed myocardial contractility, which may result from organic heart disease, cardiac surgery. *Pregnancy category:* C; PB: UK; $t_{\frac{1}{2}}$: 2 min
Isoetharine HCl (Bronkosol) Beta₂	A: IPPB: 0.5–1.0 mL of 0.5% solu OR 0.5 mL of 1% sol diluted in 3 mL of NSS A: inhal: 1–2 puffs	To control asthma and chronic obstructive pulmonary disease (COPD) by dilating the bronchial tubes. *Pregnancy category:* C; PB: UK; $t_{\frac{1}{2}}$: UK
Terbutaline sulfate (Brethine, Brethaire, Bricanyl) Beta₂	*Bronchodilator:* A: PO: 2.5–5 mg t.i.d. OR q8h; SC: 0.25 mg initially; no more than 0.5 mg in 4 h Inhal: 2 puffs q4–6h C >12 y: PO: 2.5 mg t.i.d. OR q8h *Premature labor:* A: PO: 2.5 mg q4–6h; IV: 10 μg/min, gradually increase; *max:* 80 μg/min	Primary use is to correct bronchospasm. Unofficial use is during premature labor to prevent premature-term birth. *Pregnancy category:* B; PB: 25%; $t_{\frac{1}{2}}$: 3–11 h
Ritodrine HCl (Yutopar) Beta₂ and some beta₁	A: PO: Initially 10 mg q2h for first 24 h; maint: 10–20 mg q4–6h; *max:* 120 mg/d IV: 50–100 μg/min; dose may gradually increase to 300 μg/min	Used to decrease and/or stop uterine contraction. To be effective, the heart rate must be over 100 beats per minute (bpm). Because there are many side effects, the drug is not used as frequently in controlling premature labor as it once was. *Pregnancy category:* C; PB: UK; $t_{\frac{1}{2}}$: 1.6–2.6 h

KEY: A: adult; C: child; PO: by mouth; IV: intravenous; PB: protein-binding; $t_{\frac{1}{2}}$: half-life; UK: unknown; SC: subcutaneous; Inf: infusion; inhal: inhalation; OTC: over-the-counter; NSS: normal saline solution; IM: intramuscular; PRN: as needed; >: greater than; <: less than.

NURSING PROCESS
ADRENERGIC AGONIST

Assessment

- Obtain vital signs (VS) for future comparison. Epinephrine stimulates the alpha$_1$ (increases blood pressure), beta$_1$ (increases heart rate), and beta$_2$ (dilates bronchial tubes) receptors. Isoproterenol (Isuprel) stimulates the beta$_1$- and beta$_2$-receptors. Albuterol (Proventil) stimulates the beta$_2$-receptor.
- Assess the drugs the client is taking and report possible drug-drug interaction. Beta blockers decrease the effect of epinephrine.
- Assess the medical history. Most adrenergic drugs are contraindicated if the client has cardiac dysrhythmias, narrow-angle glaucoma, or cardiogenic shock.
- Assess the results of laboratory values and compare with future laboratory findings.

Potential Nursing Diagnoses

- Risk for impaired tissue integrity
- Decreased cardiac output

Planning

- Client's VS will be closely monitored and will be within normal or acceptable ranges.

Nursing Interventions

- Monitor the client's VS. Report signs of increasing blood pressure and increasing pulse rate. If the client is receiving an alpha-adrenergic drug intravenously for shock, the blood pressure should be checked every 3 to 5 min or as indicated to avoid severe hypertension.
- Report side effects of adrenergic drugs, such as tachycardia, palpitations, tremors, dizziness, and increased blood pressure.
- Check the client's urinary output and assess for bladder distention. Urinary retention can result from high drug dose or continuous use of adrenergic drugs.
- For cardiac resuscitation, administer epinephrine 1:1000 IV (1 mg/mL), which may be diluted in 10 mL of saline solution (as prescribed).
- Check IV site frequently when administering norepinephrine bitartrate (Levarterenol) or dopamine (Intropin) because infiltration of these drugs causes tissue necrosis. These drugs should be diluted sufficiently in IV fluids. An antidote for norepinephrine (Levophed) and dopamine is phentolamine mesylate (Regitine) 5 to 10 mg, diluted in 10 to 15 mL of saline infiltrated into the area.
- Offer food when giving adrenergic drugs to avoid nausea and vomiting.
- Monitor laboratory test results. Blood glucose levels may be increased.

Client Teaching

General
- Instruct the client to read labels on all over-the-counter (OTC) drugs for cold symptoms and diet pills. Many of these have properties of sympathetic (adrenergic, sympathomimetics) drugs and should not be taken if the client is hypertensive or has diabetes mellitus, cardiac dysrhythmias, or coronary artery disease.
- Instruct mothers not to take drugs containing sympathetic drugs while nursing infants. These drugs pass into the breast milk.
- Explain to the client that continuous use of nasal sprays or drops that contain adrenergics may result in nasal congestion rebound (inflamed and congested nasal tissue).

Self-Administration
- Instruct the client and family how to administer cold medications by spray or drops in the nostrils. Spray should be used with head in upright position. The use of nasal spray

Nursing process continued on following page

lying down can cause systemic absorption. Coloration of nasal spray or drops might indicate deterioration.
- Instruct the client not to use bronchodilator sprays in excess. If the client is using a nonselective adrenergic drug that affects beta₁- and beta₂-receptors, tachycardia may occur.

Side Effects
- Instruct the client to report side effects to health care provider, that is, rapid heart rate, palpitations, or dizziness.

Evaluation

- Evaluate the client's response to the adrenergic drug. Continue monitoring the client's VS and report abnormal findings.

receptors are alpha₁, beta₁, and beta₂. Table 21–3 lists the effects of alpha- and beta-blockers.

Alpha-Adrenergic Blockers

Drugs that block or inhibit a response at the alpha-adrenergic receptor site are called alpha-adrenergic blockers, or more commonly, **alpha blockers.** Alpha blocking agents are divided into two groups: selective alpha blockers that block alpha₁ and nonselective alpha blockers that block alpha₁ and alpha₂. Because alpha-adrenergic blockers can cause orthostatic hypotension and reflex tachycardia, many of these drugs are not as frequently prescribed as the beta blockers. The alpha blockers are helpful in decreasing symptoms of benign prostatic hypertrophy (BPH).

The alpha blockers promote vasodilation, thus causing a decrease in blood pressure. If the vasodilation is longstanding, orthostatic hypotension can result. Dizziness may also be a symptom of a drop in

blood pressure. As the blood pressure decreases, pulse rate usually increases to compensate for the low blood pressure and inadequate blood flow. The alpha blockers can be used to treat peripheral vascular disease, such as Raynaud's disease. Vasodilation occurs, permitting more blood flow to the extremities. The alpha blockers are also discussed in Chapter 40.

Beta-Adrenergic Blockers

Beta-adrenergic blockers, commonly referred to as **beta blockers,** decrease heart rate; a decrease in blood pressure usually follows. Some of the beta blockers are nonselective, blocking both beta₁ and beta₂ receptors. Not only does the pulse rate decrease because of beta₁ blocking, but bronchoconstriction also occurs. Nonselective beta blockers (beta₁ and beta₂) should be used with extreme caution in any client who has chronic obstructive pulmonary disease (COPD) or asthma. If the desired effect is to decrease pulse rate and blood pressure, then a selective beta₁-blocker, such as metoprolol tartrate (Lopressor), may be ordered.

An intrinsic sympathomimetic activity (ISA) causes partial stimulation of beta-receptors. Certain nonselective beta blockers (block beta₁ and beta₂) that have ISA are carteolol, carvedilol, penbutolol, and pindolol. The selective blocker (blocks beta₁ only) that has ISA is acebutolol. It is reported that these agents cause fewer serious side effects and are helpful to those clients experiencing severe bradycardia.

Propranolol hydrochloride (Inderal) was the first beta blocker prescribed for treating angina, cardiac dysrhythmias, and hypertension. Although it is still prescribed today, it has many side effects, partly due to its nonselective response in blocking both beta₁ and beta₂ receptors. It is contraindicated for clients with asthma or second- or third-degree heart block. Propranolol is extensively metabolized by the liver, hepatic first-pass; thus, a small amount of the drug

Table 21–3	
Effects of Adrenergic Blockers at Receptors	
RECEPTOR	**RESPONSES**
Alpha₁	Vasodilation: Decreases blood pressure. Reflex tachycardia might result. Miosis: Constricts the pupil. Suppresses ejaculation. Reduces contraction of the smooth muscles in the bladder neck and prostate.
Beta₁	Decreases heart rate. Reduces force of contractions.
Beta₂	Constricts bronchioles; contracts uterus; inhibits glycogenolysis, which can decrease blood sugar.

Chart 21-3.   Adrenergic Blocker (Sympatholytic)

BETA$_1$- AND BETA$_2$-BLOCKER

Drug Name

Propranolol HCl
    (Inderal), ♥ Apo-Propranolol, Detensol, No-
    vopranolol
Pregnancy Category: C

Dosage

See Antihypertension (Chapter 39), antianginal
(Chapter 37), and antidysrhythmics (Chapter 37)
A: PO: Initially: 20–40 mg, b.i.d., titrate up to
    160–240 mg/d in 2–3 divided doses
    SR: 120–160 mg/d
C: PO: 2–4 mg/kg/d in 2 divided doses

Contraindications

Congestive heart failure, secondary heart block,
cardiogenic shock, bronchial asthma, bronchospasm
Caution: Renal or hepatic dysfunction

Drug-Lab-Food Interactions

Increase atrioventricular block with digoxin, cal-
cium channel blockers
Increase hypotensive effect with phenothiazines,
diuretics, antihypertensives
Decrease absorption with antacids
Lab: *Increase* serum potassium, uric acid, AST,
ALT, ALP; *decrease* blood sugar

Pharmacokinetics

Absorption: PO: Well absorbed
Distribution: PB: 93%
Metabolism: t$\frac{1}{2}$: 2–4 h
Excretion: 90% excreted in urine as metabolites

Pharmacodynamics

PO: Onset: 30 min
    Peak: 1–1.5 h (SR: 6 h)
    Duration: 6 h
IV: Onset: Immediate
    Peak: 5 min
    Duration: UK

Therapeutic Effects/Uses

To treat cardiac dysrhythmias, hypertension, angina pectoris, myocardial infarction.

Mode of Action: Blocks beta$_1$- (cardiac) and beta$_2$- (pulmonary) adrenergic receptor sites.

Side Effects

Bradycardia, confusion, drowsiness, fatigue, vertigo, pruritus, dry mouth, nasal stuffiness,
brown discoloration of the tongue (rare)

Adverse Reactions

Visual hallucinations, thrombocytopenia
Life-threatening: Laryngospasm, atrioventricular heart block, agranulocytosis

Sidebar (vertical): Assessment and Planning · Interventions · Evaluation · NURSING PROCESS

KEY: A: adult; C: child; PO: by mouth; IV: intravenous; PB: protein-binding; t$\frac{1}{2}$: half-life; UK: unknown; SR: sustained release; ♥: Canadian
drug names, ALP: alkaline phosphatase, ALT: alanine aminotransferase, AST: asparate aminotransferase

reaches the systemic circulation. Chart 21–3 describes
the pharmacologic behavior of propranolol.

PHARMACOKINETICS

Propranolol is well absorbed from the GI tract. It
crosses the blood–brain barrier and the placenta and

is found in breast milk. It is metabolized by the liver
and has a short half-life of 3 to 6 h.

PHARMACODYNAMICS

By blocking both types of beta receptors, propranolol
decreases heart rate and, secondarily, the blood pres-

Table 21–4
Adrenergic Blockers

GENERIC (BRAND)	ROUTE AND DOSAGE	USES AND CONSIDERATIONS
Tolazoline (Priscoline HCl) Alpha$_1$	A: SC/IM/IV: 10–50 mg q.i.d. *Pulmonary hypertension:* NB: IV: 1–2 mg/kg infused over 10 min, followed by 1–2 mg/kg/h, for 24–48 h	For peripheral vascular disorder and for persistent pulmonary hypertension in the newborn. Also for emergency hypertension. *Pregnancy category:* C; PB: UK; t$\frac{1}{2}$: 3–10 h
Phentolamine mesylate (Regitine) Alpha$_1$	A: IM/IV: 2.5–5 mg, repeat q5min until controlled, then q2–3h PRN C: IM/IV: 0.05–0.1 mg/kg, repeat if needed	Management of peripheral vascular disorder and hypertensive emergency. Antidote for dopamine infiltration. *Pregnancy category:* C; PB: UK; t$\frac{1}{2}$: 20 min
Doxazosin mesylate (Cardura) Alpha$_1$	A: PO: 1 mg/d, titrate dose up to *max:* 16 mg/d; maint: 4–8 mg/d	For mild to moderate hypertension and BPH. Check for orthostatic hypotension. Dizziness, headache, syncope may occur. *Pregnancy category:* C; PB: 98%; t$\frac{1}{2}$: 9–12 h
Prazosin HCl (Minipress) Alpha$_1$	A: PO: 1 mg b.i.d./t.i.d.; maint: 3–15 mg/d; *max:* 20 mg/d in divided doses	Management of mild to moderate hypertension. May be used in combination with other antihypertensive drugs. *Pregnancy category:* C; PB: 95%; t$\frac{1}{2}$: 3 h
Terzosin HCl (Hytrin) Alpha$_1$	A: PO: 1 mg/h.s., maint: 1–5 mg in 1–2 divided doses; *max:* 20 mg/d	For hypertension. May be used in combination with diuretic or other antihypertensive drugs. May also be used for BPH. May cause dizziness, headache, edema, orthostatic hypotension. *Pregnancy category:* C; PB: UK; t$\frac{1}{2}$: 9–12 h
Carteolol HCl (Cartrol) Beta$_1$ and beta$_2$	A: PO: 2.5–5.0 mg/d	For hypertension and glaucoma. Primarily blocks beta$_1$-adrenergic receptor; however, in large doses it blocks beta$_2$. *Pregnancy category:* C; PB: 23%–30%; t$\frac{1}{2}$: 4–6 h
Carvedilol (Coreg) Alpha$_1$, beta$_1$, and beta$_2$	A: PO: 6.25 mg b.i.d. May increase to 12.5 mg b.i.d. *max:* 50 mg/d	For treatment of hypertension. Can be used alone or with a thiazide diuretic. Used also for mild to moderate heart failure. *Pregnancy category:* C; PB: UK; t$\frac{1}{2}$: 7–10 h
Labetalol (Normodyne, Trandate) Alpha$_1$, beta$_1$, and beta$_2$	A: PO: 100 mg b.i.d.; dose may be increased; *max:* 2.4 g/d A: IV: 20 mg OR 1–2 mg/kg; repeat 20–80 mg at 10-min interval; *max* 300 mg/d	To treat mild to severe hypertension; angina pectoris; used during surgery to manage blood pressure. *Pregnancy category:* C; PB: 50%; t$\frac{1}{2}$: 6–8 h
Penbutolol (Levatol) Beta$_1$ and beta$_2$	A: PO: 10–20 mg/d; *max:* 80 mg/d	To treat mild to moderate hypertension. Clients with asthma should avoid taking the drug. *Pregnancy category:* C; PB: 80%–98%; t$\frac{1}{2}$: 5 h
Propranolol HCl (Inderal) Beta$_1$ and beta$_2$	See Chart 21–3	Treatment of hypertension, cardiac dysrhythmias, angina pectoris, postmyocardial infarction. Contraindicated in asthma and COPD. *Pregnancy category:* C; PB: 93%; t$\frac{1}{2}$: 2–4 h
Nadolol (Corgard) Beta$_1$ and beta$_2$	A: PO: 40–80 mg/d; *max:* 320 mg/d	Management of hypertension and angina pectoris. Contraindicated in bronchial asthma and severe COPD because it blocks beta$_2$. *Pregnancy category:* C; PB: 30%; t$\frac{1}{2}$: 10–24 h
Pindolol (Visken) Beta$_1$ and beta$_2$	A: PO: 5 mg b.i.d./t.i.d.; maint: 10–30 mg in divided doses; *max:* 60 mg/d in divided doses	Management of hypertension and angina pectoris. Contraindicated in asthma, COPD, and second-third-degree heart block. *Pregnancy category:* B; PB: 40%; t$\frac{1}{2}$: 3–4 h
Sotalol (Betapace) Beta$_1$ and beta$_2$	A: PO: 80 mg b.i.d., may increase gradually. Average: 240–320 mg/d	To treat life-threatening ventricular arrhythmias; chronic angina pectoris. *Pregnancy category:* B; PB: 0; t$\frac{1}{2}$: 12 h

Table 21–4 *Continued*
Adrenergic Blockers

GENERIC (BRAND)	ROUTE AND DOSAGE	USES AND CONSIDERATIONS
Timolol maleate (Blocadren) Beta$_1$ and beta$_2$	A: PO: Initially 10 mg b.i.d.; maint: 20–40 mg/d in 2 divided doses; *max:* 60 mg/d	Management of mild to moderate hypertension, dysrhythmias, and post-myocardial infarction. Also may be used as prophylaxis of migraine headache. For ophthalmic use to treat IOP. Use with caution for clients with asthma or COPD. *Pregnancy category:* C; PB: <10%; t$\frac{1}{2}$: 3–4 h
SELECTIVE BETA ADRENERGICS		
Metoprolol tartrate (Lopressor) Beta$_1$	*Hypertension:* A: PO: 50–100 mg/d in 1–2 divided doses; maint: 100–450 mg/d in divided doses; *max:* 450 mg/d in divided doses *Myocardial infarction:* A: IV: 5 mg q2min × 3 doses, then PO: 100 mg b.i.d.	Management of hypertension, angina pectoris, postmyocardial infarction. Bradycardia, dizziness, gastrointestinal distress may occur. *Pregnancy category:* C; PB: 12%; t$\frac{1}{2}$: 3–4 h
Atenolol (Tenormin) Beta$_1$	A: PO: 25–100 mg/d	Treatment of mild to moderate hypertension and angina pectoris. May be used in combination with antihypertensive drugs. Bradycardia, dizziness, and hypotension may occur. *Pregnancy category:* C; PB: 6%–16%; t$\frac{1}{2}$: 6–7 h
Acebutolol HCl (Sectral) Beta$_1$	A: PO: Initially: 200–400 mg/d A: PO: maint; 200–800 mg/d in 1–2 divided doses; *max:* 1200 mg/d	Treatment for mild to moderate hypertension, angina pectoris, and supraventricular dysrhythmias. Check apical pulse; do not give if <60 bpm. *Pregnancy category:* B; PB: 26%; t$\frac{1}{2}$: 3–13 h
Betaxolol (Kerlone) Beta$_1$	A: PO: 10–20 mg/d. Also for ophthalmic use: glaucoma	For hypertension and glaucoma. Ophthalmic preparation is used to decrease intraocular pressure (IOP). *Pregnancy category:* C; PB: UK; t$\frac{1}{2}$: 14–22 h
Bisoprolol fumarate (Zebeta) Beta$_1$	A: PO: Initially: 5 mg/d; maint: 2.5–20 mg/d	For hypertension and angina pectoris. Long-acting beta-blocker. Heart rate and blood pressure may be decreased. *Pregnancy category:* C; PB: <30%; t$\frac{1}{2}$: 9–12 h
Esmolol HCl (Brevibloc) Beta$_1$	A: IV: Loading dose: 500 μ/kg/min for 1 min; then 50 μg/kg/min for 4 min	For treatment of supraventricular tachycardia, atrial fibrillation/flutter, and hypertension. *Contraindications:* heart block, bradycardia, cardiogenic shock, uncompensated congestive heart failure (CHF). *Pregnancy category:* C; PB: UK; t$\frac{1}{2}$: 9 min

KEY: *A: adult; C: child; PO: by mouth; IM: intramuscular; IV: intravenous; NB: newborn; PRN: as necessary; UK: unknown; bpm: beats per minute; COPD: chronic obstructive pulmonary disease; PB: protein-binding; t$\frac{1}{2}$: half-life; BPH: benign prostatic hypertrophy; IOP: intraocular pressure.*

sure. It also causes the bronchial tubes to constrict and the uterus to contract. It is available orally in tablets and sustained-release capsules, and intravenously. The onset of action of the sustained-release preparation is longer than that of the tablet; peak time and duration of action are also longer for the sustained-release formulation. This form is effective for dosing once a day, especially for clients who do not comply with drug doses of several times a day.

DRUG INTERACTIONS

Many drugs interact with propranolol. Phenytoin, isoproterenol, nonsteroidal antiinflammatory drugs (NSAIDs), barbiturates, and xanthines (caffeine, theoph-

NURSING PROCESS
ADRENERGIC BLOCKERS

Adrenergic alpha and beta blockers are also presented within the antihypertensive, antianginal, and antidysrhythmia sections.*

Assessment

- Obtain baseline vital signs (VS) and ECG for future comparison. Bradycardia and decrease in blood pressure are common cardiac effects of adrenergic beta-blockers. Adrenergic beta-blockers are frequently referred to as beta-blockers, blocking beta$_1$ and beta$_2$ (nonselective) or beta$_1$ (cardiac selective).
- Assess whether the client is having respiratory problems by listening for signs of wheezing or noting dyspnea (difficulty in breathing). If the beta-blocker is nonselective, not only does the pulse rate decrease but also bronchoconstriction can result. Clients with asthma should take a beta$_1$ blocker, such as metoprolol (Lopressor), and avoid nonselective beta-blockers.
- Assess the drugs the client is currently taking. Report if any are phenothiazines, digoxin, calcium channel blockers, or other antihypertensives.
- Assess the client's urine output and use for future comparison.

Potential Nursing Diagnoses

- Decreased cardiac output
- Impaired tissue integrity

Planning

- The client will comply with the drug regimen.
- The client's VS will be within desired range.

Nursing Interventions

- Monitor the client's VS. Report marked changes such as marked decrease in blood pressure and pulse rate.
- Administer IV propranolol undiluted or diluted in D$_5$W.
- Report any complaints of excessive dizziness or lightheadedness.

Nursing process continued on following page

ylline) decrease the drug effect of propranolol. When propranolol is taken with digoxin or a calcium blocker, atrioventricular (AV) heart block may occur. The blood pressure can be decreased if propranolol is taken with another antihypertensive (this may be desirable).

Beta blockers are useful in treating cardiac dysrhythmias, mild hypertension, mild tachycardia, and angina pectoris. The use of beta blockers as antihypertensives, antidysrhythmics, and drugs for angina is discussed in Chapters 37 and 39. Table 21–4 lists the alpha and beta blockers, their dosages, uses, and considerations.

SIDE EFFECTS AND ADVERSE REACTIONS

General side effects of *alpha-adrenergic blockers* include dysrhythmias, flushing, hypotension, and reflex tachy-cardia. The side effects commonly associated with *beta blockers* are bradycardia, dizziness, hypotension, headaches, hyperglycemia, intensified hypoglycemia, and agranulocytosis. Usually the side effects are dose-related.

Adrenergic Neuron Blockers

Drugs that block the release of norepinephrine from the sympathetic terminal neurons are called **adrenergic neuron blockers,** which are classified as a subdivision of the adrenergic blockers. The clinical use of neuron blockers is to decrease blood pressure. Guanethidine monosulfate (Ismelin) and guanadrel sulfate (Hylorel), examples of the adrenergic neuron blockers, are potent antihypertensive agents.

- Report any complaint of stuffy nose. Vasodilation results from use of alpha-adrenergic blockers, and nasal congestion can occur.
- Report if the client is a diabetic and receiving an adrenergic beta blocker; insulin dose or oral hypoglycemic may need to be adjusted.
- Clients taking beta-blockers do not have normal compensatory mechanisms in shock states. To resuscitate such clients, glucagon must be given in high doses to counteract the sympatholytic effects of beta-blockers.

Client Teaching

General
- Advise the client to avoid abruptly stopping a beta-blocker; rebound hypertension, rebound tachycardia, or an angina attack could result.
- Instruct the client to comply with the drug regimen.
- Advise clients on insulin therapy that early warning signs of hypoglycemia (i.e., tachycardia, nervousness) may be masked by the beta-blocker.
- Advise clients on insulin therapy to carefully monitor their blood sugar and follow diet orders.

Self-Administration
- Instruct the client and family how to take pulse and blood pressure.

Side Effects
- Instruct the client to avoid orthostatic (postural) hypotension, such as by slowly rising from supine or sitting to standing positions.
- Inform the client and family of possible mood changes when taking beta-blockers. Mood changes can include depression, nightmares, and suicidal tendencies.
- Advise the male client that certain beta-blockers, such as propranolol, metoprolol, and pindolol, and alpha-blockers, such as prazosin, may cause impotence or a decrease in libido. Usually the problem is dose related.

Evaluation

- Evaluate the effectiveness of the adrenergic blocker. VS must be stable within desired range.

*Chapter 39: Antihypertensives; Chapter 37: Antianginals and antidysrhythmics

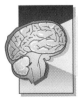

Critical Thinking in Action

V. T., 79 years old, has asthma. An adrenergic drug is being selected.

1. What are the drug advantages and disadvantages associated with the use of ephedrine, isoproterenol, metaproterenol, albuterol, and terbutaline for V. T.?
2. Is age a factor in drug selection? Explain.

H. P., 69 years old, has hypertension and asthma. An adrenergic blocker is being selected.

1. What are the drug advantages and disadvantages associated with the use of doxazosin, prazosin, propranolol, metoprolol, atenolol, and acebutolol for H. P.? Explain.
2. What needs to be included in teaching H. P. about using an adrenergic blocker?

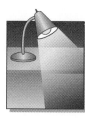

Study Questions

1. What are the adrenergic receptors? What are the major physiologic responses of each?

2. What is the difference between selective adrenergic drugs and nonselective drugs? Give examples of each.

3. What are the major side effects of adrenergic drugs? What are the implications for client teaching?

4. What drugs are selective and nonselective adrenergic blockers? What are the uses of alpha-blockers and beta-blockers?

5. What are the side effects of adrenergic blockers?

6. What are the nursing interventions associated with the use of adrenergic drugs?

Cholinergics and Anticholinergics 22

Objectives

- Name the two cholinergic receptors.
- Describe the responses of cholinergic drugs and anticholinergic drugs.
- Differentiate between direct-acting and indirect-acting cholinergic drugs.
- List the major side effects of cholinergic and anticholinergic drugs.
- Describe the uses of cholinergics and anticholinergics.
- Explain the nursing process, including client teaching, associated with cholinergics and anticholinergics.

Terms

acetylcholine
anticholinergics
anticholinesterases
cholinergic
cholinergic blocking agents

cholinesterase
direct-acting cholinergics
indirect-acting cholinergics
miosis
muscarinic receptors

mydriasis
nicotinic receptors
parasympathomimetics
parasympatholytics

INTRODUCTION

The two groups of drugs that affect the parasympathetic nervous system are (1) the cholinergics (parasympathomimetics) and (2) the anticholinergics (parasympatholytics). Drugs in these groups are discussed in this chapter. The parasympathetic nervous system (parasympathomimetics and parasympatholytics), along with the sympathetic nervous system, is discussed and compared in Chapter 20.

CHOLINERGICS

Drugs that stimulate the parasympathetic nervous system are called **cholinergic drugs,** or **parasympathomimetics,** because they mimic the parasympathetic neurotransmitter acetylcholine. Cholinergic drugs are also called cholinomimetics, cholinergic stimulants, or cholinergic agonists. **Acetylcholine (ACh)** is the neurotransmitter located at the ganglions and the parasympathetic terminal nerve endings and innervates the receptors in organs, tissues, and glands. There are two types of cholinergic receptors: (1) **muscarinic receptors,** which stimulate smooth muscle and slow the heart rate, and (2) **nicotinic receptors** (neuromuscular), which affect the skeletal muscles. Many cholinergic drugs are nonselective because they can affect both the muscarinic and the nicotinic receptors. However, there are selective cholinergic drugs for the muscarinic receptors that do not have an effect on the nicotinic receptors. Figure 22–1 illustrates the effects of parasympathetic or cholinergic stimulation.

There are direct-acting cholinergic drugs and indirect-acting cholinergic drugs. **Direct-acting** cholinergic drugs act on the receptors to activate a tissue response (Fig. 22–2A). **Indirect-acting** cholinergic drugs inhibit the action of the enzyme **cholinesterase** (acetylcholinesterase) by forming a chemical complex,

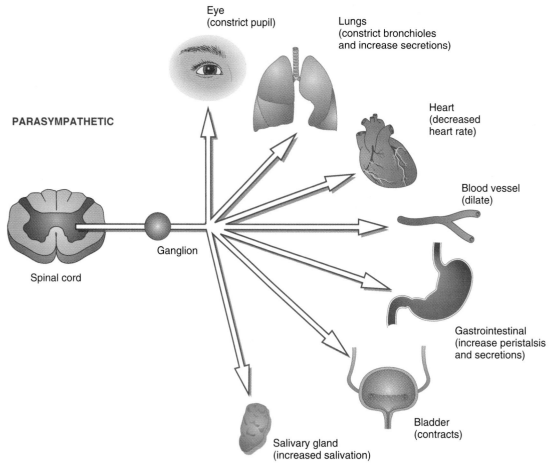

Figure 22–1

Parasympathetic responses. Stimulation of the parasympathetic nervous system or use of parasympathomimetic drugs causes the pupils to constrict, bronchioles to constrict and increase bronchial secretions, heart rate to decrease, blood vessels to dilate, peristalsis and gastric secretions to increase, bladder muscle to contract, and salivation to increase.

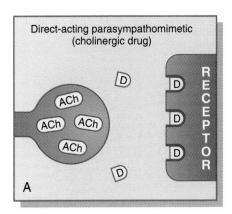
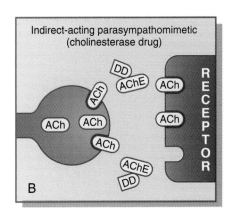

Figure 22–2

(A) Direct-acting parasympathomimetic (cholinergic drugs). Cholinergic drugs resemble acetylcholine and act directly on the receptor. (B) Indirect-acting parasympathomimetic (cholinesterase inhibitors). Cholinesterase inhibitors inactivate the enzyme acetylcholinesterase (cholinesterase), thus permitting acetylcholine to react to the receptor. D: cholinergic drug; DD: cholinesterase inhibitor (anticholinesterase); AChE: acetylcholinesterase or cholinesterase; ACh: acetylcholine.

thus permitting acetylcholine to persist and attach to the receptor (see Fig. 22–2B). A drug that inhibits cholinesterase is called a **cholinesterase inhibitor,** or an **anticholinesterase drug.** Cholinesterase may destroy acetylcholine before it reaches the receptor or after it has attached to the site. By inhibiting or destroying the enzyme cholinesterase, more acetylcholine is available to stimulate the receptor and remain in contact with it longer.

The cholinesterase inhibitors (anticholinesterases) can be separated into reversible inhibitors and irreversible inhibitors. The reversible inhibitors bind the enzyme, cholinesterase, for several minutes to hours, and the irreversible inhibitors bind the enzyme permanently. The resulting effects vary with the amount of time the cholinesterase is bound.

The major responses of cholinergic drugs are to stimulate bladder and gastrointestinal (GI) tone, constrict pupils of the eyes **(miosis),** and increase neuromuscular transmission. Other effects of cholinergic drugs include decreased heart rate and blood pressure and increased salivary, GI, and bronchial glandular secretions. Table 22–1 lists the functions of direct- and indirect-acting cholinergic drugs.

Direct-Acting Cholinergics

Many drugs in this category are primarily selective to the muscarinic receptors but are nonspecific because the muscarinic receptors are located in the smooth muscles of the GI and genitourinary tracts, glands, and heart. Bethanechol chloride (Urecholine), a direct-acting cholinergic drug, acts on the muscarinic (cholinergic) receptor and is used primarily to increase urination. Chart 22–1 details the pharmacologic behavior of bethanechol.

PHARMACOKINETICS

Bethanechol chloride (Urecholine) is poorly absorbed from the GI tract. The percentage of protein-binding and the half-life are unknown. The drug is most likely to be excreted in the urine.

PHARMACODYNAMICS

The principal use of bethanechol is to promote micturition (urination) by stimulating the muscarinic cholinergic receptors to increase urine output. The client voids approximately 30 min to 1.5 h after taking an oral dose of bethanechol because of the increased

Table 22–1
Effects of Cholinergic Drugs

BODY TISSUE	RESPONSE
Cardiovascular*	Decreases heart rate, lowers blood pressure due to vasodilation, and slows conduction of atrioventricular node.
Gastrointestinal†	Increases the tone and motility of the smooth muscles of the stomach and intestine. Peristalsis is increased and the sphincter muscles are relaxed.
Genitourinary	Contracts the muscles of the urinary bladder, increases tone of the ureters, and relaxes the bladder's sphincter muscles. Stimulates urination.
Eye†	Increases pupillary constriction, or miosis (pupil becomes smaller), and increases accommodation (flattening or thickening of eye lens for distant or near vision).
Glandular*	Increases salivation, perspiration, and tears.
Bronchi (lung)*	Stimulates bronchial smooth muscle contraction and increases bronchial secretions.
Striated muscle†	Increases neuromuscular transmission and maintains muscle strength and tone.

Tissue responses to large doses of cholinergic drugs.
†Major tissue responses to normal doses of cholinergic drugs.

Chart 22–1. Cholinergic

CHOLINERGIC/PARASYMPATHOMIMETIC

Drug Name

Bethanechol Chloride
(Urecholine), 🍁Duvoid, Urecholine
Pregnancy Category: C

Dosage

A: PO: 10–50 mg b.i.d./t.i.d./q.i.d.; *max:*
120 mg/d
SC: 2.5–5 mg, repeat at 15–30 min intervals;
PRN
Do *NOT* give IM or IV

Contraindications

Severe bradycardia or hypotension, chronic obstructive pulmonary disease, asthma, peptic ulcer, parkinsonism, hyperthyroidism

Drug-Lab-Food Interactions

Decrease bethanechol effect with antidysrhythmics
Lab: *Increase* AST, bilirubin, amylase, lipase

Pharmacokinetics

Absorption: PO: Poorly absorbed
Distribution: PB: UK
Metabolism: t½: UK
Excretion: In urine

Pharmacodynamics

PO: Onset: 0.5–1.5 h
    Peak: 1–2 h
    Duration: 4–6 h
SC: Onset: 5–15 min
    Peak: 0.5 h
    Duration: 2 h

Therapeutic Effects/Uses

To treat urinary retention, abdominal distention.

Mode of Action: Stimulation of the cholinergic (muscarinic) receptor. Promote contraction of the bladder; increase GI peristalsis, GI secretion, pupillary constriction, and bronchoconstriction.

Side Effects

Nausea, vomiting, diarrhea, salivation, sweating, flushing, frequent urination, rash, miosis, blurred vision, abdominal discomfort

Adverse Reactions

Orthostatic hypotension, bradycardia, muscle weakness
Life-threatening: Acute asthmatic attack, heart block, circulatory collapse, cardiac arrest

Assessment and Planning

Interventions

Evaluation

NURSING PROCESS

KEY: A: adult; C: child; PO: by mouth; SC: subcutaneous; PB: protein-binding; t½: half-life; UK: unknown; GI: gastrointestinal; PRN: as needed; AST: adenosine triphosphate; 🍁: Canadian drug names.

tone of the detrusor urinae muscle. Bethanechol also increases peristalsis in the GI tract. The drug should be taken on an empty stomach, and it should not be administered intramuscularly or intravenously. Bethanechol can be given subcutaneously, and micturition usually occurs within 15 min. Duration of action for oral administration is 4 to 6 h; for the subcutaneous route it is 2 h.

SIDE EFFECTS AND ADVERSE REACTIONS: DIRECT-ACTING MUSCARINIC CHOLINERGIC AGONISTS

Mild to severe side effects of most muscarinic agonists such as bethanechol include hypotension, bradycardia, excessive salivation, increased secretion of gastric acid, abdominal cramps, diarrhea, bronchoconstriction, and, in some cases, cardiac dysrhythmias.

NURSING PROCESS
CHOLINERGIC, DIRECT ACTING: BETHANECHOL (URECHOLINE)

Assessment

- Obtain baseline vital signs (VS) for future comparison.
- Assess urine output that should be >600 mL/d. Report decrease in urine output.
- Obtain a history from the client of health problems, such as peptic ulcer, urinary obstruction, or asthma. Cholinergics can aggravate symptoms of these conditions.

Potential Nursing Diagnoses

- Urinary retention
- Anxiety

Planning

- Client will have increased bladder and GI tone after taking cholinergics.
- Client will have increased neuromuscular strength.

Nursing Interventions

Direct Acting
- Monitor the client's VS. Pulse rate and blood pressure decrease when large doses of cholinergics are taken. Orthostatic hypotension is a side effect of a cholinergic such as bethanechol.
- Monitor fluid intake and output. Decreased urinary output should be reported because it may be related to urinary obstruction.
- Give cholinergics 1 h before or 2 h after meals. If the client complains of gastric pain, the drug may be given with meals.
- Check serum enzyme values for amylase and lipase, as well as aspartate aminotransferase (AST) and bilirubin levels. These laboratory values may increase slightly when taking cholinergics.
- Observe the client for side effects, such as gastric pain or cramping, diarrhea, increased salivary or bronchial secretions, bradycardia, and orthostatic hypotension.
- Auscultate for bowel sounds. Report decreased or hyperactive bowel sounds.
- Auscultate breath sounds for rales (cracking sounds from fluid congestion in lung tissue) or rhonchi (rough sounds resulting from mucus secretions in lung tissue). Cholinergic drugs can increase bronchial secretions.
- Have IV atropine sulfate (0.6 mg) available as an antidote for overdosing of cholinergics. Early signs of overdosing include salivation, sweating, abdominal cramps, and flushing.
- Note that diaphoresis (excessive perspiration) may occur; linens should be changed as needed.

Indirect Acting
- Beware of the possibility of cholinergic crisis (overdose); symptoms include muscular weakness and increased salivation.

Client Teaching

Direct Acting: General
- Instruct the client to take the cholinergic as prescribed. Compliance with the drug regimen is essential.

Side Effects
- Instruct the client to report severe side effects, such as profound dizziness or a decrease in pulse rate to below 60.
- Instruct the client to arise from a lying position slowly to avoid dizziness; this is most likely a result of orthostatic hypotension.

Nursing Process continued on following page

- Encourage the client to maintain effective oral hygiene if excess salivation occurs.
- Advise the client to report any difficulty in breathing as a result of respiratory distress.

Indirect Acting: See Drugs for Myasthenia Gravis

- Instruct the client to take the drug on time to avoid respiratory muscle weakness.
- Instruct the client to assess changes in muscle strength. Cholinesterase inhibitors (anticholinesterases) increase muscle strength.

Evaluation

- Evaluate the effectiveness of the cholinergic or anticholinesterase drug.
- Evaluate the stability of the client's VS, and note the presence of side effects or adverse reactions.

This group of agents should be prescribed cautiously for clients with low blood pressure and heart rate. Muscarinic agonists are contraindicated for clients having intestinal or urinary tract obstruction, and for clients with active asthma.

DIRECT-ACTING CHOLINERGIC: EYE

Pilocarpine is a direct-acting cholinergic drug that constricts the pupils of the eyes, thus opening the canal of Schlemm to promote drainage of aqueous humor (fluid). This drug is used to treat glaucoma by relieving fluid (intraocular) pressure in the eye. Pilocarpine also acts on the nicotinic receptor. Carbachol acts on the nicotinic receptors. These agents are discussed in more detail in Chapter 43.

Indirect Acting Cholinergics

The indirect-acting cholinergic drugs do not act on receptors; instead they inhibit or inactivate the enzyme cholinesterase, thus permitting acetylcholine to accumulate at the receptor sites (see Fig. 22–2B). This action gives them the name **cholinesterase inhibitors,** or **anticholinesterases,** of which there are two types: reversible and irreversible.

The function of the enzyme, cholinesterase (ChE) is to break down acetylcholine (ACh) into choline and acetic acid. This process occurs when binding ACh to ChE or splitting of ACh, which permits regeneration of free ChE. A small amount of cholinesterase can break down a large amount of acetylcholine in a short period of time. A cholinesterase inhibitor drug binds with cholinesterase, thus allowing the acetylcholine to activate the muscarinic and nicotinic cholinergic receptors. This action permits skeletal muscle stimulation, which increases the force of muscular contraction. Because of this action, the cholinesterase inhibitors are useful for increasing muscle tone for clients with myasthenia gravis. By increasing acetylcholine, additional effects occur such as increase in GI motility, bradycardia, miosis, bronchial constriction, and increased micturition.

REVERSIBLE CHOLINESTERASE INHIBITORS

These inhibitors are used (1) to produce pupillary constriction in the treatment of glaucoma, and (2) to increase muscle strength in clients with **myasthenia gravis** (a neuromuscular disorder). Drug effects persist for several hours. Drugs used to increase muscular strength in myasthenia gravis include neostigmine (Prostigmin: short-acting), pyridostigmine bromide (Mestinon: moderate-acting), ambenonium chloride (Mytelase: long-acting), and edrophonium chloride (Tensilon: short-acting for diagnostic purposes). These drugs are discussed in more detail in Chapter 23. A reversible ophthalmic anticholinesterase drug is physostigmine (Eserine). Ophthalmic agents are further discussed in Chapter 43.

The primary use of cholinesterase inhibitors is to treat myasthenia gravis. Other uses for ChE inhibitors are to treat glaucoma, Alzheimer's disease, and muscarinic antagonist poisoning. Tacrine (Cognex) is frequently prescribed for clients with Alzheimer's disease.

SIDE EFFECTS

Caution in taking reversible cholinesterase inhibitors is required for clients who have bradycardia, asthma, peptic ulcers, or hyperthyroidism. ChE inhibitors are contraindicated for clients with intestinal or urinary obstruction.

IRREVERSIBLE CHOLINESTERASE INHIBITORS

Irreversible inhibitors are potent agents because of their long-lasting effect. The enzyme cholinesterase must be regenerated before the drug effect diminishes, a process that may take days or weeks. These drugs are used to produce pupillary constriction and for manufacture of organophosphate insecticides.

With irreversible cholinesterase inhibitors, the bond between the irreversible ChE inhibitor and cholinesterase is considered permanent; however, this bond can be broken with the use of the drug, pralidoxime (Protopam). Pralidoxime is an antidote to reverse the irreversible organophosphate. The effect is at the neu-

Table 22–2
Cholinergics

GENERIC (BRAND)	ROUTE AND DOSAGE	USES AND CONSIDERATIONS
DIRECT-ACTING CHOLINERGICS		
Bethanechol Cl (Urecholine)	See Chart 22–1	To increase urination; can stimulate gastric motility. Contraindicated in bronchial asthma, mechanical GI and urinary obstruction, and pronounced bradycardia. *Pregnancy category:* C; PB: UK; t½: UK
Carbachol (Miostat)	Ophthalmic: 0.75%–3%, 1–2 gtt, t.i.d.	To reduce intraocular pressure, miosis. See Chapter 43.
Pilocarpine HCl (Pilocar)	Ophthalmic: 0.5%–4%, 1 gt	To reduce intraocular pressure, miosis. See Chapter 43.
CHOLINESTERASE INHIBITOR		
Tacrine HCl (Cognex)	*For Alzheimer's disease:* A: PO: 10 mg, q.i.d., increase dose at 6-wk intervals. A: PO: 40–160 mg/d p.c.; *max:* 160 mg/d	To improve memory in mild to moderate Alzheimer's dementia. Drug enhances cholinergic function. *Pregnancy category:* C; PB: 55%; t½: 1.5–3.5 h
Velnacrine (Mentane)	A: PO: 150–225 mg/d in divided doses	To treat Alzheimer's disease. Clinical trial drug. *Pregnancy category:* C; PB: UK; t½: 2–3 h
INDIRECT-ACTING CHOLINERGICS OR CHOLINESTERASE INHIBITORS FOR THE EYE		
Demecarium bromide (Humorsol)	0.125%–0.25%, 1 gt q12–48h	To reduce intraocular pressure in glaucoma, long-acting miotic. See Chapter 43.
Echothiophate iodide (Phospholine Iodide)	0.03%–0.25%, 1 gt daily or b.i.d.	To reduce intraocular pressure, long-acting miotic. See Chapter 43.
Isoflurophate (Floropryl)	0.25%, ointment q8–72h	To treat glaucoma. Apply to the conjunctival sac. See Chapter 43.
REVERSIBLE CHOLINESTERASE INHIBITORS: MYASTHENIA GRAVIS		
Ambenonium Cl (Mytelase)	A: PO: 2.5–5.0 mg t.i.d./q.i.d.; dose may be increased; maint: 5–25 mg t.i.d./q.i.d.	To increase muscle strength in myasthenia gravis; long-acting. May be used with glucocorticoids. *Pregnancy category:* C; PB: UK; t½: UK
Edrophonium Cl (Tensilon)	A: IV: 2 mg; then 8 mg if no response IM: 10 mg; may repeat with 2 mg in 30 min C < 34 kg: IV: 1 mg; repeat in 30–45 sec if no response; *max:* 5 mg C > 34 kg: IV: 2 mg; repeat with 1 mg if no response; *max:* 10 mg	To diagnose myasthenia gravis; very short-acting. *Pregnancy category:* C; PB: UK; t½: 1.2–2 h
Neostigmine (Prostigmin) Neostigmine methylsulfate (injectable form)	A: PO: Initially 15 mg t.i.d.; maint: 150 mg/d in divided doses; range: 15–375 mg/d IM/IV: 0.5–2.5 mg as needed C: PO: 2 mg/kg/d in 6 divided doses	To increase muscle strength in myasthenia gravis; short-acting. Used also to prevent or treat postoperative urinary retention. *Pregnancy category:* C; PB: 15%–25%; t½: 1–1.5 h
Physostigmine salicylate (Eserine Salicylate)	0.25%–0.5%, 1 gt daily or q.i.d.	To reduce intraocular pressure, miosis, short-acting.
Pyridostigmine bromide (Mestinon)	A: PO: 60–120 mg t.i.d./q.i.d.; maint: 600 mg/d in 3–4 divided doses; *max:* 1.5 g/d SR: 180–540 mg daily or b.i.d. IM/IV: 2 mg q2–3 h C: PO: 7 mg/kg/d in 5–6 divided doses	To increase muscle strength in myasthenia gravis; moderate-acting. Prevents the destruction of the neurotransmitter acetylcholine. *Pregnancy category:* C; PB: <10%; t½: 3–4 h

Table continued on following page

Table 22–2 *Continued*
Cholinergics

GENERIC (BRAND)	ROUTE AND DOSAGE	USES AND CONSIDERATIONS
ANTIDOTE FOR IRREVERSIBLE AND REVERSIBLE CHOLINESTERASE INHIBITORS		
Pralidoxime Cl (Protopam)	A: IM: 1–2 g, repeat in 1–2 h, then 10 to 12 h intervals. A: PO: 1–3 g, repeat in 5 h as needed. C: IM: 20–50 mg/kg/dose; repeat in 1–2 h; 10- to 12-h intervals if necessary.	To treat overdose of organophosphate pesticides that cause muscle paralysis and to treat an overdose of a ChE inhibitor for myasthenia gravis. *Pregnancy category:* C; PB: UK; t½: 1–2.7 h

KEY: A: adult; C: child; PO: by mouth; IM: intramuscular; IV: intravenous; gt: drop; gtt: drops; UK: unknown; SR: sustained-release; >: greater than; IOP: intraocular pressure; PB: protein-binding; t½: half-life; maint: maintenance; GI: gastrointestinal; <: less than.

romuscular junction. Examples of all types of cholinergic drugs, their standard dosages, and common uses are in Table 22–2.

ANTICHOLINERGICS

Drugs that inhibit the actions of acetylcholine by occupying the acetylcholine receptors are called **anticholinergics** or **parasympatholytics.** Other names for anticholinergics are **cholinergic blocking agents,** cholinergic or muscarinic antagonists, antiparasympathetic agents, antimuscarinic agents, or antispasmodics. The major body tissues and organs affected by the anticholinergic group of drugs are the heart, respiratory tract, GI tract, urinary bladder, eye, and exocrine glands. By blocking the parasympathetic nerves, the sympathetic (adrenergic) nervous system is allowed to dominate. Anticholinergic and adrenergic drugs produce many of the same responses.

Anticholinergic and cholinergic drugs have opposite effects. The major responses to anticholinergics are a decrease in GI motility, a decrease in salivation, dilation of the pupils of the eyes **(mydriasis),** and an increase in pulse rate. Other effects of anticholinergics include decreased bladder contraction, which can result in urinary retention, and decreased rigidity and tremors related to neuromuscular excitement. Anticholinergics can act as an antidote to the toxicity caused by cholinesterase inhibitors and organophosphate ingestion. The various effects of anticholinergics are described in Table 22–3.

Muscarinic receptors, also known as cholinergic receptors, are involved in tissue and organ responses to anticholinergics, because anticholinergics inhibit the actions of acetylcholine by occupying these receptor sites. Figure 22–3 illustrates this action of anticholinergic drugs. Anticholinergic drugs may block the effect of direct-acting parasympathomimetics, such as

bethanechol and pilocarpine, and of indirect-acting parasympathomimetics, such as physostigmine and neostigmine.

Atropine sulfate, first derived from the belladonna plant *(Atropa belladonna)* and purified in 1831, is a classic anticholinergic, or muscarinic antagonist drug.

Table 22–3
Effects of Anticholinergic Drugs

BODY TISSUES	RESPONSES
Cardiovascular	Increases heart rate with large doses. Small doses can decrease heart rate.
Gastrointestinal (GI)	Relaxes smooth muscle tone of GI tract, decreasing GI motility and peristalsis. Decreases gastric and intestinal secretions.
Urinary tract	Relaxes the bladder detrusor muscle and increases constriction of the internal sphincter. Urinary retention can result.
Eye	Dilates pupils of the eye (mydriasis) and paralyzes ciliary muscle (cycloplegia), causing a decrease in accommodation.
Glandular	Decreases salivation, sweating, and bronchial secretions.
Lung	Dilates the bronchi and decreases bronchial secretions.
Central nervous system	Decreases tremors and rigidity of muscles. Drowsiness, disorientation, and hallucination can result from large doses.

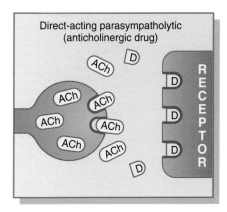

Figure 22–3
Anticholinergic response. The anticholinergic drug is occupying the receptor sites, thus blocking acetylcholine. D: anticholinergic drug; ACh: acetylcholine.

Scopolamine was the second belladonna alkaloid produced. Atropine and scopolamine act on the muscarinic receptor, but they have little effect on the nicotinic receptor. Atropine is useful as a preoperative medication to decrease salivary secretions, as an antispasmodic drug for treating peptic ulcers because it relaxes the smooth muscles of the GI tract and decreases peristalsis, and for increasing heart rate when bradycardia is present. Atropine can be used as an antidote for muscarinic agonist poisoning caused by an overdose of a muscarinic drug such as bethanechol or from a cholinesterase inhibitor. However, if a client is on atropine or an atropine-like drug (antihistamine) for any long period, side effects can occur. Chart 22–2 details the pharmacologic behavior of atropine.

Synthetic anticholinergic drugs are also used as antispasmodics to treat peptic ulcers and intestinal spasticity. One example of such a drug is propantheline bromide (Pro-Banthine), which has been available for several decades. It decreases gastric secretions and GI spasms. Since the introduction of the histamine blockers (H_2), anticholinergic agents such as propantheline are not used as frequently to decrease gastric secretions.

Pharmacokinetics

Atropine sulfate is well absorbed orally and parenterally. It crosses the blood–brain barrier and exerts its effect on the central nervous system (CNS). The protein-binding is unknown; it crosses the placenta. Atropine has a short half-life; therefore, there is little cumulative effect. Most of absorbed atropine is excreted in the urine (75% to 95%).

Pharmacodynamics

Atropine sulfate blocks acetylcholine by occupying the muscarinic receptor. It increases heart rate by blocking vagus stimulation, and promotes dilation of the pupil by paralyzing the iris sphincter. The two most frequent uses of atropine are preoperatively to decrease salivation and respiratory secretions, and to treat sinus bradycardia by increasing the heart rate. Atropine also is used ophthalmically for mydriasis and cycloplegia before eye refraction and to treat inflammation of the iris (iritis) and uveal tract.

Its onset of action orally is between 0.5 to 1 h and peaks at 2 to 4 h. For the intramuscular route, the onset of action is 10 to 30 min and peaks at 30 min. Duration time for both oral and intramuscular routes is 4 h. Intravenously, the onset of action is immediate and peak action is at 5 min.

Side Effects and Adverse Reactions

Anticholinergic drugs have many side effects. The common side effects of atropine and atropine-like drugs include dry mouth, decreased perspiration, blurred vision, tachycardia, constipation, and urinary retention. Other side effects and adverse reactions are nausea, headache, dry skin, abdominal distention, hypotension or hypertension, impotence, photophobia, and coma.

Antiparkinsonism-Anticholinergic Drugs

At one time, atropine was given to clients with Parkinson's disease to decrease salivation and drooling. It was also found to have some effect on the motor manifestation of this disease by decreasing tremors and rigidity. Additional studies indicated that anticholinergic (antimuscarinic) agents affect the central nervous system (CNS) as well as the parasympathetic nervous system. These anticholinergic drugs affect the CNS by suppressing the tremors and muscular rigidity of parkinsonism, but they have little effect on mobility and muscle weakness. As the result of these findings, several anticholinergic drugs were developed, such as trihexyphenidyl hydrochloride (Artane), procyclidine (Kemadrin), biperiden (Akineton), and benztropine (Cogentin), for the treatment of Parkinson's disease. These drugs can be used alone in early stages of parkinsonism. These drugs may be used in combination with levodopa for controlling parkinsonism or used singly to treat pseudoparkinsonism resulting from the side effects of the phenothiazines in antipsychotic drugs. Drugs for parkinsonism are described in more detail in Chapter 23. Chart 22–3 lists the drug data related to trihexyphenidyl, which is used for pseudoparkinsonism.

Chart 22–2. Anticholinergic

ANTICHOLINERGIC/PARASYMPATHOLYTIC

Drug Name

Atropine SO$_4$
(Atropine), 🍁 Atropair
Atropisol (Optic)
Pregnancy Category: C

Dosage

A: PO/IM/IV: 0.4–0.6 mg q4–6h PRN
C: PO/IM/IV: 0.01 mg/kg/dose; *max:* 0.4 mg/dose, q4–6h, PRN

Contraindications

Narrow-angle glaucoma, obstructive GI disorders, paralytic ileus, ulcerative colitis, tachycardia, benign prostatic hypertrophy, myasthenia gravis, myocardial ischemia
Caution: Renal or hepatic disorders, chronic obstructive pulmonary disease (COPD), congestive heart failure

Drug-Lab-Food Interactions

Increase anticholinergic effect with phenothiazines, antidepressants, MAOIs, amantadine; may *increase* effects of atenolol

Pharmacokinetics

Absorption: PO/IM: Well absorbed
Distribution: PB: UK; crosses the placenta
Metabolism: t$\frac{1}{2}$: 2–3 h
Excretion: >75% excreted in urine

Pharmacodynamics

PO: Onset: 0.5–1 h
   Peak: 1–2 h
   Duration: 4 h
IM: Onset: 10–30 min
   Peak: 0.5 h
   Duration: 4 h
IV: Onset: Immediate
   Peak: 5 min
   Duration: UK
Instill: Onset: 20–30 min
    Peak: 30–40 min
    Duration: days

Therapeutic Effects/Uses

Preoperative medication to reduce salivation, increase heart rate, dilate pupils of the eye.

Mode of Action: Inhibition of acetylcholine by occupying the receptors; increase heart rate by blocking vagus stimulation; promote dilation of the pupil by blocking iris sphincter muscle.

Side Effects

Dry mouth, nausea, headache, constipation, rash, dry skin, flushing, blurred vision, photophobia

Adverse Reactions

Tachycardia, hypotension, pupillary dilatation, abdominal distention, palpitations, nasal congestion
Life-threatening: Paralytic ileus, coma

(Assessment and Planning · Interventions · Evaluation · NURSING PROCESS)

KEY: A: adult; C: child; PO: by mouth; IM: intramuscular; IV: intravenous; PB: protein-binding; t$\frac{1}{2}$: half-life; UK: unknown; instill: instillation; MAOIs: monoamine oxidase inhibitors; GI: gastrointestinal; >: greater than; PRN: as necessary; 🍁: Canadian drug names.

Chart 22–3.   Antiparkinsonism: Anticholinergic

ANTIPARKINSONISM ANTICHOLINERGIC

Drug Name

Trihexyphenidyl HCl (Artane, Aphen, Hexaphen, Trihexane, Trihexy), 🍁 Aparkane, Apo-Trihex, Novohexidyl
Pregnancy Category: C

Dosage

Parkinsonism:
A: PO: Initially 1–2 mg/d; increase to 6–10 mg/d in divided doses
Extrapyramidal symptoms: Drug induced:
A: PO: 1 mg/d; increase to 5–15 mg/d in divided doses

Contraindications

Narrow-angle glaucoma, GI obstruction, urinary retention, severe angina pectoris, myasthenia gravis
Caution: Tachycardia, benign prostatic hypertrophy, children, elderly, during lactation

Drug-Lab-Food Interactions

Increase anticholinergic effect with phenothiazines, antihistamines, tricyclic antidepressants, amantadine, quinidine
Decrease trihexyphenidyl absorption with antacids

Pharmacokinetics

Absorption: PO: Well absorbed
Distribution: PB: UK
Metabolism: t½: 5–10 h
Excretion: In urine

Pharmacodynamics

PO: Onset: 1 h
Peak: 2–3 h
Duration: 6–12 h
SR/PO: Onset: UK
Peak: UK
Duration: 12–24 h

Assessment and Planning / Interventions / Evaluation — NURSING PROCESS

Therapeutic Effects/Uses

To decrease involuntary symptoms of parkinsonism or drug-induced parkinsonism by inhibiting acetylcholine.

Mode of Action: Blocks cholinergic (muscarinic) receptors: thus decreases involuntary movements.

Side Effects

Nausea, vomiting, dry mouth, constipation, anxiety, restlessness, headache, dizziness, blurred vision, photophobia, pupil dilation, dysphagia

Adverse Reactions

Tachycardia, palpitations, urticaria, postural hypotension, urinary retention
Life-threatening: Paralytic ileus

KEY: A: adult; PO: by mouth; PB: protein-binding; SR: sustained-release; t½: half-life; UK: unknown; 🍁: Canadian drug names.

PHARMACOKINETICS

Trihexyphenidyl is well absorbed from the GI tract. Its protein-binding percentage and half-life are unknown. It is excreted in the urine.

PHARMACODYNAMICS

Trihexyphenidyl decreases involuntary movement and diminishes the signs and symptoms of tremors and muscle rigidity that occur with Parkinson's disease and pseudoparkinsonism. It is available in tablet, elixir, and sustained-release capsule. The duration of action of the sustained-release preparation is twice as long as that for the oral and elixir forms. Alcohol, narcotics, amantadine, phenothiazines, and antihistamines may increase the effect of trihexyphenidyl. The side effects are similar to other anticholinergic drugs.

Table 22–4
Anticholinergics

GENERIC (BRAND)	ROUTE AND DOSAGE	USES AND CONSIDERATIONS
ANTICHOLINERGICS: GI OR CHOLINERGIC BLOCKERS		
Atropine sulfate	See Chart 22–2	Presurgery to decrease salivary and bronchial secretions. Increases heart rate with doses ≥0.5 mg. *Pregnancy category:* C; PB: UK; t$\frac{1}{2}$: 2–3 h
Dicyclomine HCl (Bentyl, Antispas, Di-Spaz)	A: PO: 10–20 mg t.i.d./q.i.d. IM: 20 mg q6h C > 2 y: PO: 10 mg t.i.d./q.i.d.	For irritable bowel syndrome. Avoid taking drug for those with narrow-angle glaucoma, severe ulcerative colitis, paralytic ileus. *Pregnancy category:* B; PB: UK; t$\frac{1}{2}$: 9–10 h
Glycopyrrolate (Robinul)	*GI disorders:* A: PO: 1–2 mg b.i.d./t.i.d. IM/IV: 0.1–0.2 mg t.i.d./q.i.d. *Preoperative:* A: IM: 4.4 µg/kg 30 min–1 h before surgery	Presurgery to reduce secretions and for peptic ulcer. Contraindicated in narrow-angle glaucoma, obstructive GI tract, and ulcerative colitis. *Pregnancy category:* B; PB: UK; t$\frac{1}{2}$: 1–4.5 h
Hyoscyamine SO$_4$ (Cystospaz, Anaspaz, Levsin)	A: PO/SL: 0.125–0.25 mg t.i.d./q.i.d. a.c. & h.s. SR: 0.375–0.75 mg/q12h SC/IM/IV: 0.25–0.5 mg b.i.d./q.i.d. C: 2–10 y: one-half of the adult dose or individualized	Treatment of peptic ulcer and irritable bowel syndrome. Controls gastric secretion and spastic bladder. Contraindicated in narrow-angle glaucoma and severe ulcerative colitis. *Pregnancy category:* C; PB: 50%–60%; t$\frac{1}{2}$: 3.5 h
Isopropamide iodide (Darbid)	A: PO: 5 mg b.i.d. or q12h; may increase to 10 mg b.i.d.	To treat peptic ulcer and irritable bowel syndrome. Not for use in children under 12 y. *Pregnancy category:* C; PB: UK; t$\frac{1}{2}$: UK
Mepenzolate bromide (Cantil)	A: PO: 25–50 mg t.i.d. with meals and h.s.	To treat peptic ulcer, irritable bowel syndrome. Efficacy not established in children. *Pregnancy category:* C; PB: UK; t$\frac{1}{2}$: UK
Methscopolamine bromide (Pamine)	A: PO: 2.5 mg a.c., and 2.5–5.0 mg, h.s. C: PO: 0.2 mg/kg q.i.d.	Treatment of peptic ulcer and irritable bowel syndrome. Avoid use with prostatic hypertrophy and intestinal atony. *Pregnancy category:* C; PB: UK; t$\frac{1}{2}$: UK
Oxyphencyclimine HCl (Daricon)	A: PO: 5–10 mg b.i.d., t.i.d.	For peptic ulcer and irritable bowel syndrome. Not for use in children under 12 y. *Pregnancy category:* C; PB: UK; t$\frac{1}{2}$: UK
Propantheline bromide (Pro-Banthīne)	A: PO: 15 mg a.c. t.i.d.; 30 mg h.s.; *max:* 120 mg/d Elderly: 7.5 mg a.c. t.i.d.	Antispasmodic for peptic ulcer and irritable bowel syndrome. Also used for pancreatitis and urinary bladder spasm. *Pregnancy category:* C; PB: UK; t$\frac{1}{2}$: 9 h
Scopolamine hydrobromide (also hyoscine hydrobromide)	*Preoperative:* A: PO: 0.5–1.0 mg SC/IM/IV: 0.3–0.6 mg C: SC: 0.006 mg/kg or 0.2 mg/m²; *max:* 0.3 mg *Motion sickness:* A: PO: 0.3–0.6 mg; transderm patch: 1 patch behind ear q 72h	For preanesthetic drug, irritable bowel syndrome, motion sickness, and to treat delirium. Contraindicated in narrow-angle glaucoma, obstructive GI disease, severe ulcerative colitis, and paralytic ileus. *Pregnancy category:* C; PB: <30%; t$\frac{1}{2}$: 8 h
CHOLINERGIC ANTAGONISTS: EYE		
Cyclopentolate HCl (Cyclogyl)	0.5%–2%, sol, 1–2 gtt	For mydriasis and cycloplegia for eye examination. See Chapter 43.
Homatropine (Isopto Homatropine)	2%–5% sol, 1–2 gtt	For mydriasis and cycloplegia (paralysis of ciliary muscle resulting in loss of accommodation) for eye examination. See Chapter 43.

Table continued on following page

Side Effects

- Advise the client of common side effects from long-term use of anticholinergics, such as dry mouth, decrease in urination, and constipation.
- Instruct the client to increase fluid intake to prevent constipation when taking anticholinergics for a prolonged period of time.
- Instruct the client to urinate before taking the anticholinergic. Urinary retention can be a problem. The client should report a marked decrease in urine output.
- Suggest that the client use hard candy, ice chips, or chewing gum and maintain effective oral hygiene if the client's mouth is dry. Anticholinergics decrease salivation.
- Encourage the client to use Artificial Tears (eye drops) for dry eyes that result from decreased lacrimation (tearing).

Evaluation

- Evaluate the client's response to the anticholinergic.
- Determine whether constipation, urine retention, or increased pulse rate is or remains a problem.

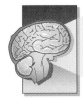

Critical Thinking in Action

J. S., age 56, is scheduled for surgery for removal of gallstones. He has been in good health and his only other clinical problem is glaucoma. Preoperative medications, meperidine 75 mg and atropine sulfate 0.4 mg, were given intramuscularly 1 hour before surgery.

1. What are the advantages of giving atropine sulfate before surgery?
2. If J. S. received an atropine-like drug for several months, what assessments should be made related to the effects of the atropine-like drug?
3. How does atropine sulfate differ from bethanechol chloride?

J. S. is receiving ophthalmic pilocarpine drops for controlling glaucoma.

4. How does pilocarpine differ from physostigmine? Explain.
5. What client teaching should the nurse include related to the use of pilocarpine?

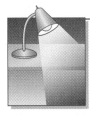

Study Questions

1. What are the actions of cholinergic drugs and anticholinergic drugs? Differentiate between direct-acting and indirect-acting cholinergic drugs.
2. What are the major side effects of cholinergic and anticholinergic drugs? What are the implications for client teaching for each of these classes of drugs?
3. What are the general uses and indications for cholinergic and anticholinergic drugs?
4. What are the nursing implications associated with the use of cholinergic and anticholinergic drugs?
5. Your client has glaucoma. What should you instruct the client regarding OTC drugs? The same client is to have surgery and atropine has been ordered. What are your nursing responsibilities?

Drugs for Neuromuscular Disorders: Parkinsonism, Myasthenia Gravis, Multiple Sclerosis, Alzheimer's Disease, and Muscle Spasms

23

Outline

Objectives

- Define parkinsonism, myasthenia gravis, multiple sclerosis, and Alzheimer's disease.
- Describe the actions of anticholinergic drugs and dopaminergic drugs in the treatment of parkinsonism.
- Describe the side effects of antiparkinsonism drugs.
- Identify the drug group for the treatment of myasthenia gravis and Alzheimer's disease.
- Differentiate between centrally acting and peripherally acting muscle relaxants. Give an example of a drug from each group.
- Describe the nursing interventions, including client teaching, of drugs used in the treatment of parkinsonism, myasthenia gravis, muscle spasms, and Alzheimer's disease.
- Explain the treatment strategies for multiple sclerosis (MS).

Terms

acetylcholinesterase inhibitor
bradykinesia
cholinergic crisis
dopamine agonist
dyskinesia

dystonic movement
multiple sclerosis
muscle relaxants
muscle spasms
myasthenia crisis

myasthenia gravis
parkinsonism
pseudoparkinsonism

INTRODUCTION

Four types of neuromuscular disorders and the drugs used to treat them are discussed in this chapter: parkinsonism, myasthenia gravis, multiple sclerosis, and muscle spasms. Alzheimer's disease, a neurological problem, is also discussed in this chapter.

Parkinsonism (Parkinson's disease), a chronic neurologic disorder that affects the extrapyramidal motor tract (which controls posture, balance, and locomotion), is considered a syndrome (combination of symptoms) because of its three major features: rigidity, **bradykinesia** (slow movement), and tremors. Rigidity (abnormally increased muscle tone) increases with movement. Postural changes caused by rigidity and bradykinesia include the chest and head thrust forward with the knees and hips flexed, a shuffling gait, and the absence of arm swing. Other characteristic symptoms are masked facies (no facial expression), involuntary tremors of the head and neck, and pill-rolling motions of the hands. The tremors may be more prevalent at rest.

Myasthenia gravis, a lack of nerve impulses and muscle responses at the myoneural (nerves in muscle endings) junction, causes fatigue and muscular weakness of the respiratory system, facial muscles, and extremities. Because of cranial nerve involvement, ptosis (drooping eyelid) and difficulty in chewing and swallowing occur. Respiratory arrest may result from respiratory muscle paralysis. Myasthenia gravis is caused by an inadequate secretion of acetylcholine or a loss of acetylcholine because of an increase of the enzyme acetylcholinesterase, which destroys acetylcholine at the myoneural junction.

Multiple sclerosis (MS) treatment strategies for acute, remissions and exacerbations, and chronic progressive phases of MS are described in Table 23–5. This neuromuscular disorder is difficult to diagnose; therefore, pharmacologic treatment is necessary to control the symptoms of this disorder.

Muscle spasms have various causes, including injury or motor neuron disorders, resulting in conditions such as cerebral palsy, multiple sclerosis, spinal cord injuries (paraplegia—paralysis of the legs), and cerebral vascular accident (stroke) or hemiplegia (paralysis of one side of the body). Spasticity of muscles can be reduced with the use of skeletal muscle relaxants.

PARKINSONISM

Dr. James Parkinson in 1817 described six patients as having "shaking palsy." Three symptoms were described by Dr. Parkinson: (1) involuntary tremors of the limbs, (2) rigidity of muscles, and (3) slowness of movement. In the United States, there are approximately one million persons with parkinsonism and 50,000 new cases diagnosed each year. Because parkinsonism generally affects clients between the ages of 50 and 70 years and older, many consider the health problem as part of the aging process caused by the loss of neurons. Usually, the symptoms have a gradual onset.

There are different types of parkinsonism. Pseudoparkinsonism frequently occurs as an adverse reaction to many antipsychotic drugs, especially the phenothiazines. Also, parkinsonism symptoms could result from poisonings, such as from carbon monoxide or manganese, and from arteriosclerosis and Wilson's disease (hepatolenticular degeneration).

Pathophysiology

Parkinsonism is caused by an imbalance of the neurotransmitters dopamine and acetylcholine. Parkinson's disease is marked by degeneration of neurons that originate in the substantia nigra of the midbrain and terminate at the basal ganglia of the extrapyramidal motor tract. The reason for the degeneration of neurons is unknown.

There are two neurotransmitters within neurons of the striatum of the brain: dopamine (DA), an inhibitory neurotransmitter, and acetylcholine (ACh), an excitatory neurotransmitter. Dopamine is released from the dopaminergic neurons; acetylcholine is released from the cholinergic neurons. Dopamine normally maintains control of acetylcholine and inhibits its excitatory response. With Parkinson's disease (parkinsonism), there is a degeneration of the dopaminergic neurons (cause unknown); thus, an imbalance between dopamine and acetylcholine occurs. With less dopamine production, acetylcholine is unopposed, thereby causing the excitation and stimulation of the neurons that release gamma-aminobutyric acid (GABA). With the increased stimulation of GABA-ergic neurons, movement disorders that are seen in parkinsonism occur.

By the time early symptoms of Parkinson's disease appear, 80% of the striatal dopamine has been depleted. The remaining striatal neurons synthesize the dopamine from levodopa and release dopamine as needed. Before the next dose of levodopa, symptoms (slow walking, loss of dexterity) return or worsen; 30 to 60 minutes after the dose, the client's functioning is much improved.

The drugs used to treat parkinsonism by reducing the symptoms or replacing the dopamine deficit fall into two categories: (1) anticholinergics, which block the cholinergic receptors, and (2) dopaminergics, which stimulate the dopamine receptors. Table 23–1 compares the various drugs used to treat parkinsonism.

Table 23–1
Comparison of Drugs to Treat Parkinson's Disease

DRUG	PURPOSE
DOPAMINERGICS	
Levodopa Carbidopa-levodopa	Decrease symptoms of parkinsonism. Carbidopa, a decarboxylase inhibitor, permits more levodopa to reach the striatum nerve terminals (where levodopa is converted to dopamine). With the use of carbidopa, less levodopa is needed.
DOPAMINE AGONISTS	
Amantadine	Amantadine was first used as an antiviral drug for influenza A. It decreases symptoms of parkinsonism. It can be given as an early treatment for Parkinson's disease, which could delay the use of levodopa. Amantadine is effective in treating drug-induced parkinsonism and has fewer side effects than anticholinergics.
Bromocriptine	A D_2 dopamine receptor agonist. Bromocriptine may be used for early treatment of Parkinson's disease. With increasing motor symptoms, bromocriptine can be given with levodopa therapy.
Pergolide	A D_1 and D_2 dopamine receptor agonist. It is more potent than bromocriptine and may be used for early treatment of Parkinson's disease. Pergolide can be used with levodopa.
MAO-B INHIBITOR	
Selegiline	Inhibits the catabolic enzymes of dopamine. Monoamine oxidase-B inhibitor extends the action of dopamine. It can be given in the early diagnosed phase of Parkinson's disease. If the drug is given with levodopa, the dosage of levodopa is usually decreased.
ANTICHOLINERGICS; ANTIPARKINSONISM	
	Anticholinergics were the first group of drugs used to treat Parkinson's disease before levodopa and dopamine agonists were introduced. Anticholinergics are useful in decreasing tremors related to Parkinson's disease. The major use of these agents currently is to treat drug-induced parkinsonism. Treatment should start with low dosages and then the dose should gradually be increased. The elderly are more susceptible to the many side effects of anticholinergics. Those clients with memory loss or dementia should *not* be on anticholinergic therapy.

Anticholinergics

Anticholinergic drugs reduce the rigidity and some of the tremors characteristic of parkinsonism but have minimal effect on the bradykinesia. The anticholinergics are parasympatholytics that inhibit the release of acetylcholine. Anticholinergics are still used to treat drug-induced parkinsonism **(pseudoparkinsonism),** a side effect of the antipsychotic drug group phenothiazines. Examples of anticholinergics used for parkinsonism include trihexyphenidyl (Artane), benztropine (Cogentin), biperiden (Akineton), procyclidine (Kemadrin), ethopropazine (Parsidol), and orphenadrine (Norflex). The latter two drugs are the newer anticholinergics.

Table 23–2 lists the anticholinergics, their dosages, uses, and considerations. Nursing process for anticholinergics for antiparkinsonism is presented according to assessment, potential nursing diagnoses, planning, nursing interventions, and evaluation. Anticholinergics used to treat parkinsonism are also discussed in Chapter 22.

Diphenhydramine (Benadryl), an antihistamine, has similar anticholinergic properties. It is sometimes used for treating mild parkinsonism and for the elderly who may not be able to tolerate levodopa or the dopamine agonist group of drugs.

Dopaminergics

LEVODOPA

The first dopaminergic drug was levodopa (L-dopa), introduced in 1961. Levodopa is the most effective drug for diminishing the symptoms of Parkinson's disease. The major benefit with the use of levodopa products is the client's increased mobility. Because dopamine cannot cross the blood–brain barrier, levodopa, a precursor of dopamine that can cross the blood–brain barrier, was developed. The enzyme dopa decarboxylase converts levodopa to dopamine in the brain. However, this enzyme is also found in the peripheral nervous system, thereby allowing 99% of levodopa to be converted to dopamine before it

Table 23-2
Antiparkinsonism Drugs: Anticholinergics

GENERIC (BRAND)	ROUTE AND DOSAGE	USES AND CONSIDERATIONS
Benztropine mesylate (Cogentin)	*Parkinsonism:* A: PO: Initially 0.5–1.0 mg/d in 1–2 divided doses (larger dose at h.s.); maint: 0.5–6 mg/d in 1–2 divided doses *Extrapyramidal syndrome:* A: PO: 1–4 mg/d in 1–2 divided doses IM/IV: 1–2 mg/d	For parkinsonism and drug-induced parkinsonism to reduce dystonia. May be taken with other antiparkinsonism drugs. Contraindicated in glaucoma, GI obstruction, severe ulcerative colitis, prostatic hypertrophy, myasthenia gravis. *Pregnancy category:* C; PB: UK; t½: UK
Biperiden HCl (Akineton)	*Parkinsonism:* A: PO: 2 mg t.i.d./q.i.d. IM/IV: 2 mg every 30 min to 4 doses; *max:* 8 mg/d C: IM/IV: 0.04 mg/kg or 1.2 mg/m², repeat if necessary	For parkinsonism and drug-induced parkinsonism (extrapyramidal symptoms [EPS]). With prolonged use, drug tolerance may occur. Similar contraindications as benztropine. Avoid taking drug with alcohol or CNS depressants. Dry mouth, blurred vision, drowsiness, muscle weakness and constipation may occur. *Pregnancy category:* C; PB: UK; t½: UK
Ethopropazine HCl (Parsidol)	*Parkinsonism:* A: PO: Initially 50 mg daily/b.i.d.; maint: 100–400 mg/d in divided doses; *max:* 600 mg/d in divided doses	For all types of parkinsonism. A phenothiazine derivative with anticholinergic and antihistamine effects. Common side effects include dry mouth, drowsiness, dizziness, confusion, urinary retention, constipation. Contraindications: glaucoma, GU obstruction, prostatic hypertrophy. *Pregnancy category:* C; PB: UK; t½: UK
Orphenadrine HCl or citrate (Disipal, Norflex, Banflex)	A: PO: 50 mg t.i.d. or 100 mg b.i.d.	For parkinsonism. It is an antihistamine with some anticholinergic effects. Has slight CNS stimulation and can cause euphoria. *Pregnancy category:* C; PB: UK; t½: 14 h
Procyclidine HCl (Kemadrin)	*Parkinsonism:* A: PO: 2.5 mg p.c. t.i.d. *Extrapyramidal syndrome:* A: PO: Initially 2.5 mg p.c. t.i.d.; maint: 2.5–5 mg p.c. t.i.d.	For parkinsonism and drug-induced parkinsonism. Relieves rigidity more than tremors. May be taken with other antiparkinsonism drugs. Contraindicated in glaucoma. *Pregnancy category:* C; PB: UK; t½: UK
Trihexyphenidyl HCl (Artane)	See Chart 22–3	For all types of parkinsonism. Most widely used antiparkinsonism drug. Contraindicated in narrow-angle glaucoma. Common side effects include nausea, dry mouth, nervousness, dizziness, blurred vision, constipation, urinary hesitancy. *Pregnancy category:* C; PB: UK; t½: 5 to 10 h

KEY: *A: adult; C: child; IM: intramuscular; IV: intravenous; PB: protein-binding; PO: by mouth: t½: half-life; UK: unknown; GI: gastrointestinal; CNS: central nervous system; GU: genitourinary; p.c.: after meals.*

reaches the brain. Because only about 1% of levodopa is converted to dopamine in the brain, large doses of the drug are needed to achieve a pharmacologic response. Many side effects occur because of these high doses, including nausea, vomiting, dyskinesia, orthostatic hypotension, cardiac dysrhythmias, and psychosis. Levodopa has a short half-life (1 to 2 h), so the drug is taken three to four times a day. The drug is initially administered in low doses for a week and gradually increased over a period of weeks. It usually takes 2 to 4 months to achieve the maximum effect of the drug.

CARBIDOPA AND LEVODOPA

Because of the side effects of levodopa and the fact that so much of the levodopa is metabolized before it reaches the brain, an alternative drug, carbidopa, was developed that inhibits the enzyme dopa decarboxylase. By inhibiting the enzyme in the periphery, more levodopa reaches the brain. The carbidopa is combined with levodopa in a ratio of 1 part carbidopa to 10 parts levodopa. Figure 23–1 illustrates the comparative action of levodopa and carbidopa-levodopa.

The advantages of combining levodopa with carbidopa are

NURSING PROCESS
ANTIPARKINSONISM: ANTICHOLINERGIC

Assessment

- Obtain a medical history. Report if the client has a history of glaucoma, gastrointestinal (GI) dysfunction, urinary retention, angina pectoris, or myasthenia gravis. All anticholinergics are contraindicated if the client has glaucoma.
- Obtain a drug history. Report if a drug-drug interaction is probable. Phenothiazines, tricyclic antidepressants, and antihistamines increase the effect of trihexyphenidyl.
- Assess baseline vital signs (VS) for future comparisons. Pulse rate may increase.
- Determine usual urinary output as a baseline for comparison. Urinary retention may occur with continuous use of anticholinergics.

Potential Nursing Diagnoses

- Impaired physical mobility
- Risk for activity intolerance

Planning

- Client will have decreased involuntary symptoms caused by parkinsonism or drug-induced parkinsonism.

Nursing Interventions

- Monitor VS, urine output, and bowel sounds. Increased pulse rate, urinary retention, and constipation are side effects of anticholinergics.
- Observe for involuntary movements.

Client Teaching

General
- Advise the client to avoid alcohol, cigarette smoking, caffeine, and aspirin to decrease gastric acidity.

Diet
- Encourage the client to ingest foods that are high in fiber and to increase fluid intake to prevent constipation.

Side Effects
- Suggest that the client relieve dry mouth with hard candy, ice chips, or sugarless chewing gum. Anticholinergics decrease salivation.
- Suggest that the client use sunglasses in direct sun because of possible photophobia.
- Advise the client to void before taking the drug to minimize urinary retention. This is especially important if urine retention is present.
- Advise the client taking an anticholinergic to control symptoms of parkinsonism to have routine eye examinations to determine the presence of increased intraocular pressure, which indicates glaucoma. Clients who have glaucoma should *not* take anticholinergics.

Evaluation

- Evaluate the client's response to trihexyphenidyl or benztropine mesylate to determine whether parkinsonism symptoms are controlled.

- More dopamine reaches the basal ganglia.
- A single dose per day is administered instead of multiple doses.
- Smaller doses of levodopa are required to achieve the desired effect.

The disadvantage of the carbidopa-levodopa combination is that with more available levodopa, more side effects may be noted, including nausea, vomiting, **dystonic movements** (involuntary abnormal movements), and psychotic behavior. The drug is

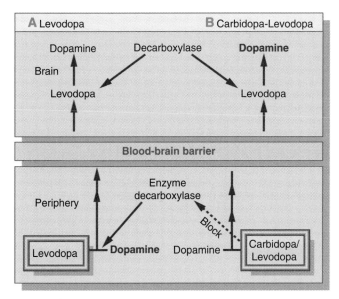

Figure 23–1
Levodopa and carbidopa-levodopa. (A) Levodopa. Ninety-nine percent of levodopa has been converted to dopamine in the periphery, and 1% of levodopa reaches the brain. (B) Carbidopa-levodopa. Carbidopa in this combination of carbidopa-levodopa inhibits the enzyme decarboxylase in the periphery; thus, more levodopa reaches the brain.

usually not prescribed for drug-related parkinsonism (antipsychotics). The peripheral side effects of levodopa are not as prevalent; however, cardiac dysrhythmia, palpitations, and orthostatic hypotension may occur. Chart 23–1 lists the pharmacologic behavior of carbidopa-levodopa.

Dopamine Agonists

Other dopaminergics called **dopamine agonists** stimulate the dopamine receptors. For example, amantadine hydrochloride (Symmetrel) is an antiviral drug that acts on the dopamine receptors. It may be taken as the only drug for parkinsonism or taken in combination with levodopa or an anticholinergic drug. Initially, amantadine produces improvement in symptoms of parkinsonism in approximately two-thirds of the clients; however, the improvement is usually not sustained because of the development of drug tolerance. Amantadine can be used for drug-induced parkinsonism.

Bromocriptine mesylate (Parlodel) acts directly on the dopamine receptors in the central nervous system (CNS), cardiovascular system, and GI tract. Bromocriptine is more effective than amantadine and the anticholinergics; however, it is not as effective as levodopa in alleviating parkinsonian symptoms. Clients who do not tolerate levodopa are frequently given bromocriptine. It is thought that dopamine receptors affected by bromocriptine are different from those affected by levodopa. Bromocriptine may be given with levodopa or carbidopa-levodopa.

The enzyme monoamine oxidase-B (MAO-B) causes catabolism (breakdown) of dopamine. Selegiline inhibits MAO-B, thus prolonging the action of levodopa. It may be ordered for newly diagnosed clients with Parkinson's disease. This drug could delay levodopa therapy by a year.

Large doses of selegiline may inhibit MAO-A, an enzyme that promotes the metabolism of tyramine in the gastrointestinal tract. Ingestion of foods high in tyramine, such as aged cheese, red wine, and bananas, if they are not metabolized by MAO-A, can cause a hypertensive crisis. Severe adverse drug interactions can occur between selegiline and various tricyclic antidepressants (TCA) or selective serotonin uptake inhibitors (SSUI).

Table 23–3 lists dopaminergics, dopamine agonists, and MAO-B inhibitors, their dosages, and uses and considerations.

SIDE EFFECTS AND ADVERSE REACTIONS

The common side effects of anticholinergics include dry mouth and dry secretions, urinary retention, constipation, blurred vision, and an increase in pulse rate. Mental effects, such as restlessness and confusion, may occur in the older adult.

The side effects of levodopa are numerous. GI disturbances are common because dopamine stimulates the chemoreceptor trigger zone (CTZ) in the medulla, which stimulates the vomiting center. Nausea and vomiting can be decreased by taking the drug with food or at mealtime; however, food will slow the absorption rate. **Dyskinesia** (impaired voluntary movement) may occur with high levodopa dosages. Cardiovascular side effects include orthostatic hypotension and increased heart rate during early use of levodopa. Cardiac dysrhythmias may occur as the levodopa dosages are increased. Psychosis (paranoia) and increased libido are additional side effects of increased levodopa dosages.

Amantadine has few side effects, but they can intensify when the drug is combined with other antiparkinsonism drugs. Orthostatic hypotension, confusion, urinary retention, and constipation are common side effects of amantadine. Side effects from bromocriptine are more common than from amantadine and include GI disturbances (nausea), orthostatic hypotension, palpitations, chest pain, edema in the lower extremities, nightmares, delusions, and confusion. If bromocriptine is taken with levodopa, usually the drug dosages are reduced and side effects and drug intolerance decrease.

NURSING PROCESS
ANTIPARKINSONISM: DOPAMINERGIC AGENT: CARBIDOPA-LEVODOPA

Assessment

- Obtain the client's VS to use for future comparison.
- Assess the client for signs and symptoms of parkinsonism, including stooped forward posture, shuffling gait, masked facies, and resting tremors.
- Obtain a history from the client of glaucoma, heart disease, peptic ulcers, kidney or liver disease, and psychosis.
- Report if drug-drug interaction is probable. Drugs that should be avoided or closely monitored are levodopa, bromocriptine, and anticholinergics.
- Obtain a drug history.

Potential Nursing Diagnoses

- Impaired physical mobility
- Risk for activity intolerance

Planning

- Symptoms of parkinsonism will be decreased or absent after 1 to 4 wk of drug therapy.

Nursing Interventions

- Monitor the client's VS and electrocardiogram (ECG). Orthostatic hypotension may occur during early use of levodopa and bromocriptine. Have the client rise slowly to avoid faintness.
- Check for weakness, dizziness, or syncope, which are symptoms of orthostatic hypotension.
- Administer carbidopa-levodopa (Sinemet) with low-protein foods. High-protein diets interfere with drug transport to the CNS.
- Observe for parkinsonism symptoms.

Client Teaching

General
- Advise the client not to abruptly discontinue the medication. Rebound parkinsonism (increased symptoms of parkinsonism) can occur.
- Inform the client that urine may be discolored and will darken with exposure to air. Perspiration also may be dark. Explain that both are harmless but that clothes may be stained.

Nursing Process continued on following page

CONTRAINDICATIONS

Anticholinergics or any drugs that have anticholinergic effects are contraindicated for persons with glaucoma. Persons with severe cardiac, renal, or psychiatric health problems should avoid levodopa drugs because of adverse reactions. Clients with chronic obstructive lung diseases, such as emphysema, can have dry, thick mucous secretions resulting from large doses of anticholinergic drugs.

DRUG-DRUG INTERACTIONS

Pyridoxine (vitamin B_6) increases dopa decarboxylase action, which metabolizes levodopa in the peripheral

nervous system to dopamine. Foods rich in pyridoxine such as beans (lima, navy, and kidney) and certain cereals should therefore be avoided. Antipsychotic drugs block the receptors for dopamine. Levodopa taken with a MAO inhibitor antidepressant can cause a hypertensive crisis.

MYASTHENIA GRAVIS

Myasthenia gravis (MG) is mainly caused by an autoimmune disease that affects approximately 1 in 10,000 persons. This disorder involves an antibody response

- Advise the diabetic client that the blood sugar level should be checked with an over-the-counter (OTC) reagent strip (Hemastix or Chemstrip bG) and not done through urine testing. With Clinitest, a false-positive test result can occur; with Tes-Tape or Clinistix, a false-negative test result can occur.

Diet
- Suggest to the client that taking levodopa with food may decrease GI upset; however, food will slow the drug absorption rate.
- Advise the client to avoid vitamins that contain vitamin B_6 (pyridoxine) and foods rich in vitamin B_6, such as beans (lima, navy, kidney) and cereals that contain the vitamin.
- Advise the client taking high doses of selegiline to avoid foods high in tyramine, such as aged cheese, red wine, cream, yogurt, chocolate, bananas, and raisins. Encourage the client to check with a dietitian in regard to these foods.

Side Effects
- Instruct the client to report side effects and symptoms of dyskinesia. Explain to the client that it may take weeks or months before the symptoms are controlled.

Amantadine and Bromocriptine
- Suggest that the client taking amantadine report any signs of skin lesions, seizures, or depression. A history of these health problems should have been reported to the health care provider.
- Advise the client taking bromocriptine to report symptoms of lightheadedness when changing positions (a symptom of orthostatic hypotension).
- Advise the client to avoid alcohol when taking bromocriptine.
- Teach the client to check heart rate and to report changes in rate or irregularity. The client should know baseline heart rate.
- Instruct the client not to abruptly stop the drug without first notifying the health care provider. Any adverse reactions should be reported immediately.

Cultural Considerations
- Recognize that various cultural groups will need guidance in understanding the disease process of parkinsonism. Support the client and family member who may be dismayed about the symptoms of parkinsonism and lack knowledge of the disease process.
- An interpreter may be needed for clients who speak little or no English, to understand drug doses and schedules and to recognize severe side effects that need to be reported to the health care provider.

Evaluation

- Evaluate the effectiveness of the drug therapy in controlling the symptoms of parkinsonism.
- Determine that there is an absence of side effects.

against an alpha subunit of the acetylcholine receptor (AChR) site in the skeletal muscle. The response leads to a degradation of the acetylcholine receptors. About 90% of clients with MG have anti-AChR antibodies, which are detected through serum testing. Myasthenia gravis has been associated with abnormalities of the thymus gland. Thymectomy has been an option for clients younger than age 50.

Myasthenia gravis results from a lack of acetylcholine reaching the cholinergic receptors. This health problem is characterized by weakness and fatigue of the skeletal muscles. Another theory is that the decrease in acetylcholine (ACh) is caused by the enzyme acetylcholinesterase (AChE) destroying the ACh. Early reported symptoms of myasthenia gravis are ptosis and diplopia. Other characteristics of MG include muscle weakness, dysphagia, dysarthria, and respiratory muscle weakness. The group of drugs for controlling myasthenia gravis is the AChE inhibitors, also known as cholinesterase inhibitors and anticholinesterase, which inhibit the action of the enzyme. As the result of this action, more ACh activates the cholinergic receptors and promotes muscle contraction. The **AChE inhibitors** are classified as parasympathomimetics.

If muscle weakness persists after taking AChE inhibitors, the reason may be due to inadequate drug dosing. The client may be experiencing **myasthenia**

Chart 23–1.   Antiparkinsonism: Dopaminergic

CARBIDOPA-LEVODOPA

Drug Name

Carbidopa-Levodopa (Sinemet)
Pregnancy Category: C

Dosage

A: PO: 1:10 ratio; initially 10 carbidopa/100 levodopa t.i.d.; maint: 25/250 mg t.i.d.

Contraindications

Narrow-angle glaucoma; severe cardiac, renal, or hepatic disease
Caution: peptic ulcer, psychiatric disorders

Drug-Lab-Food Interactions

Drug: *Increase* hypertensive crisis with MAOIs
Decrease levodopa effect with anticholinergics, phenytoin, tricyclic antidepressants, pyridoxine
Lab: May *increase* BUN, AST, ALT, ALP, LDH
Food: Avoid foods containing pyridoxine (vitamin B_6)

Pharmacokinetics

Absorption: PO: Well absorbed
Distribution: PB: Carbidopa: 36%; levodopa: UK
Metabolism: $t\frac{1}{2}$: 1–2 h
Excretion: In urine as metabolites

Pharmacodynamics

PO: Onset: 15 min
        Peak: 1–3 h
        Duration: 5–12 h

Therapeutic Effects/Uses

To treat parkinsonism, to relieve tremors and rigidity.

Mode of Action: Transmission of levodopa to brain cells for conversion to dopamine; carbidopa blocks the conversion of levodopa to dopamine in the periphery.

Side Effects

Anorexia, nausea, vomiting, dysphagia, fatigue, dizziness, headache, dry mouth, bitter taste, twitching, blurred vision, insomnia

Adverse Reactions

Involuntary choreiform movements, palpitations, orthostatic hypotension, urinary retention, psychosis, severe depression, hallucinations

Life-threatening: Agranulocytosis, hemolytic anemia, cardiac dysrhythmias, leukopenia

Assessment and Planning · *Interventions* · *Evaluation* — **NURSING PROCESS**

KEY: A: adult; PO: by mouth; PB: protein-binding; $t\frac{1}{2}$: half-life; MAOIs: monoamine oxidase inhibitors; UK: unknown; BUN: blood urea nitrogen; AST: aspartate aminotransferase; ALT: alanine aminotransferase; ALP: alkaline phosphatase; LDH: lactic dehydrogenase.

crisis. If the muscle weakness remains untreated, death could result from paralysis of the respiratory muscle. Neostigmine, a fast-acting AChE inhibitor, can relieve myasthenia crisis. Overdosing with AChE inhibitors may cause cholinergic crisis.

Acetylcholinesterase Inhibitors

The first drug used to manage myasthenia gravis was neostigmine (Prostigmin). It is a short-acting AChE inhibitor with a half-life of 0.5 to 1 h. The drug is given every 2 to 4 h and must be given on time to prevent muscle weakness. The AChE inhibitor, pyridostigmine bromide (Mestinon), has an intermediate

action and is given every 3 to 6 h. Ambenonium chloride (Mytelase) is a long-acting AChE inhibitor and is usually prescribed when the client does not respond to neostigmine or pyridostigmine. Chart 23–2 presents drug data related to pyridostigmine. The cholinesterase (AChE) inhibitors are also discussed in Chapter 22.

PHARMACOKINETICS

Pyridostigmine is poorly absorbed from the GI tract. Fifty percent of the sustained-release capsule is absorbed readily and the balance is poorly absorbed. The half-life of oral pyridostigmine is 3.5 to 4 h, and intravenously it is 2 h. Because of its short half-life, it

Table 23–3
Antiparkinsonism: Dopaminergics

GENERIC (BRAND)	ROUTE AND DOSAGE	USES AND CONSIDERATIONS
DOPAMINERGICS		
Carbidopa-Levodopa (Sinemet)	See Chart 23–1	For parkinsonism. More levodopa reaches the brain; carbidopa blocks dopa decarboxylase in the periphery. Lower doses of levodopa are needed; thus fewer side effects. *Pregnancy category:* C; PB: 36% (carbidopa); $t\frac{1}{2}$: 1–2 h
Levodopa (or L-dopa) (Dopar, Larodopa)	A: PO: 0.5–1.0 g/d in 2–4 divided doses; increase dose gradually; average maint: 3–6 g/d with food, in divided doses; *max:* 8 mg/d	For parkinsonism. *Not* for drug-induced parkinsonism. Can cause GI upset; drug should be taken with food. Has many side effects, such as nausea, vomiting, orthostatic hypotension, cardiac dysrhythmias, and psychosis. *Pregnancy category:* C; PB: UK; $t\frac{1}{2}$: 1–3 h
DOPAMINE AGONISTS		
Amantadine HCl; (Symmetrel)	*Parkinsonism:* A: PO: 100 mg b.i.d.; may increase dose; *max:* 400 mg/d	For early onset parkinsonism, drug-induced parkinsonism, and influenza a respiratory virus. Effective for rigidity and bradykinesia; less effective for decreasing tremors. May be used alone or in combination. Has fewer side effects than anticholinergic drugs. *Pregnancy category:* C; PB: 60–70%; $t\frac{1}{2}$: 12–24 h
Bromocriptine mesylate (Parlodel)	A: PO: Initially 1.25–2.5 mg/d; may gradually increase dose; maint: 30–60 mg/d in 3 divided doses; *max:* 100 mg/d	For parkinsonism. Response is better than amantadine. Can be taken in adjunct with levodopa or carbidopa-levodopa. Hypotension, lightheadedness, and syncope are major side effects. Initially, small doses are given and then gradually increased over several weeks. *Pregnancy category:* C; PB: 90%–96%; $t\frac{1}{2}$: 6–8 h: terminal phase: 50 h
Pergolide mesylate (Permax)	A: PO: Initially 0.05 mg/d × 2 d; increase by 0.1–0.15 mg q3d × 12 d; *max:* 5 mg/d	For parkinsonism. Usually used as adjunct with levodopa or carbidopa-levodopa. It is more potent than bromocriptine. Same side effects as bromocriptine. *Pregnancy category:* B; PB: 90%; $t\frac{1}{2}$: UK
Pramipexole dihydrochloride (Mirapex)	A: PO: Initially: 0.375 mg/d in 3 divided doses; *maint:* 1.5–4.5 mg/d in 3 divided doses	New drug. Stimulates dopamine receptors in striatum. *Pregnancy category:* UK; PB: UK $t\frac{1}{2}$: UK
Ropinirole HCl (Requip)	A: PO: Initially: 0.25 mg, t.i.d.; *max:* 24 mg/d	New drug. Stimulates dopamine receptors in striatum. *Pregnancy category:* UK; PB: UK; $t\frac{1}{2}$: UK
MAO-B INHIBITOR		
Selegiline HCl (Eldepryl)	A: PO: 10 mg/d in 2 divided doses	For early onset parkinsonism. May delay the use of levodopa therapy by 1 year. It can be given with levodopa preparations; dose of levodopa would need to be decreased. *Pregnancy category:* C; PB: >90%; $t\frac{1}{2}$: 2–20 h
OTHERS		
Tolcapone (Tasmar)	A: PO: 50–400 mg, t.i.d.	To potentiate dopamine activity by inhibiting the enzyme COMT. It is used in conjunction with levodopa/carbidopa (Sinemet) and prolongs the action of levodopa. *Pregnancy category:* UK; PB: UK; $t\frac{1}{2}$: 2–3 h.

KEY: A: adult; PB: protein-binding; PO: by mouth; $t\frac{1}{2}$: half-life; UK: unknown; ×: times; GI: gastrointestinal.

Chart 23-2.   Myasthenia Gravis (Drugs for)

CHOLINESTERASE INHIBITOR

Drug Name

Pyridostigmine Bromide (Mestinon)
Pregnancy Category: C

Dosage

A: PO: 60–120 mg t.i.d./q.i.d.; *max:* 1.5 g/d
SR: 180–540 mg q.d. or b.i.d.
IM/IV: 2 mg q2–3h
C: PO: 7 mg/kg/d in 5–6 divided doses

Contraindications

GI and GU obstruction, severe renal disease
Caution: Asthma, bradycardia, peptic ulcer, cardiac dysrhythmias, pregnancy

Drug-Lab-Food Interactions

Drug: *Decrease* pyridostigmine effect with atropine, muscle relaxants, antidysrhythmics, magnesium

Pharmacokinetics

Absorption: PO: Poorly absorbed; SR: 50% absorbed
Distribution: PB: UK
Metabolism: t½: PO: 3.5–4 h; IV: 2 h
Excretion: In urine and by liver

Pharmacodynamics

PO:	Onset:	30–45 min
	Peak:	UK
	Duration:	3–6 h
PO SR:	Onset:	0.5–1 h
	Peak:	UK
	Duration:	6–12 h
IM:	Onset:	15 min
	Peak:	UK
	Duration:	2–4 h
IV:	Onset:	2–5 min
	Peak:	UK
	Duration:	2–3 h

Therapeutic Effects/Uses

To control and treat myasthenia gravis.

Mode of Action: Transmission of neuromuscular impulses by preventing the destruction of acetylcholine.

Side Effects

Nausea, vomiting, diarrhea, headache, dizziness, abdominal cramps, sweating, rash, miosis

Adverse Reactions

Hypotension, urticaria

Life-threatening: Respiratory depression, bronchospasm, cardiac dysrhythmias, seizures

Assessment and Planning

Interventions

Evaluation

NURSING PROCESS

KEY: A: adult; C: child; PO: by mouth; SR: sustained-release; IM: intramuscular; IV: intravenous; max: maximum; PB: protein-binding; t½: half-life; UK: unknown; GI: gastrointestinal; GU: genitourinary.

must be administered several times a day. The drug is metabolized by the liver and excreted in the urine.

PHARMACODYNAMICS

Pyridostigmine increases muscle strength of clients with muscular weakness resulting from myasthenia gravis. The onset of action of oral preparations is 0.5 to 1 h. The duration of action is longer with the sustained-release drug capsule. One-thirtieth of the oral dose of pyridostigmine can be administered intravenously. Overdosing of pyridostigmine can result in signs and symptoms of **cholinergic crisis** (extreme muscle weakness, increased salivation, tears, sweating, and miosis); thus, the antidote, atropine sulfate, should be available. This crisis requires emergency medical intervention.

Table 23-4
Acetylcholinesterase (AChE) Inhibitors: Myasthenia

GENERIC (BRAND)	ROUTE AND DOSAGE	USES AND CONSIDERATIONS
Ambenonium (Mytelase)	A: PO: 2.5–5.0 mg t.i.d./q.i.d.; dose may be increased; maint: 5–40 mg t.i.d./q.i.d.	For myasthenia gravis. A long-acting acetylcholinesterase (AChE) inhibitor. It is 6 times more potent than neostigmine. Frequently used when client cannot take neostigmine or pyridostigmine because of the bromide component. It can be taken in adjunct with glucocorticoid drug. *Pregnancy category:* C; PB: UK; t½: UK
Edrophonium Cl (Tensilon)	A: IV 2 mg; then 8 mg if no response IM: 10 mg, may repeat with 2 mg in 30 min C <34 kg: IV: 1 mg, repeat in 30–45 sec if no response; *max:* 5 mg C >34 kg: IV: 2 mg, repeat with 1 mg if no response; *max:* 10 mg	For diagnosing myasthenia gravis. Ptosis should be absent in 1–5 min. Very short-acting drug. *Pregnancy category:* C; PB: UK; t½: 1.2–2 h
Neostigmine bromide (Prostigmin) Neostigmine methyl-sulfate (injectable form)	A: PO: 150 mg/d in divided doses; *range:* 15–375 mg/d IM/IV: 0.5–2.5 mg as needed C: PO: 2 mg/kg/d in divided doses or 10 mg/m² q4h	For controlling myasthenia gravis. Must be given on time to prevent myasthenia crisis. Parenteral route is used if chewing, swallowing, and breathing are affected. Because of its short half-life, dose is usually given in 3 to 6 divided doses. Overdose can cause cholinergic reaction; nausea, abdominal cramps, excessive salivation, sweating. *Pregnancy category:* C; PB: 15%–25%; t½: 1–1.5 h
Pyridostigmine bromide (Mestinon)	See Chart 23–2	For myasthenia gravis. Also used to reverse postoperative muscle paralysis caused by a neuromuscular blocker. *Pregnancy category:* C; PB: UK; t½: 3.5–4 h

KEY: A: adult; C: child; PO: by mouth; IM: intramuscular; IV: intravenous; PB: protein-binding; t½: half-life; UK: unknown; <: less than; >: greater than.

Edrophonium chloride (Tensilon) is a drug used in diagnosing myasthenia gravis. It is a very short-acting AChE inhibitor that increases muscle strength during its duration of action (5 to 20 min). If ptosis (droopy eyelid) is immediately corrected after administration of this drug, the diagnosis is most likely myasthenia gravis. Table 23–4 lists the acetylcholinesterase inhibitors.

Overdosing and underdosing of AChE inhibitors have similar symptoms, such as muscle weakness, dyspnea (difficulty breathing), and dysphagia (difficulty swallowing). Additional symptoms that may be present with overdosing are increased salivation (drooling), bradycardia, abdominal cramping, and increased tearing and sweating. All doses of AChE inhibitors should be administered *on time* because late administration of the drug could result in muscle weakness.

Edrophonium (Tensilon) is an ultrashort-acting AChE inhibitor that may be used to distinguish between myasthenia crisis and cholinergic crisis. These two different crises have a similar major symptom, severe muscle weakness. After edrophonium is administered, if the symptoms are alleviated because of an increase in acetylcholine, the cause is myasthenia crisis. However, if the muscle weakness becomes more severe, the cause is cholinergic crisis caused by drug overdosing.

Side Effects and Adverse Reactions

Side effects and adverse reactions of AChE inhibitors include GI disturbances (nausea, vomiting, diarrhea, abdominal cramps), increased salivation and tearing, miosis (constricted pupil of the eye), and possible hypertension.

MULTIPLE SCLEROSIS

Multiple sclerosis (MS) is characterized by multiple lesions of the myelin sheath called plaques. It is a condition in which there are remissions and exacerbations of multiple symptoms (sensory and cerebellar)

NURSING PROCESS
MYASTHENIA GRAVIS (DRUGS FOR): PYRIDOSTIGMINE (MESTINON)

Assessment

- Obtain a drug history of drugs that the client is currently taking. Report if a drug-drug interaction is likely. Client should avoid atropine, atropine-like drugs, and muscle relaxants.
- Obtain baseline VS for future comparison.
- Assess the client for signs and symptoms of **myasthenia crisis,** such as muscle weakness with difficulty breathing and swallowing.

Potential Nursing Diagnoses

- Inability to sustain spontaneous ventilation
- Risk for activity intolerance
- Anxiety related to possible recurrence of myasthenia crisis

Planning

- The client's symptoms of muscle weakness and difficulty breathing and swallowing caused by myasthenia gravis will be eliminated or reduced in 2 to 3 d.

Nursing Interventions

- Monitor the effectiveness of drug therapy (acetylcholinesterase [AChE] inhibitors). Muscle strength should be increased. Both depth and rate of respirations should be assessed and maintained within normal range.
- Administer IV pyridostigmine undiluted at rate of 0.5 mg/min. Do *not* add the drug to IV fluids.
- Observe the client for signs and symptoms of cholinergic crisis caused by overdosing, including muscle weakness, increased salivation, sweating, tearing, and miosis.
- Have readily available an antidote for cholinergic crisis (atropine sulfate).

Client Teaching

General
- Instruct the client to take the drugs as prescribed to avoid recurrence of symptoms.
- Encourage the client to wear a medical ID bracelet or necklace (e.g., MedicAlert) indicating the health problem and the drugs taken.

Diet
- Instruct the client to take the drug before meals for best drug absorption. If gastric irritation occurs, take the drug with food.

Side Effects
- Advise the client to report to the health care provider recurrence of symptoms of myasthenia gravis. Drug therapy may need to be modified.

Evaluation

- Evaluate the effectiveness of the drug therapy. Muscle strength should be maintained.
- Determine the absence of respiratory distress.

---

such as motor weakness, spasticity, or diplopia. MS is difficult to diagnose because there is no specific diagnostic test. Available laboratory tests that may suggest MS include elevated IgG in the cerebrospinal fluid, increased IgG/albumin ratio, and multiple lesions on magnetic resonance imaging (MRI). A study, cited by Noronha and Arnason, of monthly MRI scans of clients with MS indicated that the MRI scans identified four times the frequency of new lesions, suggestive of MS attacks, without clients having clinical symptoms. Having a scheduled treatment protocol to avoid clinical MS attacks is not recommended because of the side effects of the drugs used, such as glucocorticoids.

There are treatment strategies for three types or phases of MS: the acute attack, remission-exacerbation, and chronic progressive MS. Table 23–5 describes these three phases of MS. Goals for treatment strategies are to decrease the inflammatory process of nerve fibers and to improve conduction of demyelinating axons.

Drugs that the client with MS should avoid include histamine (H_2) blockers such as cimetidine and ranitidine, indomethacin (an NSAID), and beta-blockers such as propranolol. Various drug regimens for treating MS are currently in research and development.

ALZHEIMER'S DISEASE

Alzheimer's disease is an incurable dementing illness characterized by chronic, progressive neurodegenerative conditions with marked cognitive dysfunction. The onset occurs between ages 45 and 65 (Table 23–6). It affects about 4 million Americans, and about 250,000 new cases are diagnosed annually. Approximately 50% of clients in nursing homes were admitted with Alzheimer's disease. This health problem is the fourth leading cause of death in adults. The annual cost for caring for clients with Alzheimer's is around $85 billion dollars.

Pathophysiology

Many physiologic changes contribute to Alzheimer's disease. Currently, the theories related to the changes causing Alzheimer include (1) degeneration of the cholinergic neuron and deficiency in acetylcholine, (2) neuritic plaques that form mainly outside the neurons and in the cerebral cortex, (3) beta-amyloid protein accumulation in high levels that may contribute to neuronal injury, and (4) presence of neurofibrillary tangles with twists inside the neurons. Figure 23–2 illustrates the normal neuron and the neuron affected by Alzheimer's disease. Other factors thought to influence the occurrence of Alzheimer's are slow virus or infection that attacks brain cells and genetic predisposition.

Symptoms of Alzheimer's disease progress from confusion to memory loss, to dementia (Table 23–7). With loss of memory, loss of logical thinking and judgment and time disorientation occur. As the disease progresses, memory loss becomes more severe, personality changes occur, and tendency to wander,

Table 23–5
Treatment Strategies for the Three Phases of Multiple Sclerosis

PHASES OF MULTIPLE SCLEROSIS	CHARACTERISTICS	TREATMENT STRATEGIES
Acute attack	Fatigue; motor weakness; optic neuritis	• Tapering course of glucocorticoids (prednisone) • Adrenocorticotropic hormone (ACTH) stimulates the adrenal cortex to secrete cortisol. • ACTH can be given IM or IV. (1) Aqueous ACTH, 80 units in 500 mL of D_5W for 1–5 d (2) Tapering doses of ACTH gel, IM for 25–30 d, starting with 40 units, b.i.d. • 6-alpha methylprednisolone sodium succinate (MP) (1) MP 1 g/d, IV, for 5–7 d (2) Tapering doses of oral glucocorticoid
Remission-exacerbation	Recurrence of clinical MS symptoms; spasticity	• Biologic (immune) response modifiers (BRM); see Chapter 34. Betaseron, an interferon-β (IFN-β), 0.25 mg (8 mIU) every other day. It reduces spasticity and improves muscle movement. • Immunosuppressant drug azathioprine (Imuran). Reduces exacerbation (relapses). Used for MS to decrease steroid use.
Chronic progressive	Progressive MS symptoms (wheelchair bound)	• Immunosuppressant cyclophosphamide (Cytoxan) *Possible treatment protocol* (1) Cytoxan 600 mg/m² in 250 mL of D_5W, every other day × 5 doses. Monitor WBC values. (2) ACTH, tapering doses for 14 d. Starting with 40 units, IM, b.i.d.

KEY: IM: intramuscular; IV: intravenous; m²: square meter (body surface area); WBC: white blood count.

Table 23–6
Percentage of Persons in United States Having Alzheimer's Disease

AGE (YEARS)	PERCENTAGE
45–65	2
65–74	3–5
75–84	19
>85	47

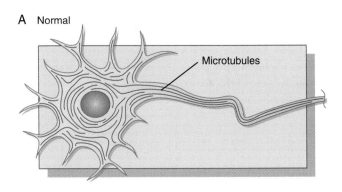

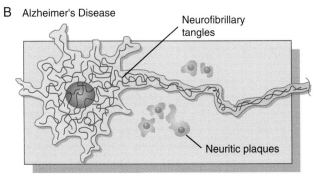

Figure 23–2
Histologic changes in Alzheimer's disease. (A) Healthy neuron. (B) Neuron affected by Alzheimer's disease, showing characteristic neuritic plaques and cellular neurofibrillary tangles. (Adapted from Lehne, R. A. *Pharmacology for Nursing Care*, 3/E. Philadelphia: WB Saunders, 1998.)

hyperactivity, hostility, paranoia, and inability to speak or express oneself result. Custodial care becomes necessary.

Acetylcholinesterase Inhibitors

There are no known medications to cure Alzheimer's disease. Two medications approved by the Food and Drug Administration (FDA) are ergoloid mesylate (Hydergine), which has not been that successful for treating memory loss, and tacrine (Cognex), which is helpful in diminishing memory loss. A new AChE inhibitor that has recently been approved by the FDA is donepertl (Aricept), which permits more acetylcholine in the neuron receptors. Doneperil is useful to treat mild to moderate Alzheimer's disease. Several drugs are under investigation for treating Alzheimer's. Some of these are certain NSAIDs (piracetam, indomethacin), calcium blockers, MAO-B inhibitors (selegiline), serotonin antagonists, CNS stimulants (methylphenidate [Ritalin]), and angiotensin-converting enzyme (ACE) inhibitors.

Table 23–7
Stages and Phases of Alzheimer's Disease

STAGE	CLINICAL PHASE	SYMPTOMS
1	Mild (early confusion)	Early cognitive decline in one or more areas; memory loss, decreased ability to function in work situation, name-finding deficit, some decrease in social functioning, recall difficulties, anxiety
2	Moderate	Unable to perform complex tasks such as managing personal finances, planning a dinner party, concentration, and knowledge of current events
3	Moderately severe (early dementia)	Usually needs assistance for survival; reminders to bathe, help in selecting clothes, and other daily functions; may be disoriented as to time and recent events although this can fluctuate; may become tearful
4	Severe (dementia)	Needs assistance with dressing, bathing, and toilet functions (e.g., flushing), may forget spouse, family, and caregivers' names, details of their personal life, and generally be unaware of their surroundings; incontinence of urine and feces may occur in this stage; increase in central nervous system disturbances such as agitation, delusions, paranoia, obsessive anxiety, and increased potential for violent behavior
5	Very severe (late dementia)	Unable to speak (speech limited to 5 words or less), person may scream or make other sounds; unable to ambulate, sit up, smile, or feed self; unable to hold head erect, will ultimately slip into stupor or coma

Data from McKenry, L M., and Salerno, E. Pharmacology in Nursing, 20/E. St. Louis: C.V. Mosby, p. 469, 1998.

Chart 23–3. Alzheimer's Disease (Drugs for)

ACETYLCHOLINESTERASE INHIBITOR

Drug

Tacrine (Cognex)
Pregnancy Category: C

Dosage

A: PO: Initially: 10 mg, q.i.d.; after 6 wk: 20 mg, q.i.d.; after 12 wk: 30 mg, q.i.d.; after 16 wk: 40 mg, q.i.d.; *max:* 160 mg/d

Contraindications

Liver and renal diseases

Drug-Lab-Food Interactions

Drug: *Increase* effect of theophylline
Increase effect with cimetidine
Lab: *Increase* ALT, AST

Pharmacokinetics

Absorption: PO: Food decreases absorption rate
Distribution: PB: 50%
Metabolism: t½: 3 h
Excretion: In urine

Pharmacodynamics

PO: Onset: 0.5 h
       Peak: 2 h
       Duration: 24–36 h

Therapeutic Effects/Uses

Improves memory loss.

Mode of Action: Elevates acetylcholine concentration.

Side Effects

Anorexia, nausea, vomiting, diarrhea, dizziness, headache, constipation, rhinitis, depression

Adverse Reactions

Life threatening: Hepatotoxicity

(Nursing Process side labels: Assessment and Planning; Interventions; Evaluation; NURSING PROCESS)

KEY: PO: by mouth; PB: protein-binding; t½: half-life; ALT: alanine aminotransferase; AST: aspartate aminotransferase.

Table 23–8
Acetylcholinesterase (AChE) Inhibitors for Alzheimer's Disease

GENERIC (BRAND)	ROUTE AND DOSAGE	USES AND CONSIDERATIONS
Donepezil (Aricept)	A: PO: 5–10 mg/d	New AChE inhibitor. To treat mild to moderate phase of Alzheimer's disease. *Pregnancy category:* UK; PB: UK; t½: UK
Ergoloid mesylates (Hydergine)	A: PO: Initially, 1 mg	To increase cognitive function. The actual improvement is uncertain. *Pregnancy category:* C; PB: UK; t½: 3.5 h
Tacrine HCl (Cognex)	See Chart 23–3	To treat mild to moderate phase of Alzheimer's disease. It increases the acetylcholine concentration and helps to increase memory. *Pregnancy category:* C; PB: 50%; t½: 3 h

KEY: A: adult; PO: by mouth; PB: protein-binding; t½: half-life; UK: unknown.

NURSING PROCESS
ALZHEIMER'S DISEASE (DRUGS FOR): TACRINE

Assessment

- Assess client's mental and physical abilities. Note limitation of cognitive function and self-care.
- Obtain a history of liver or renal disease or dysfunction.
- Assess for memory and judgment losses. Elicit from family members a history of behavioral changes, such as memory loss, declining interest in people, home, difficulty in following through with simple activities, and tendency to wander from home.
- Observe for signs of behavioral disturbances such as hyperactivity, hostility, wandering.
- Check for signs of aphasia or difficulty in speech.
- Determine client's motor function.
- Determine family members' ability in coping with client's mental and physical changes.

Potential Nursing Diagnoses

- Altered thought processes
- Impaired physical mobility
- Self-care deficit: dressing, feeding, toileting
- Chronic confusion
- Altered family processes
- Ineffective family coping
- Risk for injury
- Altered nutrition: less than body requirement

Planning

- Client's loss of memory will proceed slower with the medication AChE inhibitor than without medication.
- Client can maintain self-care of body functions with assistance.

Nursing Interventions

- Maintain consistency in care.
- Assist client in ambulation and activity.
- Check for side effects related to the continuous use of AChE inhibitors.

Nursing Process continued on following page

Tacrine (Cognex), an AChE inhibitor, is prescribed to improve cognitive function for clients with mild to moderate Alzheimer's disease (Chart 23–3). This drug increases the amount of acetylcholine (ACh) at the cholinergic synapses. Tacrine tends to slow the disease process. Only 30% of clients have an effective response to tacrine, and for those it has a short-lasting effect. Table 23–8 lists the drugs used for treating Alzheimer's disease.

PHARMACOKINETICS

Tacrine is absorbed faster through the gastrointestinal tract without food. Because it has a relatively short half-life, tacrine is given four times a day, and the dose is gradually increased. The protein-binding power is average.

PHARMACODYNAMICS

Tacrine has been somewhat successful in improving memory in early phase Alzheimer's disease. The onset of action and peak time are average: ½ to 1½ hours for onset and 2 hours for peak action. However, the duration of action is prolonged to 24 to 36 hours, thus side effects should be closely monitored. This drug is contraindicated for clients with liver disease because hepatotoxicity may occur. Cumulative drug effect is likely to occur in the "older" elderly, and those with liver and renal dysfunction.

SKELETAL MUSCLE RELAXANTS

Muscle relaxants relieve muscular spasms and pain associated with traumatic injuries and chronic debili-

- Check vital signs periodically. Note signs of bradycardia and hypotension.
- Monitor client's behavioral changes and record improvement or decline.

Client Teaching

General
- Explain to client and family members the purpose for the prescribed drug therapy.
- Explain to the family member who is responsible for the client's medications, the time for drug dosing and the schedule for increasing drug dosing.
- Instruct the family member in such techniques as placing obstacles away from the client's foot path, and so on, so that the client can avoid injury from wandering.
- Inform the family member of support groups that are available, such as Alzheimer's Disease and Related Disorders Association.

Side Effects
- Inform client and family member that the client should rise slowly to avoid dizziness and loss of balance.

Diet
- Instruct family member about foods that may be prepared for client's consumption and tolerance.

Cultural Considerations
- Recognize that various cultural groups may need guidance in understanding the disease process of Alzheimer's disease.
- Explain to family members from various cultural backgrounds that their family member is not "crazy" but has a neurologic problem that may be part of the aging process. Explain how the symptoms may become more progressive.

Evaluation

- Evaluate the effectiveness of drug regimen by determining whether client's mental and physical status shows improvement from drug therapy.

tating disorders, such as multiple sclerosis, strokes (cerebrovascular accident [CVA]), cerebral palsy, and spinal cord injuries. Spasticity results from increased muscle tone from hyperexcitable neurons caused by increased stimulation from the cerebral neurons or lack of inhibition in the spinal cord or at the skeletal muscles. Muscle relaxants are divided into two major groups: centrally acting and peripherally acting. The centrally acting muscle relaxants depress neuron activity in the spinal cord or brain, and the peripherally acting muscle relaxants act directly on the skeletal muscles.

Centrally Acting Muscle Relaxants

The centrally acting muscle relaxants are used to treat acute spasms from muscle trauma. This group of muscle relaxants is not as effective against chronic neurologic disorders as the peripherally acting muscle relaxants, with the exceptions of diazepam (Valium) and baclofen (Lioresal). Examples of centrally acting muscle relaxants include carisoprodol (Soma), chlorphenesin carbamate (Maolate), chlorzoxazone (Paraflex), cyclobenzaprine (Flexeril), metaxalone (Skelaxin), methocarbamol (Robaxin), orphenadrine citrate (Norflex), and baclofen (Lioresal). Baclofen acts on the spinal cord. These drugs are similar in their action, side effects, and adverse reactions. The choice of drug is usually personal.

The centrally-acting muscle relaxants decrease pain and increase range of motion. They have a sedative effect and should not be taken concurrently with CNS depressants, such as barbiturates, narcotics, and alcohol. The centrally acting muscle relaxants are described in Table 23–9.

Two anxiolytics, diazepam (Valium) and meprobamate (Equanil), may be effective in decreasing muscle spasms resulting from acute traumatic injury or chronic neurologic disorders. Diazepam may also be

Table 23–9
Muscle Relaxants (Skeletal)

GENERIC (BRAND)	ROUTE AND DOSAGE	USES AND CONSIDERATIONS
ANXIOLYTICS		
Diazepam (Valium) CSS IV	A: PO: 2–10 mg b.i.d./q.i.d. IM/IV: 5–10 mg; may repeat	Diazepam has many uses, one of which is to relieve muscle spasms associated with paraplegia and cerebral palsy. Contraindicated in narrow-angle glaucoma. *Pregnancy category:* D; PB: 98%; $t_{\frac{1}{2}}$: 20–50 h
Meprobamate (Equanil, Miltown) CSS IV	A: PO: 400 mg–1.2 g/d in divided doses	This anxiolytic has a muscle relaxant effect. *Pregnancy category:* D; PB: UK; $t_{\frac{1}{2}}$: 10–12 h
CENTRALLY ACTING MUSCLE RELAXANTS		
Baclofen (Lioresal)	A: PO: Initially 5 mg t.i.d.; may increase dose; maint: 10–20 mg t.i.d./q.i.d.; *max:* 80 mg/d	For muscle spasms caused by multiple sclerosis and spinal cord injury. Overdose may cause CNS depression. Drowsiness, dizziness, nausea, hypotension may occur. *Pregnancy category:* C; PB: 30%; $t_{\frac{1}{2}}$: 3–4 h
Carisoprodol (Soma)	See Chart 23–4	For muscle spasms and other painful musculoskeletal disorders. It is available in compound form with aspirin and aspirin with codeine. Same side effects as baclofen. *Pregnancy category:* C; PB: UK; $t_{\frac{1}{2}}$: 8 h
Chlorphenesin carbamate (Maolate)	A: PO: Initially 800 mg t.i.d.; maint: 400 mg q.i.d.	For muscle spasm. For short-term treatment of acute spasm. *Pregnancy category:* C; PB: UK; $t_{\frac{1}{2}}$: 3–4 h
Chlorzoxazone (Paraflex, Parafon Forte)	A: PO: 250–750 mg t.i.d./q.i.d.; *max:* 3 g/d C: PO: 20 mg/kg/d or 600 mg m²/d in 3–4 divided doses	For acute or severe muscle spasms. Not effective for cerebral palsy. Take with food to decrease GI upset. *Pregnancy category:* C; PB: UK; $t_{\frac{1}{2}}$: 1 h
Cyclobenzaprine HCl (Flexeril, Cycoflex)	A: PO: 10 mg t.i.d.; may increase dose; *max:* 60 mg/d	For short-term treatment of muscle spasms. Not effective for relieving cerebral or spinal cord disease. Take with food or milk to decrease GI upset. *Pregnancy category:* B; PB: 93%; $t_{\frac{1}{2}}$: 1–3 d
Methocarbamol (Robaxin, Delaxin, Marbaxin)	A: PO: Initially 1.5 g q.i.d.; maint: 1 g q.i.d. IM/IV: 0.5–1 g q8h; *max:* 3 g/d	For acute muscle spasms; drug used for treatment of tetanus. Has CNS depressant effects (sedation). Avoid taking alcohol or CNS depressants. Urine may be green, brown, or black. Drowsiness that may occur usually decreases with continued drug use. *Pregnancy category:* C; PB: UK; $t_{\frac{1}{2}}$: 1–2 h
Orphenadrine citrate (Norflex, Flexon)	A: PO: 100 mg b.i.d. IM/IV: 60 mg daily/b.i.d.	For acute muscle spasm. It can be toxic with a mild overdose. Used in combination with aspirin and caffeine (Norgesic). *Pregnancy category:* C; PB: <20%; $t_{\frac{1}{2}}$: 14 h
DEPOLARIZING MUSCLE RELAXANTS (ADJUNCT TO ANESTHESIA)		
Pancuronium bromide (Pavulon)	A: IV: 0.04–0.1 mg/kg; then 0.01 mg/kg every 30–60 min as needed C >10 y: same as for adult.	Used in surgery for relaxation of skeletal muscle (e.g., abdominal wall). It is considered to be 5 times as potent as tubocurarine chloride. It does not cause hypotension or bronchospasm. *Pregnancy category:* C; PB: <10%; $t_{\frac{1}{2}}$: 2 h
Succinylcholine Cl (Anectine Cl, Quelicin, Sucostrin)	A: IM: 2.5–4 mg/kg; *max:* 150 mg; IV: 0.3–1.1 mg/kg; *max:* 150 mg C: IM/IV: 1–2 mg/kg; *max:* IM: 150 mg	Used in surgery with anesthesia for skeletal muscle relaxation. Also used in endoscopy and intubation. *Pregnancy category:* C; PB: UK; $t_{\frac{1}{2}}$: UK

Table continued on following page

Table 23–9 *Continued*
Muscle Relaxants (Skeletal)

GENERIC (BRAND)	ROUTE AND DOSAGE	USES AND CONSIDERATIONS
Vecuronium bromide (Norcuron)	A or C >9 y: IV: Initially 0.08–0.1 mg/kg/dose; maint: 0.05–0.1 mg/kg/h as needed	Use is similar as succinylcholine chloride. It can be used for clients having asthma, renal disease or with limited cardiac reserve. Given after general anesthesia has been started. *Pregnancy category:* C; PB: 60%–80%; $t_{\frac{1}{2}}$: 1–1.5 h
Recuronium bromide	*Anesthesia intubation:* A: IV: Initially: 0.45–0.6 mg/kg C: IV: 0.6 mg/kg *During surgery:* A: IV bolus: 0.9–1.2 mg/kg *Postoperative:* A: IV: 0.01–0.012 mg/kg/min	Similar to vecuronium. *Pregnancy category:* B; PB: 30%: $t_{\frac{1}{2}}$: 2–18 min
PERIPHERALLY ACTING MUSCLE RELAXANT		
Dantrolene sodium (Dantrium)	A: PO: Initially 25 mg/d; increase gradually; maint: 100 mg b.i.d.–q.i.d. C: PO: Initially 0.5 mg/kg b.i.d.; increase dose gradually by 0.5 mg/kg t.i.d./q.i.d.; *max:* 100 mg q.i.d.	For chronic neurologic disorders causing spasms such as spinal cord injuries, stroke, multiple sclerosis. Start with low doses and increase every 4 to 7 d. Avoid taking with alcohol and CNS depressants. *Pregnancy category:* C; PB: 95%; $t_{\frac{1}{2}}$: 8 h

KEY: *A: adult; C: child; CSS: Controlled Substance Schedule; PO: by mouth; IM: intramuscular; IV: intravenous; PB: protein-binding; $t_{\frac{1}{2}}$: half-life; UK: unknown; >: greater than; CNS: central nervous system.*

used as an adjunctive agent in the relief of muscle spasms.

Peripherally Acting Muscle Relaxants

Dantrolene sodium (Dantrium), a peripherally acting muscle relaxant, acts on the muscles directly and has minimal effect on the CNS. This drug is most effective for spasticity or muscle contractions of neurologic origin (multiple sclerosis, CVA). The centrally acting muscle relaxant baclofen is also effective in treating muscle spasms caused by multiple sclerosis. However, high doses of dantrolene may cause hepatotoxicity, so liver enzyme blood tests should be monitored. Chart 23–4 compares the drug data of the centrally acting muscle relaxant carisoprodol and the peripherally acting muscle relaxant dantrolene.

PHARMACOKINETICS

Carisoprodol is well absorbed from the GI tract, but only 35% of dantrolene is absorbed. Both carisoprodol and dantrolene have moderate half-lives. The half-life for intravenous dantrolene is shorter than that for the oral preparation. The protein-binding percentage for carisoprodol is unknown; that for dantrolene is 90%. Signs and symptoms of drug accumulation of dantrolene should be assessed. Both drugs are metabolized in the liver and excreted in the urine.

PHARMACODYNAMICS

Carisoprodol alleviates muscle spasm associated with acute painful musculoskeletal conditions. Dantrolene acts directly on the skeletal muscles and decreases the release of calcium, thereby aiding in the reduction of muscle spasticity. Both drugs have similar drug interactions. When these drugs are taken with alcohol, sedative-hypnotics, barbiturates, or tricylic antidepressants, increased CNS depression occurs.

The onset of action, peak concentration time, and duration of action for carisoprodol are shorter than those for dantrolene. Dantrolene can be administered intravenously as well as orally, and the onset of action and peak time occur rapidly.

Chart 23–4. Muscle Relaxants

MUSCLE RELAXANTS

Assessment and Planning

Drug Name

Centrally Acting Muscle Relaxant
Carisoprodol *(C)* (Soma, Soprodol)
Pregnancy Category: C

Peripherally Acting Muscle Relaxant
Dantrolene *(D)* (Dantrium)
Pregnancy Category: C

Dosage

(C):
A: PO: 350 mg, t.i.d., h.s.
C >5y: PO 25 mg/kg/d in 4 divided doses.
(D):
A: PO: Initially: 25 mg/d; increase to 25 mg,
b.i.d. to q.i.d. and in increments of 25 mg up to
100 mg, b.i.d.–q.i.d.
IV: 2.5 mg/kg before surgery
C >5y: Initially: 0.5 mg/kg, b.i.d.; increase to
0.5 mg/kg t.i.d. or q.i.d. *max:* 100 mg. q.i.d.

Contraindications

(C & D): Severe liver or renal disease
(D): Severe heart disease

Drug-Lab-Food Interactions

Drug: *(C & D):* Increase CNS depression with
alcohol, narcotics, sedative-hypnotics, antihistamines, tricyclic antidepressants. May increase
risk of ventricular fibrillation with calcium
channel blockers

Interventions

Pharmacokinetics

Absorption: PO: *(C):* well absorbed; *(D):* 35%
absorbed
Distribution: PB: *(C):* UK; *(D):* 90%
Metabolism: t½: *(C):* 8 h; *(D):* 8–9 h; IV: 4–8 h
Excretion: *(C & D):* in the urine

Pharmacodynamics

(C):
PO: Onset: 30 min
       Peak: 3–4 h
       Duration: 4–6 h
(D):
PO: Onset: 1 h
       Peak: 5 h
       Duration: 8 h
IV: Onset: rapid
       Peak: rapid
       Duration: 6–8 h

NURSING PROCESS

Evaluation

Therapeutic Effects/Uses

(C): To relax skeletal muscles; *(D):* To treat spasticity associated with stroke, spinal cord injury,
multiple sclerosis, cerebral palsy

Mode of Action: *(C):* Blocks interneuronal activity. *(D):* Produces direct relaxation of the spastic
muscle by interfering with the release of the calcium ion.

Side Effects

(C): Nausea, vomiting, dizziness, weakness, insomnia
(D): Muscle weakness, anorexia, vomiting,
drowsiness, dizziness, diarrhea, sweating, photosensitivity, insomnia

Adverse Reactions

(C): Asthmatic attack, tachycardia, hypotension,
diplopia
(D): Pleural effusions, tachycardia, hypotension,
palpitations

KEY: PO: by mouth; IV: intravenous; UK: unknown; PB: protein-binding; t½: half-life; >: greater than; CNS: central nervous system.

NURSING PROCESS
MUSCLE RELAXANT: CARISOPRODOL

Assessment

- Obtain a medical history. Carisoprodol is contraindicated if the client has severe renal or liver disease.
- Obtain baseline VS for future comparison.
- Obtain the client's history to identify the cause of muscle spasm and to determine whether it is acute or chronic.
- Obtain a drug history. Report if a drug-drug interaction is probable.
- Note if there is a history of narrow-angle glaucoma or myasthenia gravis. Cyclobenzaprine and orphenadrine are contraindicated with these health problems.

Potential Nursing Diagnoses

- Impaired physical mobility
- Activity intolerance

Planning

- Client will be free of muscular pain within 1 wk.

Nursing Interventions

- Monitor serum liver enzyme levels of clients taking dantrolene and carisoprodol. Report elevated levels of liver enzymes, such as alkaline phosphatase (ALP), alanine aminotransferase (ALT), and gamma-glutamyl transferase (GGT).
- Monitor VS. Report abnormal results.
- Observe for CNS side effects (e.g., dizziness).

Client Teaching

General
- Inform the client that the muscle relaxant should not be abruptly stopped. Drug should be tapered over 1 wk to avoid rebound spasms.
- Advise the client not to drive or operate dangerous machinery when taking muscle relaxants. These drugs have a sedative effect and can cause drowsiness.
- Inform the client that most of the centrally acting muscle relaxants for acute spasms are usually taken for no longer than 3 wk.
- Advise the client to avoid alcohol and CNS depressants. If muscle relaxants are taken with these drugs, CNS depression may be intensified.
- Inform the client that these drugs are contraindicated during pregnancy or by lactating mothers. Check with the health care provider.

Diet
- Advise the client to take muscle relaxants with food to decrease GI upset.

Side Effects
- Instruct the client to report side effects of the muscle relaxant, such as nausea, vomiting, dizziness, faintness, headache, and diplopia. Dizziness and faintness are most likely due to orthostatic (postural) hypotension.

Evaluation

- Evaluate the effectiveness of the muscle relaxant to determine whether the client's muscular pain has decreased or disappeared.

SIDE EFFECTS AND ADVERSE REACTIONS

The side effects from centrally acting muscle relaxants include drowsiness, dizziness, lightheadedness, headaches, and occasional nausea, vomiting, diarrhea, and abdominal distress. Cyclobenzaprine and orphenadrine have anticholinergic effects.

The side effects from peripherally acting muscle relaxants include liver toxicity (increased liver enzymes), drowsiness, photosensitivity, and occasional anorexia, nausea, and vomiting. Avoid use if the client has a history of breast cancer, because mammary malignancy could recur.

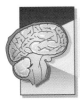

Critical Thinking in Action

T. R., age 79 years, was diagnosed as having parkinsonism 10 years ago. During early treatment of parkinsonism, he was taking levodopa (L-dopa). The drug dosage had to be increased in order to alleviate symptoms.

1. How does levodopa alleviate symptoms of parkinsonism?
2. What assessments should be made before and during the time T. R. is taking L-dopa?

Because numerous side effects and adverse reactions to levodopa developed, the health care provider changed the drug to carbidopa-levodopa (Sinemet). The client asks the nurse why the drug was changed.

3. What are the similarities and differences between L-dopa and Sinemet? What would be an appropriate response to the question about changing the drug for parkinsonism?
4. How does the dose for carbidopa-levodopa differ from that for levodopa? What are the advantages of carbidopa-levodopa?

The client's family say that they know a person with parkinsonism taking the antiviral drug amantadine (Symmetrel). The family asks whether Symmetrel is the same as Sinemet and, if so, shouldn't the client take that drug instead of a drug containing levodopa.

5. What is the effect of amantadine on parkinsonism symptoms?
6. What would be an appropriate response to the family's question concerning the use of Symmetrel for T. R.?
7. Explain the uses for dopamine agonists.
8. Certain anticholinergic drugs may be used for controlling parkinsonism symptoms. What is the action of these drugs and what are their side effects? These anticholinergic drugs are usually prescribed for parkinsonism symptoms resulting from what?

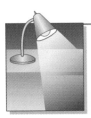

Study Questions

1. A 66-year-old man was recently diagnosed with parkinsonism. What are four physical characteristics associated with parkinsonism?
2. This gentleman was instructed to take 250 mg of levodopa three times a day. At what time of the day should the drug be taken? What are three side effects of the drug? Why should vitamin B_6 (pyridoxine) be avoided in foods and vitamin supplements?
3. Because of the side effects, the drug therapy was changed to bromocriptine. How do these two drugs differ? Explain.
4. Selected anticholinergics are prescribed for parkinsonism. What are their effects on parkinsonism symptoms? What are the side effects of anticholinergics?

5. An AChE inhibitor is used in the treatment of myasthenia gravis. What is its action?

6. What teaching should be included concerning drug compliance and drug dose intervals?

7. Centrally acting muscle relaxants are used for what type of muscle spasms? What is the major side effect of this group of drugs?

8. The client with multiple sclerosis has muscle spasms. What are two muscle relaxants that are used to reduce this spasticity?

9. Acetylcholinesterase inhibitors are presently used to treat Alzheimer's disease. For what purpose are these agents used in the treatment of Alzheimer's, and how effective are they? What other drugs are being considered for treating Alzheimer's disease?

Unit V

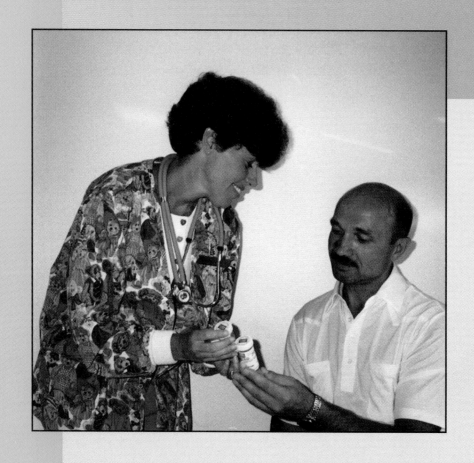

Antiinflammatory and Antiinfective Agents

INTRODUCTION

Unit V discusses agents prescribed for alleviating an inflammatory process and combating disease-producing microorganisms (pathogens). Included in this unit are antiinflammatory drugs; antibacterials-antibiotics (penicillins, cephalosporins, macrolides, tetracyclines, aminoglycosides, and fluoroquinolones); sulfonamides; peptides; antitubercular, antifungal, antiviral, anthelmintic, and antimalarial drugs; and urinary antiseptics.

INFLAMMATION

Inflammation is a reaction to tissue injury due to the release of chemical mediators that cause both a vascular response and fluid and cells (leukocytes, or WBCs) to migrate to the injured site. The chemical mediators are (1) histamines, (2) kinins, and (3) prostaglandins. Histamine, the first mediator in the inflammatory process, causes dilation of the arterioles and increases capillary permeability, allowing fluid to leave the capillaries and flow into the injured area. The kinins, such as bradykinin, also increase capillary permeability and the sensation of pain. Prostaglandins are released, causing an increase in vasodilation, capillary permeability, pain, and fever. The antiinflammatory drugs, such as nonsteroidal antiinflammatory drugs (NSAIDs) and steroids (cortisone preparations), inhibit chemical mediators, thus decreasing the inflammatory process. Figure V–1 illustrates the process of chemical mediators acting on the injured tissues. The five responses to tissue injury are referred to as the cardinal signs of inflammation: redness, swelling, pain, heat, and loss of function.

Inflammation may or may not be the result of an infection. Only a small percentage of inflammations are due to infections; other causes include trauma, surgical interventions, extreme heat or cold, and caustic chemical agents. Antiinflammatory drugs reduce fluid migration and pain, thus lessening loss of function and increasing the client's mobility and comfort.

INFECTION

Disease-producing organisms may be gram-positive or gram-negative bacteria, viruses, or fungi. The degree to which they are pathogenic depends on the microorganism and its virulence. The cell walls of bacteria differ in their structure: bacilli are elongated, cocci are spherical, and spirilla are helical.

Viruses are very small organisms that do not have an organized cellular structure. There are numerous families of virus, including herpesviruses, cytomegalovirus, adenovirus, papovavirus, and the human immunodeficiency virus (HIV). HIV agents are discussed in Chapter 31. Today, an increasing number of antiviral drugs seek to inhibit viral replication to control the virus.

The fungi are divided into yeasts and molds. The few fungi that produce disease usually affect the skin and subcutaneous tissues in such conditions as athlete's foot and ringworm. Serious fungal infections are systemic and usually need aggressive drug therapy. Opportunistic fungal infections commonly result from prolonged antibiotic and steroidal therapies and debilitating diseases, such as cancer. The yeast *Candida albicans* is a cause of common infections of the mucous membranes of the mouth, gastrointestinal tract, vagina, and skin. *Candida*, like most fungi, is resistant to penicillin-type antibiotics because of its rigid cell wall structure. Chapter 28 describes the variety of topical and systemic drugs used in treating yeast and mold infections.

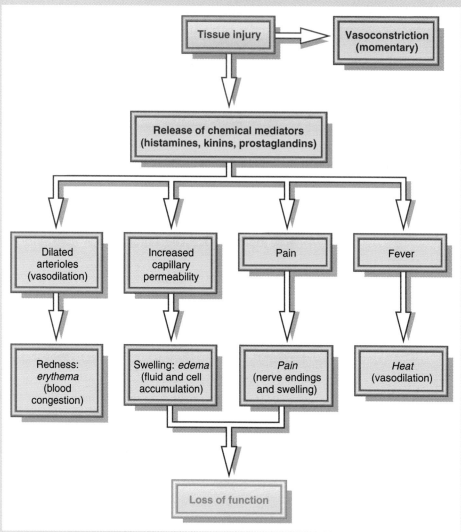

Figure V–1
Chemical mediator response to tissue injury.

Antiinflammatory Drugs

24

Outline

Objectives

- Describe the action of nonsteroidal antiinflammatory drugs (NSAIDs).
- List the major side effects of NSAIDs.
- Explain the use of disease-modifying antirheumatic drugs (DMARDs).
- Identify several side effects and adverse reactions of DMARDs.
- Give nursing process, including client teaching, associated with NSAIDs and DMARDs.
- Discuss the use of antigout drugs.

Terms

chrysotherapy
DMARDs
gout

immunosuppressives
infection
inflammation

NSAIDs
prostaglandins
uricosuric

INTRODUCTION

Inflammation is a response to tissue injury and infection. When the inflammatory process occurs, a vascular reaction takes place in which fluid, elements of blood, white blood cells (leukocytes), and chemical mediators accumulate at the injured tissue or infection site. The process of inflammation is a protective mechanism in which the body attempts to neutralize and destroy harmful agents at the site of injury and to establish conditions for tissue repair.

Although there is a relationship between inflammation and infection, these terms should *not* be used interchangeably. **Infection** is caused by microorganisms and results in inflammation, but *not* all inflammations are caused by infections.

CARDINAL SIGNS OF INFLAMMATION

The five characteristics of inflammation, referred to as the cardinal signs of inflammation, are redness, heat, swelling (edema), pain, and loss of function (Table 24–1). The two phases of inflammation are the vascular phase, which occurs 10 to 15 min following an injury, and the delayed phase. The vascular phase is associated with vasodilation and increased capillary permeability, during which blood substances and fluid leave the plasma and go to the injured site. The delayed phase occurs when leukocytes infiltrate the inflamed tissue.

Various chemical mediators are released during the inflammation process. Prostaglandins that have been isolated from the exudate at inflammatory sites are among them. **Prostaglandins** (chemical mediators) have many effects, including vasodilation, relaxation of smooth muscle, increased capillary permeability,

and sensitization of nerve cells to pain. Drugs, such as aspirin, inhibit the biosynthesis of prostaglandins and therefore are referred to as prostaglandin inhibitors. Because prostaglandin inhibitors affect the inflammatory process, they are also referred to as antiinflammatory agents.

Antiinflammatory agents have additional properties, such as relief of pain (analgesic), reduction of an elevated body temperature (antipyretic), and inhibition of platelet aggregation (anticoagulant). Aspirin is the oldest antiinflammatory drug, but was first used for its analgesic and antipyretic properties. As a result of searching for a more effective drug with fewer side effects, many other antiinflammatory agents, or prostaglandin inhibitors, have been discovered. Although these drugs have potent antiinflammatory effects that mimic the effects of corticosteroids (cortisone), they are *not* chemically related and therefore are referred to as **nonsteroidal antiinflammatory drugs,** or **NSAIDs.**

NONSTEROIDAL ANTIINFLAMMATORY DRUGS

NSAIDs are aspirin and "aspirin-like" drugs that inhibit the enzyme cyclooxygenase that is needed for the biosynthesis of prostaglandins (see Chapter 17 and Fig. 17–1). These drugs may be called prostaglandin inhibitors, with varying degrees of analgesic and antipyretic effects, but are used primarily as antiinflammatory agents for relieving inflammation and pain. When administering NSAIDs for pain relief, the dosage is usually higher than for treatment of inflammation. Their antipyretic effect is less than their antiinflammatory effect. With the exceptions of aspirin and ibuprofen, NSAID preparations are not suggested for use in alleviating mild headaches and mild ele-

Table 24–1
Cardinal Signs of Inflammation

SIGNS	DESCRIPTION AND EXPLANATION
Erythema (redness)	Redness occurs in the first phase of inflammation. Blood accumulates in the area of tissue injury due to release of the body's chemical mediators (kinins, prostaglandins, and histamine). Histamine dilates the arterioles.
Edema (swelling)	Swelling is the second phase of inflammation. Plasma leaks into the interstitial tissue at the injury site. Kinins dilate the arterioles, increasing capillary permeability.
Heat	Heat at the inflammatory site can be due to increased blood accumulation and may result from pyrogens (substances that produce fever) that interfere with the temperature-regulating center in the hypothalamus.
Pain	Pain is due to tissue swelling and the release of chemical mediators.
Loss of function	Function is lost due to the accumulation of fluid at the tissue injury site and to pain, which decreases mobility at the affected area.

Table 24–2

Antiinflammatory: Nonsteroidal Antiinflammatory

GENERIC (BRAND)	ROUTE AND DOSAGE	USES AND CONSIDERATIONS
SALICYLATES		
Aspirin (ASA, Bayer, Ecotrin)	A: PO: 325–650 mg PRN See Chart 24–1	Requires large dose for inflammation, rheumatoid arthritis. GI upset and ulceration can occur. Alcohol can increase GI effects. *Pregnancy category:* D; PB: 59%–90%; $t_{\frac{1}{2}}$: 2–3 h (low doses), 2–20 h (high doses)
Diflunisal (Dolobid)	A: PO: Initially: 1 g (1000 mg); maint: 500 mg q8–12h	Relief of mild to moderate pain; used to treat osteoarthritis and rheumatoid arthritis. Acts by inhibiting prostaglandin synthesis. Avoid if hypersensitive to aspirin. Do not use during third trimester of pregnancy. *Pregnancy category:* C; PB: 99%; $t_{\frac{1}{2}}$: 1 h
ACETIC ACID GROUP		
Para-Chlorobenzoic Acid (Indoles)		
Indomethacin (Indocin)	A: PO: 25–50 mg b.i.d./t.i.d. with food; SR: 75 mg q.d./b.i.d.; *max:* 200 mg/d C: PO: 1–2 mg/kg/d in 2–4 divided doses; may increase to 4 mg/kg/d; *max:* 150–200 mg/d	For moderate to severe arthritic conditions. Potent drug. GI upset and ulceration are common. Take drug with food. Avoid indomethacin if allergic to aspirin. *Pregnancy category:* B (D near term); PB: 90%–99%; $t_{\frac{1}{2}}$: 3–120 h
Sulindac (Clinoril)	A: PO: 150–200 mg b.i.d.	For acute and chronic arthritis, bursitis, and tendinitis. Not as potent as indomethacin. Give with food. *Pregnancy category:* C; PB: 93%; $t_{\frac{1}{2}}$: 7–18 h
Tolmetin (Tolectin)	A: PO: Initially: 400 mg t.i.d.; maint: 600–1800 mg/d in divided doses; *max:* 2 g/d C >2 y: PO: 20 mg/kg/d in divided doses; *max:* 30 mg/kg/d	For acute and chronic arthritis, including juvenile rheumatoid arthritis. Less potent than indomethacin; more effective than aspirin. Take drug with food. *Pregnancy category:* B (D near term); PB: 99%; $t_{\frac{1}{2}}$: 1–1.5 h
Phenylacetic Acid		
Bromfenac sodium (Duract)	A: PO: 25 mg, q6–8h; *max:* 150 mg/d	NSAID for short-term treatment to alleviate pain. It inhibits prostaglandin synthesis and reduces inflammatory response. *Pregnancy category:* UK; PB: UK; $t_{\frac{1}{2}}$: UK.
Diclofenac sodium (Voltaren)	A: PO: 25–50 mg t.i.d./q.i.d. or 75 mg b.i.d.	For rheumatoid arthritis, osteoarthritis, and spondylitis. Also for acute gout, juvenile rheumatoid arthritis, bursitis, and tendinitis. If GI distress occurs, take with food. *Pregnancy category:* B; PB: 90%–99%; $t_{\frac{1}{2}}$: 2 h
Etodolac (Lodine)	A: PO: 200–400 mg q6–8h PRN; *max:* 1200 mg/d	Used for acute pain, rheumatoid arthritis, and osteoarthritis. Take with food or antacid to avoid GI distress. *Pregnancy category:* C; PR: 99%; $t_{\frac{1}{2}}$: 6–7 h
Ketorolac tromethamine (Toradol)	A: <50 kg: IM: LD: 30 mg; maint: 15 mg q6h A: >50 kg: IM: LD: 30–60 mg; maint: 15–30 mg PRN	First injectable NSAID. For short-term management of pain. Also available for ophthalmic use to relieve itching due to allergic conjunctivitis. *Pregnancy category:* B; PB: 99%; $t_{\frac{1}{2}}$: 5–6 h
PYRAZOLONE		
Phenylbutazone (Butazolidin)	A: PO: 100–400 mg/d in divided doses; *max:* 600 mg/d	For acute rheumatoid arthritis, osteoarthritis, and gouty arthritis. Potent drug. Severe side effects can occur. Take with food. Very long half-life. *Pregnancy category:* C; PB: 98%; $t_{\frac{1}{2}}$: 50–100 h
PROPIONIC ACID		
Fenoprofen calcium (Nalfon)	A: PO: 300–600 mg t.i.d./q.i.d.; *max:* 3.2 g/d	Treatment of mild to moderate pain. Also for arthritic conditions. Most effective after 2–3 weeks of therapy. Take with food. *Pregnancy category:* B (D at term); PB: 90%; $t_{\frac{1}{2}}$: 3 h

Table continued on following page

Table 24–2 *Continued*
Antiinflammatory: Nonsteroidal Antiinflammatory

GENERIC (BRAND)	ROUTE AND DOSAGE	USES AND CONSIDERATIONS
Flurbiprofen sodium (Ansaid, Ocufen)	A: PO: 50–300 mg/d in 2–4 divided doses; *max:* 300 mg/d *Ophthalmic use:* 0.03% sol	Treatment of acute and chronic arthritis. Take drug with food. *Pregnancy category:* C; PB: UK; $t\frac{1}{2}$: 5 h
Ibuprofen (Motrin, Advil, Nuprin, Medipren)	See Chart 24–2	Relief of mild to moderate pain; used to reduce fever (adult and children) and also for arthritic conditions. Similar effect as aspirin. Can increase bleeding time. GI upset can occur. Take with food, milk, or antacids if GI discomfort occurs. *Pregnancy category:* B; PB: 98%; $t\frac{1}{2}$: 2–4 h
Ketoprofen (Orudis)	*Inflammatory:* A: PO: 150–300 mg/d in 3–4 divided doses *Mild-moderate pain:* A: PO: 25–50 mg q6–8h PRN; *max:* 300 mg/d	Relief of mild to moderate pain and acute and chronic arthritis. Take with food or 8 ounces of water to avoid GI upset. *Pregnancy category:* B (D at term); PB: 99%; $t\frac{1}{2}$: 3–4 h
Naproxen (Naprosyn)	A: PO: 250–500 mg b.i.d. C: PO: 5–10 mg/kg/d in 2 divided doses	Relief of mild to moderate pain. Also for arthritic, gout, bursitis conditions. Similar OTC drug: Aleve. Take with food or with a full glass of water. *Pregnancy category:* B; PB: 99%; $t\frac{1}{2}$: 10–15 h
Oxaprozin (Daypro)	A: PO: Initially: 1200 mg/d; maint: 600 mg/d; *max:* 1800 mg/d in divided doses	Treatment of acute and chronic arthritis. Take with food for GI discomfort. *Pregnancy category:* C; PB: 99%; $t\frac{1}{2}$: 40 h
ANTHRANYLIC ACIDS (FENAMATES)		
Meclofenamate (Meclomen)	A: PO: 200–400 mg in 3–4 divided doses	For acute and chronic arthritis. GI symptoms can be severe. Used when other NSAIDs are not effective. Take with food to avoid GI upset. *Pregnancy category:* B (D at term); PB: 99%; $t\frac{1}{2}$: 3 h
Mefenamic acid (Ponstel)	A: PO: Initially: 500 mg; then 250 mg q6h PRN; *max:* 1 g/d	For acute and chronic arthritis. Diarrhea is common problem. Usually discontinued after 7 days. *Pregnancy category:* C; PB: 90%; $t\frac{1}{2}$: 2–4 h
OXICAMS		
Piroxicam (Feldene)	A: PO: 10 mg b.i.d. or 20 mg q.d.	For arthritic conditions. Long half-life; effective at 2 weeks. GI upset may occur. *Pregnancy category:* C; PB: 99%; $t\frac{1}{2}$: 30–86 h

KEY: A: adult; C: child; PO: by mouth; IM: intramuscular; IV: intravenous; >: greater than; <: less than; LD: loading dose; PRN: as necessary; PB: protein-binding; $t\frac{1}{2}$: half-life; sol: solution; SR: sustained-release; maint: maintenance; GI: gastrointestinal; NSAID: nonsteroidal antiinflammatory drug; OTC: over the counter.

vated temperature. The choice of drugs for headaches and fever are aspirin, acetaminophen, and ibuprofen (given to children and adults with high fever). NSAIDs are more appropriate for reducing swelling, pain, and stiffness in joints.

NSAIDs cost more than aspirin. Other than aspirin, the only NSAIDs that can be purchased over-the-counter (OTC) are ibuprofen (Motrin, Nuprin, Advil, Medipren) and naproxen (Aleve). Ibuprofen is also available in generic form of 200 mg per tablet or capsule. All other NSAIDs must be ordered with a prescription. If a client can take aspirin for the inflammatory process without gastrointestinal (GI) upset, then the salicylate products are usually recommended.

There are eight groups of NSAIDs:

• Salicylates related to aspirin (see Chapter 17)
• *Para*-chlorobenzoic acid derivatives, or indoles
• Pyrazolone derivatives
• Propionic acid derivatives
• Fenamates
• Oxicams
• Phenylacetic acids
• Selective COX-2 inhibitors

Table 24–2 provides dosage information and considerations for use for the most commonly used NSAIDs. The half-lives of NSAIDs differ greatly—

Chart 24–1.   Analgesic and Antiinflammatory Drug: Aspirin

SALICYLATE

Drug Name

Aspirin (A.S.A., Bayer, Astrin, Ecotrin, Alka Selt-zer [in some], Empirin) ❧ Ancasal, Astrin, En-trophen, Novasen
Pregnancy Category: D

Dosage

Analgesic:
A: PO: 325–650 mg q4h PRN; *max:* 4 g/d
C: PO: 40–65 mg/d in 4–6 divided doses; *max:* 3.5 g/d
TIA and thromboembolic condition:
A: PO: 325–650 mg/d or b.i.d.
Arthritis:
A: PO: 3.6–5.4 g/d in divided doses
TDM: 15–30 mg/dL; 150–300 μg/mL

Contraindications

Hypersensitivity to salicylates or NSAIDs, flu or virus symptoms in children, third trimester of pregnancy
Caution: Renal or hepatic disorders

Drug-Lab-Food Interactions

Drug: *Increase* risk of bleeding with anticoagu-lants; *increase* risk of hypoglycemia with oral hypoglycemic drugs; *increase* ulcerogenic effect with glucocorticoids
Lab: *Decrease* cholesterol and potassium, T_3, T_4 levels; *increase* PT, bleeding time, uric acid

Pharmacokinetics

Absorption: PO: 80%–100%
Distribution: PB: 59%–90%, crosses placenta
Metabolism: t½: 2–3 h (low dose); 2–20 h (high dose)
Excretion: 50% in urine

Pharmacodynamics

PO: Onset: 15–30 min
          Peak: 1–2 h
          Duration: 4–6 h
Rectal: Onset: 1–2 h
          Peak: 3–5 h
          Duration: 4–7 h

Therapeutic Effects/Uses

To reduce pain and inflammatory symptoms; to decrease body temperature; to inhibit platelet aggregation.

Mode of Action: Inhibition of prostaglandin synthesis, inhibition of hypothalamic heat-regulator center.

Side Effects

Anorexia, nausea, vomiting, diarrhea, dizziness, confusion, hearing loss, heartburn, rash, stom-ach pains, drowsiness

Adverse Reactions

Tinnitus, urticaria, ulceration
Life-threatening: Agranulocytosis, hemolytic anemia, bronchospasm, anaphylaxis, thrombocy-topenia, hepatotoxicity, leukopenia

Assessment and Planning · Interventions · Evaluation · NURSING PROCESS

KEY: A: adult; C: child; PO: by mouth; TDM: therapeutic drug monitoring; UK: unknown; PB: protein-binding; t½: half-life; PRN: as necessary; PT: prothrombin; ❧: Canadian drug names.

some have a short half-life, others have a moderate to long half-life with a general range of 8 to 24 h. Aspi-rin and an NSAID should *not* be taken together be-cause of the side effects. Also, combined therapy does not increase effectiveness.

Salicylates

Aspirin comes from the family of salicylates derived from salicylic acid. Aspirin is also called acetylsali-cylic acid (ASA) after the acetyl group used in the

NURSING PROCESS
ANALGESIC AND ANTIINFLAMMATORY DRUG: ASPIRIN

Assessment

- Obtain a medical history. Determine whether there is any history of gastric upset, gastric bleeding, or liver disease. Aspirin can cause gastric irritation. It prolongs bleeding time by inhibiting platelet aggregation.
- Obtain a drug history. Report if a drug-drug interaction is probable.

Potential Nursing Diagnoses

- Risk for injury
- Pain

Planning

- Client will be free of mild pain in 12 to 24 hours and mild inflammation within 1 week. Aspirin may be ordered for mild to severe arthritic condition, pain relief, antiinflammatory effects, fever reduction, and inhibition of platelet aggregation.

Nursing Interventions

- Monitor serum salicylate (aspirin) level when the client is taking high doses of aspirin for chronic conditions such as arthritis. The normal therapeutic range is 15 to 30 mg/dL. Mild toxicity occurs at serum level of >30 mg/dL, and severe toxicity occurs at >50 mg/dL.
- Observe the client for signs of bleeding, such as dark (tarry) stools, bleeding gums, petechiae (round red spots), ecchymosis (excessive bruising), and purpura (large red spots) when the client is taking high doses of aspirin.

Client Teaching

General

- Advise the client not to take aspirin with alcohol or drugs that are highly protein-bound, such as the anticoagulant warfarin (Coumadin). Aspirin displaces drugs such as warfarin from the protein-binding site, causing more free anticoagulant.

Nursing Process continued on opposite page

composition of aspirin. The abbreviation frequently used for aspirin is ASA.

Aspirin is the oldest antiinflammatory agent, developed in 1899 by Dr. Bayer. A prostaglandin inhibitor that decreases the inflammatory process, aspirin was the most frequently used antiinflammatory agent before the introduction of ibuprofen. Because high doses of aspirin are generally needed to relieve inflammation, gastric distress is a common problem. In such cases, enteric-coated tablets may be used.

There are two enzyme forms of cyclooxygenase: COX-1 and COX-2. COX-1 protects the stomach lining and regulates blood platelets, and COX-2 triggers inflammation and pain. Aspirin and other NSAIDs inhibit COX-1, which decreases the protection of the stomach lining, and COX-2, which decreases inflammation and pain. Aspirin decreases inflammation and pain by inhibiting COX-2; however, when COX-1 is decreased, the stomach lining is not protected; thus,

stomach ulcers and bleeding may occur. Aspirin is a choice drug for alleviating inflammation and pain in arthritic conditions, but when given in high doses, severe gastrointestinal problems develop in approximately 20% of clients. Many pharmaceutical companies are developing antiinflammatory and analgesic drugs that inhibit only COX-2 (see Chapter 17).

Aspirin should not be taken with other NSAIDs because it decreases the blood level and the effectiveness of the NSAID. Aspirin is also considered an antiplatelet drug for clients having cardiac or cerebrovascular disorders by decreasing platelet aggregation, thus decreasing blood clotting.

PHARMACOKINETICS
Aspirin is well absorbed from the GI tract (Chart 24–1). It can cause GI upset; therefore, it should be taken

- Suggest that the client inform the dentist before a dental visit if the client is taking high doses of aspirin.
- With the health care provider's approval, instruct the client to discontinue aspirin 3 to 7 d before surgery to reduce the risk of bleeding.
- Keep aspirin bottle out of reach of small children.
- Instruct the parent to call the poison control center immediately if a child has taken a large or unknown amount of aspirin (also acetaminophen).
- Instruct the client *not* to administer aspirin for virus or flu symptoms in children. Reye's syndrome (vomiting, lethargy, delirium, and coma) has been linked with aspirin and viral infections. Acetaminophen is usually prescribed for cold and flu symptoms.
- Inform the client that old aspirin tablets can cause GI distress.
- Inform the client with dysmenorrhea to take acetaminophen instead of aspirin 2 d before and 2 d during the menstrual period.

Diet
- Instruct the client to take aspirin (also ibuprofen) with food, at mealtime, or with plenty of fluids. Enteric-coated aspirin avoids GI disturbance.

Side Effects
- Instruct the client to report side effects such as drowsiness, tinnitus (ringing in the ears), headaches, flushing, dizziness, GI symptoms (bleeding, heartburn), visual changes, and seizures.

Evaluation

- Evaluate the effectiveness of aspirin in relieving pain. If pain persists, another analgesic such as ibuprofen may be prescribed.
- Determine whether the client is having any side effects to aspirin.

---

with water, milk, or food. The enteric-coated (EC) or buffered form can decrease gastric distress. Gastric irritation can be decreased if aspirin and other NSAIDs are taken with food and at mealtimes. The EC tablet should not be crushed or broken.

Aspirin has a short half-life. It should not be taken during the last trimester of pregnancy because it could cause premature closure of ductus arteriosus in the fetus. Aspirin should not be taken by children with flu symptoms because it may cause the potentially fatal Reye's syndrome.

PHARMACODYNAMICS
Aspirin, like other NSAIDs, inhibits prostaglandin synthesis by inhibiting COX-1 and COX-2; thus, it decreases inflammation and pain. The onset of action for aspirin is within 30 min. It peaks in 1 to 2 h, and the duration of action is an average of 4 to 6 h. The action for the rectal preparation of aspirin can be erratic because of blood supply and fecal material in the rectum; it may take a week or more for a therapeutic antiinflammatory effect.

HYPERSENSITIVITY TO SALICYLATE PRODUCTS
Clients may be hypersensitive to aspirin. Tinnitus (ringing in the ears), vertigo (dizziness), and broncho-spasm—especially in asthmatic clients—are symptoms of aspirin overdose or hypersensitivity to aspirin. Clients should not take diflunisal if they are hypersensitive to aspirin. Diflunisal is a derivative of salicylic acid, although it is not converted to salicylic acid in the body.

Salicylates are present in numerous foods such as prunes, raisins, and licorice and in spices, such as curry powder and paprika.

Para-Chlorobenzoic Acid

One of the first NSAIDs introduced was indomethacin (Indocin). It is used for rheumatoid, gouty, and osteoarthritis and is a potent prostaglandin inhibitor. It is a highly protein-bound drug (90%) and displaces other protein-bound drugs, resulting in potential toxicity. It has a moderate half-life (4 to 11 h). Indomethacin is very irritating to the stomach and should be taken with meals or food.

Two other *para*-chlorobenzoic acid derivatives—sulindac (Clinoril) and tolmetin (Tolectin)—produce less severe adverse reactions than indomethacin. Tolmetin is not as highly protein-bound as indomethacin and sulindac and has a short half-life. This group of NSAIDs may decrease blood pressure and cause sodium and water retention.

Pyrazolone Derivatives

The pyrazolone group of NSAIDs, like the *para*-chlorobenzoic acid group, is highly protein-bound. Phenylbutazone (Butazolidin), 96% protein-bound, has been used for years to treat rheumatoid arthritis and acute gout. It has a very long half-life, 50 to 65 h, so adverse reactions are common and drug accumulation may occur. Gastric irritation occurs in 10% to 45% of clients.

The most dangerous adverse reactions to this group of drugs are blood dyscrasias, such as agranulocytosis and aplastic anemia. Phenylbutazone should be reserved for the treatment of arthritis and other severe inflammatory conditions when other less toxic NSAIDs have been used without success.

Propionic Acid Derivatives

The propionic acid group represents a relatively new group of NSAIDs. These drugs are aspirin-like but have stronger effects and create less GI irritation. Drugs in this group are highly protein-bound, so drug interactions might occur, especially when given with another highly protein-bound drug. Ibuprofen (Motrin) is the most widely used NSAID and in lower doses (200 mg) it may be purchased OTC. These NSAIDs are better tolerated than other NSAIDs. Gastric upset occurs but it is not as severe as it is with aspirin, indomethacin, and phenylbutazone. Severe adverse reactions, such as blood dyscrasias, are *not* frequently seen. Chart 24–2 details the pharmacologic behavior of ibuprofens. Five other propionic acid agents are fenoprofen calcium (Nalfon), naproxen (Naprosyn), suprofen (Profenal); ketoprofen (Orudis), and flurbiprofen (Ansaid).

PHARMACOKINETICS

Ibuprofens are well absorbed from the GI tract. These drugs have a short half-life but are highly protein-bound. If ibuprofen is taken with another highly protein-bound drug, severe side effects may occur. The drug is metabolized in the liver to inactive metabolites and is excreted as inactive metabolites in the urine.

PHARMACODYNAMICS

Ibuprofens inhibit prostaglandin synthesis and are therefore effective in alleviating inflammation and pain. They have a short onset of action, peak concentration time, and duration of action. It may take several days for the antiinflammatory effect to be evident.

There are many drug interactions associated with ibuprofen. It can increase the effects of Coumadin, sulfonamides, many of the cephalosporins, and phenytoin. When taken with aspirin, its effect can be de-

creased. Hypoglycemia may result when ibuprofen is taken with insulin or an oral hypoglycemic drug. There is high risk of toxicity when ibuprofen is taken concurrently with calcium blockers.

Fenamates

The fenamate group includes potent NSAIDs used for acute and chronic arthritic conditions. Like most NSAIDs, gastric irritation is a common side effect of fenamates, and clients with a history of peptic ulcer should avoid taking this group of drugs. Other side effects include edema, dizziness, tinnitus, and pruritus. Two fenamates are meclofenamate sodium monohydrate (Meclomen) and mefenamic acid (Ponstel).

Oxicams

Piroxicam (Feldene) is indicated for long-term arthritic conditions, such as rheumatoid and osteoarthritis. It is well tolerated, and its major advantage over the others is its long half-life, which allows it to be dosed only once daily. It also can cause gastric problems, such as ulceration and epigastric distress, but the incidence is lower than for some of the other NSAIDs.

Full clinical response to piroxicam may take a week or two. This drug is also highly protein-bound and may interact with another highly protein-bound drug if taken together. Piroxicam should not be taken with aspirin or other NSAIDs.

Phenylacetic Acid Derivatives

Diclofenac sodium (Voltaren) has a plasma half-life of 8 to 12 h. Its analgesic and antiinflammatory effects are similar to those of aspirin, but it has minimal to no antipyretic effect. It is indicated for rheumatoid arthritis, osteoarthritis, and ankylosing spondylitis. Adverse reactions are similar to those of other NSAIDs.

Ketorolac (Toradol) is the first injectable nonsteroidal antiinflammatory agent. Like other NSAIDs, it inhibits prostaglandin synthesis, but it has greater analgesic properties than other antiinflammatory agents. Ketorolac is recommended for short-term management of pain. For postsurgical pain it has shown analgesic efficacy equal or superior to that of opioid analgesics. It is administered intramuscularly in doses of 30 to 60 mg q6h for adults.

GENERAL SIDE EFFECTS AND ADVERSE REACTIONS

Most NSAIDs tend to have fewer side effects than aspirin when taken at antiinflammatory doses, but

Chart 24–2. Antiinflammatory: Nonsteroidal Antiinflammatory Drug (NSAID)

NSAID

Drug Name *Ibuprofen* (Motrin, Advil, Nuprin, Medipren, Rufen) 🍁 Amersol Proprionic acid derivative *Pregnancy Category:* B	**Dosage** A: PO: 200–800 mg t.i.d./q.i.d.; *max:* <3.2 g/d (<3200 mg/d) C: PO: Average: 5–10 mg/kg/d; *max:* 40 mg/kg/d 1–4 y: 400 mg/d in divided doses 5–7 y: 600 mg/d in divided doses >8 y: 800 mg/d in divided doses	**Assessment and Planning**
Contraindications Severe renal or hepatic disease, asthma, peptic ulcer *Caution:* Bleeding disorders, early pregnancy, lactation, systemic lupus erythematosus (SLE)	**Drug-Lab-Food Interactions** **Drug:** *Increase* bleeding time with oral anticoagulants; *increase* effects of phenytoin, sulfonamides, warfarin; *decrease* effect with aspirin; may *increase* severe side effects of lithium	

Pharmacokinetics
 	
Absorption: PO: Well absorbed
Distribution: PB: 98%
Metabolism: t½: 2–4 h
Excretion: In urine, mostly as inactive metabolites; some in bile
	Pharmacodynamics
	
	PO: Onset: 0.5 h
	       Peak: 1–2 h
	       Duration: 4–6 h
		Interventions

Therapeutic Effects/Uses

To reduce inflammatory process; to relieve pain; antiinflammatory effect for arthritic conditions and reduce fever.

Mode of Action: Inhibition of prostaglandin synthesis, thus relieving pain and inflammation.

Side Effects Anorexia, nausea, vomiting, diarrhea, edema, rash, purpura, tinnitus, fatigue, dizziness, lightheadedness, anxiety, confusion	**Adverse Reactions** GI bleeding **Life-threatening:** Blood dyscrasias, cardiac dysrhythmias, nephrotoxicity, anaphylaxis

(Evaluation) • NURSING PROCESS

KEY: A: adult; C: child; PO: by mouth; PB: protein-binding; t½: half-life; <: less than; >: greater than; 🍁: Canadian drug name.

---

gastric irritation is still a common problem when NSAIDs are taken without food. Also, sodium and water retention may occur with phenylbutazone. Alcoholic beverages consumed with NSAIDs may increase gastric irritation and should be avoided.

Selective COX-2 Inhibitors

Selective inhibitors of COX-2 used to decrease inflammation and pain are becoming available. Most NSAIDs are nonselective inhibitors that inhibit COX-1

and COX-2. By inhibiting COX-1, protection of the stomach lining is decreased, and the clotting time is also decreased, which may benefit the client with cardiovascular and coronary artery disease (CAD). When clients need to take large doses of NSAIDs for arthritic conditions, peptic ulcer and gastric bleeding may occur. The selected COX-2 inhibitors become the choice drug for clients with severe arthritic conditions who need high doses of an antiinflammatory drug.

In the next few years, more COX-2 inhibitors will become available. Currently there is one drug, nabu-

NURSING PROCESS
ANTIINFLAMMATORY: NONSTEROIDAL ANTIINFLAMMATORY DRUG

Assessment

- Check the client's history of allergy to NSAIDs, including aspirin. If an allergy is present, notify the health care provider.
- Obtain a drug history and report any possible drug-drug interaction. NSAIDs can increase the effects of phenytoin (Dilantin), sulfonamides, and warfarin. Most NSAIDs are highly protein-bound and can displace other highly protein-bound drugs, such as warfarin (Coumadin).
- Obtain a medical history. NSAIDs are contraindicated if the client has a severe renal or liver disease, peptic ulcer, or bleeding disorder.
- Assess the client for GI upset and peripheral edema, which are common side effects of NSAIDs.

Potential Nursing Diagnoses

- Impaired tissue integrity
- Risk for activity intolerance

Planning

- The inflammatory process will subside in 1 to 3 wk.

Nursing Interventions

- Observe the client for bleeding gums, petechiae, ecchymoses, or black (tarry) stools. Bleeding time can be prolonged when NSAIDs are taken, especially with a highly protein-bound drug such as warfarin (anticoagulant).
- Report if the client is having GI discomfort. Administer the NSAIDs at mealtime or with food to prevent GI upset.
- Monitor vital signs (VS) and check for peripheral edema, especially in the morning.

Nursing Process continued on following page

metone, that could be classified as a COX-2 inhibitor. This drug has a strong affinity to inhibit COX-2 more than COX-1. Two new COX-2 inhibitors, celecoxib and vioxx, are awaiting final approval from the Food and Drug Administration. Table 24–3 lists selective COX-2 inhibitors.

CORTICOSTEROIDS

Corticosteroids, such as prednisone, prednisolone, and dexamethasone, are frequently used as antiinflammatory agents. This group of drugs can control inflammation by suppressing or preventing many of the components of the inflammatory process at the injured site. Corticosteroids have been widely prescribed for arthritic conditions, and although they are not the drug of choice for arthritis because of their numerous side effects, they are frequently used to control arthritic flare-ups.

The half-life of corticosteroids is long, greater than 24 h, and with a large prescribed dose, the steroid is administered once a day. When discontinuing steroid therapy, the dosage should be tapered over a period of 5 to 10 days. Steroids are discussed in more detail in Chapter 45.

DISEASE-MODIFYING ANTIRHEUMATIC DRUGS

When NSAIDs do not control immune-mediated arthritic disease sufficiently, other drugs, although more toxic, can be prescribed to alter the disease process. The **disease-modifying antirheumatic drug (DMARD) group** includes gold drug therapy, immunosuppressive agents, and antimalarials.

Gold

Gold drug therapy, referred to as **chrysotherapy** or heavy metal therapy, is the most frequently used DMARD. It is used to arrest progression of rheumatoid arthritis and to prevent deformities caused by

Client Teaching

General
- Instruct the client not to take aspirin and acetaminophen with NSAIDs. Taking an NSAID with aspirin could cause GI upset and possible GI bleeding.
- Instruct the client to avoid alcohol when taking NSAIDs. GI upset or gastric ulcer may result.
- Advise the client to inform the dentist or surgeon before a procedure when taking ibuprofen or other NSAIDs for a continuous period of time.
- Advise women not to take NSAIDs 1 to 2 d before menstruation to avoid heavy menstrual flow. If discomfort occurs, acetaminophen is usually prescribed.
- Advise women in the third trimester of pregnancy to avoid NSAIDs. If delivery occurs, excess bleeding might result from use of NSAIDs.
- Inform the client that it may take several weeks to experience the desired drug effect of some NSAIDs and disease-modifying antirheumatic drugs (DMARDs).

Diet
- Instruct the client to take NSAIDs with meals or food to reduce GI upset.

Side Effects
- Advise the client of the common side effects of NSAIDs. Nausea, vomiting, peripheral edema, GI upset, purpura or petechiae, and/or dizziness might occur. Report occurrences of side effects.

Cultural Considerations
- Recognize that clients from various cultural backgrounds respond to pain and inflammation in various ways. In some cultures, the use of drugs to alleviate pain and inflammation is not acceptable to members of the culture. They may use methods such as herbal medicine and acupuncture to alleviate pain.
- Be supportive of the client's methods for pain control. Explain the purpose of medications and their action and side effects.

Evaluation

- Evaluate the effectiveness of the drug therapy, such as a decrease in pain and in swollen joints and an increase in mobility.

Table 24–3		
Selective COX-2 Inhibitors		
GENERIC (BRAND)	**ROUTE AND DOSAGE**	**USES AND CONSIDERATIONS**
Nabumetone (Relafen)	A: PO: 500–1000 mg/d or in 2 divided doses	To treat chronic inflammation and pain especially for arthritic conditions, such as rheumatoid arthritis. Inhibits cyclooxygenase, particularly COX-2 more than COX-1, therefore causing fewer GI problems. *Pregnancy category:* C; PB: UK: t½: 22–30 h.
Celecoxib (Soon to be marketed)		A potent COX-2 inhibitor that suppresses inflammation and causes minimal side effects. It may be given in higher doses than other NSAIDs.

KEY: A: adult; PO: by mouth; PB: protein-binding; GI: gastrointestinal; NSAIDs: nonsteroidal antiinflammatory drugs; t½: half-life; UK: unknown.

Chart 24–3. Antiinflammatory Agent: Gold

GOLD PREPARATION

Drug Name

Auranofin (Ridaura)
Pregnancy Category: C

Dosage

A: PO: 6 mg/d in single or divided doses; may increase dose to 9 mg/d
C: Initial: 0.1 mg/kg/d in 1–2 divided doses; *maint:* 0.15 mg/kg/d in 1–2 divided doses; *max:* 0.2 mg/kg/d in 1–2 divided doses

Contraindications

Severe renal or hepatic disease, colitis, systemic lupus erythematosus (SLE), pregnancy, blood dyscrasias
Caution: Diabetes mellitus, CHF

Drug-Lab-Food Interactions

Drug: With anticancer drugs, may cause bone marrow depression
Lab: Slightly *increase* liver enzyme tests

Pharmacokinetics

Absorption: PO: 25% absorbed
Distribution: PB: 60%
Metabolism: t½: 26 d in blood; 40–120 d in tissue
Excretion: >60% in urine (may appear for 15 mon); in feces

Pharmacodynamics

PO: Onset: UK
      Peak: 1–2 h
      Duration: Months

Therapeutic Effects/Uses

To alleviate inflammation and pain of rheumatoid arthritis.

Mode of Action: Inhibition of prostaglandin synthesis and decreased phagocytosis.

Side Effects

Anorexia, nausea, vomiting, diarrhea, stomatitis, abdominal cramps, pruritus, dizziness, headache, metallic taste, rash, dermatitis, photosensitivity

Adverse Reactions

Corneal gold deposits, urticaria, hematuria, proteinuria, bradycardia
Life-threatening: Nephrotoxicity, agranulocytosis, thrombocytopenia, interstitial pneumonitis

Assessment and Planning / Interventions / Evaluation / NURSING PROCESS

KEY: A: adult; C: child; PO: by mouth; PB: protein-binding; t½: half-life; UK: unknown; CHF: congestive heart failure; >: greater than.

the disease. It depresses migration of leukocytes and suppresses prostaglandin activity. Gold preparations are thought to inhibit destructive lysosomal enzymes that are contained in leukocytes, which are released in the joints. The effect of gold on the immune mechanism is limited.

Gold is not used in early arthritis unless the illness is progressing rapidly and is unresponsive to other therapy, nor is it used in far-advanced arthritis. It is used for palliative (relief of symptoms) and not for curative effects. Response in alleviating symptoms is slow; with injectable gold, it could take up to 2 months and, for oral dosage of gold, it could take 3 to 6 months for clinical response. The half-life of gold is 7 to 25 days, and gold drugs are highly protein-bound. Blood should be monitored for blood dyscrasia before and during parenteral or oral gold therapy.

The newest gold salt is auranofin (Ridaura). It is the only gold preparation that can be administered orally. The two parenteral gold salts are aurothioglucose (Solganal) and gold sodium thiomalate (Myochrysine). Oral gold may be absorbed erratically; thus, parenteral gold may be advisable. Switching from parenteral to oral gold preparations may be necessary for long-term use. Chart 24–3 presents drug data for the gold preparation auranofin (Ridaura).

PHARMACOKINETICS

Twenty-five percent of auranofin is absorbed from the GI tract. It is moderately highly protein-bound. Its half-life is long, both in the blood (26 days) and in the body tissues (40 to 120 days). Sixty percent of auranofin is excreted in the urine, and the drug may be present in the urine up to 15 months after it has been discontinued.

PHARMACODYNAMICS

Auranofin is prescribed to relieve inflammation and pain from rheumatoid arthritis when NSAIDs and other measures are ineffective. The therapeutic effect may take 3 to 6 months; steady state (the average therapeutic effect that is maintained) of the drug is achieved after 2 to 4 months. Side effects and adverse reactions need to be closely monitored.

Table 24–4 details dosages and considerations for the three gold drugs used as antiinflammatory agents for rheumatoid arthritis.

SIDE EFFECTS AND ADVERSE REACTIONS

Approximately 25% to 45% of clients receiving gold therapy experience side effects. The side effects may occur anytime during or several months after therapy. The numerous possible side effects include dermatitis, urticaria (hives), erythema, alopecia (loss of hair), stomatitis (mouth ulcers), pharyngitis, gastritis, colitis, hepatitis, severe blood dyscrasias (agranulocytosis, aplastic anemia), and even anaphylactic shock.

CONTRAINDICATIONS

Gold therapy is contraindicated for clients with eczema, urticaria, colitis, hemorrhagic conditions, and systemic lupus erythematosus.

Immunosuppressive Agents

Immunosuppressives are used to treat refractory rheumatoid arthritis; that is, arthritis that does not respond to antiinflammatory drugs. In low doses, selected immunosuppressive agents have been effective in the treatment of rheumatoid arthritis. Drugs such as azathioprine (Imuran), cyclophosphamide (Cytoxan), and methotrexate (Mexate) are used primarily to suppress cancer growth and proliferation. These drugs might be used in suppressing the inflammatory process of rheumatoid arthritis when other treatments fail. In one study of clients receiving cyclophosphamide, few new erosions of joint cartilage were present, which suggests that the disease process is not active. These agents are not the first or second choice drugs for treatment of rheumatoid arthritis.

Antimalarials

Antimalarial drugs may be used in treatment of rheumatoid arthritis when other methods of treatment fail.

Table 24–4
Antiinflammatory Drugs: Gold Preparations

GENERIC (BRAND)	ROUTE AND DOSAGE	USES AND CONSIDERATIONS
Auranofin (Ridaura)	See Chart 24–3	For rheumatoid arthritis when unresponsive to NSAIDs. Start with low dose. Check laboratory values, especially white blood cell count, hemoglobin, and hematocrit. Check renal and liver function. *Pregnancy category:* C; PB: 60%; $t_{\frac{1}{2}}$: 26 d
Aurothioglucose (Solganal)	Increase dose weekly: A: IM: 10, 25, 50 mg (sol in oil)	Same considerations as auranofin. *Pregnancy category:* C; PB: 95%; $t_{\frac{1}{2}}$: 3–27 d
Gold sodium thiomalate (Myochrysine)	Increase dose weekly: A: IM: 10, 25, 50 mg (aqueous sol) until 1 g cumulative dose; maint: 25–50 mg q2–3 wk C: TD: 10 mg, followed by 1 mg/kg/wk × 20 wk; maint: 1 mg/kg/dose every 2–4 wk	Same considerations as auranofin. Contains 50% gold. *Pregnancy category:* C; PB: 95%; $t_{\frac{1}{2}}$: 3–27 d

Key: A: adult; C: child; IM: intramuscular; TD: test dose; PB: protein-binding; $t_{\frac{1}{2}}$: half-life; sol: solution; maint: maintenance; NSAIDs: nonsteroidal antiinflammatory drugs.

NURSING PROCESS
ANTIINFLAMMATORY: GOLD

Assessment

- Obtain the client's health history. Usually, gold drugs such as auranofin are contraindicated if there is renal or hepatic dysfunction, marked hypertension, congestive heart failure, systemic lupus erythematosus (SLE), or uncontrolled diabetes mellitus.
- Check for proteinuria and hematuria before giving initial gold dose and during gold therapy.
- Observe the client for 30 min after gold injection for possible allergic reaction after the first and second injections. It takes approximately 10 to 15 min for a serious allergic reaction (anaphylaxis) to occur.
- Obtain baseline vital signs (VS) and hematology laboratory findings for future comparisons.

Potential Nursing Diagnoses

- Impaired physical mobility
- Pain
- Risk for impaired skin integrity

Planning

- The client will be free of inflammation and pain while taking the gold treatment without adverse drug reaction.

Nursing Interventions

- Monitor the client's VS. Report abnormal findings.
- Monitor laboratory tests, for example, complete blood count (CBC). Report abnormal findings.
- Check periodically for signs of side effects and adverse reactions to gold therapy. Side effects may include anorexia, nausea, vomiting, diarrhea, gingivitis, stomatitis, rash, itching, and decreased urine output. Most gold drugs have a long half-life; thus, a cumulative effect can result. Auranofin causes less severe adverse reactions than other gold preparations.

Nursing Process continued on following page

The mechanism of action of antimalarials in suppression of rheumatoid arthritis is unclear. The effect may take 4 to 12 weeks to become apparent, and antimalarials are usually used in combination with NSAIDs in clients whose arthritis is not under control.

ANTIGOUT DRUGS

Gout has been called the "disease of Kings" because, in the past, royalty ate "rich foods" and drank wine and alcohol and suffered from gout. It was also referred to as the "unwalkable disease." Hippocrates (460–357 B.C.) referred to gout as *podagra* (foot seizure). He recognized gout as affecting other joints of the large toe, hand, elbow, knee, and shoulder. Hippocrates' recommendation of treatment included purgatives (strong laxatives). Galen (131–200 A.D.) attributed gout to "intemperance" and heredity.

Gout is an inflammatory condition that attacks joints, tendons, and other tissues. The most common site of acute gouty inflammation is at the joint of the big toe. Also it may be referred to as gouty arthritis. Gout is characterized by a uric acid metabolism disorder and a defect in purine (products of certain proteins) metabolism, resulting in an increase in urates (uric acid salts) and an accumulation of uric acid (hyperuricemia) or an ineffective clearance of uric acid by the kidneys. Uric acid solubility is poor in acid urine and urate crystals may form, causing urate calculi. Gout may appear as bumps or "tophi" in the subcutaneous tissue of earlobes, elbows, hands, and the base of the large toe. The complications of untreated or prolonged periods of gout include tophi, gouty arthritis, urinary calculi, and gouty nephropathy.

Fluid intake should be increased while taking antigout drugs, and the urine should be alkaline. Acetaminophen should be taken for discomfort instead of aspirin (salicylic acid) to reduce acidity. Foods rich in

Client Teaching

General

- Instruct the client to perform frequent dental hygiene, including brushing the teeth with a soft toothbrush and flossing to prevent or control gingivitis and stomatitis. Use of diluted hydrogen peroxide can be helpful in mild stomatitis.
- Instruct the client to adhere to scheduled laboratory blood tests and appointments with the health care provider so any adverse reactions can be monitored.
- Inform the client that the desired therapeutic effect may take as long as 3 to 4 months to occur.

Diet

- Suggest high-fiber diet or antidiarrheal drugs to control diarrhea. If diarrhea is continuous or severe for a prolonged time, the gold drug is usually discontinued.

Side Effects

- Advise the client to report early symptoms of possible gold toxicity such as a metallic taste or pruritus. A rash may occur. These symptoms should be reported to the health care provider.
- Teach the client the side effects and to report them immediately. (See Chart 24–3 for a list of side effects and adverse reactions.)
- Instruct the client to avoid direct sunlight because the gold drug may cause photosensitivity. Use of sunblock is necessary.
- Instruct the client to report skin conditions such as dermatitis, bruising, and petechiae. Bleeding gums and blood in the stools should be reported to the health care provider.

Evaluation

- Evaluate the effectiveness of the gold therapy by determining whether the client has less pain and inflammation.
- Evaluate the client for present or repeated side effects. The gold therapy regimen may need to be changed or discontinued.

---

purine, including wine, alcohol, organ meats, sardines, salmon, and gravy, should be avoided.

Antiinflammatory Gout Drug: Colchicine

The first drug to treat gout was colchicine, introduced in 1936. The antiinflammatory drug colchicine inhibits the migration of leukocytes to the inflamed site. It is effective in alleviating acute symptoms of gout but it is not effective in decreasing inflammation occurring in other inflammatory disorders. It does not inhibit uric acid synthesis and does not promote uric acid excretion. It should not be used if the client has a severe renal, cardiac, or GI problem. Gastric irritation is a common problem; therefore, colchicine should be taken with food. With high doses of colchicine, nausea, vomiting, diarrhea, or abdominal pain occurs in approximately 75% of clients taking the drug.

Colchicine is well absorbed in the GI tract, and its peak concentration time is within 2 h. Most of the drug is excreted in the feces, but 10% to 20% is excreted in the urine.

Uric Acid Inhibitor

Allopurinol (Zyloprim), marketed in 1963, is not an antiinflammatory drug; instead, it inhibits the final steps of uric acid biosynthesis and therefore lowers serum uric acid levels, preventing the precipitation of an attack. It is a choice drug for clients with chronic tophaceous gout. This drug is frequently used for prevention (prophylaxis) of gout. Allopurinol is also indicated for gout clients with renal impairment. It is useful for clients who have renal obstructions caused by uric acid stones, and for clients with blood disorders such as leukemia and polycythemia vera. It is also given to clients who do not respond well to uricosuric drugs such as probenecid. Increased fluid intake is recommended to promote diuresis and pre-

Chart 24–4. Antigout

URIC ACID BIOSYNTHESIS INHIBITOR

Drug Name

Allopurinol (Zyloprim) 🍁 Alloprin, Apo-Allo-purinol, Novopurinol
Pregnancy Category: C

Dosage

A: PO: 200–300 mg/d (for mild gout); 400–600 mg/d (for severe gout)
C: PO: 10 mg/kg/d in 2–3 divided doses
<6 y: 150 mg/d in 3 divided doses

Contraindications

Hypersensitivity, severe renal disease
Caution: Hepatic disorder

Drug-Lab-Food Interactions

Drug: *Increase* effect of warfarin, phenytoin, theophylline, anticancer drugs, ACE inhibitors; *increase* rash with ampicillin, amoxicillin; *increase* toxicity with thiazide diuretics; *decrease* allopurinol effect with antacids
Lab: Increase AST, ALT, BUN

Pharmacokinetics

Absorption: PO: 80% absorbed
Distribution: PB: UK
Metabolism: $t\frac{1}{2}$: Drug: 2–3 h
Metabolite: 20–24 h
Excretion: 10%–20% in urine; 80%–90% in feces

Pharmacodynamics

PO: Onset: 0.5–1 h
     Peak: 2–4 h
     Duration: 18–30 h

Therapeutic Effects/Uses

To treat gout and hyperuricemia; prevent urate calculi.

Mode of Action: Reduction of uric acid synthesis.

Side Effects

Anorexia, nausea, vomiting, diarrhea, stomatitis, dizziness, headache, rash, pruritus, malaise, metallic taste

Adverse Reactions

Cataracts, retinopathy
Life-threatening: Bone marrow depression, aplastic anemia, thrombocytopenia, agranulocytosis, leukopenia

Assessment and Planning

Interventions

Evaluation

NURSING PROCESS

KEY: A: Adult; C: child; PO: by mouth; UK: unknown; PB: protein-binding; ACE: angiotensin-converting enzyme; $t\frac{1}{2}$: half-life; <: less than; 🍁: Canadian drug names; ALT: alanine aminotransferase; AST: aspartate aminotransferase; BUN: blood urea nitrogen.

vent alkalinization of the urine. Chart 24–4 presents the pharmacologic behavior of allopurinol.

PHARMACOKINETICS

Eighty percent of allopurinol is absorbed from the GI tract. Biosynthesis of uric acid occurs in the liver in pure form and active metabolites. The half-life of the drug itself is 2 to 3 h, and of its active metabolites is 20 to 24 h. The protein-binding percentage is unknown. Most of the drug and its metabolite are excreted in feces and some in urine.

PHARMACODYNAMICS

Allopurinol inhibits the production of uric acid by inhibiting the enzyme xanthine oxidase, which is needed in the synthesis of uric acid. Allopurinol also improves the solubility of uric acid. Its onset of action occurs within 30 to 60 min; its peak time is average, 2 to 4 h; and it has a long duration of action.

Alcohol, caffeine, and thiazide diuretics increase the uric acid level. Use of ampicillin or amoxicillin with allopurinol increases the risk of rash formation.

Allopurinol can increase the effect of coumadin and oral hypoglycemic drugs.

Uricosurics

Uricosurics increase the rate of uric acid excretion by inhibiting its reabsorption. This group of drugs is effective in alleviating chronic gout, but they should *not* be used during acute attacks. Probenecid (Benemid) is a uricosuric that has been available since 1945. It blocks the reabsorption of uric acid and promotes its excretion. Probenecid can be taken with colchicine. To begin initial therapy for relieving symptoms of gout and inhibiting uric acid reabsorption, small doses of colchicine should be given before adding probenecid. If gastric irritation occurs, probenecid should be taken with meals. It has an average half-life of 8 to 10 h and is 85% to 95% protein-bound. Caution should be taken when administering this drug with other highly protein-bound drugs.

Another uricosuric is sulfinpyrazone (Anturane). This drug is a metabolite of phenylbutazone and is more potent than probenecid. Sulfinpyrazone should be taken with meals or with antacids to prevent gastric irritation. Severe blood dyscrasias might occur, especially with a history of blood dyscrasia. Table 24–5 gives dosages and considerations for the commonly used antigout drugs.

SIDE EFFECTS AND ADVERSE REACTIONS
Side effects may include flushed skin, sore gums, and headache. Kidney stones, resulting from the uric acid, could be prevented by increasing water intake and maintaining a urine pH above 6.0. Blood dyscrasias occur rarely. Aspirin use should be avoided because it causes uric acid retention.

Other Drugs

Indomethacin (Indocin), an antiinflammatory agent, can be used for short-term management of symptoms of acute gouty arthritis. It has little to no effect on the serum uric acid levels. It may be used in early stages of gout to decrease leukocytic phagocytosis of urate crystals.

Table 24–5 Antigout Drugs		
GENERIC (BRAND)	**ROUTE AND DOSAGE**	**USES AND CONSIDERATIONS**
ANTIINFLAMMATORY GOUT DRUG		
Colchicine (Novocolchine, Colsalide)	A: PO: Initially: 0.5–1.2 mg; then 0.5–0.6 mg q1–2h for pain relief; *max:* 4 mg/d; IV: Initially: 2 mg; then 0.5 mg q6h PRN; *max:* 4 mg/d	Treatment of acute gout and prophylaxis of recurrent gouty arthritis. Not for clients with renal or gastric disorders. Take with food. *Pregnancy category:* C; PB: 10%–30%; $t_{\frac{1}{2}}$: 20–30 min
URIC ACID BIOSYNTHE-SIS INHIBITOR		
Allopurinol (Zyloprim)	See Chart 24–4	Treatment for hyperuricemia by preventing uric acid synthesis. Prevents acute gouty attack. Keep urine alkaline; increase fluid intake. *Pregnancy category:* C; PB: UK; $t_{\frac{1}{2}}$: 2–3 h
URICOSURICS		
Probenecid (Benemid)	A: PO: First week: 250 mg b.i.d.; maint: 500 mg b.i.d.; *max:* 2 g/d C <50 kg: PO: 25–40 mg/kg/d in 4 divided doses	Treatment for hyperuricemia; promotes urinary excretion of uric acid. For gout and gouty arthritis. Alkaline urine helps to prevent renal stones. Increase fluid intake. *Pregnancy category:* B; PB: 90%; $t_{\frac{1}{2}}$: 4–10 h
Sulfinpyrazone (Anturane)	A: PO: First week: 100–200 mg b.i.d.; maint: 200–400 mg b.i.d.; may reduce to 200 mg/d; *max:* 800 mg/d	Used in the management of hyperuricemia; decreases gouty attacks. Can cause GI distress. Take with food. *Pregnancy category:* C; PB: 90%; $t_{\frac{1}{2}}$: 3 h

KEY: A: adult; C: child; PO: by mouth; IV: intravenous; UK: unknown; <: less than; PRN: as necessary; PB: protein-binding; $t_{\frac{1}{2}}$: half-life; maint: maintenance.

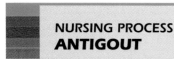

NURSING PROCESS
ANTIGOUT

Assessment

- Obtain a medical history from the client of any gastric, renal, cardiac, or liver disorders. Antigout drugs are excreted via kidneys, so sufficient renal function is needed. Drug dosage and drug selection might need to be changed.
- Obtain a drug history. Report possible drug-drug interactions. (See drug-laboratory-food interaction list in Chart 24–4.)
- Assess the serum uric acid value to be used for future comparisons.
- Assess the urine output. Use the initial urine output for future comparison.
- Obtain laboratory tests (BUN, serum creatinine, ALP, AST, ALT, LDH) and compare with future laboratory test results.

Potential Nursing Diagnoses

- Impaired tissue integrity
- Pain

Planning

- Client's "gouty pain" is absent or controlled without side effects.

Nursing Interventions

- Report GI symptoms, gastric pain, nausea, vomiting, or diarrhea when taking antigout drugs. Take these drugs with food to alleviate gastric distress.
- Monitor the client's urine output. Because the drugs and uric acid are excreted through the urine, kidney stones might occur, so both water intake and urine output should be increased.
- Monitor laboratory tests for renal and liver function; that is, BUN, serum creatinine, ALP, AST, and ALT.

Client Teaching

General
- Encourage the client to keep medical appointments and to have regular scheduled laboratory tests for renal, liver, and blood cell (CBC) functions. Some antigout drugs may cause blood dyscrasias; blood tests should be monitored.
- Instruct the client to increase fluid intake; it will increase drug and uric acid excretion.

Diet
- Advise the client to avoid alcohol and caffeine because they can increase uric acid levels.
- Suggest to the client not to take large doses of vitamin C while taking allopurinol; kidney stones may occur.

Nursing Process continued on following page

Phenylbutazone (Butazolidin), a pyrazoline derivative, has some uricosuric effect. It promotes renal excretion of uric acid. It has been used to treat acute attacks of gouty arthritis.

A new drug, etanercept (Enbrel), has been recently approved by the FDA for the treatment of advanced rheumatoid arthritis. Enbrel appears to cause few serious side effects. It does not cure rheumatoid arthritis, and if the drug is stopped, symptoms reappear. In a recent study, it helped 59% of clients with advanced rheumatoid arthritis and, when the drug was combined with methotrexate, 71% of the clients reported decreased symptoms. Rheumatoid arthritis affects 2 million persons in the United States.

- Instruct the client not to ingest foods that are high in purine content, such as organ meats, salmon and sardines, gravies, and legumes. Purine foods increase the uric acid levels.
- Instruct the client to report any gastric distress. Encourage the client to take antigout drugs with food or at mealtime.

Side Effects
- Instruct the client to report side effects of antigout drugs, such as anorexia, nausea, vomiting, diarrhea, stomatitis, dizziness, rash, pruritus, and metallic taste, to the health care provider.
- Advise the client to have a yearly eye examination because visual changes can result from prolonged use of allopurinol.

Cultural Considerations
- Provide additional explanation as needed to clients and their families from various cultural groups related to the disease process, and the purpose of the drug and its side effects.
- Suggest follow-up by a community nurse to determine the client's compliance to the drug regimen and the effectiveness of the prescribed drug therapy.

Evaluation

- Evaluate the client's response to the antigout drug. If pain persists, the drug regimen may need modification.
- Determine the presence of adverse reactions. Drug therapy for gout pain may need to be changed.

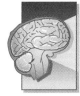

Critical Thinking in Action

P. Q., 72 years old, had taken 650 mg of aspirin four times a day for 8 months to alleviate her chronic symptoms of pain and inflammation associated with arthritis. Four weeks ago, a peptic ulcer developed.

1. Explain the process in which P. Q. could have a peptic ulcer. What ways could this have been prevented?
2. How does aspirin differ from other NSAIDs?
3. What client teaching points should P. Q. receive before and during the time she is taking aspirin?
4. How would the new COX-2 inhibitors prevent the development of a peptic ulcer?
5. Would the DMARD group be more helpful to alleviate P. Q.'s symptoms? Explain your rationale.

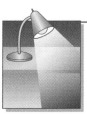

Study Questions

1. What is the action of nonsteroidal antiinflammatory drugs (NSAIDs)? Give examples of common NSAIDs.

446 Unit V • Antiinflammatory and Antiinfective Agents

2. What are the major side effects of NSAIDs?
3. What are the uses of disease-modifying antirheumatic drugs (DMARDs)?
4. What are the side effects and adverse reactions of DMARDs?
5. What are the nursing interventions associated with the use of NSAIDs and DMARDs?
6. What drugs are used to treat gout? What are the nursing considerations?

Antibacterials: Penicillins and Cephalosporins

25

Outline

Objectives

- Explain the mechanisms of action of antibacterial drugs.
- Differentiate between bacteria that are naturally resistant and those that have acquired resistance to an antibiotic.
- Identify several adverse effects associated with antibacterial drugs.
- Differentiate between narrow-spectrum and broad-spectrum antibiotics.
- Give an example each of natural, broad-spectrum (extended), penicillinase-resistant, and antipseudomonal penicillins.
- Explain the expected effects of the first, second, and third generations of cephalosporins.
- Describe specific nursing interventions and the client teaching that relate to the administration of penicillins and cephalosporins.

Terms

acquired resistance

antibacterials

antimicrobials

bactericidal

bacteriostatic

broad-spectrum antibiotics

cross-resistance

immunoglobulins

inherent resistance

microorganisms

narrow-spectrum antibiotics

nephrotoxicity

nosocomial infection

superinfection

INTRODUCTION

Although the terms *antibacterial, antimicrobial,* and *antibiotic* are frequently used interchangeably, there are some subtle differences in meaning. **Antibacterial** and **antimicrobial drugs** are substances that inhibit the growth of or kill bacteria or other **microorganisms** (microscopic organisms including bacteria, viruses, fungi, protozoa, and rickettsiae). Technically, the term *antibiotic* refers to chemicals that are produced by one kind of microorganism that inhibits the growth of or kills another. For practical purposes, however, these terms may be used interchangeably. Several drugs, including antiinfective and chemotherapeutic agents, have actions similar to those of the antibacterial and antimicrobial agents. Antibacterial drugs do not act alone in destroying bacteria. Natural body defenses, surgical procedures to excise infected tissues, and dressing changes may be needed along with antibacterial drugs to eliminate the infecting bacteria.

Antibacterial drugs are obtained from natural sources or are manufactured. The use of moldy bread on wounds to fight infection dates back 3500 years. In 1928, Alexander Fleming, a British bacteriologist, noted that "mold" was contaminating the bacterial cultures and inhibiting the bacterial growth. Fleming called the mold *Penicillium notatum.* In 1939, Howard Florey continued with Fleming's findings and purified the penicillin so that it could be used commercially. Penicillin was used during World War II and became widely marketed in 1945. Sulfonamide, a synthetic antibacterial, was introduced in 1935. Sulfonamides are discussed in greater detail in Chapter 27.

Bacteriostatic drugs inhibit the growth of bacteria, whereas **bactericidal** drugs kill bacteria. Some antibacterial drugs, such as tetracycline and sulfonamides, have a bacteriostatic effect, whereas other antibacterials, such as penicillins and cephalosporins, have a bactericidal effect. Depending on the drug dose and serum level, certain drugs can have both bacteriostatic and bactericidal effects. Drug serum levels should be monitored.

Peaks and troughs of serum antibiotic levels are monitored for drugs with a narrow therapeutic index, such as aminoglycosides, to determine whether the drug is within the therapeutic range for its desired effect. If the serum peak level is too high, drug toxicity could occur. If the serum trough level, drawn minutes before the next drug dose, is below the therapeutic range, the client is not receiving an adequate antibiotic dose to kill the microorganism.

ANTIBACTERIAL DRUGS

Antibacterial drugs are currently grouped into 10 categories: penicillins, cephalosporins, macrolides, tetra-

cyclines, lincosamides, vancomycin, aminoglycosides, chloramphenicol, fluoroquinolones, and peptides. Penicillins and cephalosporins are discussed in this chapter. Antibacterials and antibiotics II (macrolides, tetracyclines, aminoglycosides, and fluoroquinolones) are described in Chapter 26. Sulfonamides are presented in Chapter 27. Antitubercular drugs, antifungal drugs, and peptides are covered in Chapter 28. Antivirals, antimalarials, and anthelmintics are discussed in Chapter 29. Most antibiotics are produced semisynthetically or synthetically.

Mechanisms of Antibacterial Action

Five mechanisms of antibacterial action are responsible for the inhibition of growth or destruction of microorganisms: (1) inhibition of bacterial cell wall synthesis, (2) alteration of membrane permeability, (3) inhibition of protein synthesis, (4) inhibition of the synthesis of bacterial RNA and DNA, and (5) interference with metabolism within the cell (Table 25–1).

Antibacterial drugs must not only penetrate the bacterial cell wall in sufficient concentration but also the drug must have an affinity to the binding sites on the bacterial cell. The time that the drug remains at the binding sites increases the effect of the antibacterial action. The time is controlled by the pharmacokinetics (distribution, half-life, and elimination) of the drug. Antibacterials that have a longer half-life usually maintain a greater concentration at the binding site, and frequent dosing is not required. Most antibacterials are not highly protein-bound, with the exception of a few (i.e., oxacillin, ceftriaxone, cefoperazone, cefonicid, cefprozil, cloxacillin, nafcillin, and clindamycin). Thus, protein binding does not have a major influence on the effectiveness of the drug dose. The steady state of the antibacterial drug occurs after the fourth to fifth half-lives, and the drug is eliminated from the body after the seventh half-life.

Antibacterial drugs are used to achieve the minimum effective concentration (MEC) necessary to halt the growth of a microorganism—a concentration that depends on the drug's pharmacokinetics (absorption, distribution, metabolism, and excretion). However, when minimum effective concentration is desired, a considerably greater concentration of drug is usually needed, so the client should be monitored and assessed for drug toxicity.

Pharmacodynamics of Antibacterials

The drug concentration at the site or the exposure time for the drug plays an important role in bacteria eradication. Many antibacterials have a bactericidal effect against the pathogen when the drug concentra-

Table 25-1
Mechanisms of Actions of Antibacterial Drugs

ACTION	EFFECT	DRUGS
Inhibitions of cell wall synthesis	Bactericidal effect. Enzyme breakdown of the cell wall. Inhibition of the enzyme in the synthesis of the cell wall.	Penicillin Cephalosporins Bacitracin Vancomycin
Alteration in membrane permeability	Bacteriostatic or bactericidal effect. Membrane permeability is increased. The loss of cellular substances causes lysis of the cell.	Amphotericin B Nystatin Polymyxin Colistin
Inhibition of protein synthesis	Bacteriostatic or bactericidal effect. Interferes with protein synthesis without affecting normal cell. Inhibits the steps of protein synthesis.	Aminoglycosides Tetracyclines Erythromycin Lincomycins
Inhibition of synthesis of bacterial RNA and DNA	Inhibits synthesis of RNA and DNA in bacteria. It binds to the nucleic acid and to the enzymes, which are needed for nucleic acid synthesis.	Fluoroquinolones
Interference with cellular metabolism	Bacteriostatic effect. Interferes with steps of metabolism within the cells.	Sulfonamides Trimethoprim Isoniazid (INH) Naldixic acid Rifampin

tion remains constantly above the MEC during the dosing interval. Duration of time for use of the antibacterial varies according to the type of pathogen, site of infection, and immunocompetence of the host. With some severe infections, a continuous infusion regimen is more effective than an intermittent dosing because of constant drug concentration and time exposure. Once-daily antibacterial dosing (e.g., aminoglycosides) has been effective in eradicating pathogens and, in most of those cases, has not caused severe adverse reactions (ototoxicity, nephrotoxicity). In addition, once- or twice-daily drug dosing increases the client's adherence to the drug regimen.

Figure 25-1 illustrates the effect of three methods of drug dosing. The drug dose is effective while it remains above the MEC.

Body defenses and antibacterial drugs work together to stop the infectious process. The effect that antibacterial drugs have on an infection depends not only on the drug but also on the host's defense mechanisms. Factors such as age, nutrition, immunoglobulins, white blood cells, organ function, and circulation influence the body's ability to fight infection. If the host's natural body defense mechanisms are inadequate, drug therapy might not be as effective. As a result, drug therapy may need to be closely monitored or revised. When circulation is impeded, an antibacterial drug may not be distributed properly to the infected area. In addition, **immunoglobulins,** such as IgG and IgM (a protein with antibody activity,

part of the immune response system) and white blood cells needed to combat infections may be depleted in individuals with poor nutritional status.

Resistance to Antibacterials

Bacteria may be sensitive or resistant to certain antibacterials. When bacteria are sensitive to the drug, the organism is inhibited or destroyed. If bacteria are resistant to an antibacterial, the organism continues to grow despite administration of that antibacterial drug.

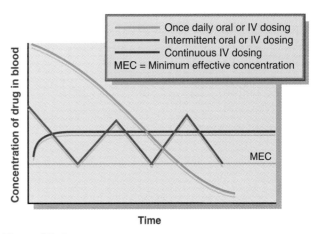

Figure 25-1
Effects of concentrated drug dosing.

Bacterial resistance may result naturally (inherent), or it may be acquired. A **natural, or inherent, resistance** occurs without previous exposure to the antibacterial drug. For example, the gram-negative (non–gram-staining) bacterium *Pseudomonas aeruginosa* is resistant to penicillin G. An **acquired resistance** is caused by prior exposure to the antibacterial. For example, although *Staphylococcus aureus* was once sensitive to penicillin G, previous exposures have caused this organism to become resistant to penicillin G. Penicillinase, an enzyme produced by the microorganism, is responsible for causing penicillin resistance. This enzyme metabolizes penicillin G, causing the drug to be ineffective. Currently available are penicillinase-resistant penicillins that are effective against *S. aureus.*

In large health care institutions, there is a tendency toward drug resistance to bacteria. Mutant strains of organisms have developed, thus increasing the resistance to the antibiotics that were once effective. Infections that are acquired while clients are hospitalized are called **nosocomial infections.** Many of these infections are caused by drug-resistant bacteria and can prolong hospitalization, which is costly to the client.

Antibiotic resistance is a major problem. In the early 1980s pharmaceutical companies thought that enough antibiotics were on the market, so these companies concentrated on developing antiviral and antifungal drugs. Fewer new antibiotics were developed during the 1980s. Antibiotic resistance continues to occur when antibiotics are used frequently. As the bacteria reproduce, some mutation occurs and eventually the mutant bacteria survive the effects of the drug. One explanation is that the mutant bacteria strain may have grown a thicker cell wall.

Another problem related to antibiotic resistance is that bacteria can transfer their genetic instruction to another bacterial species; thus, the other bacterial species becomes resistant to that antibiotic as well. It can pass its high resistance to a more virulent and aggressive bacterium, such as *Staphylococcus aureus* and enterococci. One of the biggest resistance problems is vancomycin-resistant enterococci (VRE), which can cause death in many persons with weakened immune systems. The incidence of VRE in hospitals increased from 0.3% in 1989 to 14.2% in 1996. Staphylococcal bacteria tend to be resistant to every drug except vancomycin. If VRE transfers to *Staphylococcus* its resistance to vancomycin, a major medical problem could result.

One antibiotic after another is ineffective against new resistant strains of bacteria. As new drugs are developed, drug resistance will probably develop as well. Pharmaceutical companies and biotechnical firms are working on new classes of drugs to "beat" the problem of bacterial resistance to antibiotics. Recently, the new everninomicin class antibiotic Ziracin

has been approved, although it is not yet on the U.S. market. Another class of antibiotics, oxazolidinones, was discovered by a pharmaceutical company in 1988, but the company could not overcome toxicity problems in this class of drug. Another pharmaceutical company has taken the compound and has made it less toxic. The new antibiotic, Linezolid, is effective against methicillin-resistant staphylococci, vancomycin-resistant enterococci, and penicillin-resistant streptococci. Linezolid should be available soon in the United States.

Another way to attack antimicrobial resistance is to develop drugs that disable the antibiotic-resistant mechanism in the bacteria. Clients would take the antibiotic-resistance disabler along with the antibiotic already on the market, making it effective again. Developing bacterial vaccine is another way to combat bacteria and lessen the need for antibiotics. The bacterial vaccine against pneumococcus has been effective in decreasing the occurrence of pneumonia and meningitis among various age groups. An important way to decrease antibiotic resistance is to prevent antibiotic abuse. Antibiotic abuse is a major problem. Consumer education is important because many clients "demand" antibiotics for viral conditions. Antibiotics are ineffective against virus. However, viral infections that persist could decrease the body's immune system, thus promoting a bacterial infection.

Cross-resistance can also occur between antibacterial drugs that have similar actions, such as the penicillins and cephalosporins. The organism causing the infection can be determined by culture, and the antibiotics sensitive to the organism are determined by culture and sensitivity (C & S). To determine the effect antibacterial drugs have on a specific microorganism, C & S or antibiotic susceptibility testing is performed. The susceptibility or resistance of one microorganism to several antibacterials can be determined by this method. Multiantibiotic therapy (daily use of several antibacterials) delays the development of microorganism resistance.

Use of Antibiotic Combinations

Combination antibiotics should not be routinely prescribed or administered except for specific uncontrollable infections. Usually a single antibiotic will successfully treat a bacterial infection. When there is a severe infection that persists and is of unknown origin or has been unsuccessfully treated with several single antibiotics, a combination of two or three antibiotics may be suggested. Before antibiotic therapy, a culture or cultures should be taken to identify the bacteria.

When two antibiotics are combined, the result is additive, potentiative, or antagonistic. The additive effect is equal to the sum of the effects of two antibiotics. The potentiative effect occurs when one antibiotic potentiates the effect of the second antibiotic, increasing their effectiveness. The antagonistic result would be a combination of a drug that is bactericidal, such as penicillin, and a drug that is bacteriostatic, such as tetracycline. When these two drugs are used together, the desired effect may be greatly reduced.

General Adverse Reactions to Antibacterials

Three major adverse reactions associated with the administration of antibacterial drugs are allergic (hypersensitivity) reactions, superinfection, and organ toxicity. Table 25–2 describes these adverse reactions, all of which require close monitoring of the client.

Narrow-Spectrum and Broad-Spectrum Antibiotics

Antibacterial drugs are either narrow spectrum or broad spectrum. The **narrow-spectrum antibiotics** are primarily effective against one type of organism. For example, penicillin and erythromycin are used to treat infections caused by gram-positive bacteria. **Broad-spectrum antibiotics,** such as tetracycline and the cephalosporins, are effective against both gram-positive and gram-negative organisms. Because narrow-spectrum antibiotics are selective, they are more

active against those single organisms than the broad-spectrum antibiotics. Broad-spectrum antibiotics are frequently used to treat infections when the offending microorganism has not been identified by culture and sensitivity.

PENICILLINS

Penicillin, a natural antibacterial agent obtained from the mold genus *Penicillium,* was introduced to the military during World War II and is considered to have saved many soldiers' lives. It became widely used in 1945 and was labeled the "miracle" drug. With the advent of penicillin, many clients survived who would have died from wound and severe respiratory infections.

Penicillin's beta-lactam structure (beta-lactam ring) interferes with bacterial cell wall synthesis by inhibiting the bacterial enzyme that is necessary for cell division and cellular synthesis. The bacteria die of cell lysis (cell breakdown). The penicillins can be both bacteriostatic and bactericidal depending on the drug and dosage. Penicillin G is primarily bactericidal.

Penicillins are mainly referred to as beta-lactam antibiotics. Bacteria can produce a variety of enzymes, beta-lactamases, that can inactivate penicillin and other beta-lactam antibiotics such as the cephalosporins. The beta-lactamases, which attack penicillins, are referred to as penicillinases.

Table 25–2
General Adverse Reactions to Antibacterial Drugs

TYPE	CONSIDERATIONS
Allergy or hypersensitivity effect	Allergic reactions to drugs may be mild or severe. Examples of mild reactions are rash, pruritus, and hives. An example of a severe response is anaphylactic shock. Anaphylaxis results in vascular collapse, laryngeal edema, bronchospasm, and cardiac arrest. Shortness of breath is frequently the first symptom of anaphylaxis. Severe allergic reaction generally occurs within 20 min. Mild allergic reaction is treated with an antihistamine; anaphylaxis requires treatment with epinephrine, bronchodilators, and antihistamines.
Superinfection	Superinfection is a secondary infection that occurs when the normal microbial flora of the body are disturbed during antibiotic therapy. Superinfections can occur in the mouth, respiratory tract, intestine, genitourinary tract, or skin. Fungus infections frequently result in superinfections, although bacterial organisms, such as *Proteus, Pseudomonas,* and staphylococci may be the offending microorganisms. Superinfections rarely develop when the drug is administered for less than a week. They occur more commonly with the use of broad-spectrum antibiotics. For fungal infection of the mouth, nystatin is frequently used.
Organ toxicity	Organs, such as the liver and kidney, are involved in drug metabolism and excretion. Antibacterials may result in damage to these organs. For example, aminoglycosides can be ototoxic and nephrotoxic.

Penicillin G was the first penicillin administered orally and by injection. With oral administration, only about one-third of the dose is absorbed. Because of its poor absorption, penicillin G given by injection (intramuscular and intravenous) is more effective in achieving a therapeutic serum penicillin level. Aqueous penicillin G has a short duration of action, and the intramuscular injection is very painful because it is an aqueous drug solution. Therefore, a longer-acting form of penicillin, procaine penicillin (milky color), was produced to extend the activity of the drug. Procaine in the penicillin decreases the pain related to injection of this medication.

Penicillin V was the next type of penicillin produced. Although two-thirds of the oral dose is absorbed by the gastrointestinal (GI) tract, it is a less potent antibacterial drug than penicillin G. Penicillin V is effective against mild to moderate infections.

Initially, penicillin was overused. It was first introduced for the treatment of staphylococcal infections, but after a few years, mutant strains of *Staphylococcus* developed that were resistant to penicillins G and V because of the bacterial enzyme penicillinase that destroys penicillin, rendering it ineffective. This led to the development of new broad-spectrum antibiotics with structures similar to penicillin to combat infections that are resistant to penicillins G and V.

Food may decrease the absorption of some penicillins that are taken orally; therefore, those penicillins should be taken with a full glass of water 1 hour before food intake or 2 hours after mealtime. Table 25–3 indicates how the oral penicillins are affected when taken with food.

Broad-Spectrum Penicillins (Aminopenicillins)

The broad-spectrum penicillins are used to treat both gram-positive and gram-negative bacteria. They are not, however, as "broadly" effective against all microorganisms as they were once considered to be. This group of drugs is costlier than penicillin and therefore should not be used when ordinary penicillins, such as penicillin G, are effective. The broad-spectrum penicillins are effective against some gram-negative organisms, such as *Escherichia coli*, *Haemophilus influenzae*, *Shigella dysenteriae*, *Proteus mirabilis*, and *Salmonella*; however, these drugs are not penicillinase-resistant. They are readily inactivated by beta-lactamases, thus becoming ineffective against *Staphylococcus aureus*. Examples of this group are ampicillin, amoxicillin, bacampicillin, and cyclacillin (Table 25–4). Amoxicillin is the most prescribed penicillin derivative for adults and children.

Table 25–3
The Effect of Food on Oral Penicillin Absorption

DRUG (GENERIC/BRAND)	EFFECT ON ABSORPTION
BASIC PENICILLINS	
Penicillin G (Pentids)	Decreases
Penicillin V (V-Cillin K, Veetids)	Slightly decreases
BROAD-SPECTRUM PENICILLINS	
Amoxicillin (Amoxil)	None
Amoxicillin-clavulanate (Augmentin)	None
Ampicillin (Omnipen, Polycillin)	Decreases
Bacampicillin HCl (Spectrobid)	None
PENICILLINASE-RESISTANT PENICILLINS	
Cloxacillin (Cloxapen, Tegopen)	Decreases
Dicloxacillin sodium (Dynapen, Dycill)	Decreases
Nafcillin (Nafcin, Unipen)	Decreases
Oxacillin (Prostaphlin, Bactocill)	Decreases
EXTENDED-SPECTRUM PENICILLINS	
Carbenicillin indanyl (Geocillin, Geopen)	Increases

Penicillinase-Resistant Penicillins (Antistaphylococcal Penicillins)

The penicillinase-resistant penicillins (antistaphylococcal penicillins) are used for treating penicillinase-producing *Staphylococcus aureus*. Cloxacillin and dicloxacillin are oral preparations of these antibiotics; methicillin, nafcillin, and oxacillin are intramuscular and intravenous preparations. This group of drugs is not effective against gram-negative organisms, and they are less effective than penicillin G against gram-positive organisms. Chart 25–1 compares the similarities and differences of the broad-spectrum penicillin amoxicillin and the penicillinase-resistant penicillin cloxacillin.

Extended-Spectrum Penicillins (Antipseudomonal Penicillins)

The antipseudomonal penicillins are a group of broad-spectrum penicillins. This group of drugs is effective against *Pseudomonas aeruginosa*, a gram-negative bacillus that is difficult to eradicate. These drugs are also useful against many gram-negative orga-

Table 25–4
Antibacterials: Penicillins

GENERIC (BRAND)	ROUTE AND DOSAGE	USES AND CONSIDERATIONS
BASIC PENICILLINS		
Penicillin G procaine (Crysticillin, Wy-cillin)	A: IM: 600,000–1.2 million U/d in 1–2 divided doses C: IM: 300,000–600,000 U/d in 1–2 divided doses NB: IM: 50,000 U/kg/d	For moderately serious infections. Slow IM absorption with prolonged action. The solution is milky. *Pregnancy category:* B; PB: 65%; t½: 0.5 h
Penicillin G benza-thine (Bicillin)	A: IM: 1.2 million U as a single dose C: IM: >27 kg: 900,000 U/dose IM: <27 kg: 50,000 U/kg/dose or 300,000–600,000 U/dose	Long-acting penicillin when given by injection. Used as a prophylaxis for rheumatic fever. *Pregnancy category:* B; PB: 65%; t½: 1 h
Penicillin G so-dium/potassium (Pentids, Pfizerpen)	A: PO: 200,000–500,000 U q6h IM: 500,000–5 million U/d in divided doses IV: 4–20 million U/d in divided doses, diluted in IV fluids C: PO: 25,000–90,000 U/d in divided doses IV: 50,000–100,000 U/kg/d in divided doses	Poorly absorbed orally due to gastric acidity and food. Take before or after meals. Penicillin G is available in salts (potassium [K] and sodium [Na]). With high doses, electrolyte levels should be monitored. Injectable solution is clear. *Pregnancy category:* B; PB: 60%; t½: 0.5–1 h
Penicillin V potas-sium (V-Cillin K, Veetids, Betapen VK)	A: PO: 125–500 mg q6h C: PO: 15–50 mg/kg/d in 3–4 divided doses	Acid-stable and less active than penicillin G against some bacteria. Not recommended in renal failure. Take drug after meals. *Pregnancy category:* B; PB: 80%; t½: 0.5 h
BROAD-SPECTRUM PENICILLINS		
Amoxicillin (Amoxil)	See Chart 25–1	Effective against throat, nose, ear, skin, and genitourinary infections. Eighty percent is absorbed from the GI tract. Food does not prevent absorption.
Amoxicillin-clavu-lanate (Augmentin)	See Chart 25–1	Same as amoxicillin. Clavulanic acid prevents amoxicillin breakdown. *Pregnancy category:* B; PB: 25%; t½: 1–1.5 h
Ampicillin (Polycil-lin, Omnipen)	A: PO: 250–500 mg q6h IM/ IV: 2–8 g/d in divided doses C: PO: 50–100 mg/kg/d in divided doses IM/IV: 50–200 mg/kg/d in divided doses	First broad-spectrum penicillin. Fifty percent of drug is absorbed by GI tract. Effective against gram-negative and gram-positive bacteria. Individuals with penicillin allergies may also be allergic to ampicillin. *Pregnancy category:* B; PB: 15%–28%; t½: 1–2 h
Ampicillin-sulbac-tam (Unasyn)	A: IV: 1.5–3.0 g q6h C: IV: 100–200 mg/kg/d, divided q6h	Same as ampicillin. Sulbactam inhibits beta lactamase, thus extending the spectrum. *Pregnancy category:* B; PB; 28%–38%; t½: 1–2 h
Bacampicillin HCl (Spectrobid)	A: PO: 400–800 mg q12h C: PO: 25–50 mg/kg/d in divided doses	Same as ampicillin. Ninety percent is absorbed. It is hydrolyzed to ampicillin during absorption from the GI tract. *Pregnancy category:* B; PB: 17%–20%; t½: 1 h
PENICILLINASE-RESISTANT PENICILLINS		
Cloxacillin (Tego-pen)	A: PO: 250–500 mg q6h C: PO: 50–100 mg/kg/d in 4 divided doses	For penicillin-resistant staphylococci. Take before or after meals. *Pregnancy category:* B; PB: 90%; t½: 0.5–1 h
Dicloxacillin sodium (Dynapen)	A: PO: 125–500 mg q6h C: PO: 12.5–25 mg/kg/d in 4 divided doses	For systemic infection. Used against penicillin-resistant staphylococci. Has bactericidal effect. *Pregnancy category:* B; PB: 95%; t½: 0.5–1 h
Methicillin (Staph-cillin)	A: IM: 1 g q6h IV: 1–2 g q6h diluted in NSS C: IM/IV: 100–300 mg/kg/d in 4–6 divided doses	First penicillinase-resistant penicillin. Used to treat staphylococcal infection. *Pregnancy category:* B; PB: 25%–40%; t½: 0.5–1 h

Table continued on following page

Table 25–4 *Continued*
Antibacterials: Penicillins

GENERIC (BRAND)	ROUTE AND DOSAGE	USES AND CONSIDERATIONS
Nafcillin (Nafcin, Unipen)	A: PO: 250 mg–1 g q4–6h IM: 250–500 mg q6h IV: 500 mg–1 g q4–6h C: PO: 25–100 mg/kg/d in 4 divided doses IM: 25 mg/kg b.i.d. IV: 50–200 mg/kg/d in divided doses	Highly effective against penicillin G-resistant *Staphylococcus aureus*. Not recommended for oral use due to its instability in gastric juices. *Pregnancy category:* B; PB: 90%; $t_{\frac{1}{2}}$: 0.5–1.5 h
Oxacillin sodium (Prostaphlin, Bactocil)	A: PO: 250–1 g q4–6h IM/IV: 500 mg–2 g q4h; *max:* IM/IV: 12 g C: PO/IM/IV: 50–100 mg/kg/d in divided doses; *max:* IM/IV: 300 mg/kg/d	For penicillin-resistant staphylococci. As effective as methicillin. *Pregnancy category:* B; PB: 95%; $t_{\frac{1}{2}}$: 0.5–1 h
EXTENDED-SPECTRUM PENICILLINS		
Carbenicillin indanyl (Geocillin, Geopen)	A: PO: 1.5–3.0 g/d in divided doses IM: 1–2 g q6h or 200 mg/kg/d in 4 divided doses IV: 4–6 g q4–6h C: PO: 30–50 mg/kg/d in divided doses; *max:* 2–3 g/d IM: 50–200 mg/kg/d in divided doses IV: 50–500 mg/kg/d in divided doses	The first penicillin-like drug developed to treat infections due to *Pseudomonas aeruginosa* and *Proteus* spp. It contains large amounts of sodium. Use with caution when administering to clients with hypertension or congestive heart failure. *Pregnancy category:* B; PB: 50%; $t_{\frac{1}{2}}$: 1–1.5 h
Mezlocillin sodium (Mezlin)	A: IM/IV: 3–4 g q6h or 100–300 mg/kg/d in 4 divided doses; *max:* 24 g/d C: IM/IV: 50 mg/kg q4h	For serious infections, especially due to *Pseudomonas aeruginosa*. It can be given in combination with aminoglycosides and cephalosporins to obtain synergistic effect. *Pregnancy category:* B; PB: 30%–40%; $t_{\frac{1}{2}}$: 1 h
Piperacillin sodium (Pipracil)	A: IM/IV: 2–4 g q6h or 100–300 mg/kg/d in divided doses; *max:* 24 g/d C: <12 y: IM/IV: 100–300 mg/kg/d in 4–6 divided doses	For serious infections. Can be given prior to and following surgery. Primarily used for gram-negative organisms. Treatment for septicemia; bone, joint, respiratory, and urinary tract infections. *Pregnancy category:* B; PB: 16%–22%; $t_{\frac{1}{2}}$: 0.6–1.5 h
Piperacillin-tazobactam (Zosyn)	A: IV: 3.375 g, q6h over 30 min, 7–10 d. Reduce for renal insufficiency	To treat severe appendicitis, skin infections, pneumonia, beta-lactamase–producing bacteria. Tazobactam is a beta-lactamase inhibitor. *Pregnancy category:* B; PB: UK; $t_{\frac{1}{2}}$: 0.7–1.2 h
Ticarcillin disodium (Ticar)	A: IM/IV: 1–2 g q6h C: IM/IV: 50–200 mg/kg/d in 4 divided doses *Systemic infections:* Dose is increased	Effective against gram-positive and gram-negative bacilli. Used to treat respiratory, urinary, reproductive, skin, and soft tissue infections. It can be given in combination with aminoglycosides for synergistic effect. *Pregnancy category:* C; PB: 45%–65%; t½: 1–1.5 h
Ticarcillin-clavulanate (Timentin)	A: IV: 3.1 g q6h C: >12 y: IV: 200–300 mg/kg/d in 4–6 divided doses	Clavulanic acid protects ticarcillin from degradation by beta-lactamase enzymes. Effective for treating lower respiratory tract, urinary tract, skin, bone, and joint infections, and also septicemia. *Pregnancy category:* B; PB: 45–65%; $t_{\frac{1}{2}}$: 1.1–1.5 h

KEY: A: *adult;* C: *child;* PO: *by mouth;* IM: *intramuscular;* IV: *intravenous;* NB: *newborn;* NSS: *normal saline solution;* PB: *protein-binding;* $t_{\frac{1}{2}}$: *half-life;* >: *greater than;* <: *less than.*

Chart 25-1. Penicillin Derivations: Amoxicillin and Cloxacillin

PENICILLINS

Drug Name

Broad-Spectrum Penicillins
Amoxicillin trihydrate (A), (Amoxil),
🍁 Apo-Amoxi
Amoxicillin-clavulanate (Augmentin),
🍁 Clavulin
Pregnancy Category: B
Penicillinase-Resistant Penicillin
Cloxacillin sodium (C) (Tegopen),
🍁 Apo-Cloxi, Novocloxin
Pregnancy Category: B

Contraindications

(A&C) Allergic to penicillin
(A) Severe renal disorder
Caution: (A&C)
Hypersensitivity to cephalosporins

Dosage

(A) A: PO: 250–500 mg, q8h
    C: PO: 20–40 mg/kg/d; in 3 divided doses

(C) A: PO: 250–500 mg, q6h
    C: PO: 12.5–25 mg/kg/d in 4 divided doses

Drug-Lab-Food Interactions

(A&C) **Drug:** *Increase* effect with aspirin, probenecid; *decrease* effect with tetracycline, erythromycin
Lab: *Increase* serum AST, ALT

Pharmacokinetics

Absorption: PO:
(A) >80% in intestine
(C) 40%–60% GI tract
Distribution: PB:
(A) 20%
(C) 90%–95%
Metabolism: $t\frac{1}{2}$:
(A) 1–1.5 h
(C) 0.5–1 h
Excretion:
(A) 70% in urine; clavulanate: 30%–40% in urine
(C) Excreted in bile and urine

Pharmacodynamics

(A)
PO: Onset: 0.5 h
    Peak: 1–2 h
    Duration: 6–8 h
(C)
PO: Onset: 0.5 h
    Peak: 1–2 h
    Duration: 6 h

Therapeutic Effects/Uses

(A) To treat respiratory tract infection, urinary tract infection, otitis media, sinusitis. (C) To treat *Staphylococcus aureus* infection.

Mode of Action: (A&C) Inhibition of the enzyme in cell wall synthesis. Bactericidal effect.

Side Effects

(A&C) Nausea, vomiting, diarrhea, rash
(A) Edema, stomatitis
(C) Lethargy, twitching, depression, increased bleeding time

Adverse Reaction

(A&C) Superinfections (vaginitis)
Life-threatening:
(A&C) Blood dyscrasias, hemolytic anemia, bone marrow depression
(A) Respiratory distress
(C) Agranulocytosis

Assessment and Planning / **Interventions** / **Evaluation** / **NURSING PROCESS**

KEY: A: adult; C: child; PO: by mouth; PB: protein-binding; $t\frac{1}{2}$: half-life; 🍁: Canadian drug names; AST: aspartate aminotransferase; ALT: alanine aminotransferase.

NURSING PROCESS
ANTIBACTERIALS: PENICILLINS

Assessment

- Assess for allergy to penicillin or cephalosporins. The client who is hypersensitive to amoxicillin should not take any type of penicillin products. Severe allergic reaction could occur. A small percentage of clients who are allergic to penicillin could also be allergic to a cephalosporin product.
- Check laboratory results, especially liver enzymes. Report elevated ALP, ALT, or AST.
- Assess urine output. If the amount is inadequate (<30 mL/h or <600 mL/d), drug or drug dosage may need to be changed.

Potential Nursing Diagnoses

- Risk for infection
- Risk for impaired tissue integrity
- Noncompliance with drug regimen

Planning

- Client's infection will be controlled and later eliminated.

Nursing Interventions

- Send a sample of material from the infectious area to the laboratory for culture to determine antibiotic susceptibility (also known as C & S) before antibiotic therapy is started.
- Check for signs and symptoms of superinfection, especially for clients taking high doses of the antibiotic for a prolonged time. Signs and symptoms include stomatitis (mouth ulcers), genital discharge (vaginitis), and anal or genital itching.
- Check the client for allergic reaction to the penicillin product, especially after the first and second doses. This may be a mild reaction, such as a rash, or a severe reaction, such as respiratory distress or anaphylaxis.
- Have epinephrine available to counteract a severe allergic reaction.

Nursing Process continued on following page

nisms such as *Proteus* spp., *Serratia* spp., *Klebsiella pneumoniae*, *Enterobacter* spp., and *Acinetobacter* spp. The antipseudomonal penicillins are not penicillinase-resistant. Their pharmacologic action is similar to that of aminoglycosides, but they are less toxic than the aminoglycosides.

Beta-Lactamase Inhibitors

When a broad-spectrum antibiotic such as amoxicillin is combined with a beta-lactamase (enzyme) inhibitor, clavulanic acid, this antibiotic amoxicillin-clavulanic acid (Augmentin) inhibits the bacterial beta-lactamases, thus making the antibiotic effective and extending its antimicrobial effect. There are three beta-lactamase inhibitors: clavulanic acid, sulbactam, and tazobactam. These inhibitors are not given alone but are combined with a penicillinase-sensitive penicillin such as amoxicillin, ampicillin, piperacillin, and ticar-

cillin. The combined drugs currently marketed include the following:

- *Oral use:* amoxicillin-clavulanic acid (Augmentin)
- *Parenteral use:* ampicillin-sulbactam (Unasyn), piperacillin-tazobactam (Zosyn), and ticarcillin-clavulanic acid (Timentin)

Pharmacokinetics

Amoxicillin is well absorbed from the GI tract, whereas cloxacillin is only partially absorbed. Protein-binding power differs between the two drugs—amoxicillin is 25% protein-bound and cloxacillin is highly protein-bound (>90%). Drug toxicity may result when other highly protein-bound drugs are used with cloxacillin. Both of these drugs have short half-lives. Seventy percent of amoxicillin is excreted in the urine; cloxacillin is excreted in the bile and urine.

- Check the client for bleeding if high doses of penicillin are being given; a decrease in platelet aggregation (clotting) may result.
- Monitor body temperature and infectious area.
- Dilute the antibiotic for IV use in an appropriate amount of solution as indicated in the drug circular.

Client Teaching

General

- Instruct the client to take all of the prescribed penicillin product such as amoxicillin until the bottle is empty. If only a portion of the penicillin is taken, drug resistance to that antibacterial agent may develop in the future.
- Advise the client who is allergic to penicillin to wear a medical alert (Medic-Alert) bracelet or necklace and carry a card that indicates the allergy. The client should notify the health care provider during history taking of his or her allergy to penicillin.
- Keep drugs out of reach of small children. Request child safety cap bottle.
- Inform the client to report any side effects or adverse reaction that may occur while taking the drug.
- Encourage the client to increase fluid intake; it will aid in decreasing the body temperature and in excreting the drug.
- Instruct the client or child's parent that chewable tablets must be chewed or crushed before swallowing.

Diet

- Advise the client to take medication with food if gastric irritation occurs and to take oral penicillin 1 h before or 2 h after meals to avoid delay in drug absorption.

Cultural Considerations

- Recognize that clients and family members from various cultural backgrounds have various alternatives for alleviating infections. Accept their alternative methods if they are not harmful to the client. Explain the purpose of the antibiotic.
- If the client does not speak English, request a translator to obtain a history of symptoms related to the infection and any allergies to antibiotics.

Evaluation

- Evaluate the effectiveness of the antibacterial agent by determining whether the infection has ceased and whether any side effects, including superinfection, have occurred.

Pharmacodynamics

Both amoxicillin and cloxacillin are penicillin derivatives and are bactericidal. These drugs interfere with bacterial cell wall synthesis, causing cell lysis. Amoxicillin may be produced with or without clavulanic acid, an agent that prevents the breakdown of amoxicillin by decreasing resistance to the antibacterial drug. The addition of clavulanic acid intensifies the effect of amoxicillin. The amoxicillin-clavulanic acid preparation (Augmentin) and amoxicillin trihydrate (Amoxil) have similar pharmacokinetics and pharmacodynamics, as well as similar side effects and adverse reactions.

When aspirin and probenecid are taken with amoxicillin or cloxacillin, the serum antibacterial levels may be increased. The effects of amoxicillin and cloxacillin are decreased when taken with erythromycin and tetracycline. The onset of action, serum peak concentration time, and duration of action for amoxicillin and cloxacillin are very similar.

Side Effects and Adverse Reactions

Common adverse reactions to penicillin administration are hypersensitivity and **superinfection** (occurrence of a secondary infection when the flora of the body is disturbed) (see Table 25–2). Nausea, vomiting, and diarrhea are common GI disturbances. Rash is an indicator of a mild to moderate allergic reaction. Severe allergic reaction leads to anaphylactic shock. Allergic effects occur in 5% to 10% of persons receiving penicillin compounds; therefore, close monitoring during the first dose and subsequent doses of penicillin is essential.

CEPHALOSPORINS

In 1948, a fungus called *Cephalosporium acremonium* was discovered from seawater at a sewer outlet off the coast of Sardinia. This fungus was found to be active against gram-positive and gram-negative bacteria and resistant to beta-lactamase (enzyme that acts against beta-lactam structure of penicillin). In the early 1960s, cephalosporins were used with clinical effectiveness. For the cephalosporins to be effective against numerous organisms, their molecules were chemically altered and semisynthetic cephalosporins were produced. Like penicillin, the cephalosporins have a beta-lactam structure and act by inhibiting the bacterial enzyme that is necessary for cell wall synthesis. Lysis to the cell occurs, and the bacterial cell dies.

First-, Second-, Third- and Fourth-Generation Cephalosporins

Cephalosporins are a major antibiotic group used in hospitals and in health care offices. These drugs are bactericidal with action similar to penicillin. For antibacterial activity, the beta-lactam ring of cephalosporins is necessary.

Four groups of cephalosporins have been developed, identified as *generations*. Each generation is effective against a broader spectrum of bacteria (Table 25–5).

Not all cephalosporins are affected by the beta-lactamases. The first-generation cephalosporins are destroyed by beta-lactamases, but not all of the second generation is affected by beta-lactamases. Third-generation cephalosporins are resistant to beta-lactamases. A new generation of cephalosporins, the fourth generation, is more effective in treating gram-positive beta-lactamase bacteria than those in the third generation. The drug in this generation is cefepime (Maxipime).

Approximately 10% of persons allergic to penicillin are also allergic to cephalosporins because both groups of antibacterials have similar molecular structures. If a client is allergic to penicillin and is taking a cephalosporin, the nurse should watch for a possible allergic reaction to the cephalosporin, even though the likelihood of a reaction is small.

Only a few cephalosporins are administered orally. These include cephalexin (Keflex), cefadroxil (Duricef), cephradine (Velosef), cefaclor (Ceclor), cefuroxime acetoxyethyl ester (Ceftin), cefuroxime sodium (Zinacef), cefdinir (Omnicef), ceftibuten (Cedox), and cefixime (Suprax). The rest of the cephalosporins are administered intramuscularly and intravenously. Chart 25–2 compares the similarities of and differences between a first-generation cephalosporin, cefazolin sodium (Ancef, Kefzol), and a second-generation cephalosporin, cefaclor (Ceclor).

Pharmacokinetics

Cefazolin is administered intramuscularly and intravenously, and cefaclor is given orally. The protein-

Table 25–5
Activity of the Four Generations of Cephalosporins

GENERATION	ACTIVITY
First	Effective against gram-positive bacteria, such as streptococci and most staphylococci. Effective against most gram-negative bacteria, such as *Escherichia coli* and species of *Klebsiella, Proteus, Salmonella,* and *Shigella.*
Second	Same effectiveness as the first generation. These antibiotics possess a broader spectrum against other gram-negative bacteria, such as *Haemophilus influenzae, Neisseria gonorrhoeae, Neisseria meningitidis, Enterobacter* spp., and several anaerobic organisms.
Third	Same effectiveness as the first and second generations. Also effective against gram-negative bacteria, such as *Pseudomonas aeruginosa, Serratia* spp., and *Acinetobacter* spp. Less effective against gram-positive bacteria.
Fourth	Similar to the third generations. Resistant to most beta-lactamase bacteria. Has a broader gram-positive coverage than the third generations. Effective against *E. coli, Klebsiella, Proteus,* streptococci, certain staphylococci, and *P. aeruginosa.*

binding power of cefazolin is greater than that of cefaclor. The half-life of each drug is short, and the drugs are excreted 60% to 80% unchanged in the urine.

Pharmacodynamics

Cefazolin and cefaclor inhibit bacterial cell wall synthesis and produce a bactericidal action. For intramuscular and intravenous use of cefazolin, the onset of action is almost immediate, and the peak concentration time is 5 to 15 minutes for intravenous use. The peak concentration time for an oral dose of cefaclor is 30 to 60 minutes.

When probenecid is administered with either of these drugs, the urine excretion of cefazolin or cefaclor is decreased, which increases the action of the drug. The effects of cefazolin and cefaclor can be decreased if the drug is given with tetracyclines or erythromycin. These drugs can cause false-positive

Chart 25-2. Cephalosporins

CEPHALOSORINS

Assessment and Planning — NURSING PROCESS

Drug Name

First-Generation Cephalosporin
Cefazolin (A) (Ancef, Kefzol)
Pregnancy Category: B

Second-Generation Cephalosporin
Cefaclor (C) (Ceclor)
Pregnancy Category: B

Dosage

(A)
A: IM/IV: 250 mg–2 g, q6–8h; *max:* 12 g/d
C: IM/IV: 25–100 mg/kg/d in 3 divided doses;
max: 4 g/d
(C)
A: PO: 250–500 mg, q8h; *max:* 4 g/d
C: PO: 20–40 mg/kg/d in 3 divided doses; *max:*
1 g/d

Contraindications

(A&C) Hypersensitivity to cephalosporins
Caution: (A&C): Hypersensitivity to penicillins;
renal disease, lactation

Drug-Lab-Food Interactions

(A&C) Drug: *Increase* effect with probenecid; *increase* toxicity with loop diuretics, aminoglycosides, colisitin, vancomycin; *decrease* effect with tetracyclines, erythromycin
Lab: May *increase* BUN, serum creatinine, AST, ALT, ALP, LDH, bilirubin

Pharmacokinetics

Absorption:
(A) IM, IV
(C) PO: well absorbed
Distribution: PB:
(A) 75%–85%
(C) 25%
Metabolism: $t\frac{1}{2}$:
(A) 1.5–2.5 h
(C) 0.5–1 h
Excretion:
(A) 70% excreted unchanged in urine
(C) 60%–80% excreted unchanged in urine

Pharmacodynamics

(A)
IM: Onset: rapid
    Peak: 0.5–2 h
    Duration: UK
IV: Onset: immediate
    Peak: 5–15 min
    Duration: UK
(C)
PO: Onset: rapid
    Peak: 0.5–1 h
    Duration: UK

Interventions — NURSING PROCESS

Therapeutic Effects/Uses

(A&C) To treat respiratory, urinary, and skin infections.
(A) To treat bone and joint infection, genital infections, and endocarditis.
(C) To treat ear infection, ampicillin-resistant strains, and certain gram-negative organisms, *E. coli*,
Proteus, H. influenzae, and gram-positive strains, *Streptococcus pneumoniae, S. pyogenes,* and *S. aureus.*

Mode of Action: Inhibition of cell wall synthesis, causing cell death; bactericidal effect.

Side Effects

(A&C) Anorexia, nausea, vomiting, diarrhea,
rash
(A) Abdominal cramps, fever
(C) Pruritus, headaches, vertigo, weakness

Adverse Reactions

(A&C) Superinfections, urticaria
Life-threatening:
(A) Seizures (high doses), anaphylaxis
(C) Renal failure

Evaluation — NURSING PROCESS

KEY: A: adult; C: child; PO: by mouth; IM: intramuscular; IV: intravenous; PB: protein-binding; $t\frac{1}{2}$: half-life; UK: unknown; BUN: blood urea nitrogen; AST: aspartate aminotransferase; ALT: alanine aminotransferase; ALP: alkaline phosphatase; LDH: lactic dehydrogenase.

Table 25–6
Antibacterials: Cephalosporins

GENERIC (BRAND)	ROUTE AND DOSAGE	USES AND CONSIDERATIONS
FIRST GENERATION		
Cefadroxil (Duricef)	A: PO: 500 mg–2 g/d in 1–2 divided doses C: PO: 30 mg/kg/d in 2 divided doses	To treat urinary tract infections, beta-hemolytic streptococcal infections, and staphylococcal skin infection. It is well absorbed by the gastrointestinal tract and is not affected by food. *Pregnancy category:* B; PB: 20%; t½: 1–2 h
Cefazolin sodium (Ancef, Kefzol)	A: IM/IV: 250 mg–1 g q6–8h; *max:* 12 g/d C: IM/IV: 25–100 mg/kg/d in 3 divided doses; *max:* 6 g/d	Similar to cephalothin but more effective against *Escherichia coli* and *Klebsiella*. *Pregnancy category:* B; PB: 75%–85%; t½: 1.5–2.5 h
Cephalexin (Keflex)	*Infection:* A: PO: 250–500 mg q6h C: PO: 25–50 mg/kg/d in 3–4 divided doses *Otitis media:* C: PO: 25–100 mg/kg/d in 4 divided doses	First acid-stable cephalosporin sufficiently absorbed from the GI tract. Useful for treating urinary tract infections. *Pregnancy category:* B; PB: 10%–15%; t½: 0.5–1.2 h
Cephalothin (Keflin)	A: IM/IV: 500 mg–1 g q4–6h C: IM/IV: 20–40 mg/kg q6h	To treat respiratory, GI, genitourinary, bone, joint, skin, soft tissue infections; septicemia; endocarditis; meningitis. Cephalothin is the first cephalosporin used clinically. It is usually given IV. *Pregnancy category:* B; PB: 65%–80%; t½: 0.5–1 h
Cephapirin sodium (Cefadyl)	A: IM/IV: 500 mg–1 g q4–6h C: IM/IV: 40–80 mg/kg/d in 4 divided doses	Treatment is the same as for cephalothin. *Pregnancy category:* B; PB: 40%–50%; t½: 0.5–1 h
Cephradine (Velosef)	A: PO: 250–500 mg q6h or 500 mg–1 g q12h IM/IV: 500 mg–1 g q6–12h C: PO: 25–50 mg/kg/d in 4 divided doses IM/IV: 50–100 mg/kg/d in 4 divided doses	Treatment is the same as for cephalothin. The oral drug is similar to cephalexin. Well absorbed from GI tract. *Pregnancy category:* B; PB: 20%; t½: 1–2 h
SECOND GENERATION		
Cefaclor (Ceclor)	See Chart 25–2	Used to treat respiratory infections and otitis media, especially in children. Also effective for urinary tract and skin infections. Well absorbed by GI tract. *Pregnancy category:* B; PB: 25%; t½: 0.5–1 h
Cefamandole (Mandol)	A: IM/IV: 500 mg–1 g q4–8h	Used to treat infections of the bone, joint, and respiratory tract, as well as septicemia. *Pregnancy category:* B; PB: 60%–75%; t½: 1 h
Cefmetazole sodium (Zefazone)	A: IV: 2 g q6–12h	For treatment of lower respiratory and urinary tract infections. Also used for preoperative prophylaxis for surgery. *Pregnancy category:* B; PB: 68%; t½: 1.5–3 h
Cefonicid sodium (Monocid)	A: IM/IV: 500 mg–2 g/d single dose or b.i.d.	Similar to cefamandole. Also used for surgical prophylaxis. *Pregnancy category:* B; PB: 98%; t½: 4.5 h
Ceforanide (Precef)	A: IM/IV: 500 mg–1 g q12h C: IM/IV: 20–40 mg/kg/d in 2 divided doses	For treatment of respiratory, urinary, skin, bone, and joint infections. Also used to treat septicemia, endocarditis, cardiovascular surgery, and prosthetic arthroplasty. *Pregnancy category:* B; PB: 80%; t½: 3 h
Cefotetan (Cefotan)	A: IM/IV: 500 mg–2g q12h	Effective against some gram-negative organisms, except *Pseudomonas aeruginosa*. *Pregnancy category:* B; PB: 85%; t½: 3–5 h

Table continued on following page

Table 25–6 *Continued*
Antibacterials: Cephalosporins

GENERIC (BRAND)	ROUTE AND DOSAGE	USES AND CONSIDERATIONS
Cefoxitin sodium (Mefoxin)	A: IM/IV: 1–2 g q6–8h; *max:* 12 g/d C: IM/IV: 80–160 mg/kg/d in divided doses	Used to treat severe infections and septicemia. *Pregnancy category:* B; PB: 70%; t½: 45 min–1 h
Cefprozil monohydrate (Cefzil)	A: PO: 250–500 mg daily or q12h C: PO: 15 mg/kg q12h × 10 d	Effective against gram-positive bacilli including *Staphylococcus aureus.* With impaired renal function, dose is usually decreased by 50%. *Pregnancy category:* B; PB: 99%; t½: 1–2 h
Cefuroxime (Ceftin, Zinacef)	A: PO: 250–500 mg q12h IM/IV: 750 mg–1.5 g q8h C: PO: 125–250 mg q12h IM/IV: 50–100 mg/kg/d in divided doses	Similar to cefamandole. Effective in treating meningitis and septicemia and for cardiothoracic procedures and surgical prophylaxis. *Pregnancy category:* B; PB: 50%; t½: 1.5–2 h
Loracarbef (Lorabid)	A: PO: 200 mg qd × 7 d C: PO: 15 mg/kg q12h × 7 d	A carbacephen. For treatment of respiratory, urinary, and skin infections. Effective against gram-positive bacteria. If creatinine clearance is <50 mL/min, drug dose is reduced by 50%. *Pregnancy category:* B; PB: UK; t½: 1 h

THIRD GENERATION

GENERIC (BRAND)	ROUTE AND DOSAGE	USES AND CONSIDERATIONS
Cefixime (Suprax)	A: PO: 400 mg/d in 1–2 divided doses C: <12 y: PO: 8 mg/kg/d in 1–2 divided doses	Effective against most gram-positive and gram-negative bacilli: minimal effect against staphylococci and ineffective against *P. aeruginosa.* Food does not affect drug dose. *Pregnancy category:* B; PB: 65%; t½: 2.5–4 h
Cefoperazone (Cefobid)	A: IM/IV: 2–4 g/d in 2 divided doses C: IV: 25–100 mg/kg q12h	To treat respiratory, urinary tract, and female genital tract infections. Most effective against pseudomonas. *Pregnancy category:* B; PB: 70%–80%; t½: 2.5 h
Cefotaxime (Claforan)	A: IM/IV: 1–2 g q8–12h C: IM/IV: 50–200 mg/kg/d in 4–6 divided doses *Life-threatening infection:* 2 g q4h	First of the third generation. Effective against *P. aeruginosa.* Also used in treating gram-negative meningitis. *Pregnancy category:* B; PB: 30%–40%; t½: 1–1.5 h
Cefpodoxime (Proxetil, Vantin)	A: PO: 100–400 mg q12h × 1–2 wk C 6 mo–12 y: PO: 10 mg/kg/d in 2 divided doses	To treat respiratory and urinary tract infection, and otitis media. Food enhances drug absorption. *Pregnancy category:* B; PB: 20%–40%; t½: 2–3 h
Ceftazidime (Fortaz, Tazicef)	A: IM/IV: 500 mg–2 g q8–12h C: IV: 50 mg/kg q8h; *max:* 6 g/d	Most effective against *Pseudomonas* spp. *Pregnancy category:* B; PB: 10%–17%; t½: 1–2 h
Ceftriaxone (Rocephin)	A: IM/IV: 500 mg–2 g in single dose or q12h C: IM/IV: 50–75 mg/kg/d in 2 divided doses	Similar to ceftizoxime and cefotaxime. It has a very long half-life, so is given once or twice a day. It is used against neisseria and gonococcal infections and in the treatment of Lyme disease. *Pregnancy category:* B; PB: 85%–95%; t½: 8 h
Ceftizoxime sodium (Cefizox)	A: IM/IV: 500 mg–2 g q8–12h C: IV: 50 mg/kg q6–8h; *max:* 200 mg/kg/d	For treatment of respiratory, urinary tract, skin, bone, and joint infections. For surgical prophylaxis. *Pregnancy category:* B; PB: 30%–60%; t½: 2 h
Cefdinir (Omnicef)	A: PO: 300 mg q12h or 600 mg/d C: PO: 7 mg/kg q12h or 14 mg/kg/d Preferred: q12h dosing due to short half-life	New third-generation cephalosporin. To treat otitis media, acute sinusitis, chronic bronchitis, pharyngitis, pneumonia, and skin infections. Active for *Haemophilus influenzae, Neisseria gonorrhoeae,* and many strains of enteric gram-negative bacilli. *Not* active for *P. aeruginosa,* enterococcus, *Legionella, Chlamydia. Pregnancy category:* UK; PB: UK; t½: 1.7 h

Table continued on following page

Table 25–6 *Continued*
Antibacterials: Cephalosporins

GENERIC (BRAND)	ROUTE AND DOSAGE	USES AND CONSIDERATIONS
Ceftibuten (Cedax)	A: PO: 400 mg/d	Treatment for chronic bronchitis, pharyngitis, and tonsillitis. Active against gram-positive and gram-negative bacteria, *H. influenzae,* and *Streptococcus penumoniae* and *Streptococcus pyogenes.* Poor activity against staphylococci and pneumococci. *Pregnancy category:* B; PB: UK; $t\frac{1}{2}$: 1.5–3 h
Moxalactam disodium (Moxam)	A: IM, IV; 2–6 g/d in 2–3 divided doses; *max:* 4 g q8h	For lower respiratory, urinary tract, bone, and joint infection. Also for septicemia and meningitis. Less active against gram-positive cocci, *S. aureus,* and streptococci. Active against *E. coli, Klebsiella pneumoniae,* and *Serratia.* Variable activity for *P. aeruginosa.* Can be used with an aminoglycoside. *Pregnancy category:* C; PB: UK; $t\frac{1}{2}$: 2–3.5 h
Meropenem (Merrem)	A: IV: 1–2 g q8h C >3 mo: 20–40 mg/kg q8h	A carbapenem antibiotic with many characteristics similar to cephalosporins. It is highly resistant to most beta-lactamase bacteria. It is effective for complicated appendicitis, peritonitis, meningitis, and skin and soft tissue infections. *Pregnancy category:* B; PB: UK; $t\frac{1}{2}$: 0.8–1h
FOURTH GENERATION		
Cefepime (Maxipime)	A: IM: IV: 0.5–1g q12h	Similar to third-generation cephalosporins. Resistant to most beta-lactamase bacteria. Effective against pneumonia, *E. coli, Klebsiella, Proteus,* streptococci, certain staphylococci, and *P. aeruginosa.* It has a broader gram-positive coverage than the third-generation cephalosporins. *Pregnancy category:* B; PB: UK; $t\frac{1}{2}$: 2 h

KEY: A: adult; C: child; PO: by mouth; IM: intramuscularly; IV: intravenously; PB: protein-binding; $t\frac{1}{2}$: half-life; <: less than; >; more than.

laboratory results for proteinuria and glucosuria, especially when they are taken in large doses.

Table 25–6 lists the drugs in their designated generation, dosages, and considerations.

Side Effects and Adverse Reactions

The side effects and adverse reactions to cephalosporins include GI disturbances (nausea, vomiting, and diarrhea), alteration in blood clotting time (increased bleeding) with administration of large doses, and **nephrotoxicity** (toxicity to the kidney) in individuals with a preexisting renal disorder.

Drug Interactions

Drug interactions can occur with certain cephalosporins and ingestion of alcohol. For example, consuming alcohol while taking cefamandole, cefoperazone, or moxalactam may cause flushing, dizziness, headache, nausea and vomiting, and muscular cramps. Uricosuric drugs taken concurrently can decrease the excretion of cephalosporins, greatly increasing serum levels.

ANTIBACTERIALS: CEPHALOSPORINS

Assessment

- Assess for allergy to cephalosporins. If allergic to one type or class of cephalosporin, the client should not receive any other type of cephalosporin.
- Assess vital signs (VS) and urine output. Report abnormal findings, which may include an elevated temperature or a decrease in urine output.
- Check laboratory results, especially those that indicate renal and liver function, such as BUN, serum creatinine, AST, ALT, ALP, and bilirubin. Report abnormal findings. Use these laboratory results for baseline values.

Potential Drug Diagnoses

- Risk for infection
- Noncompliance with drug regimen

Planning

- Client's infection will be controlled and later eliminated.

Nursing Interventions

- Culture the infectious area before cephalosporin therapy is started. The organism causing the infection can be determined by culture, and the antibiotics sensitive to the organism are determined by C & S. (Antibiotic therapy may be started before culture result is reported. The antibiotic may need to be changed after C & S test results are received.)
- Check for signs and symptoms of a superinfection, especially if the client is taking high doses of a cephalosporin product for a prolonged period of time. Superinfection is usually caused by the fungal organism *Candida* in the mouth (mouth ulcers) or in the genital area, such as the vagina (vaginitis).
- Refrigerate oral suspensions. For IV cephalosporins, dilute in an appropriate amount of IV fluids (50–100 mL) according to the drug circular.
- Administer IV cephalosporins over 30–45 min 2–4 times a day.
- Monitor VS, urine output, and laboratory results. Report abnormal findings.

Client Teaching

General
- Keep drugs out of reach of small children. Request child safety cap bottle.
- Instruct the client to report signs of superinfection, such as mouth ulcers or discharge from the anal or genital area.
- Advise the client to ingest buttermilk or yogurt to prevent superinfection of the intestinal flora with long-term use of a cephalosporin.
- Instruct the diabetic client not to use Clinitest tablets for urine glucose testing because false test results may occur. Tes-Tape or Clinistix may be used for urine testing, or Chemstrip bG may be used for blood glucose testing.
- Instruct the client to take the complete course of medication even when symptoms of infection have ceased.

Diet
- Advise the client to take medication with food if gastric irritation occurs.

Side Effects
- Instruct the client to report any side effects from use of oral cephalosporin drug; they may include anorexia, nausea, vomiting, headache, dizziness, itching, and rash.

Evaluation

- Evaluate the effectiveness of the cephalosporin by determining if the infection has ceased and no side effects, including superinfection, have occurred.

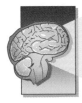

Critical Thinking in Action

S. A., who is 6 years old, has otitis media. The health care provider ordered amoxicillin 250 mg q8h. The nurse asks S. A.'s mother if S. A. is allergic to any drugs, and her mother says she is allergic to penicillin.

1. What are the similarities and differences of penicillin and amoxicillin? Explain.
2. What nursing action should the nurse take? Why?

The health care provider changed the amoxicillin order to cefaclor (Ceclor) 250 mg q8h. The therapeutic dosage for children is 20–40 mg/kg/d in three divided doses. S. A. weighs 40 lb.

3. What are the similarities and differences of amoxicillin and cefaclor? Explain.
4. Is the prescribed cefaclor dosage for S. A. within safe parameters? Explain.
5. Explain the significance of the nurse asking about allergies to antibiotics such as penicillin. What is the relationship of penicillin and cefaclor in regard to allergies?
6. What should the nurse include in client teaching for S. A. and her mother?

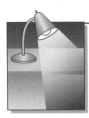

Study Questions

1. What is the action of a bacteriostatic drug? Of a bactericidal drug?
2. What is a nosocomial infection?
3. What is meant by cross-resistance? Give an example of how it can occur.
4. When do superinfections occur? What is the nurse's role?
5. Your client is taking ampicillin. What type/category is ampicillin? Explain the drug effect against pathogens.
6. What is the severe adverse reaction associated with penicillin? What is an early symptom of such an adverse reaction? What emergency intervention is required?
7. Your client is taking cephalexin (Keflex) for a urinary tract infection. What generation of cephalosporin is cephalexin? What is its route of administration?
8. What antibiotics are used as penicillin substitutes?

Antibacterials: Macrolides, Tetracyclines, Aminoglycosides, Fluoroquinolones

26

Outline

Objectives

- Describe the pharmacokinetics and pharmacodynamics of erythromycin.
- Differentiate between bacteriostatic and bactericidal drugs. Give examples of each.
- Explain the nursing process for tetracyclines including the adverse reactions.
- Describe the nurse's role in detecting ototoxicity and nephrotoxicity associated with the administration of aminoglycosides.
- Discuss the reasons for ordering serum aminoglycosides for peak and trough concentration levels.
- Explain the mechanism of action of fluoroquinolones (quinolones).
- Describe the nursing interventions, including client teaching, for each of the drug categories.

Terms

bactericidal

bacteriostatic

hepatotoxicity

nephrotoxicity

ototoxicity

pathogen

photosensitivity

superinfection

INTRODUCTION

The groups of antibacterials discussed in this chapter include macrolides (erythromycin, clarithromycin, azithromycin, dirithromycin), lincosamides, vancomycin, tetracyclines, aminoglycosides, and fluoroquinolones (quinolones). The macrolides, lincosamides, and tetracyclines are primarily bacteriostatic drugs and may be bactericidal, depending on drug dose or pathogen. Vancomycin, aminoglycosides, and fluoroquinolones are **bactericidal** drugs.

MACROLIDES, LINCOSAMIDES, AND VANCOMYCIN

These three groups of drugs are discussed together, because although they differ in structure, they have similar spectrums of antibiotic effectiveness to penicillin. Drugs from these groups are used as penicillin substitutes, especially in individuals who are allergic to penicillin. Erythromycin is the drug frequently prescribed if the client has a hypersensitivity to penicillin.

Macrolides: Erythromycin

Macrolides are broad-spectrum antibiotics, so named to reflect their large size. Erythromycin, derived from the fungus-like bacterium *Streptomyces erythraeus*, was first introduced as a macrolide in the early 1950s. Erythromycin inhibits protein synthesis. At low to moderate drug doses, it has a **bacteriostatic** effect, and with high drug doses, the effect is bactericidal. Erythromycin can be administered orally or intravenously. Because gastric acid destroys the drug, various salts of erythromycin (e.g., ethylsuccinate, stearate, and estolate) are used to decrease dissolution (breakdown in small particles) in the stomach and to allow absorption in the intestine. For intravenous use, the compounds erythromycin lactobionate and erythromycin gluceptate are used to increase drug absorption. Table 26–1 lists the erythromycins.

Erythromycin is active against most gram-positive bacteria, except *Staphylococcus aureus,* and it is moderately active against some gram-negative bacteria. Resistant organisms may emerge during treatment. It is often prescribed as a penicillin substitute. It is a drug of choice for mycoplasmal pneumonia and legionnaires' disease. Chart 26–1 details the pharmacologic behavior of erythromycin-based antibiotics.

PHARMACOKINETICS

Erythromycin oral preparations are well absorbed from the gastrointestinal (GI) tract. The drug is available intravenously, but should be diluted in 100 mL of saline or 5% dextrose in water solution to prevent phlebitis or burning sensations at the injection site. It has a short half-life and a moderate protein-binding effect. The drug is excreted in bile, feces, and to some degree, in the urine. Because a small amount is excreted in the urine, renal insufficiency is not a contraindication for erythromycin use.

PHARMACODYNAMICS

Erythromycin suppresses bacterial protein synthesis. The onset of action of the oral preparation is 1 h, peak concentration time is 4 h, and the duration of action is 6 h.

SIDE EFFECTS AND ADVERSE REACTIONS

Side effects and adverse reactions to erythromycin include GI disturbances such as nausea, vomiting, diarrhea, and abdominal cramping. Allergic reactions to erythromycin are rare. **Hepatotoxicity** (liver toxicity) can occur if the drug is taken in high doses with other hepatotoxic drugs, such as acetaminophen (high doses), phenothiazines, and sulfonamides. Erythromycin estolate (Ilosone) appears to have more toxic effects on the liver than the other erythromycins. Liver damage is usually reversible when the drug is discontinued. Erythromycin should not be taken with clindamycin or lincomycin because they compete for receptor sites.

DRUG INTERACTIONS

Erythromycin can increase the serum levels of theophylline (bronchodilator), carbamazepine (anticonvulsant), and warfarin (anticoagulant). If these drugs are given with erythromycin, their drug serum levels should be closely monitored. Erythromycin should not be used with other macrolides to avoid severe toxic effects.

EXTENDED MACROLIDE GROUP

New derivatives of erythromycin have been effective in the treatment of numerous organisms. Like erythromycin, they inhibit protein synthesis. Many of these macrolides have a longer half-life and are administered once a day. The first extended macrolide group after erythromycin is clarithromycin (Biaxin), which has been effective against many bacterial infections. Clarithromycin is administered twice a day. Two recently released macrolides are azithromycin (Zithromax) and dirithromycin (Dynabac). These two drugs have long half-lives, up to 40 to 50 hours; therefore, they are only prescribed once a day for 5 days. Elimination of these drugs is via bile and feces. Azithromycin is frequently prescribed for upper and lower respiratory infections, uncomplicated skin infections, and sexually transmitted diseases (Fig. 26–1). Dirithromycin is usually prescribed to treat chronic bronchitis, community-acquired pneumonia, and uncom-

Chart 26–1. Antibacterials: Erythromycin

MACROLIDE

Drug Name

Erythromycin (E-Mycin, Erythrocin, Erythrocin Lactobionate [IV]), ✹ Novorythro, Erythromid, Apo-Erythro-S
Pregnancy Category: B

Dosage

A: PO: 250–500 mg q6h
   IV: 1–4 g/d in divided doses
C: PO: 30–50 mg/kg/d in 4 divided doses
   IV: 20–50 mg/kg/d in 4–6 divided doses

Contraindications

Severe hepatic disease
Caution: Hepatic dysfunction, lactation

Drug-Lab-Food Interactions

Drug: *Increase* effect of digoxin, carbamazepine, theophylline, cyclosporine, warfarin, triazolam; *decrease* effect of penicillins, clindamycin

Pharmacokinetics

Absorption: PO: Well absorbed
Distribution: PB: 65%
Metabolism: t½: PO: 1–2 h; IV: 3–5 h
Excretion: In bile, feces, and small amount in urine

Pharmacodynamics

PO: Onset: 1 h
     Peak: 4 h
     Duration: 6 h
IV: Onset: UK
     Peak: UK
     Duration: UK

Therapeutic Effects/Uses

To treat gram-positive and some gram-negative organisms; for clients who are allergic to penicillin. To treat respiratory infections, legionnaires' disease, and prevent recurrence of rheumatic fever.

Mode of Action: Inhibition of the steps of protein synthesis, bacteriostatic or bactericidal effect.

Side Effects

Anorexia, nausea, vomiting, diarrhea, tinnitus, abdominal cramps, pruritus, rash

Adverse Reactions

Superinfections, vaginitis, urticaria, stomatitis, hearing loss
Life-threatening: Hepatotoxicity, anaphylaxis

KEY: A: adult; C: child; PO: by mouth; IV: intravenous; PB: protein-binding; t½: half-life; UK: unknown; ✹: Canadian drug names.

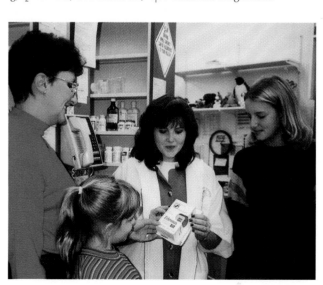

Figure 26–1
The pharmacist discusses the use of azithromycin with the family of an 8-year-old child for whom it was prescribed. What would be the recommended dosage for this child?

Table 26-1

Antibacterials: Macrolides, Lincosamides, and Vancomycin

GENERIC (BRAND)	ROUTE AND DOSAGE	USES AND CONSIDERATIONS
MACROLIDES		
Azithromycin (Zithromax)	A: PO: Initially: 500 mg × 1 dose; maint: 250 mg/d for 4 d A: IV: 500 mg for 2 d C: PO: 10 mg/kg for 1 d, then 5 mg/kg for 4 d	For treatment of mild to moderate streptococcal infections, lower respiratory tract infections, bacterial infections, gonorrhea, chancroid, and infection with *Streptococcus pneumoniae, Haemophilus influenzae,* and *Staphylococcus aureus.* Food decreases absorption of drug by 50%. *Caution:* renal and hepatic impairment. *Pregnancy category:* C; PB: 50%; $t_\frac{1}{2}$: 11–55 h
Clarithromycin (Biaxin)	A: PO: 250–500 mg q12h × 7–14 d C: PO: 15 mg/kg/d in 2 divided doses	For treatment of upper and lower respiratory infections, skin and soft tissue infections, *Helicobacter pylori* and mycobacterial species, and gram-positive and negative organisms. Report persistent diarrhea. *Pregnancy category:* C; PB: 65%–75%; $t_\frac{1}{2}$: 3–6 h
Dirithromycin (Dynabac)	A: PO: 500 mg/d C >12 y: PO: same as adult	To treat chronic bronchitis, pneumonia, pharyngitis, tonsillitis, and uncomplicated skin infections. Effective against *H. pylori, Legionella,* and *Chlamydia trachomatis.* Not effective against *Pseudomonas aeruginosa,* methicillin-resistant *S. aureus,* or *H. influenzae. Pregnancy category:* C; PB: UK; $t_\frac{1}{2}$: 20–50 h
Erythromycin base (E-Mycin, Ilotycin) Erythromycin estolate (Ilosone) Erythromycin ethylsuccinate (E.E.S., E-Mycin E, Pediamycin)	See Chart 26–1	Enteric-coated tablet to prevent gastric acid from destroying the drug. Higher doses are needed for severe infections. Available in liquid, chewable tablet, tablet, and capsule forms. Hepatotoxicity is associated with the estolate salt. Not affected by food. Available in liquid form, chewable tablets, and coated tablets.
Erythromycin lactobionate (Erythrocin Lactobionate IV)		For intravenous administration.
Erythromycin stearate (Erythrocin)		Acid-stable. It should not be taken with food. It comes in coated tablet form. *Pregnancy category:* B; PB: 65%; $t_\frac{1}{2}$: PO: 1–2 h, IV: 3–5 h
LINCOSAMIDES		
Clindamycin HCl (Cleocin)	A: PO: 150–450 mg q6–8h; *max:* 1800 mg/d	For serious infections. Available in capsule form. Taken with a full glass of water. Not affected by food. *Pregnancy category:* B; PB: 94%; $t_\frac{1}{2}$: 2–3 h
Clindamycin palmitate (Cleocin Pediatric)	C: PO: 25–40 mg/kg/d in 3–4 divided doses	Available in suspension for children and elderly.
Clindamycin phosphate (Cleocin Phosphate)	A: IM/IV: 300–900 mg q6–8h; *max:* 2700 mg/d C: IM/IV: 20–30 mg/kg/d in 3–4 divided doses	For treatment of serious infections, such as septicemia caused by gram-negative organism. *Not* to be given as a bolus. *Pregnancy category:* B; PB: 94%; $t_\frac{1}{2}$: 2–3 h
Lincomycin (Lincorex)	A: PO: 500 mg q6–8h; *max:* 8 g/d IM: 600 mg daily–q12h IV: 600 mg–1 g q8–12h; dilute in 100 mL of IV fluids C: PO: 30–60 mg/kg/d in 3–4 divided doses IV: 10–20 mg/kg/d in 2–3 divided doses, dilute in IV fluids	In most situations, this drug has been replaced by clindamycin. *Pregnancy category:* B; PB: 70%–75%; $t_\frac{1}{2}$: 4–6 h
VANCOMYCIN		
Vancomycin HCl (Vancocin)	A: IV: 500 mg q6h or 1 g q12h C: IV: 40 mg/kg/d in 4 divided doses; dilute in IV fluids; run for 1–1.5 h	For *S. aureus*-resistant infections and cardiac surgical prophylaxis in clients with penicillin allergy. Adverse reactions include possible ototoxicity, nephrotoxicity, vascular collapse. *Pregnancy category:* C; PB: 10%; $t_\frac{1}{2}$: 5–11 h

KEY: A: adult; C: child; PO: by mouth; IM: intramuscular; IV: intravenous; PB: protein-binding; $t_\frac{1}{2}$: half-life; max: maximum; >: greater than.

ANTIBACTERIALS: MACROLIDES: ERYTHROMYCIN

Assessment

- Assess vital signs (VS) and urine output. Report abnormal findings.
- Check laboratory tests for liver enzyme values to determine liver function. Liver enzyme tests should be periodically ordered for clients taking large doses of erythromycin for a continuous period.
- Obtain a history of drugs the client is currently taking. Erythromycin can increase the effects of digoxin, oral anticoagulants, theophylline, carbamazepine, and cyclosporine. Dosing for these drugs may need to be decreased.

Potential Nursing Diagnoses

- Risk for infection
- Risk for impaired tissue integrity

Planning

- Client's infection will be controlled and later eliminated.

Nursing Interventions

- Obtain a sample from the infected area and send to the laboratory for culture and sensitivity (C & S) test *before* starting erythromycin therapy. Antibiotic can be initiated after obtaining culture sample.
- Monitor VS, urine output, and laboratory values, especially liver enzymes: ALP, ALT, AST, and bilirubin.
- Monitor the client for liver damage resulting from prolonged use and high dosage of macrolides, such as erythromycin. Signs of liver dysfunction include elevated liver enzyme levels and jaundice.
- Monitor bleeding times if the client is receiving an oral anticoagulant.
- Administer oral erythromycin 1 h before meals or 2 h after meals. Give with a full glass of water and not fruit juice. Give the drug with food if GI upset occurs. Chewable tablets should be chewed and not swallowed whole.
- For IV erythromycin, dilute in an appropriate amount of solution as indicated in the drug circular.

Client Teaching

General

- Instruct the client to take the full course of antibacterial agent as prescribed. Drug compliance is most important for all antibacterials (antibiotics).

Side Effects

- Instruct the client to report side effects, including adverse reactions. Encourage the client to report nausea, vomiting, diarrhea, abdominal cramps, and itching. Superinfection, a secondary infection resulting from drug therapy, such as stomatitis or vaginitis, may occur.
- Instruct the client to report any symptoms of hearing impairment, such as tinnitus, vertigo, or roaring noises.

Cultural Considerations

- Recognize that the client and family members from various cultural backgrounds may need a written drug schedule as to when the drug should be taken. The nurse should either give a detailed explanation or write out the possible side effects that should be reported to the health care provider.

Evaluation

- Evaluate the effectiveness of erythromycin by determining whether the infection has been controlled or has ceased and no side effects, including superinfection, have occurred.

plicated skin infections. Table 26–1 lists the drugs that were developed from the derivatives of erythromycin.

Common side effects of clarithromycin and dirithromycin are nausea, diarrhea, and abdominal discomfort. With azithromycin, the side effects of nausea, diarrhea, and abdominal pain are occasional, not common.

Lincosamides

Clindamycin and lincomycin are examples of lincosamides. Like erythromycin, they inhibit bacterial protein synthesis and have both bacteriostatic and bactericidal actions, depending on drug dosage. Clindamycin is more widely prescribed than lincomycin because it is active against most gram-positive organisms, including *Staphylococcus aureus* and anaerobic organisms. It is not effective against the gram-negative bacteria, such as *Escherichia coli, Proteus,* and *Pseudomonas.* Clindamycin is absorbed better than lincomycin through the GI tract and maintains a higher serum drug concentration. Clindamycin is considered to be more effective than lincomycin and has fewer toxic effects. Table 26–1 lists the lincosamides.

SIDE EFFECTS AND ADVERSE REACTIONS
Side effects and adverse reactions to clindamycin and lincomycin include GI irritation, such as nausea, vomiting, and stomatitis. Also, rash may occur. Severe adverse reactions include colitis and anaphylactic shock.

DRUG INTERACTIONS
Clindamycin and lincomycin are incompatible with aminophylline, phenytoin (Dilantin), barbiturates, and ampicillin.

Vancomycin

Vancomycin, a glycopeptide bactericidal antibiotic, was widely used in the 1950s to treat staphylococcal infections. The use of the drug was almost abandoned because of the many reports of nephrotoxicity and ototoxicity. **Ototoxicity** results in damage to the auditory or vestibular branch of the eighth cranial nerve. Such damage can result in permanent hearing loss (auditory branch) or temporary or permanent loss of balance (vestibular branch). Vancomycin is still being used against drug-resistant *S. aureus* and in cardiac surgical prophylaxis for individuals with penicillin allergies. Serum vancomycin levels are usually drawn on clients receiving this drug so that toxic effects can be minimized.

TETRACYCLINES

The tetracyclines, isolated from *Streptomyces aureofaciens* in 1948, were the first broad-spectrum antibiotics effective against gram-positive and gram-negative bacteria and many other organisms, such as mycobacteria, rickettsiae, spirochetes, and chlamydiae. Tetracyclines act by inhibiting bacterial protein synthesis and have a bacteriostatic effect. Tetracyclines are not effective against *Staphylococcus aureus* (except for the newer tetracyclines), *Pseudomonas,* or *Proteus.* They can be used against *Mycoplasma pneumoniae.*

Tetracycline in combination with metronidazole and bismuth subsalicylate is useful in treating *Helicobacter pylori,* a bacterium in the stomach that can cause a peptic ulcer. For years, oral and topical tetracycline has been used to treat severe acne vulgaris. Low doses are usually prescribed to minimize the toxic effect of the drug.

Continuous use of tetracyclines has resulted in bacterial resistance to the drugs. Tetracycline resistance has increased in the treatment of pneumococci and gonococci infections; therefore, tetracyclines are not as useful in treating these infections.

The tetracyclines are frequently prescribed for oral use, although they are also available for intramuscular and intravenous use (Chart 26–2). Because intramuscular administration of tetracycline causes pain on injection and tissue irritation, this route of administration is seldom used. The intravenous route is used to treat severe infections. The newer oral preparations of tetracyclines, doxycycline, minocycline, and methacycline, are more rapidly and completely absorbed. Tetracyclines should not be taken with magnesium and aluminum preparations (antacids), milk products containing calcium, or iron-containing drugs because all of these substances bind with tetracycline and prevent absorption of the drug. It is suggested that tetracyclines, except for doxycycline and minocycline, be taken on an empty stomach 1 h before or 2 h after meals. The absorption of minocycline and doxycycline is improved with food ingestion. Table 26–2 describes the tetracycline preparations, their dosages, uses, and considerations. The tetracyclines are listed according to short-acting, intermediate-acting, and long-acting. The short-acting tetracyclines have a shorter half-life than the long-acting ones.

Although tetracyclines are widely used, they have numerous side effects, adverse reactions, toxicities, and drug interactions.

Side Effects and Adverse Reactions

GI disturbances such as nausea, vomiting, and diarrhea are side effects of tetracyclines. **Photosensitivity**

Chart 26-2. Antibacterials: Tetracyclines

TETRACYCLINE

Drug Name

Tetracycline (Achromycin, Tetracyn, Panmycin, Sumycin), ❦ Novotetra
Pregnancy Category: D (includes child <8 y)

Dosage

Systemic infection:
A: PO: 250–500 mg q6h–12 h
   IM: 250 mg/d; 300 mg/d in 2–3 divided doses
C: >8 y: PO: 25–50 mg/kg/d in 4 divided doses
   IM: 15–25 mg/kg/d in 2–3 divided doses; *max:* 250 mg/dose

Contraindications

Hypersensitivity, pregnancy, severe hepatic or renal disease
Caution: History of allergies, renal and hepatic dysfunction, myasthenia gravis

Drug-Lab-Food Interactions

Drug: May *increase* or *decrease* effects of anticoagulants; *decrease* tetracycline absorption with antacids, iron, and zinc; *decrease* effects of oral contraceptives
Lab: *Decrease* serum potassium level
Food: Dairy products (milk, cheese) *decrease* effect

Pharmacokinetics

Absorption: PO: 75%–80% absorbed
Distribution: PB: 20–60 h
Metabolism: t½: 6–12 h
Excretion: Unchanged in the urine

Pharmacodynamics

PO: Onset: 1–2 h
     Peak: 2–4 h
     Duration: 6 h
IV: Onset: Rapid
     Peak: 0.5–1 h
     Duration: UK

Therapeutic Effects/Uses

To treat infections due to uncommon gram-positive and gram-negative organisms, skin infections or disorders, chlamydial infection, gonorrhea, syphilis, rickettsial infection.

Mode of Action: Inhibition of the steps of protein synthesis. Bacteriostatic or bactericidal

Side Effects

Nausea, vomiting, diarrhea, rash, flatulence, abdominal discomfort, headache, photosensitivity, pruritus, epigastric distress, heartburn

Adverse Reactions

Superinfections, (candidiasis)
Life-threatening: Blood dyscrasias, hepatotoxicity, nephrotoxicity, exfoliative dermatitis, intracranial hypertension

Assessment and Planning

Interventions

NURSING PROCESS

Evaluation

KEY: A: adult; C: child; PO: by mouth; IM: intramuscular; IV: intravenous; PB: protein-binding; t½: half-life; UK: unknown; >: greater than; ❦: Canadian drug name.

(sunburn reaction) may occur in persons taking tetracyclines, especially demeclocycline. Pregnant women should not take tetracycline during the first trimester of pregnancy because of possible teratogenic effects. Women in the last trimester of pregnancy and children younger than 8 should *not* take tetracycline because it irreversibly discolors the permanent teeth. Minocycline can cause damage to the vestibular part of the inner ear, which may result in difficulty maintaining balance. Tetracyclines should be taken 1 h before or 2 h after meals because food, especially milk products, impairs absorption. Outdated tetracy-

ANTIBACTERIALS: TETRACYCLINES

Assessment

- Assess VS and urine output. Report abnormal findings.
- Check laboratory results, especially those that indicate renal and liver function, such as BUN, serum creatinine, AST, ALT, APT, and bilirubin.
- Obtain a history of dietary intake and drugs the client is currently taking. Dairy products and antacids decrease drug absorption.

Potential Nursing Diagnoses

- Risk for infection
- Noncompliance with drug regimen
- Risk for impaired skin integrity

Planning

- Client's infection will be controlled and later eliminated.

Nursing Interventions

- Obtain a sample for culture from the infected area and send to the laboratory for C & S test. Antibiotic therapy can be started after the culture sample has been taken.
- Administer tetracycline 1 h before meals or 2 h after meals for absorption.
- Monitor laboratory values for liver and kidney functions; these include liver enzymes, BUN, and serum creatinine.
- Monitor VS and urine output.

Client Teaching

General
- Instruct the client to store tetracycline out of the light and extreme heat. Tetracycline decomposes in light and heat, causing the drug to become toxic.
- Advise the client to check the expiration date on the bottle of tetracycline; out-of-date tetracycline can be toxic.
- Advise a woman who is contemplating pregnancy who has an infection to inform her health care provider and to avoid taking tetracycline because of possible teratogenic effect.
- Inform parents that children less than 8 years old should not take tetracycline because it can cause discoloration of permanent teeth.
- Instruct the client to take the complete course of tetracycline as prescribed.

Diet
- Instruct the client to avoid milk products, iron, and antacids. Tetracycline should be taken 1 h before meals or 2 h after meals with a full glass of water. If GI upset occurs, drug can be taken with nondairy foods.

Side Effects
- Instruct the client to use sunblock/protective clothing during sun exposure. Photosensitivity is associated with tetracycline.
- Instruct the client to report signs of a superinfection (mouth ulcers, anal or genital discharge).
- Advise client to use additional contraceptive techniques and not to rely on oral contraceptives when taking drug because effectiveness may decrease.
- Advise the client to use effective oral hygiene several times a day to prevent or alleviate mouth ulcers (stomatitis).

Cultural Considerations

- Recognize that the client and family members from various cultural backgrounds may need a written drug schedule as to when the drug should be taken. Explain how dairy

Nursing Process continued on following page

products should not be taken with specific tetracyclines but that food helps with the absorption of minocycline and doxycycline.
• Provide a detailed explanation orally or in written form of the possible side effects that should be reported to the health care provider.

Evaluation

• Evaluate the effectiveness of tetracycline by determining whether the infection has been controlled or has ceased and there are no side effects.

Table 26–2
Antibacterials: Tetracyclines

GENERIC (BRAND)	ROUTE AND DOSAGE	USES AND CONSIDERATIONS
SHORT-ACTING		
Tetracycline (Achromycin, Tetracyn, Sumycin, Panmycin)	See Chart 26–2	Used for respiratory and urinary tract infections. For acne, the usual dose is 250 mg, b.i.d. Milk products and antacids should not be taken with tetracyclines. Should *not* be taken in the last trimester of pregnancy or before a child is 8 years old to prevent discoloration of the teeth. Also used to treat stage I of Lyme disease. Photosensitivity is a problem; wear protective clothing or sunscreen when in sunlight. *Pregnancy category:* D; PB: 20%–60%; $t_{\frac{1}{2}}$: 6–12 h
Oxytetracycline HCl (Terramycin)	A: PO: 250–500 mg q6–12h IM: 200–300 mg/d in 2–3 divided doses IV: 250–500 mg in 2 divided doses C >8 y: PO: 25–50 mg/kg/d in 4 divided doses IM: 15–25 mg/kg/d in 2–3 divided doses; *max:* 250 mg/dose IV: 10–20 mg/kg/d in 2 divided doses	Used for urinary tract infections. Administered primarily by the oral route. *Pregnancy category:* D; PB: 20%–40%; $t_{\frac{1}{2}}$: 6–10 h
INTERMEDIATE-ACTING		
Demeclocycline HCl (Declomycin)	A: PO: 150 mg q6h or 300 mg q12h C: >8 y: PO: 6–12 mg/kg/d in 2–4 divided doses	Used for gram-positive and gram-negative bacteria. Photosensitivity may occur. *Pregnancy category:* D; PB: 35%–90%; $t_{\frac{1}{2}}$: 10–17 h
Methacycline HCl (Rondomycin)	A: PO: 600 mg, q12h C: PO: 6–12 mg/kg	It is a costly tetracycline. It has similar actions as demeclocycline. The side effects are similar to other tetracyclines. *Pregnancy category:* UK; PB: UK; $t_{\frac{1}{2}}$: UK
LONG-ACTING		
Doxycycline hyclate (Vibramycin)	A: PO: 100 mg q12–24h IV: 100–200 mg/d C >8 y: PO/IV: 2–4 mg/kg/d in 1–2 divided doses	Smaller doses are effective against bacteria and microorganisms. Also used for legionella syndrome. Chances of tooth discoloration are less with this drug. Should take with food. *Pregnancy category:* D; PB: 25%–92%; $t_{\frac{1}{2}}$: 20 h
Minocycline HCl (Minocin)	A: PO/IV: 100 mg q12h or 50 mg q6h C >8 y: PO/IV: 4 mg/kg/d in 2 divided doses	Effective against bacterial infections and acne. Should not be administered to clients with renal insufficiency. Should take with food. *Pregnancy category:* D; PB: 55%–88%; $t_{\frac{1}{2}}$: 11–20 h

KEY: A: adult; C: child; PO: by mouth; IV: intravenous; PB: protein-binding; $t_{\frac{1}{2}}$: half-life; >: greater than; max: maximum.

Chart 26–3.   Antibacterials: Aminoglycosides

AMINOGLYCOSIDES

Drug Name

Gentamicin sulfate (G)
(Garamycin)
Pregnancy Category: C

Netilmicin sulfate (N)
(Netromycin)
Pregnancy Category: D

Dosage

(G)
A: IM: 30 mg/kg/d in 3–4 divided doses
IV: 3–5 mg/kg/d in 3–4 divided doses
C: IM/IV: 2–2.5 mg/kg, q8–12 h
TDM: 5–10 μg/mL; peak: 10–12 μg/mL;
trough: 0.5–2 μg/mL
(N)
A: IM/IV: 3–6 mg/kg/d in 3 divided doses
C: IM/IV: 5–8 mg/kg/d in 3 divided doses
TDM: Peak: 0.5–10 μg/mL; trough: <4 μg/mL

Contraindications

(G & N)
Hypersensitivity, severe renal disease, pregnancy, and breast feeding
Caution: (G & N) Renal disease, neuromuscular disorders (myasthenia gravis, parkinsonism), heart failure, elderly, neonates

Drug-Lab-Food Interactions

(G & N)
Drug: *Increase* risk of ototoxicity with loop diuretics, methoxyflurane; *increase* risk of nephrotoxicity with amphotericin B, polymyxin, cisplatin, furosemide, vancomycin
Lab: *Increase* BUN, serum AST, ALT, LDH, bilirubin, creatinine; *decrease* serum potassium and magnesium

Pharmacokinetics

Absorption: Both: IM, IV
Distribution: PB: (G) UK, (N) 10%
Metabolism: t½: (G) 2 h, (N) 2–3 h
Excretion: (G) unchanged in urine, (N) 90% excreted unchanged in urine

Pharmacodynamics

(G)
IM/IV: Onset: rapid
         Peak: 1–2 h
         Duration: 6–8 h
(N)
IM: Onset: rapid
         Peak: 0.5–1.5 h
         Duration: UK
IV: Onset: immediate
         Peak: 0.5–1 h
         Duration: UK

Assessment and Planning

Interventions

NURSING PROCESS

Therapeutic Effects/Uses

(G & N) To treat serious infections caused by gram-negative organisms, such as *Pseudomonas aeruginosa, Proteus*; to treat pelvic inflammatory disease (PID).
(G) Effective against methicillin-resistant *Staphylococcus aureus* infections. (N) Effective against gentamicin-resistant bacteria.

Mode of Action: Inhibition of bacterial protein synthesis. Bactericidal effect.

Side Effects

(G & N) Anorexia, nausea, vomiting, rash, numbness, visual disturbances, tremors, tinnitus, pruritus, muscle cramps or weakness, photosensitivity

Adverse Reactions

(G & N) Oliguria, urticaria, palpitation, superinfection
Life-threatening: (G & N) Ototoxicity, nephrotoxicity, thrombocytopenia, agranulocytosis, neuromuscular blockade, liver damage

Evaluation

KEY: G: gentamicin sulfate; N: netilmicin sulfate; A: adult; C: child; IM: intramuscular; IV: intravenous; PB: protein-binding; t½: half-life; UK: unknown; TDM: therapeutic drug monitoring; <: less than; >: more than; BUN: blood urea nitrogen; AST: aspartate aminotransferase; ALT: alanine aminotransferase; LDH: lactic dehydrogenase.

Table 26-3
Antibacterials: Aminoglycosides

GENERIC (BRAND)	ROUTE AND DOSAGE	USES AND CONSIDERATIONS
Amikacin SO$_4$ (Amikin)	A&C: IM/IV: 15 mg/kg/d in 2–3 divided doses; *max:* 1.5 g/d NB: IV: 7.5 mg/kg q12h TDM: Peak: 15–30 mg/mL; trough: 5–10 mg/mL	Synthetic derivative of kanamycin. Effective against *Pseudomonas* spp. Hearing changes should be monitored. *Pregnancy category:* C; PB: 4%–11%; t$\frac{1}{2}$: 2–3 h
Gentamicin SO$_4$ (Garamycin)	See Chart 26-3	Effective against gram-negative bacteria, including *Pseudomonas* spp. Urinary output should be monitored. *Pregnancy category:* C; PB: UK; t$\frac{1}{2}$: 2 h
Kanamycin SO$_4$ (Kantrex)	A: PO: 1 g q6h *Hepatic coma:* 8–12 g/d in divided doses IM/IV: 15 mg/kg/d in 2 divided doses C: IV: Same as adult	Used orally for hepatic coma. Effective against gram-negative bacteria with the exception of *Pseudomonas aeruginosa.* Monitor for hearing loss and urinary output. *Pregnancy category:* D; PB: 10%; t$\frac{1}{2}$: 2–3 h
Neomycin SO$_4$ (Mycifradin)	A: PO: GI surgery: 1 g qh for 4 doses; then 1 g q4h For 24 h or other regimens *Hepatic coma:* 4–12 g/d in divided doses IM: 15 mg/kg/d in 4 divided doses; *max:* 1 g/d C: PO: 10 mg/kg q4–6h for 3 d	Decreases bacteria in the bowel and is used as a preoperative bowel antiseptic. It is also available as a topical antibiotic ointment. *Pregnancy category:* C; PB: 10%; t$\frac{1}{2}$: 2–3 h
Netilmicin (Netromycin)	A: IM/IV: 3–6 mg/kg/d in 3 divided doses C: IM/IV: 5–8 mg/kg/d in 3 divided doses TDM: Peak: 0.5–10 μg/mL; trough: <4 μg/mL	This newer aminoglycoside is effective against gram-negative bacteria and has fewer side effects. Similar to gentamicin and tobramycin. *Pregnancy category:* D; PB: 10%; t$\frac{1}{2}$: 2–3 h
Paromomycin (Humatin)	*Intestinal amebiasis:* A&C: PO: 25–35 mg/kg/d in 3 divided doses for 5–10 d	Used in treating hepatic coma and parasitic infections. Hearing changes and urinary output should be monitored. Is not systemically absorbed. *Pregnancy category:* C; PB: UK; t$\frac{1}{2}$: UK
Streptomycin SO$_4$	*Tuberculosis:* A: IM: 1 g daily for 2–3 mo; then 1 g 3 × wk *Endocarditis:* A: IM: 1 g q12h for 1 wk; dose may be decreased	First aminoglycoside. Used with antituberculosis drugs in treatment of tuberculosis. Ototoxicity is a major problem. *Pregnancy category:* C; PB: 30%; t$\frac{1}{2}$: 2–3 h
Tobramycin SO$_4$ (Nebcin)	A: IM/IV: 3–5 mg/kg/d in 3 divided doses C: IM/IV: 4.5–7.5 mg/kg/d in 3–4 divided doses TDM: Peak: 10–12 μg/mL; trough: 0.5–2 μg/mL	Very effective against *Pseudomonas aeruginosa.* Hearing changes and urinary output should be monitored. Toxic effects are less than for other aminoglycosides. *Pregnancy category:* D; PB: 10%; t$\frac{1}{2}$: 2–3 h

KEY: *A:* adult; *C:* child; *PO:* by mouth; *IM:* intramuscular; *IV:* intravenous; *NB:* newborn; *PB:* protein-binding; t$\frac{1}{2}$: half-life; *TDM:* therapeutic drug monitoring; *UK:* unknown; *<:* less than; *max:* maximum.

clines should always be discarded because the drug breaks down into a toxic byproduct. **Nephrotoxicity** results when the tetracycline is given in high doses with other nephrotoxic drugs. **Superinfection** is another problem that might result because tetracycline can disrupt the microbial flora of the body.

AMINOGLYCOSIDES

Aminoglycosides act by inhibiting bacterial protein synthesis. The aminoglycoside antibiotics are used against gram-negative bacteria, such as *Escherichia coli, Proteus* spp., and *Pseudomonas* spp. Some gram-positive cocci are resistant to aminoglycosides, so penicillins or cephalosporins may be used.

Streptomycin sulfate, derived from the bacterium *Streptomyces griseus* in 1944, was the first aminoglycoside available for clinical use and was used in the treatment of tuberculosis. Because of its ototoxicity and the bacterial resistance that can develop, it is infrequently used today.

Aminoglycosides are for serious infections. Aminoglycosides cannot be absorbed from the GI tract and cannot cross into the cerebrospinal fluid. These agents are primarily administered intravenously except for a few aminoglycosides (neomycin and paromomycin), which may be given orally to decrease the bacteria and other organisms in the bowel. Paromomycin is useful in treating intestinal amebiasis and tapeworm infestation. Neomycin is frequently used as a preoperative bowel antiseptic.

The aminoglycosides that are currently used to treat *Pseudomonas aeruginosa* infection include gentamicin (1963), tobramycin (1970), amikacin (1970s), and netilmicin (1980s). Netilmicin is one of the latest aminoglycosides, and the occurrence of toxicities from this drug is not as frequent or as intense as those from other aminoglycosides. *P. aeruginosa* is resistant to gentamicin. Amikacin may be used when there is bacterial resistance to gentamicin and tobramycin. Gentamicin is less costly than the other aminoglycosides. Chart 26–3 lists the drug data related to the aminoglycosides gentamicin (Garamycin) and netilmicin (Netromycin).

Pharmacokinetics

Gentamicin and netilmicin are administered intramuscularly and intravenously. Both drugs have a short half-life, and drug dose can be given 3 to 4 times a day. Netilmicin has a low protein-binding power. Excretion of these drugs is primarily unchanged in the urine.

Pharmacodynamics

Gentamicin and netilmicin inhibit bacterial protein synthesis and both have a bactericidal effect. Although netilmicin is the newer aminoglycoside, its pregnancy category is D, whereas gentamicin has a pregnancy category of C. The onset of action for both drugs is similar (rapid or immediate). The peak action for netilmicin is 30 minutes faster than gentamicin.

Aminoglycosides are not readily absorbed through the GI tract; thus, they are administered intramuscularly and intravenously. To ensure a desired blood level, the drug is usually administered intravenously. The aminoglycosides can be given with penicillins and cephalosporins, but should not be mixed together in the same administered container. When combinations of antibiotics are given intravenously, the IV line is flushed after each antibiotic has been administered to ensure that the antibiotic is completely delivered.

Side Effects and Adverse Reactions

The serious adverse reactions to aminoglycosides include ototoxicity and nephrotoxicity. Nephrotoxicity might occur, depending on renal function, drug dose, and age (young and elderly). Careful drug dosing is especially important with young and old clients. The nurse must assess changes in clients' hearing, balance, and urinary output. Prolonged use of aminoglycosides could result in a superinfection. Specific serum aminoglycoside levels should be closely monitored to avoid adverse reactions. Table 26–3 lists the aminoglycosides, their dosages, uses, and considerations.

FLUOROQUINOLONES (QUINOLONES)

The mechanism of action of fluoroquinolones is to interfere with the enzyme DNA gyrase, which is needed for the synthesis of bacterial DNA. Their antibacterial spectrum includes both gram-positive and gram-negative organisms. They are bactericidal. Nalidixic acid and cinoxacin are the earliest derivatives of the fluoroquinolone group, which is prescribed primarily for urinary tract infection caused by common gram-negative organisms, such as *Escherichia coli*. The fluoroquinolones are effective against some gram-positive organisms, such as *Streptococcus pneumoniae*, and against *Haemophilus influenzae*, *Pseudomonas aeruginosa*, *Salmonella*, and *Shigella*. This group of antibiotics is useful in the treatment of urinary tract, bone, and joint infections, bronchitis, pneumonia, gastroenteritis, and gonorrhea. Table 26–4 lists the various fluoroquinolones.

Ciprofloxacin and norfloxacin are synthetic antibacterials related to nalidixic acid. These two fluoroquinolones have a broad spectrum of action on gram-positive and gram-negative organisms, including *Pseudomonas aeruginosa*. Norfloxacin is indicated for urinary tract infections, and ciprofloxacin has FDA approval for urinary tract infections; lower respiratory tract infections; and skin, soft tissue, bone, and joint infections.

The use of fluoroquinolones as urinary antibiotics is discussed in Chapter 30. Chart 26–4 lists the drug data related to ciprofloxacin. Ciprofloxacin's use is not limited to urinary tract infections but is equally effective for treating bone, joint, and soft tissue infections.

NURSING PROCESS
ANTIBACTERIALS: AMINOGLYCOSIDES

Assessment

- Assess VS and urine output. Compare these results with future VS and urine output. An adverse reaction to most aminoglycosides is nephrotoxicity.
- Assess laboratory results to determine renal and liver functions, including BUN, serum creatinine, ALP, ALT, AST, and bilirubin. Serum electrolytes should also be checked. Aminoglycosides may decrease the serum potassium and magnesium levels.
- Obtain a medical history related to renal or hearing disorders. Large doses of aminoglycosides could cause nephrotoxicity or ototoxicity.

Potential Nursing Diagnoses

- Risk for infection
- Risk for impaired tissue integrity
- Risk for altered tissue perfusion: renal

Planning

- Client's infection will be controlled and later eliminated.

Nursing Interventions

- Send a sample from the infected area to the laboratory for culture to determine organism and antibiotic sensitivity (C & S) before aminoglycoside is started.
- Monitor intake and output. Urine output should be at least 600 mL/d. Immediately report if urine output is decreased. Urinalysis may be ordered daily. Check results for proteinuria, casts, blood cells, or appearance.
- Check for hearing loss. Aminoglycosides can cause ototoxicity.
- Check laboratory results and compare with baseline values. Report abnormal results.
- Monitor VS. Note if body temperature has decreased.
- For IV use, dilute the aminoglycoside in 50–200 mL of normal saline solution (NSS) or D$_5$W solution and administer in 30–60 min.
- Check that therapeutic drug monitoring (TDM) has been ordered for peak and trough drug levels. The TDM for gentamicin is 5–10 μg/mL. Blood should be drawn 45–60 min after drug has been administered for peak levels and minutes before the next drug dosing for trough levels. Drug peak values should be 10–12 μg/mL, and trough values should be 0.5–2 μg/mL.
- Monitor for signs and symptoms of superinfection, such as stomatitis (mouth ulcers), genital discharge (vaginitis), and anal or genital itching.

Client Teaching

General
- Unless fluids are restricted, encourage the client to increase fluid intake.
- Instruct the client never to take leftover antibiotics.

Side Effects
- Instruct the client to report side effects resulting from the aminoglycosides, including nausea, vomiting, tremors, tinnitus, pruritus, and muscle cramps.
- Instruct the client to use sunblock lotion and protective clothing during sun exposure. Photosensitivity can be caused by aminoglycosides.

Evaluation

- Evaluate the effectiveness of the aminoglycoside by determining whether the infection has ceased and no side effects have occurred.

Table 26-4
Antibacterials: Fluoroquinolones (Quinolones) and Unclassified

GENERIC (BRAND)	ROUTE AND DOSAGE	USES AND CONSIDERATIONS
FLUOROQUINOLONES		
Cinoxacin (Cinobac)	A: PO: 1 g/d 2-4 divided doses for 1-2 wk C >12 y: Same as adult	For acute and chronic urinary tract infections (UTIs). Effective against gram-negative organisms except for *Pseudomonas*. Absorbed in prostatic tissue. More effective than nalidixic acid. *Pregnancy category:* B; PB: 60%-80%; t½: 1.5 h
Ciprofloxacin HCl (Cipro)	See Chart 26-4	Has a broad-spectrum antibacterial effect. For UTI, skin and soft tissue infections, and bone and joint infections. Antacid inhibits drug absorption. *Pregnancy category:* C (X at term); PB: 20%; t½: 3-4 h
Enoxacin (Penetrex)	A: PO: 200-400 mg b.i.d. 7-14 d	To treat UTI including those caused by *Escherichia coli, Proteus, Pseudomonas. Pregnancy category:* C; PB: 40%; t½: 3-6 h
Grepafloxacin HCl (Raxar)	A: PO: 400-600 mg/d for 10 d	To treat mild to moderate infections, chronic bronchitis, community-acquired pneumonia (CAP), cervicitis, and uncomplicated gonorrhea. *Pregnancy category:* UK; PB: UK; t½: UK
Levofloxacin (Levaquin)	A: PO: IV: 500 mg/d for 7-14 d	To treat respiratory tract infection, such as pneumonia, chronic bronchitis, and for skin infections. *Pregnancy category:* C; PB: 50%; t½: 6 h
Lomefloxacin HCl (Maxaquin)	A: PO: 200-400 mg/d × 7-14 d	For complicated and uncomplicated UTIs, transurethral surgery, lower respiratory infections. Drug dose is reduced for clients with a low creatinine clearance. *Pregnancy category:* C; PB: UK; t½: 6-8 h
Nalidixic acid (NegGram)	A: PO: 1 g q.i.d. for 1-2 wk; 1 g b.i.d. for long-term use C: PO: 55 mg/kg/d in 4 divided doses for 1-2 wk; 33 mg/kg/d for long-term use	For acute and chronic UTIs. Drug resistance may occur. Is not distributed in prostatic fluid. *Pregnancy category:* B; PB: 95%; t½: 2-6 h
Norfloxacin (Noroxin)	A: PO: 400 mg b.i.d., a.c. or p.c. for 1-3 wk	For acute and chronic UTIs. Most potent drug of the fluoroquinolone group. Food may inhibit drug absorption. *Pregnancy category:* C; PB: 10%-15%; t½: 3-4 h
Ofloxacin (Floxin)	A: PO: 200-400 mg q12h × 10 d	For respiratory and UTIs, prostatitis, and skin infections. Not to be given with meals. Superinfection may result. Avoid excessive sunlight. *Pregnancy category:* C; PB: 20%; t½: 5-8 h
Sparfloxacin (Zagam)	A: PO: 400 mg for 1 d, 200 mg/d for 2nd to 10th day	To treat CAP, chronic bronchitis, and skin disorders. Side effects include gastrointestinal disturbances and photosensitivity. Clients should use sunscreen when in the sun. *Pregnancy category:* UK; PB: UK; t½: UK
Trovafloxacin (Trovan)	PO: IV: 100-300 mg/d, for 7-10 d	To treat acute sinusitis, chronic bronchitis, UTIs, and skin infections. *Pregnancy category:* UK; PB: UK; t½: UK
UNCLASSIFIED		
Aztreonam (Azactam)	*Urinary tract infections:* A: IM/IV: 0.5-1.0 g q8-12h *Severe infections:* A: IM/IV: 1.0-2.0 g q6-8h; *max:* 8 g/d	For treatment of gram-negative infections of the lower respiratory tract, UTIs, and skin and gynecologic infections. May be used in combination with other antibacterials. *Pregnancy category:* B; PB: 56%; t½: 1.7-2.1 h
Chloramphenicol (Chloromycetin)	A&C: PO/IV: 50 mg/kg/d in 4 divided doses (q6h) NB: 25 mg/kg/d in 4 divided doses (q6h)	For treatment of severe infections. Drug can be toxic. *Pregnancy category:* C; PB: 50%-60%; t½: 1.5-4.0 h
Imipenem-cilastatin (Primaxin)	A: IM: 500-750 mg q12h IV: 250 mg-1 g q6-8h C: IV: 15-25 mg/kg q6h	For treatment of severe infections of the lower respiratory tract, UTIs, skin, bones, joints, and septicemia. *Pregnancy category:* C; PB: 20%; t½: 1 h
Spectinomycin HCl (Trobicin)	A: IM: 2 g as single dose or 2 g q12h for severe infection	Has a bacteriostatic effect. Effective against *Neisseria gonorrhoeae*. Ineffective against syphilis. *Pregnancy category:* B; PB: 10%; t½: 1-3 h

KEY: A: adult; C: child; PO: by mouth; IM: intramuscular; IV: intravenous; NB: newborn; PB: protein-binding; t½: half-life; UTI: urinary tract infection; max: maximum; >: greater than.

Chart 26–4.   Antibacterials: Fluoroquinolones (Quinolones)

FLUOROQUINOLONE

Drug Name

Ciprofloxacin (Cipro)
Quinolone, fluoroquinoline
Pregnancy Category: C (X at term), breast feeding

Dosage

A: PO: 250–500 mg q12h
Severe infections:
A: PO: 500–750 mg q12h; IV: 200 mg q12h
Mild to moderate infections:
A: IV: 400 mg q12h

Contraindications

Severe renal disease, hypersensitivity to other quinolones, pregnancy and breast feeding
Caution: Seizure disorders, renal disorders, children <14 y, elderly, clients receiving theophylline

Drug-Lab-Food Interactions

Drug: *Increase* effect with probenecid; *increase* effect of theophylline, caffeine; *decrease* drug absorption with antacids, iron
Lab: *Increase* AST, ALT

Pharmacokinetics

Absorption: PO: 70% absorbed
Distribution: PB: 20%
Metabolism: t½: 3–4 h
Excretion: 50% unchanged in urine

Pharmacodynamics

PO: Onset: 0.5–1 h
Peak: 1–2 h
Duration: UK

Therapeutic Effects/Uses

To treat lower respiratory tract, renal, bone, and joint infections.

Mode of Action: Interference with the enzyme DNA gyrase, which is needed for bacterial DNA synthesis. Bactericidal effect.

Side Effects

Nausea, vomiting, diarrhea, abdominal cramps, flatulence, headache, dizziness, fatigue, restlessness, insomnia, rash, flushing, tinnitus, photosensitivity

Adverse Reactions

Urticaria, oral candidiasis, crystalluria, hematuria, seizures

Assessment and Planning
Interventions
Evaluation
NURSING PROCESS

KEY: A: adult; PB: protein-binding; t½: half-life; PO: by mouth; IV: intravenous; <: less than; UK: unknown; AST: aspartate aminotransferase; ALT: alanine aminotransferase.

The number of new fluoroquinolones has increased in the past few years. These new agents included grepafloxacin (Raxar), levofloxacin (Levaquin), sparfloxacin (Zagam), and trovafloxacin (Trovan). These drugs are primarily given to treat respiratory problems, such as community-acquired pneumonia (CAP), chronic bronchitis, urinary tract infections, and uncomplicated skin infections. These drugs are included in Table 26–4.

Pharmacokinetics

Approximately 70% of ciprofloxacin hydrochloride (Cipro) is absorbed from the GI tract. It has a low protein-binding effect and a moderately short half-life of 3 to 4 h. About one-half of the drug is excreted unchanged in the urine.

Pharmacodynamics

Ciprofloxacin inhibits bacterial DNA synthesis by inhibiting the enzyme DNA gyrase. The drug has a high tissue distribution. If possible, it should be taken before meals since food slows the absorption rate. Antacids also decrease absorption rate. When taking probenecid with ciprofloxacin, the drug action of ciprofloxacin is increased. Ciprofloxacin prolongs the drug action of theophylline.

NURSING PROCESS
ANTIBACTERIALS: FLUOROQUINOLONES

Assessment

- Assess VS and intake and urine output. Compare these results with future VS and urine output. Fluid intake should be at least 2000 mL/d.
- Assess laboratory results to determine renal function: BUN and serum creatinine.
- Obtain a drug and diet history. Antacids and iron preparations decrease absorption of fluoroquinolones such as ciprofloxacin (Cipro). Ciprofloxacin can increase the effects of theophylline and caffeine.

Potential Nursing Diagnoses

- Risk for infection
- Risk for impaired tissue integrity
- Noncompliance with drug regimen

Planning

- Client's infection will be controlled and later eliminated.

Nursing Interventions

- Obtain specimen from the infected site and send to the laboratory for C & S before initiating antibacterial drug therapy.
- Monitor intake and output. Urine output should be at least 750 mL/d. Client should be well hydrated, and fluid intake should be >2000 mL/d to prevent crystalluria. Urine pH should be <6.7.
- Monitor VS. Report abnormal findings.
- Check laboratory results, especially BUN and serum creatinine. Elevated values may indicate renal dysfunction.
- Administer ciprofloxacin 1 h before or 2 h after meals or 2 h before or after antacids and iron products for absorption. Give with a full glass of water. If GI distress occurs, drug may be taken with food.
- For IV ciprofloxacin, dilute the antibiotic in an appropriate amount of solution as indicated in the drug circular. Infuse over 60 min.
- Check for signs and symptoms of superinfection such as stomatitis (mouth ulcers), furry black tongue, anal or genital discharge, and itching.
- Monitor serum theophylline levels. Ciprofloxacin can increase theophylline levels. Check for symptoms of central nervous system (CNS) stimulation: nervousness, insomnia, anxiety, and tachycardia.

Client Teaching

General
- Instruct the client to drink at least 6 to 8 glassfuls (8 oz) of fluid daily.
- Instruct the client to avoid caffeinated products.

Side Effects
- Advise the client to avoid operating hazardous machinery or operating a motor vehicle while taking the drug or until drug stability has occurred due to possible drug-related dizziness.
- Advise the client that photosensitivity is a side effect of most fluoroquinolones. The client should use sunglasses, sunblock, and protective clothing when in the sun.
- Instruct the client to report side effects, such as dizziness, nausea, vomiting, diarrhea, flatulence, abdominal cramps, tinnitus, and rash. Older adults are more likely to develop side effects.

Evaluation

- Evaluate the effectiveness of the fluoroquinolone by determining if the infection has ceased and the body temperature has returned within normal range.

Ciprofloxacin has an average onset of action of 0.5 to 1.0 h, and the peak concentration time is 1 to 2 h. The duration of action is unknown.

UNCLASSIFIED ANTIBACTERIAL DRUGS

Several antibacterials, such as chloramphenicol, spectinomycin, imipenem-cilastatin, and aztreonam, do not belong to any major drug group. Chloramphenicol (Chloromycetin) was discovered in 1947 and has a bacteriostatic action by inhibiting bacterial protein synthesis. Because of the toxic effects of chloramphenicol, including blood dyscrasias related to bone marrow suppression, it is used only for treatment of serious infections. It is effective against gram-negative and gram-positive bacteria, and many other microorganisms, such as rickettsiae, mycoplasmas, and *Haemophilus influenzae*.

Spectinomycin hydrochloride (Trobicin), introduced in 1971, is used against *Neisseria gonorrhoeae*, the microbe that causes gonorrhea. It is also prescribed for persons allergic to penicillins, cephalosporins, or tetracyclines. It is administered intramuscularly as a single dose.

Imipenem with cilastatin sodium (Primaxin) is a new antibacterial introduced in 1986. It is effective against gram-positive bacteria, including *Staphylococcus aureus* and *Pseudomonas aeruginosa*.

Aztreonam (Azactam) is a monobactam antibacterial. Though aztreonam has the same beta lactam structure as penicillin and cephalosporins, it has a different spectrum of activity. It is not effective against gram-positive bacteria but is effective against the gram-negative bacteria *Neisseria gonorrhoeae* and *Haemophilus influenzae*.

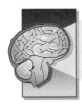

Critical Thinking in Action

A. J. N., 46 years old, has a wound infection. The culture report stated that the infection was due to *Pseudomonas aeruginosa*. A. J. N.'s temperature was 104°F (40°C). Amikacin sulfate (Amikin) is to be administered intravenously in 100 mL of D₅W over 45 min, every 8 h. Dosage is 15 mg/kg/d in three divided doses. A. J. N. weighs 165 lb.

1. What is the drug classification of amikacin? How many milligrams of amikacin should A. J. N. receive every 8 h?
2. What type of intravenous infusion should be used? What would be the IV flow rate?
3. When should a wound culture be obtained to determine the appropriate antibacterial agent? Give your rationale.
4. What are the similarities of amikacin to other aminoglycosides such as gentamicin? Would one aminoglycoside be preferred over another one? Explain.

The nurse assessed A. J. N. for hearing and urinary function before and during amikacin therapy.

5. What should a hearing assessment include?
6. A. J. N.'s urine output in the last 8 h was 125 mL. Explain the possible cause for the amount of urine output. What nursing action should be taken?
7. What laboratory tests monitor renal function?
8. The health care provider requests peak and trough serum amikacin levels. When should the blood samples to determine peak serum level and trough serum level be drawn?

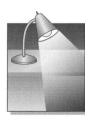

Study Questions

1. Name two groups of drugs that are classified as bacteriostatic drugs.
2. What antibacterial drugs are used as penicillin substitutes?
3. Give an example of a macrolide.
4. What is the nurse's role in client teaching about tetracycline?
5. What types of antibacterial drugs are aminoglycosides?
6. What two types of toxicities are related to aminoglycosides? What signs and symptoms should the nurse assess?
7. Fluoroquinolones are used to treat what health problems?
8. Name four GI problems associated with a fluoroquinolone such as ciprofloxacin.

Antibacterials: Sulfonamides

27

Outline

Objectives

- Differentiate between short-acting and intermediate-acting sulfonamides.
- Describe the uses, side effects, and adverse reactions to all the sulfonamides and co-trimoxazole.
- Explain the nursing interventions, including client teaching, related to sulfonamides.

Terms

bacteriostatic

cross-sensitivity

crystalluria

erythema multiforme

exfoliative dermatitis

photosensitivity

synergistic effect

INTRODUCTION

Sulfonamides are one of the oldest antibacterial agents used to combat infection. When penicillin was marketed initially, the sulfonamide drugs were not widely prescribed because penicillin was considered the "miracle drug." However, new sulfonamides and the combination drug of sulfonamide with an antibacterial agent in such preparations as trimethoprim-sulfamethoxazole (Bactrim, Septra) have increased the usage of sulfonamides.

SULFONAMIDES

Sulfonamides were first isolated from the coal tar analine compound in the early 1900s and were produced for clinical use against coccal infections in 1935. It was the first group of drugs used against bacteria. Sulfonamides are not classified as an antibiotic because they were not obtained from biologic substances. The sulfonamides are **bacteriostatic,** acting by inhibiting bacterial synthesis of folic acid, which is essential for bacterial growth. Humans do not synthesize folic acid but acquire it through diet; therefore, sulfonamides selectively inhibit bacterial growth without affecting normal cells. Folic acid (folate) is required by cells for biosynthesis of RNA, DNA, and proteins.

The clinical usefulness of sulfonamides has decreased because the availability and effectiveness of penicillin and other antibiotics has increased and bacterial resistance to some sulfonamides can develop. Sulfonamides may be an alternative drug for clients who are allergic to penicillin. They are still used in treating urinary tract and ear infections and may be used for newborn eye prophylaxis. Sulfonamides are not effective against viruses and fungi.

Sulfonamides are approximately 90% effective against *Escherichia coli;* therefore, they are frequently a preferred treatment for urinary tract infections, which are often caused by *E. coli.* They are also useful in the treatment of meningococcal meningitis, and the organisms *Chlamydia* and *Toxoplasma gondii.*

Pharmacokinetics and Pharmacodynamics

Many of the sulfonamides are for oral administration because they are absorbed readily by the gastrointestinal (GI) tract. They also are available in solution and ointment for ophthalmic use and in cream form, silver sulfadiazine (Silvadene) and mafenide acetate (Sulfamylon), for burns. Sulfonamide drugs are well distributed to body tissues and the brain. The liver metabolizes the sulfonamide drug, and the kidneys excrete it.

Most of the early sulfonamides were highly protein-bound and displaced other drugs by competing for protein sites. There are two categories of sulfonamides, classified according to their duration of action:

- Short-acting sulfonamides (rapid absorption and excretion rate)
- Intermediate-acting sulfonamides (moderate to slow absorption and a slow excretion rate)

Sulfisoxazole (Gantrisin) is a water-soluble sulfonamide that is effective in treating most uncomplicated urinary tract infections. It is also useful, along with sulfadiazine, in prophylaxis treatment of streptococcal infections in clients with rheumatic fever who are hypersensitive to penicillin. Sulfadiazine is poorly soluble in urine and can cause crystallization, which could damage the kidneys if there is insufficient fluid

Table 27–1
Pharmacokinetics of Selected Sulfonamides

DRUG	PROTEIN-BINDING (%)	HALF-LIFE	SOLUBILITY IN URINE
SHORT-ACTING			
Sulfadiazine (Microsulfon)	20–60	17 h	+1
Sulfamethizole (Thiosulfil)	90	2.5 h	+3
Sulfisoxazole (Gantrisin)	90	5–7.5 h	+3
INTERMEDIATE-ACTING			
Sulfamethoxazole (Gantanol)	85–90	11 h	+1
Sulfasalazine (Azulfidine)	99	5–10 h	+1
Trimethoprim-sulfamethoxazole	50–65	8–12 h	+1–2

and water intake. Sulfamethoxazole (Gantanol), an intermediate-acting sulfonamide, has a longer duration of action than other sulfonamides; however, it has poorer water solubility than sulfisoxazole. Table 27–1 lists the protein-binding, half-life, and solubility in urine of most of the sulfonamide group.

The only combination of sulfonamides that is still marketed but infrequently used is trisulfapyrimides. This triple sulfa drug is a combination of low doses of sulfadiazine, sulfamerazine, and sulfamethazine. The three drugs have an additive effect, which increases the potency of the drug. It has a longer duration of action than other sulfonamides and is considered to be poorly soluble in water. With the low doses of the three drugs, crystal formation in the urine is less likely to occur. Older sulfonamides, such as sulfadiazine, have low solubility and may cause crystallization in the urine. The current sulfonamides have a greater water solubility, such as sulfisoxazole; therefore, crystal formations in the urine and renal damage are unlikely. Table 27–2 lists and describes the sulfonamides.

Table 27–2
Antibacterials: Sulfonamides

GENERIC (BRAND)	ROUTE AND DOSAGE	USES AND CONSIDERATIONS
SHORT-ACTING		
Sulfadiazine (Microsulfon)	A: PO: LD: 2–4 g; then 2–4 g/d in 4 divided doses C: PO: LD: 75 mg/kg or 2 g/m²; then 150 mg/kg/d in 4–6 divided doses	For treatment of systemic infections. This drug could be classified as a short–immediate-acting sulfonamide. When taking this drug, increase the fluid intake to >2000 mL/d. *Pregnancy category:* C; PB: 20%–30%; $t_\frac{1}{2}$: 8–12 h
Sulfamethizole (Sulfasol, Thiosulfil Forte)	A: PO: 0.5–1 g in 3–4 divided doses C: PO: 30–45 mg/kg/d in 4 divided doses	For treatment of urinary tract infections. It is highly soluble. Fluid intake should be at least 2000 mL/d. *Pregnancy category:* C; PB: 90%; $t_\frac{1}{2}$: 1.5 h
Sulfisoxazole (Gantrisin)	A: PO: LD: 2–4 g; then 4–8 g/d in 4–6 divided doses C: PO: LD: 75 mg/kg or 2 g/m²; then 150 mg/kg/d in 4–6 divided doses	Popular drug for treating urinary tract infections because it is more soluble in urine. Rapidly absorbed from GI tract. Used for treatment and prophylaxis of otitis media. Often ordered with a one-time initial loading dose. Fluid intake ≥2000 mL/d. *Pregnancy category:* C; PB: 85%–95%; $t_\frac{1}{2}$: 4.5–7.5 h
INTERMEDIATE-ACTING		
Sulfamethoxazole (Gantanol)	A: PO: LD: 2 g; then 2–3 g/d in 2–3 divided doses for 7–10 d C: PO: LD: 50–60 mg/kg; then 25–30 mg/kg q12h; *max:* 75 mg/kg/d	For urinary tract infections, otitis media, and meningococcal A strain meningitis prophylaxis. Similar to Gantrisin, except it is absorbed and excreted slowly. Fluid intake should be at least 2000 mL/d. *Pregnancy category:* C; PB: 60%–70%; $t_\frac{1}{2}$: 7–12 h
Sulfasalazine (Azulfidine, Salazoprine)	A: PO: Initially: 1 g q6–8h; maint: 2 g q6h C: >2 y: PO: Initially: 40–60 mg/kg/d in 4–6 divided doses; maint: 20–30 mg/kg/d in 4 divided doses; *max:* 2 g/d	For treatment of ulcerative colitis, Crohn's disease, rheumatoid arthritis (some cases). Take after eating. Side effects include nausea, vomiting, bloody diarrhea. *Pregnancy category:* C (near term: D); PB: 99%; $t_\frac{1}{2}$: 5.5 h
Trimethoprim-sulfamethoxazole: co-trimoxazole (Bactrim, Septra)	See Chart 27–1	For urinary tract and ear infections. Single-strength tablet contains 80 mg of trimethoprim (T) and 400 mg of sulfamethoxazole (S). Drug of choice for treating *Pneumocystis carinii* pneumonia. Most frequently used as a sulfonamide. *Pregnancy category:* C (near term: D); PB: 50%–65%; $t_\frac{1}{2}$: 8–12 h
LONG-ACTING		
Sulfamethoxypyridazine (Kynex, Midicel)		No longer used owing to very slow excretion rate and toxicity.
Sulfameter (Sulla)		Same as for sulfamethoxypyridazine

KEY: A: adult; C: child; LD: loading dose; PB: protein-binding; PO: by mouth; (S): sulfamethoxazole; (T): trimethoprim; $t_\frac{1}{2}$ half-life; >: greater than.

NURSING PROCESS
ANTIBACTERIALS: SULFONAMIDES

Assessment

- Assess the client's renal function by checking urinary output (>600 mL/d), blood urea nitrogen (BUN) (normal, 8 to 25 mg/dL), and serum creatinine (normal, 0.5 to 1.5 mg/dL).
- Obtain a medical history from the client. Sulfonamides such as co-trimoxazole (trimethoprim-sulfamethoxazole [Bactrim, Septra]) are contraindicated for clients with severe renal or liver disease.
- Assess whether the client is hypertensive to sulfonamides. An allergic reaction can include rash, skin eruptions, and itching. A severe hypersensitivity reaction includes **erythema multiforme** (erythematous macular, papular, or vesicular eruption; if severe, can cover the entire body) or **exfoliative dermatitis** (desquamation, scaling, and itching of skin).
- Obtain a drug history of drugs the client is currently taking. Oral antidiabetic drugs (sulfonylureas) with sulfonamides increase the hypoglycemic effect; the use of warfarin with sulfonamides increases the anticoagulant effect.
- Assess baseline laboratory results, especially complete blood count (CBC). Blood dyscrasias may occur as a result of high doses of sulfonamides over a continuous period of time, causing life-threatening conditions.

Potential Nursing Diagnoses

- Risk for infection
- Risk for impaired tissue integrity
- Altered patterns of urinary elimination

Planning

- Client's infection will be controlled and later alleviated.

Nursing Interventions

- Administer sulfonamides with a full glass of water. Extra fluid intake can prevent crystalluria and kidney stone formation.
- Monitor the client's intake and output. Urine output should be at least 1200 mL/d to decrease the risk of crystalluria. The sulfonamides sulfadiazine and sulfamethoxazole are more likely to cause crystalluria than are sulfisoxazole (Gantrisin) and combination drugs. Fluid intake should be at least 2000 mL/d.

Nursing Process continued on following page

Side Effects and Adverse Reactions

The side effects of sulfonamides may include an allergic response, such as skin rash and itching. Anaphylaxis is not common. Blood disorders, such as hemolytic anemia, aplastic anemia, and low white blood cell and platelet counts, could result from prolonged use and high dosages. GI disturbances (anorexia, nausea, and vomiting) may also occur. The early sulfonamides were insoluble in acid urine; thus, **crystalluria** (crystals in urine) and hematuria were common problems. Crystalluria occurs less commonly with sulfisoxazole (Gantrisin) than it does with sulfadiazine and sulfamethoxazole. Increasing fluid intake dilutes the drug, which helps to prevent crystalluria from occur-

ring. **Photosensitivity** can occur, so the client should avoid sunbathing and excess ultraviolet light. **Cross-sensitivity** might occur with the different sulfonamides, but does not occur with other antibacterial drugs. Sulfonamides should be avoided during the third trimester of pregnancy.

Trimethoprim and Co-Trimoxazole

Trimethoprim (Proloprim, Trimpex) is an antibacterial agent that interferes with bacterial folic acid synthesis similarly to sulfonamides. Trimethoprim is classified as a urinary tract antiinfective that may be used alone for uncomplicated urinary tract infections. This drug

- Monitor vital signs (VS). Note if the client's temperature has decreased.
- Observe the client for hematologic reaction that may lead to life-threatening anemias. Early signs are sore throat, purpura, and decreasing white blood cell and platelet counts. Check the client's CBC and compare with baseline findings.
- Check for signs and symptoms of superinfection (secondary infection caused by a different organism than the primary infection). Symptoms include stomatitis (mouth ulcers), furry black tongue, anal or genital discharge, and itching.

Client Teaching

General
- Instruct the client to drink several quarts of fluid daily while taking sulfonamides to avoid the complication of crystalluria.
- Advise the pregnant woman to avoid sulfonamides during the last 3 months of pregnancy.
- Instruct the client not to take antacids with sulfonamides because antacids decrease the absorption rate.
- Advise the client who has an allergy to one sulfonamide that all sulfonamide preparations should be avoided, with the health care provider's approval, because of the possibility of cross-sensitivity. Observe the client for rash or any skin eruptions.

Self-Administration
- Instruct the client to take the sulfonamide 1 h before or 2 h after meals with a full glass of water.

Side Effects
- Instruct the client to report bruising or bleeding that could be a result of drug-induced blood disorder. Advise the client to have blood cell count monitored on a regular basis.
- Advise the client to avoid direct sunlight and to use sunblock and protective clothing to decrease the risk of photosensitive reactions.

Cultural Considerations

- Respect cultural beliefs and values regarding alternative methods for treating infections. Explain the purpose of the drug therapy and how often the drug should be taken.
- Communicate that the client should increase fluid intake to 10 to 12 glasses per day. Written instructions may be necessary if the client's cultural background prevents understanding of the health problem and drug regimen.

Evaluation
- Evaluate the effectiveness of the sulfonamide by determining whether the infection has been alleviated and the blood cell count is within normal range.

---

is effective against the gram-negative bacteria *Proteus* spp., *Klebsiella* spp., and *E. coli.* In the 1970s, it was combined with the sulfonamide sulfamethoxazole (an intermediate-acting sulfonamide) to prevent bacterial resistance to sulfonamide drugs and to obtain a better response against many organisms. Giving both drugs together in one compound form causes bacterial resistance to develop much more slowly than if one of the drugs were used alone. This combination drug, trimethoprim-sulfamethoxazole (TMP-SMX) (co-trimoxazole; Bactrim, Septra) is commonly used. The drug ratio is 1:5; one part trimethoprim and 5 parts sulfamethoxazole. The two drugs have a **synergistic effect,** increasing the desired drug response.

Co-trimoxazole is effective in treating urinary, intestinal, and lower respiratory tract infections; otitis media; prostatitis; and gonorrhea; and in preventing *Pneumocystis carinii* in clients with AIDS. Increased fluid intake is highly recommended to prevent any complication such as crystallization in the urine. Chart 27–1 describes the pharmacologic behavior of co-trimoxazole.

PHARMACOKINETICS
Co-trimoxazole (Bactrim, Septra) is well absorbed from the gastrointestinal (GI) tract and is moderately

Chart 27–1.   Antibacterials: Sulfonamides (Trimethoprim-Sulfamethoxazole)

CO-TRIMOXAZOLE

Drug Name	**Dosage**	**Assessment and Planning**

Drug Name

Co-trimoxazole (Bactrim, Septra)
Sulfonamide: trimethoprim (TMP)–sulfamethox-azole (SMZ)
Pregnancy Category: C

Dosage

A: PO: 160/800 mg q12h (160 mg [TMP]/800 mg [SMZ])
C: PO: 8/40 mg q12h (8 mg [TMP]/40 mg [SMZ])
Dosing is based on trimethoprim component

Contraindications

Severe renal or hepatic disease, hypersensitivity to sulfonamides

Drug-Lab-Food Interactions

Drug: *Increase* anticoagulant effect with warfarin; *increase* hypoglycemic effect with an oral hypoglycemic drug
Lab: May *increase* BUN, serum creatinine, AST, ALT, ALP

Pharmacokinetics

Absorption: PO: Well absorbed
Distribution: PB: 50%–65%; crosses placenta
Metabolism: t½: 8–12 h
Excretion: In urine as metabolites

Pharmacodynamics

PO: Onset: 0.5–1 h
        Peak: 2–4 h
        Duration: UK
IV: Onset: Immediate
        Peak: 0.5–1 h
        Duration: UK

NURSING PROCESS — Interventions

Therapeutic Effects/Uses

To treat urinary tract infection, otitis media, bronchitis, pneumonia, *Pneumocystis carinii* infection, rheumatic fever, burns.

Mode of Action: Inhibition of protein synthesis of nucleic acids. Bactericidal effect.

Side Effects

Anorexia, nausea, vomiting, diarrhea, rash, stomatitis, fatigue, depression, headache, vertigo, photosensitivity

Adverse Reactions

Life-threatening: Leukopenia, thrombocytopenia, increased bone marrow depression, hemolytic anemia, aplastic anemia, agranulocytosis, Stevens-Johnson syndrome, renal failure

Evaluation

Note: Sulfa drugs should *not* be used in infants <2 mo.
KEY: TMP: trimethoprim; SMZ: sulfamethoxazole; A: adult; C: child; PO: by mouth; UK: unknown; IV: intravenous; PB: protein-binding; t½: half-life; BUN: blood urea nitrogen; AST: aspartate aminotransferase; ALT: alanine aminotransferase; ALP: alkaline phosphatase.

protein-bound. Its half-life is 8 to 12 h; thus, it is administered twice a day. It is excreted as unchanged metabolites in the urine.

PHARMACODYNAMICS

Co-trimoxazole is a combination of trimethoprim and sulfamethoxazole. Trimethoprim, a nonsulfonamide antibiotic, enhances the activity of the drug combination. Co-trimoxazole blocks steps in bacterial synthe-

sis of protein and nucleic acid, producing a bactericidal effect.

Co-trimoxazole can be administered orally or intravenously. Orally, the drug has a moderately rapid onset of action, and intravenously the drug action is immediate. Serum peak concentration time for oral use is 2 to 4 h and shorter for intravenous use, 0.5 to 1.0 h. Co-trimoxazole, when taken with an oral hypoglycemic agent sulfonylurea, increases the hypoglycemic response. It can also increase the activity of oral anticoagulants.

SIDE EFFECTS AND ADVERSE REACTIONS

Side effects of co-trimoxazole may include mild to moderate rashes, anorexia, nausea, vomiting and diarrhea, stomatitis, crystalluria, and photosensitivity. Serious adverse reactions are rare; however, agranulocytosis, aplastic anemia, and allergic myocarditis have been reported as possible life-threatening conditions.

Topical and Ophthalmic Sulfonamides

Sulfonamides can be administered for topical and ophthalmic uses. Topical use of sulfonamides can cause hypersensitivity reactions; therefore, they are not frequently used. Mafenide acetate (Sulfamylon) is

a sulfonamide derivative prescribed for second- and third-degree burns to prevent sepsis. Silver sulfadiazine (Silvadene) is another topical sulfonamide used in treatment of burns. Both of these drugs are discussed in more detail in Chapter 44.

Sulfacetamide sodium (AK-Sulf, Cetamide, Isopto Cetamide, Sodium Sulamyd, Sulf-10) is a sulfonamide for ophthalmic and topical uses. For the ophthalmic preparations (liquid/drop and ointment), sulfacetamide sodium is used to treat conjunctivitis and corneal ulcers, and is used as prophylactic treatment after eye injury or removal of a foreign body. Do *not* use ointment for the eye unless it has "ophthalmic" printed on the drug label. This drug is discussed in more detail in Chapter 43.

Topical sulfacetamide sodium for the skin is an ointment and is used to treat seborrheic dermatitis and secondary bacterial skin infections. This form is *not* used for the eye.

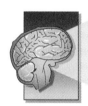

Critical Thinking in Action

R. M., age 46 years, has a severe urinary tract infection (UTI). She is taking co-trimoxazole 160 mg/800 mg, every 6 hours.

1. Is the drug dose within recommended drug dose and dosing interval? What is the nurse's responsibility?
2. What are the similarities and differences of trimethoprim-sulfamethoxazole (co-trimoxazole) and sulfisoxazole?
3. What are the signs of thrombocytopenia, hemolytic anemia, and agranulocytosis for clients who are on high doses of sulfonamides? Explain the assessment and nursing interventions in regard to these severe adverse reactions to sulfonamides.

Client teaching is an important part of nursing interventions. Explain the nurse's role in regard to client teaching concerning the following:

4. The required amount of daily fluid intake that should be taken
5. Cross-sensitive effects if allergic to other sulfonamide preparations; allergic reaction may include _____.
6. The time of day for taking the sulfonamide
7. Reporting bruising, bleeding. Why?

8. Protective measures to take to prevent effects from possible photosensitive reaction

R. M. is taking the anticoagulant Coumadin 7.5 mg daily.

9. What effect does co-trimoxazole have on warfarin and what is the nursing responsibility? Should R. M.'s Coumadin dosage be increased or decreased? Explain.

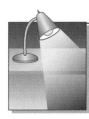

Study Questions

1. Why would a nurse instruct a client taking a sulfonamide to increase fluid intake? Why is the use of sunblock lotion indicated for sun exposure for a client taking a sulfonamide drug?

2. If your client is allergic to a sulfonamide drug, what should you advise the client about the use of other sulfonamides?

3. What is the generic name for Gantrisin? What is its main clinical use? Is it classified as a short-acting, intermediate-acting, or long-acting sulfonamide?

4. What is the purpose of the drug trimethoprim-sulfamethoxazole/co-trimoxazole (Bactrim, Septra)?

5. Your client is taking a sulfonylurea (oral hypoglycemic to promote insulin production). What effect may co-trimoxazole have on the sulfonylurea? What is the nurse's responsibility if the client is receiving both drugs?

6. What effects can co-trimoxazole have on the following laboratory tests: AST, ALT, ALP, BUN, serum creatinine?

7. What hematologic conditions can occur because of excessive or long-term use of sulfonamides such as co-trimoxazole?

Antitubercular Drugs, Antifungal Drugs, Peptides, and Metronidazole

28

Outline

Objectives

- Differentiate between first-line and second-line antitubercular drugs and give examples of each.
- Name the three classes of antifungal drugs.
- Identify examples of polyenes and explain their uses.
- Describe the adverse reactions of antitubercular, antifungal, and peptide drugs.
- Describe the nursing interventions, including client teaching, for clients taking antitubercular drugs, antifungal drugs, and peptides.

Terms

AIDS

antifungal drugs

antimycotic

antitubercular drugs

first-line drugs

hepatotoxicity

HIV infection

neurotoxicity

opportunistic infection

paresthesias

peptides

prophylaxis

second-line drugs

INTRODUCTION

Antitubercular, antifungal, and peptide drugs are presented in this chapter. Although these categories of drugs differ from each other, these drugs inhibit or kill organisms that cause diseases.

This chapter includes a drug table and nursing process for each of the three categories of drugs. Prototype drugs for antitubercular drugs and antifungal drugs are included.

TUBERCULOSIS

Tuberculosis (TB) is caused by the acid-fast bacillus *Mycobacterium tuberculosis.* The pathogen is frequently referred to as the tubercle bacillus. TB is one of the major health problems in the world and kills more persons than any other infectious disease. More than 1½ billion people in the world have tuberculosis and many do not know it. Each year there are more than 8 million new cases of tuberculosis. The occurrence of TB had decreased in the United States until the 1980s. The increase in TB can be attributed, in part, to the increased number of persons with **acquired immunodeficiency syndrome (AIDS)** in whom active tuberculosis has developed because of their compromised immune system. Also, the increasing incidence is partly due to the increasingly crowded living conditions in urban areas. Clients susceptible to TB are those with alcohol addiction, those with AIDS, and those with debilitative conditions. Since 1993, there has been a slight decline in the reported numbers of clients with active tuberculosis.

Tuberculosis is transmitted from one person to another by droplets dispersed in the air through coughing and sneezing. The organisms are inhaled into the alveoli (air sacs) of the lung. The tubercle bacilli can spread from the lungs to other organs of the body via the blood and lymphatic system. If the body's immune system is strong or intact, the phagocytes stop the multiplication of the tubercle bacilli. When the immune system is compromised, the tubercle bacilli spread in the lungs and to other organs. Dissemination of tuberculosis bacilli can be found in the liver, kidneys, spleen, and other organs. Symptoms of tuberculosis include anorexia, cough and sputum production, increased fever, night sweats, weight loss, and positive acid-fast bacilli in the sputum.

ANTITUBERCULAR DRUGS

Before 1944, many people died from tuberculosis because of the absence of drug therapy. Streptomycin, a parenteral antibiotic, was the first drug used for treating TB. Isoniazid (INH) was discovered in 1952 and was the first oral drug preparation effective against the tubercle bacillus. Group names for drugs used in treating tuberculosis include antimycobacterial agents and **antitubercular drugs.**

Prophylactic antitubercular therapy is suggested for persons who have been in close contact with those with TB and human immunodeficiency virus (HIV)-positive persons who have a positive TB skin test or close contact with a person with TB. Clients who have converted from a negative to a positive TB skin test should be considered candidates for prophylactic INH therapy. Young children who have been in contact with persons with active TB are at high risk and should receive prophylactic antitubercular therapy. When a person is given the diagnosis of tuberculosis, the family members are usually given prophylactic doses of isoniazid (INH) for 6 months to a year.

Table 28–1
Various Possible Drug Regimens for the Treatment of Tuberculosis

PHASE	EXAMPLE I	EXAMPLE II	EXAMPLE III	EXAMPLE IV
First phase (2 mo)*	Isoniazid, rifampin	Isoniazid rifampin, pyrazinamide	Isoniazid, rifampin, streptomycin	Isoniazid, rifampin, pyrazinamide, kanamycin or ciprofloxacin
Second phase (4–7 mo)	Isoniazid, rifampin	Isoniazid, rifampin, ethambutol	Isoniazid, rifampin, capreomycin or cycloserine	Isoniazid, rifampin, ethambutol, streptomycin or kanamycin or ciprofloxacin or clarithromycin or capreomycin

If there is bacterial resistance to isoniazid (INH), then the first phase of the drug regimen may be rifampin, ethambutol, and pyrazinamide. Adjust drug regimen according to drug susceptibility. The health care provider determines which antitubercular drug and how many combinations to use. Symptoms for drug toxicity should be closely monitored. Examples III and IV may be used in various combinations for multidrug resistance.

Chart 28–1. Antitubercular Drugs

ISONIAZID

NURSING PROCESS

Assessment and Planning

Drug Name

Isoniazid (INH, Nydrazid, Laniazid), 🍁 Isotamine, PMS, Isoniazid
Pregnancy Category: C

Dosage

A: PO/IM: 5–10 mg/kg/d in a single dose; *max:* 300 mg/d
Prophylaxis: 300 mg/d
C: PO/IM: 10–20 mg/kg/d in a single dose; *max:* 300 mg/d
Prophylaxis: 10 mg/kg/d in a single dose

Contraindications

Severe renal or hepatic disease, alcoholism, diabetic retinopathy

Drug-Lab-Food Interactions

Drug: *Increase* effect with alcohol, rifampin, cycloserine
Lab: *Increase* AST, ALT, bilirubin

Interventions

Pharmacokinetics

Absorption: PO: Well absorbed
Distribution: PB: 10%
Metabolism: $t\frac{1}{2}$: 1–4 h
Excretion: 50% unchanged in urine

Pharmacodynamics

PO: Onset: 0.5 h
Peak: 1–2 h
Duration: PO: 6–8 h
IM: 6 h

Evaluation

Therapeutic Effects/Uses

To treat tuberculosis; prophylactic measure against tuberculosis.

Mode of Action: Inhibition of bacterial cell wall synthesis.

Side Effects

Drowsiness, tremors, rash, blurred vision, photosensitivity

Adverse Reactions

Psychotic behavior, peripheral neuropathy, vitamin B_6 deficiency
Life-threatening: Blood dyscrasias, thrombocytopenia, seizures, agranulocytosis, hepatotoxicity

KEY: A: adult; C: child; PO: by mouth; IM: intramuscular; PB: protein-binding; $t\frac{1}{2}$: half-life; 🍁: Canadian drug name; ALT: alanine aminotransferase; AST: aspartate aminotransferase.

Prophylactic therapy is contraindicated for those persons with liver disease. Isoniazid is the primary drug used and may cause isoniazid-induced liver damage. Other antitubercular drugs may also cause liver damage if given in high doses over an extended period of time.

Single-drug therapy with isoniazid proved to be ineffective in treating tuberculosis because resistance to the drug developed in a short time. It was discovered that, by using a combination of antitubercular drugs, bacterial resistance did not occur. In fact, the duration of treatment was reduced from 2 years to 6 to 9 months. Different combinations of drugs can be used, for example, isoniazid and rifampin, or isoniazid, rifampin, and ethambutol, or isoniazid, rifampin, and pyrazinamide. Rifampin and ethambutol were discovered in the early 1960s and either drug given alone is not effective against the tubercle bacillus. In fact, if rifampin is taken alone, bacterial resistance occurs quickly.

Multidrug therapy against tuberculosis is more effective. The treatment regimen is divided into two phases, the first or the initial phase is for 2 months, and the second phase is the next 4 to 7 months. The total treatment plan is for 6 to 9 months and depends on the response to the antitubercular therapy. Table 28–1 gives examples of various drug treatment regimens for treating tuberculosis.

Table 28-2
Antitubercular Drugs

GENERIC (BRAND)	ROUTE AND DOSAGE	USES AND CONSIDERATIONS
FIRST-LINE DRUGS		
Ethambutol HCl (Myambutol)	A: PO: 15 mg/kg as a single dose *Retreatment* A: PO: 25 mg/kg as a single dose for 2 mo; then decrease to 15 mg/kg/d C: >12 y: same as adult	Used as a combination drug for active tuberculosis. Decrease dose if renal insufficiency is present. *Pregnancy category:* C; PB: 10%–20%; $t_{\frac{1}{2}}$: 3–4 h (8 h with renal dysfunction)
Isoniazid (INH, Nydrazid)	See Chart 28-1	Used in combination drug therapy against active tuberculosis. For prophylactic use against tuberculosis, vitamin B_6 frequently given to prevent peripheral neuropathy and when isoniazid is given on an extended basis. *Pregnancy category:* C; PB: 10%; $t_{\frac{1}{2}}$: 1–4 h
Pyrazinamide (Tebrazid; Canadian drug)	A: PO: 20–35 mg/kg/d in 3–4 divided doses; *max:* 3 g/d	Second-line antitubercular drug. Used in combination with other antitubercular drugs for short-term and initial phase of therapy. Promote fluid intake. *Pregnancy category:* C; PB: 10%–20%; $t_{\frac{1}{2}}$: 9.5 h
Rifampin (Rifadin, Rimactane)	A: PO: 600 mg/d as a single dose C: PO: 10–20 mg/kg/d as a single dose; *max:* 600 mg/d	Used as a combination drug for active tuberculosis. For selective gram-positive and gram-negative bacteria, including *Neisseria meningitidis*. Liver enzymes should be monitored. *Pregnancy category:* C; PB: 85%–90%; $t_{\frac{1}{2}}$: 3 h
Streptomycin SO_4	A: IM: 1 g daily or 7–15 mg/kg/d for 2–3 mo, then 2–3 × wk C: IM: 20–40 mg/kg/d in divided doses	Used against tuberculosis as the third drug with isoniazid and rifampin or with isoniazid and ethambutol. First drug use to treat tuberculosis. *Pregnancy category:* C; PB: 30%; $t_{\frac{1}{2}}$: 2–3 h
SECOND-LINE DRUGS		
Aminosalicylate sodium, P.A.S. sodium	A: PO: 14–16 g/d in 2–3 divided doses C: PO: 275–420 mg/kg/d in 3–4 divided doses; take with food	Second-line antitubercular drug. To treat pulmonary and extrapulmonary tuberculosis. Used in combination with other antitubercular drugs. Take after meals to reduce gastric irritation. *Pregnancy category:* C; PB: 15%; $t_{\frac{1}{2}}$: 1 h
Capreomycin (Capastat)	A: IM: 1 g/d for 2–4 mo, then 1 g, 2–3 × per week C: IM: 15 mg/kg/d	It is sensitive to the bacillus *Mycobacterium tuberculosis*. It should be used in combination with other antitubercular drugs; it is not effective when used alone. It is useful when the first-line drug is resistant to the bacilli. Hearing loss is an adverse reaction. Client should take pyridoxine (vitamin B_6) to avoid peripheral neuropathy. *Pregnancy category:* C; PB: UK; $t_{\frac{1}{2}}$: 3–6 h
Cycloserine (Seromycin)	A: PO: 200 mg q12h for 2 wks; *max:* 1 g/d C: PO: 10–20 mg/kg/d in divided doses	Broad-spectrum antimycobacterial drug for the treatment of tuberculosis. It is a second-line drug and used when first-line drugs fail. Cycloserine should be used in combination with other antitubercular drugs. *Pregnancy category:* C; PB: UK; $t_{\frac{1}{2}}$: 10 h
Ethionamide (Trecator-SC)	A: PO: 250 mg, q8–12h C: PO: 4–5 mg/kg/q8h	Like INH, it is effective against the tubercle bacilli. It is used when the first-line drugs fail. Client should take pyridoxine to avoid peripheral neuropathy. Side effects include GI discomfort. Use with *caution* in persons with diabetes mellitus, alcoholism, and hepatic disorder. *Pregnancy category:* D; PB: UK; $t_{\frac{1}{2}}$: 2–3 h

Table continued on following page

Table 28–2 *Continued*
Antitubercular Drugs

GENERIC (BRAND)	ROUTE AND DOSAGE	USES AND CONSIDERATIONS
Rifabutin (Mycobutin)	A: PO: 300 mg/d in 1 or 2 divided doses	To treat *Mycobacterium tuberculosis* infection; to prevent disseminated *Mycobacterium avium* complex (MAC) disease in clients with advanced HIV infection. *Pregnancy category:* B; PB: 85%; $t_{\frac{1}{2}}$: 16–69 h

OTHER SECOND-LINE DRUGS

Kanamycin, amikacin, ciprofloxacin, and ofloxacin are effective against the tubercle bacilli when used in combination with antitubercular drugs. See Chapter 26.

KEY: A: adult; C: child; PO: by mouth; IM: intramuscular; PB: protein-binding; $t_{\frac{1}{2}}$: half-life; >: greater than.

If multidrug resistance to the tubercle bacilli persists, then other antibacterial drugs such as the aminoglycosides (streptomycin, kanamycin, amikacin) or the fluoroquinolones (ciprofloxacin, ofloxacin) may be given as part of the multidrug therapy. Susceptibility testing to determine drug resistance should be performed before drug therapy. At times susceptibility testing of the sputum and antitubercular drugs is performed only if the client has not responded to the drug therapy regimen.

Mycobacterium tuberculosis strains that are resistant to streptomycin can be sensitive to kanamycin. An aminoglycoside should not be taken if renal dysfunction is present. When antibacterial agents that are used continuously or at high doses are prescribed, the serum drug level should be closely monitored to avoid drug toxicity.

Isoniazid (INH) is the most frequently prescribed antitubercular drug for treating tuberculosis. Chart 28–1 lists the drug data for isoniazid.

Pharmacokinetics

Isoniazid is well absorbed from the gastrointestinal (GI) tract. It can also be administered intramuscularly and intravenously. It has a very low protein-binding rate (10%), and its half-life is 1 to 4 h. Isoniazid is metabolized by the liver, and 75% to 95% of the drug is excreted in the urine.

Pharmacodynamics

Isoniazid inhibits cell wall synthesis of the tubercle bacillus. It is usually prescribed with other antitubercular agents. The onset of action and peak concentration time for oral and intramuscular routes of isoniazid are the same. Peripheral neuropathy is an adverse reaction to isoniazid; thus, *pyridoxine, vitamin B_6,* is usually taken with isoniazid to decrease the probability of neuropathy. Alcohol ingestion with the

drug can increase the incidence of peripheral neuropathy. If phenytoin is taken with isoniazid, the effect of phenytoin may be decreased. Antacids decrease isoniazid absorption.

Antitubercular drugs in the treatment of TB are divided into two categories, first-line and second-line drugs. **First-line drugs** (isoniazid, rifampin, ethambutol, and streptomycin) are considered to be more effective and less toxic than second-line drugs in treating TB. **Second-line drugs** (*para*-aminosalicylic acid, kanamycin, cycloserine, ethionamide, capreomycin, pyrazinamide, and others) are not as effective as first-line drugs and some can be more toxic. Second-line drugs may be used in combination with first-line drugs, especially to treat disseminated TB. First-line drugs and some second-line drugs are described in Table 28–2.

Side Effects and Adverse Reactions

Side effects and adverse reactions differ according to the drug prescribed. For isoniazid, peripheral neuropathy can be a problem, especially to the malnourished, those with diabetes mellitus, and alcoholics. Peripheral neuropathy can be prevented by giving pyridoxine (vitamin B_6). **Hepatotoxicity** is an adverse reaction to isoniazid, from which hepatitis can result. Clients with liver disorders should not take isoniazid or isoniazid and rifampin unless liver enzymes are closely monitored. Rifampin can increase liver enzyme levels.

ANTIFUNGAL DRUGS

Antifungal drugs, also called **antimycotic drugs,** are used to treat two types of fungal infections. (1) superficial fungal infections of the skin or mucous membrane and (2) systemic fungal infections of the lung or central nervous system. Fungal infections may be

NURSING PROCESS
ANTITUBERCULAR DRUGS

Assessment

- Obtain a history from the client of any past instances of tuberculosis, last purified protein derivative (PPD) tuberculin test and reaction, last chest x-ray and result, and allergy to any of the antitubercular drugs if taken previously.
- Obtain a medical history from the client. Most antitubercular drugs are contraindicated if the client has a severe hepatic disease.
- Check laboratory tests for liver enzyme values, bilirubin, blood urea nitrogen (BUN), and serum creatinine. These baseline values can be compared with future laboratory test results.
- Assess the client for signs and symptoms of peripheral neuropathy, such as numbness or tingling of the extremities.
- Check the client for hearing changes if the antitubercular drug regimen includes streptomycin. Ototoxicity is an adverse reaction to streptomycin.

Potential Nursing Diagnoses

- Risk for infection
- Risk for impaired tissue integrity

Planning

- Client's sputum test for acid-fast bacilli will be negative in 2 to 3 mo after the prescribed antitubercular therapy.

Nursing Interventions

- Administer the commonly ordered antitubercular drug isoniazid (INH) 1 h before or 2 h after meals. Food decreases absorption rate.
- Administer pyridoxine (vitamin B$_6$) as prescribed with isoniazid to prevent peripheral neuropathy.
- Monitor serum liver enzyme levels, especially if the client is taking isoniazid or rifampin. Elevated levels may indicate liver toxicity.
- Collect sputum specimens for acid-fast bacilli early in the morning. Usually three consecutive morning sputum specimens are sent to the laboratory, and the routine is repeated several weeks later.
- Have eye examinations performed on clients taking isoniazid and ethambutol. Visual disturbances may result in clients taking these antitubercular drugs.
- Emphasize the importance of complying with drug regimen.

mild, such as tinea pedis (athlete's foot), or severe, as in pulmonary conditions or meningitis. Fungi, such as *Candida* spp. (yeast), are part of the normal flora of the mouth, skin, intestine, and vagina. Candidiasis might occur as an opportunistic infection when the body's defense mechanisms are impaired, allowing for overgrowth of the fungus. Drugs such as antibiotics, oral contraceptives, and immunosuppressives may also alter the body's defense mechanisms. Opportunistic fungal infections can be mild (yeast infection in the vagina) or severe (systemic fungal infection).

The antifungal drugs are classified into four groups (Table 28–3):

- Polyenes, including amphotericin B and nystatin
- Imidazoles, which include ketoconazole, miconazole, and clotrimazole
- The antimetabolic antifungal flucytosine
- Antiprotozoal agents

Polyenes

The polyene antifungal drug of choice for treating severe systemic infection is amphotericin B. Introduced in 1956 and used currently with close supervision because of its toxicity, amphotericin B is effective

Client Teaching

General
- Instruct the client to take the antitubercular drug such as isoniazid 1 h before meals or 2 h after meals for better absorption.
- Instruct the client to take the antitubercular drugs as prescribed. Ineffective treatment of tuberculosis might occur if the drugs are taken intermittently or discontinued when symptoms are decreased or when the client is feeling better. Compliance with the drug regimen is a must.
- Instruct the client not to take antacids while taking antitubercular drugs because they decrease the drug absorption. The client should also avoid alcohol because it may increase the risk of hepatotoxicity.
- Advise the client to keep medical appointments and to participate in sputum testing. Sputum testing is important to determine the effectiveness of the drug regimen.
- Advise the woman contemplating pregnancy to first check with her health care provider about taking the antitubercular drugs ethambutol and rifampin.

Side Effects
- Instruct the client to report any numbness, tingling, or burning of the hands and feet. Peripheral neuritis is a common side effect of isoniazid. Vitamin B$_6$ prevents peripheral neuropathy. Neuritis may not occur if the client eats a balanced diet daily.
- Advise the client to avoid direct sunlight to decrease the risk of photosensitivity. Client should use sunblock while in the sun.
- Inform the client taking rifampin that urine, feces, saliva, sputum, sweat, and tears may be a harmless red-orange color. Soft contact lenses may be permanently stained.
- Advise the client receiving ethambutol to take daily single doses to avoid visual problems. Divided doses of ethambutol may cause visual disturbances.

Cultural Considerations

- Explain to the clients from various cultural backgrounds having active tuberculosis that their family members should get a tubercular skin test and may receive prophylactic drug for 6 months to 1 year. Emphasize the importance of their family members seeking medical care.
- Provide a written sheet for their drug and treatment regimens. Explain the importance of good hygiene, such as discarding tissues that contain sputum, and separating dishes or using a dishwasher to clean dishes.

Evaluation

- Evaluate the effectiveness of the antitubercular drugs. Sputum specimen for acid-fast bacilli should be negative after taking antitubercular drugs for several weeks to months.

---

against numerous fungal diseases, including histoplasmosis, cryptococcosis, coccidioidomycosis, aspergillosis, blastomycosis, and candidiasis (systemic infection). Amphotericin B is not absorbed from the GI tract; therefore, it is administered intravenously in low doses for treating systemic fungal infections.

Amphotericin B is highly protein-bound and has a long half-life, and only 5% of the drug is excreted in the urine. Renal disease does not affect the excretion of amphotericin B.

SIDE EFFECTS AND ADVERSE REACTIONS
Side effects of and adverse reactions to amphotericin B include flushing, fever, chills, nausea, vomiting, hy-potension, paresthesias, and thrombophlebitis. Amphotericin B is considered *highly toxic* and can cause nephrotoxicity and electrolyte imbalance, especially hypokalemia and hypomagnesemia (low serum potassium and magnesium levels). Urinary output, BUN, and serum creatinine levels need to be closely monitored.

Nystatin (Mycostatin), a polyene antifungal drug, is administered orally or topically to treat candidal infection. It is available in suspensions, cream, ointment, and vaginal tablets. Nystatin is poorly absorbed via the GI tract; however, the oral tablet form is used for intestinal candidiasis. The more common use of nystatin is in oral suspension for candidal infection in

Table 28-3
Antifungal Drugs

GENERIC (BRAND)	ROUTE AND DOSAGE	USES AND CONSIDERATIONS
POLYENES		
Amphotericin B (Fungizone)	*Test dose:* A: IV: 0.25–1.0 mg in 20 mL of D$_5$W infused over 20–30 min A: IV: 0.25–1.0 mg/kg/d in D$_5$W or 1.5 mg/kg q.o.d.: *max:* 1.5 mg/kg/d C: IV: Same as adult, except dilution and infuse time differ	For treatment of a variety of systemic fungal (mycotic) infections, such as aspergillosis, blastomycosis, coccidioidomycosis, cryptococcosis, histoplasmosis. Nephrotoxicity may occur when given in high doses. Hypokalemia might occur. *Pregnancy category:* B; PB: 95%; t$\frac{1}{2}$: 24 h
Nystatin (Mycostatin)	See Chart 28–2	For oral and intestinal candidiasis. Absorption is poor. Oral tablets are for intestinal candidiasis. Liquid form is for oral candidiasis; use by swish and swallow or expectorate. *Pregnancy category:* C; PB: UK; t$\frac{1}{2}$: UK
IMIDAZOLES		
Butoconazole nitrate (Femstat)	2% vaginal cream, Apply h.s. × 3 d; extend for 3 days as needed	Used for the treatment of vulvovaginal candidiasis. It is not recommended during the first trimester of pregnancy. *Pregnancy category:* C; PB: UK; t$\frac{1}{2}$: 21–24 h
Clotrimazole (Femcare, Mycelex, Gyne Lotrimin)	A: topical cream 1%, Vaginal tablet: 100 mg h.s. × 7 d or 500 mg h.s. × 1 day only A: PO: 1 troche (lozenge) 5 × d for 14 d	Used to treat candidiasis of the skin, mouth, and vagina and for dermal infections such as tinea pedis, tinea cruris, tinea corporis. Also for oropharyngeal candidiasis. Mild burning may occur with vaginal use. *Pregnancy category:* B (topical use) and C (troche); PB: UK; t$\frac{1}{2}$: UK
Econazole (Spectazole)	A: topical cream 1%, Apply 2 × d for 2–4 wk	Used to treat superficial candidiasis and the tinea infections (pedis, cruris, corporis). *Pregnancy category:* C; PB: UK; t$\frac{1}{2}$: UK
Fluconazole (Diflucan)	A: PO/IV: 50–400 mg/d; maint: 100–200 mg/d C: PO/IV: 3–6 mg/kg/d	For a variety of fungal infections. Highly selective inhibitor of fungal cytochrome P-450. Used to treat cryptococcal meningitis in AIDS clients and oropharyngeal and systemic candidiasis. *Pregnancy category:* C; PB: 12%; t$\frac{1}{2}$: 20–40 h
Itraconazole (Sporanox)	A: PO: Loading dose: 200 mg q8h × 3 d: maint: 200 mg/d: *max:* 400 mg/d in 2 divided doses	Effective against various systemic fungal infections, particularly blastomycosis and histoplasmosis. *Pregnancy category:* C; PB: 99%; t$\frac{1}{2}$: 21–42 h
Ketoconazole (Nizoral)	A: PO: 200–400 mg/d as a single dose C: PO: 3.3–6.6 mg/kg/d as single dose C: <20 kg: PO: 50 mg daily	For infections by *Candida* spp., histoplasmosis, blastomycosis, and others. Treatment could last 1–6 months for systemic infections. Take with food to avoid GI discomfort. *Pregnancy category:* C; PB: 95%; t$\frac{1}{2}$: 2–8 h
Miconazole nitrate (Monistat, Micatin)	A: IV: 200–3,600 mg/d in D$_5$W in 3 divided doses; infuse IV over 30–60 min C: IV: 20–40 mg/kg/d in divided doses; *max:* 15 mg/kg per inf A: Supp: 100 mg vag h.s. for 7 d Available: Vaginal cream 2%; lotion	For fungal meningitis and fungal bladder infections. Also for vaginal fungal infections. *Pregnancy category:* B; PB: 92%; t$\frac{1}{2}$: 2–24 h
Oxiconazole (Oxistat)	Cream applied once daily in the evening for 2–4 wk	For topical treatment for tinea pedis, tinea cruris, and tinea corporis. *Pregnancy category:* B; PB: UK; t$\frac{1}{2}$: UK
Sulconazole (Exelderm)	Cream and solution forms, apply once daily for 2–4 wk	Broad-spectrum antifungal drug to treat tinea infections. *Pregnancy category:* UK; PB: UK; t$\frac{1}{2}$: UK

Table continued on following page

Table 28–3 *Continued*
Antifungal Drugs

GENERIC (BRAND)	ROUTE AND DOSAGE	USES AND CONSIDERATIONS
Terconazole (Terazol-3)	A: Vaginal suppository h.s. × 3 d Vaginal cream 0.4% and 0.8%. Apply h.s. × 3 d (0.8%) or × 7 d (0.4%).	To treat vulvovaginal candidiasis. Not recommended during the first trimester of pregnancy. *Pregnancy category:* C; PB: UK; $t_{\frac{1}{2}}$: 4–11 h
Tioconazole (Vagistat)	A: Vaginal ointment 6.5%; apply h.s. × 1 d	To treat vulvovaginal candidiasis. Not recommended during the first trimester of pregnancy. *Pregnancy category:* C; PB: UK; $t_{\frac{1}{2}}$: UK
Terbinafine HCl (Lamisil)	A & C: Topical: Cream 1%, apply 1–2 × per day	For treatment of superficial mycosis; i.e., tinea pedis, tinea cruris, and tinea corporis. *Pregnancy category:* B; PB: NA; $t_{\frac{1}{2}}$: NA
ANTIMETABOLITES		
Flucytosine (Ancobon)	A: PO: 50–150 mg/kg/d in 4 divided doses C: <50 kg: PO: 1.5–4.5 g/m²/d in 4 divided doses	Use with amphotericin B may increase therapeutic action as well as toxicity. Fungal resistance occurs if the drug is given alone. *Pregnancy category:* C; PB: UK; $t_{\frac{1}{2}}$: 3–6 h
ANTIPROTOZOAL		
Atovaquone (Mepron)	A: PO: 750 mg t.i.d. with food × 21 d	For treatment of mild to moderate *Pneumocystis carinii* pneumonia. *Pregnancy category:* C; PB: 99%; $t_{\frac{1}{2}}$: 2–3 d

KEY: A: adult; C: child; PO: by mouth; IV: intravenous; PB: protein-binding; Supp: suppository; AIDS: acquired immunodeficiency syndrome; $t_{\frac{1}{2}}$: half-life; UK: unknown; Vag: vaginal; >: greater than; <: less than.

the mouth. The client is instructed to swish the liquid within the mouth to have contact with the mucous membrane, and then to swallow the liquid after a few minutes. If the throat area is involved, instruct the client to gargle with nystatin after swishing and before swallowing. Chart 28–2 describes the pharmacologic behavior of nystatin.

PHARMACOKINETICS
Nystatin is poorly absorbed. Its protein-binding power and half-life are unknown. The drug is excreted unchanged in feces.

PHARMACODYNAMICS
Nystatin increases permeability of the fungal cell membrane, thus causing the fungal cell to become unstable and to discharge the content. This drug has a fungistatic and fungicidal action. The onset of action for both suspension and tablet is rapid. The onset of action for vaginal tablet or cream is approximately 24 or more hours.

Imidazole Group

The imidazole group is effective against candidiasis (superficial and systemic), coccidioidomycosis, crypto-

coccosis, histoplasmosis, and paracoccidioidomycosis. Ketoconazole is the first effective antifungal drug that is orally absorbed. Fluconazole and itraconazole are two imidazole drugs for systemic fungal infection. These two antifungals can be taken orally, unlike amphotericin B, which is only administered intravenously.

There are numerous imidazoles (zoles) used to treat candidiasis and the tinea infections. These are topical medications, available in forms of vaginal tablet, cream, ointment, and solution. The group of antifungal-imidazole agents to treat candidiasis include clotrimazole (Femcare, Mycelex, Gyne-Lotrimin), butoconazole nitrate (Femstat), econazole (Spectazole), terconazole (Terazol-3), and tioconazole (Vagistat). The antifungal-imidazole group that is used to treat the tinea infections (tinea pedis [ringworm of foot], tinea cruris ["jock itch"], tinea corporis [ringworm of the body]) are clotrimazole (Mycelex), econazole (Spectazole), oxiconazole (Oxistat), and sulconazole (Exelderm). The last imidazole is miconazole (Monistat), and is for intravenous and topical use. Topically, it is frequently used in the treatment of vaginitis. Intravenously, it is used to treat bladder infections and meningitis. These agents are discussed in Table 28–3.

Chart 28–2. Antifungals

NYSTATIN

Assessment and Planning

Drug Name

Nystatin (Mycostatin), ✦ Nadostine, Nyaderm
Antifungal
Pregnancy Category: C

Dosage

A: Topical use as directed
Intestinal infections:
A: PO: 500,000–1,000,000 U t.i.d. or q8h
Oral candidiasis:
A: PO: 400,000–600,000 U q6–8h
Neonate (<7 d): PO: 100,000 U q.i.d.
C: PO: 250,000–500,000 U q.i.d.

Contraindications

Hypersensitivity
Vag: Pregnancy

Drug-Lab-Food Interactions

None significant known

Interventions

Pharmacokinetics

Absorption: PO: Poorly absorbed
Distribution: PB: UK
Metabolism: $t\frac{1}{2}$: UK
Excretion: In feces unchanged

Pharmacodynamics

PO: Onset: Rapid
Peak: UK
Duration: 6–12 h
Vaginally: Onset: 24–72 h
Peak: UK
Duration: UK

Evaluation

Therapeutic Effects/Uses

To treat *Candida* infections.

Mode of Action: Increase permeability of the fungal cell membrane.

Side Effects

PO: Anorexia, nausea, vomiting, diarrhea (large doses), stomach cramps, rash
Vag: Rash, burning sensation

Adverse Reactions

None known

NURSING PROCESS

KEY: A: adult; C: child; PO: by mouth; <: less than; Vag: Vaginal; UK: unknown; PB: protein-binding; $t\frac{1}{2}$: half-life; ✦: Canadian drug names.

Antimetabolite

The antimetabolite flucytosine has antifungal action. It is well absorbed from the GI tract. Flucytosine is used in combination with other antifungal drugs, such as amphotericin B, see Table 28–3.

Antiprotozoal

Atovaquone (Mepron), an antiprotozoal agent, is used to treat mild to moderate *Pneumocystis carinii* pneumonia.

PEPTIDES

The two groups of **peptides** used as antibiotics are the polymyxins and bacitracin. Polymyxins were one of the early groups of antibacterials, but many of the early drugs were discontinued because of nephrotoxicity. Two polymyxins, colistin and polymyxin B, are approved for pharmaceutical use. Polymyxins produce a bactericidal effect by interfering with the cellular membrane of the bacterium, thereby causing cell death. They affect most gram-negative bacteria, such as *Pseudomonas aeruginosa, Escherichia coli, Klebsiella* spp., and *Shigella* spp.

NURSING PROCESS
ANTIFUNGALS

Assessment

- Obtain a medical history from the client of any serious renal or hepatic disorder. Antifungal agents such as amphotericin B, fluconazole (Diflucan), flucytosine (Ancobon), and ketoconazole (Nizoral) are contraindicated if the client has a serious renal or liver disease.
- Check laboratory tests for liver enzyme values (ALP, ALT, AST, GGT), BUN, bilirubin, and serum creatinine. Elevated levels can indicate liver or renal dysfunction. These test results may be used for future comparisons.
- Obtain baseline vital signs (VS) for future comparison.

Potential Nursing Diagnoses

- Risk for infection
- Risk for impaired tissue integrity

Planning

- Client's fungal infection will be resolved.

Nursing Interventions

- Obtain a culture to determine the fungus; e.g., *Candida*.
- Monitor the client's urinary output; many of the antifungal drugs may cause nephrotoxicity.
- Monitor the laboratory results and compare with baseline findings (i.e., BUN, serum creatinine, ALP, ALT, AST, bilirubin, and electrolytes). Certain antifungals could cause hepatotoxicity as well as nephrotoxicity when taking high doses over a prolonged period of time.
- Monitor VS. Compare with baseline findings.
- Observe for side effects and adverse reactions to antifungal drugs (antimycotics), such as nausea, vomiting, headache, phlebitis, and signs and symptoms of electrolyte imbalance (hypokalemia with amphotericin B).

Client Teaching

General
- Instruct the client to take the drug as prescribed. Compliance is of utmost importance since discontinuing the drug too soon may result in a relapse.
- Advise the client to obtain laboratory testing as indicated. Serum liver enzymes, BUN, creatinine, and electrolytes should be monitored.
- Advise the client taking ketoconazole not to consume alcohol.

Self-Administration
- Instruct the client on the administration of nystatin (Mycostatin) suspension. Place the nystatin dose, usually 1 to 2 teaspoons, in the mouth. Swish the solution in the mouth and swallow (swish and swallow), or after swishing, have the client expectorate the solution (check with health care provider).

Side Effects
- Advise the client to avoid operating hazardous equipment or a motor vehicle when taking amphotericin B, ketoconazole, or flucytosine because these drugs may cause visual changes, sleepiness, dizziness, or lethargy.
- Instruct the client to report side effects, such as nausea, vomiting, diarrhea, dermatitis, rash, dizziness, tinnitus, edema, and flatulence. These symptoms may occur when taking certain antifungal drugs.

Nursing Process continued on following page

Cultural Considerations

- Recognize that clients from various cultures may have a lack of understanding of the purpose and procedure for the use of vaginal tablets or creams. A detailed explanation may be needed.
- Respect the client's apprehensions and fear concerning the use of the topical antifungal drugs and the desire to use alternative methods. Evaluate the client's method for topical administration in regard to safe practice. If the method is considered unsafe, explain why and suggest modifications, and, if appropriate, involve other persons for clarification.

Evaluation

- Evaluate the effectiveness of the antifungal (antimycotic) drug by noting the absence of the fungal infection (e.g., decreased itching, redness, and rawness).

Table 28–4
Antibacterials: Peptides

GENERIC (BRAND)	ROUTE AND DOSAGE	USES AND CONSIDERATIONS
Bacitracin (Bactrin USP)	C <2.5 kg: IM: <900 U/kg/d in 2–3 divided doses C >2.5 kg: IM: <1000 U/kg/d in 2–3 divided doses. Available in topical and ophthalmic ointment	It is seldom used parenterally except for children. Topical ointment for skin infection and ophthalmic ointment for infections of the eye. *Pregnancy category:* C; PB: <20%; t½: UK
Colistin (PO) (Coly-Mycin S, Polymyxin E)	A & C: PO: 5–15 mg/kg/d in 3 divided doses	For treating *Pseudomonas aeruginosa* infection. For gastroenteritis due to *Shigella* spp. *Pregnancy category:* C; PB: UK; t½: 2–3 h
Colistimethate sodium (IM/IV) (Coly-Mycin M)	IM/IV: 2.5–5 mg/kg/d in divided doses	For treating *Pseudomonas aeruginosa* infection. *Pregnancy category:* C; PB: UK; t½: 2–3 h
Polymyxin B SO₄ (Aerosporin)	A: IM: 25,000 U/kg/d in divided doses IV: 15,000–25,000 U/kg/d in 2 divided doses (q12h) C >2 y: Same as adult	For systemic use; also available in ointment form. May cause nephrotoxicity if given with aminoglycosides or amphotericin. *Pregnancy category:* B; PB: UK; t½: 4.5–6 h

ADDITIONAL ANTIBACTERIAL AGENT

Metronidazole (Flagyl, Flagyl-ER, MetroGel, Protostat)	*Amebiasis:* A: PO: 500–750 mg, t.i.d. for 5–10 d C: PO: 35–50 mg/kg/d in 3 divided doses *Anaerobic infections:* A: PO: 7.5 mg/kg, q6h; *max:* 4 g/d A: IV: 15 mg/kg loading dose, then 7.5 mg/kg, q6h *Bacterial vaginosis:* A: PO: ER preparation: 750 mg/d × 7 d *Perioperative prophylaxis:* A: IV: 1 g, 1 h before surgery, 500 mg, 6 and 12 hours after first dose *Rosacea:* Thin application 2 × d to affected areas Available: vaginal and topical gel	For treatment of intestinal amebiasis, trichomoniasis, inflammatory bowel disease, *H. pylori* infection causing peptic ulcers, bacterial vaginosis, and anaerobic infections and perioperative prophylaxis in colorectal surgery. Side effects may include GI discomfort, headache, depression, although not common. Not recommended during the first trimester of pregnancy. *Pregnancy category:* B; PB: UK; t½: 6–8 h

KEY: A: adult; C: child; IM: intramuscular; IV: intravenous; PB: protein-binding; t½: half-life; UK: unknown; >: greater than; <: less than.

Except for colistin, which exerts action on the colon and is excreted in the feces, the polymyxins are not absorbed through the oral route. Intramuscular injection of polymyxins produces marked pain at the injection site. Intravenous administration of polymyxins at a slow infusion rate is, therefore, the suggested method. Table 28–4 lists the polymyxins, their dosage, and uses.

High serum levels of polymyxins can cause nephrotoxicity and neurotoxicity. With nephrotoxicity, the blood urea nitrogen (BUN) and serum creatinine levels are elevated; however, when the serum drug level decreases, renal toxicity is usually reversed. Signs and symptoms of **neurotoxicity** are numbness and tingling of the extremities, **paresthesias** (abnormal sensation), and dizziness. Neurotoxicity is usually reversible when the drug is discontinued.

Bacitracin has a polypeptide structure and acts by inhibiting bacterial cell wall synthesis and damaging the cell wall membrane. The drug action can be bacteriostatic or bactericidal. Bacitracin is not absorbed by the GI tract and, if given orally, is excreted in the feces. It is, therefore, given intravenously or intramuscularly. It crosses the blood–brain barrier and, thus, is effective in treating meningitis. Bacitracin is effective against most gram-positive bacteria and some gram-negative bacteria. Over-the-counter (OTC) bacitracin ointment is available for application to the skin.

Side Effects and Adverse Reactions

The side effects of bacitracin include nausea and vomiting. Severe adverse reactions are renal damage, respiratory paralysis, blood dyscrasias (life-threatening anemias), and mild to severe allergic reactions, ranging from hives to anaphylaxis.

METRONIDAZOLE

Metronidazole (Flagyl) is used primarily for the treatment of various disorders associated with organisms in the gastrointestinal tract. It is prescribed to treat intestinal amebiasis, trichomoniasis, inflammatory bowel disease, anaerobic infections, and bacterial vaginosis and as perioperative prophylaxis in colorectal surgery. Metronidazole is commonly used with other agents to treat *Helicobacter pylori*, which is associated with frequent recurrent peptic ulcers. Table 28–4 includes data related to metronidazole.

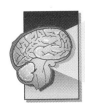

Critical Thinking in Action

C. J., 41 years old, has had a constant cough and night sweats for several months. He consumes 1 pint of whiskey per day. Sputum is positive for acid-fast (tubercle) bacillus. The health care provider orders a 6- to 9-month antitubercular drug regimen (time of therapy to be determined according to sputum and x-ray test results). For 2 months, C. J. is prescribed isoniazid, rifampin, and pyrazinamide daily. The next 4 to 7 months, C. J. receives isoniazid and rifampin biweekly.

1. What could be the contributing causes for C. J.'s contracting tuberculosis? Give other contributing causes for contracting tuberculosis.
2. C. J. received first-line antitubercular drugs for treatment of tuberculosis. How can the health professional determine whether the drugs are effective in eradicating the tubercle bacilli? Explain.
3. What is the nurse's role in client teaching concerning the drug regimen?
4. Name at least two serious adverse reactions that can occur when antitubercular drugs are given over an extended period of time.
5. What laboratory tests should be monitored while C. J. is taking isoniazid and rifampin? Why?

The health care provider ordered pyridoxine to be given daily.

6. Give your rationale for the use of pyridoxine. What type of drug is it? What is its purpose and when should it be administered?
7. What health agencies may the nurse suggest that could be helpful to C. J. during and after therapy?

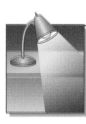

Study Questions

1. What is the purpose of combination drug therapy in the treatment of tuberculosis?

2. What is a common side effect of isoniazid? Why should some clients receive pyridoxine (vitamin B$_6$) while taking isoniazid? What are the signs and symptoms of peripheral neuropathy?

3. What is a potential adverse reaction to the use of isoniazid and rifampin? Would the problem be intensified if the drugs were taken by an alcoholic or a client with a liver disorder? Explain.

4. Your client is to receive nystatin or an oral fungal infection. How would you instruct the client to use the oral suspension of nystatin?

5. What is the type of electrolyte imbalance associated with the use of amphotericin B? What other adverse effect might result from the use of amphotericin B?

6. Two new oral antifungal drugs that may be taken for systemic fungal infections are _____ and _____ . How do these drugs differ from one another according to their protein-binding and half-life? What are the advantages of these drugs over amphotericin B?

7. Why should kidney function be assessed with polymyxin administration? Against what bacteria are polymyxins and colistin effective?

Antiviral, Antimalarial, and Anthelmintic Drugs

29

Outline

Objectives

- Name several antiviral and antimalarial drugs and explain their uses.
- Identify the various helminths and the human body sites for their infestation.
- Describe the action of anthelmintics.
- Explain the side effects of and adverse reactions to antiviral, antimalarial, and anthelmintic drugs.
- Identify several nursing interventions, including client teaching, for antiviral, antimalarial, and anthelmintic drug therapy.

Terms

AIDS

anthelmintic drugs

antimalarial drugs

antiviral drugs

erythrocytic phase

helminths

helminthiasis

opportunistic infection

prophylaxis

tissue phase

trichinosis

ANTIVIRAL DRUGS

Viruses are more difficult to eradicate than most types of bacteria. Viruses depend on the biochemical processes of the host cells for viral reproduction. The growth cycle of viruses depends on the host cell enzymes and cell substrates for viral replication. Antiviral drug development has been slower than the prolific antibacterial drug production. This may be partly because of the toxic effects of some antivirals to the body cells, related to their inability to differentiate viral from host cells.

Antiviral drugs are used to destroy, prevent, or delay the spread of a viral infection. A virus replicates itself in several steps. The purpose of antiviral drugs is to prevent the replication of the virus by inhibiting one of these steps, thus preventing it from reproducing. This group of drugs is effective against influenza, herpes species, and human immunodeficiency virus (HIV).

Amantadine hydrochloride (Symmetrel) has been used to treat parkinsonism and has also been found to be effective against the virus that causes influenza A. The drug is used prophylactically during epidemics and in minimizing influenza symptoms following early diagnosis. However, amantadine is *not* effective against influenza B. The drug is excreted unchanged in the urine, so adequate urinary output and renal function are essential. Dosages of amantadine might need to be decreased if renal function is impaired. Rimantadine HCl is a relatively new antiviral drug to treat influenza A. As with amantadine HCl, the client's renal and hepatic function should be monitored.

Antiviral Non-HIV Drugs

Before 1994, there were four antiviral drugs. Currently, there are 10 approved antivirals and more are in the experimental stages for controlling the human immunodeficency virus (HIV). Those that are marketed for systemic non-HIV antivirals include acyclovir (Zovirax), amantadine (Symmetrel), cidofovir (Vistide), famciclovir (Famvir), foscarnet (Foscavir), ganciclovir sodium (Cytovene), ribavirin (Virazole), rimantadine hydrochloride (Flumadine), valacyclovir (Valtrex), and vidarabine monohydrate (Vira-A). The three topical drugs are idoxuridine (Herplex Liquifilm, Stoxil), penciclovir (Denavir), and trifluridine (Viroptic). These non-HIV antiviral drugs are used to combat herpes simplex virus 1 (HSV-1), herpes simplex virus 2 (HSV-2, genital herpes), influenza A and B viruses, herpes zoster (shingles), varicella zoster virus (VZV), and cytomegalovirus (CMV).

Vidarabine was first introduced as an antineoplastic drug for the treatment of leukemia. In 1964, it was discovered that vidarabine exerts an antiviral effect against herpes simplex type I, herpes zoster, varicella zoster, and cytomegalovirus. Although it is not effective against genital herpes simplex II, vidarabine has been used effectively in treating herpes simplex viral encephalitis.

The antiviral drug ribavirin was marketed in 1986. It is being used to treat respiratory syncytial virus (RSV) in children and respiratory infections caused by the influenza A and B viruses in the aged. Ribavirin is administered by aerosol.

Acyclovir was introduced as an antineoplastic drug and was later found to be effective against herpesvirus, especially genital herpes simplex II, but also against herpes simplex I, herpes zoster (shingles), and cytomegalovirus (which can cause congenital defects). There has been reported resistance to acyclovir as a result of the lack of viral-producing enzyme (thymidine kinase) needed to convert the drug to an effective antiviral compound. Chart 29–1 lists the drug data for acyclovir.

PHARMACOKINETICS

Acyclovir is slowly absorbed, depending on the dose, and is widely distributed to body and organ tissues. Fifty percent passes into the cerebrospinal fluid. Ten to 30 percent of the drug is protein-bound. The half-life is 2 to 3 h with normal renal function. Acyclovir is excreted unchanged in the urine.

PHARMACODYNAMICS

Acyclovir interferes with the viral synthesis of DNA, thereby short-circuiting its replication. The onset of action for the oral preparation is unknown and for the intravenous route is rapid. The peak concentration time is within 2 h for both routes of administration, and the duration of action for both is similar.

Probenecid can increase the effect of acyclovir. If aminoglycoside or amphotericin B is taken with acyclovir, the incidence of nephrotoxicity is increased.

Valacyclovir (Valtrex) is converted to acyclovir, which has inhibitory activity against HSV-1, HSV-2, and VZV or herpes zoster. With herpes zoster, valacyclovir had a greater decrease in pain and an increase in healing time (40 to 43 days) than with acyclovir (59 days). Famciclovir (Famvir), an antiviral drug developed before valacyclovir, is equally effective as acyclovir for treating acute herpes zoster. Ganciclovir (Cytovene, Vitrasert) is effective in treating the herpesviruses and cytomegalovirus (CMV). It has serious adverse reactions—thrombocytopenia and granulocytopenia; therefore, it is used primarily to treat CMV infections. Table 29–1 lists the commonly used antiviral drugs, their dosages, uses, and considerations.

Chart 29-1. Antivirals

ACYCLOVIR SODIUM

Drug Name

Acyclovir sodium (Zovirax) Antiviral
Pregnancy Category: C

Dosage

Herpes simplex virus
A: PO: 200 mg q4h, 3–5×/d
IV: 5 mg/kg q8h × 5d (diluted in D_5W)
Herpes zoster virus
A: PO: 800 mg q4h 5 × d for 5–7 d
Herpes simplex encephalitis:
A: IV: 10 mg/kg, q8h × 10d.
C: IV: 500 mg/m², q8h × 7d.

Contraindications

Hypersensitivity, severe renal or hepatic disease
Caution: Electrolyte imbalance, lactation

Drug-Lab-Food Interactions

Drug: *Increase* nephro-neurotoxicity with aminoglycosides, probenecid, interferon
Lab: May *increase* AST, ALT, BUN

Pharmacokinetics

Absorption: PO: Slowly absorbed
Distribution: PB: 10%–30%
Metabolism: $t_{\frac{1}{2}}$: PO: 2–3 h
Excretion: 95% unchanged in urine

Pharmacodynamics

PO: Onset: UK
       Peak: 1.5–2 h
       Duration: 4–8 h
IV: Onset: Rapid
       Peak: 1–2 h
       Duration: 4–8 h

Therapeutic Effects/Uses

To treat herpes simplex I, genital herpes II.

Mode of Action: Interference with viral synthesis of DNA.

Side Effects

Nausea, vomiting, diarrhea, headache, tremors, lethargy, rash, pruritus, increased bleeding time, phlebitis at IV site

Adverse Reactions

Urticaria, anemia, gingival, hyperplasia
Life-threatening: Nephrotoxicity (large doses), neuropathy, bone marrow depression, granulocytopenia, thrombocytopenia, leukopenia, seizure, acute renal failure

Assessment and Planning

Interventions

Evaluation

NURSING PROCESS

KEY: A: adult; C: child; PO: by mouth; IV: intravenous; <: less than; PB: protein-binding; $t_{\frac{1}{2}}$: half-life; BUN: blood urea nitrogen; AST: aspartate aminotransferase; ALT: alanine aminotransferase.

SIDE EFFECTS AND ADVERSE REACTIONS
Amantadine and Rimantadine

The side effects of and adverse reactions to amantadine include central nervous system (CNS) effects, such as insomnia, depression, anxiety, confusion, and ataxia; orthostatic hypotension; neurologic problems, such as weakness, dizziness, slurred speech; and gastrointestinal (GI) disturbances, including anorexia, nausea, vomiting, and diarrhea. The CNS side effects of rimantadine occur less often than with amantadine.

Vidarabine, Acyclovir, and Ganciclovir

The side effects of and adverse reactions to vidarabine, ganciclovir, and acyclovir include GI disturbances (nausea, vomiting, diarrhea). With vidarabine, there might be CNS disturbances, such as weakness, malaise, tremors, and confusion. Adverse reactions can include a decrease in hemoglobin, white blood cells, and platelets; liver involvement (transient); and thrombophlebitis. With acyclovir, there might be headache, dizziness, and hematuria. Insomnia, de-

Table 29-1
Antivirals

GENERIC (BRAND)	ROUTE AND DOSAGE	USES AND CONSIDERATIONS
SYSTEMIC NON-HIV ANTIVIRALS		
Amantadine HCl (Symmetrel)	*Influenza A:* A: PO: 200 mg/d in 1–2 divided doses C 1–8 y: PO: 4.4–8.8 mg/kg/d in 2–3 divided doses C 9–12 y: PO: 100–200 mg/d in 1–2 divided doses	Primary use is prophylaxis against influenza A. Well absorbed by the GI tract. *Pregnancy category:* C; PB: UK; $t_{\frac{1}{2}}$: 24 h
Acyclovir (Zovirax)	See Chart 29–1	For treatment of herpes simplex viruses (HSV-1, HSV-2). Food does not affect oral absorption. Renal function should be monitored. *Pregnancy category:* C; PB: 10%–30%; $t_{\frac{1}{2}}$: 2–3 h
Cidofovir (Vistide)	A: IV: 5 mg/kg once wk for 2 wk, then 5 mg/kg every other week. Take probenecid, 2 g, 3 h before infusion and 1 g 8 h after infusion	For treatment of CMV retinitis especially in clients with AIDS. Kidney damage may occur; monitor kidney function. *Pregnancy category:* C; PB: UK; $t_{\frac{1}{2}}$: 17–65 h
Famciclovir (Famvir)	*Herpes zoster:* A: PO: 500 mg q8h × 7 d	For treatment of herpes zoster. *Pregnancy category:* C; PB: UK; $t_{\frac{1}{2}}$: UK
Foscarnet (Foscavir)	*CMV retinitis:* A: IV: Induction: 60 mg/kg infused over 1 h, q8h, for 2 to 3 wk. *Maint:* 90–120 mg/kg/d infused over 2 h *Herpes simplex infections: AIDS:* A: IV: 40–60 mg/kg, q8h, for 2–3 wk; may include: 50 mg/kg/d for 5 to 7 d/wk up to 15 wk	For treatment of herpesviruses (HSV-1 and 2, VZV) and CMV retinitis. It is expensive. It does not cause granulocytopenia or thrombocytopenia. It can cause kidney damage and hyperphosphatemia. Monitor kidney function closely. *Pregnancy category:* C; PB: UK; $t_{\frac{1}{2}}$: 3–4 h
Ganciclovir sodium (Cytovene)	A & C: IV: Initially: 5 mg/kg q12h × 14–21 d; *maint:* 5 mg/kg/d × 7 d or 6 mg/kg/d × 5 d	For treatment of CMV systemic infection in immunocompromised clients. *Pregnancy category:* C; PB: 1%–2%; $t_{\frac{1}{2}}$: 2.5–6 h
Ribavirin (Virazole)	A & C: By aerosol inhalation administration	For respiratory syncytial viral infection in infants and children. *Pregnancy category:* X; PB: NA; $t_{\frac{1}{2}}$: 24 h
Rimantadine HCl (Flumadine)	A: PO: 200 mg/d in 1 or 2 divided doses C: PO: 5–7 mg/kg/d	For prophylaxis and treatment against influenza A virus. Drug dose is usually reduced for clients with severe hepatic or renal impairment. *Pregnancy category:* C; PB: 40%; $t_{\frac{1}{2}}$: 33 h
Valacyclovir HCl (Valtrex)	*Herpes zoster:* A: PO: 1 g t.i.d. × 7 d *Recurrent genital herpes:* A: PO: 500 mg b.i.d. 5 d	It is converted to acyclovir during intestinal and liver metabolism. It is effective against VZV causing herpes zoster (shingles) and recurrent genital herpes. Monitor kidney function. GI disturbances and headaches are common side effects. *Pregnancy category:* B; PB: UK; $t_{\frac{1}{2}}$: 2.5–3.5 h
Vidarabine monohydrate (Vira-A)	A: IV: 10–15 mg/kg/d infused over 12–24 h	Effective against serious herpes simplex 1 (HSV-1), herpes zoster, and varicella zoster. *Pregnancy category:* C; PB; 20%–30%, $t_{\frac{1}{2}}$: 1.5–3 h
TOPICAL NON-HIV ANTIVIRALS		
Idoxuridine (Herplex Liquifilm, Stoxil)	0.5% ointment: q4h during day. *Solution:* Instill 1 gt during day and q2h at night. Time interval can be decreased.	Used primarily for HSV-1 keratitis. *Pregnancy category:* C; PB: UK; $t_{\frac{1}{2}}$: UK
Penciclovir (Denavir)	1% cream: apply q2h during the day for 4 days.	For treatment of recurrent herpes labialis (cold sores) of lips. *Pregnancy category:* B; PB: UK; $t_{\frac{1}{2}}$: UK
Trifluridine (Viroptic)	1% ophthalmic solution: 1 gt q2h during the day; *max:* 9 gtt/d	Used primarily for keratoconjunctivitis because of herpes simplex virus. *Pregnancy category:* C; PB: UK; $t_{\frac{1}{2}}$: UK

KEY: *A: adult; C: child; IV: intravenous; m²: body surface area; PB: protein-binding; PO: by mouth; $t_{\frac{1}{2}}$: half-life; <: less than; >: more than; gt: drop; gtt: drops; CMV: cytomegalovirus; HIV: human immunodeficiency virus; AIDS: acquired immunodeficiency syndrome; VZV: varicella zoster virus.*

NURSING PROCESS
ANTIVIRALS

Assessment

- Obtain a medical history of any serious renal or hepatic disease.
- Obtain baseline vital signs (VS) and a complete blood count (CBC). Use these findings for comparison with future results.
- Assess baseline laboratory results, particularly BUN, serum creatinine, liver enzymes, bilirubin, and electrolytes. Use these results for future comparisons.
- Assess baseline VS and urine output. Report abnormal findings.

Potential Nursing Diagnoses

- Risk of infection
- Risk for impaired tissue integrity

Planning

- Symptoms of viral infections will be eliminated or diminished.

Nursing Interventions

- Monitor the client's CBC. Report abnormal results, such as leukopenia, thrombocytopenia, and low hemoglobin and hematocrit.
- Monitor other laboratory tests, such as BUN, serum creatinine, and liver enzymes, and compare with baseline values.
- Monitor the client's urinary output. An antiviral drug such as acyclovir can affect renal function.
- Monitor VS, especially blood pressure. Acyclovir and amantadine may cause orthostatic hypotension.
- Observe for signs and symptoms of side effects. Most antiviral drugs have many side effects; see Chart 29–1.
- Check for superimposed infection (superinfection) caused by high dose and prolonged use of an antiviral drug such as acyclovir.
- Administer oral acyclovir as prescribed. Oral dose can be taken at mealtime.
- For IV use, dilute the antiviral drug in an appropriate amount of solution as indicated in the drug circular. Administer the IV drug over 60 min. *Never* give acyclovir as a bolus (IV push).

Client Teaching

General
- Advise the client to maintain an adequate fluid intake to ensure sufficient hydration for drug therapy and to increase urine output.
- Instruct the client with genital herpes to avoid spreading the infection by practicing sexual abstinence or the use of a condom. Advise these women to have a Pap test done every 6 months or as indicated by the health care provider. Cervical cancer is more prevalent in women with genital herpes simplex.
- Instruct clients taking zidovudine to have blood cell count monitored.

Side Effects
- Instruct the client to perform oral hygiene several times a day. Gingival hyperplasia (red, swollen gums) can occur with prolonged use of antiviral drugs.
- Instruct the client to report adverse reactions, including decrease in urine output and CNS changes such as dizziness, anxiety, or confusion.
- Advise the client with dizziness resulting from orthostatic hypotension to arise slowly from a sitting to a standing position.
- Instruct the client to report any side effects associated with the antiviral drug, such as nausea, vomiting, diarrhea, increased bleeding time, rash, urticaria, or menstrual abnormalities.

Nursing Process continued on following page

Cultural Considerations

- Teach the non–English-speaking client and family members how to use ophthalmic preparations. Using pictures may be helpful.

Evaluation

- Evaluate the effectiveness of the antiviral drug in eliminating the virus or in decreasing symptoms.
- Determine whether side effects are absent.

pression, and hypotension, although infrequent, can also occur. Elevated blood urea nitrogen (BUN) and serum creatinine levels can result from renal involvement; such involvement is usually transient.

Ganciclovir can cause thrombocytopenia and granulocytopenia. Because of the possible serious adverse reactions, this drug should be prescribed primarily for severe systemic cytomegalovirus infections for immunocompromised clients.

Gamma Globulin (Immune Globulin)
Gamma globulin (IgG) is rich in antibodies found in the blood. It provides a passive form of immunity to a virus by blocking the penetration of a virus into the host cell. It is administered during the early infectious stage to prevent a viral invasion in the body.

The human immune globulin (Gamastan) is administered intramuscularly. A single-dose injection protects for approximately 2 to 3 weeks; it may be repeated in 2 to 3 weeks. For clients who need an immediate increase in immune globulin levels, intravenous immune globulin (Gamimune) may be administered.

Antiviral HIV Drugs
The microbe of human immunodeficiency virus (HIV) is the cause of acquired immunodeficiency syndrome (**AIDS**). HIV is a retrovirus. There are two classes of antiretroviral drugs: (1) reverse transcriptase inhibitors and (2) protease inhibitors. Antiviral drugs that are classified as reverse transcriptase inhibitors include delavirdine (Rescriptor), didanosine (Videx), lamivudine (Epivir), nevirapine (Viramune), stavudine (Zerit), zalcitabine (Hivid), and zidovudine (Retrovir, AZT). These drugs aid in inhibiting viral replication. Zidovudine was one of the first retroviral drugs approved by the Food and Drug Administration (FDA). It inhibits the action of viral reverse transcriptase, thus preventing the synthesis of DNA and allowing the T_4 lymphocytes to increase initially.

The protease inhibitor group includes indinavir (Crixivan), nelfinavir (Viracept), ritonavir (Norvir), and saquinavir (Invirase). This group of antivirals inhibits the replication of retroviruses (HIV-1 and -2). When a protease inhibitor is used in combination with a reverse transcriptase inhibitor, these drugs may greatly reduce the viral level to the point that it is undetectable. The combination of drugs helps to decrease HIV drug resistance. The antiviral drugs for suppressing HIV are discussed in Chapter 31.

ANTIMALARIAL DRUGS

Malaria, caused by the protozoan parasites *Plasmodium* spp. that are carried by an infected *Anopheles* mosquito, is still one of the most prevalent protozoan diseases. After the mosquito infects the human, the protozoan parasite passes through two phases, the tissue phase and the erythrocytic phase. The **tissue phase** produces no clinical symptoms in the human, but the **erythrocytic phase** (invasion of the red blood cells) causes symptoms of chills, fever, and sweating.

There are approximately 50 species of *Plasmodium;* four types of the species cause malaria: *P. malariae, P. ovale, P. vivax,* and *P. falciparum. P. vivax* is the most prevalent type; *P. falciparum* is the most severe type. In the world there are about 200 million cases of malaria, but in the United States malaria is confined mainly to those who enter the country from elsewhere.

Treatment of malaria depends on the type of *Plasmodium* and the organism's life cycle. Quinine was the only antimalarial drug available from 1820 until the early 1940s. Synthetic **antimalarial drugs** have since been developed that are as effective as quinine and cause fewer toxic effects. When drug-resistant malaria occurs, combinations of antimalarials are used to facilitate effective treatment. Chloroquine is a commonly prescribed drug for malaria. If drug resistance to chloroquine occurs, quinine may be used in combination with an antibiotic such as tetracycline. Various combinations may be used when drug resistance occurs. Three methods used to eradicate malaria are

Chart 29–2. Antimalarials: Chloroquine HCl

ANTIMALARIAL

Drug Name

Chloroquine HCl (Aralen HCl)
Pregnancy Category: C

Dosage

Acute Malaria:
A: PO: 600 mg base/dose; then 6 h later: 300 mg/dose; then at 24 and 48 h: 300 mg/dose
IM: 200 mg/base q6h, PRN
C: PO: 10 mg base/kg/dose, then 6 h later: 5 mg base/kg/dose; then 5 mg base/kg/d for 2 d; IM: 5 mg base/kg q12h
Prophylaxis:
2 wk before and 6–8 wk after exposure
A & C: PO: 5 mg/kg/wk; *max:* 300 mg base/wk

Contraindications

Hypersensitivity to 4-aminoquinolones, renal disease, psoriasis, retinal changes
Caution: Alcoholism; liver dysfunction; G-6-PD deficiency; GI, neurologic, and hematologic disorders

Drug-Lab-Food Interactions

Drug: *Increase* effects of digoxin, anticoagulants, neuromuscular blocker; *decrease* absorption with antacids and laxatives
Lab: *Decrease* red blood cell (RBC) count, hemoglobin, hematocrit

Pharmacokinetics

Absorption: well absorbed from GI tract
Distribution: PB: 50%–65%
Metabolism: $t\frac{1}{2}$: 1–2 months
Excretion: excreted slowly in urine

Pharmacodynamics

PO: Onset: rapid
    Peak: 3.5 h
    Duration: days to weeks
IM: Onset: Rapid
    Peak: 0.5 h
    Duration: days to weeks

Therapeutic Effects/Uses

To treat acute malaria and for prophylaxis.

Mode of Action: Increased pH in the malaria parasite inhibits parasitic growth.

Side Effects

Anorexia, nausea, vomiting, diarrhea, abdominal cramps, fatigue, pruritus, nervousness, visual disturbances (blurred vision)

Adverse Reactions

ECG changes, hypotension, psychosis
Life-threatening: Agranulocytosis, aplastic anemia, thrombocytopenia, ototoxicity, cardiovascular collapse

(Side bar:) Assessment and Planning · Interventions · Evaluation · NURSING PROCESS

KEY: A: adult; C: child; PO: by mouth; IM: intramuscular; PB: protein-binding; $t\frac{1}{2}$: half-life; G-6-PD: glucose-6-phosphate dehydrogenase; GI: gastrointestinal; ECG: electrocardiographic.

prophylaxis for the prevention of malaria, treatment for the acute attack, and prevention of relapse. Many of the synthetic antimalarials, such as chloroquine, primaquine, and pyrimethamine-sulfadoxine are used prophylactically. Chloroquine and mefloquine are frequently used to treat an acute malarial attack. Chart 29–2 lists the drug data for chloroquine HCl.

Pharmacokinetics

Chloroquine HCl is well absorbed from the GI tract. It is moderately protein-binding, and the drug has a long half-life. The first two doses have a loading dose effect. Because of the long half-life, the next dose is given on the second day, and the fourth dose is given

Table 29–2
Antimalarials

GENERIC (BRAND)	ROUTE AND DOSAGE	USES AND CONSIDERATIONS
Chloroquine HCl (Aralen HCl)	*Acute malaria:* A: PO: 600 mg base/dose; then 6 h later: 300 mg/dose; then at 24 and 48 h: 300 mg/dose IM: 200 mg/base q6h PRN C: PO: 10 mg base/kg/dose, then 6 h later: 5 mg base/kg/dose; 24–48 h later: 5 mg base/kg/dose. IM: 5 mg base/kg q12h *Prophylaxis:* 2 wk before and 6–8 wk after exposure A & C: PO: 5 mg/kg/wk; *max:* 300 mg base/wk	Treatment of acute malaria. For prophylactic use, the drug should be taken 2 weeks before possible exposure and after the return visit. Chloroquine is considered to be the drug of choice; however, it can be combined with primaquine. *Pregnancy category:* C; PB: 50%–65%; $t_{\frac{1}{2}}$: 2.5–5 d
Hydroxychloroquine SO$_4$ (Plaquenil SO$_4$)	*Acute malaria:* A: PO: 800 mg/dose; 6 h later: 400 mg; then 400 mg daily for 2 d C: PO: 10 mg base/kg/dose, 6 h: 5 mg base/kg; 5 mg base/kg daily for 2 d *Prophylaxis:* 1 wk before and 6–8 wk after exposure A & C: PO: 5 mg base/kg/wk; *max:* 300 mg base/wk	Alternative to chloroquine. Dosage varies for treating malaria. Can be used adjunctively with primaquine. Give drug with meals to reduce the occurrence of GI distress. *Pregnancy category:* C; PB: 55% $t_{\frac{1}{2}}$: 2.5–5 d
Mefloquine HCl (Lariam)	A: PO: Single dose: 1250 mg; then 250 mg q wk × 4 wk	New antimalarial drug. Action is similar to chloroquine HCl. *Pregnancy category:* C; PB: 98%; $t_{\frac{1}{2}}$: 21 d
Primaquine phosphate	*Malaria prophylaxis:* A: PO: 15 mg/d for 14 d (single doses) C: PO: 0.3 mg/kg/d for 14 d (single doses)	Prophylaxis against certain *Plasmodium* spp. (*P. vivax* and *P. ovale*) and for relapse. Can affect white blood cell production (granulocytopenia). *Pregnancy category:* C; PB: UK; $t_{\frac{1}{2}}$: 3.7–9.6 h
Pyrimethamine (Daraprim)	*Malaria prophylaxis:* A & C: >10 y: PO: 25 mg/wk C <4 y: PO: 6.25 mg/wk C 4–10 y: PO: 12.5 mg/wk	Prophylaxis use for malaria. For treatment of chloroquine-resistant *Plasmodium falciparum* infections. May be used with quinacrine, quinine, or chloroquine. *Pregnancy category:* C; PB: 80%; $t_{\frac{1}{2}}$: 1.5–2 d
Quinacrine HCl (Atabrine HCl)	*Malaria suppression:* A: PO: 100 mg/d C: PO: 50 mg/d	For treating *Plasmodium malariae* and *Plasmodium vivax* infections. *Pregnancy category:* C; PB: UK; $t_{\frac{1}{2}}$: UK
Quinine SO$_4$ (Quin-260, Quiphile)	*Acute malaria:* A: PO: 650 mg q8h for 3–7 d C: PO: 25 mg/kg/d in 3 divided doses (q8h) for 3–7 d	Used in combination drug therapy or for chloroquine-resistant malaria. Used to treat nocturnal leg cramps. *Pregnancy category:* X; PB: 70%–95%; $t_{\frac{1}{2}}$: 6–14 h

KEY: A: adult; C: child; PB: protein-binding; PO: by mouth; IM: intramuscular; $t_{\frac{1}{2}}$: half-life; UK: unknown; >: greater than; <: less than.

on the third day. Chloroquine is metabolized in the liver to active metabolites and excreted in the urine.

Pharmacodynamics

Chloroquine HCl inhibits the malaria parasite's growth by interfering with its protein synthesis.

Whether the drug is taken orally or given intramuscularly, the onset of action is rapid. The peak effect is slower when given orally. The duration of effect of the drug is very long—days to weeks.

Table 29–2 lists commonly ordered antimalarial drugs, their dosage, uses, and considerations. (*Note:* Quinine and quinidine are *not* the same drug. Qui-

NURSING PROCESS
ANTIMALARIAL DRUGS

Assessment

- Assess the client's hearing, especially if taking quinine or chloroquine. These drugs may affect the eighth cranial nerve.
- Assess the client for visual changes. Clients on chloroquine and hydroxychloroquine should have frequent ophthalmic examinations.

Potential Nursing Diagnoses

- Risk of infection
- Risk for impaired tissue integrity

Planning

- Client will be free of malarial symptoms.

Nursing Interventions

- Monitor the client's urinary output and liver function by checking the urine output (>600 mL/d) and the liver enzymes. Antimalarial drugs concentrate first in the liver; serum liver enzyme levels should be checked especially if the person drinks considerable amounts of alcohol or has a liver disorder.
- Report if the client's serum liver enzymes are elevated.

Client Teaching

- Advise clients traveling to malaria-infested countries to receive prophylactic doses of antimalarial drug before leaving, during the visit, and upon return.
- Instruct the client to take oral antimalarial drugs with food or at mealtime if GI upset occurs.
- Monitor the client returning from a malaria-infested area for malarial symptoms.
- Instruct the client on chloroquine or hydroxychloroquine to report vision changes immediately.
- Advise the client to avoid consuming large quantities of alcohol.

Cultural Considerations

- If a client from a malaria-infested country complains of chills, high fever, and profuse sweating, the client's serum should be tested for malaria. The client may receive an antimalarial drug as a prophylactic measure or for treatment of an acute attack. Explanation is necessary so the client complies with the drug regimen.

Evaluation

- Evaluate the effectiveness of the antimalarial drug by determining that the client is free of symptoms.

nine is an antimalarial drug and quinidine is an antidysrhythmic drug).

Side Effects and Adverse Reactions

General side effects of and adverse reactions to antimalarials include GI upset, eighth cranial nerve involvement (quinine and chloroquine), renal impairment (quinine), and cardiovascular effects (quinine).

ANTHELMINTIC DRUGS

Helminths are large organisms (parasitic worms) that feed on host tissue. The most common site for **helminthiasis** (worm infestation) is the intestine. Other sites for parasitic infestation are the lymphatic system, blood vessels, and liver.

There are four groups of helminths: (1) cestodes (tapeworms), (2) trematodes (flukes), (3) intestinal

Table 29–3
Anthelmintic Drugs

DRUG	DOSAGE	USES AND CONSIDERATIONS
Bithional (Actamer)	Dose: UK	Effective against flukes. Treatment of *Paragonimus westermani* (lung fluke).
Diethylcarbamazine (Hetrazan)	A: PO: 2–3 mg/kg/t.i.d.	Treatment for nematode-filariae
Ivermectin (Mectizan)	A: C >15 kg: PO: 200 μg/kg/1 dose	A broad-spectrum antiparasitic drug. Causes paralysis to the parasite. Highly active against various mites. *Pregnancy category:* C; PB: UK; $t\frac{1}{2}$: 12–16 h
Mebendazole (Vermox)	A: PO: 100 mg b.i.d. × 3 d Repeat in 2–3 wk if necessary C >2y: PO: same as adult	Treatment for giant roundworm, hookworm, pinworm, whipworm. *Pregnancy category:* C
Niclosamide (Niclocide)	A: PO: 2 g, single dose C >34 kg: PO: 1.5 g, single dose C 11–34 kg: PO: 1 g, single dose A: PO: 2 g/d × 1 wk C >34 kg: PO: 1.5 g, single dose, then 1 g/d × 6 days	Treatment for beef and fish tapeworms. *Pregnancy category:* B Treatment of dwarf tapeworms.
Oxamniquine (Vansil)	A: PO: 15 mg/kg/b.i.d. for 1–2 d C: PO: 10–15 mg/kg/b.i.d. for 1–2 d	Treatment against mature and immature worms. *Pregnancy category:* C
Piperazine citrate (Antepar, Vermizine)	*Roundworm:* A: PO: 3.5 g/d × 2 d C: PO: 75 mg/kg/d × 2 d *max:* 3.5 g/d *Pinworms:* A & C: 65 mg/kg/d × 7 d *max:* 2.5 g/d	Treatment of roundworms and pinworms. *Pregnancy category:* B
Praziquantel (Biltricide)	A & C: PO: 10–20 mg/kg single dose A & C: PO: 20 mg/kg, t.i.d., × 1 d A & C: 25 mg/kg, t.i.d., 1–2 d	Treatment for beef, pork, fish tapeworms. Treatment for blood flukes. Treatment for liver, lung, and intestinal flukes. *Pregnancy category:* B; PB: UK; $t\frac{1}{2}$: 0.8–1.5 h
Pyrantel pamoate (Antiminth)	A & C: PO: 11 mg/kg single dose Repeat in 2 wks if necessary	Treatment of giant roundworm, hookworm, pinworm. *Pregnancy category:* C
Thiabendazole (Mintezol, Minzolum)	A & C: PO: 25 mg/kg, for 2–5 d Repeat in 2 d if necessary	Treatment of threadworm and pork worm. *Pregnancy category:* C

KEY: A: adult; C: child; PB: protein-binding; PO: by mouth: $t\frac{1}{2}$: half-life; UK: unknown; >: greater than; <: less than.

nematodes (roundworms), and (4) tissue-invading nematodes (tissue roundworms and filariae). The cestodes (tapeworms) are segmented and enter the intestine via contaminated food. There are four species of cestodes: *Taenia solium* (pork tapeworm), *Taenia saginata* (beef tapeworm), *Diphyllobothrium latum* (fish tapeworm), and *Hymenolepis nana* (dwarf tapeworm). The segmented cestodes have heads and have hooks or suckers that attach to the tissue.

The trematodes (flukes) are flat, nonsegmented parasites that feed on the host. Four types of trematodes exist: *Fasciola hepatica* (liver fluke), *Fasciolopsis*

buski (intestinal fluke), *Paragonimus westermani* (lung fluke), and *Schistosoma* species (blood fluke). Five types of nematodes may feed on the intestinal tissue; these include *Ascaris lumbricoides* (giant roundworm), *Necator americanus* (hookworm), *Enterobius vermicularis* (pinworm), *Strongyloides stercoralis* (threadworm), and *Trichuris trichiura* (whipworm). Two types of nematodes that are tissue invading include *Trichinella spiralis* (pork roundworm) and *Wuchereria bancrofti* (filariae). The pork roundworm or *T. spiralis* can cause **trichinosis,** which can be diagnosed by a muscle biopsy. By thoroughly cooking pork, the roundworm, if present, is destroyed.

NURSING PROCESS
ANTHELMINTICS

Assessment

- Obtain a history of foods the client has eaten, especially meat and fish, and how the food was prepared.
- Note if any other person in the household has been checked for helminths (worms).
- Assess baseline vital signs (VS) and collect a stool specimen.

Potential Nursing Diagnoses

- Altered comfort related to GI symptoms
- Activity intolerance related to dizziness, headache, drowsiness

Planning

- The client will be free of helminths.
- The client will understand how to prepare foods properly to avoid recurrence.

Nursing Interventions

- Collect a stool specimen in a clean container. Avoid having the stool come in contact with water, urine, or chemicals, which could destroy parasitic worms.
- Administer the prescribed anthelmintics after meals to prevent or minimize the occurrence of GI distress.
- Report to the health care provider if the client has any side effects.

Client Teaching

- Explain to the client the importance of washing hands before eating and after going to the toilet. The parasite can be transferred within the family if proper hygiene is not used.
- Instruct the client to take daily showers and *not* baths.
- Instruct the client to change sheets, bedclothes, towels, and underwear daily.
- Explain to the client that, if the problem persists after therapy, a second course of anthelmintics may be necessary.
- Emphasize the importance of taking the prescribed drug at designated times and to keep health care appointments.
- Alert the client that drowsiness may occur and that he or she should avoid operating a car or machinery if drowsiness occurs.
- Instruct the client to report any side effects to the health care provider.

Evaluation

- Evaluate the effect of the anthelmintics and the absence of side effects.
- Determine whether the client is using proper hygiene to avoid spread of parasitic worms.

Table 29–3 lists eight anthelmintic drugs that are prescribed to treat various types of parasitic worms.

Side Effects and Adverse Reactions

The common side effects of anthelmintics include GI upset such as anorexia, nausea, vomiting, and occasionally diarrhea and stomach cramps. The neurologic problems associated with anthelmintics are dizziness, weakness, headache, and drowsiness. Adverse reactions do not occur frequently because the drugs are usually given only for a short period of time (1 to 3 days), except for niclosamide for treatment of dwarf tapeworms, piperazine for treatment of pinworms, and thiabendazole for treatment of threadworms and pork worms. Thiabendazole should be avoided if the client has liver disease.

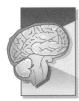

Critical Thinking in Action

T. P., 75 years old, has shingles. She complains of pain and blisters (vesicular eruptions), which partially surround her waist. The health care provider prescribed acyclovir, 800 mg, q4h, 5 times a day for 7 days.

1. In history taking, what should the nurse ask T. P.?
2. How does herpes zoster differ from varicella-zoster virus (VZV)? Explain who would be more susceptible to contracting herpes zoster virus infection.
3. How is acyclovir effective for relieving T. P.'s symptoms?
4. Is the prescribed acyclovir dose correct? If so explain why?
5. How does acyclovir differ from famciclovir and amantadine?
6. What comfort measures would you suggest to T. P.?
7. What should the nurse inform T. P. about being around other people?

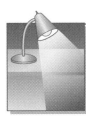

Study Questions

1. Amantadine is an antiviral drug. For what other disease is this drug used? What are some side effects of and adverse reactions to amantadine?

2. Vidarabine and acyclovir are antiviral antimetabolites. How are these drugs similar and how do they differ in their uses?

3. What three antiviral drugs may be prescribed for advanced HIV infection?

4. Your client is to receive chloroquine as a prophylactic against malaria. How does chloroquine act to prevent malaria? What is the schedule for administration when it is used prophylactically? Discuss the significance of protein-binding and half-life of chloroquine HCl.

5. The client's hematology tests should be monitored while the client is taking chloroquine HCl. Why?

6. Concerning the use of antimalarials, what should be included in client teaching?

7. What are helminths? Most types of helminths are concentrated in what part of the body?

8. Trichinosis is caused by what organism? How can this health problem be prevented? How is it diagnosed?

9. What client teaching instructions should be included for a client diagnosed as having helminths?

Drugs for Urinary Tract Disorders 30

Outline

Objectives

- Identify the groups of drugs that are urinary antiseptics and antiinfectives.
- Describe the side effects of and adverse reactions to urinary antiseptics and antiinfectives.
- Give uses for a urinary analgesic, a urinary stimulant, and a urinary antispasmodic.
- Describe the nursing process, including client teaching, regarding urinary antiseptic/antiinfective drugs and urinary analgesics.

Terms

acute cystitis
acute pyelonephritis
bactericidal
bacteriostatic

micturition
urinary analgesics
urinary antiseptics/antiinfectives

urinary antispasmodics
urinary stimulants
urinary tract infection (UTI)

INTRODUCTION

The largest number of urinary tract disorders are due to **urinary tract infections (UTIs).** UTIs may result from an upper urinary tract infection, such as pyelonephritis, or from a lower urinary tract infection, such as cystitis, urethritis, or prostatitis. A group of drugs called **urinary antiseptics/antiinfectives** prevent bacterial growth in the kidneys and bladder but are not effective for systemic infections. Urinary antiseptics/antiinfectives have a **bacteriostatic** effect when given in lower dosages. They also have a **bactericidal** effect when given in higher dosages.

Urinary antiseptics/antiinfectives, urinary stimulants, urinary antispasmodics, and urinary analgesics are presented in this chapter. Antibacterials/antibiotics and sulfonamides that are used in treating urinary tract infections are discussed in Chapters 25, 26, and 27. Diuretics are discussed in Chapter 38.

Acute cystitis, a lower UTI, frequently occurs in female clients because of their shorter urethra. It is more common in women of childbearing age, elderly women, and young girls. Acute cystitis is commonly caused by *Escherichia coli*. Other bacterial causes include the gram-positive *Staphylococcus saprophyticus* and gram-negative *Klebsiella, Proteus,* and *Pseudomonas*. Symptoms of cystitis include pain and burning on urination, and urinary frequency and urgency. A urine culture is obtained before the start of any antiinfective/antibiotic drug therapy. In males, a lower UTI is most likely to be prostatitis with symptoms similar to cystitis.

Acute pyelonephritis, an upper UTI, is commonly seen in women of childbearing age, elderly women, and young girls. *E. coli* is the most common organism causing pyelonephritis. Symptoms include chills, high fever, flank pain, pain during urination, urinary frequency and urgency, and pyuria. The bacterial count in the urine is greater than 100,000 bacteria/mL. In severe cases, the client may be hospitalized and receive intravenous antibiotics such as an aminoglycoside, ticarcillin/clavulanic acid, or piperacillin/tazobactam.

The most commonly used agents for treating UTIs are trimethoprim-sulfamethoxazole (co-trimoxazole, Bactrim, Septra), nitrofurantoin, and the fluoroquinolones such as cinoxacin, nalidixic acid, and norfloxacin. Treatment may consist of either a single double-strength dose of the chosen drug, a short-term 3-day course, or the traditional method of 7 to 14 days of drug dosing. Fosfomycin tromethamine (Monurol), a nitrofurantoin prototype drug, is effective as a single dose treatment for UTIs. Other agents used to treat UTIs include oral amoxicillin/clavulanic acid (Augmentin), oral third-generation cephalosporins (cefixime, cefpodoxime proxetil, or ceftibuten). With severe UTIs, intravenous drug therapy followed by oral drug therapy is usually recommended.

URINARY ANTISEPTICS/ ANTIINFECTIVES AND ANTIBIOTICS

Urinary antiseptics/antiinfectives are limited to the treatment of UTIs. The drug action occurs in the renal tubule and bladder, and thus is effective in reducing bacterial growth. A urinalysis and culture and sensitivity test are usually performed before the initiation of drug therapy. The groups of urinary antiseptics/antiinfectives are nitrofurantoin, methenamine, trimethoprim, and the fluoroquinolones.

Nitrofurantoin

Nitrofurantoin (Furolan, Macrodantin) was first prescribed for UTI in 1953. Nitrofurantoin is bacteriostatic or bactericidal, depending on drug dosage, and is effective against many gram-positive and gram-negative organisms, especially *E. coli*. It is used in the treatment of acute and chronic UTIs. The drug data for nitrofurantoin are given in Chart 30–1.

PHARMACOKINETICS

Nitrofurantoin is well absorbed from the gastrointestinal (GI) tract. The drug is usually taken with food to decrease GI distress. Decreased absorption occurs when the drug is taken with antacids. Nitrofurantoin is moderately protein-bound. With normal renal function, the drug is rapidly eliminated because of a short half-life of 20 minutes; however, it accumulates in the serum with urinary dysfunction.

PHARMACODYNAMICS

When nitrofurantoin is given in low doses for prophylactic use, the drug has a bacteriostatic effect. High concentration of nitrofurantoin causes a bactericidal effect. Nitrofurantoin is effective against many gram-positive and gram-negative organisms such as *E. coli, Neisseria,* streptococci, *Staphylococcus aureus,* and others. It is not as effective against *Pseudomonas aeruginosa, Proteus* species, and some species of *Klebsiella*. The onset and duration of action are unknown. Peak action occurs one-half hour after absorption. If sudden onset of dyspnea, chest pain, cough, fever, and chills develops, the client should contact the health care provider. Symptoms resolve after discontinuing the drug.

Methenamine

Methenamine (Hiprex) produces a bactericidal effect when the urine pH is less than 5.5. It is available

Chart 30–1. Urinary Antiinfectives

ANTIINFECTIVE

Drug Name

Nitrofurantoin
(Furalan, Furan, Macrodantin),
❦ Apo-nitrofurantoin, Novofuran
Pregnancy Category: B

Dosage

Initial/recurrent UTI:
A: PO: 50–100 mg q.i.d. with meals and h.s.;
take with food
C: PO: >1 mo: 5–7 mg/kg in 4 divided doses
Long-term prophylaxis:
A: PO: 50–100 mg h.s.
A: PO: 1–2 mg/kg in 1–2 divided doses

Contraindications

Hypersensitivity, moderate to severe renal impairment, oliguria, anuria, Cl_{cr} <40 mL/min, infants <1 mo, term pregnancy, lactation with infant suspected of having G-6-PD deficiency
Caution: Vitamin B deficiency, electrolyte imbalance, diabetes mellitus

Drug-Lab-Food Interactions

Drug: *Decrease* effect with probenecid; *decrease* absorption with antacids

Pharmacokinetics

Absorption: Well absorbed from GI tract; enhanced with food
Distribution: PB: 60%, crosses placenta and enters breast milk
Metabolism: $t\frac{1}{2}$: 20–60 min
Excretion: In urine; small amounts in bile

Pharmacodynamics

PO: Onset: UK
Peak: 30 min
Duration: UK

Therapeutic Effects/Uses

To treat acute and chronic UTIs.

Mode of Action: Inhibits bacterial enzymes and metabolism.

Side Effects

Anorexia, nausea, vomiting, rust/brown discoloration of urine, diarrhea, rash, pruritus, dizziness, headache, drowsiness

Adverse Reactions

Superinfection, peripheral neuropathy, hemolytic anemia, agranulocytosis
Life-threatening: Anaphylaxis, hepatotoxicity, Stevens-Johnson syndrome

Assessment and Planning
Interventions
Evaluation
NURSING PROCESS

KEY: A: adult; C: child; PO: by mouth; UK: unknown; PB: protein-binding; $t\frac{1}{2}$: half-life; >: greater than; <: less than; Cl_{cr}: creatinine clearance; UTI: urinary tract infection; G-6-PD: glucose-6-phosphate dehydrogenase; GI: gastrointestinal; ❦: Canadian drug names.

as mandelate salt (short-acting) and as hippurate salt. Methenamine is effective against gram-positive and gram-negative organisms, especially *E. coli* and *P. aeruginosa*. It is used for chronic UTIs. Methenamine should not be taken with sulfonamides because crystalluria would likely occur. It is absorbed readily from the GI tract, and approximately 90% of the drug is excreted unchanged. Methenamine forms ammonia and formaldehyde in acid urine; therefore, the urine needs to be acidified to exert a bactericidal action. Cranberry juice (several 8-ounce glasses per day),

ascorbic acid, and ammonium chloride can be taken to decrease the urine pH.

Trimethoprim and Trimethoprim-Sulfamethoxazole

Trimethoprim (Proloprim, Trimpex) can be used alone (although frequently it is not) for the treatment of UTIs or in combination with a sulfonamide, sulfamethoxazole (the combined preparation is generically

Table 30–1
Antiseptics and Urinary Antiinfectives

GENERIC (BRAND)	ROUTE AND DOSAGE	USES AND CONSIDERATIONS
Fosfomycin tromethamine (Monurol)	A and C >12 y: PO: 1–3 g packet dissolved in 4 oz water, as a single dose	To treat uncomplicated UTIs in women. Has a bactericidal effect against most gram-negative and gram-positive bacteria. Side effects include headaches and diarrhea. *Pregnancy category:* B; PB: 0; $t\frac{1}{2}$: 5.7 h
Methenamine mandelate (Mandelamine, Mandameth)	A: PO: 1 g q.i.d. p.c. C 6–12 y: PO: 0.5 g q.i.d. p.c. C <6 y: PO: 50 mg/kg in 4 divided doses p.c.	For chronic UTIs. Urine pH should be acidic (<5.5). It should not be used with sulfonamides. May cause crystalluria, so push fluids. It can cause GI irritation, so take the drug with meals. *Pregnancy category:* C; PB: UK; $t\frac{1}{2}$: 3–6 h
Methenamine hippurate (Hiprex, Urex)	A: PO: 1 g b.i.d. C 6–12 y: 0.5–1 g b.i.d.	Same as above
Nitrofurantoin (Furalan, Macrodantin, Nitrofan)	See Chart 30–1	For acute and chronic UTIs. A normal creatinine clearance ensures the effectiveness of the drug. Peripheral neuropathy is an adverse effect. It may cause GI irritation. Taking with food decreases GI upset. *Pregnancy category:* B; PB: 40%; $t\frac{1}{2}$: 20–60 min
Trimethoprim (Proloprim, Trimpex)	A: PO: 100 mg q12h or 200 mg q24h; if Cl_{cr} (CrCl) is 15–30 mL/min: 50 mg q12h; if Cl_{cr} <15 mL/min: do not use	For prevention and treatment of acute and chronic UTIs in both males and females. High doses can cause GI upset. Drug can be combined with sulfamethoxazole (Bactrim). *Pregnancy category:* C; PB: UK; $t\frac{1}{2}$: 8–11 h
SULFONAMIDES		
Co-trimoxazole or sulfamethoxazole-trimethoprim (Bactrim, Septra)	See sulfonamides, Chapter 27 (Chart 27–1)	Effective for serious UTIs. Useful for otitis media. See Chapter 27. *Pregnancy category:* C; PB: 60%–70%; $t\frac{1}{2}$: 9 h
QUINOLONES (FLUOROQUINOLONES)		
Cinoxacin (Cinobac)	A: PO: 1 g/d in 2–4 doses for 1–2 wk *Renal dysfunction:* Initially: 500 mg; if Cl_{cr} is >80 mL/min: 500 mg b.i.d.; 80–50 mL/min: 250 mg t.i.d.; 50–20 mL/min: 250 mg b.i.d.; <20 mL/min: 250 mg q.d. Not recommended for infants or prepubertal children	For acute and chronic UTIs. More effective than nalidixic acid. Absorbed in prostatic tissue. Can cause dizziness and photosensitivity. Avoid excessive exposure to sunlight. *Pregnancy category:* C; PB: 60%–80%; $t\frac{1}{2}$: 1.5 h
Ciprofloxacin (Cipro)	A: PO: mild to moderate: 250 mg q12h; severe/complicated: 250–500 mg q12h *Renal dysfunction:* If Cl_{cr} >50 mL/min (PO); Cl_{cr} >30–50 mL/min: 250–500 mg q/2 h (IV); Cl_{cr} 5–29 mL/min: 250–500 mg q18h (PO) or 200–400 mg q24h (IV) *Hemo or peritoneal dialysis:* 250–500 mg q24h after dialysis	Has a broad-spectrum antibacterial effect. For UTI, skin and soft tissue infections, and bone and joint infections. Antacid inhibits drug absorption. Use with caution in clients with seizure disorders. Can be taken without food. Photosensitivity can occur. Avoid excessive exposure to sunlight. *Pregnancy category:* C; PB: 20%–40%; $t\frac{1}{2}$: 4–6 h
Enoxacin (Penetrex)	*Uncomplicated UTI:* A: PO: 200 mg q12h for 7 d *Complicated or severe UTI:* A: PO: 400 mg q12h for 14 d If Cl_{cr} <30 mL/min, reduce dose by 50%	Effective against complicated and uncomplicated UTIs. Fluid intake should be increased. Take before or after meals. Phototoxicity may occur. *Pregnancy category:* C (pregnant: X); PB: UK; $t\frac{1}{2}$: 3–6 h

Table continued on following page

Table 30–1 *Continued*
Antiseptics and Urinary Antiinfectives

GENERIC (BRAND)	ROUTE AND DOSAGE	USES AND CONSIDERATIONS
Lomefloxacin (Maxaquin)	A: PO: 400 mg/d × 10 d	For UTIs and transurethral surgery prophylaxis. *Pregnancy category:* C; PB: UK; $t\frac{1}{2}$: 6.25–7.75 h
Nalidixic acid (NegGram)	A: PO: 1 g q.i.d. for 1–2 wk; 1 g b.i.d. for long-term use C: PO: 55 mg/kg/d in 4 divided doses for 1–2 wk; 33 mg/kg/d for long-term use C: <3 mo: *Do not use*	For acute and chronic UTIs. Resistance to drug may occur. Highly protein-bound. Not distributed in prostatic fluid. Take with food to avoid GI upset. Photosensitivity can occur. Avoid excessive exposure to sunlight. Contact health care provider if seizures or severe headaches occur. *Pregnancy category:* B; PB: 93%; $t\frac{1}{2}$: 1–2 h (elderly: 12 h)
Norfloxacin (Noroxin)	A: PO: 400 mg b.i.d. for 1–2 wk on empty stomach *Uncomplicated cystitis caused by E. coli, K. pneumoniae, P. mirabilis:* 400 mg b.i.d. × 3 d *Uncomplicated caused by any other organism:* 400 mg b.i.d. × 7–10 d *Complicated:* 400 mg b.i.d. × 10–21 d *Renal impairment (Cl_{cr} <30 mL/min):* 400 mg q.d.	For acute and chronic UTIs. Most potent drug of the quinolone group. Food may inhibit drug absorption. *Pregnancy category:* C; PB: 10%–15%; $t\frac{1}{2}$: 3–4 h
Ofloxacin (Floxin)	A: PO: IV: 200 mg q12h × 10 d	For UTIs, respiratory tract and skin infections. May cause headaches, dizziness, insomnia. *Pregnancy category:* C; PB: 20%–32%; $t\frac{1}{2}$: 5–7.5 h
OTHER		
Aztreonam (Azactam)	A: IM/IV: 500 mg–1 g q8–12h	Treatment of UTIs caused by gram-negative organisms. Also useful for low respiratory infection, septicemia. *Pregnancy category:* B; PB: 56%–60%; $t\frac{1}{2}$: 1.5–2 h
Imipenem/cilastatin sodium (Primaxin)	A: IV: 250 mg–1 g q6h *max:* 4 g/d or 50 mg/kg/d, whichever is the lesser amount C: Safety and efficacy not established Dosing adjustment with renal impairment	Treatment of serious UTIs. Also useful for lower respiratory, bone, and joint infections; and septicemia and endocarditis. *Pregnancy category:* C; PB: 20%–40%; $t\frac{1}{2}$: 1 h
Methylene blue (Urolene Blue)	*Cystitis, urethritis:* A: PO: 60–125 mg b.i.d./t.i.d. p.c. with glass of water	For urinary calculi. Urine, sweat, and/or stool may be blue-green due to the dye in the drug. *Pregnancy category:* C; PB: UK; $t\frac{1}{2}$: UK
Polymyxin B SO$_4$ (Aerosporin)	A&C: IV: 15,000–25,000 U/kg/d in divided doses q12h	Effective for UTIs and to prevent bacteriuria occurring from indwelling catheter. Can cause nephrotoxicity. Monitor renal function (BUN, serum creatinine). *Pregnancy category:* B; PB: UK; $t\frac{1}{2}$: 4–6 h

KEY: *A: adult; C: child; PO: by mouth; IM: intramuscular; IV: intravenous; UK: unknown, Cl_{cr}: creatinine clearance; >: greater than; <: less than; PB: protein-binding; $t\frac{1}{2}$: half-life; GI: gastrointestinal; UTI: urinary tract infection; BUN: blood urea nitrogen; p.c.: after meals.*

referred to as co-trimoxazole), to prevent the occurrence of trimethoprim-resistant organisms. It produces slow-acting bactericidal effects against most gram-positive and gram-negative organisms. Co-trimoxazole (Bactrim, Septra) is discussed in detail in Chapter 27. Trimethoprim is used in the treatment and prevention of acute and chronic UTIs. The amount of trimethoprim in the prostatic fluid is about two to three times greater than the amount in the vascular fluid. The half-life of trimethoprim is nor-

NURSING PROCESS
URINARY ANTIINFECTIVE: NITROFURANTOIN

Assessment

- Obtain a history from the client of clinical problems with urinary tract infection (UTI) or other urinary tract disorders.
- Assess the client for signs and symptoms of UTI, such as pain or burning sensation on urination and frequency and urgency of urination.
- Assess complete blood count (CBC) on clients with long-term therapy; monitor regularly.
- Assess renal and hepatic function.
- Assess urine pH; 5.5 is desired; however, alkalinization of the urine is *not* recommended.

Potential Nursing Diagnoses

- Altered; comfort, pain
- Risk for infection

Planning

- Client will be free of signs and symptoms of UTI within 10 d.

Nursing Interventions

- Monitor the client's output. Careful attention to output is required when administering urinary antiseptics to clients with anuria and oliguria. Report promptly any decrease in urine output.
- Before the start of drug therapy, obtain a urine culture to determine the organism causing the UTI.
- Observe the client for side effects of and adverse reactions to urinary antiseptic drugs. Peripheral neuropathy (tingling, numbness of extremities) may result from renal insufficiency (inability to excrete drug) or long-term use of nitrofurantoin. Peripheral neuropathy may be irreversible.
- Dilute intravenous (IV) nitrofurantoin in 500 mL of IV solution before administering; reconstitute in sterile water without preservative.

Client Teaching

General
- Advise the client not to crush tablets or open capsules.
- Advise the client to rinse mouth thoroughly after taking oral nitrofurantoin. This drug can stain the teeth.

Nursing Process continued on following page

mally 9 to 11 h; the half-life is longer with renal dysfunction.

Fluoroquinolones (Quinolones)

Fluoroquinolones are one of the newest groups of urinary antiseptics and are effective against lower UTIs. Nalidixic acid (NegGram) was developed in 1964, and cinoxacin (Cinobac), norfloxacin (Noroxin), and ciprofloxacin hydrochloride (Cipro) were marketed in the 1980s. Enoxacin was marketed in the late 1980s or early 1990s; ofloxacin in 1990; and lomefloxacin in 1992. The newer fluoroquinolones (norfloxacin, ciprofloxacin, enoxacin, ofloxacin, and lomefloxacin) are effective against a wide variety of UTIs. Drug dosage should be decreased when renal dysfunction is present. The half-lives of these drugs are 2 to 4 h but are prolonged with renal dysfunction. Table 30–1 lists the urinary antiseptics/antiinfectives, their dosages, uses, and considerations.

Side Effects and Adverse Reactions

The side effects of and adverse reactions to urinary antiseptics are listed herein by category.

- Avoid antacids because they interfere with drug absorption.
- Instruct client to shake suspension well before taking and protect it from freezing.
- Advise client not to drive a motor vehicle or operate dangerous machinery; drug may cause drowsiness.
- Advise the diabetic client not to use Clinitest to test for glucose because a false-positive result may occur.

Diet
- Instruct the client to increase fluids and take the drug with food; this minimizes GI upset.

Side Effects
- Advise the client that urine may turn a harmless brown.
- Advise the client to report any signs of secondary fungal or bacterial infection (superinfection), such as stomatitis or anogenital discharge or itching.

Methenamine
- Advise the client to drink cranberry juice or take vitamin C with approval of the health care provider in order to keep the urine acidic. Foods that are alkaline, such as milk and some vegetables, may increase the urine pH. The urine pH should be less than 5.5 for the antiseptic to be effective.

Fluoroquinolones
- Advise the client to avoid operating hazardous machinery or driving a car while taking the drug, especially if dizziness is present.
- Instruct the client to take the drug with food and to avoid antacids because they interfere with drug absorption.
- Advise the client that the urine may turn a harmless brown because of the drug.
- Advise the client to report any signs of superinfection or a secondary fungal or bacterial infection.
- Instruct the client to avoid excessive exposure to sunlight.

Cultural Considerations

- Alleviate fear or concerns of a client from a different cultural background by explaining the treatment regimen for a UTI. An interpreter may be necessary. The use of pamphlets could help the client to understand the urinary tract problem.
- A detailed explanation of use of preventive measures of UTIs could be helpful. Proper use of toilet paper after defecation should be emphasized.

Evaluation

- Evaluate the effectiveness of the urinary antiinfectives in alleviating the UTI. Client is free of side effects and adverse reactions to drug.

NITROFURANTOIN
Side effects of nitrofurantoin use include GI disturbances such as anorexia, nausea, vomiting, diarrhea, and abdominal pain, and pulmonary reactions such as dyspnea, chest pain, fever, and cough.

METHENAMINE
Methenamine use also has GI side effects, including nausea, vomiting, and diarrhea. There are some allergic reactions to the dye in Hiprex. Bladder irritation and crystalluria (with large doses) may occur.

TRIMETHOPRIM
GI symptoms, including nausea and vomiting, and skin problems, such as rash and pruritus, can accompany trimethoprim use.

FLUOROQUINOLONES
Nalidixic acid use can have the following side effects: headaches, dizziness, syncope (fainting), peripheral neuritis, visual disturbances, and rash. Nausea, vomiting, diarrhea, headaches, and visual disturbances can occur with cinoxacin and norfloxacin use. Photosensitivity is a common side effect associated with fluoroquinolones.

Drug-Drug Interactions

The following drug-drug interactions can occur.

- Nalidixic acid enhances the effects of warfarin.
- Antacids decrease nitrofurantoin absorption.
- Most urinary antiseptics cause false-positive Clini-

Chart 30–2.   Urinary Analgesic

ANTIPRURITIC, LOCAL ANESTHETIC

Drug Name

Phenazopyridine
(Pyridium, Urodine);
✦ Phenazo, Pyronium
Pregnancy Category: B

Dosage

A: PO: 100–200 mg t.i.d. p.c. × 2 d
C: PO: 12 mg/kg in 3 divided doses

Contraindications

Severe liver or renal disease, pregnancy or breast feeding

Drug-Lab-Food Interactions

Lab: May interfere with urinalysis color reactions, urinary glucose, ketones, proteins, steroids

Pharmacokinetics

Absorption: PO: Well absorbed
Distribution: PB: UK
Metabolism: t½: UK
Excretion: In urine

Pharmacodynamics

PO: Onset: UK
Peak: 5–6 h
Duration: 6–8 h

Therapeutic Effects/Uses

For relief of UTI from infection, trauma, and surgery (use with urinary antiseptic).

Mode of Action: Produces analgesia/local anesthesia on urinary tract mucosa. Exact mechanism of action unknown.

Side Effects

Anorexia, nausea, vomiting, diarrhea, heartburn, red-orange discoloration of urine, rash, pruritus, headache, vertigo

Adverse Reactions

Life-threatening: Agranulocytosis, hepatotoxicity, nephrotoxicity, thrombocytopenia, leukopenia, hemolytic anemia

(Assessment and Planning / Interventions / Evaluation — NURSING PROCESS)

KEY: A: adult; C: child; PO: by mouth; UK: unknown; PB: protein-binding; t½: half-life; UTI: urinary tract infection; ✦: Canadian drug names.

test results.
• Sodium bicarbonate inhibits the action of methenamine.
• Methenamine taken with sulfonamides increases the risk of crystalluria.

The nursing process for nitrofurantoin is applicable for other urinary antiseptics/antiinfectives.

URINARY ANALGESICS

Phenazopyridine

Phenazopyridine hydrochloride (Pyridium), an azo dye, is a **urinary analgesic** that has been available for almost 40 years. It is used to relieve pain, burning sensation, and the frequency and urgency of urination that are symptomatic of lower UTIs. The drug can cause GI disturbances, hemolytic anemia, nephrotoxicity, and hepatotoxicity. The urine becomes a harmless reddish orange color because of the dye. Phenazopyridine can alter the glucose urine test (Clinitest), so a blood test should be used to monitor glucose levels. Chart 30–2 describes the pharmacologic behavior of phenazopyridine.

PHARMACOKINETICS

Phenazopyridine is well absorbed from the GI tract. Its protein-binding percentage and half-life are unknown. Phenazopyridine is metabolized by the liver and excreted in the urine, which is colored a reddish orange because of the harmless dye in the drug.

NURSING PROCESS
URINARY ANALGESIC: PHENAZOPYRIDINE (PYRIDIUM)

Assessment

- Obtain a history from the client of clinical problems with the urinary tract.
- Obtain a drug history; report probable drug-drug interactions.
- Assess the client for signs and symptoms of UTI such as pain or burning sensation on urination and frequency and urgency of urination.
- Assess hepatic function studies, especially serum liver enzymes, with long-term therapy.

Potential Nursing Diagnoses

- Altered patterns of urinary elimination
- Pain due to renal problem

Planning

- The client will be free of urinary tract pain within 3 d.

Nursing Interventions

- Administer drug with food or milk to decrease gastric distress. Chewable tablets should be chewed.
- Observe client for side effects of and adverse reaction to urinary analgesic.

Client Teaching

General
- Instruct client to take medication exactly as ordered; recommended dosage should not be exceeded. Advise client to take with food or milk.

Side Effects
- Advise the client that urine will be harmless reddish orange but that the dye does permanently stain clothing and tears will stain contact lenses.
- Instruct client to report signs of hepatotoxicity, including yellowing of skin or sclera, clay-colored stools, abdominal pain, diarrhea, dark urine, or fever.

Bethanechol
- Instruct the client to report abdominal discomfort, diarrhea, nausea, vomiting, increased salivation, urgency, flushing, or sweating.

Evaluation

- Evaluate the effectiveness of the drug in alleviating the urinary tract pain. Client is free of side effects and adverse reactions to drug.

PHARMACODYNAMICS

Phenazopyridine has been available for decades for decreasing urinary pain and discomfort. It has an anesthetic effect on the urinary tract mucosa; exact action is unknown. The serum peak concentration time for this drug is 5 h, and its duration of action is 6 to 8 h. Phenazopyridine is usually administered several times a day. With severe liver or renal diseases, hepatotoxicity or nephrotoxicity, respectively, may occur.

URINARY STIMULANTS

When bladder function is decreased or lost as a result of a neurogenic bladder (a dysfunction caused by a lesion of the nervous system), as a result of a spinal cord injury (paraplegia, hemiplegia), or as a result of severe head injury, a parasympathomimetic may be used to stimulate **micturition** (urination). The drug of choice, bethanechol chloride (Urecholine), is a **urinary stimulant,** also known as a direct-acting parasym-

Table 30–2
Urinary Analgesic, Stimulant, and Antispasmodics

GENERIC (BRAND)	ROUTE AND DOSAGE	USES AND CONSIDERATIONS
URINARY ANALGESIC		
Phenazopyridine HCl (Pyridium, Urodine)	See Chart 30–2	For chronic cystitis to alleviate pain and burning sensation during urination. Urine will be reddish orange. Can be taken concurrently with an antibiotic. It treats only symptoms, not the underlying cause of the pain; therefore, do not use long term for undiagnosed urinary tract pain. *Pregnancy category:* B; PB: UK; $t_{\frac{1}{2}}$: UK
URINARY STIMULANT		
Bethanechol Cl (Urecholine, Duvoid, Urabeth)	A: PO: 10–50 mg t.i.d./q.i.d. 1 h a.c. or 2 h p.c. SC: 2.5–10 mg t.i.d./q.i.d. PRN C: PO: 0.6 mg/kg/d in 3–4 divided doses	For hypotonic or atonic bladder. Should not be taken if peptic ulcer is present. Can cause epigastric distress, abdominal cramps, nausea, vomiting, diarrhea, and flatulence. Can cause dizziness, lightheadedness, and fainting, especially when standing up from lying or sitting position. *Pregnancy category:* C; PB: UK; $t_{\frac{1}{2}}$: UK
URINARY ANTISPAS-MODICS		
Dimethyl sulfoxide (DMSO, Rimso-50)	*Bladder instillation:* 50 mL of 50% sol retained for 15 min; repeat q2wk until relief	For cystitis. Administered into the bladder to remain for 15 min. Additional effects are antiinflammatory, anesthetic, and bacteriostatic. Can cause a garlic-like taste and odor on breath/skin for up to 72 hours. *Pregnancy category:* C; PB: UK; $t_{\frac{1}{2}}$: UK
Flavoxate HCl (Urispas)	A: PO: 100–200 mg t.i.d. or q.i.d.	For urinary tract spasms. To be avoided by persons with glaucoma. Cautious use by the elderly. Side effects include nausea, vomiting, dry mouth, drowsiness, blurred vision. *Pregnancy category:* B; PB: UK; $t_{\frac{1}{2}}$: UK
Oxybutynin Cl (Ditropan)	A: PO: 5 mg b.i.d. or t.i.d. C: >5 y: PO: 5 mg b.i.d. C 1–5 y: PO: 0.2 mg/kg b.i.d.–q.i.d.	For urinary tract spasms. Contraindicated for persons with cardiac, renal, hepatic, and prostate problems. Side effects include drowsiness, blurred vision, dry mouth. *Pregnancy category:* B; PB: UK; $t_{\frac{1}{2}}$: 1–3 h
Propantheline bromide (Pro-Banthine)	A: PO: 15 mg t.i.d. 30 min a.c. and 30 mg h.s.; *max:* 120 mg/d Elderly: 7.5 mg t.i.d./q.i.d. C: PO: 2–3 mg/kg/d in divided doses	Effective for ureteral and urinary bladder spasm. Frequent dosing may cause urinary hesitancy or retention. Have client void before each dose. *Pregnancy category:* C; PB: UK; $t_{\frac{1}{2}}$: 1.5 h

KEY: A: adult; C: child; PO: by mouth; SC: subcutaneous; >: greater than; <: less than; a.c.: before meals; p.c.: after meals; UK: unknown; PB: protein-binding; $t_{\frac{1}{2}}$: half-life; sol: solution.

pathomimetic (cholinomimetic). The drug action is to increase bladder tone by increasing tone of the detrusor urinal muscle, which produces a contraction strong enough to stimulate urination. Bethanechol is discussed in detail in Chapter 22.

URINARY ANTISPASMODICS

Urinary tract spasms resulting from infection or injury can be relieved with **antispasmodics** that have a direct action on the smooth muscles of the urinary tract. This group of drugs (dimethyl sulfoxide [also called DMSO], oxybutynin, and flavoxate) is contraindicated for use if urinary or GI obstruction is present or if the client has glaucoma. Antispasmodics have the same effects as antimuscarinics, parasympatholytics, and anticholinergics (discussed in Chapter 22). Side effects include dry mouth, increased heart rate, dizziness, intestinal distention, and constipation. Table 30–2 lists drugs that are urinary analgesics, stimulants, and antispasmodics.

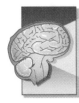

Critical Thinking in Action

F. L., 29 years old, is married and has a 3-year-old child. F. L. complained to her health care provider of painful urinary frequency and urgency. The client has an elevated temperature. The urine specimen indicated that the client had an urinary tract infection (UTI). Co-trimoxazole D.S. (double-strength, T-160 mg/S-800 mg) tablet twice a day for 14 days is prescribed.

1. What other information should the health care provider obtain from the client?
2. What other dose of co-trimoxazole could be prescribed? Explain.
3. Explain what the health care provider should discuss with the client in regard to taking the drug and its possible side effects. What other information should F. L. receive?
4. What preventive measures should be discussed with the client to prevent future occurrences of UTIs?
5. Explain the recommended follow-up care for F. L.
6. What other drugs might be used instead of co-trimoxazole? Would one urinary anti-infective drug be more effective than another antiinfective drug? Explain.

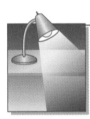

Study Questions

1. What are the symptoms of UTIs? What group of drugs is used to alleviate these symptoms?
2. What is the major group of side effects associated with most urinary antiseptics/antiinfectives. How can they be prevented?
3. What type of drug is phenazopyridine and what is its purpose? What are two nursing interventions related to this drug?
4. What are the side effects of urinary antispasmodics? Why? Why should a person with glaucoma avoid taking a drug from this group?

Unit VI

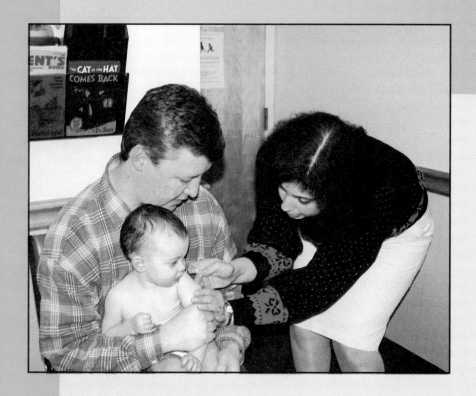

Immunologic Agents

Immunity comprises functions that protect people from the effects of invasion of the body by microscopic organisms: bacteria, viruses, molds, spores, pollens, protozoa, and cells from other people or animals. A person remains in harmony with these organisms as long as the organisms do not enter the body's internal environment. The body has various defenses (e.g., skin) to prevent microorganisms from gaining access to the internal environment. But these defenses are not infallible, and invasion of the body's internal environment by microorganisms occurs often. A properly functioning immune system neutralizes, eliminates, or destroys the invading microorganisms. To do this without harming the body, immune system cells use defensive actions against only *nonself* proteins and cells. Therefore, immune system cells can differentiate between the body's own, healthy *self* cells and other *nonself* proteins and cells.

Nonself proteins and cells include infected or debilitated body cells, self cells that have undergone malignant transformation into cancer cells, and all foreign cells and microorganisms. This ability to recognize self versus nonself, necessary to prevent healthy body cells from being destroyed along with the invaders, is called *self-tolerance*. The immune system cells are the only body cells capable of recognizing self and nonself.

Unique proteins on the surface of all body cells of each individual serve as a personal identification code for that person. The cell-surface proteins of one person are recognized as "foreign" by the immune system of another person. These are antigens, proteins capable of stimulating an immune response.

Immune function is generally most efficient when people are in their 20s and 30s; it slowly declines with increasing age. The elderly have marginal immune function, causing increased susceptibility to a variety of pathologic conditions.

IMMUNE SYSTEM STRUCTURE

The immune system is not confined to any one organ or body area. Instead, immune system cells originate in the bone marrow. Some of these cells mature in the bone marrow; others leave the bone marrow and mature in different specific body sites. After maturation, most immune system cells are released into the blood, to circulate throughout the body and exert specific effects.

IMMUNE SYSTEM FUNCTION

The three processes necessary for immunity and the cells involved in these responses can be categorized as inflammation, antibody-mediated immunity (humoral immunity), and cell-mediated immunity.

Inflammation is discussed in the introduction to Unit V. Full immunity, or immunocompetence, requires the adequate function and interaction of all three processes, even though some functions of each overlap. Long-lasting immune actions are those generated by antibody-mediated immunity and cell-mediated immunity.

Antibody-Mediated Immunity

Antibody-mediated immunity (AMI), also known as humoral immunity, involves antigen-antibody interactions to neutralize, eliminate, or destroy foreign proteins. Antibodies for these interactions are produced by populations of B lymphocytes.

ANTIGEN-ANTIBODY INTERACTIONS

Antigen-antibody interactions occur in the body's internal environment. To make an antibody that can exert its effects on a specific antigen, the body must first be exposed to that antigen to the degree that the antigen enters the body. Even when exposure includes penetration, not all exposures result in the stimulation of antibody production. Invasion by the antigen must occur in such large numbers that some of the antigen either evades detection by the normal nonspecific defenses or overwhelms the abilities of the inflammatory response to neutralize, eliminate, or destroy the invader.

ACQUIRING ANTIBODY-MEDIATED IMMUNITY

The two broad categories of immunity are innate immunity and acquired immunity. *Innate immunity* is a genetically determined characteristic of an individual, group, or species. A person either has or does not have innate immunity. For example, people have many innate immunities to viruses and other microorganisms that cause specific diseases in animals. As a result, humans are not susceptible to such diseases as mange, distemper, hog cholera, or any of a variety of animal afflictions. This type of immunity cannot be developed or transferred from one person to another and is not an adaptive response to exposure or invasion by foreign proteins.

Acquired immunity is the immunity that every person's body makes (or can receive) as an adaptive response to invasion by foreign proteins. Antibody-mediated immunity is an acquired immunity. Acquired immunity occurs either naturally or artificially and can be either active or passive. *Active immunity* occurs when antigens enter the body and the body responds by making specific antibodies against the antigen. This type of immunity is active, because the body takes an active part in making the antibodies. Active immunity can occur under conditions that are either natural or artificial. *Natural active immunity* occurs when an antigen enters the body without human assistance, and the body responds by actively making antibodies against that antigen (e.g., chickenpox virus). Most of the time, the first invasion of the body by this antigen results in the person's manifesting signs and symptoms of the disease. However, processes occurring in the body at the same time allow the person to acquire immunity to that antigen so that he or she will not become ill after a second exposure to the same antigen. This type of immunity is the most effective and the longest lasting.

Artificial active immunity is a type of protection developed against illnesses that produce such serious side effects that total avoidance of the disease is most desirable. Small amounts of specific antigens are deliberately placed (as a vaccination) in the body so that the body responds by actively making antibodies against the antigen. Because antigens used for this procedure have been specially processed to make them less likely to proliferate within the body, this exposure does not in itself cause the disease.

Examples of diseases for which artificially acquired active immunity can be obtained include tetanus, diphtheria, measles, smallpox, mumps, and rubella, among others. This type of immunity lasts many years, although repeated but smaller doses of the original antigen are required as a "booster" for maintaining complete protection against the antigen.

Passive immunity occurs when antibodies against a specific antigen are in a person's body but the person did not actively generate these antibodies. These antibodies are made in the body of another person or animal and then transferred to the body of a specific individual. Because these antibodies are foreign to the individual, the body recognizes the antibodies as nonself and takes steps to eliminate them relatively quickly. For this reason, passive immunity can provide only immediate, short-term protection against a specific antigen.

Cell-Mediated Immunity

Cell-mediated immunity (CMI), or cellular immunity, involves many leukocyte actions, reactions, and interactions that range from the simple to the complex. This type of immunity is provided by committed lymphocyte stem cells that mature in the secondary lymphoid tissues of the thymus and pericortical areas of lymph nodes. Certain CMI responses influence and regulate the activities of antibody-mediated immunity and inflammation by producing and releasing cytokines. Therefore, total immunocompetence relies on optimal CMI function.

The leukocytes playing the most important roles in cell-mediated immunity include several specific T-lymphocyte subsets along with a special population of cells known as natural killer cells (NK cells). T lymphocytes further differentiate into a variety of subsets, each of which has a specific function. The three T-lymphocyte subsets that are crucial for the development and continuation of cell-mediated immunity are helper/inducer T cells, suppressor T cells, and cytotoxic/cytolytic T cells.

PROTECTION PROVIDED BY CELL-MEDIATED IMMUNITY

Specific components of cell-mediated immunity (CMI) assist in providing protection to the body by their highly developed abilities to differentiate self from nonself. The nonself cells most easily recognized by CMI are those self cells that are infected by organisms that live within host cells and those self cells mutated at the DNA level and no longer normal. CMI provides a surveillance system for ridding the body of self cells that might potentially harm the body. CMI is critically important in preventing development of cancer and metastasis after exposure to carcinogens.

31 HIV and AIDS-Related Agents

Patricia S. Lincoln and Robert Kizior

Outline

Objectives

- Define antiretroviral therapy.
- Describe the life cycle of the human immunodeficiency virus (HIV).
- List the three classifications of antiretroviral therapy with examples of medications in each group.
- Explain prophylactic treatment for opportunistic infections.
- Describe postexposure prophylaxis for health care workers.
- Identify implications of the related drugs for pregnancy.
- Describe specific factors related to adherence/compliance with the medication regimen.

Terms

antibody

antigen

antiretroviral

CD4+ T cells

compliance/adherence

HAART

immune response

immune system

integrase

postexposure prophylaxis (PEP)

protease inhibitors

resistance

reverse transcriptase inhibitors: nucleoside analogues and nonnucleoside analogues

viral load

INTRODUCTION

In 1981, a group of young predominantly homosexual men were diagnosed with a syndrome that was later named acquired immunodeficiency syndrome (AIDS). Worldwide by early 1998, there were 42 million people infected with human immunodeficiency virus (HIV), and approximately 11.7 million people have died of AIDS-related diseases.

PATHOLOGY

HIV was identified to be the causative agent of AIDS in 1983. HIV is a retrovirus that causes a gradual deterioration of immune function. AIDS is characterized by profound immunologic deficits, opportunistic infection (OI), secondary infections, and malignant neoplasms.

Once a person is infected with HIV, crucial immune cells called **CD4+ T cells** are disabled and killed. During the course of infection, the numbers of CD4+ T cells progressively decline. CD4+ T cells play a crucial role in the **immune response,** signaling other cells in the **immune system** to perform their special function.

There are three modes of transmission of HIV infection: injection of infected blood or blood products, sexual contact, and maternal-fetal transmission. Occupational exposure accounts for a small number of infected individuals; the majority of such infections are from needlestick injury.

LABORATORY AND DIAGNOSTIC TESTS

A healthy, uninfected person usually has 800 to 1200 CD4+ T cells per cubic millimeter (mm³) of blood.

When severe damage from the HIV infection causes the CD4+ T-cell count to decrease to 200 mm³ or equal to or less than 14%, the person is particularly vulnerable to opportunistic infections and cancers, and the person is then classified as having AIDS. Table 31–1 lists the 1993 AIDS surveillance case definition. In addition to the T-cell count, a second test used to evaluate the status of the patient's immune system is the **viral load (VL).** HIV RNA (viral particles) are counted; the higher the number, the higher the viral burden.

HIV is a retrovirus. HIV uses three different enzymes to genetically encode, replicate, and assemble new virus within the cells (HIV can replicate only inside cells). These three enzymes are reverse transcriptase, integrase, and protease.

The virus enters the cell through the CD4 molecule on the cell surface. The virus uncoats with the help of the **reverse transcriptase** enzyme, and a single-stranded viral RNA is converted into DNA, the form in which the cell carries its genes. The viral DNA migrates to the nucleus of the cell, where it is spliced into the host DNA with the help of the second enzyme, **integrase.** Once incorporated, HIV DNA is called the provirus and is duplicated together with the cell genes every time the cell divides. **Protease,** the third enzyme, assists in the assembly of newly formed viral particles (Fig. 31–1).

As of 1995, monotherapy with any antiretroviral agent was no longer recommended. Combination therapy known as **highly active antiretroviral therapy (HAART)** is the current treatment recommendation. Medications designed to slow or inhibit these enzymes are called **antiretroviral** medications. In 1987, the Food and Drug Administration (FDA) approved the first reverse transcriptase (RT) inhibitor and, in 1995, approved the first protease inhibitor. To date, no integrase inhibitors have been approved.

The goals of HAART include decreasing the viral

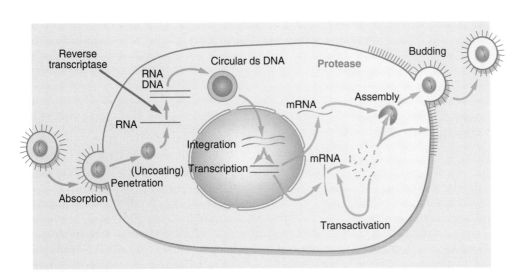

Figure 31–1
The life cycle of human immunodeficiency virus.

Table 31–1A
A. Classification System for HIV-Infection*

CD4⁺ T-CELL CATEGORIES	CLINICAL CATEGORIES FOR ADULTS		
	(A) Asymptomatic, Acute (Primary) HIV or PGM	(B) Symptomatic, not (A) or (C) Conditions	(C) AIDS-Indicator Conditions
(1) ≥500/μL	A1	B1	C1
(2) 200–499/μL	A2	B2	C2
(3) <200/μL AIDS-indicator T-cell count	A3	B3	C3

*The revised CDC classification system for HIV-infected adolescents and adults categorizes persons on the basis of CD4⁺ T-lymphocyte counts and clinical conditions associated with HIV infection. The system is based on three ranges of CD4⁺ T-lymphocyte counts and three clinical categories, represented by a matrix of nine mutually exclusive categories.

CD4⁺ T-Lymphocyte Categories

HIV-infected persons should be classified based on existing guidelines for the medical management of HIV-infected persons. Thus, the lowest accurate CD4⁺ T-lymphocyte count should be used (but not necessarily the most recent) for classification purposes.

Clinical Categories

Category A

Category A consists of one or more of the following conditions in an adolescent or adult (13 years of age or older) with documented HIV infection. Conditions listed in categories B and C must not have occurred.

• *Asymptomatic HIV infection*
• *Persistent generalized lymphadenopathy*
• *Acute (primary) HIV infection with accompanying illness or history of acute HIV infection*

Category B

Category B consists of symptomatic conditions in a HIV-infected adolescent or adult that are not included in category C and are attributed to HIV infection or are considered to have a clinical course complicated by HIV infection. Examples of conditions in category B include, but are not limited to, the following:

• *Bacillary angiomatosis*
• *Candidiasis, oropharyngeal (thrush)*
• *Candidiasis, vulvovaginal; persistent, frequent, or poorly responsive to therapy*
• *Cervical dysplasia (moderate or severe)/cervical carcinoma in situ*
• *Constitutional symptoms, such as fever (38.5°C) or diarrhea lasting >1 month*
• *Hairy leukoplakia, oral*
• *Herpes zoster (shingles), involving at least two distinct episodes or more than one dermatome*
• *Idiopathic thrombocytopenic purpura*
• *Listeriosis*
• *Pelvic inflammatory disease, particularly if complicated by tubo-ovarian abscess*
• *Peripheral neuropathy*

For classification purposes, category B conditions take precedence over category A conditions.

Category C

Category C includes the clinical conditions listed in the AIDS surveillance case definition. For classification purposes, once a category C condition occurs, the person remains in category C.
KEY: PGM: persistent generalized lymphadenopathy.
From DHHS and Henry J. Kaiser Family Foundation (Dec. 1, 1998). Panel on Practices for Treatment of HIV Infection. Guidelines for the Use of Antiretroviral Agents in HIV-Infected Adults and Adolescents.

load to undetectable levels, preserving and increasing the number of CD4⁺ T cells, preventing resistance, having the client in good clinical condition, and preventing secondary infections and cancers. HIV viral load testing has been approved by the FDA only for the RT-PCR assay (Roche) and only for determining disease prognosis. To obtain and maintain the goals of HAART therapy, the patient must have excellent adherence/compliance skills. Failure to take combination therapy as directed can lead to resistance to or

failure of antiretroviral agents. Additionally, the clinical management of the HIV/AIDS patient must include measures to minimize associated opportunistic infections and malignancies. Aggressive prophylaxis and treatment of opportunistic infections are suggested. Nutritional therapy, complementary therapy, and supportive care are also necessary.

It is recommended that antiretroviral therapy be offered to those with less than 500 CD4⁺ T cells mm³ or plasma HIV RNA levels greater than 10,000 cop-

Table 31–1B
B. Pediatric Human Immunodeficiency Virus (HIV) Classification*

IMMUNOLOGIC CATEGORIES	CLINICAL CATEGORIES			
	N: No Signs/ Symptoms	A: Mild Signs/ Symptoms	B:† Moderate Signs/ Symptoms	C:† Severe Signs/ Symptoms
1: No evidence of suppression	N1	A1	B1	C1
2: Evidence of moderate suppression	N2	A2	B2	C2
3: Severe suppression	N3	A3	B3	C3

**Children whose HIV infection status is not confirmed are classified by using the above grid with a letter E (for perinatally exposed) placed before the appropriate classification code (e.g., EN2).*
†*Both category C and lymphoid interstitial pneumonitis in category B are reportable to state and local health departments as acquired immunodeficiency syndrome.*
KEY: PGM: persistent generalized lymphadenopathy.
From DHHS and Henry J. Kaiser Family Foundation (Dec. 1, 1998). Panel on Practices for Treatment of HIV Infection. Guidelines for the Use of Antiretroviral Agents in HIV-Infected Adults and Adolescents.

ies/mL (B-DNA assay) or 20,000 copies/mL (RT-PCR assay).

Therapy should be considered for all HIV-infected patients with detectable HIV RNA in plasma. The patient's willingness to accept therapy and the probability of adherence to the prescribed therapeutic regimen **(compliance/adherence)** provide the basis for treatment of asymptomatic individuals. The risks and benefits of early initiation of antiretroviral therapy in the asymptomatic HIV-infected patient are listed in Table 31–2.

Management of HIV is evolving rapidly. The most current information is found on the HIV/AIDS Treatment Information Service website, http://www:hivatis.org. Recommendations are updated on a regular basis.

ANTIRETROVIRAL THERAPY

Currently, reverse transcriptase inhibitors (RT inhibitors) and protease inhibitors (PI) make up the classification of drugs known as antiretroviral therapy. RT inhibitors are divided into nucleoside and nonnucleoside analogues. Protease inhibitors have changed the prognosis for millions of patients infected with HIV. Protease inhibitors combined with RT inhibitors can reduce viral plasma levels to undetectable levels, thus offering significant clinical benefit.

Antiretroviral Agents

Currently, three classes of agents are used in the treatment of HIV infection: nucleoside analogues, nonnucleoside analogues, and protease inhibitors. Nucleoside and nonnucleoside analogues act by inhibiting HIV reverse transcriptase (HIV-RT), which is re-

sponsible for viral replication early in the virus life cycle. These agents prevent HIV infection of new cells but cannot prevent the production of new infections by already infected cells. Thus, these agents have limited effects. The protease inhibitors block protease, an

Table 31–2
Risks and Benefits of Early Initiation of Antiretroviral Therapy in the Asymptomatic HIV-Infected Patient

POTENTIAL BENEFITS

- Control of viral replication and mutation; reduction of viral burden
- Prevention of progressive immunodeficiency; potential maintenance or reconstruction of a normal immune system
- Delayed progression to acquired immunodeficiency syndrome and prolongation of life
- Decreased risk of selection of resistant virus
- Decreased risk of drug toxicity
- Possible decreased risk of viral transmission

POTENTIAL RISKS

- Reduction in quality of life from adverse drug effects and inconvenience of current maximally suppressive regimens
- Earlier development of drug resistance
- Transmission of drug-resistant virus
- Limitation in future choices of antiretroviral agents as a result of development of resistance
- Unknown long-term toxicity of antiretroviral drugs
- Unknown duration of effectiveness of current antiretroviral therapies

From DHHS and Henry J. Kaiser Family Foundation (Dec. 1, 1998). Panel on Practices for Treatment of HIV Infection. Guidelines for the Use of Antiretroviral Agents in HIV-Infected Adults and Adolescents.

enzyme required for viral replication late in the virus life cycle. They suppress production of infectious virions in infected cell populations. The emergence of protease inhibitors has changed the prognosis for millions of persons infected with HIV. When combined with nucleoside or nonnucleoside agents, protease inhibitors can reduce viral plasma levels to undetectable levels, thus offering significant clinical benefit. Several different combinations are currently being used, but the most effective combination is still not yet established.

Drug Class-Related Adverse Effects

Several class-related adverse effects have been recognized with antiretroviral drugs during the post-marketing period. For nucleoside analogue reverse transcriptase inhibitors (NRTIs), lactic acidosis with hepatomegaly and hepatic steatosis has been reported. For protease inhibitors, reports of hyperglycemia/diabetes mellitus, increased bleeding episodes in patients with hemophilia, and fat redistribution with and without serum lipid abnormalities have been received. Because these effects were identified from spontaneous reports and other uncontrolled data, their actual incidence and the causal association with these drugs have not been definitively established. Controlled and/or population-based epidemiologic studies evaluating these potential class-related adverse effects are warranted.

Nucleoside Reverse Transcriptase Inhibitors

Zidovudine (AZT, ZDV, Retrovir) was the first nucleoside reverse transcriptase inhibitor (NRTI) approved in 1987. Zidovudine improves CD4 counts, improves survival rates and survival times, and decreases disease progression. Zidovudine penetrates the central nervous system and may be useful in the treatment of HIV dementia and thrombocytopenia. Additionally, it is effective in preventing infection of infants both in utero and during delivery from HIV-infected women.

PHARMACOKINETICS

Zidovudine is absorbed rapidly and well from the gastrointestinal tract, peaking in 30 to 90 minutes. Absorption shows considerable interclient variation (range: 42%–95%). It is widely distributed, crossing the blood–brain barrier with good levels in cerebrospinal fluid. Tablets are best taken on an empty stomach, swallowed whole with plenty of water. The capsules may be taken with or without regard to food (taking with food decreases nausea, but high-fat meals impair absorption). Intravenous administration should be over at least 60 minutes. Zidovudine is primarily excreted in the urine.

PHARMCODYNAMICS

Zidovudine, like other nucleoside analogues, inhibits viral enzyme reverse transcriptase, an enzyme necessary for viral HIV replication early in the viral life cycle. Zidovudine must be converted intracellularly to be active. It slows HIV replication, reducing the progression of HIV infection.

Chart 31–1 presents the pharmacologic data for zidovudine.

Nonnucleoside Reverse Transcriptase Inhibitors

Nevirapine (NVP, Viramune) was the first nonnucleoside reverse transcriptase inhibitor (NNRTI) approved by the FDA. Nevirapine improves CD4 counts and reduces viral load. Resistance is problematic with the NNRTIs; therefore, nevirapine should be used only in combination with at least one other nucleoside analogue.

PHARMACOKINETICS

Nevirapine is readily absorbed following oral administration, with peak concentrations achieved in 4 hours. It is widely distributed (crosses placenta, found in cerebrospinal fluid [CSF]). Nevirapine is metabolized in the liver and is primarily excreted in the urine. Tablets may be taken with or without food.

PHARMACODYNAMICS

Nevirapine inhibits catalytic reaction of reverse transcriptase (enzyme necessary for viral HIV replication) independent of nucleotide binding. Its action occurs early in the viral life cycle. Nevirapine slows HIV replication, reducing progression of HIV infection (must be used in combination therapy).

Chart 31–2 presents the pharmacologic data for nevirapine.

Protease Inhibitors: Saquinavir (Invirase)

Saquinavir was the first protease inhibitor approved by the FDA. It is well tolerated and is less likely to confer cross-resistance to other protease inhibitors.

PHARMACOKINETICS

Saquinavir is poorly absorbed from the GI tract and should not be taken on an empty stomach (taking with a high-fat meal increases absorption). Saquinavir is minimally absorbed in the CSF. It is metabolized in the liver and is primarily eliminated in feces. It should be taken with a full meal; grapefruit juice increases its bioavailability.

Chart 31–1.   Zidovudine

NUCLEOSIDE REVERSE TRANSCRIPTASE INHIBITOR

Drug Name

Zidovudine
  (ZDV, AZT, Retrovir)
Pregnancy Category: C
FDA approved 1987
Estimated annual cost: $2830

Contraindications

Life-threatening allergies to zidovudine or components of preparation.
Caution: Bone marrow compromise, renal and hepatic dysfunction, decreased hepatic blood flow

Drug-Lab-Food Interactions

Drug: Ganciclovir and trimethoprim/sulfamethoxazole may increase risk of neutropenia; probenecid may increase concentration, risk of toxicity.
Lab: May increase mean corpuscular volume

Dosage

Prophylaxis vertical transmission HIV
Maternal therapy: PO: 100 mg 5x/d PACTG 076
Initiated at 14–34 wk of gestation through pregnancy
Intrapartum: IV: 2 mg/kg loading dose over 30–60 min followed by continuous infusion of 1 mg/kg/h until the cord is clamped
Newborn (Syrup): PO: 2 mg/kg q6h; IV: 1.5 mg/kg over 30 minutes q6h
Treatment
A: PO: 200 mg q8h or 300 mg q12h; IV: 1 mg/kg q4h
C: PO: premature birth to 2 wk: 1.5 mg/kg q12h, increasing to 2 mg/kg q8h after 2 weeks of age; neonatal: 2 mg/kg q6h; <12 y: 160 mg/m^2 q8h; >12 y: adult dose
C: IV: neonatal: 1.5 mg/kg q6h; <12 y: intermittent infusion: 120 mg/m^2 q6h; *max* 160 mg/m^2 per dose; continuous infusion: 20 mg/m^2/h

Assessment and Planning

Pharmacokinetics

Absorption: PO: 66%–70%
Distribution: PB: 25%–38%, crosses blood–brain barrier, crosses placenta, peak serum levels: 30–90 minutes
Metabolism: t½: 60 min; extensive first pass effect in liver
Excretion: Urine (63%–95%)

Pharmacodynamics

Not applicable

Interventions

NURSING PROCESS

Therapeutic Effects/Uses

Management of clients with HIV infection; prevention of maternal-fetal HIV transmission.

Mode of Action: Inhibits viral enzyme reverse transcriptase, an enzyme necessary for viral HIV replication.

Side Effects

Numbness, tingling, burning and pain in lower extremities, abdominal pain, rash, GI intolerance, fever, sore throat, headache, pruritus, muscle pain, difficulty swallowing, arthralgia, insomnia, confusion, mental changes, bluish-brown bands on fingernails.

Adverse Reactions

Nausea, vomiting, anemia (pale skin, unusual fatigue or weakness), neutropenia (fever, chills, sore throat), seizures

Evaluation

KEY: A: adult; C: child; PO: by mouth; IV: intravenous; PB: protein-binding; t½: half-life; >: greater than; <: less than; GI: gastrointestinal; CSF: cerebrospinal fluid.

PHARMACODYNAMICS

Saquinavir blocks protease, an enzyme required for viral replication late in the virus life cycle. Saquinavir reduces viral plasma levels, slows HIV replication, and reduces the progression of HIV infection. It must be used in combination therapy.

Chart 31–3 presents the pharmacologic data for saquinavir.

Chart 31–2.   Nevirapine

NONNUCLEOSIDE REVERSE TRANSCRIPTASE INHIBITOR

Drug Name

Nevirapine
  (Viramune)
Pregnancy Category: C
FDA approved 1996
Estimated annual cost: $2515

Dosage

Treatment
A: PO: Initially, 200 mg/d for 14 d; then 200 mg 2 times a day.
C: PO: <3 mo: start with 5 mg/kg once daily for 14 d, followed by 120 mg/m² q12h for 14 d, followed by 200 mg/m² q12h; >3 months: start with 120 mg/m² once daily for 14 d, increasing to 120–200 mg/m² q12h if there is no rash or other untoward effects

Contraindications

Life-threatening allergies to nevirapine or components of preparation.
Caution: Renal or hepatic function impairment

Drug-Lab-Food Interactions

Drug: Affects levels of protease inhibitors (PI), which may require PI dosage adjustment; may *decrease* concentration of oral contraceptives, rifabutin or rifampin
Lab: May *increase* SGPT (ALT), SGOT (AST), bilirubin, GGT; may *decrease* Hgb, platelets, neutrophil count.

Pharmacokinetics

Absorption: PO: 93%
Distribution: PB: 60%, widely distributed (crosses placenta, found in CSF)
Metabolism: t½: 45 h; metabolized in liver
Excretion: Urine (81%)

Pharmacodynamics

Not applicable

Therapeutic Effects/Uses

Management of clients with HIV infection (in combination with other antiretroviral therapy). Never give as monotherapy.

Mode of Action: Inhibits viral enzyme reverse transcriptase, an enzyme necessary for viral HIV replication.

Side Effects

Rash, fever, headache, abnormal liver function tests, stomatitis (sores or ulcers in mouth), numbness, muscle pain, hepatitis (yellow skin, diarrhea, nausea, headache)

Adverse Reactions

Rash may become severe and life threatening.

Assessment and Planning
Interventions
Evaluation
NURSING PROCESS

KEY: A: adult; C: child; PO: by mouth; IV: intravenous; PB: protein-binding; t½: half-life; <: less than; >: greater than; CSF: cerebrospinal fluid. ALT: alanine aminotransferase; AST: asparate aminotransferase.

Drugs that should not be used with protease inhibitors are listed in Table 31–3. Drug interactions between protease inhibitors and other drugs (requiring dose modifications) are listed in Table 31–4. Table 31–5 presents drug interactions: protease inhibitors and nonnucleoside reverse transcriptase inhibitors.

Summary of Antiretroviral Agents

A list of the antiretroviral agents (nucleoside analogues, nonnucleoside analogues, and protease inhibitors) are presented in Table 31–6 with their respective routes and dosage, and considerations.

Chart 31-3. Protease Inhibitor

PROTEASE INHIBITOR

Drug Name

Saquinavir
   (Invirase, Fortovase)
Pregnancy Category: B
FDA approved 1997
Estimated annual cost: $4829

Dosage

Treatment
A: PO: Invirase: 600 mg t.i.d.; Fortovase: 1200 mg t.i.d.

Contraindications

Life-threatening allergies to saquinavir or components of preparation.
Caution: Impaired hepatic function

Drug-Lab-Food Interactions

Drug: Ketoconazole increases saquinavir concentration; rifampin, phenobarbital, phenytoin, dexamethasone, carbamazepine may reduce plasma concentrations of saquinavir; may *increase* astemizole, calcium channel blockers, clindamycin, dapsone, quinidine, triazolam plasma concentrations.
Lab: May *increase* liver function tests, decrease glucose level, and alter CPK
Food: Grapefruit juice *increases* absorption

Pharmacokinetics

Absorption: PO: 4%
Distribution: PB: 98%, poor CSF penetration
Metabolism: t½: 13 h; extensive first pass effect in liver, metabolized in liver
Excretion: Primarily fecal elimination

Pharmacodynamics

Not applicable

Therapeutic Effects/Uses

Management of clients with HIV infection.

Mode of Action: Inhibits protease, a process occurring late in viral replication.

Side Effects

Nausea, diarrhea, ulcers in mouth, abdominal discomfort, abdominal pain, burning or prickling sensation, skin rash, weakness, headache; may increase blood glucose (symptoms include increased thirst, hunger, and urination, weight loss, fatigue, dry skin, itching)

Adverse Reactions

None significant

Assessment and Planning

Interventions

Evaluation

NURSING PROCESS

KEY: A: adult; PO: by mouth; PB: protein-binding; t½: half-life; CPK: creatine phosphokinase.

OTHER DRUGS FOR HIV

A welcome and unexpected newcomer drug in the treatment of HIV infection and AIDS is Hydrea. Currently, Hydrea is not FDA approved for the treatment of AIDS. Table 31–7 presents additional data on Hydrea.

Adefovir dipivoxil (Preveon) is a nucleotide reverse transcriptase inhibitor. It is available to clients in whom at least two NRTIs and one protease inhibitor have failed. This availability is only through an expanded access protocol. The primary adverse effect of adefovir has been mild to moderate nephrotoxicity. Side effects include nausea, diarrhea, asthenia, and aminotransferase activity. There are no reports of interactions with other drugs. This drug awaits FDA approval.

Table 31-3
Drugs that Should Not Be Used with Protease Inhibitors

DRUG CATEGORY	INDINAVIR	RITONAVIR*	SAQUINAVIR (given as Invirase or Fortovase)	NELFINAVIR	ALTERNATIVES
Analgesics	None	Meperidine Piroxicam Propoxyphene	None	None	ASA Oxycodone Acetaminophen
Cardiac	None	Amiodarone Encainide Flecainide Propafenone Quinidine	None	None	Limited experience
Antimycobacterial	Rifampin	Rifabutin†	Rifampin Rifabutin	Rifampin	For rifabutin (as alternative for mycobacterium avium infection (MAI) treatment): clarithromycin, ethambutol (treatment, not prophylaxis), or azithromycin
Ca²⁺ channel blocker	None	Bepridil	None	None	Limited experience
Antihistimine	Astemizole Terfenadine	Astemizole Terfenadine	Astemizole Terfenadine	Astemizole Terfenadine	Loratadine
Gastrointestinal	Cisapride	Cisapride	Cisapride	Cisapride	Limited experience
Antidepressant	None	Bupropion	None	None	Fluoxetine Desipramine
Neuroleptic	None	Clozapine Pimozide	None	None	Limited experience
Psychotropic	Midazolam Triazolam	Clorazepate Diazepam Estazolam Flurazepam Midazolam Triazolam zolpidem	Midazolam Triazolam	Midazolam Triazolam	Temazepam Lorazepam
Ergot alkaloids (vasoconstrictor)	Dihydroergotamine (DHE 45) Ergotamine‡ (various forms)	Dihydroergotamine (DHE 45) Ergotamine‡ (various forms)	Dihydroergotamine (DHE 45) Ergotamine‡ (various forms)	Dihydroergotamine (DHE 45) Ergotamine‡ (various forms)	Limited experience

*The contraindicated drugs listed are based on theoretical considerations. Thus, drugs with low therapeutic indices yet with suspected major metabolic contribution from cytochrome P450 3A, CYP2D6, or unknown pathways are included in this table. Actual interactions may or may not occur in patients.
† Reduce rifabutin dose to one fourth of the standard dose.
‡ This is likely a class effect.
From DHHS and Henry J. Kaiser Family Foundation (Dec. 1, 1998). Panel on Practices for Treatment of HIV Infection. Guidelines for the Use of Antiretroviral Agents in HIV-Infected Adults and Adolescents.

ADHERENCE TO DRUG REGIMEN

Adherence to the therapeutic regimen is a major concern and issue with clients on antiretroviral therapy. Relative to this, the nurse must be knowledgeable about ways to promote adherence to the regimen. Nonadherence will result in HIV viral replication, increased viral loads, and deterioration of the immune

Table 31-4
Drug Interactions Between Protease Inhibitors and Other Drugs

DRUG INTERACTIONS REQUIRING DOSE MODIFICATIONS

	Indinavir	Ritonavir	Saquinavir*	Nelfinavir
Fluconazole	No dosage change	No dosage change	No data	No dosage change
Ketoconazole and itraconazole	Decrease dose to 600 mg q8h	Increases ketoconazole >3-fold; dose adjustment required	Increases saquinavir levels 3-fold; no dose change†	No dose change
Rifabutin	Reduce rifabutin to half dose: 150 mg/d	Consider alternative drug or reduce rifabutin dose to one fourth	Not recommended with either Invirase or Fortovase	Reduce rifabutin to half dose: 150 mg/d
Rafampin	Contraindicated	Unknown†	Not recommended with either Invirase or Fortovase	Contraindicated
Oral contraceptives	Modest increase in Ortho-Novum levels; no dose change	Ethinyl estradiol levels decreased; use alternative or additional contraceptive method	No data	Ethinyl estradiol and norethindrone levels decreased; use alternative or additional contraceptive method
Miscellaneous	Grapefruit juice reduces indinavir levels by 26%	Desipramine increased 145%: reduce dose Theophylline levels decreased: increase dose	Grapefruit juice increases saquinavir levels†	

Several drug interaction studies have been completed with saquinavir given as Invirase or Fortovase. Results from studies conducted with Invirase may not be applicable to Fortovase.

†Conducted with Invirase.

‡Rifampin reduces ritonavir 35%. Increased ritonavir dose or use of ritonavir in combination therapy is strongly recommended. The effect of ritonavir on rifampin is unknown. Used concurrently, there may be increased liver toxicity. Therefore, patients on ritonavir and rifampin should be monitored closely.

From DHHS and Henry J. Kaiser Family Foundation (Dec. 1, 1998). Panel on Practices for Treatment of HIV Infection. Guidelines for the Use of Antiretroviral Agents in HIV-Infected Adults and Adolescents.

system. Development of resistant viral strains, enhanced with subtherapeutic levels of antiretroviral agents, is a serious current and long-term threat for clients with AIDS. Reasons commonly identified by clients for missing medications include forgetting to take them, feeling too sick, or not having the medicine with them. Also, there are public health implications of nonadherence with the expanding pool of drug-resistant viruses.

The following suggestions are offered to promote client adherence to the therapeutic regimen. Clients' understanding of their drug regimen is crucial to adherence, including the purpose of each medication, dosage schedule, food and fluid restrictions, recommended food choices, and storage of medications (e.g., refrigeration). Pictorial representation of the medications may be helpful to the clients along with a pillbox designed for medications to be taken four times a day. Additional helpful hints to promote adherence are associating taking medications with a daily routine such as brushing teeth or feeding the pet; having a buddy to remind the client to take the medication; using a medications calendar to check off medications taken; and using the pharmacist as a resource.

Clients need to have the telephone number of a contact person for questions. Discussion of anticipated side effects of the medications and how to manage their occurrence is necessary. A trusting client-provider relationship is essential. Long-term adherence to the regimen remains a major challenge and requires an interdisciplinary team approach.

OPPORTUNISTIC INFECTIONS AND KAPOSI'S SARCOMA

Once the CD4 count decreases to less than 200/mm³, many opportunistic infections are more likely to develop. The lower the CD4 count, the greater are the risk and number of infections. In most instances, with all the microorganisms, there is breakthrough and

Text continued on page 547

Table 31–5
Protease Inhibitors and Nonnucleoside Reverse Transcriptase Inhibitors: Effect of Drug on Levels/Dose

DRUG AFFECTED	INDINAVIR	RITONAVIR	SAQUINAVIR*	NELFINAVIR	NEVIRAPINE	DELAVIRDINE	EFAVIRENZ
Indinavir (IDV)	—	No data	Levels: IDV no effect SQV ↑ 4–7x‡ Dose: No data	Levels: IDV ↑ 50% NFV ↑ 80% Dose: No data	Levels: IDV ↓ 28% Dose: Standard	Levels: IDV ↑ 40% Dose: IDV 600 mg q8h	Levels: IDV ↓ 31% Dose: IDV 1000 mg q8h
Ritonavir (RTV)	No data	—	Levels: RTV no effect SQV ↑ 20x‡ Dose: Invirase or Fortovase 400 mg b.i.d. + RTV: 400 mg b.i.d.	Levels: RTV no effect NFV ↑ 1.5x Dose: No data	Levels: RTV ↓ 11% Dose: Standard	Levels: RTV ↑ 70% Dose: No data	Levels: RTV ↑ 18% Dose: RTV 600 mg b.i.d. (500 mg b.i.d. for intolerance)
Saquinavir (SQV)	Levels: SQV ↑ 4–7x IDV no effect‡ Dose: No data	Levels: SQV ↑ 20x† RTV no effect Dose: Invirase or Fortovase 400 mg b.i.d. + RTV: 400 mg b.i.d.	—	Levels: SQV ↑ 3–5x NFV ↓ 20%‡ Dose: Standard NFV Fortovase 800 mg t.i.d.	Levels: SQV ↓ 25% Dose: No data	Levels: SQV ↑ 5x† Dose: Standard for Invirase (monitor transaminase levels)	Levels: SQV ↓ 62%+ Coadministration not recommended
Nelfinavir (NFV)	Levels: NFV ↑ 80% IDV ↑ 50% Dose: No data	Levels: NFV ↑ 1.5x RTV no effect Dose: No data	Levels: NFV ↑ 20% SQV ↑ 3–5x‡ Dose: Standard NFV Fortovase 800 mg t.i.d.	—	Levels: NFV ↑ 10% Dose: Standard	Levels: NFV ↑ 2x DLV ↓ 50% Dose: Standard (monitor for neutropenic complications)	Levels: NFV ↑ 20% Dose: Standard
Nevirapine (NVP)	Levels: IDV ↓ 28% Dose: Standard	Levels: RTV ↓ 11% Dose: Standard	Levels: SQV ↓ 25%+ Dose: No data	Levels: NFV ↑ 10% Dose: Standard	—	Do not use together	Coadministration not recommended
Delavirdine (DLV)	Levels: IDV ↑ 40% Dose: IDV 600 q8h	Levels: RTV ↑ 70% Dose: No data	Levels: SQV ↑ 5x† Dose: Standard for Invirase. Monitor transaminase levels	Levels: NFV ↑ 2x DLV ↓ 50% Dose: Standard (monitor for neutropenic complications)	Do not use together	—	Coadministration not recommended
Efavirenz (EFV)	Levels: EFV no effect Dose: Standard	Level: EFV ↑ 21% Dose: Standard	Levels: EFV ↓ 12%‡ Coadministration not recommended.	Levels: EFV no effect Dose: Standard	Coadministration not recommended	Coadministration not recommended	—

* Several drug interaction studies have been completed with saquinavir given as Invirase or Fortovase. Results from studies conducted with Invirase may not be applicable to Fortovase.
‡ Conducted with Invirase.
† Conducted with Fortovase.
From DHHS and Henry J. Kaiser Family Foundation (Dec. 1, 1998). Panel on Practices for Treatment of HIV Infection. Guidelines for the Use of Antiretroviral Agents in HIV-Infected Adults and Adolescents.

NURSING PROCESS
ANTIRETROVIRAL THERAPY

Assessment

- Assess whether client needs HIV testing.
- Refer as appropriate for anonymous or confidential testing.
- Assess for renal and hepatic disorders; use of oral contraceptives.
- Assess for signs and symptoms related to clinical progression toward a depressed immune system including profound involuntary weight loss, chronic diarrhea, chronic weight loss, intermittent or constant fever.
- Assess use of other prescription and OTC medications.
- Refer high-risk clients who test negative to counseling.
- Assess needs and refer to medical care and psychological support.
- Obtain client history for clients who test positive for HIV.

Potential Nursing Diagnoses

- Altered health maintenance related to knowledge deficit about HIV/AIDS
- Fear related to potential outcome of HIV screening, powerlessness, and/or threat to well-being
- Altered nutrition; less than body requirements
- Ineffective individual and/or family coping related to situational crises (positive HIV screening outcome)
- Risk for infection
- Body image disturbance
- Knowledge deficit
- Alteration in sleep pattern, memory loss

Planning

- Client's viral load will be undetectable.
- Client's CD4 count will be as high as possible.
- Client will not experience secondary infections.
- Client will participate in medical treatment and in spiritual and psychological support.

Nursing Intervention

- Promote adherence/compliance to the therapeutic regimen.
- Promote meticulous handwashing; apply standard precautions.
- Administer increased fluids, up to 2400 mL/d unless contraindicated.
- Monitor laboratory reports for indications of decreasing $CD4^+$ T-lymphocyte cell counts; inform health care provider.
- Refer client for preventive care measures including annual PAP exams, eye examinations and dental examinations.
- Refer client for nutritional counseling.
- Refer client for spiritual support.

Client Teaching

General
- Explain how the virus may cause severe damage to the immune system.
- Describe the modes of transmission of the virus.
- Explain the emotional response.
- Explain the need for monitoring of health practices.
- Emphasize protective precautions to decrease risk of infection as necessary.
- Advise client not to visit anyone with any type of respiratory infection.
- Provide personal drug therapy plan in writing.
- Establish client/family partnership in the plan.

Nursing Process continued on following page

NURSING PROCESS *Continued*
ANTIRETROVIRAL THERAPY

Self-Administration
- Assist client to develop a system for taking the correct dose of the correct medications at the correct time. A drug organizer is of practical help for many clients.
- Instruct client of importance of having adequate supply of medication so there is no interruption in the schedule. Omission of drugs may result in deterioration of client's condition.

Diet
- Advise client to eat a variety of foods.
- Advise client how to minimize side effects (e.g., take specific drug with food).
- Discuss BRAT diet (banana, rice, applesauce, and tea) for management of diarrhea.

Side Effects
- Advise the client about what symptoms to promptly report to the health care provider.
- Discuss possible side effects and strategies to manage them.
- Provide suggestions for managing diarrhea.

Cultural Considerations

- Know that there is an oral history that the drug AZT may be harmful to certain groups of people.
- Some cultures pressure women to reproduce regardless of health status and the implications for future generations.
- AIDS is a highly stigmatized disease.

Evaluation

- Evaluate the effectiveness of the antiretroviral therapy.
- Determine whether the viral load is undetectable or as low as possible.

Table 31–6
Antiretroviral Agents

GENERIC (BRAND)	ROUTE AND DOSAGE	CONSIDERATIONS
NUCLEOSIDE REVERSE TRANSCRIPTASE INHIBITORS		
NUCLEOSIDE ANALOGUES		
Abacavir (Ziagen) FDA approved 1998 Estimated annual cost: $3540	A: PO: 300 mg b.i.d.	No dietary restrictions. Hypersensitivity reaction in 3%–5% of clients on this drug (fever, GI symptoms, malaise, occasionally rash). Symptoms resolve when drug is stopped. However, if given drug again, more severe symptoms occur more rapidly, including hypotension and respiratory distress. FDA mandates that clients receive detailed description of these symptoms and carry a wallet-sized card with a description of hypersensitivity reaction with them at all times. No reports of adverse reactions with other drugs. Pregnancy Category: UK; PB: UK; $t_{\frac{1}{2}}$: UK.

Table continued on following page

Table 31–6 *Continued*
Antiretroviral Agents

GENERIC (BRAND)	ROUTE AND DOSAGE	CONSIDERATIONS
NUCLEOSIDE ANALOGUES		
Didanosine (ddI) (Videx) FDA approved 1991 Estimated annual cost: $1875	A: PO: (>60 kg): tablets: 200 mg q12h; powder: 250 mg q12h; (<60 kg): tablets: 125 mg q12h; powder: 167 mg q12h C: PO: (<90 d): 50 mg/m² q12h; (>90 d): 90–150 mg/m² q12h	Give on empty stomach. Tablets chewed, crushed, or dispersed in water (when dispersed, use within 1 h); powder should be mixed in drinking water only. Pediatric powder mixed by pharmacist and is stable for 30 d refrigerated. Avoid within 2 h of dapsone. Give in combination, never as monotherapy. *Pregnancy category:* B; PB: <5%; t½: 1.6 h
Lamivudine (3TC, Epivir) FDA approved 1995 Estimated annual cost: $2275	A: PO: (>50 kg): 150 mg b.i.d.; (<50 kg): 2 mg/kg b.i.d. C: PO: (<30 d): 2 mg/kg q12h; (>30 d): 4 mg/kg q12h	Give in combination; never as monotherapy. May take without regard to food. Avoid alcohol. Report persistent, severe abdominal pain, nausea, vomiting, numbness or tingling. *Pregnancy category:* C; PB: <36%; t½: 5–7 hrs
Stavudine (Zerit) FDA approved 1992 Estimated annual cost: $2365	A: PO: (>60 kg): 40 mg q12h; (<60 kg): 30 mg q12h C: PO: 1 mg/kg q12h (up to 30 kg)	Compounded with lactose; lactose intolerant clients can take LactAid tablets prior to stavudine. May take without regard to food. Avoid alcohol. Report tingling, burning, pain, or numbness of hands or feet. *Pregnancy Category:* C; PB: negligible; ½: 1.44 h
Zalcitabine (ddC, Hivid) FDA approved 1992 Estimated annual cost: $2099	A: PO: 0.75 mg q8h C: PO: 0.005–0.01 mg/kg q8h	Best given on empty stomach. Swallow tablets whole with plenty of water. *Pregnancy category:* C; PB: <4%; t½: 1–3 h
Zidovudine (ZDV, AZT, Retrovir) FDA approved 1986 Estimated annual cost: $2830	*Prophylaxis vertical transmission HIV* Maternal therapy: PO: 100 mg 5x/d Intrapartum: IV: 2 mg/kg loading dose over 30–60 min followed by continuous infusion of 1 mg/kg/h until the cord is clamped Newborn (syrup): PO: 2 mg/kg q6h; IV: 1.5 mg/kg over 30 min q6h *Treatment* A: PO: 200 mg q8h or 300 mg q12h; IV: 1 mg/kg q4h C: PO: premature birth to 2 wk: 1.5 mg/kg q12h, increasing to 2 mg/kg q8h after 2 wk of age; neonatal: 2 mg/kg q6h; <12 y: 160 mg/m² q8h; >12 y: adult dose C: IV: neonatal: 1.5 mg/kg q6h; <12 y: intermittent infusion: 120 mg/m² q6h; *max:* 160 mg/m² per dose; continuous infusion: 20 mg/m²/h	Protect from light. May take without regard to food. Take with food to decrease nausea; avoid high-fat meal, which decreases absorption. Infusion given over at least 60 min. *Pregnancy category:* C; PB: 34%–38%; t½: 1 h
NONNUCLEOSIDE ANALOGUES		
Delavirdine (Rescriptor) FDA approved 1997 Estimated annual cost: $2204	A: PO: Initially, 200 mg t.i.d. for 14 d then 400 mg t.i.d.	May take without regard to food. *Pregnancy category:* C; PB: 98%; t½: 2–11 h
Nevirapine (Viramune) FDA approved 1996 Estimated annual cost: $2515	*Treatment* A: PO: Initially, 200 mg/d for 14 d; then 200 mg 2 times a day. C: PO: <3 mo: start with 5 mg/kg once daily for 14 d, followed by 120 mg/m² q12h for 14 d, followed by 200 mg/m² q12h; >3 mo: start with 120 mg/m² once daily for 14 d, increasing to 120–200 mg/m² q12h if there is no rash or other untoward effects	Give in combination, never as monotherapy. May take without regard to food. *Pregnancy category:* C; PB: 60%; t½: 25–30 h

Table continued on following page

Table 31–6 *Continued*
Antiretroviral Agents

GENERIC (BRAND)	ROUTE AND DOSAGE	CONSIDERATIONS
Efavirenz (EFV) (Sustiva) FDA approved 1998 Estimated annual cost: $3920	A: PO: 600 mg/d usually hs	Take with or without food. Avoid high-fat meal, which may increase drug absorption, resulting in increased side effects. About 40% of clients have problems with CNS effects: dizziness, insomnia, trouble concentrating, vivid dreams, nightmares. Usually these side effects disappear within 2 wk. Rash is not serious. Contraindicated in pregnancy. PB: UK; $t_{\frac{1}{2}}$: 40–52 h
PROTEASE INHIBITORS		
Indinavir (Crixivan) FDA approved 1996 Estimated annual cost: $4290	A: PO: 800 mg q8h or 1200 mg q12h C: PO: 500 mg/m² q8h	Give in combination, never as monotherapy. May take with a light meal (avoid high-fat, high-calorie, high-protein meal). If given with didanosine, give at least 1 h before or after didanosine. Drink at least 1500 mL water daily. Compounded with lactose; lactose intolerant clients can take LactAid tablets before taking indinavir. Extremely moisture sensitive; keep in original container with desiccants; do not keep in bathroom. Monitor blood glucose. *Pregnancy category:* C; PB: 60%; $t_{\frac{1}{2}}$: 1.8 h
Nelfinavir (Viracept) FDA approved 1997 Estimated annual cost: $5535	A: PO: 750 mg t.i.d. or 1250 mg b.i.d. C: PO: (2–13 y): 20–30 mg/kg q8h	Give in combination, never as monotherapy. Oral powder may be mixed with small amount of water, milk, or dietary supplement and use within 6 h. Give with food for optimal absorption. Monitor blood glucose. *Pregnancy category:* B; PB: >98%; $t_{\frac{1}{2}}$: 3.5–5 h
Ritonavir (Norvir) FDA approved 1996 Estimated annual cost: $5942	A: PO: Initially, 300 mg q12h, increasing by 100 mg q12h to maximum of 600 mg q12h (when given with saquinavir, ritonavir dosage is 400 mg q12h) C: PO: Initially, 250 mg/m² q12h, increasing by 50 mg/m² q12h over 5 d to maximum of 400 mg/m² q12h	Store capsules, solution in refrigerator; protect from light. Refrigeration of solution not necessary if used within 30 d of reconstitution, but store below 77°F. Take with food. Review other medications before initiating them; there are many drug interactions. Give in combination, never as monotherapy. Monitor blood glucose. *Pregnancy category:* B; PB: 98%–99%; $t_{\frac{1}{2}}$: 3 h
Saquinavir (Invirase, Fortovase) FDA approved 1997 Estimated annual cost: $4829	A: PO: *Invirase:* 600 mg t.i.d.; *Fortovase:* 1200 mg t.i.d.	Compounded with lactose; lactose intolerant clients can take LactAid tablets before giving saquinavir. Take with full meal or within 2 h of a meal. Taking with grapefruit juice increases absorption. Photosensitivity can occur; use sunscreen or protective clothing. Monitor blood glucose. *Pregnancy category:* B; PB: 98%; $t_{\frac{1}{2}}$: 5 h

KEY: A: adult; C: child; PO: by mouth; IV: intravenous; PB: protein-binding; $t_{\frac{1}{2}}$: half-life; >: greater than; <: less than; Gi: gastrointestinal; hs: bedtime; CNS: central nervous system.

Table 31–7 Hydrea	
Generic name	Hydrea
Trade name	Hydroxyurea
Form	500 mg capsules
Dose	500 mg b.i.d.
Classification	Hydroxyurea is used for sickle cell disease and is not FDA approved for HIV. It is currently thought of as a possible drug for salvage therapy. In vitro studies show synergistic activity when combined with didanosine (ddI).
Oral bioavailability	Well absorbed
Major toxicity	Dose-dependent bone marrow suppression with leukopenia, anemia, and thrombocytopenia. Gastrointestinal intolerance may be severe, including stomatitis, nausea, vomiting, anorexia, diarrhea, and constipation.

progression. There are no cures, and lifelong treatment is required to prevent recurrence.

CANDIDIASIS. Fungal infection. Symptoms: patches of inflammation with or without ulceration. May cause difficulty swallowing, nausea, sternal pain. Women may have thick vaginal discharge and pruritus. Diagnosis by KOH-scraping from mucous membranes.

CRYPTOCOCCUS. Fungal infection. Symptoms: fever, malaise, headache, cough, GI disturbances. May localize in CNS (meningitis, encephalitis), memory loss, confusion. Diagnosis by culture of cerebrospinal fluid (CSF).

CYTOMEGALOVIRUS. Viral infection. Symptoms: painless, progressive loss of vision, sometimes complicated by retinal detachment. In the GI tract, causes nausea, vomiting, weight loss. Diagnosis by funduscopic examination.

HERPES SIMPLEX. Viral infection (HSV-1 and HSV-2). Symptoms: orolabial, genital, anorectal (pain, itching, painful defecation), mucocutaneous lesions, esophagitis, encephalitis (less common). Diagnosis by viral culture.

HISTOPLASMOSIS. Fungal infection. Symptoms: often asymptomatic, may cause flulike symptoms, high fever, weight loss, liver and spleen enlargement. Diagnosis by fungal cultures.

MYCOBACTERIUM AVIUM **COMPLEX (MAC).** Bacterial infection. Symptoms: high spiking fevers, diarrhea, night sweats, malaise, weight loss, anemia, neutropenia. Diagnosis by blood cultures or biopsy of liver, bone marrow, and lymph nodes.

PNEUMOCYSTIS CARNII **PNEUMONIA (PCP).** Protozoal/fungal infection. Symptoms: fever, dyspnea, tachypnea with or without rales or rhonchi, and nonproductive or mildly productive cough, chills, sweats. Diagnosis: by bronchial washings or open lung biopsy.

SALMONELLA. Bacterial infection. Symptoms: fever, chills, night sweats. Diagnosis by blood cultures.

TOXOPLASMOSIS GONDII. Parasite infection. Primarily infects the brain and eye. Symptoms: fever, headache, seizures, focal neurologic abnormalities, and mental status changes. Diagnosis is presumptive or based on computed tomography (CT) or magnetic resonance imaging (MRI).

TUBERCULOSIS. Bacterial infection. Symptoms: Cough, fever, sweating, malaise, fatigue, weight loss, nonpleuritic chest pain, dyspnea. Diagnosis by TB smear, culture.

KAPOSI'S SARCOMA. Symptoms: red-blue blotches or nodules ranging in size from a few millimeters to several centimeters in diameter. The lesion may bleed. Nodules may appear in the mouth or in the viscera. Diagnosis made by biopsy. Rarely seen in women.

Therapies for common opportunistic infections and Kaposi's sarcoma are presented in Table 31–8.

ANTIRETROVIRAL THERAPY IN PREGNANCY

One of the most significant research studies in the history of HIV/AIDS was the ACTG 076 study (AIDS Clinical Trials Group Protocol, the 76th study), a phase III, randomized, double-blind, placebo-controlled clinical trial. The goal of the trial was to evaluate whether AZT (zidovudine, ZDV) administered to HIV-infected pregnant women and their infants could reduce the rate of transmission from mother to infant. Approximately 7000 infants are born to HIV-infected women in the United States each year. The study was halted in February 1994 when the review board found a 67.5% reduction in HIV maternal/fetal transmission.

The protocol for HIV-infected pregnant women/newborns from this study (*MMWR*, August 5, 1994/Vol 43/No. RR-11. Recommendations of the US Public Health Service Task Force on the Use of Zidovudine to Reduce Perinatal Transmission of Human Immunodeficiency Virus) is as follows:

PREGNANT WOMEN

• Oral administration of 100 mg of ZDV five times daily, initiated at 14 to 34 weeks of gestation and continued throughout the pregnancy.

Table 31-8
Therapies for Common Opportunistic Infections and Conditions

CLINICAL DISEASE	PROPHYLACTIC AGENTS	AGENTS—ACUTE INFECTION

Candida	Clotrimazole troches
	Fluconazole
	Ketoconazole
	Nystatin
		Oral
		  Clotrimazole
		  Nystatin
		Esophageal
		  Fluconazole
		  Ketoconazole

Cryptococcus	Fluconazole	Amphotericin +/− flucytosine, followed by flu-conazole
Cytomegalovirus	Oral ganciclovir	Ganciclovir (IV) Foscarnet
Herpes simplex	Oral acyclovir	Oral acyclovir
Histoplasma	—	Amphotericin Itraconazole

Kaposi's sarcoma	—	Individualized
		  Bleomycin
		  Doxorubicin
		  Etoposide
		  Interferon alpha
		  Vinblastine
		  Vincristine

Mycobacterium avium complex (MAC)	Azithromycin Clarithromycin Rifabutin	Clarithromycin + ethambutol (may add rifampin) Clotazimine Ciprofloxacin
Pneumocystis carinii pneumonia	Trimethoprim-sulfamethoxazole Dapsone Pentamidine (aerosol)	Trimethoprim-sulfamethoxazole (IV) Atovaquone (mild case)
Salmonella	—	Ciprofloxacin Trimethoprim-sulfamethoxazole
Toxoplasma gondii	Trimethoprim-sulfamethoxazole Dapsone + pyrimethamine	Pyrimethamine + sulfadiazine + folinic acid
Tuberculosis	Isoniazid Rifampin	Isoniazid + rifampin + pyrazinamide + etham-butol or streptomycin

- During labor, intravenous administration of ZDV in a 1-hour loading dose of 2 mg per kg of body weight, followed by a continuous infusion of 1 mg per kg of body weight per hour until delivery.

  NEWBORNS
- Oral administration of ZDV to the newborn (ZDV syrup at 2 mg per kg of body weight per dose every 6 hours) for the first 6 weeks of life, beginning 8 to 12 hours after birth.
- Consider referring all pregnant clients to the national Antiretroviral Therapy registry. The telephone number is 1-800-258-4263; FAX 1-800-800-1052.

The US Public Health Service Task Force recommendations for use of antiretroviral agents during pregnancy for maternal health and reduction of perinatal transmission of HIV (*MMWR*, 47 RR-2, 1998) include the use of combination antiretroviral therapy. There are some early reports of increased numbers of premature births with HIV-infected pregnant women receiving combination therapy.

POSTEXPOSURE PROPHYLAXIS FOR HEALTH CARE WORKERS

As of June 1997, a total of 52 health care workers in the United States had acquired HIV infection from occupational exposure. Needlestick injuries carried a 0.33% chance of transmission; mucosal surface exposure carried a 0.09% chance of transmission. There were no transmissions from skin exposures. Of the 52 confirmed cases, nurses and laboratory technicians made up the majority of the cases; all cases involved blood or bloody body fluids (three were laboratory workers exposed to HIV viral cultures). To date, there are no confirmed cases in surgeons and no transmissions attributed to exposure to a suture needle.

Table 31–9
Basic and Expanded Postexposure Prophylaxis Regimens

REGIMEN CATEGORY	APPLICATION	DRUG REGIMEN
Basic	Occupational HIV exposures for which there is a recognized transmission risk	4 wk (28 d) of both zidovudine 600 mg every day in divided doses (i.e., 300 mg twice a day, 200 mg three times a day, or 100 mg every 4 h) *and* lamivudine 150 mg twice a day.
Expanded	Occupational HIV exposures that pose an increased risk for transmission (e.g., larger volume of blood and/or higher virus titer in blood)	Basic regimen plus *either* indinavir 800 mg every 8 h *or* nelfinavir 750 mg three times a day*

Indinavir should be taken on an empty stomach (i.e., without food or with a light meal) and with increased fluid consumption (i.e., drinking six 8-oz glasses of water throughout the day); nelfinavir should be taken with meals.

From DHHS and Henry J. Kaiser Family Foundation (Dec. 1, 1998). Panel on Practices for Treatment of HIV Infection. Guidelines for the Use of Antiretroviral Agents in HIV-Infected Adults and Adolescents.

The policy for postexposure prophylaxis (PEP) needs to be institution specific and available to all employees. The basic and expanded postexposure regimens are described in Table 31–9. HIV postexposure prophylaxis resources and registries are presented in Table 31–10.

A comprehensive reference for PEP is Public Health Service Statement on the Management of Occupational Exposures to HIV and Recommendations for Postexposure Prophylaxis, *MMWR*, May 15, 1998, Vol. 47/No. RR - 7.

THE FUTURE OF HIV/AIDS-RELATED AGENTS

HIV/AIDS is a prime area of clinical investigations. Multiple vaccines have been tested; only one has been approved for large clinical trials. Table 31–11 lists the drugs available through treatment investigational new drug protocols.

Table 31–10
Postexposure Prophylaxis Resources and Registries

RESOURCE OR REGISTRY	CONTACT INFORMATION	
National Clinicians' Postexposure Hotline	Telephone:	(888) 448-4911
HIV Postexposure Prophylaxis Registry	Telephone:	(888) 737-4448 ([888] PEP4HIV)
	Write:	1410 Commonwealth Drive Suite 215 Wilmington, NC 28405
Antiretroviral Pregnancy Registry	Telephone:	(800) 258-4263
	Fax:	(800) 800-1052
	Write:	1410 Commonwealth Drive Suite 215 Wilmington, NC 28405
Food and Drug Administration (for reporting unusual or severe toxicity to antiretroviral agents)	Telephone:	(800) 332-1088
CDC (for reporting HIV seroconversions in health care workers who received PEP)	Telephone:	(404) 639-6425

From DHHS and Henry J. Kaiser Family Foundation (Dec. 1, 1988). Panel on Practices for Treatment of HIV Infection. Guidelines for the Use of Antiretroviral Agents in HIV-Infected Adults and Adolescents.

Table 31–11
Drugs Available Through Treatment Investigational New Drug Protocols

DRUG	ADEFOVIR (PREVEON)	ABACAVIR (1592-U89)	AMPRENAVIR (AGENERASE; 141W94)
Source	Gilead 800-GILEAD-5	Glaxo-Wellcome 800-501-4672	Vertex; Glaxo-Wellcome 800-248-9757
Class	Nucleotide RT Inhibitor	Nucleoside RT Inhibitor	Protease Inhibitor
Usual dose	60 mg po qd or 120 mg po qd + L-carnitine 500 mg po qd	300 mg po b.i.d.	1200 mg po b.i.d.
Side effects (major)	Proximal renal tubular dysfunction, nausea, elevated liver function tests	Hypersensitivity: 2%–5% usually in first 4 wk (fever, nausea, vomiting, morbilliform rash) *Do not rechallenge*	Nausea, diarrhea, rash, headache
Comments	Activity against HBV, CMV, HSV	Good CNS penetration; non CY450-mediated metabolism	Unique resistance profile; clinical significance unknown
Enrollment criteria	Failure or intolerance with current therapy; absence of clinically significant renal dysfunction and no concurrent use of nephrotoxic drugs	Failure or intolerance with current therapy	Failure or intolerance with current therapy

KEY: HBV: hepatitis B virus; CMV: cytomegalovirus; HSV: herpes simplex virus; CNS: central nervous system.
From DHHS and Henry J. Kaiser Family Foundation (Dec. 1, 1998). Panel on Practices for Treatment of HIV Infection. Guidelines for the Use of Antiretroviral Agents in HIV-Infected Adults and Adolescents.

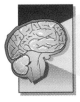

Critical Thinking in Action

R. S. was diagnosed with HIV infection in 1994 and began zidovudine (AZT) therapy in 1994. In 1995, 3TC (Epivir, Lamivudine) was added to the ZDV.

In the early part of 1996, the laboratory reported R. S.'s viral load (VL) at 120,000. At that time, ritonavir was added. The VL decreased to 3500 and the CD4$^+$T cells increased from 06 mm^3 to 96 mm^3.

R. S. reports that it is hard to "always be taking medicine" and states, "Now that I'm back to work and going out again, I sometimes forget my pills." Additionally, there is a complaint of increased fatigue, VL increased to 8500, and CD4$^+$ T cells decreased to 70 mm^3.

It is believed that R. S. has become resistant to RT inhibitors and is started on dual PIs. In 6 weeks, the VL is undetectable and the CD4$^+$ T cells are 85 mm^3.

1. Missing doses of protease inhibitors can be very harmful to the client. Given the client's history, what can the nurse do to assist R. S. with issues related to adherence/compliance?
2. What is the rationale for including 3TC in R. S.'s therapeutic plan?
3. What action should the nurse take to facilitate R. S.'s understanding of the consequences of her nonadherence to the drug regimen?
4. Explain the danger of missing doses of protease inhibitors.

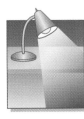

Study Questions

1. Identify at least two side effects of NRTIs.

2. What are the two modes of action of nevirapine (Viramune)?

3. What is the major problem with NRTIs that requires they be used only in combination with a nucleoside analogue?

4. NNRTIs do affect the concentration of oral contraceptives.
   _____ True
   _____ False

5. What was the first protease inhibitor approved by the FDA?

6. What is a toxic effect of efavirenz (EFV) that affects about 40% of clients that take this drug?

7. What are at least eight general factors to be included in client teaching about antiretroviral therapy?

8. What suggestions related to diet would you share with a client newly diagnosed with AIDS and starting on a therapeutic plan?

32 Vaccines

Lynette M. Wachholz

Outline

Objectives

- Describe the differences between active and passive immunity.
- Describe the differences between active natural and active acquired immunity.
- List infectious diseases for which vaccines are currently available.
- Outline the currently recommended childhood immunization schedule.
- Identify vaccines routinely administered to adults.
- Discuss contraindications to administration of varicella vaccine.
- Explain the nursing interventions, including client teaching, related to the administration of vaccines.

Terms

anaphylaxis
antibodies
antigen
immunity: acquired, active, natural, passive

immunization
pathogens
seroconversion

toxoids
vaccines: attenuated, conjugate, recombinant

INTRODUCTION

Vaccination is a wise investment. For each dollar spent on vaccinations, an estimated $14 in future health care costs is saved. Thus, universal vaccination is a national goal. Nationwide, more than one child in three is not current with the recommended immunizations by the age of 2 years.

The Childhood Immunization Initiative of 1993 focuses on preventing epidemics such as the measles epidemic of 1989–1991 in which 130 people died, more than half of whom were children, of the 55,000 cases reported.

Active Immunity

The human immune response is activated when a **pathogen** such as a bacterium or virus invades the body. The body recognizes this pathogen as a foreign substance and promptly begins producing **antibodies** and other infection-fighting cells whose responsibility it is to attempt to rid the body of this foreign substance. On the first exposure to the pathogen, the immune response is relatively slow, and is typically accompanied by signs and symptoms of disease. However, the immune system retains memory of this pathogen. If this same pathogen invades the body again, the immune response, including the increased production of pathogen-specific antibodies, occurs much more rapidly and generally prevents disease. This active **natural immunity** may be present for the remaining life of the individual.

Active protection against disease may also be provoked through **immunization.** Vaccination involves the administration of a small amount of **antigen,** which, although capable of stimulating an immune response, does not typically produce disease. The antigen in vaccines may be produced in a number of ways. Traditional vaccines contain the whole or components of an inactivated (killed) microorganism. Others are composed of live, **attenuated** (weakened) microorganisms. **Toxoids** are inactivated toxins, the harmful disease-causing substance produced by some microorganisms.

Some newer vaccines are called **conjugate** vaccines. Such vaccines require the linking of a protein or toxoid from an unrelated organism to the outer coat of the disease-causing microorganism to create a substance that can be recognized by the immature immune system of young infants. *Haemophilus influenzae* type b is an example.

Recombinant subunit vaccines involve the insertion of some of the genetic material (DNA) of a pathogen into another cell or organism, where the antigen is then produced in massive quantities. These antigens are then used as a vaccine in place of the whole pathogen. Examples of these vaccines are hepatitis B and LYMErix for Lyme disease (see later discussion).

Regardless of the composition of the vaccine, all are designed to stimulate an immune response against a specific pathogen. Booster doses are sometimes required to maintain sufficient immunity. Because the immune system retains memory, the vaccinated individual who is later exposed to the actual pathogen mounts a rapid immune response, thus preventing disease. This active artificially **acquired** immunity is the focus of this chapter.

Passive Immunity

Passive immunity occurs when an individual receives antibodies against a particular pathogen from another source. Newborn infants naturally receive passive immunity via the transfer of maternal antibodies across the placenta. Passive immunity may also be acquired via the administration of antibodies pooled from a number of human or animal sources that have been exposed to disease-causing pathogens. Alternatively, antibodies may be produced using recombinant DNA technology.

Whether natural or acquired, passive immunity is transient, lasting no more than several weeks to a few months. The recipient does not mount his or her own immune response. However, passive immunity is important. It helps young infants who, because of their immature immune systems, are poorly equipped to protect themselves against disease. Acquired passive immunity is important when time does not permit active vaccination alone, when the exposed individual is at high risk for complications of the disease, or when the person suffers from an immune system deficiency that renders that person unable to produce an effective immune response.

VACCINE-PREVENTABLE DISEASES

In the United States, there are more than 20 infectious diseases that may be prevented by active vaccination. Many of these vaccines are routinely administered to healthy children and adults. Others are reserved for special populations such as military personnel, travelers to certain foreign countries, or the chronically ill. Table 32–1 provides an overview of the disease manifestations and vaccine information including route of administration. Vaccine-preventable diseases include adenovirus, cholera, diphtheria, *Haemophilus influenzae* type b (Hib), hepatitis A, hepatitis B, influenza, Japanese encephalitis, Lyme disease, measles, meningococcal disease, mumps, pertussis, plague, pneumococcal disease, poliomyelitis, rabies, rotavirus, rubella, tetanus, tuberculosis, typhoid, varicella, and yellow fever.

Tables 32–2 to 32–5 summarize the latest recom-

Table 32–1
Vaccine-Preventable Diseases

DISEASE	MANIFESTATIONS	VACCINE	ROUTE OF ADMINISTRATION AND STORAGE TEMPERATURE
Adenovirus	• Respiratory infection, which may involve the upper and/or lower respiratory tracts • May also cause vomiting and diarrhea	• Live virus • Administration limited to military personnel	PO
Cholera	• Severe watery diarrhea • May be accompanied by vomiting and dehydration	• Inactivated bacteria • Occasionally administered to foreign travelers	SC, IM, ID
Diphtheria	• Respiratory infection • May result in heart failure or paralysis if left untreated	• Toxoid • Contained in DTP, DTaP, DT, and Td vaccines	IM
Haemophilus influenzae type b (Hib)	• Causes meningitis, pneumonia, sepsis, arthritis, and skin and throat infections • Most serious in children younger than 1 year	• Bacterial conjugate • Contained in Hib, Hib-DTP, Hib-DTaP, and Hib-hepatitis B vaccines	IM
Hepatitis A	• Fever, malaise, jaundice, anorexia, and nausea • Acute, self-limited illness	• Inactivated virus • Administered to high-risk populations and persons traveling to certain foreign countries	IM 35°–46°F 2°–8°C
Hepatitis B	• Malaise, anorexia, arthralgias, arthritis, jaundice • Chronic infection can occur leading to liver cirrhosis, liver cancer, and death	• Recombinant viral antigen • Contained in hepatitis B and hepatitis B-Hib vaccines • Infants have routinely been vaccinated against hepatitis B since approximately 1990	IM 35°–46°F 2°–8°C
Influenza	• Fever, chills, headaches, malaise, myalgias, nasal congestion, and cough • Occasionally causes croup and pneumonia	• Inactivated whole virus or viral components	IM 35°–46°F 2°–8°C
Japanese encephalitis	• Headache, fever, myalgias, encephalitis	• Inactivated virus • Administered to some foreign travelers	SC
Lyme disease	• Fever, malaise, rash, cranial nerve palsies, meningitis, arthralgias, arthritis, carditis	• Recombinant bacterial antigen • Newly licensed vaccine • Administered to certain populations in areas that have a high incidence of Lyme disease	IM
Measles	• Rash, fever, cough, nasal congestion, conjunctivitis, pneumonia • Occasionally results in encephalitis	• Live virus • Contained in measles, MR, and MMR vaccines	SC 35°–46°F 2°–8°C
Meningococcal disease	• Fever, sepsis, rash, meningitis	• Portions of meningococcus bacterial capsule • Sometimes administered to persons exposed to known cases of meningococcal disease, travelers to certain foreign countries, military personnel, and certain high-risk groups	SC

Table continued on following page

Table 32–1 *Continued*
Vaccine-Preventable Diseases

DISEASE	MANIFESTATIONS	VACCINE	ROUTE OF ADMINISTRATION AND STORAGE TEMPERATURE
Mumps	• Swelling of salivary glands, fever, and headache • Rarely causes encephalitis, inflamed testicles, or permanent hearing loss	• Live virus • Contained in mumps and MMR vaccines	SC 35°–46°F 2°–8°C
Pertussis ("whooping cough")	• Severe coughing spasms • Rarely causes pneumonia, seizures, encephalitis, and death • Symptoms more severe in infants and young children	• Inactivated whole-cell bacteria or antigenic components of inactivated bacteria (acellular) • Contained in pertussis, DTP, DTP-Hib, DTaP, and DTaP-Hib vaccines	IM
Plague	• Fever and painful, swollen lymph nodes	• Inactivated bacteria • Recommended only for persons whose occupation puts them at high risk for exposure to plague-infected rodents (e.g., field biologists and animal laboratory workers) and for persons traveling to areas with epidemic plague	IM
Pneumococcal disease	• Ear infections, sinus infections, pneumonia • Occasionally causes sepsis and meningitis	• Portions of pneumococcal bacterial capsules • Administered to elderly and certain other high-risk populations	IM, SC 35°–46°F 2°–8°C
Poliomyelitis	• Mild form causes fever, sore throat, nausea, and headaches • Severe form causes paralysis and death	• Available as both live (OPV) and inactivated (IPV) virus vaccines	PO, SC IPV 35°–46°F 2°–8°C
Rabies	• Anxiety, difficulty swallowing, seizures, and, invariably, progresses to death	• Inactivated virus • Administered to high-risk groups (e.g., veterinarians and animal handlers) and to persons traveling to areas where rabies is common	IM, ID
Rotavirus	• Vomiting, diarrhea, fever • May lead to dehydration, especially in young children	• Live virus • Newly licensed vaccine • Recommended for infants younger than 1 year of age	IM, PO
Rubella ("German measles")	• Rash, fever • Birth defects if acquired by pregnant women	• Live virus • Contained in rubella, MR, and MMR vaccines	SC 35°–46°F 2°–8°C
Tetanus ("lock jaw")	• Headache, irritability, muscle spasms (jaw, neck, arms, legs, back, and abdomen)	• Toxoid • Contained in tetanus, DTP, DTaP, DTP-Hib, DTaP-Hib, DT, and Td vaccines	IM 35°–46°F 2°–8°C
Tuberculosis ("TB")	• Highly contagious respiratory infection • May also cause meningitis and bone, joint, and skin infections	• Live bacteria • Referred to as BCG (bacillus Calmette-Guérin) vaccine • Not routinely administered in the U.S. • Prevents severe disease but does not prevent infection with the bacterium	ID, SC

Table continued on following page

Table 32–1 *Continued*
Vaccine-Preventable Diseases

DISEASE	MANIFESTATIONS	VACCINE	ROUTE OF ADMINISTRATION AND STORAGE TEMPERATURE
Typhoid	• Fever, headache, anorexia, abdominal pain, enlarged liver and spleen, constipation, and later, diarrhea	• Available as live bacteria, inactivated bacteria, or components of typhoid bacterial capsule • Recommended only for travelers to certain countries	SC, PO
Varicella ("chickenpox")	• Fever and rash, consisting of a few to hundreds of itchy, blister-like lesions • Symptoms more severe in older children and adults • Complications may include encephalitis, bacterial skin infections, pneumonia, Reye's syndrome, and death	• Live virus	SC 5°F–15°C or colder
Yellow fever	• Fever, jaundice, and gastrointestinal hemorrhage	• Live virus • Recommended for travelers to foreign countries with high yellow fever rates • Required by international regulations for travel to and from certain countries	SC

PO = oral, SC = subcutaneous, IM = intramuscular, ID = intradermal

mendations for childhood and adult immunizations. Please note that those recommendations change regularly; check with the Centers for Disease Control and Prevention (CDC), website www.cdc.gov.

CHILDHOOD IMMUNIZATIONS

Table 32–2 outlines the recommended immunization schedule for infants and children up to 16 years of age. The 1998 recommendations include the following vaccines: hepatitis B; diphtheria, tetanus, pertussis; *H. influenza* type B; polio; rotavirus, measles, mumps, rubella; and varicella. Children who have not been immunized during infancy are referred to the schedule in Table 32–3. This table has two sections: the first is for children younger than 7 years of age; the second section is the schedule for children 7 to 12 years of age. Immunization tables are reviewed and updated annually to reflect changes in national immunization recommendations.

A summary of Rules for Childhood Immunizations (Table 32–4) is located at the website:

http://www.immunize.org. Helpful information about each vaccine includes route of administration, age usually given, minimum dosing intervals, and contraindications to their use. DTaP, tetanus and diphtheria (Td), polio, varicella, MMR, Hib, and HepB are the recommended vaccines.

ADULT IMMUNIZATIONS

Whereas much emphasis is placed on regularly immunizing infants and children, adult immunizations are frequently overlooked. However, they are equally important to the health and well-being of this population. Recommended vaccines for adults may include influenza, pneumococcal, hepatitis B, hepatitis A, tetanus, diphtheria, measles, mumps, rubella, varicella, and polio. The CDC suggests review of adult immunization record on decade birthdays (eg., 30, 40, 50). Table 32–5 summarizes the recommendations for adult immunization, minimum dosing intervals, and contraindications to vaccination.

Text continued on page 569

Table 32–2
Recommended Childhood Immunization Schedule, United States, January–December 1999

Vaccines[1] are listed under routinely recommended ages. | Bars | indicate range of recommended ages for immunization. Any dose not given at the recommended age should be given as a "catch-up" immunization at any subsequent visit when indicated and feasible. (Ovals) **indicate vaccines to be given if previously recommended doses were missed or given earlier than the recommended minimum age.**

AGE ▶ VACCINE ▼	Birth	1 mo	2 mos	4 mos	6 mos	12 mos	15 mos	18 mo	4–6 yrs	11–12 yrs	14–16 yrs
Hepatitis B[2]	Hep B										
		Hep B			Hep B					Hep B	
Diphtheria, tetanus, Pertussis[3]			DTaP	DTaP	DTaP		DTaP[3]		DTaP	Td	
H. influenzae type b[4]			Hib	Hib	Hib	Hib					
Polio[5]			IPV	IPV	Polio[5]				Polio		
Rotavirus[6]			Rv[6]	Rv[6]	Rv[6]						
Measles, Mumps, Rubella[7]						MMR			MMR[7]	MMR[7]	
Varicella[8]						Var				Var[8]	

Approved by the Advisory Committee on Immunization Practices (ACIP), the American Academy of Pediatrics (AAP), and the American Academy of Family Physicians (AAFP).

[1] *This schedule indicates the recommended ages for routine administration of currently licensed childhood vaccines. Combination vaccines may be used whenever any components of the combination are indicated and its other components are not contraindicated. Providers should consult the manufacturers' package inserts for detailed recommendations.*

[2] ***Infants born to HBsAg-negative mothers*** *should receive the 2nd dose of hepatitis B (Hep B) vaccine at least one month after the 1st dose. The 3rd dose should be administered at least 4 months after the 1st dose and at least 2 months after the 2nd dose, but not before 6 months of age for infants.*
Infants born to HBsAG-positive mothers *should receive hepatitis B vaccine and 0.5 mL hepatitis B immune globulin (HBIG) within 12 hours of birth at separate sites. The 2nd dose is recommended at 1–2 months of age and the 3rd dose at 6 months of age.*
Infants born to mothers whose HBsAg status is unknown *should receive hepatitis B vaccine within 12 hours of birth. Maternal blood should be drawn at the time of delivery to determine the mother's HBsAg status; if the HBsAg test is positive, the infant should receive HBIG as soon as possible (no later than 1 week of age).*
All children and adolescents (through 18 years of age) who have not been immunized against hepatitis B may begin the series during any visit. Special efforts should be made to immunize children who were born in or whose parents were born in areas of the world with moderate or high endemicity of hepatitis B virus infection.

[3] *DTaP (diphtheria and tetanus toxoids and acellular pertussis vaccine) is the preferred vaccine for all doses in the immunization series, including completion of the series in children who have received 1 or more doses of whole-cell DTP vaccine. Whole-cell DTP is an acceptable alternative to DTaP. The 4th dose (DTP or DTaP) may be administered as early as 12 months of age, provided 6 months have elapsed since the 3rd dose and if the child is unlikely to return at age 15–18 months. Td (tetanus and diphtheria toxoids) is recommended at 11–12 years of age if at least 5 years have elapsed since the last dose of DTP, DTaP or DT. Subsequent routine Td boosters are recommended every 10 years.*

[4] *Three Haemophilus influenzae type b (Hib) conjugate vaccines are licensed for infant use. If PRP-OMP (PedvaxHIB or ComVax [Merck]) is administered at 2 and 4 months of age, a dose at 6 months is not required. Because clinical studies in infants have demonstrated that using some combination products may induce a lower immune response to the Hib vaccine component, DTaP/Hib combination products should not be used for primary immunization in infants at 2, 4 or 6 months of age, unless FDA-approved for these ages.*

[5] *Two poliovirus vaccines currently are licensed in the United States: inactivated poliovirus (IPV) vaccine and oral poliovirus (OPV) vaccine. The ACIP, AAP and AAFP now recommend that the first two doses of poliovirus vaccine should be IPV. The ACIP continues to recommend a sequential schedule of two doses of IPV administered at ages 2 and 4 months, followed by two doses of OPV at 12–18 months and 4–6 years. Use of IPV for all doses also is acceptable and is recommended for immunocompromised persons and their household contacts. OPV is no longer recommended for the first two doses of the schedule and is acceptable only for special circumstances such as: children of parents who do not accept the recommended number of injections, late initiation of immunization which would require an unacceptable number of injections, and imminent travel to polio-endemic areas. OPV remains the vaccine of choice for mass immunization campaigns to control outbreaks due to wild poliovirus.*

[6] *Rotavirus (Rv) vaccine is shaded and italicized to indicate: 1) health-care providers may require time and resources to incorporate this new vaccine into practice; and 2) the AAFP feels that the decision to use rotavirus vaccine should be made by the parent or guardian in consultation with their physician or other health care provider. The first dose of Rv vaccine should not be administered before 6 weeks of age, and the minimum interval between doses is 3 weeks. The Rv vaccine series should not be initiated at 7 months of age or older, and all doses should be completed by the first birthday.*

Table continued on following page

Table 32–2 *Continued*

Recommended Childhood Immunization Schedule, United States, January–December 1999

^{7} The 2nd dose of measles, mumps, and rubella (MMR) vaccine is recommended routinely at 4–6 years of age but may be administered during any visit, provided at least 4 weeks have elpased since receipt of the 1st dose and that both doses are administered beginning at or after 12 months of age. Those who have not previously received the second dose should complete the schedule by the 11- 12-year-old visit.

^{8} Varicella (Var) vaccine is recommended at any visit on or after the first birthday for susceptible children, i.e., those who lack a reliable history of chickenpox (as judged by a health care provider) and who have not been immunized. Susceptible persons 13 years of age or older should receive 2 doses, given at least 4 weeks apart.

Table 32–3

Recommended Immunization Schedules for Children Not Immunized in the First Year of Life*

RECOMMENDED TIME/AGE	IMMUNIZATION(S)†‡	COMMENTS
YOUNGER THAN 7 YEARS		
First visit	DTaP (or DTP), Hib, HBV, MMR, OPV¶	If indicated, tuberculin testing may be done at same visit. If child is 5 y of age or older, Hib is not indicated in most circumstances.
Interval after first visit 1 mo (4 wk)	DTaP (or DTP), HBV, Var§	The second dose of OPV may be given if accelerated poliomyelitis vaccination is necessary, such as for travelers to areas where polio is endemic.
2 mo	DTaP (or DTP), Hib, OPV¶	Second dose of Hib is indicated only if the first dose was received when younger than 15 mo.
≥8 mo	DTaP (or DTP), HBV, OPV¶	OPV and HBV are not given if the third doses were given earlier.
Age 4–6 y (at or before school entry)	DTaP (or DTP), OPV,¶ MMR**	DTaP (or DTP) is not necessary if the fourth dose was given after the fourth birthday; OPV is not necessary if the third dose was given after the fourth birthday.
Age 11–12 y	See Table 32–2	
7–12 YEARS		
First visit	HBV, MMR, Td, OPV¶	
Interval after first visit 2 mo (8 wk)	HBV, MMR,** Var,§ Td, OPV¶	OPV also may be given 1 mo after the first visit if accelerated poliomyelitis vaccination is necessary.
8–14 mo	HBV,†† Td, OPV¶	OPV is not given if the third dose was given earlier.
Age 11–12 y	See Table 32–2	

* Table is not completely consistent with all package inserts. For products used, also consult manufacturer's package insert for instructions on storage, handling, dosage, and administration. Biologics prepared by different manufacturers may vary, and package inserts of the same manufacturer may change from time to time. Therefore, the physician should be aware of the contents of the current package insert.

Vaccine abbreviations: HBV indicates hepatitis B virus vaccine; Var, varicella vaccine; DTP, diphtheria and tetanus toxoids and pertussis vaccine; DTaP, diphtheria and tetanus toxoids and acellular pertussis vaccine; Hib, Haemophilus influenzae type b conjugate vaccine; OPV, oral poliovirus vaccine; IPV, inactivated poliovirus vaccine; MMR, live measles-mumps-rubella vaccine; Td, adult tetanus toxoid (full dose) and diphtheria toxoid (reduced dose), for children ≥7 years and adults.

† If all needed vaccines cannot be administered simultaneously, priority should be given to protecting the child against those diseases that pose the greatest immediate risk. In the United States, these diseases for children younger than 2 years usually are measles and Haemophilus influenzae type b infection; for children older than 7 years, they are measles, mumps, and rubella. Before 13 years of age, immunity against hepatitis B and varicella should be ensured.

‡ DTaP, HBV, Hib, MMR, and Var can be given simultaneously at separate sites if failure of the patient to return for future immunizations is a concern.

¶ IPV is also acceptable. However, for infants and children starting vaccination late (i.e., after 6 months of age), OPV is preferred in order to complete an accelerated schedule with a minimum number of injections.

§ Varicella vaccine can be administered to susceptible children any time after 12 months of age. Unvaccinated children who lack a reliable history of chickenpox should be vaccinated before their 13th birthday.

** Minimal interval between doses of MMR is 1 month (4 weeks).

†† HBV may be given earlier in a 0-, 2-, and 4-month schedule.

Table compiled from various Centers for Disease Control and Prevention sources.

Table 32-4

Summary of Rules for Childhood Immunization*

VACCINE	AGES USUALLY GIVEN, OTHER GUIDELINES	IF CHILD FALLS BEHIND— MINIMUM INTERVALS	CONTRAINDICATIONS (Remember, Mild Illness is not a Contraindication)
DTaP contains acellular pertussis DTP or DTwP contains whole cell pertussis Give IM	• DTaP is preferred for all doses in the series but DTwP is acceptable. • Give at 2m, 4m, 6m, 15–18m, 4–6yrs of age. • May give #1 as early as 6wks of age. • May give #4 as early as 12m of age if 6m has elapsed since #3 and the child is unlikely to return at age 15–18m. • If started with DTwP, may complete series with DTaP. • Do not give DTaP or DTwP to children ≥7 yrs of age (give Td). • DTaP/DTwP may be given with all other vaccines but at a separate site. • It is preferable but not mandatory to use the same DTaP product for all doses.	• #2 & #3 may be given 4wks after previous dose. • #4 may be given 6m after #3. • If #4 is given before 4th birthday, wait at least 6m for #5. • If #4 is given after 4th birthday, #5 is not needed. • Don't restart series, no matter how long since previous dose.	(DTaP and DTwP have the same contraindications and precautions.) • Anaphylactic reaction to a prior dose or to any vaccine component. • Moderate or severe acute illness. Don't postpone for minor illness. • Previous encephalopathy within 7 days after DTwP/DTaP. • Undiagnosed progressive neurologic problem. **Precautions:** The following are precautions not contraindications. Generally when these conditions are present, the vaccine shouldn't be given. But, there are situations when the benefit outweighs risk so vaccination should be considered (e.g., pertussis outbreak). • Previous rxn of T ≥ 105°F (40.5°C) within 48 hrs after dose. • Previous continuous crying lasting 3 or more hours within 48 hrs after dose. • Previous convulsion within 3 days after immunization. • Previous pale or limp episode, or collapse within 48 hrs after dose.
DT Give IM	• Give to children <7yrs of age if the child has had a serious reaction to the "p" in DTaP/DTwP, or if the parents refuse the pertussis component. • DT can be given with all other vaccines but at a separate site.	For children who have fallen behind, use information in box directly above.	• Anaphylactic reaction to a prior dose or to any vaccine component. • Moderate or severe acute illness. Don't postpone for minor illness.
Td Give IM	• Use for persons ≥ 7yrs of age. • A booster dose is now recommended for children 11–12yrs of age if 5yrs have elapsed since previous dose. Then boost every 10 years. • Td may be given with all other vaccines but at a separate site.	For those never vaccinated or behind, or if the vaccination history is unknown, give dose #1 now; dose #2 4wks later; dose #3 6m after #2; and then boost every 10 years.	• Anaphylactic reaction to a prior dose or to any vaccine component. • Moderate or severe acute illness. Don't postpone for minor illness.

Table continued on following page

Table 32-4 *Continued*
Summary of Rules for Childhood Immunization*

VACCINE	AGES USUALLY GIVEN, OTHER GUIDELINES	IF CHILD FALLS BEHIND— MINIMUM INTERVALS	CONTRAINDICATIONS (Remember, Mild Illness is not a Contraindication)
Polio IPV and OPV Give IPV SQ or IM Give OPV PO	• Give at 2m, 4m, 6–18m, and 4–6yrs of age. • Give IPV for doses #1 and #2 (except in special circumstances, e.g., parent's refusal, imminent travel to polio-endemic area). • ACIP says for dose #3, give OPV at 12–18m, and for dose #4, give OPV at 4–6yrs. An all-IPV schedule is also acceptable. If an all-IPV or all-OPV schedule is used, dose #3 may be given as early as 6m of age. • AAP/AAFP say give either IPV or OPV for doses #3 and #4. Dose #3 is given at 6–18m of age and dose #4 at 4–6yrs. • ACIP/AAP/AAFP say IPV is acceptable for all 4 doses. • Not routinely given to anyone ≥18yrs of age (except certain travelers). • IPV may be given with all other vaccines but at a separate site. • OPV may be given with all other vaccines.	• #1, #2, & #3 (IPV or OPV) should be separated by at least 4wks. • All IPV: a 6m interval is preferred between dose #2 and #3 for best response. • #4 (IPV or OPV) is given between 4–6yrs of age. • If #3 of an all-IPV or all-OPV series is given at ≥4yrs of age, dose #4 is not needed. • Children who receive any combination of IPV and OPV doses must receive all 4 doses, regardless of the age when first initiated. • Don't restart series, no matter how long since previous dose.	• Anaphylactic reaction to a prior dose or to any vaccine component. • Moderate or severe acute illness. Don't postpone for minor illness. • Use IPV when an adult in the household or other close contact has never been vaccinated against polio. • In pregnancy, neither OPV nor IPV is recommended, but if immediate protection is needed, see the ACIP recommendations on the use of polio vaccine. **The following are contraindications for OPV so use IPV in these situations:** • Cancer, leukemia, lymphoma, immunodeficiency, including HIV/AIDS. • Taking a drug that lowers resistance to infection, e.g., anticancer, high-dose steroids. • Someone in the household has any of the above medical problems.
Varicella Var Give SQ	• Routinely give at 12–18m. • Vaccinate all children ≥12m of age including adolescents who have not had prior infection with chickenpox. • If Var and MMR (and any other live virus vaccine polio) are not given on the same day, space them ≥28d apart. • Var may be given with all other vaccines but at a separate site.	• Do not give to children <12m of age. • Susceptible children ≤12yrs of age receive 1 dose. • Susceptible persons ≥13yrs of age receive 2 doses 4–8wks apart. • Don't restart series, no matter how long since previous dose.	• Anaphylactic reaction to a prior dose or to any vaccine component. • Moderate or severe acute illness. Don't postpone for minor illness. • Pregnancy, or possibility of pregnancy within 1 month. • If blood, plasma, or immune globulin (IG or VZIG) were given in past 5 months, see ACIP recs or AAP's 1997 *Red Book* (p. 353) re: time to wait before vaccinating. • Immunocompromised persons due to cancer, leukemia, lymphoma, immunodeficiency, including HIV/AIDS. Note: For patients on high-dose immunosuppressive therapy, consult ACIP recommendations regarding delay time. Note: Manufacturer recommends "no salicylates" for 6wks following this vaccine.

MMR

- ACIP, AAP, and AAFP recommend 2 doses of MMR for <u>all</u> children up to 18 years of age.
- Give #1 at 12–15m. Give #2 at 4–6yrs.
- Can give as early as 6m of age in an outbreak, but two routine doses will still need to be given at ≥12m of age.
- If a dose was given before 12m of age, give #1 at 12–15m of age with a minimum interval of 1m between these doses.
- If MMR and Var (and any other live virus vaccine except polio) are not given on the same day, space them ≥28d apart.
- May give with all other vaccines but at a separate site.

- Give whenever behind. Exception: If MMR and Var (and any other live virus vaccine except polio) are not given on the same day, space them ≥28d apart.
- There should be a minimum interval of 28 days between MMR #1 and MMR #2.
- Dose #2 can be given at any time if at least 28days have elapsed since dose #1, and both doses are administered after 1 year of age. This also applies if dose #2 is given before 4–6 years of age.
- Don't restart series, no matter how long since previous dose.

- Anaphylactic reaction to a prior dose or to any vaccine component.
- Pregnancy or possible pregnancy within next 3m (use contraception).
- Moderate or severe acute illness. Don't postpone for minor illness.
- If blood products or immunoglobulin have been administered during the past 11 months, consult ACIP recommendations or *AAP's 1997 Red Book* (page 353) regarding time to wait before vaccinating.
- HIV positivity is NOT a contraindication to MMR except for those who are severely immunocompromised.
- Immunocompromised persons, e.g., cancer, leukemia, lymphoma

Note: For patients on high-dose immunosuppressive therapy, consult ACIP recommendations regarding delay time.

Note: MMR is not contraindicated if a PPD test was done recently, but PPD should be delayed if MMR was given 1–30 days before the PPD.

Give SQ

Hib

- HibTITER (HbOC) & ActHib (PRP-T): give at 2m, 4m, 6m, 12–15m.
- PedvaxHiB (PRP–OMP): give at 2m, 4m, 12–15m.
- Dose #1 of all Hib vaccines may be given as early as 6 wks of age but do NOT give it any earlier than 6 wks of age.
- May give with all other vaccines but at a separate site.

Rules for all Hib vaccines:

- If the child is ≥15m of age, only 1 dose is given.
- Not routinely given to children ≥5yrs of age.
- Give booster dose a minimum of 2m after previous dose.
- Don't restart series, no matter how long since previous dose.

- Anaphylactic reaction to a prior dose or to any vaccine component.
- Moderate or severe acute illness. Don't postpone for minor illness.

Table continued on following page

Table 32–4 *Continued*
Summary of Rules for Childhood Immunization*

VACCINE	AGES USUALLY GIVEN, OTHER GUIDELINES	IF CHILD FALLS BEHIND— MINIMUM INTERVALS	CONTRAINDICATIONS (Remember, Mild Illness is not a Contraindication)
Give IM	• All Hib products licensed for the primary series are interchangeable. • Any Hib vaccine may be used for the booster dose. • Hib is not routinely given to children ≥5yrs of age.	**Rules for HbOC (HibTITER) & PRP-T (ActHib) only:** • If #1 is given up to 7m, give #2 & #3 spaced 1–2m after previous dose and boost at 12–15m. • If #1 is given at 7–11m only 3 doses are needed: #2 given 1–2m after #1, then boost at 12–15m. • If #1 is given at 12–14m, give a booster dose in 2m. **Rules for PRP-OMP (PedvaxHiB) only:** • If #1 is given at 3–11m of age, give #2 1–2m later and boost at 12–15m. • If #1 is given at 12–14m, boost 2m later.	• Anaphylactic reaction to a prior dose or to any vaccine component • Moderate or severe acute illness. Don't postpone for minor illness.
Hep-B **Give IM**	• ACIP, AAP, and AAFP say to vaccinate **ALL** children 0–18 years of age. • For infants, give at 0–2m, 1–4m, 6–18m of age. • For older children/teens, spacing options include: 0m, 1m, 6m; 0m, 2m, 4m; or 0m, 1m, 4m. • Children who were born or whose parents were born in countries of high HBV endemicity or who have other risk factors should be vaccinated as soon as possible. • **If mother is HBsAg positive:** give HBIG and hep-B #1 within 12 hrs of birth, #2 at 1–2m, and #3 at 6m of age. • **If mother's HBsAg status is unknown:** give hep B #1 within 12 hrs of birth, #2 at 1–2m, and #3 at 6m of age. If mother is later found to be HBsAg-positive, her infant should receive the additional protection of HBIG within the first 7 days of life. • **If mother is not chronically infected but is from an endemic area:** complete series by 6m of age. • May give with all other vaccines but at a separate site.	• **Don't restart series, no matter how long since previous dose.** • 3-dose series can be started at any age. • Minimum spacing for children and teens: 4 wks between #1 & #2, and 2m between #2 & #3. Overall there must be 4m between #1 and #3. • Dose #3 should not be given earlier than 6 months of age. **Dosing of hepatitis B vaccine:** Engerix-B: 1) 10μg=dose for 0–19 yr olds. 2) 20μg=dose for those ≥20 yrs. old. Recombivax HB: 1) 5μg=dose for 0–19 yr olds. 2) 10μg=dose for ages ≥20 yrs old. NOTE: Engerix-B and Recombivax-HB have different packaging and concentrations. Read the package insert to determine the volume of vaccine to administer.	

Rotavirus		
Rv Give PO	• Give at 2m, 4m, and 6m. • Dose #1 should not be given before 6wks or at ≥7m. • No dose should be given on or after the first birthday. • Do not readminister a regurgitated dose. • May give with all other vaccines.	• Minimum interval is 3wks between doses. • Use minimum intervals to achieve protection prior to rotavirus season or if behind schedule. • Don't restart the series no matter how long since previous dose.	• Moderate or severe acute illness, including persistent vomiting. Don't postpone for minor illness. • Anaphylactic reaction to a prior dose or to any vaccine component. • Known or suspected altered immunity, including infants born to HIV+ mothers unless it is known that the child is not HIV infected. • For infants with pre-existing chronic GI conditions, see ACIP statement.

Adapted from ACIP, AAP, and AAFP by the Immunization Action Coalition, March 1999.

Table 32-5
Summary of Recommendations for Adult Immunization

VACCINE NAME AND STORAGE TEMPERATURE	FOR WHOM IT IS RECOMMENDED	WHAT IS THE USUAL SCHEDULE?	SCHEDULE FOR THOSE WHO HAVE FALLEN BEHIND	CONTRAINDICATIONS AND PRECAUTIONS	RULES OF SIMULTANEOUS ADMINISTRATION	ROUTE
Influenza *"flu shot"* 35–46°F 2–8°C	• People who are 65 years of age or older. • People under 65 with medical problems such as heart disease, lung disease, diabetes, renal dysfunction, hemoglobinopathies, immunosuppression, and/or those living in chronic care facilities. People (≥6mo of age) working or living with these people should be vaccinated as well. • All health care workers. • Healthy pregnant women who will be in their 2nd or 3rd trimesters during the influenza season. • Pregnant women who have underlying medical conditions should be vaccinated before the flu season, regardless of the trimester. • Anyone who wishes to reduce the likelihood of becoming ill with influenza.	• October–November is optimal time to receive a flu shot to maximize protection, but the vaccine may be given at any time during the influenza season, (typically December–March).	May be given anytime during the influenza season, including the winter months, as long as cases are still occurring in the community.	• Previous anaphylactic reaction to this vaccine, to any of its components, or to eggs. • Moderate or severe acute illness.	Can give with all others but at a separate site.	IM
Pneumococcal *"pneumococcal shot"* 35–46°F 2–8°C	• All adults 65 years of age and older. • People under 65 who have chronic illness or other high risk factors including chronic cardiac and pulmonary diseases, anatomic or functional asplenia (including sickle cell disease), chronic liver disease, alcoholism, diabetes mellitus, CSF leaks. Others at high risk include immunocompromised persons including those with HIV infection, leukemia, lymphoma, Hodgkin's disease, multiple myeloma, generalized malignancy, chronic renal failure, or nephrotic syndrome, those receiving immunosuppressive chemotherapy (including corticosteroids), and those who received an organ or bone marrow transplant.	• Routinely given as a one-time dose. • One-time revaccination is recommended 5 years later for people at highest risk of fatal pneumococcal infection, or if the 1st dose was given prior to age 65 and ≥5 years since previous dose.	Give as soon as need is recognized.	• Previous anaphylactic reaction to this vaccine or to any of its components. • Moderate or severe acute illness.	Can give with all others but at a separate site.	IM or SC

| Hepatitis B (Hep-B) (HBV) 35–46°F 2–8°C | • Many high-risk adults need vaccination including: household contacts and sexual partners of hepatitis B carriers; users of illicit injectable drugs; heterosexuals with more than one sexual partner in 6 months; men who have sex with men; people with recently diagnosed STDs; patients in hemodialysis units; recipients of certain blood products; health care workers and public safety workers who are exposed to blood; clients and staff of institutions for the developmentally disabled; inmates of long-term correctional facilities, and certain international travelers.
• All adolescents.
Note: In 1997, the NIH Consensus Development Conference, a panel of national experts, recommended that hepatitis B vaccination be given to all persons infected with hepatitis C virus.
Note: Prior serologic testing may be recommended depending on the specific level of risk and/or likelihood of previous exposure.
Ed. note: It is prudent to screen individuals who have emigrated from endemic areas. When HBsAg "carriers" are identified, offer them appropriate disease management. In addition, their household members and intimate contacts should be screened and, if found susceptible, vaccinated. | • Commonly used timing options for vaccination:
0, 1, 6 months
0, 2, 4 months
0, 1, 4 months
• There must be one month between doses #1 and #2, and two months between doses #2 and #3. Overall there must be at least four months between doses #1 and #3.
• If the series is delayed between doses, do not start the series over. Simply continue from where you left off. | • Previous anaphylactic reaction to this vaccine or to any of its components.
• Moderate or severe acute illness. | Can give with all others but at a separate site.

IM |

Table continued on following page

Table 32–5 *Continued*
Summary of Recommendations for Adult Immunization

VACCINE NAME AND STORAGE TEMPERATURE	FOR WHOM IT IS RECOMMENDED	WHAT IS THE USUAL SCHEDULE?	SCHEDULE FOR THOSE WHO HAVE FALLEN BEHIND	CONTRAINDICATIONS AND PRECAUTIONS	RULES OF SIMULTANEOUS ADMINISTRATION	ROUTE
Hepatitis A (Hep-A) 35–46°F 2–8°C Brands may be used interchangeably.	• Adults who travel outside of the U.S. (except for Northern and Western Europe, New Zealand, Australia, Canada, and Japan). • People with chronic liver disease; all people with hepatitis C virus infection; people with hepatitis B who have chronic liver disease; illicit drug users; men who have sex with men; people with clotting disorders; people who work with hepatitis A virus in experimental lab settings (does not refer to routine medical labs); and food handlers where health authorities or private employers determine vaccination to be cost-effective. Note: Prevaccination testing is likely to be cost effective for persons >40 years and for younger persons in certain groups with a high prevalence of HAV infection.	• Two doses are needed • The minimum interval between dose #1 and #2 is 6 months.	If dose #2 is delayed, do not repeat dose #1. Just give dose #2.	• Previous anaphylactic reaction to this vaccine or to any of its components. • Moderate or severe acute illness. • Safety during pregnancy has not been determined, so benefits must be weighed against potential risk.	Can give with all others but at a separate site.	IM
Td (Tetanus, diphtheria) 35–46°F 2–8°C	After the primary series has been completed, a booster dose is recommended every 10 years. Make sure your patients have received a primary series of 3 doses.	Booster dose every 10 years after completion of the primary series of 3 doses.	The primary series is: • #1 • #2 given 1 month later • #3 given 6–12 months after #2.	• Previous anaphylactic reaction to this vaccine or to any of its components. • Moderate or severe acute illness.	Can give with all others but at a separate site.	IM

MMR Measles, Mumps, Rubella 35–46°F 2–8°C				SC
• Adults born in 1957 or later need one dose of the MMR if no serologic proof of immunity or documentation of a dose given on or after 1st birthday. • Adults in high-risk groups, (health care workers, students entering post secondary schools, and international travelers) may need a second dose. • All women of childbearing age (i.e., adolescent girls and premenopausal women) without acceptable evidence of rubella immunity or vaccination. Note: Adults born before 1957 are considered immune but proof of immunity may be required for health care workers.	• #1 • #2, if recommended, is given no sooner than 1 month after #1. #2 may be given as early as 1 month after dose #1.	• Previous anaphylactic reaction to this vaccine, or to any of its components. (An-aphylactic reaction to eggs is not a contraindication to MMR, so skin testing isn't needed prior to vaccination.) • Pregnancy or possibility of pregnancy within 3 months. • HIV positivity is NOT a contraindication to MMR except if severely immunocompromised. • Immunocompromised: includes cancer, leukemia, lymphoma, immunosuppressive drug therapy, including high dose steroids or radiation therapy. • If blood products or immune globulin have been administered during the past 11 months, consult the ACIP recommendations regarding time to wait before vaccinating. • Moderate or severe acute illness. Note: MMR is NOT contraindicated if a PPD test was done recently. PPD should be delayed for 4–6 weeks after an MMR has been given.	Can give with all others but at a separate site. If varicella is not given at the same time, space varicella and MMR at least 30 days apart.

Table continued on following page

Table 32–5 *Continued*
Summary of Recommendations for Adult Immunization

VACCINE NAME AND STORAGE TEMPERATURE	FOR WHOM IT IS RECOMMENDED	WHAT IS THE USUAL SCHEDULE?	SCHEDULE FOR THOSE WHO HAVE FALLEN BEHIND	CONTRAINDICATIONS AND PRECAUTIONS	RULES OF SIMULTANEOUS ADMINISTRATION	ROUTE
Varicella "Chickenpox shot" (Var) 5°F –15°C or colder	• All susceptible adults should be vaccinated. Special efforts should be made to vaccinate: susceptible persons who have close contact with persons at high risk for serious complications (e.g., health care workers and family contacts of immunocompromised persons) and susceptible persons who are at high risk of exposure (e.g., teachers of young children, day care employees, residents and staff in institutional settings such as colleges and correctional institutions, as well as nonpregnant women of childbearing age, and international travelers who do not have evidence of immunity). Note: Adults with reliable histories of chickenpox (self or parental report of disease) are assumed to be immune. For those who have no reliable history, serologic testing may be cost effective to determine immunity since most adults are immune.	All adults need two doses. Give dose #2 4–8 weeks after dose #1.	• Give #2 no sooner than 4 weeks after #1.	• Previous anaphylactic reaction to this vaccine or to any of its components. • Pregnancy, or possibility of pregnancy within 1 month. • Immunocompromised persons due to malignancies and primary or acquired immunodeficiency including HIV/AIDS. Note: For those on high dose immunosuppressive therapy, consult ACIP recommendations regarding delay time. • If blood products or immune globulin have been administered during the past 5 months, consult the ACIP recommendations regarding time to wait before vaccinating. • Moderate or severe acute illness. Note: Manufacturer recommends that salicylates be avoided for 6 weeks after receiving varicella vaccine.	Can give with all others but at a separate site. If MMR is not given on the same day, space MMR and varicella at least 30 days apart.	SC
Polio vaccine IPV 35–46°F 2–8°C	Not routinely recommended for adults ≥18 years of age. Note: Adults living in the U.S. who never received or completed a primary series of polio vaccine, need not be vaccinated, unless they intend to travel to areas where exposure to wild-type virus is likely. Health care workers need a completed primary series. Previously vaccinated adults need one booster dose if traveling to polio endemic areas.	Refer to ACIP recommendations regarding unique situations, schedules, and dosing information. If polio vaccine is indicated for adults, IPV is generally preferred.		• Refer to ACIP recommendations.	Can give with all others but at a separate site.	SC or IM

Adapted from the Advisory Committee on Immunization Practices (ACIP) by the Immunization Action Coalition with review by ad hoc team—October 1998.

IMMUNIZATION PRIOR TO FOREIGN TRAVEL

Foreign travel warrants the administration of all routine vaccines that may be indicated based on age and/or immunization history. Foreign travel also requires consideration of additional vaccines depending on the client's travel itinerary. These may include yellow fever, typhoid, meningococcal, rabies, and Japanese encephalitis vaccines. A country-specific review of vaccinations is beyond the scope of this chapter. However, current vaccine recommendations and related travel information are available from the CDC. To receive CDC travel information by FAX, telephone (888-232-3299) or download this information from the travel website at www.cdc.gov/travel. Shoreland, Inc., also provides travel information including vaccine recommendations at www.shoreland.com.

REPORTING OF DISEASES AND ADVERSE REACTIONS

Health care providers are responsible for reporting cases of vaccine-preventable diseases to public health officials who make weekly reports to the Centers for Disease Control and Prevention (CDC). These data identify whether an outbreak is occurring, and the impact of immunization policies and procedures.

Vaccines are generally safe. Common mild reactions include swelling at the injection site and fever. Awareness of the contraindications for use of vaccines decreases the incidence of serious adverse reactions. Absolute contraindications include anaphylactic reaction to a specific vaccine or component of another vaccine or moderate or severe illness. In general, vaccines may be given if the client has the following: mild acute illness or convalescent phase of illness, antimicrobial therapy, exposure to infectious disease, and prematurity.

Health care providers must report adverse reactions to the Vaccine Adverse Events Reporting System (VAERS). Information and forms are available at (800) 822-7967. The Childhood Vaccine Injury Act of 1986 set forth the National Vaccine Injury Compensation Program (NVICP). Under this program, negligence is not a requirement, and it provides compensation for injury/death caused by the vaccination. Call NVICP for additional information (800) 338-2382.

VARICELLA VACCINE

Chart 32–1 provides pharmacologic data for varicella vaccine.

Pharmacokinetics

Biologic products such as vaccines do not undergo the pharmacokinetic processes associated with other drug therapy.

Pharmacodynamics

Seroconversion is defined as the acquisition of detectable levels of antibodies in the bloodstream. In the case of varicella vaccine, seroconversion occurs in 97% of 12-month to 12-year-old recipients at approximately 4 to 6 weeks after vaccination. Susceptible 13-year-olds and older receiving two doses of varicella vaccine 4 to 8 weeks apart show a seroconversion rate of approximately 75% of 4 weeks after the first dose and of 99% 4 weeks after the second dose. The immune response appears to persist indefinitely after vaccination. No booster is currently indicated.

Contraindications

Varicella vaccine should be avoided in clients with a history of previous anaphylaxis to this vaccine or to any of its components, including gelatin and neomycin. It is also contraindicated in the presence of moderate to severe acute illness or active untreated tuberculosis.

The possible effects of the vaccine on fetal development are currently unknown. However, chickenpox can sometimes cause fetal harm. Therefore, varicella vaccine is contraindicated during pregnancy. Pregnancy should also be avoided for at least one month after each dose of the vaccine. Note: this differs from the product package insert, which suggests a three-month delay.

Clients who are immunocompromised because of malignancies should avoid varicella vaccine. Likewise, the vaccine is contraindicated in the presence of primary or acquired immunodeficiencies, including human immunodeficiency virus (HIV).

Drug Interactions

Frequently, a client is eligible for several immunizations at any given visit. A client receiving varicella vaccine may receive all other vaccines concurrently as long as they are administered at separate sites. If measles-mumps-rubella (MMR) vaccine in not given the same day as varicella vaccine, administration of the two vaccines should be spaced at least 4 weeks apart.

If a client has received a transfusion of blood or blood products, including immune globulin, varicella vaccine should be deferred for at least 5 months. Likewise, such products should, if possible, be avoided for at least 2 months after vaccination. Blood products and immune globulin interfere with the body's production of antibodies specific to chicken-

Chart 32–1.   Vaccines: Varicella

VACCINE

Drug Name

Varicella (Varivax)
Pregnancy Category: C

Dosage

C: 12 mo–12 y: SC: 0.5 ml × 1 dose
C: ≥13 y: SC: 0.5 ml × 2 doses given 4–8 wk apart

Contraindications

Previous anaphylaxis to this vaccine or to any of its components; pregnancy or possibility of pregnancy within 1 mo; immunocompromised vaccine recipient; presence of moderate to severe acute illness; active untreated tuberculosis

Drug-Lab-Food Interactions

Drug: Separate from MMR vaccine by 4 wk, if not given on same day; delay VV for at least 5 mo after blood transfusion or Ig; delay Ig for 2 mo after VV; high dose immunosuppressant medications; avoid salicylates for 6 wk after VV

Pharmacokinetics

N/A

Pharmacodynamics

Seroconversion rates:
12 mo–12 y: 97% at 4–6 wk after vaccination
≥13 y: 75% 4 wk after first dose and 99% 4 wk after second dose
No booster indicated at this time

Therapeutic Effects/Uses

Prevention of chickenpox. When administered to susceptible individuals, vaccine results in complete protection from chickenpox for majority. For the minority in whom breakthrough chickenpox develops after vaccination, the disease is typically very mild.

Mode of Action: Stimulates active immunity against natural disease.

Side Effects

Pain and redness at injection site, fever, chickenpox-like rash (generalized or confined to area surrounding injection site)

Adverse Reactions

Anaphylaxis, thrombocytopenia, encephalitis, SJS

Assessment and Planning

Interventions

Evaluation

NURSING PROCESS

KEY: SC: subcutaneous; MMR: measles-mumps-rubella; VV: varicella vaccine; Ig: immune globulin; SJS: Stevens-Johnson syndrome.

pox, thereby decreasing the likelihood that active immunity will develop.

Reye's syndrome has occasionally occurred in children following natural chickenpox infection. The majority of these children were also receiving salicylate medications (e.g., aspirin). Therefore, it is recommended that clients avoid salicylates for 6 weeks after vaccination.

RECENT DEVELOPMENTS AND THE FUTURE OF VACCINES

Currently there are new vaccines and delivery systems in development. Potential warfare tactics have increased the level of awareness of the vaccine for anthrax.

Anthrax, as a biological weapon, is highly lethal—it is easily produced, stored, and spread over large areas. Proper vaccination is an essential part of protection against this disease. Approved by the FDA in 1970, anthrax vaccine has been routinely and safely administered to laboratory personnel, livestock farmers, veterinarians, and military personnel deployed during the Gulf War. The vaccine requires 6 injections: three given 2 weeks apart followed by three additional doses at 6, 12, and 18 months. There have been no reports of serious side effects; contraindicated during pregnancy. Additional information is available at http://www.defenselink.mil/other_info/protection.html#Anthrax.

NURSING PROCESS
VACCINES

Assessment

- Obtain medical history including history of malignancy or other immune deficiency.
- Obtain history of pregnancy or possible pregnancy within the next month. Do not administer vaccines to pregnant individuals.
- Obtain drug history, including high-dose immunosuppressants, blood transfusions, and immune globulin.
- Obtain complete allergy history, including drugs, vaccines, food, and environmental allergies.
- Assess for adverse reactions (other than allergic) to previous doses of vaccine or any vaccine component.
- Assess for symptoms of moderate to severe acute illness with or without fever.
- Screen for unvaccinated or immunodeficient household contacts.
- Obtain immunization history to determine current vaccine needs.

Potential Nursing Diagnoses

- Knowledge deficit: vaccine-preventable diseases, risks and benefits of vaccination
- Altered health maintenance

Planning

- Client will adhere to recommended immunization schedule for vaccine-preventable diseases.
- Client will be free of adverse reactions.

Nursing Interventions

- Strictly adhere to individual vaccine storage requirements to ensure potency of the product.
- Upon preparation, including reconstitution of a given vaccine, administer within time limits stated in package insert to ensure potency.
- At time of visit, administer at separate sites all vaccines for which a client is eligible. Do *not* mix vaccines in the same syringe.
- Observe clients for signs and symptoms of adverse reactions to vaccines.
- Keep epinephrine readily available for immediate use in case of anaphylactic reaction.
- Provide client with a record of immunizations administered.

Client Teaching

General

- Discuss with client and/or client's family the manifestations of and risk of contracting vaccine-preventable diseases.
- Instruct female clients of childbearing age to avoid pregnancy for one month depending on the vaccines to be administered.
- Instruct clients to avoid contact with immunocompromised persons depending on vaccines to be administered.
- In accordance with federal law, provide client or client's family with current Vaccine Information Statements (VISs), available from the CDC, for each vaccine administered. The following data must be documented in the client's record: date of vaccination, route and site; vaccine type, manufacturer, lot number, and expiration date; name, address, and title of individual administering vaccine.
- Remind client or client's family to bring immunization record to all visits.
- Provide client or client's family with date upon which to return for next vaccination.

Nursing Process continued on following page

NURSING PROCESS *Continued*
VACCINES

Side Effects

- Discuss common side effects of vaccines such as injection site soreness, fever, and side effects specific to individual vaccines.
- Instruct client or client's family to contact the health care provider if signs of a serious reaction are noted.

Evaluation
- Evaluate client's or client's family's understanding of rationale for immunizations.
- Evaluate client adherence to recommended immunization schedule.

LYMErix, FDA approved in late 1998, is used to treat an infection caused by *Borrelia burgdorferi*, a spirochete transmitted by the deer tick. LYMErix does not prevent Lyme disease in individuals with undetermined infection at the time of vaccination. A series of three injections over a year is required; it is not for children under 15 years old. Efficacy is 79% after three doses. Individuals should be cautioned of the need to practice strategies of personal protection against tick bites.

In addition, there is work in progress on an HIV vaccine.

New delivery systems for vaccines are currently in development to replace the "needle." Watch for mucosal vaccines, via a nasal spray, for influenza in both adults and children. Timed-release pills have the potential to offer lifetime immunity to a specific disease in a one-time dose. With this, the need for a booster is eliminated. In addition, skin patches may be used to administer tetanus and flu vaccines.

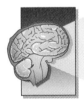

Critical Thinking in Action

J. W., a 29-year-old woman, is seen at the immunization clinic with her 2-month-old daughter and her son, who just turned 5 years old last month. She reports they all need shots.

1. J. W. will soon be returning to work at a long-term care facility for developmentally disabled adults. She reports that her new employer is encouraging her to be immunized against hepatitis B. She wonders how long it will take her to complete the vaccine series. What is your response?
2. You administer J. W.'s first dose of hepatitis B vaccine today. When should she return for the next dose?
3. You ask J. W. about her vaccine history. She says she does not have an immunization card but remembers last receiving a "booster when I stepped on a nail at my high school graduation picnic." What "booster" did she likely receive? At what point is another booster due?
4. J. W. says her daughter needs her "regular baby shots." The infant received her first hepatitis B vaccine while in the newborn nursery. Against what vaccine-preventable illnesses will you plan to vaccinate this infant today?

Continued on following page

5. When would this baby be due for a next round of immunizations?
6. J. W. asks you about chickenpox vaccine. She would like her daughter to be vaccinated against chickenpox as soon as possible because she does not want her to suffer through chickenpox as her brother did. You inform J. W. that the earliest age at which her daughter can receive varicella vaccine is _____.
7. J. W. says she has heard that you can get chickenpox from the shot. How would you respond to this comment?
8. J. W. has brought her son's immunization card. It shows he received hepatitis B vaccine at birth, at 2 months, and at 9 months. He received DTP, Hib, and OPV vaccines at 2 months, 4 months, and 6 months. She is worried that he will need to start his immunizations over because "he's so far behind." How would you respond to her concern?
9. For what vaccines is he due today?

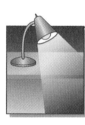

Study Questions

1. Describe the difference between active natural and active acquired immunity.
2. Describe the difference between active and passive immunity.
3. What vaccines are typically indicated for children up to 16 years of age?
4. For what age group is pneumococcal vaccine typically indicated?
5. If a 2-month-old infant experiences redness and tenderness at the DTaP injection site associated with fever of 100.8 degrees Fahrenheit, what vaccine would you administer at the next visit in 6 to 8 weeks?
6. List contraindications to the use of varicella vaccine.
7. Describe nursing interventions related to vaccine administration.

Unit VII

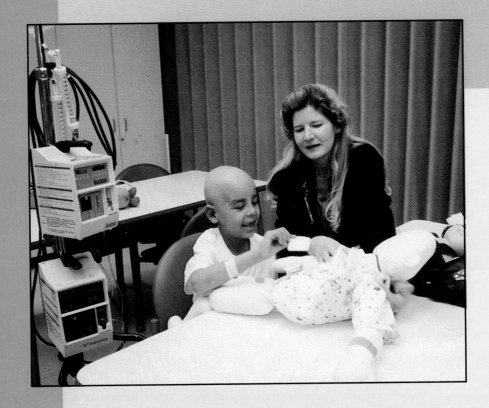

Antineoplastic
Agents

Cancer continues to be a major health problem in our society. Causes of some cancers may be attributed to the environment (chemicals, radiation, and infections) and to genetic background. Cancer (malignant) cells are characterized by (1) fast growth, (2) undifferentiated tissue mass, and (3) spread, or metastasis, to other body cells and organs. Cancer cells that divide rapidly respond more effectively to anticancer therapy than the slow-growing cells or solid tumors.

CELL CYCLE

The cell cycles of normal and cancer cells are similar. In the cell cycle there are five phases; four of the phases are directed to cell replication, and a fifth phase is the resting phase. The cycle begins with G_1, which is the presynthesis phase in preparing for DNA synthesis. The S phase is when DNA synthesis actually occurs. G_2 phase is the postsynthesis, and cell division occurs in the M phase. Cells that are in G_0 or resting phase may remain there, die, or reenter the cell cycle going through the phases to cell division. The cell cycle is demonstrated in Figure VII–1, and the phases are described in Table VII–1.

GROWTH FRACTION

Growth fraction plays a major role in the cancer cell response to the anticancer drug therapy. Growth fraction is the percentage of the cancer cell that is actively dividing. A high growth fraction occurs when the cell is rapidly dividing, and a low growth fraction occurs when the cell divides slowly. In general, anticancer drugs are more effective against the cancer cells that have a high growth fraction.

DOUBLING TIME

Doubling time is related to the growth fraction. It is the time required for a number of cancer cells to double their mass. When the tumor ages and enlarges, its growth fraction decreases and its doubling time increases. Compare, for example, breast cancer, whose growth fraction is 1% and whose doubling time is 55 days, and lymphocytic leukemia, whose growth fraction is 50% and whose doubling time is 4 days.

In the past two decades, more advances have been made to control and eradicate cancer through the use of numerous anticancer drugs, research, and treatment protocols that include select combinations of anticancer drugs. Nurses are taking an

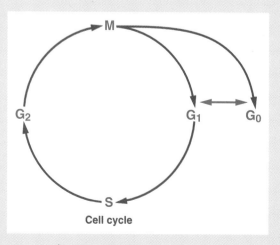

Cell cycle

Figure VII–1
Cell cycle. G_1 phase (postmitotic gap): Production of enzyme for DNA synthesis. The G_1 phase lasts 15 to 18 hours. S phase (synthesis): The DNA is doubled. The S phase lasts 10 to 20 hours. G_2 phase (premitotic gap): RNA synthesis for later mitosis. The G_2 phase lasts approximately 3 hours. M phase (mitosis): Cell division, producing two identical cells. The M phase lasts approximately 1 hour. G_0 phase (resting phase): Remain in this phase or return to the cell cycle for cell replication. Cells in this phase are not as sensitive to many antineoplastic drugs.

Table VII–1
Cell Cycle and Its Phases

1. G_1: enzyme production needed for DNA (deoxyribonucleic acid)
2. S, or synthesis: DNA synthesis and replication
3. G_2: RNA (ribonucleic acid) and protein synthesis
4. M, or mitosis: cell division
5. G_0: resting phase

active role in various health facilities and in the home care of clients receiving anticancer therapy. To be a resourceful participant in the care of clients with cancer, the nurse first needs to understand the type of drug therapy the client is receiving, contraindications, drug interactions, therapeutic effects, side effects, and adverse reactions.

Chapter 33 discusses how certain anticancer drugs inhibit or prevent cell reproduction. The anticancer drugs are grouped as cell-cycle specific and cell-cycle nonspecific. Drugs in these groups are presented according to their effects on the cell cycle. Alkylating compounds, antimetabolites, antitumor antibiotics, vinca alkaloids, hormones, and steroids are anticancer drug categories discussed.

Chapter 34 describes the evolving state of biologic response modifiers, which have the following functions: (1) enhance host immunologic function, (2) destroy or interfere with tumor activities, and (3) promote differentiation of stem cells.

The nursing process is used throughout these two chapters to illustrate the importance of the role of the nurse in drug therapy.

Anticancer Drugs

33

Outline

Objectives

- Differentiate between cell-cycle specific and cell-cycle nonspecific drugs.
- Identify general side effects of and adverse reactions to anticancer drugs.
- Describe the uses and considerations for the following types of drugs: alkylating compounds, antimetabolites, antitumor antibiotics, vinca alkaloids, and hormones.
- Explain the nursing implications of anticancer drugs.

Terms

alopecia
androgens
anticancer drugs
antiestrogens
antineoplastic drugs
body surface area
cell-cycle nonspecific

cell-cycle specific
chemotherapeutic agents
corticosteroids
DNA
doubling time
growth fraction
irritants

nonvesicants
progestins
RNA
stomatitis
tumoricidal
vesication
vinca alkaloids

INTRODUCTION

In the United States, cancer is the second leading cause of death, second to heart disease. It is the leading cause of death in women. In children between the ages of 1 and 15 years, cancer is the second leading cause of death after accidents. The most common types of cancer in men are prostate, lung, and colorectal. In women, the common types of cancer include breast, lung, and colorectal.

Cancer results from the alterations in DNA within the cell. The DNA is the genetic substance in the body cells. Also DNA transfers information necessary for the production of enzymes and protein synthesis.

Anticancer drugs, also called **cancer chemotherapeutic agents** or **antineoplastic drugs,** were introduced in the treatment of cancer in the 1940s. The first antineoplastic drugs included estrogen for prostatic cancer and the nitrogen mustard drug mechlorethamine hydrochloride (Mustargen). Many of the early anticancer drugs, such as methotrexate, 5-fluorouracil, 6-mercaptopurine, and cyclophosphamide, are still in use. Since the early 1970s, more anticancer drugs have been marketed, and drug protocols (detailed plans) using combinations of drugs have been proven effective in curing specific leukemias and Hodgkin's disease. Anticancer drugs are given for several reasons, including cure, control, and palliation. Chemotherapy may be used as the sole treatment of cancer or in conjunction with radiation and surgery.

CELL-CYCLE NONSPECIFIC AND SPECIFIC

In Unit VII, the cell cycle for normal and cancer cells, growth fraction, and doubling time are discussed. Refer to the unit for clarification of the cell cycle and definitions.

Anticancer drugs cause cancer cell death by interfering with cancer cell replication.

This drug group interferes with either all phases or a specific phase of the cell cycle: G_1, S, G_2, M, and G_0 (see Fig. VII–1). There are two types of anticancer drugs: **cell-cycle nonspecific** (CCNS) drugs, which act on any phase during the cell cycle, and **cell-cycle specific** (CCS) drugs, which act on a specific phase of the cell cycle. CCNS drugs (also called cell-cycle independent) kill the cell during the dividing and resting phase. CCS drugs (also called cell-cycle dependent) are effective against rapidly growing cancer cells. In general, the groups of CCNS drugs (some alkylating agents are CCS) are the alkylating drugs, antitumor antibiotics, and hormones. The CCS drugs are the antimetabolites and the vinca alkaloids. Table 33–1 identifies the types and group of drugs and phase of the cell cycle that they affect.

Growth fraction and doubling time are two factors that play a major role in the cancer cell response to the anticancer drug. Anticancer drugs are more effective against the cancer cells that have a high growth fraction. Leukemias and some lymphomas have high growth fractions and, thus, respond well to anticancer drug therapy. Carcinomas of the breast and colon and melanomas have a low growth fraction, so they respond poorly to antineoplastics. Small and early forming cancer cells and fast-growing tumors respond well to anticancer drugs. Drug therapy for cancer diagnosed in its early stage is more effective and has a higher cure rate than cancer diagnosed in the advanced stages. Solid tumors have a large percentage of the cell mass in the G_0 phase, so these tumors have a low growth fraction and are less sensitive to anticancer drugs. Higher doses of drugs result in better **tumoricidal** (tumor-killing) effects.

Table 33–1
Groups of Cell-Cycle Nonspecific (CCNS) and Cell-Cycle Specific (CCS) Drugs

DRUG TYPE	DRUG GROUP	CELL-CYCLE EFFECT
CCNS	Alkylating drugs	All phases. Act more effectively in G_1 and S phases.
	Antitumor antibiotics	All phases. Bleomycin more effective at the G_2 phase; daunorubicin and doxorubicin more effective at the S phase, and mitomycin more effective at the G_1 and S phases.
	Nitrosoureas	All phases.
	Steroids (corticosteroids, estrogen, androgens)	All phases. Act more effectively at the S and M phases.
CCS	Antimetabolites	Effective at the S phase.
	Vinca alkaloids	Effective at the M phase.
	Antitumor antibiotics	Some have CCNS effect.

Growth of cancer is usually faster in the earlier stages. As the tumor grows, the blood supply decreases and the growth rate decreases. Anticancer agents are more effective against small tumors with sufficient blood supply. When the tumor is the size of a small grape, it is usually detectable and it contains approximately 1 billion cancer cells. At that time, symptoms may appear. As the tumor enlarges, its growth fraction decreases and its doubling time increases, which decreases the effectiveness of anticancer therapy.

CANCER CHEMOTHERAPY

Tumor cells are similar to normal cells in that it is difficult for anticancer drugs to be selective in killing tumor cells and not normal cells. If large anticancer doses are given to kill malignant cells, normal cells also usually are killed; thus, the death of the client could result.

Antibacterials (antibiotics) differ from anticancer drugs because they are selective in killing bacterial cells. Antibacterials do not harm normal-functioning cells. Many of the antibacterials, such as penicillin, attack and destroy the bacterial cell walls. The bacterial cell dies and the normal cells remain. Malignant cells do not have definite cell walls. Anticancer drug research is directed toward developing a drug that will be selective in killing cancer cells only.

With antibacterial drugs, the client's immune defense mechanism aids in destroying the bacterially infected cells, whereas the anticancer drugs compromise the immune system and the drug fails to attack only cancer cells.

There are various drug protocols for successful chemotherapy. If the chemotherapy is extended too long or the doses are too high, toxicity is likely to occur. To eliminate every cancer cell can be difficult. When symptoms disappear, it had once been thought that malignant cells were eradicated, but this generally is not true, because 1 million cancer cells could still remain when there are no symptoms. It is still not fully known how long cancer therapy should be continued. With continuous research and protocol drug therapy, an answer is anticipated soon.

Anticancer/antineoplastic drugs are listed according to classification in Table 33–2.

Drug Resistance

Tumor resistance can develop against an anticancer drug because the drug is used too infrequently or the tumor's location limits the effectiveness of the drug. Brain tumors respond poorly to anticancer drugs because most drugs do not cross the blood–brain barrier. Nitrosoureas, however, do cross the blood–brain

barrier. Intraarterial infusion of the drugs at the site may be necessary.

Changes in DNA are a major cause of drug resistance, and mutation of cancer cells is also a factor in drug resistance. As the tumor ages, cancer cells mutate as they multiply; thus, the cancer cells are no longer identical. The mutated cells may differ in response to drug therapy.

Combination Chemotherapy

Single-agent drug therapy is seldom used; instead, combinations of drugs are used to enhance tumoricidal effects. CCS and CCNS drugs are often combined to maximize cell death. Use of combination drugs has the following advantages: (1) decreased drug resistance and, in general shortened and intensified drug therapeutic effect; (2) increased destruction of cancer cells by effectiveness against the various mutated cells; and (3) reduced drug toxicity because of the use of several anticancer drugs at lower doses and with less injury to normal cells.

General Side Effects and Adverse Reactions

Anticancer drugs cause adverse reactions on rapidly growing normal cells, such as those in blood and hair. These drugs can also cause disturbances of the gastrointestinal (GI) tract, mucous membrane, and reproductive system. Table 33–3 lists the general adverse reactions to anticancer drugs on the fast-growing cells of the body. Selected nursing measures and considerations are included.

Anticancer Therapy in the Home

Use of anticancer drug administration in the home has increased and has had success in the past few years. It has been proven cost-effective for providing cancer care in the home and has decreased the need for hospitalization. However, not all anticancer agents can be given in the home because of potency of the drug and the need to closely monitor the client for severe adverse reactions and provide adequate hydration. The anticancer drugs that can be administered at home include fluorouracil, methotrexate, etoposide, vincristine, and the antitumor antibiotics bleomycin, doxorubicin, and plicamycin.

Any health care provider who is qualified to administer anticancer agents follows the policies from the oncologist and the home health care agency. In preparing the client for anticancer therapy and during and following anticancer administration, the health care provider should

Table 33–2
Lists of Anticancer/Antineoplastic Agents According to Classifications

I. **ALKYLATING DRUGS**

A. **Nitrogen mustards**
Chlorambucil (Leukeran)
Cyclophosphamide (Cytoxan)
Estramustine (Emcyt)
Ifosfamide (Iflex)
Mechlorethamine HCl
Melphalan (Alkeran)
Uracil mustard

B. **Nitrosoureas**
Carmustine (BiCNU)
Lomustine (CeeNu)
Semustine
Streptozocin (Zanosar)

C. **Alkylating-like drugs**
Altretamine (Hexalen)
Carboplatin (Paraplatin)
Cisplatin (Platinol)
Decarbazine (DTIC)
Pipobroman (Vercyte)
Triethylenethiophosphoramide (Thiotepa)

D. **Alkyl sulfonates**
Busulfan (Myleran)

II. **ANTIMETABOLITES**

A. **Folic acid antagonist**
Methotrexate (MTX, Amethopterin)

B. **Pyrimidine analogues**
Capecitabine (Xeloda)
Cytarabine HCl (Cytosar-U, ARA-C)
Floxuridine (FUDR)
5-Fluorouracil (5-FU, Adrucil)
Gemcitabine HCl (Gemzar)
Procarbazine HCl (Matulane)

C. **Purine analogues**
Cladribine (Leustatin)
Fludarabine (Fludara)
6-Mercaptopurine (Purinethol)
Thioguanine

D. **Miscellaneous ribonucleotide reductase inhibitor**
Hydroxyurea (Hydrea)
Trimetrexate glucuronate (NeuTrexin)

E. **Antimicrotubule**
Docetaxel (Taxotere)
Paclitaxel (Taxol)

F. **Enzyme inhibitor**
Pentostatin (Nipent)

G. **Topoisomerase I inhibitors**
Etoposide (VePesid, VP-16)
Ironotecan HCl (Camptozar)
Teniposide (Vumon, VM-26)
Topotecan HCl (Hycamtin)

III. **ANTITUMOR ANTIBIOTICS**

Bleomycin sulfate (Blenoxane)
Dactinomycin (Actinomycin)
Daunorubicin HCl (Cerubidine)
Doxorubicin (Adriamycin)
Idarubicin (Idamycin)
Mitomycin (Mutamycin)
Mitoxantrone (Novantrone)
Plicamycin (Mithracin)

IV. **MITOTIC INHIBITORS (VINCA ALKALOIDS)**

Vinblastine sulfate (Velban)
Vincristine sulfate (Oncovin)
Vinorelbine (Navelbine)

V. **HORMONES, HORMONAL ANTAGONISTS, AND ENZYMES**

A. **Androgens**
Testolactone (Teslac)
Progesterone (Gesterol 50)

B. **Enzymes**
L-Asparaginase (Elspar)
Pegaspargase (Oncaspar)

C. **Hormonal antagonists**
Aminoglutethimide (Cytadren)
Flutamide (Eulexin)
Goserelin acetate (Zoladex)
Letrozole (Femara)
Megestrol acetate
Mitotane (Lysodren)
Polyestradiol phosphate (Estradurin)
Tamoxifen citrate (Nolvadex)
Toremifene (Fareston)

• Discuss with the client and family the anticancer drug to be administered, its desired effects, length of time per administration, and signs and symptoms that should be reported.

• Discuss the implanted venous access device that the client may have. Explain how the drug is administered using this device.

• Emphasize the importance of taking adequate fluids.

• Check that the anticancer drug has not infiltrated if it is given intravenously and not through the implanted device. Extravasation from infiltration may cause permanently damaged muscles, nerves, or tendons.

• Record client and family responses and concerns to anticancer therapy. Answer or refer questions to other health professionals.

• Determine that the client has a support system. Discuss the client's needs with family members.

To reduce exposure to the anticancer drugs, the health care provider should use latex gloves. Mask and gown are not needed if the anticancer drug was mixed and prepared by the pharmacist. All used sup-

Table 33–3
General Adverse Reactions to Anticancer Drugs

ADVERSE REACTIONS	NURSING MEASURES AND CONSIDERATIONS
BONE MARROW SUPPRESSION	
Low white blood cell (WBC) count (neutropenia)	Susceptibility to infections is probable with a decreased WBC count. Friends and family with colds or infections should take precautions (i.e., wear mask) or avoid visiting the client. Fever, chills, or sore throat should be reported. Neutrophils are the primary WBCs that fight infections.
Low platelet count (thrombocytopenia)	Petechiae, ecchymoses, bleeding of gums, and nosebleeds are signs of a low platelet count and should be reported.
GASTROINTESTINAL DISTURBANCES	
Anorexia	Loss of appetite may be due to the bitter taste in the mouth from drugs or the nausea caused by drugs.
Nausea and vomiting	Antineoplastic drugs stimulate the vomiting centers. Antiemetics are given several hours before the chemotherapy and for 12–48 h after the treatment.
Diarrhea	Hydration should be maintained. Hot foods (increase peristalsis) and high-fiber foods should be avoided.
OTHER	
Stomatitis	Good mouth care is necessary to minimize mouth ulcers. Saline or sodium bicarbonate mouth rinses may be used. If superinfection occurs, an antifungal medication may be used.
Alopecia	Varying degrees of hair loss occur after the first or second treatment. A wig should be purchased before treatment starts. After final treatment, some hair growth is apparent in several months.
Infertility	If infertility occurs, it could be irreversible. Pretreatment counseling is advised.

plies should be double bagged and returned to the agency for proper disposal. Refer to the agency policy for disposal of used equipment.

ALKYLATING DRUGS

One of the largest groups of anticancer drugs are the alkylating compounds. Alkylating drugs kill cells by forming cross-links on the DNA strands. Drugs in this group belong to the CCNS category and affect all phases of the cell cycle. Thus, they are effective against many types of cancer: acute and chronic leukemias, lymphomas, multiple myeloma, and solid tumors (in the breast, ovaries, uterus, lungs, bladder, and stomach). Drugs in this category are classified into four groups: (1) nitrogen mustards (mechlorethamine, cyclophosphamide, chlorambucil, ifosfamide, and melphalan), (2) nitrosoureas (lomustine, carmustine, semustine, streptozocin), (3) alkyl sulfonate (busulfan), and (4) alkylating-like drugs (cisplatin, carboplatin). Adverse reactions to these drugs are the same as those listed in Table 33–3.

Cyclophosphamide

Nitrogen mustard was the first alkylating drug that became available for clinical use during World War II. It is marketed as mechlorethamine and is used to treat Hodgkin's disease and solid tumors. An analogue of nitrogen mustard commonly prescribed orally and intravenously is cyclophosphamide (Cytoxan). The client should be well hydrated while taking this drug in order to prevent hemorrhagic cystitis (bleeding that results from severe bladder inflammation). Bone marrow suppression and alopecia are common side effects. Chart 33–1 details the pharmacologic behavior of cyclophosphamide.

PHARMACOKINETICS

Cyclophosphamide (Cytoxan) is well absorbed from the GI tract. Its half-life is moderate and it is moderately protein-bound. The drug is metabolized by the liver, and less than 50% is excreted unchanged in the urine.

Chart 33–1.   Antineoplastic: Alkylating Drug

ALKYLATING DRUG

Drug Name

Cyclophosphamide (Cytoxan), 🍁 Procytox
Pregnancy Category: D

Dosage

A: PO: Initially: 1–5 mg/kg over 2–5 d; maint:
1–5 mg/kg/d
IV: Initially: 40–50 mg/kg in divided doses
over 2–5 d
C: PO/IV: Initially: 2–5 mg/kg in divided doses
for 6 d; maint: 10–15 mg/kg every 7–10 d
If bone marrow depression occurs, dosage adjustment is necessary

Contraindications

Hypersensitivity, severe bone marrow
depression
Caution: Pregnancy, liver or kidney disease

Drug-Lab-Food Interactions

Drug: Thiazides, anticoagulants, digoxin, phenobarbital, rifampin
Lab: Uric acid, Pap test, purified protein derivative (PPD), mumps, candida

Pharmacokinetics

Absorption: PO: Well absorbed
Distribution: PB: 50%
Metabolism: $t_{\frac{1}{2}}$: 3–12 h
Excretion: 25%–40% in urine unchanged;
5%–20% in feces

Pharmacodynamics

Effects on blood count:
PO/IV: Onset: 7 d
Peak: 10–14 d
Duration: 21 d

Therapeutic Effects/Uses

To treat breast, lung, ovarian cancers; Hodgkin's disease; leukemias; and lymphomas; an immunosuppressant agent.

Mode of Action: Inhibition of protein synthesis through interference with DNA replication by alkylation of DNA.

Side Effects

Nausea, vomiting, diarrhea, weight loss, hematuria, alopecia, impotence, sterility, ovarian fibrosis, headache, dizziness, dermatitis

Adverse Reactions

Hemorrhagic cystitis, secondary neoplasm
Life-threatening: Leukopenia, thrombocytopenia, cardiotoxicity (very high doses), hepatotoxicity (long term)

Assessment and Planning
Interventions
Evaluation
NURSING PROCESS

KEY: A: adult; C: child; PO: by mouth; IV: intravenous; PB: protein-binding; $t_{\frac{1}{2}}$: half-life; Pap: Papanicolaou; 🍁: Canadian drug name.

PHARMACODYNAMICS

Cyclophosphamide is an early anticancer drug and is frequently used as one of the drugs for the anticancer protocols. The onset of action begins within hours; however, the desired effect may take several days. It is one of the anticancer drugs that can be administered orally.

Several drug interactions may occur with cyclophosphamide: thiazides and allopurinol can increase bone marrow depression, the effect of digoxin decreases, and the effect of insulin increases, causing hypoglycemia. Phenobarbital and rifampin may increase cyclophosphamide toxicity. Adverse reactions should be observed and reported.

Table 33–4 lists the alkylating drugs, their dosages, uses, and considerations.

Table 33–4
Antineoplastics: Alkylating Drugs

GENERIC (BRAND)	ROUTE AND DOSAGE*	USES AND CONSIDERATIONS
NITROGEN MUSTARDS		
Chlorambucil (Leukeran)	A: PO: 0.1–0.2 mg/kg/d	For treating lymphocytic leukemia, lymphomas, and cancer of the breast and ovaries. Side effects include nausea, vomiting, anorexia, diarrhea, abdominal upset, and leukopenia. *Pregnancy category:* D; PB: 99%; $t_{\frac{1}{2}}$: 1.5 h
Cyclophosphamide (Cytoxan)	See Chart 33–1	For treating lymphocytic leukemia, Hodgkin's disease, certain solid tumors. One of the major drugs for combination drug therapy. Fluids should be forced to prevent hemorrhagic cystitis. Orally, it is taken without food or with meals. *Pregnancy category:* D; PB: 50%; $t_{\frac{1}{2}}$: 3–12 h
Estramustine phosphate sodium (Emcyt)	*Palliation prostate cancer:* A: PO: 10–16 mg/kg/d in 3–4 divided doses for 28–90 d; determine if response occurred	For treatment of progressive carcinoma of prostate. Consists of estrogen and nitrogen mustard. Common side effects: nausea, peripheral edema, thrombophlebitis, breast tenderness. *Pregnancy category:* C; PB: UK; $t_{\frac{1}{2}}$: 20 h
Ifosfamide (Iflex)	A: IV: 1–2 g/m²/d for 5 d q21–28 d C: IV: 1800 mg/m²/d for 3–5 d q21–28 d	For treating testicular cancer, lymphoma, lung cancer, and sarcomas. Mesna, a uroprotective agent, is added to prevent hemorrhagic cystitis. *Pregnancy category:* D; PB: UK; $t_{\frac{1}{2}}$: 12–15 h (high dose)
Mechlorethamine HCl (Mustargen)	A: IV: 0.4 mg/kg/dose or 6–10 mg/m² as single dose or in divided doses	For treating Hodgkin's disease, solid tumors, and pleural effusion due to cancer of the lung. Similar side effects as chlorambucil. *Pregnancy category:* D; PB: UK; $t_{\frac{1}{2}}$: <1 min
Melphalan (Alkeran)	A: PO: 6 mg/d	For treating multiple myeloma, melanoma, and cancer of the breast, ovary, and testes. *Pregnancy category:* D; PB: <30%; $t_{\frac{1}{2}}$: 1.5 h
Uracil mustard	*Palliation chronic lymphocytic leukemia, non-Hodgkin's lymphoma:* A: PO: 0.15 mg/kg/wk for 4 wk C: PO: 0.30 mg/kg/wk for 4 wk	For chronic lymphocytic and myelocytic leukemia; non-Hodgkin's disease of the cervix, ovary, and lung. GI distress may occur. *Pregnancy category:* X; PB: UK; $t_{\frac{1}{2}}$: UK
NITROSOUREAS		
Carmustine (BiCNU)	A: IV: 75–100 mg/m²/d for 2 d or 200 mg/m² q6 wk as single dose or divided into 2 doses on successive days; next course is dependent on blood count	For treating Hodgkin's disease, multiple myeloma, melanoma, and central nervous system (CNS) tumors, such as brain tumors. May be used for cancer of the breast and lung. Nausea, vomiting, and stomatitis may occur. *Pregnancy category:* D; PB: UK; $t_{\frac{1}{2}}$: 15–30 min
Lomustine (CeeNu)	A: PO: 130 mg/m²/d as single dose	For treating advanced Hodgkin's disease and CNS tumors. *Pregnancy category:* D; PB: 50%; $t_{\frac{1}{2}}$: 1–2 d
Streptozocin (Zanosar)	A: IV: 500 mg/m²/d for 5 d or 1 g/m² wk	For treating pancreatic islet cell tumor and cancer of the lung. May also be used for Hodgkin's disease, colorectal cancer. Nausea, vomiting, diarrhea, and leukopenia may occur. *Pregnancy category:* C; PB: UK; $t_{\frac{1}{2}}$: 30–45 min
ALKYL SULFONATES		
Busulfan (Myleran)	A: PO: 4–8 mg/d; *max:* 12 mg/d C: PO: 0.06–0.12 mg/kg/d	For treating myelocytic leukemia. WBC should be closely monitored. May be used as preparation agent in bone marrow transplant. *Pregnancy category:* D; PB: UK; $t_{\frac{1}{2}}$: UK
ALKYLATING-LIKE DRUGS		
Altretamine (Hexalen)	A: PO: 4–12 mg/kg/d in 3–4 divided doses for 28–90 d	Primarily for ovarian cancer. Also used for breast, cervix, colon, endometrium, head/neck, and lung cancers; lymphomas. Nausea and vomiting and peripheral neuropathy may occur. *Pregnancy category:* D; PB: 6%; $t_{\frac{1}{2}}$: 13 h

Table continued on following page

Table 33–4 *Continued*
Antineoplastics: Alkylating Drugs

GENERIC (BRAND)	ROUTE AND DOSAGE*	USES AND CONSIDERATIONS
Carboplatin (Paraplatin)	A: IV: 360 mg/m² q4wk *Solid tumors:* C: 560 mg/m² once every 4 wk *Brain tumor:* C: 175 mg/m² once weekly for 4 wk	For treatment of recurrent ovarian cancer. May be used as preparation agent in bone marrow transplant. *Pregnancy category:* D; PB: 0%; t½: 2–6 h
Cisplatin (Platinol)	A: IV: 20 mg/m²/d for 5 d; then 50–70 mg/m² q3wk or 100 mg/m² q4wk	For treating ovarian and testicular cancer. Used as adjunctive treatment. Has been used for cancer of the bladder, head and neck, and endometrium. Nausea, vomiting, peripheral neuropathy, stomatitis, tinnitus, and blurred vision may occur. Ototoxicity occurs in 30% of clients. *Pregnancy category:* D; PB: >90%; t½: 58–75 h
Dacarbazine (DTIC)	*Hodgkin's disease:* A: IV: 150 mg/m² daily for 5 d; repeat course q28d or 375 mg/m² on day 1 of combination therapy: repeat course q15d *Metastatic malignant melanoma:* A: IV: 2–4.5 mg/kg daily for 10 d; repeat q28d	For metastatic malignant melanoma, sarcomas, neuroblastoma, and refractory Hodgkin's disease. May be given as an IV bolus (push) injection or by infusion. Common side effects are anorexia, nausea, and vomiting. *Pregnancy category:* C; PB: 5%–10%; t½: 5 h
Pipobroman (Vercyte)	*Chronic myelocytic leukemia:* A: PO: Initially: 1.5–2.5 mg/kg/d for 30 d; maint: 10–175 mg/d	Treatment for polycythemia and chronic myelocytic leukemia. *Pregnancy category:* D; PB: UK; t½: UK
Triethylenethiophosphoramide (thiotepa)	A: IV: 0.2 mg/kg/d for 4–5 d; then 0.3–0.4 mg/kg at 2 to 4 wk intervals	For palliation of neoplastic diseases, especially breast and ovary. *Pregnancy category:* D; PB: UK; t½: 1.5–2 h

KEY: A: adult; C: child; PO: by mouth; m²: body surface area; IV: intravenous; PB: protein-binding; t½: half-life; UK: unknown.
*For full discussion of body surface area in dosage calculation, see Chapter 4.

ANTIMETABOLITES

Antimetabolites are the oldest group of anticancer drugs, except for the original nitrogen mustard. Many of the antimetabolite drugs resemble natural metabolites; thus, they disrupt the metabolic processes and some of the agents inhibit enzyme synthesis. They are classified as cell-cycle specific and affect the S phase (DNA synthesis and metabolism). 5-Fluorouracil and floxuridine could be classified as CCNS as well as CCS. This group is subdivided into folic acid (folate) antagonists (methotrexate), pyrimidine analogues (5-fluorouracil, floxuridine, and cytarabine), and purine analogues (6-mercaptopurine and thioguanine). Other miscellaneous groups of anticancer drugs include ribonucleotide reductase inhibitor, antimicrotubule, enzyme inhibitor, and podophyllotoxin derivative.

Methotrexate was discovered in 1948 and is used for noncancer conditions, such as immunosuppression following organ transplant. Methotrexate, a folic acid antagonist, acts by substituting for folic acid, which is needed for the synthesis of proteins and DNA. Since its discovery in 1957, 5-fluorouracil (abbreviated as 5-FU) is commonly used as a single drug or in combination to cure or alleviate the symptoms of cancer.

The types of cancer that respond to antimetabolites are lymphomas, acute leukemias, cancer within the gastrointestinal tract, and breast cancer. Chart 33–2 presents the pharmacologic data of fluorouracil.

Fluorouracil

PHARMACOKINETICS

Fluorouracil is administered intravenously for carcinoma and topically for superficial basal cell carci-

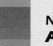

NURSING PROCESS
ALKYLATING DRUGS: CYCLOPHOSPHAMIDE

Assessment

- Assess complete blood count (CBC), differential, and platelet count weekly. Withhold drug if platelets <75,000 cells/mm³ or white blood cell (WBC) count <4000 cells/mm³; notify health care provider.
- Assess results of pulmonary function tests, chest x-rays, and renal and liver function studies during therapy.
- Assess temperature; fever may be early sign of infection.

Potential Nursing Diagnoses

- Risk for infection
- Body image disturbance

Planning

- Client will experience improved blood count status indicative of improvement/remission of the specific cancer growth.

Nursing Interventions

- Hydrate client with IV and/or oral fluids before chemotherapy starts.
- Administer antacid before oral drug.
- Administer antiemetic 30 to 60 min before giving drug.
- Monitor IV site frequently for irritation and phlebitis.
- Increase fluids to 2 to 3 L/d to reduce risk of hemorrhagic cystitis, urate deposition, or calculus formation.
- Store drug in airtight container at room temperature.

Client Teaching

General

- Advise women who are contemplating pregnancy while taking antineoplastics to first seek medical advice. There may be teratogenic effects to the fetus. Pregnancy should be

Nursing Process continued on following page

noma. Protein-binding is less than 10%, and the half-life for the intravenous route is short (10 to 20 min). A small amount of the drug is excreted in the urine and up to 80% is excreted by lungs as carbon dioxide (CO_2).

PHARMACODYNAMICS

Fluorouracil, a CCS drug, blocks the enzyme action necessary for DNA and RNA synthesis. The drug has a low therapeutic index. Fluorouracil can be used alone or in combination with other anticancer drugs.

Fluorouracil can cross the blood–brain barrier. The duration of action is 30 d.

SIDE EFFECTS AND ADVERSE REACTIONS

Side effects for fluorouracil are similar to other anticancer drugs, which include anorexia, nausea, vomiting, diarrhea, stomatitis, alopecia, photosensitivity, in-

creased pigmentation, rash, and erythema. Adverse reactions may occur 4 to 8 days after the beginning of drug therapy. These include hematologic toxic effects such as leukopenia, thrombocytopenia, and agranulocytosis.

The general side effects for antimetabolite drugs include bone marrow suppression (leukopenia, thrombocytopenia), **stomatitis** (inflammation of the oral [mouth] mucosa), and alopecia. Table 33–5 lists the antimetabolite drugs, their dosages, uses, and considerations.

ANTITUMOR ANTIBIOTICS

Antitumor antibiotics (bleomycin, dactinomycin, daunorubicin, doxorubicin, mitomycin, and plicamycin) inhibit protein and RNA synthesis and bind DNA,

avoided for 3 to 4 mo after completing antineoplastic therapy in most situations. Some sources recommend that both men and women avoid conception for 2 y after completing treatment.
• Remind client to consult health care provider before administration of any vaccination.

Diet
• Advise client to follow diet low in purines (organ meats, beans, and peas) to alkalize urine.
• Advise client to avoid citric acid.

Side Effects
• Instruct client about good oral hygiene with soft toothbrush for stomatitis; do not use toothbrush when platelet count is < 50,000 cells/mm³.
• Emphasize protective isolation precautions. Advise the client not to visit anyone with any type of respiratory infection. A decreased WBC count puts the client at high risk for acquiring an infection.
• Instruct client to report promptly signs of infection (fever, sore throat), bleeding (bleeding gums, petechiae, bruises, hematuria, blood in the stool), and anemia (increased fatigue, dyspnea, orthostatic hypotension).
• Remind female client that she may experience amenorrhea, menstrual irregularities, or sterility and remind male client that he may experience impotence.
• Advise client of possible hair loss; recommend considerations of wig or hairpiece.

Cultural Considerations

• In some cultural groups, cancer is not discussed and, in other groups, cancer is thought to be due to misdeeds of the client. Sometimes, people do not want to be close to the person with cancer for fear that they may "catch it." The health care provider should discuss facts concerning cancer with the client and family to alleviate fear and misunderstanding and to promote compliance with the planned anticancer therapy.
• The health care provider should encourage family members and friends to be part of the support system needed by the client.

Evaluation
• Client will be free of cancer as indicated by improved blood counts and free of side effects of drug.

causing fragmentation. Except for bleomycin, which has its major effect on the G_2 phase, they are classified as CCNS drugs. Dactinomycin was the first antibiotic used in the treatment of tumors in animals in the early 1940s. Bleomycin and plicamycin were introduced in 1962. These antitumor antibiotics differ from one another and are used for various cancers.

Chart 33–3 compares the similarities of and differences between doxorubicin and plicamycin.

Pharmacokinetics

Doxorubicin and plicamycin are administered intravenously. Doxorubicin is metabolized in the liver to active and inactive metabolites. The various metabolites affect the half-life, with the initial phase being 12 min, the intermediate phase 3.5 h, and the final phase 30 h.

Pharmacodynamics

The primary effects of doxorubicin and plicamycin differ although they are classified as antitumor antibiotics. Doxorubicin is prescribed in combination with other anticancer agents for treatment of cancer of the breast, ovaries, lung, and bladder, and for leukemias and lymphomas. Plicamycin may be used in combination with other anticancer agents for the treatment of testicular carcinoma. Its primary use is for correction of hypercalcemia.

Because plicamycin affects bleeding time, use of aspirin, anticoagulants, and thrombolytic agents should be avoided. The use of cyclophosphamide with doxorubicin can increase the chance of occurrence of hemorrhagic cystitis.

Table 33–6 lists the antitumor antibiotics, their dosages, uses, and considerations.

Chart 33-2. Antineoplastic: Antimetabolite

ANTIMETABOLITE

Drug Name

Fluorouracil (Adrucil, 5-FU, Efudex)
Pregnancy Category: D

Dosage

A: IV: 12 mg/kg/d × 4 d; *max:* 800 mg/d;
repeat with 6 mg/kg on day 6, 8, 10, and 12
Maint: 10–15 mg/kg/wk as single dose; *max:*
1 g/wk
Topical: 1%–2% sol/cream b.i.d. to head/neck
lesions; 5% to other body areas
Refer to specific protocol.

Contraindications

Hypersensitivity, pregnancy, severe infection,
myelosuppression, marginal nutritional status

Drug-Lab-Food Interactions

Drug: Bone marrow depressants, live virus vaccines, cimetidine, calcium
Lab: Liver function studies, albumin, AST, ALT

Pharmacokinetics

Absorption: IV and topical: 5%–10%
Distribution: PB: UK
Metabolism: t½: 10–20 min
Excretion: In urine and expired carbon dioxide

Pharmacodynamics

Effects on blood count:
IV: Onset: 1–9 d
          Peak: 9–21 d
          Duration: 30 d
Topical: Onset: 2–3 d
          Peak: 2–6 wk
          Duration: 4–8 wk

Therapeutic Effects/Uses

To treat cancer of breast, cervix, colon, liver, ovary, pancreas, stomach, and rectum. In combination
with levamisole after surgical resection in clients with Duke's Stage C colon cancer.

Mode of Action: Prevention of thymidine production, thereby inhibiting DNA and RNA synthesis.
Not phase specific.

Side Effects

Nausea, vomiting, diarrhea, stomatitis, alopecia,
rash

Adverse Reactions

Anemia
Life-threatening: Thrombocytopenia, myelosuppression, hemorrhage, renal failure

KEY: A: adult; IV: intravenous; UK: unknown; PB: protein-binding; t½: half-life, ALT: alanine aminotransferase; AST: aspartate aminotransferase.

Side Effects and Adverse Reactions

The adverse reactions to the antitumor antibiotics are
similar to the general adverse reactions to antineoplastics, which include alopecia, nausea, vomiting,
stomatitis, leukopenia, and thrombocytopenia. Most
antitumor antibiotics, except bleomycin and plicamycin, are capable of causing **vesication** (blistering of
tissue). Some antitumor antibiotics can cause organ
toxicities: bleomycin causes pulmonary toxicity, and
daunorubicin, doxorubicin, and idarubicin cause cardiac toxicity.

MITOTIC INHIBITORS (VINCA ALKALOIDS)

Mitotic inhibitors, also known as vinca alkaloids or
plant alkaloids, block cell division at the M phase of
the cell cycle. Vincristine, vinblastine, and vinorelbine
tartrate are examples of mitotic inhibitors and are
classified as cell-cycle specific.

These drugs can be used as single drugs or in
combination drug therapy. Adverse reactions include
leukopenia, partial to complete alopecia, stomatitis,

Table 33–5
Antineoplastics: Antimetabolites

GENERIC (BRAND)	ROUTE AND DOSAGE*	USES AND CONSIDERATIONS
FOLIC ACID ANTAGONIST		
Methotrexate (Amethopterin, MTX)	A: PO/IM: Induction: 3.3 mg/m^2/d for 4–6 wk; maint: 30 mg/m^2/wk in divided doses (2 × wk) C: Pediatric dosing varies with protocol and indication	For treating solid tumors, sarcomas, choriocarcinoma, leukemia. At higher doses, clients should be hydrated and keep urine pH 7.0 for drug solubility for excretion. Higher doses require use of Leucovorin as a rescue for normal cells. *Pregnancy category:* D; PB: 50%; t½: 8–16 h
PYRIMIDINE ANALOGUES		
Capecitabine (Xeloda)	A: PO: UK Available: 150-mg and 500-mg tablet	New oral antimetabolite drug for advanced metastatic breast cancer. Effective when cancer is resistant to paclitaxel. Reduces tumor size. Food decreases absorption rate. *Pregnancy category:* UK; PB: UK; t½: UK
Cytarabine HCl (Cytosar-U, ARA-C)	A: IV: 100–200 mg/m^2/d or 3 mg/kg/d as continuous 12- or 24-h infusion	For treating acute leukemias and lymphomas. Also used as an immunosuppressive drug after organ transplant. May be used in combination with other anticancer drugs. Nausea, vomiting, leukopenia, and thrombocytopenia are common side effects. *Pregnancy category:* D; PB: 15% t½: 1–3 h
Floxuridine (FUDR)	A: Intraarterial: 0.1–0.6 mg/kg/d for 14 d IV: 0.5–1 mg/kg/d for 7–15 d	For treating metastatic colon cancer and hepatomas. *Pregnancy category:* D; PB: UK; t½: 20 h
5-Fluorouracil (Adrucil, 5-FU)	See Chart 33–2	For treating solid tumors in the breast, bladder, ovaries, cervix, and gastrointestinal (GI) tract. White blood cell (WBC) count should be monitored. Can be administered by IV push or in continuous IV fluids. Common side effects are anorexia, nausea, vomiting, diarrhea, stomatitis. *Pregnancy category:* D; PB: <10%; t½: 10–20 min
Gemcitabine HCl (Gemzar)	A: IV: 1000 µg/m^2 once a week for 7 wk Dose may be increased to 1250 µg/m^2/wk or 1500 µg/m^2/wk	To treat advanced or metastatic adenocarcinoma of the pancreas. Acts at the S phase of cell cycle. To monitor leukocytes and platelet count; reduce dose if these values are extremely low. *Pregnancy category:* D; PB: UK; t½: 40–95 min
Procarbazine HCl (Matulane)	A: PO: Initially: 2–4 mg/kg/d in divided doses for 7 d; then increase to 4–6 mg/kg/d until desired leukocyte/platelet counts	Palliative treatment of advanced Hodgkin's disease and for solid tumor. May be used with other anticancer drugs. *Pregnancy category:* D; PB: UK; t½: 10 min
PURINE ANALOGUES		
Cladribine (Leustatin)	*Hairy cell leukemia:* A: IV: 0.09–0.1 mg/kg/d continuous infusion for 7 d	For treatment of hairy cell leukemia and chronic lymphocytic leukemia. Adverse reactions: bone marrow suppression, fever, nausea, vomiting, diaphoresis. *Pregnancy category:* D; PB: 20%; t½: 5.4 h
Fludarabine (Fludara)	*Chronic lymphocytic leukemia; acute leukemia:* A: IV: 25 mg/m^2/d for 5 consecutive d/q28d	For treatment of chronic lymphocytic leukemia in clients who have not responded to other alkylating drugs; low-grade non-Hodgkin's lymphoma. Anorexia, nausea, diarrhea, fever, and peripheral edema may occur. *Pregnancy category:* D; PB: UK; t½: 9 h
6-Mercaptopurine (Purinethol)	A&C: PO: 1.5–2.5 mg/kg/d; max: 5 mg/kg/d	First used in 1952 for treating acute lymphatic leukemia. Also used as an immunosuppressive drug. Adverse reactions may include hepatoxicity, bone marrow depression, hyperuricemia. *Pregnancy category:* D; PB: 19%; t½: 45 min

Table continued on following page

Table 33–5 *Continued*

Antineoplastics: Antimetabolites

GENERIC (BRAND)	ROUTE AND DOSAGE*	USES AND CONSIDERATIONS
Thioguanine	A&C: PO: 2–3 mg/kg/d	For treating acute and chronic myelogenous leukemia. Long duration of action. *Pregnancy category:* D; PB: UK; t½: 2–11 h
RIBONUCLEOTIDE REDUCTASE INHIBITOR		
Hydroxyurea (Hydrea)	*Palliation:* A: PO: 20–30 mg/kg/d or 80 mg/kg q3d C: No dosage regimens established	For treating melanoma, resistant chronic myelocytic leukemia, and ovarian cancer. Has a long duration of action. *Pregnancy category:* D; PB: UK; t½: 3–4 h
Trimetrexate glucuronate (NeuTrexin)	A: IV: 45 mg/m²/d by infusion over 1–1.5 h with Leucovorin 20 mg/m², q6h (PO or IV)	Alternative drug therapy for *Pneumocystis carinii* pneumonia; treatment for clients with AIDS. May be used for colorectal cancer. CBC should be monitored. *Pregnancy category:* D; PB: 86%–94%; t½: 11–13 h
ANTIMICROTUBULE		
Docetaxel (Taxotere)	A: IV infusion: 60–100 mg/m² over 1 h, q3wk; suggest: dexamethasone 8 mg b.i.d. × 5 d to begin 1 d before treatment.	To treat advanced or metastatic breast cancer. It inhibits mitosis in the cells. Has a greater antitumor activity with lower toxicity effect than paclitaxel (Taxol). Monitor WBC and platelet count; if low, dose may need to be decreased. *Pregnancy category:* D; PB: UK; t½: 11.1 h
Paclitaxel (Taxol)	*Ovarian cancer:* A: IV: 135 mg/m² for 24 h q3wk; shortened infusions approved for refractory breast cancer	For treating metastatic ovarian and breast cancer. Monitor vital signs and electrocardiogram. Has a long duration of action (3 wk). Peak action is 11 d. *Pregnancy category:* D; PB: 80%–90%; t½: 5–17 h
ENZYME INHIBITOR		
Pentostatin (Nipent)	*Hairy cell leukemia:* A: IV: 4 mg/m² every other wk	For treating hairy cell leukemia refractory to alpha-interferon. Causes DNA death. Has a very long duration of action. *Pregnancy category:* D; PB: UK; t½: 6 h
TOPOISOMERASE I INHIBITORS		
Etoposide (VePesid, VP-16)	A: IV: 50–100 mg/m²/d on days 1–5, q3–4 wk for 3–4 treatment therapy	For treating refractory testicular tumors, small cell lung carcinoma, Hodgkin's and non-Hodgkin's lymphomas, and acute myelogenous leukemia. Has standard chemotherapy side effects. Has a long duration of action. *Pregnancy category:* D; PB: 97%; t½: 4–11 h
Irinotecan HCl (Camptozar)	A: IV: 50–150 mg/m² once a week for 4 wk; then a rest for 2 wk	For advanced and metastatic carcinoma of the colon and rectum. Inhibits the topoisomerase enzyme that is needed for DNA and RNA synthesis. Increased fluid intake is necessary. Monitor WBC count. *Pregnancy category:* D; PB: UK; t½: 6–10 h
Teniposide (Vumon, VM-26)	*Leukemia:* C: IV: over ≥30–60 min: 165 mg/m² and cytarabine 300 mg/m² 2 × wk for 8–9 doses	For treating acute lymphoblastic leukemia (ALL) in children. Used in combination with other anticancer drugs. Severe adverse reactions include bone marrow depression and anaphylaxis. *Pregnancy category:* D; PB: 99%; t½: 5 h
Topotecan HCl (Hycamtin)	A: IV: 1.5 mg/m² over 30 min/d × 5 d (21-day course); decrease dose to 0.25 mg/m² if toxicity occurs	For advanced and metastatic carcinoma of ovary. Used when other anticancer therapy fails. It inhibits topoisomerase I enzyme required for DNA replication. Monitor WBCs. *Pregnancy category:* D; PB: 35%; t½: 2–3 h

KEY: *A: adult; C: child; PO: by mouth; IV: intravenous; >: greater than; <: less than; PB: protein-binding; t½: half-life; m²: square meter of body surface area; UK: unknown; AIDS: acquired immunodeficiency syndrome.*
For full discussion of body surface area in dosage calculation, see Chapter 4.

NURSING PROCESS
ANTIMETABOLITES: FLUOROURACIL

Assessment

- Assess the client's vital signs (VS) and use for future comparison.
- Assess CBC and platelet count weekly. Notify health care provider and withhold drug if WBC count is <3500/mm³ or platelet count is <100,000 cells/mm³.
- Assess renal function studies before and during drug therapy.
- Assess temperature every 4 to 6 h; fever may be early sign of infection.

Potential Nursing Diagnoses

- Risk for infection
- Altered nutrition; less than body requirements
- Body image disturbance

Planning

- Client will have blood tests with values in the desired range.
- Client will be free of adverse reactions to drug therapy.
- Client's neoplasm will decrease in size.

Nursing Interventions

- Handle drug with care during preparation; avoid direct skin contact with anticancer drugs. Follow protocols. Solution is colorless to light yellow.
- Administer IV dose over 1 to 2 min. Apply firm prolonged pressure to injection site if thrombocytopenia is present.
- Monitor IV site frequently. Extravasation produces severe pain. If this occurs, apply ice pack and notify health care provider.
- Administer antiemetic 30 to 60 min before drug to prevent vomiting.
- Offer the client food and fluids that may decrease nausea, such as cola, crackers, or ginger ale.
- Administer antibiotics prophylactically for infection, analgesics for pain, and antispasmodics for diarrhea, as ordered.
- Maintain strict medical asepsis.
- Encourage fluid intake of 2 to 3 L/d, unless contraindicated, to prevent dehydration.
- Support good oral hygiene; brush teeth with soft toothbrush and use waxed dental floss.
- Monitor fluid intake and output and nutritional intake. GI effects are common on the fourth day of treatment.

Client Teaching

General
- Emphasize protective precautions, as necessary.
- Teach the client to examine mouth daily and report stomatitis (ulceration in mouth). Good oral hygiene several times a day is essential. If stomatitis occurs, rinse mouth with baking soda or saline. Do not use a toothbrush when the platelet count is <50,000/mm³.
- Advise women who are contemplating pregnancy while taking antineoplastics to first seek medical advice. Teratogenic effects to the fetus can occur from antineoplastics. Pregnancy should be avoided for 3 to 4 mo after completing antineoplastic therapy in most situations. Some sources recommend that both men and women avoid conception for 2 y after completion of treatment.
- Advise the client not to visit anyone with any type of respiratory infection. A decreased WBC count puts the client at high risk for acquiring an infection.

Side Effects
- Advise the client to promptly report signs of bleeding, anemia, and infection to the health care provider.

Nursing Process continued on following page

nausea, vomiting, and neurotoxicity with vincristine and occasionally with vinblastine. Signs and symptoms of neurotoxicity might include decrease in muscular strength (numbness, tingling of fingers and toes), constipation, ptosis (drooping of the upper eyelid), hoarseness, and motor instability. Table 33–6 lists the vinca alkaloids, their dosages, uses, and considerations.

HORMONES AND HORMONE ANTAGONISTS

Hormones (steroids) are used in combination therapy for treating various cancers. The anticancer hormones have two major actions: (1) as agonists that inhibit tumor cell growth, and (2) as antagonists that compete with endogenous hormone. Examples of agonists are estrogen, progestins, androgens, and adrenocorticosteroids. Examples of antagonists are aminoglutethimide, flutamide, goserelin acetate, and tamoxifen. Table 33–7 lists the hormones, hormone antagonists, and miscellaneous anticancer drugs.

Groups of hormones are the corticosteroids (cortisone), estrogens, progestins, and androgens. **Corticosteroids** (glucocorticoids) are classified as antiinflammatory agents, suppressing the inflammatory process that occurs with tissue involvement. This hormone also suppresses leukocytes and is effective in controlling leukemia and lymphoma. It is used in conjunction with other drugs as part of an antineoplastic regimen, an example of which is the MOPP regimen (mechlorethamine, Oncovin [vincristine], procarbazine, and prednisone), which is used for Hodgkin's disease. Prednisone is a frequently prescribed, inexpensive cortisone derivative. Dexamethasone and hydrocortisone can be administered intramuscularly and intravenously. These drugs can decrease cerebral edema caused by a brain tumor (neoplasm). Cortisone drugs give the client a sense of well-being and varying degrees of euphoria.

Cortisone derivatives that are taken internally produce many side effects, such as fluid retention, potassium loss, a risk of infection, increase in blood sugar, increase in fat distribution, muscle weakness, increased bleeding tendency, and euphoria.

Estrogen therapy is a palliative treatment used in men to decrease the progression of prostatic cancer and in postmenopausal women to decrease the progression of breast cancer. Estrogen preparations suppress tumor growth, and the drug promotes remission of the cancer for 6 months to a year. Examples of this group of drugs are diethylstilbestrol (Estrobene), ethinyl estradiol (Estinyl), chlorotrianisene (Tace), and conjugated estrogens (Premarin).

Two **antiestrogens** used to treat advanced breast cancer are tamoxifen citrate (Nolvadex) and an investigative agent, nafoxidine, which act by suppressing the growth of estrogen-dependent tumors.

Progestins are prescribed for breast cancer, endometrial carcinoma, and renal cancer. These drugs—hydroxyprogesterone caproate (Duralutin), medroxyprogesterone acetate (Depo-Provera), and megestrol acetate (Megace)—act by shrinking the cancer tissues. Adverse reactions include fluid retention and thrombotic (clot) disorders.

Androgens are given to treat advanced breast cancer in premenopausal women. This male hormone promotes regression of the tumor. If androgen therapy is used for a long time, masculine secondary sexual characteristics, such as body hair growth, lowering of the voice, and muscle growth, will occur. Flutamide (Eulexin) and leuprolide acetate (Lupron) are two other androgens used in the treatment of advanced prostatic cancer.

MISCELLANEOUS ANTINEOPLASTICS

There are a number of antineoplastic drugs whose mechanism of action or chemical configuration does not allow them to be categorized as an alkylator, antimetabolite, antitumor antibiotic, vinca alkaloid, or hormone. These agents include paclitaxel (Taxol), docetaxel (Taxotere) pentostatin (Nipent), etoposide (VP-

Text continued on page 596

Chart 33–3. Antitumor Antibiotics

NURSING PROCESS

Assessment and Planning

Drug Name

Doxorubicin (Adriamycin): (D)
Pregnancy Category: D
Plicamycin (Mithracin): (P)

Pregnancy Category: X

Dosage

(D): Solid tumors:
A: IV: 60–75 mg/m²; repeat q21d, OR 25–30 mg/m²/d for 2–3 successive d, q4wk
(P) Testicular tumor:
A: IV: 25–30 μg/kg/d for 8–10 d Hypercalcemia:
A: IV: 15–25 μg/kg/d for 3–4 d
Reduce dose with renal impairment

Contraindications

(D) Pregnancy, severe cardiac disease
Caution: Hepatic and renal impairment
(P) Hypocalcemia, bleeding disorders, myelosuppression
Caution: Hepatic and renal impairment

Drug-Lab-Food Interactions

(D)
Drug: *Increase* hypercalcemia with vitamin D; *increase* cardiotoxicity with daunorubicin
Lab: ECG changes, *increase* uric acid
(P)
Drug: *Increase* hemorrhaging with aspirin, NSAIDs, anticoagulants, thrombolytic drugs, dipyridamole, sulfinpyrazone, valproic acid; *increase* serum calcium level with calcium drugs and vitamin D
Lab: *Decrease* calcium and phosphorus; *increase* BUN and creatinine, ALP

Interventions

Pharmacodynamics

Absorption: IV
Distribution: PB: (D) 80%–90%, (P) UK
Metabolism: t½: (D) 3–30 h; (P) 2–8 h
Excretion: (D) 50% in bile and 5% in urine; (P) urine

Pharmacodynamics

(D)
IV: Onset: 7–10 d
Peak: 14 d
Duration: 21 d
(P)
IV: Onset: 24 h
Peak: 48–72 h
Duration: 5–15 d

Evaluation

Therapeutic Effects/Uses

(D) To treat breast, bladder, ovarian, lung cancers, leukemias, lymphomas.
(P) To correct hypercalcemia, hypercalciuria, and to treat testicular carcinoma.

Mode of Action: (D) Inhibits DNA and RNA synthesis. Has immunosuppressant activity. (P) Inhibits hypercalcemic action of vitamin D and action by the parathyroid hormone. Inhibits DNA and RNA synthesis.

Side Effects

(D) and (P): Stomatitis, anorexia, nausea, vomiting, diarrhea, rash
(D): Alopecia
(P): Dizziness, weakness, headache, mental depression

Adverse Reactions

(D): Esophagitis, anemia, hyperpigmentation of nails, tongue, and oral mucosa, especially in blacks
(P): Nosebleeds, purpura, ecchymoses
Life-threatening:
(D) and (P): thrombocytopenia, leukopenia
(D) Cardiotoxicity, CHF, ECG severe changes, severe myelosuppression, anaphylaxis
(P) Hemorrhage

KEY: A: adult; IV: intravenous; PB: protein-binding; t½: half-life; CHF: congestive heart failure; ECG: electrocardiogram; BUN: blood urea nitrogen; NSAIDs: nonsteroidal antiinflammatory drugs; CHF: congestive heart failure; ALP: alkaline phosphatase.

Table 33-6
Antitumor Antibiotics and Vinca Alkaloids

GENERIC (BRAND)	ROUTE AND DOSAGE	USES AND CONSIDERATIONS
ANTITUMOR ANTIBIOTICS		
Bleomycin SO$_4$ (Blenoxane)	A: IM/IV: 10–20 U/m^2/wk or 0.25–0.5 U/kg/wk Reduce dose with renal impairment	For treating squamous cell-carcinomas, testicular tumor (when used with vinblastine and cisplatin), and lymphomas. Low incidence of bone marrow suppression. Total lifetime dose is 450 U. A serious adverse reaction is anaphylaxis. Has a long duration of action. *Pregnancy category:* D; PB: 1%; t$\frac{1}{2}$: 2 h
Dactinomycin (Actinomycin D, Cosmegen)	A: IV: 500 μg/m^2/d for 5 d; may repeat at 2–4 wk C: IV: 15 μg/kg/d for 5 d; may repeat at 2–4 wk; *max: 500 μg*	For treating testicular tumors. Wilms' tumor, choriocarcinoma, and rhabdomyosarcoma. Nausea and vomiting may occur during the first 24 hours. Has a long duration of action. *Pregnancy category:* C; PB: 80%–90%; t$\frac{1}{2}$: 36 h
Daunorubicin HCl (Cerubidine)	*Leukemias:* A: IV: 30–60 mg/m^2/d for 2–3 d; repeat dose in 3–4 wk Reduce dose with hepatic/renal impairment	For treating leukemias, Ewing's sarcoma, Wilms' tumor, neuroblastoma, and non-Hodgkin's lymphoma. Has a long duration of action. *Pregnancy category:* D; PB: 80%; t$\frac{1}{2}$: 19 h
Doxorubicin (Adriamycin)	*Solid tumors:* A: IV: 60–75 mg/m^2; repeat q21d Reduce dose with hepatic impairment	For treating breast, lung, and genitourinary cancers, leukemias, lymphomas, and ovarian tumors. Lower dose required when used in combinations. Total lifetime dose is 550 mg/m^2. *Pregnancy category:* D; PB: 80%–90%; t$\frac{1}{2}$: 3–22 h
Idarubicin (Idamycin)	*Solid tumor:* A: IV: 12–15 mg/m^2/d for 3 d *Leukemia:* A: IV: 10–12 mg/m^2/d for 3–4 d; repeat q3wk Reduce dose with hepatic/renal impairment	For treating acute monocytic leukemia and solid tumors. More potent than daunorubicin or doxorubicin. Vesicant, monitor complete blood count (CBC). Urine may be red. *Pregnancy category:* D; PB: 97%; t$\frac{1}{2}$: 22 h
Mitomycin (Mutamycin)	A: IV: 10–20 mg/m^2 q6–8wk Reduce dose with renal impairment	For treating disseminated adenocarcinoma of breast, stomach, and pancreas. Also used for cancer of the head, neck, cervix, and lung. Monitor temperature and CBC. *Pregnancy category:* D; PB: UK; t$\frac{1}{2}$: 12 min
Mitoxantrone (Novantrone)	*Solid tumor:* A: IV: 12 mg/m^2/d × 3. Dilute with 50 mL NSS or D$_5$W over 15–30 min	For treating acute nonlymphocytic leukemia; may be used for breast cancer. Rash, dyspnea, hypotension, facial swelling, blue urine, sclera, skin hue change may occur. Severe hepatic dysfunction with decreased total body clearance. *Pregnancy category:* D; PB: 95%; t$\frac{1}{2}$: 1.5–13 d
Plicamycin (Mithracin)	*Testicular tumor:* A: IV: 25–30 μg/kg/d for 8–10 d *Hypercalcemia:* A: IV: 15–25 μg/kg/d for 3–4 d Reduce dose with renal impairment	For treating hypercalcemia due to metastatic cancer. High doses may cause liver and renal damage. Monitor serum calcium levels. Has standard chemotherapy drug's side effects. *Pregnancy category:* D; PB: 0%; t$\frac{1}{2}$: 2–8 h
MITOTIC INHIBITORS (VINCA ALKALOIDS)		
Vinblastine SO$_4$ (Velban)	A: IV: Initial: 3.7 mg/m^2; after 7 d, increase dose weekly; *max: 18.5 mg/m^2* C: IV: Initial: 2.5 mg/m^2; increase dose weekly; *max: 12.5 mg/m^2*	For treating cancer of the testes, breast, and kidney and for treatment of lymphomas, lymphosarcomas, and neuroblastomas. Nausea, vomiting, and alopecia are common side effects. Check CBC before dosing. *Pregnancy category:* D; PB: 75%; t$\frac{1}{2}$: 25 h

Table continued on following page

Table 33–6 *Continued*
Antitumor Antibiotics and Vinca Alkaloids

GENERIC (BRAND)	ROUTE AND DOSAGE	USES AND CONSIDERATIONS
Vincristine SO$_4$ (Oncovin)	A: IV: 0.4–1.4 mg/m²/wk; *max:* 2 mg/dose C: IV: 1–2 mg/m²/wk; *max:* 2 mg/dose	For treating cancer of the breast, lungs, and cervix; multiple myelomas, sarcomas, lymphomas, Wilms' tumor. Neurologic difficulties should be assessed. Used for treating Hodgkin's disease in combination therapy, MOPP: mechlorethamine, vincristine, procarbazine, and prednisone. *Never should be given intrathecally. Pregnancy category:* D; PB: 75%; t$\frac{1}{2}$: triphasic 2–85 h
Vinorelbine (Navelbine)	A: IV: 30 mg/m² weekly as a 6- to 10-min IV infusion	For use as a first-line treatment for ambulatory clients with advanced, unresectable non-small cell lung cancer (NSCLC). May be used alone or in combination with cisplatin for stage IV NSCLC and in combination with cisplatin for stage III NSCLC. *Pregnancy category:* D; PB: UK; t$\frac{1}{2}$: UK

KEY: *A: adult; C: child; PO: by mouth; IM: intramuscular; IV: intravenous; CBC: complete blood count; m²: square meter of body surface area; UK: unknown; PB: protein-binding; t$\frac{1}{2}$: half-life; NSS: normal saline solution; D$_5$W: 5% dextrose in water.*
For full discussion of body surface area in dosage calculation, see Chapter 4.

Table 33–7
Antineoplastic: Androgens and Miscellaneous

GENERIC (BRAND)	ROUTE AND DOSAGE*	USES AND CONSIDERATIONS
ANDROGENS		
Testolactone (Teslac)	*Palliation breast carcinoma:* A: PO (females): 250 mg q.i.d.	For palliative treatment of breast carcinoma in postmenopausal women. Serum calcium levels should periodically be checked. Voice may deepen and facial hair may occur. *Pregnancy category:* D; PB: UK; t$\frac{1}{2}$: UK
Progesterone (Gesterol 50)	*Endometrial and breast cancer* A: IM: 5–10 mg/d for 6–8 d	For palliative treatment of endometrial and breast carcinoma. *Pregnancy category:* X; PB: UK; t$\frac{1}{2}$: 5 min
MISCELLANEOUS: HORMONAL ANTAGONISTS, ENZYMES		
Aminoglutethimide (Cytadren)	A: PO: 250 mg q6h; increased q2wk to 2 g/d in 2–3 divided doses to decrease nausea and vomiting	For treating adrenal carcinoma, ectopic adrenocorticotropic hormone (ACTH)-producing tumors. Drug suppresses adrenal activity. May be used in breast cancer therapy. Treatment usually used for 3 mo. *Pregnancy category:* D; PB: 20%–25%; t$\frac{1}{2}$: 7–15 h

Table continued on following page

Table 33-7 *Continued*

Antineoplastic: Androgens and Miscellaneous

GENERIC (BRAND)	ROUTE AND DOSAGE*	USES AND CONSIDERATIONS
Asparaginase (Elspar)	Start with intradermal skin test A: IV/IM: 6,000 U/m² q.o.d. for 3–4 wk or 1000–20,000 U/m² for 10–20 d or 200 IU/kg/d for 28 d	For treating acute lymphocytic leukemia. Used in combination with another anticancer drugs. Common side effects include nausea, vomiting, anorexia, leukopenia, and impaired pancreatic function. *Pregnancy category:* C; PB: 30%; t½: 8–30 h (IV)
Flutamide (Eulexin)	A: PO: 250 mg q8h *Note:* Give simultaneously with luteinizing hormone–releasing hormone (LHRH) analogue therapy, e.g., leuprolide acetate, 7.5 mg IM/mo	For treating metastatic prostatic carcinoma, usually in combination with other anticancer drugs. *Pregnancy category:* D; PB: 95%; t½: 5–10 h
Goserelin acetate (Zoladex)	*Palliation prostate cancer:* A: SC: 3.6 mg into upper abdomen q28d	For treating metastatic prostatic carcinoma. It is a synthetic luteinizing hormone-releasing analogue. May also be used in breast cancer and endometriosis. Gynecomastia, breast swelling, and hot flashes may occur. *Pregnancy category:* X; PB: UK; t½: 4–6 h
Letrozole (Femara)	A: PO: 2.5 mg/d	For treatment of advanced breast cancer in postmenopausal women. Decreases estrogen biosynthesis. May be more effective than megestrol acetate and aminoglutethimide. *Pregnancy category:* UK; PB: UK; t½: 2 d
Megestrol acetate	*Breast cancer:* A: PO: 40 mg q.i.d. *Endometrial cancer:* A: PO: 40–320 mg/d in divided doses; *max:* 800 mg/d	For palliative treatment of advanced carcinoma of the breast and endometrium. May promote weight gain by increasing appetite. *Pregnancy category:* X; PB: UK; t½: 15–20 h
Mitotane (Lysodren)	*Palliation adrenal cortical carcinoma:* A: PO: 1–6 g/d in divided doses; increasing to 8–10 g/d in 3–4 divided doses; *max:* 18 g/d	For palliative treatment of inoperable adrenal cortical carcinoma. Adverse reactions include hemorrhagic cystitis, hypouricemia, and hypercholesterolemia. Monitor vital signs. *Pregnancy category:* C; PB: UK; t½: 20–160 d
Pegaspargase (Oncaspar)	A: IV: 2500 IU/m² q14d	To treat acute lymphoblastic leukemia. It is a CCS agent affecting G₁ phase of the cell cycle. It interferes with DNA, RNA, and protein synthesis. *Pregnancy category:* C; PB: UK; t½: 1.4 to 5.2 d
Polyestradiol PO₄ (Estradurin)	*Palliation prostate cancer:* A: IM: 40 mg q2–4 wk; *max:* 80 mg	For palliative treatment of inoperable prostatic carcinoma. Estrogen derivative. Side effects may include fluid retention, nausea, vomiting, hypertension, weight change, and thromboembolic disorders. *Pregnancy category:* X; PB: UK; t½: UK
Tamoxifen citrate (Nolvadex)	*Palliation/adjunctive, treatment of breast carcinoma:* A: PO: 10–20 mg b.i.d.	For palliative treatment of advanced breast carcinoma with positive lymph nodes in postmenopausal women. Competes with estradiol at estrogen receptor sites. It decreases DNA synthesis. *Pregnancy category:* D; PB: UK; t½: 7 d
Toremifene (Fareston)	A: PO: 60 mg/d	To treat advanced breast cancer in postmenopausal women. It is an antiestrogen drug. *Pregnancy category:* UK; PB: UK; t½: 5d

KEY: *A:* adult; *C:* child; *PO:* by mouth; *IM:* intramuscular; *IV:* intravenous; *SC:* subcutaneous; *UK:* unknown; *PB:* protein-binding; *t½:* half-life.
*For full discussion of body surface area in dosage calculation, see Chapter 4.

16), and others. The miscellaneous antineoplastics are used in combination with other cancer chemotherapeutics to treat a variety of solid tumors and hematologic malignancies.

SUMMARY

The anticancer drugs act by blocking phases of the G_1, S, G_2, and M cancer cell-cycle phases. The groups of antineoplastic drugs (alkylating compounds, antimetabolites, antitumor antibiotics, vinca alkaloids, and hormones) can have either a palliative or a curative effect with single or combination drug therapy. These groups of anticancer drugs are classified as either cell-cycle specific (CCS) or cell-cycle nonspecific (CCNS). Figure 33–1 shows the phases of the cell cycle and the groups of antineoplastics that affect the different phases.

The nursing implications are to report the adverse effects and to participate as a health professional in alleviating these effects. The nurse instructs the client to use good oral hygiene for stomatitis, encourages the client to purchase a wig or use scarves for alope-

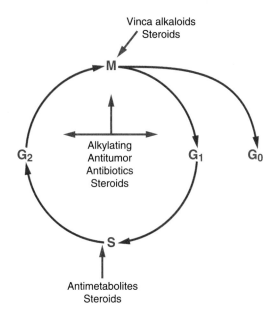

Figure 33–1
Phases and drug groups of antineoplastics.

cia, and instructs family and friends with upper or lower respiratory infections to minimize their visits with the client or use precautions, such as wearing a mask.

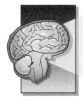

Critical Thinking in Action

A. B., age 55 years, has recently been diagnosed as having breast cancer. Cancer chemotherapy was prescribed. A. B. received 5-fluorouracil intravenously for 4 days. Also, A. B. received doxorubicin (Adriamycin) intravenously, 60 mg/m², and this dosage is to be repeated in 21 days.

1. Explain the drug actions of fluorouracil and doxorubicin. How do they differ?
2. What side effects and adverse reactions related to the two anticancer drugs should the nurse observe during A. B.'s anticancer therapy? Explain.
3. Why is a combination of antineoplastics/anticancer drugs desirable? Explain.
4. What nursing interventions and client teaching should be included in A. B.'s care?

After several months, A. B.'s serum calcium was 12.3 mEq/L. Doxorubicin and fluorouracil were discontinued. Plicamycin and cyclophosphamide (Cytoxan) were prescribed.

5. Why was plicamycin ordered? In what ways can this drug benefit A. B.?
6. What laboratory tests should be monitored while A. B. is taking plicamycin?
7. Why may cyclophosphamide be substituted for fluorouracil? What are the similarities and differences between these two drugs?
8. List the common side effects and the adverse reactions of cyclophosphamide?
9. What nursing interventions and client teaching should be included in A. B.'s care?

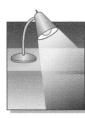

Study Questions

1. What are the five phases of the cell cycle? Name the groups of drugs that are cell-cycle specific and cell-cycle nonspecific.

2. Your client is receiving cyclophosphamide, methotrexate, and 5-fluorouracil for the treatment of breast cancer. What information would you include when teaching about self-care activities after receiving this drug?

3. What are the adverse reactions to most antineoplastic drugs? Explain.

4. What is combination drug therapy? What are its advantages?

5. What type of drug is plicamycin (Mithracin)? How is it used to correct electrolyte imbalances in clients with advanced cancer?

6. What is the action of corticosteroids, such as prednisone, in the treatment of cancer?

7. What is the definition of vesicant? List the anticancer drugs with vesicant properties.

8. What special safe handling precautions should be taken during the preparation, administration, and disposal of cancer chemotherapeutic drugs?

34 Biologic Response Modifiers

ANNE E. LARA

Outline

Objectives

* Discuss the actions of the biologic response modifiers.
* Identify two client populations who may benefit from biologic response modifiers.
* List three common side effects of interferons, colony-stimulating factors, and interleukin-2.
* Describe the nursing process, including client teaching, needed to care for clients receiving biologic response modifiers.

Terms

absolute neutrophil count
biologic response modifiers
colony-stimulating factors
erythropoietin
granulocyte
granulocyte colony-stimulating factor

granulocyte macrophage colony-stimulating factor
hybridoma technology
interferons
interleukins
lymphokines
macrophage

myelosuppressive
nadir
neumega
neutrophil
recombinant DNA
thrombocytopenia

INTRODUCTION

Biologic response modifiers (BRMs) are a class of agents used to enhance the body's immune system. Advances in biochemical technology have led to the discovery of BRMs and the identification of their clinical activities. **Recombinant DNA** (genetic engineering process to produce mass quantities of human proteins) and **hybridoma** (process to mass produce monoclonal antibodies using mice) **technology** (Figs. 34–1 and 34–2) are two advances that have led to commercial mass production of BRMs.

Interleukins, colony-stimulating factors, interferons (α, β, γ), tumor necrosis factor, and monoclonal antibodies are some currently known BRMs. With the exception of the monoclonal antibodies, BRMs are complex proteins produced by the cells of the immune system (Fig. 34–3).

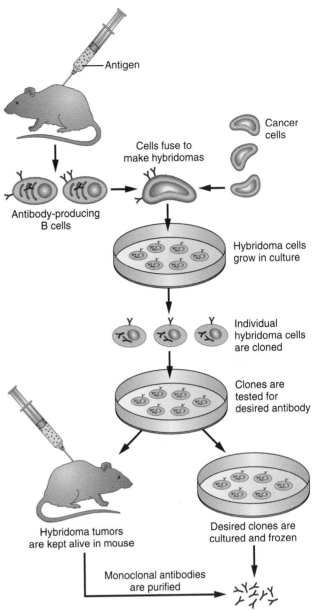

Figure 34–2
Hybridoma therapy. (Redrawn from NIH Publication No. 88-529 [1991]: Understanding the Immune System, p. 28.)

Three BRM functions have been identified:

1. Enhance host immunologic function (immunomodulation)
2. Destroy or interfere with tumor activities (cytotoxic/cytostatic effects)
3. Promote differentiation of stem cells (other biologic effects) (Table 34–1)

The indications for BRMs are currently being investigated in clinical trials. Erythropoietin, granulocyte colony-stimulating factors, granulocyte macrophage colony-stimulating factor, Neumega (oprelvekin), and interferon alpha are Food and Drug Administration (FDA) approved and commercially available. The in-

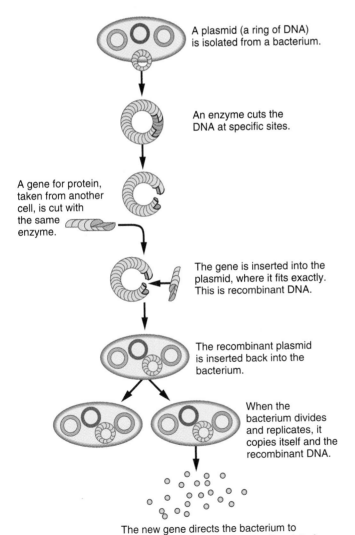

Figure 34–1
Recombinant DNA. (Redrawn from NIH Publication No. 88-529 [1991]: Understanding the Immune System, p. 29.)

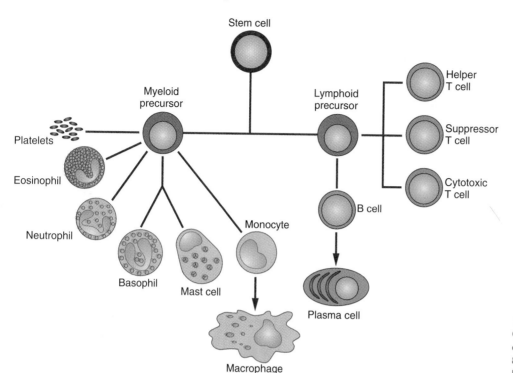

Stem cell

Myeloid precursor

Lymphoid precursor

Helper T cell

Suppressor T cell

Cytotoxic T cell

Platelets

Eosinophil

Neutrophil

Basophil

Mast cell

Monocyte

B cell

Macrophage

Plasma cell

Figure 34-3
Cells of the immune system. (Redrawn from NIH Publication No. 88-529 [1991]: Understanding the Immune System, p. 5.)

terleukins, tumor necrosis factor, and monoclonal antibodies continue to be studied in clinical trials. Only one monoclonal antibody—Trastuzumab (Herceptin)—has been approved by the FDA. Interferons, interleukins, colony-stimulating factors, and Herceptin are discussed in this chapter.

INTERFERONS

Interferons (IFNs) are a family of naturally occurring proteins that were first discovered in the 1950s. Three major types of IFNs have been identified: alpha (α) IFN, beta (β) IFN, and gamma (γ) IFN. Each type is produced by a different cell within the immune system. All three types can be manufactured using recombinant DNA technology; only IFN-α, however, is FDA approved for commercial use.

Interferon alpha is produced by B cells, T cells, macrophages, and null cells in response to the presence of viruses or tumor cells. Interferon alpha has been shown to have antiviral, antiproliferative, and immunomodulatory effects, which means that IFN-α inhibits intracellular replication of viral DNA, interferes with tumor cell growth, and enhances natural killer cell (antitumor) activity. Recombinant IFN-α is manufactured as Roferon-A and as Intron A.

In 1986, IFN-α was approved by the FDA for use in treating hairy-cell leukemia, and in 1989 it was approved for use in acquired immunodeficiency syndrome (AIDS)-related Kaposi's sarcoma. Clinically, alpha IFN has been used in the treatment of non-Hodgkin's lymphoma, multiple myeloma, chronic myelogenous leukemia, renal cell carcinoma, malignant melanoma, bladder cancer, and carcinoid (type of cancer-like disease). Intravesical administration of IFN-α has proved successful for low-grade bladder tumors, intraperitoneal administration of IFN-α has been used for ovarian cancer clients, and intralesional application of IFN-α has been used to treat melanoma and basal cell carcinoma. Benign conditions such as laryngeal papillomata and condyloma acuminata have also been treated with IFN-α. Interferon is currently being investigated in clinical trials as a chemotherapy-enhancing agent in clients with colon cancer.

Table 34–1
Action of Biologic Response Modifiers

BIOLOGIC RESPONSE MODIFIER	ACTION
Interleukins	I
Interferons	I, C
Monoclonal antibodies	C
Tumor necrosis factor	C
Colony-stimulating factors	O

KEY: I: immunomodulation; C: cytotoxic/cytostatic; O: other biologic activity.

Pharmacokinetics

Interferon is metabolized by the liver and filtered by the kidney. Approximately 80% of the dose, however, is absorbed by the body. Peak serum concentrations are reached 4 to 8 h after administration. Interferon can be administered subcutaneously, intramuscularly, and intravenously, although subcutaneous or intramuscular administration is preferred. Subcutaneous administration is recommended for clients with platelet counts below 50,000.

Roferon-A is available in both liquid and powder forms. The liquid is supplied in 3 million IU/mL vials and 18 million IU/mL vials. At a concentration of 3 million IU/0.5 mL, the powder is available as 18 million IU/vial. When mixed with 3 mL of bacteriostatic water diluent, the vial concentration is 6 million IU/mL, or 3 million IU/0.5 mL. Both the liquid and the powder should be refrigerated at 2°C to 8°C and used within 1 month. The vials should not be frozen or shaken.

Intron A is supplied as a lyophilized powder in 3, 5, 10, and 25 million IU. The powder is reconstituted with bacteriostatic water diluent. Final vial concentrations are 3 million IU/vial (3 million IU/vial with 1 mL of diluent), 5 million IU/mL (5 million IU/vial with 2 mL of diluent), and 5 million IU/mL (25 million IU/vial with 5 mL of diluent). The vials can be shaken to hasten powder dissolution. The final solution is stable for 30 days when stored at 2°C to 8°C. The IFN alphas are listed in Table 34–2 with their dosages, uses, and considerations.

Side Effects and Adverse Reactions

The major side effect of IFN-α is a flu-like syndrome. Other effects are seen in the gastrointestinal (GI), neurologic, cardiopulmonary, renal, hepatic, hematologic, and dermatologic systems.

The flu-like syndrome is characterized by fever, chills, fatigue, malaise, and myalgias. Chills can occur 3 to 6 h after IFN-α administration and may progress to rigors. A fever as high as 39°C to 40°C may occur within 30 to 90 min after the onset of chills and last for 24 h. Fatigue, malaise, and myalgias are cumulative side effects; fatigue is the dose-limiting toxicity (the side effect that would result in decrease in dose or discontinuation of drug).

GI side effects include nausea, diarrhea, vomiting,

Table 34–2
Biologic Response Modifiers: Interferons

GENERIC (BRAND)	ROUTE AND DOSAGE	USES AND CONSIDERATIONS
Interferon alfa-2a (Roferon-A)	*Hairy-cell leukemia, condylomata acuminata:* A: SC/IM: 3 million IU daily for 16–24 wk	For treating hairy-cell leukemia, condyloma acuminata, and AIDS-related Kaposi's sarcoma. Flu-like symptoms such as fatigue, aches, pain, fever, chills, headaches may occur. *Pregnancy category:* C; PB: UK; $t_\frac{1}{2}$: 2–3 h
Interferon alfa-2b (Intron A)	A: SC: 2 million IU/m² × 3 wk *Kaposi's sarcoma:* A: IM/SC/IV: Initially: 36 million IU daily for 10–12 wk; maint: 36 million IU 3 × wk	For treating hairy-cell leukemia, condyloma acuminata, AIDS-related Kaposi's sarcoma, and chronic hepatitis B and non-A hepatitis. Flu-like symptoms may occur. Monitor CBC, AST, ALT, ALP, LDH. *Pregnancy category:* C; PB: UK; $t_\frac{1}{2}$ 2 h
Interferon gamma-1b (Actimmune)	*Body surface area >0.5 m²:* A: SC: 50 μg/m² 3 × wk *Body surface area <0.5 m²;* A&C >1 y: SC: 1.5 μg/kg 3 × wk	For treating chronic granulomatous disease. Flu-like symptoms may occur. *Pregnancy category:* C; PB: UK; $t_\frac{1}{2}$: 0.5–6 h
Interferon alfa-n3 (Alferon N)	*Condylomata acuminata:* A: Inject into wart: 250,000 U (0.05 mL) twice weekly; max: 8 wk Do *not* repeat for >3 mo after end of therapy	For treating recurring condylomata acuminata (genital venereal warts). Flu-like symptoms may occur. Monitor CBC, AST, ALT, ALP, LDH. *Pregnancy category:* C; PB: UK; $t_\frac{1}{2}$: 6–8 h
Interferon beta-1b (Betaseron)	*Reduce number of clinical exacerbations of multiple sclerosis* A: >18 y: SC: 8 million U q.o.d. C: Not recommended	For treating multiple sclerosis (MS). Flu-like symptoms may occur. *Pregnancy category:* C; PB: UK; $t_\frac{1}{2}$: 8 min–4.3 h

KEY: A: adult; C: child; SC: subcutaneous; IM: intramuscular; IV: intravenous; UK: unknown; CBC: complete blood count; >: greater than; <: less than; PB: protein-binding; $t_\frac{1}{2}$: half-life; AIDS: acquired immunodeficiency syndrome; CBC: complete blood count; AST: aspartate aminotransferase; ALT: alanine aminotransferase; ALP: alkaline phosphatase; LDH: lactate dehydrogenase.

anorexia, taste alterations, and xerostomia (dry mouth). These side effects are mild, with anorexia considered to be the dose-limiting toxicity for this system.

Neurologic side effects are reversible (after the drug is stopped) and occur in 70% of clients who receive IFN-α. These effects are manifested by mild confusion, somnolence (sleepiness), irritability, poor concentration, seizures, transient aphasia (temporary loss of ability to speak), hallucinations, paranoia, and psychoses.

Cardiopulmonary side effects are dose-related and occur more frequently in the elderly and in those clients with an underlying cardiac disease. The effects include tachycardia, pallor, cyanosis, tachypnea, non-specific electrocardiographic changes, rare myocardial infarction, and orthostatic hypotension.

Renal and hepatic effects are dose-dependent and usually result in few or no symptoms. The effects are manifested by increased blood urea nitrogen (BUN) and creatinine levels, proteinuria, and elevated transaminases.

Hematologic effects are reversible and dose-limiting. Neutropenia (decreased number of neutrophils in the blood) and thrombocytopenia are manifestations of such effects. Neutropenia is usually rare and does not predispose the client to infection. Thrombocytopenia is more common in clients with hematopoietic (affecting the formation of blood cells) diseases than in those with solid tumors.

Maculopapular rashes of the trunk and extremities, pruritis, irritation at the injection site, desquamation (shedding of epithelial cells of the skin), and alopecia are dermatologic effects of IFN-α. Alopecia can occur after more than 4 months of therapy.

The administration of IFN-α is contraindicated in clients with known hypersensitivity to IFN-α, mouse immunoglobulin, or any component of the product. It should be used cautiously in clients with severe cardiac, renal, or hepatic disease, or those with seizure disorders or central nervous system dysfunction. Manufacturers recommend administering the agent to persons 18 years or older only under the supervision of a qualified physician. There have been no studies demonstrating the safety and effectiveness of IFN-α in pregnant women, nursing mothers, or children. Women of childbearing age should use contraceptives while receiving IFN-α because of the agent's effects on serum estradiol and progesterone concentrations. Studies have demonstrated no fertility or teratogenic effects in males.

It is recommended that baseline and periodic complete blood counts (CBCs) and liver function tests be performed during the course of IFN therapy. Manufacturers suggest that clients be treated for at least 6 months before a decision is made to continue treatment in those who respond or discontinue treatment

in those who do not; optimal treatment duration has not been determined. Dose reductions of 50% or drug discontinuation should be considered if adverse reactions occur. Concurrent or prior treatment with chemotherapeutic agents or radiation therapy may increase the effectiveness and the toxicity of IFN-α.

COLONY-STIMULATING FACTORS

Hematopoietic **colony-stimulating factors** (CSFs) are proteins that stimulate or regulate the growth, maturation, and differentiation of bone marrow stem cells (Fig. 34–4). The CSFs are manufactured through recombinant DNA techniques.

Although CSFs are not directly tumoricidal, they are useful in cancer treatment because they

- Decrease the length of posttreatment neutropenia (the length of time the neutrophils [a type of white blood cell] are decreased secondary to chemotherapy), thereby reducing the incidence and duration of infection.
- Permit the delivery of higher doses of drugs. Myelosuppression (suppression of bone marrow activity) is often a dose-limiting toxicity of chemotherapy. Higher, possibly tumoricidal doses of drugs cannot be administered because of potentially life-threatening side effects. CSFs can minimize the myelosuppression toxicity, thus allowing the delivery of higher doses of drugs.
- Reduce bone marrow recovery time after bone marrow transplantation.
- Enhance macrophage or granulocyte tumor-, virus-, and fungus-destroying ability.
- Prevent severe thrombocytopenia after myelosuppressive chemotherapy.

Colony-stimulating factors have been used to treat clients with neutropenia secondary to disease or treatment and can be administered both intravenously and subcutaneously. The CSFs that are FDA approved for clinical use are erythropoietin, granulocyte colony-stimulating factor (G-CSF), granulocyte macrophage colony-stimulating factors (GM-CSF), and Neumega (oprelvekin).

Erythropoietin

Erythropoietin (EPO) is a glycoprotein produced by the kidney that stimulates red blood cell production in response to hypoxia (decreased oxygen to body tissues). Specifically, EPO stimulates the division and differentiation of committed red blood cell progenitors (parent cells destined to become circulating red blood cells) in the bone marrow. EPO is currently FDA approved for use in clients with anemia secondary to chronic renal failure (CRF), AZT (zidovudine)-

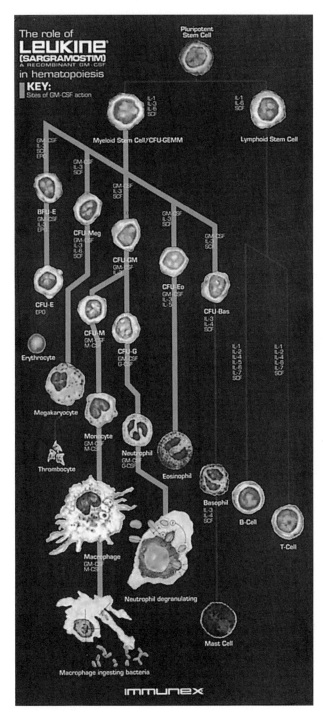

Figure 34–4

The role of Leukine (sargramostim) in hematopoiesis. (Courtesy of Immunex Corp.)

treated human immunodeficiency virus (HIV) infections, or cancer and its treatment. The use of EPO in these anemic clients may decrease the need for and frequency of red cell transfusion. Erythropoietin is marketed under the brand name Epogen.

PHARMACOKINETICS

Erythropoietin can be administered both intravenously (IV push) or subcutaneously. According to the manufacturer, intravenously administered EPO is eliminated at a rate consistent with first-order kinetics (process by which the drug is eliminated in part by hepatic and renal blood flow, with a circulating half-life ranging from approximately 4 to 13 h in clients with chronic renal failure (CRF). Plasma levels of EPO have been detected for at least 24 h. After subcutaneous administration of EPO to CRF clients, peak serum levels were achieved within 5 to 24 h after administration. The half-life of intravenously administered EPO is approximately 20% shorter in normal volunteers than in CRF clients. Pharmacokinetic studies have not been done with HIV-infected clients. See Chart 34–1.

Erythropoietin should be administered at starting doses of 50 to 100 U/kg three times a week. The dose of EPO should be reduced when the hematocrit reaches the 30% to 33% range or increases by more than four points in any 2-week period. The dosage needs to be individualized to maintain the hematocrit within the target range. Dose changes should be made in the range of 25 U/kg three times a week.

According to the manufacturer, if a client does not respond to or maintain a response, the following situations must be considered and evaluated:

1. Iron deficiency
2. Underlying infections, inflammatory or malignant processes
3. Occult blood loss
4. Underlying hematologic disease
5. Folic acid or vitamin B_{12} deficiency
6. Hemolysis
7. Aluminum intoxication
8. Osteitis fibrosa cystica (fibrous degeneration with formation of cysts and nodules secondary to hyperparathyroidism)

SIDE EFFECTS AND ADVERSE REACTIONS

The side effects of erythropoietin include hypertension, headache, arthralgias (joint pain), nausea, edema, fatigue, diarrhea, vomiting, chest pain, injection site skin reaction, asthenia (weakness), dizziness, seizures, thromboses (clots), and allergic reactions. Studies demonstrate that EPO administration was well tolerated with no reports of serious allergic reactions or anaphylaxis. Rare transient skin reactions have been reported. Blood pressure may increase in CRF clients receiving EPO during the early phase of treatment when the hematocrit (Hct) is increasing. About 25% of CRF clients receiving dialysis may re-

Chart 34–1. Biologic Response Modifiers: Erythropoietin

EPOETIN ALFA (ERYTHROPOIETIN [EPO])

Drug Name

Epoetin Alfa (Erythropoietin [EPO]) (Epogen, Procit), ❦ *Eprex*
Pregnancy Category: C

Contraindications

Uncontrolled hypertension, hypersensitivity to mammalian cell–derived products or human albumin
Caution: Pregnancy, lactation, porphyria; safety in children not known

Dosage

A: 50–100 U/kg 3 × wk
IV: Dialysis clients
IV/SC: Nondialysis, CRF clients
IV/SC: 100 U/kg 3 × wk for 8 wk in AZT-treated HIV-infected clients
Initial dose to those with EPO levels <500 mU/mL and receiving <4200 mg of AZT/wk. Clients with EPO level >500 mU/mL are unlikely to respond to EPO therapy.

Drug-Lab-Food Interactions

Drug: None known
Lab: Increase hematocrit, decreased plasma volume

Pharmacokinetics

Absorption: SC, IV
Distribution: PB: UK
Metabolism: t½: 4–13 h in clients with CRF; 20% less in those with normal renal function
Excretion: In urine

Pharmacodynamics

IV: Onset: 7–10 d
Peak: 2–4 wk
Duration: UK
SC: Onset: 7–10 d
Peak: 5–24 h
Duration: UK

Therapeutic Effects/Uses

To treat anemia secondary to CRF or AZT (zidovudine) treatment of HIV infections. Use in clients with anemia secondary to cancer or its treatment is under investigation.

Mode of Action: Increased production of RBCs, triggered by hypoxia or anemia.

Side Effects

Sense of well-being, hypertension, arthralgias, nausea, edema, fatigue, injection site reaction, rash, diarrhea, shortness of breath

Adverse Reactions

Seizures, hyperkalemia
Life-threatening: Cerebrovascular accident, myocardial infarction

KEY: A: adult; SC: subcutaneous; IV: intravenous; <: less than; >: greater than; UK: unknown; PB: protein-binding; t½: half-life. ❦: Canadian drug name; RBC: red blood cell; HIV: human immunodeficiency virus; CRF: chronic renal failure.

quire initiation of or increase in antihypertensive therapy. It is postulated that increases in blood pressure may relate to increases in Hct; therefore, it is recommended that the dose of EPO be decreased if the Hct increase exceeds four points in any 2-week period. Similarly, an increase in Hct may cause increased vascular access clotting (clots in blood vessel at connection site with artificial kidney) in hemodialysis clients. Clients may require increased heparinization during EPO therapy to prevent clotting of the artificial kidney. Seizures occurred in CRF clients receiving EPO during clinical trials; activity was particularly evident during the first 90 days of therapy.

EPO administration is contraindicated in clients with (1) uncontrolled hypertension, (2) known hypersensitivity to mammalian cell-derived products, and (3) known hypersensitivity to human albumin. Evaluation of iron stores should occur during EPO therapy. Transferrin saturation should be at least 20% and ferritin should be at least 100 ng/mL. Iron supplements may be needed to increase and maintain transferrin saturation to support EPO-stimulated erythropoiesis.

The safety and effectiveness of EPO therapy in pregnant women, nursing mothers, and children have not been established. There are no known EPO drug interactions.

The manufacturers' preparation and administration recommendations for EPO are

1. Do not shake, because shaking may denature the glycoprotein, rendering it biologically inactive.

2. Use only one dose per vial. Do not reenter the vial. Discard any unused portion because the vial contains no preservatives.

3. Store the 2000-, 3000-, 4000-, 10,000-, or 20,000-unit vials at 2°C to 8°C. Do not freeze.

4. Warm the vial to room temperature before subcutaneous (SC) administration.

5. Use the smallest volume of EPO per injection (1 mL or less per injection) to decrease injection site discomfort.

6. Use ice to numb the injection site.

7. Do not use the same needle to draw medication into the syringe and to inject the medication. Use a new needle to inject medication.

Granulocyte Colony-Stimulating Factor

Granulocyte colony-stimulating factor (G-CSF), marketed as filgrastim (Neupogen), is a human **granulocyte** (type of WBC responsible for fighting infection) colony-stimulating factor produced by recombinant DNA technology. G-CSF, which is a glycoprotein produced by monocytes (a type of WBC), fibroblasts (immature fiber-producing cells), and endothelial (cells that line the heart cavity, and blood and lymph vessels) cells, regulates the production of **neutrophils** (granular leukocytes, WBCs) within the bone marrow. G-CSF is FDA approved and commercially available to decrease the incidence of infections in clients receiving myelosuppressive chemotherapeutic agents. G-CSF has been evaluated as an adjunct to chemotherapy for both solid tumor and hematologic malignancies and in studies employing a number of different chemotherapy regimens. Chart 34–2 gives the drug data for filgrastim.

PHARMACOKINETICS

Filgrastim administration results in a two-phase neutrophil response. An early response is seen within 24 h of administration. Following the chemotherapy-induced **nadir** (low point), a second peak in circulating neutrophils is observed. The proliferation-induced increase in neutrophils usually commences 4 to 5 days after administration is initiated, but timing may vary based on the type and dose of the myelosuppressive therapy and the client's underlying disease and prior treatment history. The elimination half-life of G-CSF in both normal and cancer clients is 3.5 h. Clearance rates are approximately 0.5 to 0.7 mL/min/kg.

G-CSF can be administered subcutaneously and by intravenous infusion. Administration of G-CSF by in-travenous bolus is currently being investigated. The recommended starting dose of G-CSF is 5 μg/kg/day SC or IV infusion daily. The maximum tolerated dose has not been established. Doses may be increased in 5-μg/kg increments for each chemotherapy cycle, according to the duration and severity of the absolute neutrophil count nadir. The **absolute neutrophil count** (ANC) is determined by

Total white blood count (WBC)
    × percentage of neutrophils + percentage of bands

G-CSF should not be administered 24 h before or 24 h after the administration of therapeutic agents because of the potential sensitivity of rapidly dividing myeloid cells to chemotherapy. G-CSF may stimulate the proliferation of rapidly dividing cells, which may be destroyed by chemotherapy drugs.

G-CSF causes a transient increase in neutrophil counts 1 to 2 days after initiation of therapy. To achieve a sustained therapeutic response, however, G-CSF therapy should be continued until postchemotherapy nadir ANC is 10,000/mm^3. Premature discontinuation of G-CSF therapy before expected ANC recovery is not recommended.

SIDE EFFECTS AND ADVERSE REACTIONS

The side effects of filgrastim therapy include nausea, vomiting, skeletal pain, alopecia, diarrhea, neutropenia, fever, mucositis, fatigue, anorexia, dyspnea, headache, cough, skin rash, chest pain, generalized weakness, sore throat, stomatitis, constipation, and pain of unspecified origin. Of these reactions, bone pain was the only consistently observed reaction attributed to G-CSF therapy. The bone pain was of mild to moderate severity and well controlled with nonnarcotic analgesia. It was more frequently seen in clients receiving higher (20 to 100 μg/kg/day) intravenous doses than in clients receiving lower (3 to 10 μg/kg/day) subcutaneous doses.

G-CSF administration has no demonstrable effects on fertility in male and female rats. Its carcinogenic potential is not known. Caution should be used when G-CSF is given to pregnant women and nursing mothers. The manufacturer recommends that the benefits justify the potential risks.

Filgrastim's efficacy has not been demonstrated in children, although safety data indicate that it does not cause any greater toxicity in children than adults.

There has been no evidence of other drug interaction with filgrastim, but its administration is contraindicated in clients with known hypersensitivity to *Escherichia coli* derivant proteins.

Neupogen is supplied as 1-mL vials containing 300 μg of filgrastim or as 1.6-mL vials containing 480 μg of filgrastim. Both vials are preservative-free, and, therefore, the manufacturer recommends the vi-

Chart 34–2. Granulocyte Colony-Stimulating Factor

FILGRASTIM

Assessment and Planning

Drug Name

Filgrastim
   (Neupogen)
Granulocyte colony-stimulating factor
(G-CSF)
Pregnancy Category: C

Contraindications

Hypersensitivity to *Escherichia coli*–derived proteins; 24 h before or after cytotoxic chemotherapy
Caution: Pregnancy, lactation; safety in children not known

Dosage

A: IV inf/SC: 5 μg/kg/d
C: 5–10 μg/kg/d
Refer to specific protocols.

Drug-Lab-Food Interactions

Drug: None known
Lab: *Increase* lactic acid, LDH, alkaline phosphatase; transient *increase* in neutrophils

Interventions

Pharmacokinetics

Absorption: SC: Well absorbed
Distribution: PB: UK
Metabolism: t½: 2–3.5 h
Excretion: Probably in urine

Pharmacodynamics

IV/SC: Onset: 24 h
       Peak: 3–5 d
       Duration: 4–7 d

Evaluation

NURSING PROCESS

Therapeutic Effects/Uses

To decrease incidence of infection in clients receiving myelosuppressive chemotherapeutic agents; adjunct to chemotherapy for both solid tumor and hematologic malignancies.

Mode of Action: Increases production of neutrophils and enhances their phagocytosis.

Side Effects

Nausea, vomiting, skeletal pain, alopecia, diarrhea, fever, skin rash, anorexia, headache, cough, chest pain, sore throat, constipation

Adverse Reactions

Neutropenia, dyspnea, splenomegaly, psoriasis, hematuria
Life-threatening: Thrombocytopenia, myocardial infarction, adult respiratory distress syndrome in clients with sepsis

KEY: A: adult; C: child; IV: intravenous; UK: unknown; SC: subcutaneous; PB: protein-binding; t½: half-life; LDH: lactate dehydrogenase.

als be used one time only and that any vial left at room temperature for longer than 6 h should be discarded. Filgrastim should be stored in a refrigerator at 2°C to 8°C. Freezing and shaking of the vials should be avoided.

Granulocyte Macrophage Colony-Stimulating Factor

Granulocyte macrophage colony-stimulating factor (GM-CSF) belongs to a group of growth factors that support survival, clonal expression, and differentia-
tion (maturation) of hematopoietic progenitor cells. GM-CSF induces partially committed progenitor (parent) cells to divide and differentiate in the granulocyte macrophage (a type of WBC responsible for recognizing and destroying bacteria through phagocytosis) pathway. GM-CSF, unlike G-CSF, is a multilineage factor, promoting proliferation of myelomonocytic, megakaryocytic, and erythroid progenitors. Activated T cells, endothelial cells, and fibroblasts produce GM-CSF in vivo. Commercial production of GM-CSF is accomplished through recombinant DNA technology. GM-CSF is FDA approved for commercial use to induce and support myeloid reconstitution

Chart 34–3. Granulocyte Macrophage Colony-Stimulating Factor

SARGRAMOSTIM

Drug Name

Sargramostim
  (Leukine)
Granulocyte macrophage colony-stimulating factor (GM-CSF)
Pregnancy Category: C

Contraindications

Within 24 h of chemotherapy administration or within 12 h after last dose of radiation therapy, excessive leukemia myeloid blast cells in bone marrow, hypersensitivity to GM-CSF, yeast-derived products
Caution: Pregnancy, lactation, congestive heart failure; safety in children not established; not FDA approved for children

Dosage

A: IV 250 μg/m^2/d as a 2-h inf for 21 d after autologous BMT; a maximum tolerated dose has not been determined
Some protocols use SC administration.

Drug-Lab-Food Interactions

Lithium and steroids may *increase* effect
Lab: *Increase* in WBC and platelet counts

Pharmacokinetics

Absorption: IV: Essentially complete
Distribution: PB: UK
Metabolism: t½: 2 h
Excretion: Probably in urine

Pharmacodynamics

IV: Onset: 7–14 d
  Peak: UK
  Duration: Baseline WBC by 1 wk after administration

Therapeutic Effects/Uses

To accelerate growth and development of bone marrow and circulating blood cell activity in autologous BMT.

Mode of Action: Increased production and functional activity of eosinophils, macrophages, monocytes, and neutrophils.

Side Effects

Generally well tolerated; diarrhea, fatigue, chills, weakness, local irritation at injection site; peripheral edema, rash

Adverse Reactions

Pleural/pericardial effusion, rigors, GI hemorrhage, dyspnea

Assessment and Planning / Interventions / Evaluation — NURSING PROCESS

KEY: A: adult; IV: intravenous; UK: unknown; PB: protein-binding; t½: half-life; GI: gastrointestinal; BMT: bone marrow transplant; SC: subcutaneous; inf: infusion; FDA: Food and Drug Administration; WBC: white blood cell.

after autologous bone marrow transplant (BMT). Chart 34–3 presents the drug-data for GM-CSF (sargramostim).

PHARMACOKINETICS

GM-CSF has been found to effectively accelerate myeloid engraftment (growth and development of bone marrow and subsequent circulating blood cell activity) in autologous BMT. After autologous BMT in clients with non-Hodgkin's lymphoma, acute lymphoblastic leukemia, or Hodgkin's disease, GM-CSF administration resulted in accelerated myeloid engraftment, decreased duration of antibiotic use, reduced duration of infectious episodes, and shortened hospitalizations.

A GM-CSF product is commercially available as sargramostim: Leukine.

The recommended dose of GM-CSF is 250 μg/m^2/day for 21 days as a 2-h infusion beginning 2 to 4 h after autologous bone marrow infusion.

GM-CSF should not be administered within 24 h of chemotherapy administration or within 12 h after the last dose of radiation therapy. Manufacturers recommend dose reduction or discontinuation in the presence of a severe adverse reaction, blast cell (immature, possibly malignant cell) appearance, or underlying disease progression. GM-CSF therapy should be stopped if ANC is greater than 20,000 cells/mm^3 to avoid potential complications associated with leukocytosis.

SIDE EFFECTS AND ADVERSE REACTIONS

Side effects of GM-CSF administration include fever, mucous membrane disorder, asthenia, malaise, sepsis, nausea, diarrhea, vomiting, anorexia, liver damage, alopecia, rash, peripheral edema, dyspnea, blood dyscracias, renal dysfunction, and central nervous system disorder. GM-CSF should be administered with caution to clients with preexisting pleural or precardial effusions because it may increase fluid retention. Sequestration of granulocytes in the pulmonary circulation has been seen with GM-CSF administration. The phenomenon has resulted in dyspnea and suggests that special attention be given to respiratory symptoms during or immediately following GM-CSF infusions, a caution that is especially important for clients with underlying pulmonary disease. If dyspnea occurs, the GM-CSF infusion should be reduced by half or discontinued.

Supraventricular dysrhythmia has been observed during GM-CSF infusion, suggesting cautious administration in clients with preexisting cardiac disease. Renal and hepatic dysfunction, as indicated by elevated serum creatinine, bilirubin, and liver function tests, have occurred with GM-CSF administration. If these values become elevated, GM-CSF dosage should be reduced or therapy interrupted.

GM-CSF therapy is contraindicated in clients with excessive leukemia myeloid blast cells in the bone marrow or peripheral blood (> 10%), or in clients with known hypersensitivity to GM-CSF, yeast-derived products, or any component of the product. Because of the sensitivity of rapidly dividing hematopoietic progenitor cells to cytotoxic chemotherapy or radiologic therapy, GM-CSF should not be administered within 24 h preceding or following chemotherapy or within 12 h preceding or following radiation therapy.

GM-CSF should be administered to pregnant women or nursing mothers only if clearly indicated; that is, if the benefits outweigh the risks. Efficacy in the pediatric population has not been established.

Carcinogenic, mutagenic, or fertility effects have not been determined. Full evaluation of drug interactions have not been conducted; however, drugs that may potentiate the myeloproliferative effects of GM-CSF, such as lithium and corticosteroids, should be used with caution.

Leukine is supplied as a sterile, white, preservative-free lyophilized powder (powder that goes into solution quickly) in vials containing 250 μg or 500 μg of sargramostim. The powder is reconstituted with 1 mL of sterile water for injection. During reconstitution, the diluent should be directed at the side of the vial and contents gently swirled but not shaken. Further dilution with 0.9% sodium chloride only is performed in preparation for the 2-h intravenous infusion. The final concentration of solution should be greater than 10 μg/mL. The infusion should be completed within 6 h of preparation to ensure stability and potency. Sargramostim powder, reconstituted vials, and diluted solution should be refrigerated at 2°C to 8°C.

NEUMEGA (OPRELVEKIN)

Neumega is recombinant human interleukin-11, which is a platelet growth factor. This product, manufactured by Genetics Institute, can potentially prevent recurrent severe chemotherapy-induced thrombocytopenia. The active ingredient of Neumega is oprelvekin. Oprelvekin, according to the manufacturer, stimulates megakaryocyte and thrombocyte production. This effect results in functionally and morphologically normal circulating platelets. Neumega is advertised to be "a much needed option in patients who are receiving myelosuppressive chemotherapy." The reasons for this claim are twofold: (1) with the use of this product, chemotherapy administration does not have to be delayed because of a low platelet count, and (2) the need for potentially risk-associated platelet transfusions is reduced. Neumega, therefore, is indicated for the prevention of severe thrombocytopenia and the reduction of the need for platelet transfusions following myelosuppressive chemotherapy. Efficacy was most evident in those who had experienced severe thrombocytopenia following the previous chemotherapy cycle.

Pharmacokinetics

Neumega is available for subcutaneous administration in single-use vials containing 5 mg of oprelvekin as a sterile, lyophilized powder. When reconstituted with 1 mL of sterile water for injection, the resulting solution has a pH of 7.0 and a concentration of 5 mg/mL.

Product dosing should begin 6 to 24 h after the completion of chemotherapy. Studies have shown that daily subcutaneous dosing for 14 days increased the platelet count in a dose-dependent way. Platelet counts begin to increase between 5 and 9 days after the start of the Neumega administration. After the product was stopped, platelet counts continued to increase for up to 7 days and then returned to baseline within 14 days.

Animal studies have demonstrated that Neumega is rapidly cleared from the serum and distributed to highly perfused organs. The kidney is the primary route of elimination, although most of the product is metabolized before excretion. Neumega is contraindicated in clients with a history of hypersensitivity to the product or any of its components.

Side Effects and Adverse Reactions

The side effects of Neumega include fluid retention, cardiovascular events, ophthalmologic events, and allergic reactions. Mild to moderate fluid retention without weight gain resulted from product administration. Fluid retention, reversible within several days of product discontinuation, was manifested by peripheral edema, exertional dyspnea, and worsening of preexisting pleural effusions, ascites, and pericardial effusions. Transient atrial arrhythmias (fibrillation or flutter) have occurred in approximately 10% of clients. These arrhythmias may be related to fluid retention, advanced age, or underlying cardiac disease. Papilledema and transient visual blurring have been reported in about 1.5%. The only reported allergic reaction has been a transient rash at the injection site. There have been no reports of anaphylaxis or hypersensitivity reactions.

Drug interactions between Neumega and other medications have not been fully evaluated. No studies have been done to assess the carcinogenic potential of the product. There are no studies to determine its use in children or in pregnant or nursing mothers; its use in these situations should be carefully evaluated.

Dosing and Administration

The recommended dose of Neumega in adults is 50 μg/kg given once daily. It should be administered subcutaneously as a single injection in the thigh, abdomen, hip, or upper arm. Pediatric dosing (based on a pharmacokinetic study) should be 75 to 100 μg/kg. The first dose of Neumega should be given 6 to 24 h after the completion of chemotherapy. It is recommended that platelet counts be monitored to determine the duration of the Neumega therapy. Administration should continue until the postnadir count is >50,000 cells/μL. Dosing beyond 21 days is not recommended. Neumega should be discontinued at least 2 days before the chemotherapy is begun.

Preparation

Reconstituted Neumega is a clear, colorless, isotonic solution with pH of 7.0. During reconstitution, excessive agitation should be avoided. The sterile water for injection USP should be directed at the side of the vial and the contents gently swirled. A single-dose vial should not be reentered or reused. The parenteral drug products should be visually inspected; if they are discolored or contain particulate matter, they should be discarded.

Neumega should be used within 3 hours of reconstitution if it has been stored at either 2°C to 8°C or at room temperature up to 25°C. Neumega should not be frozen, and the reconstituted product should not be shaken.

Patient Information

Self-administration of Neumega should not be attempted until the client fully understands the health care provider's instructions about its preparation, correct dose, and proper method for injection. The injection site should not be rubbed. Dose should be given at the same time each day. If a dose is missed, the next scheduled dose should be taken.

INTERLEUKINS

Interleukins are a group of proteins that are produced by the body's white blood cells—the lymphocytes. Because interleukins are hormone-like glycoproteins manufactured by the lymphocytes, they are sometimes referred to as lymphokines. One of the most widely studied interleukins is interleukin-2 (IL-2).

This substance, first defined in 1976, has been found to have antitumor activities. The greatest antitumor effect has been identified in those with renal cell cancer or malignant melanoma.

IL-2 is produced commercially through recombinant DNA technology. It is marketed as aldesleukin (Proleukin) for use in the treatment of metastatic renal cell carcinoma.

Pharmacokinetics

IL-2, administered either by IV infusion or subcutaneous injection, is rapidly distributed to the extravascular, extracellular space and eliminated from the body by metabolism in the kidney. The serum half-life of IL-2 is short. Because of this rapid clearance, IL-2 is administered in frequent, short infusions.

Preparation

Proleukin is supplied in single-use vials, each of which contains 22×10^6 units of Proleukin. Unreconstituted vials should be stored in a refrigerator at 2°C to 8°C (36°F to 46°F). When reconstituted aseptically with 1.2 mL of sterile water for injection, each vial contains 18 million IU (1.1 mg) of Proleukin. Bacteriostatic water should not be used. The sterile water should be injected into the vial. The contents should be gently swirled, not shaken. The resulting solution should be a clear, colorless to pale yellow liquid. Any unused portion of the liquid should be discarded. The indicated dose of Proleukin should be withdrawn from the vial and diluted into a 50-mL 5% dextrose IV bag. The IV bag, if not used immediately, can be stored for 48 hours in a refrigerator. The Proleukin should be infused over a 15-min period through nonfiltered IV tubing. See Table 34–3 for dosage and administration information.

Side Effects and Adverse Reactions

The side effects most frequently reported as a result of IL-2 include hypotension, nausea, vomiting, diarrhea, mental status changes, oliguria/anuria, anemia, thrombocytopenia, fever, chills, sinus tachycardia, pulmonary congestion, dyspnea, pain at injection site, fatigue, weakness, malaise, and elevated liver function tests. See Table 34–4 for additional side effects. According to the manufacturer, Proleukin should be permanently discontinued for certain organ system toxicities (Table 34–5) and held and restarted under specific parameters for other toxicities (Table 34–6).

MONOCLONAL ANTIBODY

Trastuzumab (Herceptin) is a recombinant humanized monoclonal antibody approved by the FDA for solo treatment of metastatic breast cancer in clients whose condition is refractory to chemotherapy or in combination with paclitaxel (Taxol) for first-line treatment of metastatic breast cancer. The drug is specifically for clients with tumors that overexpress the HER2 protein found in 25% to 30% of those with metastatic breast cancer. HER2 is structurally similar to the epidermal growth factor receptor.

The metabolism and elimination of trastuzumab is unknown. Following IV infusion, the half-life is dose dependent; the half-life is about six days with a weekly maintenance dose of 2 mg/kg. The initial dose is 4 mg/kg IV over 1½ hours followed by weekly maintenance doses of 2 mg/kg over ½ hour. Estimated cost for 23 weeks of treatment for a 120-pound woman is about $14,000.

Trastuzumab can be cardiotoxic; risk of this is increased in older clients, in those with previous cardiac disease, and in those with previous exposure to an anthracycline. A flu-like symptom complex (fever, chills, nausea, vomiting, headache, asthenia, and pain) occurs in about 40% of the clients after first and sometimes later infusions. However, trastuzumab does not cause myelosuppression or alopecia.

Table 34–3 Interleukin		
DRUG	**DOSAGE**	**USES AND CONSIDERATIONS**
Interleukin-2 (Proleukin)	*Metastatic renal cancer:* A: IV: 600,000 IU/kg (0.037 mg/kg) by a 15-min IV infusion q8h for a total of 14 doses. Following 9 days of rest, the schedule is repeated for another 14 doses, for a maximum of 28 doses per course	For treating metastatic renal cancer.
	Renal cancer studies: 18 million IU/m²/d for 5 days, followed by 2 days rest, then 9 million or 18 million IU/m²/d, 5 d/wk, for 5 wk	This dosage schedule and route have also been used in renal cancer studies.
	PATIENTS RECEIVING IL-2 BY ANY ROUTE IN ANY DOSE, AND IN ANY SETTING— INPATIENT AND/OR OUTPATIENT—SHOULD BE MONITORED CLOSELY FOR SIGNS OF TOXICITY.	

KEY: A: adult; IV: intravenous; m²: square meter of body surface area.

Table 34–4
Incidence of Adverse Events to Interleukin-2

EVENTS BY BODY SYSTEM	% OF PATIENTS	EVENTS BY BODY SYSTEM	% OF PATIENTS
Cardiovascular		**Gastrointestinal**	
Hypotension	85	Nausea and vomiting	87
(requiring pressors)	71	Diarrhea	76
Sinus tachycardia	70	Stomatitis	32
Arrhythmias	22	Anorexia	27
Atrial	8	Gastrointestinal bleeding	13
Supraventricular	5	(requiring surgery)	2
Ventricular	3	Dyspepsia	7
Junctional	1	Constipation	5
Bradycardia	7	Intestinal perforation/ileus	2
Premature ventricular contractions	5	Pancreatitis	<1
Premature atrial contractions	4		
Myocardial ischemia	3	**Neurologic**	
Myocardial infarction	2	Mental status changes	73
Cardiac arrest	2	Dizziness	17
Congestive heart failure	1	Sensory dysfunction	10
Myocarditis	1	Special sensory disorders (vision, speech, taste)	7
Stroke	1	Syncope	3
Gangrene	1	Motor dysfunction	2
Pericardial effusion	1	Coma	1
Endocarditis	1	Seizure (grand mal)	1
Thrombosis	1		

Source: Proleukin: Aldesleukin for Injection: Cetus/Chiron Corp., Emeryville, CA. Printed with permission.

Table 34–5
Organ System Toxicities with Interleukin-2

ORGAN SYSTEM	PERMANENTLY DISCONTINUE TREATMENT FOR THE FOLLOWING TOXICITIES
Cardiovascular	Sustained ventricular tachycardia (≥5 beats)
	Cardiac rhythm disturbances not controlled or unresponsive to management
	Recurrent chest pain with electrocardiographic changes, documented angina or myocardial infarction
	Pericardial tamponade
Pulmonary	Intubation required >72 h
Renal	Renal dysfunction requiring dialysis >72 h
Central nervous system	Coma or toxic psychosis lasting >48 h
	Repetitive or difficult to control seizures
Gastrointestinal	Bowel ischemia/perforation/gastrointestinal bleeding requiring surgery

Source: Proleukin: Aldesleukin for Injection. Cetus/Chiron Corp., Emeryville, CA. Printed with permission.

Table 34–6
Interleukin-2 Dose Held and Given, Listed According to Organ System

ORGAN SYSTEM	HOLD DOSE FOR	SUBSEQUENT DOSES MAY BE GIVEN IF
Cardiovascular	Atrial fibrillation, supraventricular tachycardia, or bradycardia that requires treatment or is recurrent or persistent	Client is asymptomatic with full recovery to normal sinus rhythm
	Systolic bp <90 mmHg with increasing requirements for pressors	Systolic bp ≥90 mmHg and stable or improving requirements for pressors
	Any ECG change consistent with MI or ischemia with or without chest pain; suspicion of cardiac ischemia	Client is asymptomatic, MI has been ruled out, clinical suspicion of angina is low
Pulmonary	O_2 saturation <94% on room air or <90% with 2 L O_2 by nasal prongs	O_2 saturation ≥94% on room air or ≥90% with 2 L O_2 by nasal prongs
Central nervous system	Mental status changes, including moderate confusion or agitation	Mental status changes completely resolved
Systemic	Sepsis syndrome, client is clinically unstable	Sepsis syndrome has resolved, client is clinically stable, infection is under treatment
Renal	Serum creatinine ≥4.5 mg/dL or a serum creatinine of 4 mg/dL in the presence of severe volume overload, acidosis, or hyperkalemia	Serum creatinine <4 mg/dL and fluid and electrolyte status is stable
	Persistent oliguria, urine output of ≤10 mL/hour for 16 to 24 hours with rising serum creatinine	Urine output >10 mL/hour with a decrease of serum creatinine ≥1.5 mg/dL or normalization of serum creatinine
Hepatic	Signs of hepatic failure including encephalopathy, increasing ascites, liver pain, hypoglycemia	All signs of hepatic failure have resolved*
Gastrointestinal	Stool guaiac repeatedly >3–4 +	Stool guaiac negative
Skin	Bullous dermatitis or marked worsening of preexisting skin condition (avoid topical steroid therapy)	Resolution of all signs of bullous dermatitis

KEY: bp: blood pressure; ECG: electrocardiographic; MI: myocardial infarction; >: greater than; ≥: equal to or greater than; <: less than.
* Discontinue all further treatment for that course. Consider starting a new course of treatment at least 7 weeks after cessation of adverse event and hospital discharge.
Source: Proleukin: Aldesleukin for Injection. Cetus/Chiron Corp., Emeryville, CA. Printed with permission.

SUMMARY

BRM therapy is in its infancy. As clinical trial results yield more information about BRM activity and clinical efficacy, the indications for the use of BRMs will expand. As more is learned about the effect of BRMs on the quality of client life, attention will be directed toward side effect management and symptom prevention. Nurses play a key role in both the identification and management of BRM-related toxicities. Through assessment of clients receiving BRMs and a knowledge of BRM activity, nurses can develop a plan of care that will result in clients receiving BRM therapy in a safe and comfortable manner.

Text continued on page 615

NURSING PROCESS
BIOLOGIC RESPONSE MODIFIERS

Assessment

- Obtain baseline information about the client's physical status, including height, weight, vital signs (VS), laboratory values (CBC, uric acid, electrolytes, BUN, creatinine, and liver function tests), cardiopulmonary assessment, intake and output, skin assessment, daily activities status (ability to perform activities of daily living, sleep-rest cycle), nutritional status, presence or absence of underlying symptoms of disease, and the use of current or past medication and treatment.
- Assess CBC (with filgrastim, sargramostim, and Neumega) before therapy and biweekly throughout therapy to avoid leukocytosis and thrombocytosis. Assess renal and hepatic function tests in clients with dysfunction (liver enzymes, BUN, serum creatinine). With erythropoietin, assess blood pressure before start and especially early in therapy. Most clients will need supplemental iron. Desired levels are >100 ng/mL for serum ferritin and >20% for serum iron transferrin saturation.
- Obtain baseline data regarding the client's psychosocial status, including educational level, ability and desire to learn, support systems, past coping strategies, presence or absence of emotional difficulties, and self-care abilities.
- Assess the client for signs and symptoms of biologic response modifiers (BRM), such as fatigue, chills, diarrhea, and weakness. With filgrastim, be alert to changes in clients with preexisting cardiac conditions.
- Assess the client's and family's ability to administer subcutaneous BRM.
- Determine the client's and family's understanding of BRM and related side effects.

Potential Nursing Diagnoses

- Altered nutrition; less than body requirements
- High risk for infection
- High risk for fluid volume deficit
- Altered oral mucous membrane
- Fatigue
- Body image disturbance
- Anxiety
- Fear
- High risk for caregiver role strain

Planning

- Client and family will verbalize an understanding of the importance of reporting BRM-related side effects.
- Client and family will demonstrate correct and safe BRM administration.
- Client and family will identify strategies to deal with BRM-related side effects.
- Client will remain free of infection (filgrastim and sargramostim).
- Client will remain free of hemorrhage.

Nursing Interventions

- Monitor the client's temperature at the onset of chills.
- Administer prescribed meperidine 25 to 50 mg IV to decrease rigors.
- Premedicate the client with acetaminophen to reduce chills and fever and with diphenhydramine to reduce nausea.
- Cover the client with blankets to promote warmth during chills.
- Encourage the client to rest when tired and to notify health care provider if profound fatigue or anorexia occurs.

Nursing Process continued on following page

Encourage the client to drink at least 2 L of fluid a day to promote excretion of cellular breakdown products.
- Administer antiemetic as necessary. Premedicate the client with antiemetic and administer antiemetic around the clock for 24 h after BRM administration to further delay nausea or vomiting.
- Consult the dietitian, social worker, and physical or occupational therapist as necessary.
- Provide the client and family the opportunity to discuss the effect of BRM therapy on the quality of life.
- Refer the client and family to a financial counselor if reimbursement of BRM therapy is problematic.
- Administer BRM at bedtime to decrease the consequences of fatigue.
- Continue with the same brand of BRM, and notify the health care provider if you are considering changing the brand.
- Remember, with sargramostim, use only one dose per vial; be alert for expiration date. Avoid shaking vial. Reconstituted solutions are clear; use within 6 h and discard unused portion. Recall that albumin may be added, depending on drug concentration, to prevent adsorption of drug to components of the drug delivery system.
- Remember, with filgrastim, drug vials are for one-time use; any vial left at room temperature for more than 6 h should be discarded. Drug vials are preservative free. Store in refrigerator at 2°C to 8°C. Avoid shaking vials.
- Remember, with Neumega, avoid excessive agitation during preparation. Use only one dose per vial. Inspect the parenteral product and discard if it is discolored or has particulate matter. Use within 3 h of reconstitution if stored at 2°C to 8°C. Avoid freezing or shaking the drug.

Client Teaching

General
- Explain to the client and family the rationale for BRM therapy.
- Explain the frequency and rationale for studies and procedures during BRM therapy.
- Inform the client and family that most BRM side effects disappear within 72 to 96 h after discontinuation of therapy.
- Instruct clients of childbearing age to use contraceptives during BRM therapy and for 2 y after completion of therapy.
- Provide the client with information regarding the effect on sexuality of BRM-related fatigue.

Side Effects
- Advise the client to report episodes of difficulty in concentration, confusion, or somnolence.
- Report weight loss.
- Report dyspnea, palpitations, and signs of infection or bleeding.

Self Administration
- Demonstrate correct drug administration techniques.
- Provide the client and family with written or video instructions regarding BRM self-administration.

Evaluation

- Evaluate the client's and family's education strategies by asking them to discuss the potential effect of BRM therapy on the quality of life.
- Evaluate the client's and family's BRM self-administration technique.
- Evaluate periodically the client's and family's management of BRM-related side effects.
- There will be a decreased incidence of infection in clients after autologous bone marrow transplantation.
- There will be a decreased incidence of thrombocytopenia in clients after chemotherapy administration.

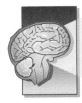

Critical Thinking in Action

J. W. is a 55-year-old man with metastatic non–small cell cancer of the lung. His past treatment regimen included external-beam chest irradiation and combination chemotherapy. Two weeks before hospitalization, J. W. received a course of carboplatin, Velban, and methotrexate as an outpatient. He was admitted to the hospital with neutropenia, **thrombocytopenia,** and anemia. Upon assessment J. W. was cachectic, weak, and able to perform activities of daily living only with assistance. Admitting laboratory data were Hgb (hemoglobin) 6.9; Hct 20.6; platelets 16,000; and WBC 600 with ANC of 96. J. W. was started on Neupogen, 480 μg SC daily; EPO, 10,000 U SC every other day; and Neumega, 50 μg/kg SC daily. Parenteral antibiotic therapy was also initiated. Nursing diagnoses for J. W. included a potential for infection related to neutropenia, fatigue related to anemia, and anxiety related to hospitalization.

Nursing interventions included

1. Maintaining good handwashing before and after client contact
2. Allowing no one with cold or infection to enter client's room
3. Obtaining vital signs and pulmonary assessment every 4 h
4. Inspecting all sites associated with a high risk for infection (venipuncture sites, oral cavity, perirectal area) every shift
5. Applying no suppositories, enemas, or urinary catheters and obtaining no rectal temperatures
6. Monitoring laboratory values daily
7. Wearing masks at all times during client contact
8. Providing bedside physical therapy
9. Giving emotional support to client and family
10. Instructing client and family in giving subcutaneous injections and about the signs and symptoms of infection.

J. W. was continued on Neupogen (filgrastim), Neumega (oprelvekin), and erythropoietin (EPO). The following laboratory data were obtained:

Lab Tests	Day 1	Day 2	Day 3	Day 4	Day 5
Hgb	6.9	6.5	7.1	7.8	7.9
Hct	20.6	19.4	21.6	22.9	22.9
Platelets	16,000	15,000	16,000	20,000	30,000
WBC/ANC	600/96	1000/0	1200/168	9400/4700	31500/18270

Neupogen was discontinued on day 5 and antibiotics were discontinued on day 4, but EPO and Neumega were continued. J. W.'s physical therapy was continued in the physical therapy department. Because J. W. refused red blood cell transfusion on the basis of religious beliefs, he was discharged to home (day 5) on EPO, 10,000 U SC every other day, and Neumega, 50 μg/kg SC daily for 7 days.

Mrs. J is a 38-year-old woman with a stage IV breast cancer diagnosed 3 years ago. When first diagnosed, she underwent lumpectomy, axillary node dissection, and breast irradiation. She recently was seen by her medical oncologist with complaints of lower back pain and dyspnea at rest. Magnetic resonance imaging (MRI) identified bone metastasis in the thoracic and lumbar spine, and chest x-ray revealed a large left-sided pleural effusion. Mrs. J. has a history of atrial fibrillation. She is on MS Contin and MSIR for back pain. She is receiving radiation to her lower thoracic and lumbar spine. She has also received two courses of chemotherapy. She tolerated the first course without incident. Ten days after the second course, however, she was seen at the emergency department with shortness of breath, fever, chills, weakness, and a 2-day history of epistaxis and bruising. Laboratory results are Hb 9.5, WBC 1000 with 30% neutrophils, 50% lymphocytes, 5% bands, platelet count 9000. She is admitted to the oncology unit with orders for IV fluid, empiric antibiotics, Neupogen, and Neumega. Mrs. J. is a single mother who lives at home with her two children, a 10-year-old son and a 6-year-old daughter.

1. Why are Neupogen and Neumega indicated? What is the patient's ANC?
2. How would the products be ordered?
3. What are the expected side effects of these agents?
4. Discuss nursing interventions for the patient's hospital stay and post discharge.
5. How long should Neupogen and Neumega be administered?
6. Discuss the use of Herceptin in this client's situation.

Study Questions

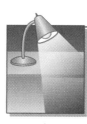

1. Identify the three functions of BRMs.
2. Describe how colony-stimulating factors exert their effect in the body.
3. List the side effects of interferon alpha, G-CSF, GM-CSF, Neumega, interleukin-2, and Herceptin.
4. Discuss client and family teaching strategies for clients receiving erythropoietin.
5. Explain how to administer EPO, G-CSF, Neumega, and GM-CSF.
6. Describe the nursing assessment for clients receiving IL-2 (discussion should include preadministration, administration, and postadministration assessments).

Unit VIII

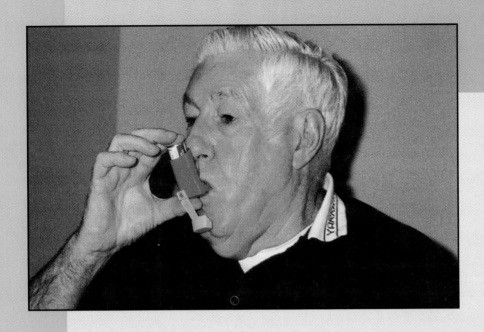

Respiratory Agents

The respiratory tract is divided into two major parts: (1) the upper respiratory tract, which consists of the nares, nasal cavity, pharynx, and larynx, and (2) the lower respiratory tract, which consists of the trachea, bronchi, bronchioles, alveoli, and alveolar-capillary membrane. Air enters through the upper respiratory tract and travels to the lower respiratory tract where gas exchanges take place. Figure VIII–1 illustrates these components.

Ventilation and *respiration* are distinct terms and should not be used interchangeably. **Ventilation** is the movement of air from the atmosphere through the upper and lower airways to the alveoli. **Respiration** is the process whereby gas exchange occurs at the alveolar-capillary membrane.

Respiration has three phases: (1) ventilation, in which oxygen passes through the airways; (2) perfusion, in which blood from the pulmonary circulation is adequate at the alveolar-capillary bed; and (3) diffusion (molecules move from higher concentration to lower concentration) of gases, in which oxygen passes into the capillary bed to be circulated and carbon dioxide leaves the capillary bed and diffuses into the alveoli for ventilatory excretion.

Perfusion is influenced by alveolar pressure. For gas exchange, the perfusion of each alveolus must be matched by adequate ventilation. Factors such as mucosal

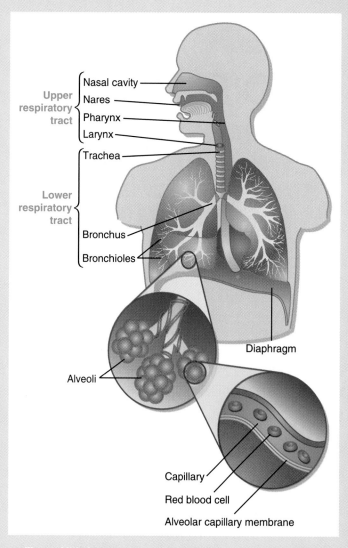

Figure VIII–1
Basic structures of the respiratory tract.

edema, secretions, and bronchospasm increase the resistance to airflow and decrease ventilation and diffusion of gases.

The chest cavity is a closed compartment bounded by 12 ribs, the diaphragm, thoracic vertebrae, sternum, neck muscles, and intercostal muscles between the ribs. The pleura is a membrane that encases the lungs. The lungs are divided into lobes: the right lung has three lobes and the left lung has two lobes. The heart, which is not attached to the lungs, lies on the midleft side in the chest cavity.

LUNG COMPLIANCE

Lung compliance (lung volume based on the unit of pressure in the alveoli) determines the lung's ability to stretch, that is, its tissue elasticity. Lung compliance is determined by (1) connective tissue (collagen and elastin) and (2) surface tension in the alveoli that is controlled by surfactant. Surfactant lowers the surface tension in the alveoli and prevents interstitial fluid from entering. Increased (high) lung compliance is present with chronic obstructive pulmonary disease (COPD), and decreased (low) lung compliance occurs with restrictive pulmonary disease. With low compliance, there is decreased lung volume, resulting from increased connective tissue or increased surface tension; the lungs become "stiff," and it takes greater than normal pressure to expand lung tissue.

CONTROL OF RESPIRATION

Oxygen (O_2), carbon dioxide (CO_2), and hydrogen (H^+) ion concentration in the blood influence respiration. Chemoreceptors are sensors that are stimulated by changes in these gases and ion. The central chemoreceptors, located in the medulla near the respiratory center and cerebrospinal fluid, respond to an increase in CO_2 and a decrease in pH by increasing ventilation. However, if the CO_2 level remains elevated, the stimulus to increase ventilation is lost.

Peripheral chemoreceptors located in the carotid and aortic bodies respond to changes in oxygen (Po_2) levels. A low blood O_2 level ($Po_2 < 60$ mmHg) stimulates the peripheral chemoreceptors, which in turn stimulate the respiratory center in the medulla, and ventilation is increased. If O_2 therapy increases the oxygen level in the blood, the Po_2 may be too high to stimulate the peripheral chemoreceptors, and ventilation will be depressed.

BRONCHIAL SMOOTH MUSCLE

The tracheobronchial tube is composed of smooth muscle whose fibers spiral around the tracheobronchial tube, becoming more closely spaced as they near the terminal bronchioles (Fig. VIII–2). Contraction of these muscles constricts the airway. The sympathetic and parasympathetic nervous systems affect the bronchial smooth muscle in opposite ways. The vagus nerve (parasympathetic nervous system) releases acetylcholine, which causes bronchoconstriction. The sympathetic nervous system releases epinephrine, which stimulates the beta$_2$ receptor in the bronchial smooth muscle, resulting in bronchodilation. These two nervous systems counterbalance each other to maintain homeostasis.

Cyclic adenosine monophosphate (cyclic AMP) in the cytoplasm of bronchial cells increases bronchodilation by relaxing the bronchial smooth muscles. The pulmonary enzyme phosphodiesterase can inactivate cyclic AMP. Drugs of the methylxanthine

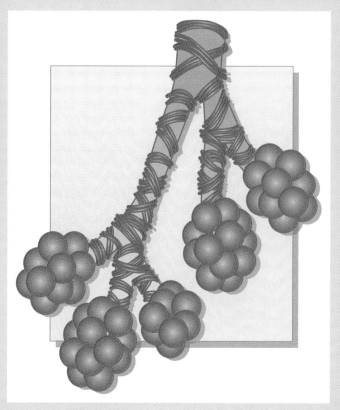

Figure VIII–2
The bronchial smooth muscle fibers become more closely spaced as they near the alveoli.

group (theophylline) inactivate phosphodiesterase, thus permitting cyclic AMP to function.

This unit includes Chapter 35, Drugs for Common Upper Respiratory Infections, and Chapter 36, Drugs for Acute and Chronic Lower Respiratory Disorders. Chapter 35 discusses drugs that are used to relieve cold symptoms, such as antihistamines, decongestants, antitussives, and expectorants. Drugs that are used to alleviate and control airway obstruction are presented in Chapter 36. These include the sympathomimetics (adrenergics), particularly the beta$_2$ adrenergics; the methylxanthines, such as theophylline; glucocorticoids; cromolyn sodium; and mucolytics. Drug charts are included in each chapter, and the nursing process with client teaching is emphasized.

Drugs for Common Upper Respiratory Infections

35

Outline

Objectives

- Define antihistamine, decongestant, antitussive, and expectorant.
- Define rhinitis, sinusitis, pharyngitis, and laryngitis.
- Identify the side effects of nasal decongestants and explain how they can be avoided.
- Describe the nursing process, including client teaching, for drugs used to treat the common cold.

Terms

acute rhinitis

allergic rhinitis

antihistamine

antitussive

common cold

decongestant

expectorant

laryngitis

pharyngitis

rebound nasal congestion

rhinorrhea

sinusitis

tonsillitis

INTRODUCTION

Upper respiratory infections (URIs) include the common cold, acute rhinitis, sinusitis, acute tonsillitis, and acute laryngitis. The common cold is the most prevalent type of URI. Adults have an average of two to four colds per year, and children have an average of four to 12 colds per year. Incidence is seasonally variable, with approximately 50% of the population having a winter cold and 25% having a summer cold. Normally, a cold is not considered to be a life-threatening illness; however, it causes physical and mental discomfort and loss of time at work and school. The common cold is a very expensive illness in the United States: over $500 million is spent each year on over-the-counter (OTC) cold and cough preparations.

COMMON COLD AND ACUTE RHINITIS

The **common cold** is caused by the rhinovirus and affects primarily the nasopharyngeal tract. **Acute rhinitis** (acute inflammation of the mucous membranes of the nose) usually accompanies the common cold. Acute rhinitis is not the same as **allergic rhinitis,** often referred to as "hay fever," which is caused by pollen or a foreign substance such as animal dander. There are increased nasal secretions in both acute rhinitis and allergic rhinitis.

A cold is most contagious 1 to 4 days before the onset of symptoms (the incubation period) and during the first 3 days of the cold. Transmission occurs more frequently from touching contaminated surfaces and then touching the nose or mouth than from viral droplets from sneezing.

There is an old saying, "Curing a cold takes 1 week with treatment or 7 days without treatment." Home remedies include rest, chicken noodle soup, hot toddy (sugar, alcohol, and tea), vitamin C (debatable), and megadoses of vitamins (controversial). The four groups of drugs used to manage cold symptoms are antihistamines (H_1 blocker), decongestants (sympathomimetic amines), antitussives, and expectorants. These drugs can be used singly or in combination preparations.

Symptoms of the common cold include **rhinorrhea** (watery nasal discharge), nasal congestion, cough, and increased mucosal secretions. If a bacterial infection secondary to the cold occurs, infectious rhinitis may result and the nasal discharge becomes tenacious, mucoid, and yellow or yellow-green in color. The nasal secretions are discolored by white blood cells and cellular debris that are byproducts of the fight against the bacterial infection.

Antihistamines

Antihistamines, or H_1 blockers, compete with histamine for receptor sites, thus preventing a histamine response. H_1 blockers are also called histamine antagonists. The two types of histamine receptors, H_1 and H_2, cause different responses. When the H_1 receptor is stimulated, the extravascular smooth muscles, including those lining the nasal cavity, are constricted. With stimulation of the H_2 receptor, an increase in gastric secretions occurs, which is a cause of peptic ulcer (see Chapter 42). These two types of histamine receptors should not be confused. Antihistamines decrease nasopharyngeal secretions by blocking the H_1 receptor.

The anticholinergic properties of most antihistamines cause dryness of the mouth and decreased secretions, making them useful in treating rhinitis caused by the common cold. Antihistamines also decrease the nasal itching and tickling that cause sneezing. Many OTC cold remedies contain an antihistamine, which can cause drowsiness. Clients should be alerted not to drive or operate dangerous machinery if they are taking a medication that contains an antihistamine.

Besides using antihistamines as cold remedies, these agents can be used for treating allergic rhinitis. Examples of antihistamines for allergic rhinitis include astemizole (Hismanal), cetirizine (Zyrtec), loratadine (Claritin), and triprolidine (Actidil). Astemizole has a long half-life that is up to 2.5 days; however, the metabolite of astemizole can extend to 14 days. Cetirizine and loratadine half-lives are between 8 and 15 hours. Astemizole, certirizine, and loratadine have fewer anticholinergic effects than diphenhydramine (Benadryl). Triprolidine has a low incidence of drowsiness.

The antihistamines are not useful in an emergency situation such as anaphylaxis. Most antihistamines are rapidly absorbed in 15 minutes, but they are not potent enough to combat anaphylaxis. The antihistamine diphenhydramine (Benadryl) has been available for years, and it is frequently combined with other ingredients in cold remedy preparations. Its primary use is to treat rhinitis. Chart 35–1 lists the pharmacologic behavior of diphenhydramine.

PHARMACOKINETICS

Diphenhydramine can be administered orally, intramuscularly, or intravenously. It is well absorbed from the gastrointestinal (GI) tract, but systemic absorption from topical use is minimal. It is highly protein-bound (98% to 99%) and has an average half-life of 2 to 7 h. Diphenhydramine is metabolized by the liver and excreted as metabolites in the urine.

Chart 35–1.   Antihistamine

ANTIHISTAMINE

Drug Name

Diphenhydramine HCl (Benadryl), 🍁 Allerdryl
Pregnancy Category: B

Dosage

A: PO: 25–50 mg q6–8h
A: IM/IV: 10–50 mg as single dose, q4–6h;
max: 400 mg/d
C: PO/IM/IV: 5 mg/kg/d in 4 divided doses;
max: 300 mg/d

Contraindications

Acute asthmatic attack, severe liver disease,
lower respiratory disease, neonate; MAOIs
Caution: Narrow-angle glaucoma, benign prostatic hypertrophy, pregnancy, newborn or premature infant, breastfeeding, urinary retention

Drug-Lab-Food Interactions

Drug: *Increase* CNS depression with alcohol,
narcotics, hypnotics, barbiturates; avoid use of
MAOIs

Pharmacokinetics

Absorption: PO: Well absorbed
Distribution: PB: 82%
Metabolism: $t\frac{1}{2}$: 2–7 h
Excretion: In urine as metabolites

Pharmacodynamics

PO: Onset: 15–45 min
    Peak: 1–4 h
    Duration: 4–8 h
IM: Onset: 15–30 min
    Peak: 1–4 h
    Duration: 4–7 h
IV: Onset: Immediate
    Peak: 0.5–1 h
    Duration: 4–7 h

Therapeutic Effects/Uses

To treat allergic rhinitis, itching; to prevent motion sickness; sleep aid; antitussive.

Mode of Action: Blocks histamine, thereby decreasing allergic response. Affects respiratory system,
blood vessels, and GI system.

Side Effects

Drowsiness, dizziness, fatigue, nausea, vomiting, urinary retention, constipation, blurred vision, dry mouth and throat, reduced secretions,
hypotension, epigastric distress, blurred vision,
hearing disturbances; excitation in children;
photosensitivity

Adverse Reactions

Life-threatening: Agranulocytosis, hemolytic
anemia, thrombocytopenia

Assessment and Planning | Interventions | Evaluation | NURSING PROCESS

KEY: A: adult; C: child; PO: by mouth; IM: intramuscular; IV: intravenous; PB: protein-binding; CNS: central nervous system; GI:
gastrointestinal; MAOIs: monoamine oxidase inhibitors; $t\frac{1}{2}$: half-life; 🍁: Canadian drug names.

PHARMACODYNAMICS

Diphenhydramine blocks the effects of histamine by
competing for and occupying H_1 receptor sites. It has
anticholinergic effects and should be avoided by clients with narrow-angle glaucoma. Drowsiness is a
major side effect of the drug, and in fact it has been
used as an ingredient in "sleep aid" products. This
drug is also used as an antitussive (for cough). Its
onset of action can occur in as few as 15 minutes
when taken orally and intramuscularly. The onset of
action is immediate with intravenous use. The duration of action is 4 to 8 h.

Table 35-1
Antihistamines for Treatment of Allergic Rhinitis

GENERIC (BRAND)	ROUTE AND DOSAGE	USES AND CONSIDERATIONS
ANTIHISTAMINES		
Astemizole (Hismanal)	A: PO: 30 mg on day 1; 20 mg on day 2, 10 mg on day 3 and thereafter; take on empty stomach C 6–12 y: PO: 5 mg/d C <6 y: PO: 0.2 mg/kg/d	Treatment of allergic rhinitis and urticaria. Has less anticholinergic effect than diphenhydramine. *Pregnancy category:* C; PB: 96%; $t\frac{1}{2}$: 2.5 d
Cetirizine (Zyrtec)	A: 5–10 mg/d	For allergic rhinitis and urticaria. Has few anticholinergic effects. *Pregnancy category:* C; PB: 93%; $t\frac{1}{2}$: 8 h
Chlorpheniramine maleate (Chlor-Trimeton, Kloromin, Phenetron, Telechlor, Teldrin)	A: PO: 2–4 mg q4–6h; *max:* 24 mg/24 h SR: 8–12 mg q8–12 h C: 6–12 y: PO: 2 mg q4–6h	For allergies including allergic rhinitis. May be in combination with nasal decongestant. *Pregnancy category:* C; PB: 72%; $t\frac{1}{2}$: 20–24 h
Diphenhydramine (Benadryl)	See Chart 35–1	For allergic rhinitis, urticaria, nausea, and vomiting due to motion sickness. May be used as a nighttime sleep aid and as an antitussive drug. *Pregnancy category:* B; PB: 82%; $t\frac{1}{2}$: 2–7 h
Loratadine (Claritin)	A: PO: 10 mg daily	Relief of allergic rhinitis and urticaria. Long-acting H_1 blocking effect. *Pregnancy category:* B; PB: UK; $t\frac{1}{2}$: 12–15 h
Triprolidine HCl (Actidil)	A: PO: 2.5 mg b.i.d. or t.i.d. C 6–12 y: PO: 1.25 mg b.i.d., or t.i.d.	For allergic rhinitis and colds. Low incidence of drowsiness. Has a rapid onset. Duration of action is 12 h. *Pregnancy category:* UK; PB: UK: $t\frac{1}{2}$: UK
PHENOTHIAZINES (ANTI-HISTAMINE ACTION)		
Promethazine HCl (Phenergan, Prometh, Prorex, V-Gan)	A: PO/IM: 12.5–25 mg q4–6h PRN a.c. & h.s.; *max:* 150 mg/d C: PO/IM: 0.5 mg/kg q4–6h Tab & suppository not recommended <2 y; *max:* 18.75 mg/d	For allergies, rhinitis, nausea, vomiting, motion sickness, and adjunct to analgesics for pain. Has a pronounced sedative effect. Avoid alcohol and CNS depressants. *Pregnancy category:* C; PB: UK; $t\frac{1}{2}$: UK
Trimeprazine tartrate (Temaril)	*Non-SR:* A: PO: 2.5 mg q.i.d. C 3–12 y: PO: 2.5 mg t.i.d. C 0.5–3 y: 1.25 mg t.i.d. *SR:* A: PO: 5 mg q12h C >6 y: PO: 5 mg/d	For allergies, rhinitis, and relief of pruritic symptoms. *Pregnancy category:* C; PB: UK; $t\frac{1}{2}$: UK
PIPERAZINE DERIVATIVE		
Hydroxyzine (Atarax, Vistaril)	A: PO: 25–100 mg t.i.d./q.i.d. C >6 y: 50–100 mg/d in divided doses; *For pruritus:* C: <6 y: PO: 50 mg/d in divided doses	For allergies, relief of tension and anxiety, and to prevent nausea and vomiting. Has a pronounced sedative effect. Avoid alcohol and CNS depressants. *Pregnancy category:* C; PB: UK; $t\frac{1}{2}$: 3 h
BUTYROPHENONE DERIVA-TIVE		
Terfenadine (Seldane)	A: PO: 60 mg b.i.d. C >6 y: PO: 30 mg b.i.d. C 3–6 y: PO: 15 mg b.i.d.	Relief of allergic rhinitis (sneezing, red itching eyes, tearing). Give with food. *Pregnancy category:* C; PB: 97%; $t\frac{1}{2}$: 20 h
ETHANOLAMINE DERIVA-TIVE		
Carbinoxamine and pseudoephedrine (Carbiset, Carbodec, Rondec)	A: PO: 5 mL q.i.d. or 1 tab q.i.d. C <18 mo: PO: 0.25–1 mL q.i.d. C 1.5–6 y: PO: 2.5 mL t.i.d./q.i.d. C >6 y: PO: 5 mL b.i.d./q.i.d.	For allergy control. Combination of an antihistamine and decongestant. *Pregnancy category:* C; PB: UK; $t\frac{1}{2}$: 10–20 h

Table continued on following page

Table 35–1 *Continued*
Antihistamines for Treatment of Allergic Rhinitis

GENERIC (BRAND)	ROUTE AND DOSAGE	USES AND CONSIDERATIONS
Clemastine fumarate (Tavist)	A: PO: 1.34–2.68 mg, b.i.d., t.i.d.; *max:* 8 mg/d C <12 y: PO: 0.67–1.34 mg, b.i.d.	For relief of allergic rhinitis and urticaria. *Pregnancy category:* C; PB: UK; $t\frac{1}{2}$: UK
ETHYLENEDIAMINE DERIVATIVE Tripelennamine HCl (Pelamine)	A: PO: 25–50 mg q4–6h or SR: 100 mg q8–12h; *max:* 600 mg/d C: PO: 5 mg/kg/d q 4–6 h in divided doses; *max:* 300 mg/d	For allergies. Has a mild CNS depressant effect. Take with food to decrease GI upset. *Pregnancy category:* B; PB: UK; $t\frac{1}{2}$: UK
PIPERIDINE DERIVATIVES Azatadine maleate (Optimine)	A: PO: 1–2 mg b.i.d., t.i.d. C <12 y: PO: not recommended	Relief of allergic rhinitis and chronic urticaria. Drowsiness, dizziness, and hypotension may occur. *Pregnancy category:* B; PB: UK; $t\frac{1}{2}$: 9–12 h
Cyproheptadine HCl (Periactin)	A: PO: 4–20 mg/d divided q8h; *max:* 0.5 mg/kg/d C >6 y: PO: 4 mg q8–12h; *max:* 16 mg/d C (2–6 y): PO: 2 mg, q8–12 h	For allergies (rhinitis, conjunctivitis, pruritus). Common side effects include drowsiness, dry mouth, dizziness, epigastric distress. *Pregnancy category:* B; PB: UK; $t\frac{1}{2}$: UK
PROPYLAMINE DERIVATIVES Brompheniramine maleate (Bromphen, Dimetane, Histaject, Nasahist B, Oraminic II)	A: PO: 4 mg q4–6h or SR: 8 mg q8–12h; *max:* 24 mg/d IM/IV/SC: 10 mg q8–12h; *max:* 40 mg/d C 6–12 y: PO: 2 mg q4–6h; *max:* 12–16 mg/d	For allergies. Also present in various cough and decongestant formulas. *Pregnancy category:* C; PB: UK; $t\frac{1}{2}$: 25–36 h
Dexchlorpheniramine maleate (Dexchlor, Poladex, Polaramine)	A: PO: 2 mg q4–6h or SR: 4–6 mg q8–12h or h.s. C >6 y: PO: 1 mg q4–6h or SR: 4 mg h.s.	Relief of allergic rhinitis. May be used with epinephrine to treat anaphylactic reaction. *Pregnancy category:* B; PB: UK; $t\frac{1}{2}$: UK
Triprolidine and pseudoephedrine (Actifed)	A: PO: 1 tab, q4–6h; *max:* 4 tab/d C >6 y: PO: $\frac{1}{2}$ tab q6–8h; *max:* 2 tab/d	For rhinitis. A combination of an antihistamine and decongestant. *Pregnancy category:* B; PB: UK; $t\frac{1}{2}$: 3 h
Triprolidine HCl (Alleract, Myidyl)	A: PO: 2.5 mg q6–8h; *max:* 10 mg/d C 6–12 y: PO: 1.25 mg q6–8h; *max:* 5 mg/d C 2–5 y: PO: 0.6 mg t.i.d./q.i.d.; *max:* 2.5 mg/d C 4 mo–2 y: PO: 0.3 mg t.i.d./q.i.d.; *max:* 1.25 mg/d	For allergies. Similar effects as other antihistamines. *Pregnancy category:* C; PB: UK; $t\frac{1}{2}$: UK
OTHER Cromolyn sodium (Intal)	*Prophylaxis bronchial asthma:* A&C >5 y: Inhal: 2 metered sprays or PO: 20 mg ≤1 h before exercise *Allergic rhinitis:* A&C >5 y: 1 spray per nostril t.i.d./q.i.d.; *max:* 6 per day	For treatment of allergic rhinitis, bronchial asthma, and prevention of bronchospasm. It is *not* an antihistamine. *Pregnancy category:* B; PB: UK; $t\frac{1}{2}$: 1.5 h
MISCELLANEOUS Methdilazine HCl (Tacaryl)	A: PO: 8 mg b.i.d./q.i.d. C >3 y: PO: 4 mg b.i.d./q.i.d.	For allergies and pruritus. *Pregnancy category:* B; PB: UK; $t\frac{1}{2}$: UK

KEY: A: adult; C: child; PO: by mouth; SC: subcutaneous; IM: intramuscular; IV: intravenous; >: greater than; <: less than; UK: unknown; PB: protein-binding; $t\frac{1}{2}$: half-life; SR: sustained-release; tab: tablet; CNS: central nervous system; inhal: inhaler.

NURSING PROCESS
ANTIHISTAMINE: DIPHENHYDRAMINE

Assessment

- Obtain baseline vital signs (VS).
- Obtain drug history; report if drug-drug interaction is probable.
- Assess for signs and symptoms of urinary dysfunction, including retention, dysuria, and frequency.
- Assess complete blood count (CBC) during drug therapy.
- Assess cardiac and respiratory status.
- If allergic reaction, obtain history of environmental exposures, drugs, recent foods, and stress.

Potential Nursing Diagnoses

- Fluid volume deficit, potential
- Sleep pattern disturbance

Planning

- Client will have improvement of histamine-associated (allergy) effects.
- Client will have improved sleep, if used as a sleep aid.

Nursing Interventions

- Give with food to decrease gastric distress.
- Administer IM in large muscle. Avoid SC injection.

Client Teaching

General
- Instruct client to avoid driving a motor vehicle and other dangerous activities if drowsiness occurs or until stabilized on drug.
- Avoid alcohol and other CNS depressants.
- Instruct client to take drug as prescribed. Notify health care provider if confusion or hypotension occurs.
- For prophylaxis of motion sickness, take drug at least 30 min before offending event and then before meals and h.s. during the event.
- Inform the breast-feeding mother that small amounts of drug pass into the breast milk. Because children are more susceptible to the side effects of antihistamines, such as unusual excitement or irritability, breastfeeding is not recommended while on these drugs.

Side Effects
- Instruct family members or parents that children are more sensitive to the effects of antihistamines; nightmares, nervousness, and irritability are more likely to occur.
- Inform older adults that they are more sensitive to the effects of antihistamines. Confusion, difficult or painful urination, dizziness, drowsiness, feeling faint, and dryness of the mouth, nose, or throat are more likely to occur in the older client.
- For temporary relief of mouth dryness, suggest using sugarless candy or gum, ice chips, or using a saliva substitute.

Evaluation

- Evaluate effectiveness of drug in relieving allergic symptoms or as a sleep aid.

Diphenhydramine can cause central nervous system depression if taken with alcohol, narcotics, hypnotics, or barbiturates.

Table 35–1 lists selected antihistamines or antihistamine-like agents that are useful for treating rhinitis.

SIDE EFFECTS AND ADVERSE REACTIONS

The most common side effects are drowsiness, dizziness, fatigue, and disturbed coordination. Skin rashes and anticholinergic symptoms, such as dry mouth, urine retention, blurred vision, and wheezing, may be seen.

Nasal and Systemic Decongestants

Nasal congestion results from dilation of nasal blood vessels due to infection, inflammation, or allergy. With this dilation, there is a transudation of fluid into the tissue spaces, resulting in swelling of the nasal cavity. Nasal **decongestants** (sympathomimetic amines) stimulate the alpha-adrenergic receptors, thus producing vascular constriction (vasoconstriction) of the capillaries within the nasal mucosa. The result is shrinking of the nasal mucous membranes and a reduction in fluid secretion (runny nose).

Nasal decongestants are administered by nasal spray or drops or in tablet, capsule, or liquid form. Frequent use of decongestants, especially nasal spray or drops, can result in tolerance and **rebound nasal congestion** (rebound vasodilation instead of vasoconstriction). The rebound nasal congestion is caused by irritation of the nasal mucosa.

The systemic decongestants (alpha-adrenergic agonists) are available in tablet, capsule, and liquid forms and are primarily used for allergic rhinitis, including hay fever, and acute coryza (profuse nasal discharge). Examples of systemic decongestants are ephedrine, phenylpropanolamine, phenylephrine, and pseudoephedrine. These agents are frequently combined with an antihistamine, analgesic, or antitussive in oral cold remedies. The advantage of systemic decongestants is that they relieve nasal congestion for a longer period of time than the nasal decongestants; however, currently, there are long-acting nasal decongestants. The nasal decongestants usually act promptly and cause fewer side effects than the systemic decongestants. Table 35–2 lists drugs, dosages, and uses and considerations of systemic and nasal decongestants.

SIDE EFFECTS AND ADVERSE REACTIONS

The incidence of side effects is low with use of topical preparations such as nose drops. Decongestants can make a client jittery, nervous, or restless. These side effects decrease or disappear as the body adjusts to the drug.

Usage of nasal decongestants longer than 5 days could result in rebound nasal congestion. Instead of the nasal membranes constricting, vasodilation occurs, causing increased stuffy nose and nasal congestion. The nurse should emphasize the importance of limiting the use of nasal sprays and drops.

As with any alpha-adrenergic drug (e.g., decongestants), blood pressure and blood glucose levels can increase. These drugs are contraindicated or to be used with extreme caution for clients having hypertension, cardiac disease, hyperthyroidism, and diabetes mellitus.

DRUG INTERACTIONS

When using decongestants with other drugs, drug interactions can occur. Pseudoephedrine may decrease the effect of beta blockers. Taking monoamine oxidase (MAO) inhibitors may increase the possibility of hypertension or cardiac dysrhythmias. The client should also stay away from caffeine (coffee, tea) in large amounts because it can increase the restlessness and palpitations caused by decongestants.

Intranasal Glucocorticoids

Intranasal glucocorticoids or steroids are effective for treating allergic rhinitis. Because these agents are steroids, they have an antiinflammatory action, thus decreasing the allergic rhinitis symptoms of rhinorrhea, sneezing, and congestion. There are six examples of intranasal steroids: beclomethasone (Beconase, Vancenase, Vanceril), budesonide (Rhinocort), dexamethasone (Decadron), flunisolide (Nasalide), fluticasone (Flonase), and triamcinolone (Nasacort). These drugs may be used alone or in combination with H_1 antihistamine. With continuous use, dryness of the nasal mucosa may occur.

It is rare for systemic effects of the steroids to occur; however, it is more likely for systemic effects to result with the use of intransal dexamethasone, which should not be used for longer than 30 days. The other intranasal glucocorticoids undergo rapid deactivation after absorption. Most allergic rhinitis is seasonal and so the drugs should be for short-term use unless otherwise indicated by the health care provider. Table 35–3 lists the intranasal glucocorticoids, their dosages, and uses and considerations.

Table 35–2
SYSTEMIC AND NASAL DECONGESTANTS (SYMPATHOMIMETIC AMINES)

GENERIC (BRAND)	ROUTE AND DOSAGE	USES AND CONSIDERATIONS
Ephedrine SO$_4$ (Ectasule, Ephedsol, Vatronol)	A: PO: 25–50 mg t.i.d./q.i.d. PRN SC/IM/IV: 25–50 mg; may repeat q10min; *max:* 150 mg/24 h	Relief of allergic rhinitis, nasal congestion, sinusitis, mild acute and chronic asthma; improves narcotic-impaired respiration; corrects hypotension. It is an alpha- and beta-adrenergic agonist. OTC drug used alone or in combination. *Pregnancy category:* C; PB: UK; t$\frac{1}{2}$: 3–6 h
Naphazoline HCl (Allerest, Albalon)	A&C >12 y: 2 gtt or 0.05% spray in each nostril; q3–6h ≤ 5 d C (6–12 y): 0.025%, 1–2 gtt in each nostril	Relief of nasal congestion, allergic rhinitis. Can cause rebound congestion, transient hypertension, bradycardia, cardiac dysrhythmias. Use only 3–5 d. *Pregnancy category:* C; PB: UK; t$\frac{1}{2}$: UK
Oxymetazoline HCl (Afrin)	A&C >6 y: 0.05% gtt or spray; 2–3 gtt or 1–2 sprays q nostril b.i.d. C 2–5 y (0.025% gtt only): 2–3 gtt b.i.d. (q10–12h)	Long-acting decongestant. Taken twice a day, morning and evening. Can cause rebound congestion. Use only 3–5 d. *Pregnancy category:* C; PB: UK; t$\frac{1}{2}$: UK
Phenylephrine HCl (Neo-Synephrine, Sinex)	A: Sol (0.25%–1%): 2–3 gtt or 1–2 sprays in each nostril q4h C 6–12 y: Sol (0.25%): 2–3 gtt or sprays in each nostril q4h C 6 mo–5 y: Sol (0.125%–0.16%): 1–2 gtt in each nostril q4h	For rhinitis. Less potent than epinephrine. Can cause transient hypertension and headaches. Do not use for longer than 3–5 d. *Pregnancy category:* C; PB: UK; t$\frac{1}{2}$: 2.5 d
Phenylpropanolamine HCl (Allerest, Dimetapp)	A: PO: 25–50 mg t.i.d./q.i.d.; *max:* 150 mg/d C 6–12 y: 12.5 mg q4h; *max:* 75 mg/d C 2–5 y: 6.25 mg q4h; *max:* 37.5 mg/d	For rhinitis. May be used to treat obesity. Various combinations. Has less CNS stimulation than ephedrine. *Pregnancy category:* B; PB: UK; t$\frac{1}{2}$: 3–4 h
Pseudoephedrine (Actified, Novafed, Sudafed)	A: PO: 60 mg q4–6h; 120 mg SR q12h; *max:* 240 mg/d C 6–12 y: 30 mg q4–6h; *max:* 120 mg/d C 2–5 y: 15 mg q4–6h; *max:* 60 mg/d	For rhinitis. Less CNS stimulation and hypertension than ephedrine. *Pregnancy category:* C; PB: UK; t$\frac{1}{2}$: 9–15 h
Tetrahydrozoline HCl (Tyzine)	A&C >6 y: 2–4 gtt (0.1%) or spray q4–6h PRN C 2–6 y: 2–3 gtt (0.05%) q4–6h PRN Direct medical supervision for use >3–5 d	Relief of nasal congestion, rhinitis, sinusitis. *Pregnancy category:* C; PB: UK; t$\frac{1}{2}$: UK
Xylometazoline HCl (Otrivin)	A&C >12 y: 1–2 gtt (0.1%) or 1–2 sprays q8–10h; *max:* 3 × in 24 h C <12 y: 2–3 gtt (0.05%) or 1 spray q8–10h; *max:* 3 × in 24 h	Relief of nasal congestion, rhinitis, sinusitis. Excessive use can cause rebound nasal congestion. *Pregnancy category:* C; PB: UK; t$\frac{1}{2}$: UK

KEY: *A: adult; C: child; PO: by mouth; SC: subcutaneous; IM: intramuscular; IV: intravenous; PRN: as necessary; gtt: drops; >: greater than; PB: protein-binding; t$\frac{1}{2}$: half-life; OTC: over-the-counter; sol: solution; SR: sustained release; CNS: central nervous system; <: less than.*

Antitussives

Antitussives act on the cough control center in the medulla to suppress the cough reflex. The cough is a protective way to clear the airway of secretions or any collected material. A sore throat may cause coughing that increases throat irritation. If the cough is nonproductive and irritating, an antitussive may be taken. Hard candy may decrease the constant, irritating cough. Dextromethorphan, a nonnarcotic antitus-

Table 35–3
Intranasal Glucocorticoids

GENERIC (BRAND)	ROUTE AND DOSAGE	USES AND CONSIDERATIONS
Beclomethasone (Beconase, Vancenase, Vanceril)	A: Inhalation: 2 puffs, b.i.d. to q.i.d. C 6–12 y: Inhalation: 1–2 puffs t.i.d.	To treat seasonal allergic rhinitis and bronchial asthma. Not for acute asthma. *Pregnancy category:* C; PB: UK; t½: 3–15 h
Budesonide (Pulmicort, Rhinocort)	A & C >6 y: Inhalation: 2 puffs b.i.d. or 4 puffs in the morning	For seasonal rhinitis in adults and children. May be used in maintenance therapy for asthma. *Pregnancy category:* C; PB: UK; t½: 2.5–3 h
Dexamethasone (Decadron)	A: Inhalation: 2 puffs b.i.d. or t.i.d. C 6–12 y: Inhalation: 1–2 puffs b.i.d.	Administered orally, intravenously, ophthalmically, topically, and intranasally. A potent steroid used for short-term therapy. May have a systemic effect. *Pregnancy category:* C; PB: UK; t½: 3–4.5 h
Flunisolide (AeroBid, Nasalide)	A: Inhalation: 2 puffs b.i.d. to t.i.d. C 6–14 y: Inhalation: 1 puff t.i.d. or 2 puffs b.i.d.	For seasonal rhinitis for adults and children. May be used for steroid-dependent asthma. *Pregnancy category:* C; PB: UK; t½: 1–2 h
Fluticasone (Flonase, Flovent)	A: Inhalation: 2 puffs q.d. or 1 puff b.i.d. C >6 y: Inhalation: 1 puff daily	For seasonal allergic rhinitis. When symptoms have decreased, reduce dose to 1 puff daily. *Pregnancy category:* C: PB: UK; t½: 3.1 h
Triamcinolone (Nasacort)	A: Inhalation: 2–4 puffs daily	For allergic rhinitis. Has many uses, such as immunosuppressant agent. *Pregnancy category:* C; PB: UK; t½: 2–5 h

sive, is widely used in OTC cold remedies. Chart 35–2 lists the drug data related to dextromethorphan.

PHARMACOKINETICS

Dextromethorphan is available in syrup or liquid form, chewable capsules, and lozenges in numerous cold and cough remedy preparations. Brand name formulations include Robitussin DM, Romilar, Pedia-Care, Contac Cold Formula, Sucrets cough formulas, and many others. The drug is rapidly absorbed and exerts its effects 15 to 30 min after oral administration. The protein-binding percentage and half-life are unknown. Dextromethorphan is metabolized by the liver.

PHARMACODYNAMICS

Dextromethorphan is a nonnarcotic antitussive that suppresses the cough center in the medulla. If the cough lasts longer than 1 week and a fever or rash is present, medical care should be sought. Clients with underlying medical conditions should seek prompt medical attention.

The onset of action for dextromethorphan is relatively fast and the duration is 3 to 6 h. Usually, preparations containing dextromethorphan can be used

several times a day. Central nervous system depression can increase if the drug is used with alcohol, narcotics, sedative-hypnotics, barbiturates, or antidepressants.

Antitussives are of three types: nonnarcotic, narcotic, or combination preparations. Usually these drugs are used in combination with other agents (Table 35–4).

Expectorants

Expectorants loosen bronchial secretions so they can be eliminated with coughing. They can be used with or without other pharmacologic agents. Expectorants are found in many OTC cold remedies along with analgesics, antihistamines, decongestants, and antitussives. The most common expectorant in such preparations is guaifenesin. Table 35–4 lists the drug data for antitussives and expectorants. Hydration is the best expectorant.

SINUSITIS

Sinusitis is an inflammation of the mucous membranes of one or more of the maxillary, frontal, eth-

Chart 35–2.   Antitussive

ANTITUSSIVE

Drug Name	**Dosage**
Dextromethorphan hydrobromide (Robitussin DM, Romilar, Sucrets Cough Control, PediCare, Benylin DM, and others); 🍁 Balminil DM, Neo-DM; Ornex DM OTC preparation *Pregnancy Category:* C	A: PO: 10–30 mg q4–8h; *max:* 120 mg/24 h C 6–12 y: PO: 5–10 mg q4–6h; *max:* 60 mg/d C 2–5 y: PO: 2.5–7.5 mg q4–8h; *max:* 30 mg/d *Sustained Action Liquid (Delsym):* A: 60 mg q12h C 6–12 y: 30 mg q12h C 2–5 y: 15 mg q12h

Assessment and Planning

Contraindications	**Drug-Lab-Food Interactions**
Chronic obstructive pulmonary disease, chronic productive cough, hypersensitivity, clients taking MAOIs	**Drug:** *Increase* effect/toxicity with MAOIs, narcotics, sedative-hypnotics, barbiturates, antidepressants, alcohol

Pharmacokinetics	**Pharmacodynamics**
Absorption: PO: Rapidly absorbed **Distribution:** PB: UK **Metabolism:** $t\frac{1}{2}$: UK **Excretion:** In urine: UK	PO: Onset: 15–30 min Peak: UK Duration: 3–6 h

Interventions

NURSING PROCESS

Therapeutic Effects/Uses

To provide temporary suppression of a nonproductive cough; to reduce viscosity of tenacious secretions.

Mode of Action: Inhibition of the cough center in the medulla.

Side Effects	**Adverse Reactions**
Nausea, dizziness, drowsiness, sedation	Hallucinations at high doses **Life-threatening:** None known

Evaluation

KEY: A: adult; C: child; PO: by mouth; PB: protein-binding; $t\frac{1}{2}$: half-life; UK: unknown; MAOIs: monamine oxidase inhibitors; 🍁: Canadian drug names.

Table 35–4
Antitussives and Expectorants

GENERIC (BRAND)	ROUTE AND DOSING	USES AND CONSIDERATIONS
NARCOTIC ANTITUSSIVES		
Codeine CSS II	A: PO: 10–20 mg q4–6h; *max:* 120 mg/d C 6–12 y: PO: 5–10 mg q4–6h; *max:* 60 mg/d C 2–5 y: PO: 2.5–4.5 mg q4–6h; *max:* 18 mg/d	Schedule II drug. Can be a Schedule V drug when combined in cough syrup. Usually mixed with an antihistamine, decongestant, and/or expectorant. Can cause drowsiness, dizziness, nausea, constipation, respiratory depression. *Pregnancy category:* C; PB: 7%; $t\frac{1}{2}$: 2.5–4 h
Guaifenesin and codeine (Cheracol, Robitussin A-C) CSS V	*Temporary relief of cough due to minor irritation:* A: PO: 5–10 mL q6–8h C 2–6 y: PO: 2.5 mL q6–8h, PRN	An expectorant that is combined with a narcotic antitussive. Also to control a cough due to the common cold or bronchitis. *Pregnancy category:* C; PB: UK; $t\frac{1}{2}$: UK

Table 35-4 *Continued*
Antitussives and Expectorants

GENERIC (BRAND)	ROUTE AND DOSING	USES AND CONSIDERATIONS
Hydrocodone bitartrate (Hycodan) CSS III	A: PO: 5–10 mg q4–6h, *max:* 15 mg/d C: PO: 0.6 mg/kg/d in 3–4 divided doses, not to exceed 10 mg/single dose	Relief of cough and pain. Has similar side effects as codeine. *Pregnancy category:* C; PB: UK; t½: 3–4 h
NONNARCOTIC ANTITUSSIVES		
Benzonatate (Tessalon)	*Relief of nonproductive cough:* A: PO: 100 mg t.i.d. or q4h; *max:* 600 mg/d C <10 y: PO: 8 mg/kg/d in 3–6 divided doses	Relief of cough. It does not decrease the respiratory center. Has few side effects. *Pregnancy category:* C; PB: UK; t½: UK
Dextromethorphan hydrobromide (Benylin, Romilar, Sucrets Cough Control, and others)	See Chart 35–2	Suppresses cough due to common cold or inhaled irritants. Nonprescription cough medication. Does not depress respiration. Does not cause physical dependence, and tolerance does not develop. *Pregnancy category:* C; PB: UK; t½: UK
Diphenhydramine (Benadryl)	See Chart 35–1	Used as a cough suppressant. Has antihistamine properties. Can cause drowsiness and dry mouth. *Pregnancy category:* B; PB: 82%; t½: 2–7 h
Promethazine with dextromethorphan	A: PO: 5 mL q4–6h; *max:* 30 mL/d C 6–12 y: PO: 2.5–5 mL q4–6h; *max:* 20 mL/d C 2–6 y: PO: 1.25–5 mL, q4–6h	For cough. A combination of a phenothiazine and a nonnarcotic antitussive. *Pregnancy category:* C; PB: UK; t½: UK
Expectorants		
Guaifenesin (Robitussin, Anti-Tuss, Glyco-Tuss)	A: PO: 200–400 mg q4h; *max:* 2.4 g/d C 6–12 y: PO: 100–200 mg q4h; *max:* 1.2 g/d C 2–5 y: PO: 50–100 mg q4h; *max:* 600 mg/d	For dry, unproductive cough. Can cause nausea, vomiting. Can be combined with other cold remedies. Take with glass of water to loosen mucus. *Pregnancy category:* C; PB: UK; t½: UK
Iodinated glycerol (Iophen)	A: PO: 60 mg q.i.d.; sol: 20 gtt q.i.d.; elix: 5 mL q.i.d. C: PO: Up to half adult dose according to weight	Same as potassium iodide. *Pregnancy category:* X; PB: UK; t½: UK
Potassium iodide (SSKI)	A: PO: 300–650 mg b.i.d., t.i.d. C: PO: 60–250 mg q8–12h	Stimulates bronchial secretions and fluids. Avoid if hyperkalemia is present. Can cause nausea and vomiting. *Pregnancy category:* D; PB: UK; t½: UK
ANTITUSSIVE/EXPECTORANT		
Guaifenesin and dextromethorphan (Robitussin-DM)	A: PO: 10 mL q6–8h C 6–12 y: PO: 5 mL q6–8h C 2–5 y: PO: 2.5 mL q6–8h	For nonproductive cough. *Pregnancy category:* C; PB: UK; t½: UK

KEY: A: adult; C: child; PO: by mouth; UK: unknown; max: maximum; PB: protein-binding; t½: half-life; CSS: Controlled Substance Schedule; PRN: as necessary; elix: elixir; <: less than.

moid, or sphenoid sinuses. A systemic or nasal decongestant may be indicated. Acetaminophen, fluids, and rest may also be helpful. For acute or severe sinusitis, an antibiotic may be prescribed.

ACUTE PHARYNGITIS

Acute pharyngitis (inflammation of the throat, or "sore throat") can be caused by a virus or by beta-

NURSING PROCESS
COMMON COLD

Assessment

- Determine whether there is a history of hypertension, especially if a decongestant is one of the ingredients of the cold remedy.
- Obtain baseline vital signs (VS). An elevated temperature of 99°F (37.2°C) to 101°F (38.3°C) may indicate a viral infection caused by a cold.

Potential Nursing Diagnoses

- Fatigue
- Sleep deprivation resulting from chronic coughing
- Risk for infection

Planning

- Client will be free of nonproductive cough. A secondary bacterial infection does not occur.

Nursing Interventions

- Monitor vital signs. Blood pressure can become elevated when a decongestant is taken. Dysrhythmias can also occur.
- Observe color of bronchial secretions. Yellow or green mucus is indicative of a bronchial infection. Antibiotics may be needed.
- Be aware that codeine preparations for cough suppression can lead to tolerance and physical dependence.

Client Teaching

- Instruct the client on proper use of a nasal spray and proper use of puff or squeeze products. Instruct client not to use more than one or two puffs, 4 to 6 times a day for 5 to 7 days. Rebound congestion can occur with overuse.
- Advise the client to read the label on OTC drugs and to check with the health care provider before taking cold remedies. This is especially important when taking other drugs or when the client has a major health problem such as hypertension or hyperthyroidism.
- Inform the client that antibiotics are not helpful in treating the common cold viruses. They may be prescribed if a secondary infection occurs.
- Advise the older client with heart disease, asthma, emphysema, diabetes mellitus, or hypertension to contact the health care provider concerning the selection of drug, including OTC drugs.
- Advise the client not to drive when starting on a cold remedy containing an antihistamine because drowsiness is common.
- Instruct the client to maintain adequate fluid intake. Fluids liquify bronchial secretions to ease elimination by coughing.
- Instruct the client not to take a cold remedy near or at bedtime. Insomnia may occur if it contains a decongestant.
- Instruct the client to drink the diluted liquid form of saturated solution of potassium iodide (SSKI) through a straw to avoid discoloration of tooth enamel.

hemolytic streptococci (strep throat) or other bacteria. It can occur alone or with the common cold and rhinitis or acute sinusitis. Symptoms include elevated temperature and cough. A throat culture should be obtained to rule out beta-hemolytic streptococcal infection. Saline gargles, lozenges, and increased fluid intake are usually indicated. Acetaminophen may be taken for the elevated temperature. A 10-day course of antibiotics is often prescribed if the throat culture is positive for beta-hemolytic streptococci. Antibiotics are not effective for viral pharyngitis.

- Encourage the client to get adequate rest.
- Instruct the client that common cold and flu viruses are transmitted frequently by hand-to-hand contact or touching a contaminated surface. Cold viruses can live on the skin for several hours and on hard surfaces for several days.
- Instruct the client to avoid environmental pollutants, smoking, and dust.
- Instruct the client/parents to have child perform three effective coughs before bedtime to promote uninterrupted sleep.
- Instruct the client/parents to keep the drug stored out of reach of small children; request child safety caps.
- Advise the client to contact the health care provider if cough persists for > 1 wk or is combined with chest pain, fever, or headache.

Self-Administration
- Instruct client about self-administration of medication such as nose drops and inhalants.
- Instruct the client to cough effectively, to take deep breaths before coughing, and to be in the upright position.

Cultural Considerations

- Accept the client's remedies for treating the common cold that may be the result of cultural practices. Discuss practices that could cause body harm.
- Present ways to care for the common cold for clients from various cultural backgrounds, such as by increasing fluid intake and rest, and using tissues to remove nasal and bronchial secretions. Advise the client to contact a health professional if the cold persists and if the body temperature is greater than 101°F.

Evaluation

- Evaluate the effectiveness of the drug therapy. Determine that the client is free of a nonproductive cough, has adequate fluid intake and rest, and is afebrile.

ACUTE TONSILLITIS

Acute tonsillitis is inflammation of the tonsils. *Streptococcus* is the usual causative microorganism. Symptoms include sore throat, pain on swallowing, chills, fever, and aching muscles. A throat culture should be obtained to determine whether the causative organism is beta-hemolytic streptococcus. Saline gargle, increased fluid intake, and antibiotics are normal treatment modalities.

ACUTE LARYNGITIS

In acute **laryngitis,** edema of the vocal cords causes the voice to be weak or husky. It may be due to stress, overuse of the vocal cords, or a respiratory infection. Drug therapy has minimal value. Voice rest is usually necessary, and smoking should be avoided.

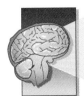

Critical Thinking in Action

G. H., 35 years old, has allergic rhinitis. Her prescriptions include loratadine (Claritin), 5 mg per day, and fluticasone, 2 nasal inhalations daily. Previously she had taken over-the-counter drugs and asked whether she should continue to take the OTC drug with her prescriptions. She has never used a nasal inhaler.

1. What additional information would be needed from G. H. in regard to her health problem?
2. What is your response to G. H. in regard to OTC drugs being taken with the prescriptive drugs?

Critical Thinking continued on page 634

3. How would you instruct G. H. to use a nasal inhaler? Explain. Refer to Chapter 3 if necessary.

4. What are the similarities and differences between loratadine and diphenhydramine? Could one of these antihistamines be more effective than the other? Explain.

5. Design a client teaching plan for G. H. in regard to medications and environmental allergens.

6. What could you suggest for decreasing allergens (dust mites) in the home?

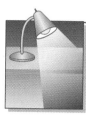

Study Questions

1. Antihistamines can be used for the common cold. What are the desired and undesired effects of antihistamines?

2. What are antitussives and expectorants? How are they administered?

3. Your client has a cold and is complaining of nasal congestion. He has been using a nasal decongestant every 3 hours for several days. He says that the nasal congestion is as bad as it had been before he started the nasal decongestant. What nursing interventions, including client teaching, should be given?

4. Your client is complaining of a "sore throat." The pharynx appears red. What nursing action should be taken?

5. P. T. states she has had a cold for 5 days and now has "lost her voice." What client teaching instructions should be included?

6. M. P. says she was with Tom the day before he "got a head cold." She asks whether she can avoid the cold by staying away from Tom. What would your response be? What client teaching is recommended?

Drugs for Acute and Chronic Lower Respiratory Disorders

36

Outline

Objectives

- Define chronic obstructive pulmonary disease (COPD) and restrictive lung disease.
- List the drug groups that are used for COPD and asthma and the desired effects of each.
- Describe the side effects of beta$_2$-adrenergic agonists and methylxanthines.
- State the therapeutic serum or plasma theophylline level and the toxic level.
- Explain the therapeutic effects of glucocorticoids, cromolyn, antihistamines, and mucolytics for asthma and COPD.
- Describe the nursing process, including client teaching, related to drugs commonly used for COPD, including asthma, and restrictive lung disease.

Terms

bronchial asthma

bronchiectasis

bronchodilator

bronchospasm

chronic bronchitis

chronic obstructive pulmonary disease (COPD)

emphysema

glucocorticoids

mucolytic

restrictive lung disease

INTRODUCTION

Chronic obstructive pulmonary disease (COPD) and restrictive pulmonary disease are the two major categories of lower respiratory tract disease. COPD is caused by airway obstruction with increased airway resistance to airflow to lung tissues. Four major pulmonary disorders cause COPD: chronic bronchitis, bronchiectasis, emphysema, and asthma. Chronic bronchitis, bronchiectasis, and emphysema frequently result in irreversible lung tissue damage. The lung tissue changes resulting from an acute asthmatic attack are normally reversible; however, if the asthma attacks are frequent and asthma becomes chronic, irreversible changes in the lung tissue may result.

Restrictive lung disease is a decrease in total lung capacity as a result of fluid accumulation or loss of elasticity of the lung. Pulmonary edema, pulmonary fibrosis, pneumonitis, lung tumors, thoracic deformities (scoliosis), and disorders affecting the thoracic muscular wall such as myasthenia gravis are among the types and causes of restrictive pulmonary disease.

Drugs discussed in this chapter are used primarily to treat COPD, particularly asthma. These drugs include bronchodilators (sympathomimetics [primarily beta$_2$-adrenergic agonists], methylxanthines [xanthines]), leukotriene antagonists, glucocorticoids, cromolyn, anticholinergics, and mucolytics. Some of these drugs may also be used for the treatment of restrictive pulmonary diseases.

CHRONIC OBSTRUCTIVE PULMONARY DISEASE

COPD includes four main lung diseases: (1) asthma, (2) chronic bronchitis, (3) emphysema, and (4) bronchiectasis. Bronchial asthma is characterized by bronchospasm (constricted bronchioles), wheezing, mucous secretions, and dyspnea. There is resistance to airflow caused by obstruction of the airway. In acute and chronic asthma, minimal to no changes are seen in the structure and function of lung tissues when the disease process is in remission. In chronic bronchitis, emphysema, and bronchiectasis, there is permanent, irreversible damage to the physical structure of the lung tissue. Symptoms are similar in these three pulmonary disorders to those of asthma, except without wheezing. Figure 36–1 displays the overlapping symptoms of COPD conditions. Frequently, there is steady deterioration over a period of years.

Chronic bronchitis is a progressive lung disease caused by smoking or chronic lung infections. Bronchial inflammation and excessive mucous secretion result in airway obstruction. Productive coughing is a response to excess mucous production and chronic

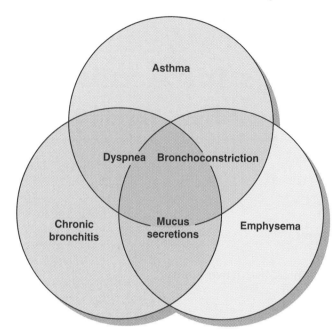

Figure 36–1
Overlapping signs and symptoms of COPD conditions.

bronchial irritation. Inspiratory and expiratory rhonchi may be heard on auscultation. Hypercapnia (increased carbon dioxide retention) and hypoxemia (decreased blood oxygen) lead to respiratory acidosis.

In **bronchiectasis,** there is abnormal dilatation of the bronchi and bronchioles secondary to frequent infection and inflammation. The bronchioles become obstructed by the breakdown of the epithelium of the bronchial mucosa. Tissue fibrosis may result.

Emphysema is a progressive lung disease caused by cigarette smoking, atmospheric contaminants, or lack of the alpha$_1$-antitrypsin protein that inhibits proteolytic enzymes that destroy alveoli (air sacs). The proteolytic enzymes are released in the lung by bacteria or phagocytic cells. The terminal bronchioles become plugged with mucus, causing a loss of fiber and elastin network in the alveoli. The alveoli enlarge as many of the alveolar walls are destroyed. Air becomes trapped in the overexpanded alveoli, leading to inadequate gas (O_2 and CO_2) exchange.

Bronchial Asthma

Bronchial asthma is a chronic obstructive pulmonary disease characterized by periods of bronchospasm resulting in wheezing and difficulty in breathing. **Bronchospasm,** or bronchoconstriction, results when the lung tissue is exposed to extrinsic or intrinsic factors that stimulate a bronchoconstrictive response. Factors that can trigger an asthmatic attack (bronchospasm) include humidity, air pressure changes, temperature changes, smoke, fumes (exhaust, perfume), stress, emotional upset, and allergies to animal dander, dust mites, food, and drugs such as aspirin, indomethacin, and ibuprofen. Reactive airway disease (RAD) is a cause of asthma resulting from sensitivity stimulation from allergens, dust, temperature changes, and cigarette smoking.

PATHOPHYSIOLOGY

Mast cells, found in connective tissue throughout the body, are directly involved in the asthmatic response, particularly to extrinsic factors. Allergens attach themselves to mast cells and basophils, resulting in an antigen-antibody reaction on the mast cells in the lung; thus, the mast cells stimulate the release of chemical mediators such as histamines, cytokines, serotonin, ECF-A (eosinophil chemotactic factor of anaphylaxis), and leukotrienes. Eosinophil counts are usually elevated during an allergic reaction, which indicates that an inflammatory process is occurring. These chemical mediators stimulate bronchial constriction, mucous secretions, inflammation, and pulmonary congestion. Histamine and ECF-A are strong bronchoconstrictors. Bronchial smooth muscles are wrapped spirally around the bronchioles, and the bronchioles contract as they are stimulated by these mediators.

Figure 36–2 shows the factors contributing to bronchoconstriction. Cyclic adenosine monophosphate (cyclic AMP, or cAMP), a cellular substance, is involved in many cellular activities and is responsible for maintaining bronchodilation. When histamine, ECF-A, and leukotrienes inhibit the action of cAMP, bronchoconstriction results. The sympathomimetic (adrenergic) **bronchodilators** and methylxanthines increase the amount of cAMP in bronchial tissue cells.

In an acute asthmatic attack, the sympathomimetics (beta-adrenergic agonists) are the first line of defense. They promote cAMP production and enhance bronchodilation. Sympathomimetics (adrenergics) are also discussed in Chapter 21.

SYMPATHOMIMETICS: ALPHA- AND BETA$_2$-ADRENERGIC AGONISTS

Sympathomimetics increase cyclic AMP, causing dilation of the bronchioles. In an acute bronchospasm caused by anaphylaxis from an allergic reaction, the nonselective sympathomimetic epinephrine (Adrenalin), which is an alpha$_1$ beta$_2$, and beta$_2$ agonist, is

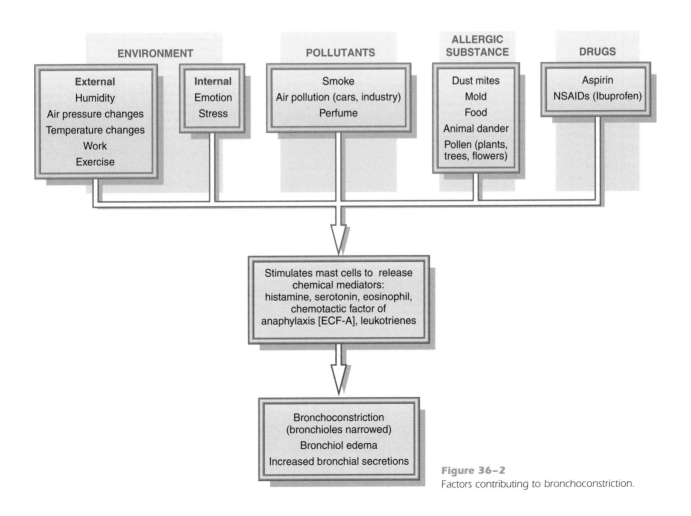

Figure 36–2
Factors contributing to bronchoconstriction.

given subcutaneously to promote bronchodilation and elevate the blood pressure. Epinephrine is administered in emergency situations to restore circulation and increase airway patency (see Chapter 52).

For bronchospasm associated with chronic asthma or COPD, selective beta$_2$-adrenergic agonists are given by aerosol or as a tablet. These drugs act primarily on the beta$_2$ receptors; therefore, the side effects are *less severe* than those of epinephrine, which acts on alpha, beta$_1$, and beta$_2$ receptors.

The first beta-adrenergic agent used for bronchospasm was isoproterenol (Isuprel), which was introduced in 1941. It has no alpha agonist properties, but it is a nonselective beta agonist because it stimulates both beta$_1$ and beta$_2$ receptors. Because the beta$_1$ receptors are stimulated, the heart rate increases and tachycardia may result. Beta$_2$ stimulation promotes bronchodilation. Isoproterenol cannot be given orally because it is metabolized in the gastrointestinal (GI) tract. It may be administered sublingually, by inhalation using an aerosol inhaler or nebulizer, or intravenously for severe asthmatic attacks. Its duration of action is short.

Metaproterenol

The second beta-adrenergic agent is metaproterenol (Alupent, Metaprel), which was first marketed in 1961. It has some beta$_1$ effect, but it is primarily used as a beta$_2$ agent. It may be administered orally or by inhalation with a metered-dose inhaler or a nebulizer.

For long-term asthma treatment, beta$_2$-adrenergic agonists are frequently administered by inhalation. Usually, more drug is delivered by inhalation directly to the constricted bronchial site. The effective inhalation drug dose is less than it would be by the oral route; there are also fewer side effects in using this route.

The onset of action of the drug is more rapid (1 to 15 min) by inhalation than orally. If the client does not receive effective relief from the inhaler, either the client's technique is faulty or the canister is empty (see Chapter 3, Fig. 3–11, to determine the amount of drug left in the canister). A spacer device may be attached to the inhaler to improve drug delivery to the lung with less deposition in the mouth (see Chapter 3, Fig. 3–12). If the client does not use the inhaler properly to deliver the drug dose, the medication may be trapped in the upper airways. Because of drug inhalation, mouth dryness and throat irritation could result. Chart 36–1 lists the pharmacologic behavior for metaproterenol.

PHARMACOKINETICS
Metaproterenol is well absorbed from the GI tract. Its protein-binding percent and half-life are unknown. It is metabolized by the liver and excreted in the urine.

PHARMACODYNAMICS
Metaproterenol reverses bronchospasm by relaxing the bronchial smooth muscle. The drug acts on the beta$_2$ receptor, promoting bronchodilation, and increases cyclic AMP.

The onset of action for oral and inhalational metaproterenol is fast and its duration is short. Excessive use of the drug by inhalation may cause tolerance and paradoxic bronchoconstriction. Because it has some beta$_1$ properties, it can cause tremor, nervousness, heart palpitations, and increased heart rate when taken in large doses. There are a few drug interactions that need to be considered. When metaproterenol is taken with a beta-adrenergic blocker, its effects are decreased. Other sympathomimetic agents increase the effects of metaproterenol.

The newer beta-adrenergic drugs for asthma are more selective for beta$_2$ receptors. High doses or overuse of the beta$_2$-adrenergic agents for asthma may cause some degree of beta$_1$ response such as nervousness, tremor, and increased pulse rate. The ideal beta$_2$ agonist is one that has a rapid onset of action, longer duration of action, and very few side effects. Albuterol (Proventil, Ventolin) is a selective beta$_2$ drug that is effective for treatment and control of asthma by causing bronchodilation.

Use of an Aerosol Inhaler*

If the beta$_2$ agonist is given by a metered-dose inhaler, correct use of the inhaler and dosage intervals need to be explained to the client. The correct method of using the inhaler is shown in Figure 36–3 and described in the Nursing Process: Bronchodilator.

Excessive use of the aerosol drug can lead to tolerance and loss of drug effectiveness. Occasionally, severe paradoxic airway resistance (bronchoconstriction) has developed with repeated, excessive use of sympathomimetic oral inhalation, especially isoproterenol. Frequent dosing can cause tremors, nervousness, and increased heart rate. Table 36–1 lists the sympathomimetics used as bronchodilators.

Side Effects and Adverse Reactions
EPINEPHRINE
The side effects and adverse reactions of epinephrine include tremors, dizziness, hypertension, tachycardia, heart palpitations, dysrhythmias, and angina. The client needs to be closely monitored when epinephrine is administered.

---

*See Chapter 3.

Chart 36–1. Bronchodilator: Adrenergic

ADRENERGIC BRONCHODILATOR

Drug Name

Metaproterenol SO₄
   (Alupent, Metaprel)
Pregnancy Category: C

Dosage

A&C >9 y and >27 kg: PO: 20 mg, q6–8 h
C 6–9 y or <27 kg: PO: 10 mg, q6–8 h
A&C >12 y: MDI 2–3 inhalations as single
   dose; wait 2 min before second dose, if necessary; use only q3–4 h to maximum of 12 inhala-
   tions/d

Contraindications

Hypersensitivity, cardiac dysrhythmias
Caution: Narrow-angle glaucoma, cardiac disease, hypertension

Drug-Lab-Food Interactions

Drug: *Increase* action with sympathomimetics;
decrease with beta blockers
Lab: *Decreased* serum potassium

Pharmacokinetics

Absorption: PO: Well absorbed
Distribution: PB: UK
Metabolism: t½: UK
Excretion: In urine as metabolites

Pharmacodynamics

PO: Onset: 15–30 min
   Peak: 1 h
   Duration: 4 h
SC: Onset: 1–5 min
   Peak: 1 h
   Duration: 3–4 h

Therapeutic Effects/Uses

To treat bronchospasm, asthma; to promote bronchodilation.

Mode of Action: Relaxation of smooth muscle of bronchi.

Side Effects

Nervousness, tremors, restlessness, insomnia,
headache, nausea, vomiting, hyperglycemia,
muscle cramping in extremities

Adverse Reactions

Tachycardia, palpitations, hypertension
Life-threatening: Cardiac dysrhythmias, cardiac
arrest, paradoxical bronchoconstriction

Assessment and Planning — Interventions — Evaluation — NURSING PROCESS

KEY: A: adult; C: child; PO: by mouth; >: greater than; <: less than; UK: unknown; MDI: metered-dose inhaler; PB: protein-binding; t½: half-life.

BETA₂-ADRENERGICS

The side effects associated with beta₂ drugs (albuterol, terbutaline) include tremors, headaches, nervousness, increased pulse rate, palpitations (high doses), and minimal lowering of the blood pressure. The beta₂ agonists may increase blood glucose levels; diabetics who take beta₂ agonists should be taught to closely monitor their serum glucose levels. Side effects of the beta₂ agonists may diminish after a week or longer. The bronchodilating effects may decrease with continued use. It is believed that tolerance to these drugs can develop; if this occurs, the dose may need to be increased. Failure to respond to a previously effective dose may indicate worsening asthma that requires reevaluation before increasing the dose.

ANTICHOLINERGICS

The beta-adrenergic agonists and methylxanthines have replaced the anticholinergic drugs in treating asthma. Recently, a new anticholinergic drug, ipratropium bromide (Atrovent), was introduced to treat asthmatic conditions by dilating the bronchioles. Unlike other anticholinergics, ipratropium has few systemic effects. It is administered by aerosol.

Clients using a beta-agonist inhalant should use it 5 minutes before using ipratropium. When using the anticholinergic agent in conjunction with an inhaled glucocorticoid (steroid) or cromolyn, the ipratropium should be used 5 minutes before the steroid or cromolyn. This causes the bronchioles to dilate so that the

Table 36-1
Sympathomimetics: Adrenergic Bronchodilators and Anticholinergics

GENERIC (BRAND)	ROUTE AND DOSAGE	USES AND CONSIDERATIONS
ALPHA- AND BETA-ADRENERGIC		
Ephedrine SO$_4$ (Ephedsol) Alpha$_1$, beta$_1$, beta$_2$	A: PO: 25–50 mg q3–4h; *max:* 150 mg/d PRN; SC/IM/IV: 12.5–25 mg PRN C >2 y: PO: 2–3 mg/kg/d in 4–6 divided doses C 6–12 y: PO: 6.25–12.5 mg q4h; *max:* 75 mg	Relief of allergic rhinitis and sinusitis; improves respiration due to narcotic excess; corrects hypotensive state. Nervousness, tachycardia, and insomnia could occur. *Pregnancy category:* C; PB: UK; t$\frac{1}{2}$: 3–6 h
Epinephrine (Adrenalin, Primatene Mist, Bronkaid Mist) Alpha$_1$, beta$_1$, beta$_2$	A: SC: 0.1–0.5 mg or mL of 1:1000 sol; may repeat q10–15 min C: SC: 0.01 mg or mL of 1:1000 sol; may repeat q20min–4h Inhal: 1–2 puffs of 1:100 q15 min × 2 doses then q3h	For acute bronchonconstriction and to combat anaphylactic reaction. It is a nonselective (alpha, beta$_1$, and beta$_2$) adrenergic drug. Used frequently by nebulizer. Side effects include nervousness, tremors, dizziness, palpitations, tachycardia, and other cardiac dysrhythmias. *Pregnancy category:* C; PB: UK; t$\frac{1}{2}$: UK
BETA-ADRENERGIC		
Albuterol (Proventil, Ventolin) Beta$_2$	A&C >6 y: Inhal: 1–2 puffs q4–6h or 2 puffs 15 min before exercise A: PO: 2–4 mg t.i.d. or q.i.d.; *max:* 8 mg q.i.d. SR: 4–8 mg q12h C 6–12 y: PO: 2 mg t.i.d./q.i.d. C 2–6 y: PO: 0.1 mg/kg t.i.d.	Treatment of acute and chronic asthma, bronchitis, and exercise-induced bronchospasm. Onset of action orally is 30 min and duration of action is 4–6 h; SR: 8–12 h. *Pregnancy category:* C; PB: UK; t$\frac{1}{2}$: 4–5 h
Bitolterol mesylate (Tornalate) Beta$_1$ (some), beta$_2$	A: Inhal: 2 (1–3 min apart), q4–6h; *max:* 12 inhal/d	Treatment of asthma and acute bronchitis. It can be used as a single-treatment therapy or in combination with theophylline or corticosteroid. Tremors, nervousness may occur. Has a longer duration of action than many other adrenergics (5–8 h) by inhalation. *Pregnancy category:* C; PB: UK; t$\frac{1}{2}$: 3 h
Isoetharine HCl (Bronkosol) Beta$_1$ (some), beta$_2$	Inhal: 1–2 puffs A: IPPB: 0.5–1.0 mL of 5% sol or 0.5 mL of 1% sol diluted in 3 mL of NSS	For bronchoconstriction and reversible obstructive pulmonary disease. Rapid onset (1–5 min); short duration of action (1–4 h). *Pregnancy category:* C; PB: UK; t$\frac{1}{2}$: UK
Isoproterenol (Isuprel) Beta$_1$ and beta$_2$	A&C: Inhal: 1–2 puffs q4–6h A: SL: 10–20 mg q6–8h C: SL: 5–10 mg q6–8h	For bronchoconstriction. Nonselective (beta$_1$ and beta$_2$). Beta$_1$ effect causes heart rate to increase. Monitor heart rate and blood pressure. The absorption of the sublingual drug can be variable and unpredictable. *Pregnancy category:* C; PB: UK; t$\frac{1}{2}$: 2–5 min
Metaproterenol sulfate (Alupent, Metaprel) Beta$_1$ (some) and beta$_2$	See Chart 36-1	Relief of bronchospasm caused by asthma, bronchitis, and emphysema. Nervousness, tremors, tachycardia, and palpitations may occur. *Pregnancy category:* C; PB: UK; t$\frac{1}{2}$: UK
Pirbuterol acetate (Maxair) Beta$_2$	*Prevention:* A&C >12 y: Inhal: 2 puffs q4–6h *Bronchospasm:* A&C >12 y: Inhal: 2 puffs (1–3 min apart) followed by 1 puff; not to exceed 12 inhalations/d	Treatment of asthma. Moderate duration of action (5 h). *Pregnancy category:* C; PB: UK; t$\frac{1}{2}$: 2–3 h

Table continued on following page

Table 36-1 *Continued*

Sympathomimetics: Adrenergic Bronchodilators and Anticholinergics

GENERIC (BRAND)	ROUTE AND DOSAGE	USES AND CONSIDERATIONS
Salmeterol (Serevent) Beta$_2$	*Maintenance bronchodilation:* A&C >12 y: Inhal: 2 puffs q12h *Prevention exercise-induced bronchospasm* A&C >12 y: Inhal: 2 puffs ≥30–60 min before exercise	Treatment for chronic asthma and exercise-induced bronchospasm. Not effective for treating acute bronchospasms. Has a long duration of action (12 h). *Pregnancy category:* C; PB: 94%–98%; t$\frac{1}{2}$: 5.5 h
Terbutaline SO$_4$ (Brethine, Bricanyl) Beta$_2$	Inhal: 1–2 puffs q4–6h A: PO: 2.5–5 mg t.i.d. SC: 0.25–0.5 mg q8h IV: 10 μg/min, gradually increase; *max:* 80 μg/min C >12 y: PO: 2.5 mg t.i.d.	To treat reversible airway obstruction caused by asthma, bronchitis, and emphysema. May cause nervousness, tremors, lightheadedness, palpitations, tachycardia if taken in excess. Slow to moderate onset (15–30 min); long oral duration (4–8 h) and moderate inhaled duration (3–6 h). *Pregnancy category:* B; PB: 25%; t$\frac{1}{2}$: 3–11 h
ANTICHOLINERGICS		
Ipratropium bromide (Atrovent)	*COPD:* A: Inhal: 2 puffs t.i.d., q.i.d. >4 h intervals; *max:* 12 inhal/d	To treat bronchospasm associated with COPD, including asthma. Use with caution in clients with narrow-angle glaucoma. *Pregnancy category:* B; PB: UK; t$\frac{1}{2}$: 1.5–2 h
Ipratropium with Albuterol (Combivent)	A: Inhalation: 2 puffs t.i.d.–q.i.d.	Anticholinergic agent combines with beta$_2$-adrenergic agonist to increase bronchodilation. With the use of this combination of drugs, the duration of action is prolonged. *Pregnancy category:* UK; PB: UK; t$\frac{1}{2}$: UK

KEY: A: adult; C: child; PO: by mouth; SR: sustained-release; SL: sublingual; IV: intravenous; COPD: chronic obstructive pulmonary disease; >: greater than; PB: protein-binding; t$\frac{1}{2}$: half-life; IPPB: intermittent positive-pressure breathing; sol: solution; NSS: normal saline solution; inhal: inhalation.

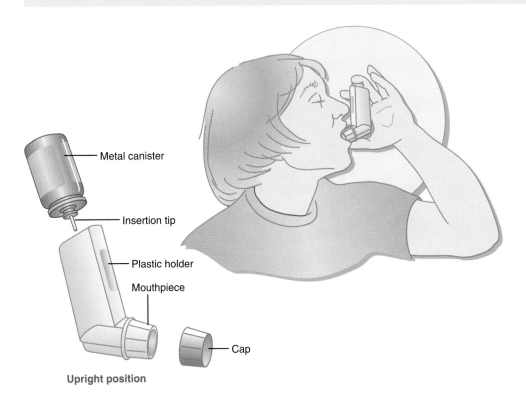

Metal canister

Insertion tip

Plastic holder

Mouthpiece

Cap

Upright position

Figure 36-3
Technique for using the aerosol inhaler.

NURSING PROCESS
BRONCHODILATOR: ADRENERGIC

Assessment

- Obtain a medical and drug history; report probable drug-drug interactions.
- Obtain baseline vital signs (VS) for abnormalities and for future comparisons.
- Assess for wheezing, decreased breath sounds, cough, and sputum production.
- Assess sensorium levels for confusion and restlessness due to hypoxia and hypercapnia.
- Assess hydration; diuresis may result in dehydration in the elderly and children.

Potential Nursing Diagnoses

- Airway clearance, ineffective
- Noncompliance with drug therapy

Planning

- Client will be free of wheezing and lung fields will be clear within 2 to 5 d.
- Client is taking oral drugs and using inhaler as prescribed.

Nursing Interventions

- Monitor VS. Blood pressure and heart rate can increase greatly. Check for cardiac dysrhythmias.
- Provide adequate hydration. Fluids aid in loosening secretions. Monitor drug therapy. Observe for side effects.
- Administer medication after meals to decrease GI distress.

Client Teaching

Self-Administration
- Instruct to correctly use the inhaler or nebulizer. Caution against overuse because side effects and tolerance may result.
  Correct use of metered-dose inhaler to deliver beta$_2$ agonist:
  1. Insert the medication canister into the plastic holder.
  2. Shake the inhaler well *before* using. Remove cap from mouthpiece.

Nursing Process continued on following page

---

steroid or cromolyn can be deposited in the bronchioles.

The combination of ipratropium bromide with albuterol sulfate (Combivent) is used to treat chronic bronchitis. The combination is more effective and has a longer duration of action than if one agent is used alone. These two agents combined increase the FEV$_1$ (forced expiratory volume), which is the parameter used to evaluate asthmatics and obstructive lung disease and to evaluate the response to bronchodilator therapy. Table 36–2 lists the nasal inhalants for asthma control.

Drug Therapy for Asthma According to Severity

Chronic asthma may be controlled through a long-term drug treatment program and by a quick-relief

program during an acute phase. Table 36–3 lists four steps for controlling chronic asthma according to the severity of the asthma. This treatment regimen was developed by the National Asthma Education and Prevention Program at the National Heart, Lung, and Blood Institute in Bethesda, MD, in 1997. The long-term drug treatment program varies according to the symptoms of the asthma and its severity. The quick-relief drug therapy is the same for all classes of asthma.

METHYLXANTHINE (XANTHINE) DERIVATIVES

The second group of bronchodilators used for asthma are the methylxanthine (xanthine) derivatives, which include aminophylline, theophylline, and caffeine.

3. Breathe *out* through the mouth. Open mouth wide and hold mouthpiece 1 to 2 inches from mouth or place inhaler mouthpiece in mouth. A spacer may be used. Discuss technique with health care provider.
4. With mouth open, take *slow deep* breath through mouth and at same time push the top of the medication canister once.
5. Hold breath for a few seconds; exhale slowly through pursed lips.
6. If a second dose is required, wait 2 min and repeat the procedure by first shaking the canister in the plastic holder with the cap on.
7. If the inhaler has not been used recently or when it is first used, "test spray" before administering the metered dose.
8. If a glucocorticoid inhalant is to be used with a bronchodilator, wait 5 min before using the inhaler containing the steroid for the bronchodilator effect.

General

* Teach client to monitor pulse rate.
* Teach client to monitor amount of medication remaining in the canister.
* Advise client not to take over-the-counter (OTC) preparations without first checking with the health care provider. Some OTC products may have an additive effect.
* Instruct the client to avoid smoking. Smoking increases drug elimination.
* Discuss ways to alleviate anxiety such as relaxation techniques and music.
* Advise client having asthma attacks to wear an ID bracelet or tags.

Cultural Considerations

* Respect the cultural beliefs of the client concerning alterative ways to treat asthma or other chronic obstructive pulmonary disease. The client should be told if these ways are unsafe and explained in terms that can be understood.
* If the client from a different cultural background does not comply with the drug regimen, the health care provider might consult a health care provider of similar background and provide a written plan.

Evaluation

* Evaluate the effectiveness of the bronchodilator. The client is breathing without wheezing and without side effects of the drug.

Xanthines also stimulate the central nervous system (CNS) and respiration, dilate coronary and pulmonary vessels, and cause diuresis. Because of their effect on respiration and pulmonary vessels, the xanthines are used in the treatment of asthma.

Theophylline

The first theophylline preparation produced was aminophylline in 1936. Aminophylline is still the treatment of choice for acute asthma when it is administered as an intravenous solution. The solution contains 85% theophylline. Theophylline relaxes the smooth muscles of the bronchi, bronchioles, and pulmonary blood vessels by inhibiting the enzyme phosphodiesterase, resulting in an increase in cyclic AMP, which promotes bronchodilation.

Theophylline has a low therapeutic index and a narrow therapeutic range of 10 to 20 μg/mL. The serum or plasma theophylline concentration level should be monitored frequently to avoid severe side effects. Toxicity is likely to occur when the serum level is greater than 20 μg/mL. Certain theophylline preparations can be given with sympathomimetic (adrenergic) drug agents, but the dose may need to be adjusted.

Chart 36–2 presents the drug data related to theophylline preparations.

PHARMACOKINETICS

Theophylline is usually well absorbed after oral administration, but absorption may vary according to the specific dosage form. Theophylline is also well absorbed from oral liquids and uncoated plain tablets. Sustained-release dosage forms are slowly absorbed. Food and antacids may decrease the rate, but not the extent, of absorption; large volumes of fluid and high-protein meals may increase the rate of absorption. The rate of absorption also can be affected by the size of the dose: larger doses are absorbed more slowly. Theophylline can be administered intravenously in IV fluids.

Table 36–2
Nasal Inhalants for Asthma Control

CATEGORIES	NASAL INHALANT AGENTS
ADRENERGICS	
Beta₁ and beta₂	Isoproterenol (Isuprel)
Beta₂ and some beta₁	Bitolterol mesylate (Tornalate)
	Isoetharine HCl (Bronkosol)
	Metaproterenol sulfate (Alupent, Metaprel)
Beta₂	Albuterol (Proventil, Ventolin)
	Pirbuterol acetate (Maxair)
	Salmeterol (Serevent)
	Terbutaline sulfate (Brethine, Bicanyl)
ANTICHOLINERGICS	Ipratropium bromide (Atrovent)
	Ipratropium and albuterol (Combivent)
ANTIINFLAMMATORY DRUGS	
Cromolyn and nedocromil	Cromolyn (Intal)
	Nedocromil (Tilade)
Glucocorticoids (Corticosteroids)	Beclomethasone (Beclovent, Vanceril)
	Budesonide (Rhinocort)
	Dexamethasone (Decadron)
	Flunisolide (Nasalide)
	Fluticasone (Flonase)
	Monetasone furoate (Elocon)
	Triamcinolone (Nasacort)

Table 36–3
Suggested Drug Therapy for Asthma According to Severity

CLASSIFICATION	LONG-TERM CONTROL DRUGS	QUICK-RELIEF DRUGS
Step I	No daily medication is needed	Short-acting inhaled B₂ agonists
Step II Mild: persistent symptoms	Nasal glucocorticoids (inhaled-low dose) OR Cromolyn or nedocromil (inhaled) OR Leukotriene antagonists	Same as step I
Step III Moderate: persistent symptoms	Inhaled glucocorticoid (medium dose) OR Inhaled glucocorticoid (low-medium dose) AND long-acting bronchodilator, such as long-acting inhaled beta₂ agonist, theophylline (sustained-release) OR long-acting beta₂ agonist tablets	Same as step I
Step IV Severe: persistent symptoms	Inhaled glucocorticoid AND long-acting bronchodilator, such as long-acting inhaled beta₂ agonist, sustained-release theophylline, or long-acting beta₂ agonist tablet, AND glucocorticoid tablet	Same as step I

Adapted from the National Asthma Education and Prevention Program: Expert Panel Report III. Bethesda, MD: National Heart, Lung, and Blood Institute, 1997.

Chart 36–2. Bronchodilator: Methylxanthine

Drug Name

Theophylline
   (Theo-Dur, Theophyllin KI, Elixophyllin-KI,
Somophyllin, Slophyllin, Slo-bid, Quibron), ✿
PMS Theophylline, Pulmophylline
Respiratory smooth muscle relaxant
Pregnancy Category: C

Contraindications

Severe cardiac dysrhythmias, hyperthyroidism,
hypersensitivity to xanthines, peptic ulcer disease, uncontrolled seizure disorder
Caution: With young children and elderly

Dosage

Bronchospasm, Bronchial Asthma:
A: PO: 250–500 mg q8–12h
C: PO: 50–100 mg q6h; max: 12 mg/kg/d
Dosing is highly individualized and is based on
therapeutic serum levels 10 and 20 μg/mL.
Monitor levels and client response.

Drug-Lab-Food Interactions

Drug: *Increase* effect with allopurinol, oral contraceptives, ciprofloxacin, cimetidine, ranitidine,
calcium blockers, erythromycin; *decrease* effects
of neuromuscular blockers, phenytoin, lithium;
decrease effect with smoking, rifampin, phenobarbital, corticosteroids, and others
Food: *Increase* metabolism with low-carbohydrate, high-protein diet; *decrease* elimination
with high-carbohydrate diet (*increase* $t\frac{1}{2}$)
Lab: Interaction with laboratory result is not
common; however, check with each laboratory

Pharmacokinetics

Absorption: PO: Well absorbed; SR: slowly ab-
sorbed
Distribution: PB: Approx 60%
Metabolism: $t\frac{1}{2}$: 7–9 h nonsmokers; 4–5 h smok-
ers
Excretion: In urine

Pharmacodynamics

PO: Onset: 30 min
       Peak: 1–2 h
       Duration: 6 h
PO-SR: Onset: 1–3 h
       Peak: 4–8 h
       Duration: 8–24 h
PO: Onset: Rapid
       Peak: UK
       Duration: 6–8 h

Therapeutic Effects/Uses

To promote bronchodilation; to treat asthma and chronic obstructive pulmonary disease.

Mode of Action: Increased cyclic AMP results in bronchodilation; diuresis; cardiac, CNS, and gastric
acid stimulation.

Side Effects

Anorexia, nausea, vomiting, restlessness, dizziness, insomnia, flushing, rash, headache

Adverse Reactions

Irritability, tremors, tachycardia, palpitations,
urticaria
Life-threatening: Seizures, cardiac dysrhythmias, convulsions

KEY: A: adult; C: child; PO: by mouth; SR: sustained release; IV: intravenous; PB: protein-binding; $t\frac{1}{2}$: half-life; UK: unknown; ✿:
Canadian drug names.

The theophylline drugs are metabolized by liver enzymes, and 90% of the drug is excreted by the kidneys. Tobacco smoking increases metabolism of theophylline drugs, thereby decreasing the half-life of the drug. The half-life is shortened in smokers and in children. With a short drug half-life, theophylline is readily excreted by the kidneys, and the drug dose may need to be increased to maintain the therapeutic serum or plasma range. In nonsmokers and older adults, the average half-life of theophylline is 7 to 9 hours, and the dose requirements may be decreased. In smokers and children, the half-life is 4 to 5 hours and the dose requirement may be increased. In premature infants, the half-life is 15 to 55 h. In clients who have congestive heart failure (CHF), cor pulmonale, COPD, or liver disease, the half-life is 12 h. Creatinine clearance may be decreased in older adults, so caution should be taken related to theophylline dosage in order to avoid drug toxicity.

PHARMACODYNAMICS

Theophylline increases the level of cyclic AMP, resulting in bronchodilation. The average time of onset of action for oral theophylline preparations is 30 minutes; for sustained-release capsules, it is 1 to 2 hours. The duration of action for the sustained-release form is 8 to 24 hours, and for other oral and intravenous theophylline preparations, approximately 6 hours.

Table 36–4 lists the theophylline preparations, their dosages, and uses and considerations.

SIDE EFFECTS AND ADVERSE REACTIONS

Side effects and adverse reactions include anorexia, nausea and vomiting, gastric pain due to increased gastric acid secretion, intestinal bleeding, nervousness, dizziness, headache, irritability, cardiac dysrhythmias, tachycardia, palpitations, marked hypotension, hyperreflexia, and seizures.

Clients should not take other xanthines while taking theophylline in order to decrease the potential for side effects. Adverse CNS reactions are often more severe in children than in adults, that is, headaches, irritability, restlessness, nervousness, insomnia, dizziness, and seizures.

Theophylline toxicity is most likely to occur when serum concentrations exceed 20 μg/mL. Theophylline can cause hyperglycemia, decreased clotting time and, rarely, increased white blood cell count (leukocytosis).

Table 36–4
Theophylline Preparations

GENERIC (BRAND)	ROUTE AND DOSAGE	USES AND CONSIDERATIONS
Aminophylline–theophylline ethylenediamine (Somophyllin)	A: PO: LD 500 mg; then 250–500 mg q6–8h IV: LD 6 mg/kg over 30 min; then 0.2–0.9 mg/kg/h C: PO: LD: 7.5 mg/kg; then 3–6 mg/kg q6–8h IV: LD 5.6 mg/kg then 1 mg/kg/h *Caution:* Individual titration is based on serum theophylline levels.	IV for acute asthmatic attack. For IV use, drug must be diluted. Oral preparations are tablets or elixirs. For oral use, give with food to avoid GI distress. Side effects include restlessness, syncope, palpitation, tachycardia, hyperventilation, cardiac dysrhythmias. *Pregnancy category:* C; PB: UK; t½: 4–9 h
Dyphylline—dihydroxypropyl theophylline (Dyline, Dilor, Lufyllin)	A: PO: 200–800 mg q.i.d. or q6h A: IM: 250–500 mg q6h C >6 y: PO: 4–7 mg/kg/d in 4 divided doses Therapeutic serum theophylline range: 10–20 μg/mL	Treatment of asthma, chronic bronchitis, and emphysema. One-tenth as potent as theophylline. *Pregnancy category:* C; PB: UK; t½: 2 h
Oxtriphylline—choline theophyllinate (Choledyl)	A: PO: 200 mg q.i.d. or q6h C: 2–12 y: PO: 4 mg/kg q6h Therapeutic serum theophylline range: 10–20 μg/mL	Relief of asthma and COPD. Useful for long-term therapy. Drug tolerance is infrequent. *Pregnancy category:* C; PB: UK; t½: 3–13 h
Theophylline	See Chart 36–2	Used for moderate to severe asthma. Also for bronchospasm due to bronchitis and emphysema. Drug comes in tablets, timed-release tablets, liquid, elixirs, suspension, and in combination with other drugs. Monitor serum theophylline levels (10–20 μg/mL). Has many side effects; see Chart 36–2. *Pregnancy category:* C; PB: 60%; t½: nonsmokers: 7–9 h; smokers: 4–5 h

KEY: A: adult; C: child; PO: by mouth; LD: loading dose; IV: intravenous; UK: unknown; >: greater than; PB: protein-binding; t½: half-life.

Because of the diuretic effect of xanthines, including theophylline, clients should be advised to avoid caffeine products such as coffee, tea, cola drinks, and chocolate and to increase their fluid intake.

Rapid intravenous administration of aminophylline (a theophylline product) can cause dizziness, flushing, hypotension, severe bradycardia, and palpitations. Intravenous theophylline preparation should be administered slowly or via an infusion pump in order to avoid severe side effects.

DRUG INTERACTIONS

Beta blockers, cimetidine (Tagamet), propranolol (Inderal), and erythromycin decrease the liver metabolism rate and increase the half-life and effects of theophylline; barbiturate and carbamazepine decrease its effects. In both situations, the theophylline dosage would need adjustment. Theophylline increases the risk of digitalis toxicity, decreases the effects of lithium, and decreases theophylline levels with phenytoin. If theophylline and beta-adrenergic agonist are given together, a synergistic effect can occur; cardiac dysrhythmias may result.

LEUKOTRIENE RECEPTOR ANTAGONISTS AND SYNTHESIS INHIBITORS

Leukotriene (LT) is a chemical mediator that can cause inflammatory changes in the lung. The group cysteinyl leukotrienes promotes an increase in eosinophil migration, mucus production, and airway wall edema, which result in bronchoconstriction. LT receptor antagonists and LT synthesis inhibitors, referred to as leukotriene modifiers, are effective in reducing the inflammatory symptoms of asthma that have been triggered by allergic and environmental stimuli. These drug groups are not recommended for the treatment of an acute asthma attack. Three leukotriene modifiers—zafirlukast (Accolate), zileuton (Zyflo), and montelukast sodium (Singulair)—are available in the United States. These drugs are listed in Table 36–5.

Zafirlukast (Accolate) was the first drug in the class of leukotriene modifers. It acts as a leukotriene receptor antagonist, thus reducing the inflammatory process and decreasing bronchoconstriction. It is administered orally and is absorbed rapidly. It has a moderate to a moderately long half-life and is given twice a day. Zileuton (Zyflo) is a leukotriene synthesis inhibitor. The result of its action is to decrease the inflammatory process and decrease bronchoconstriction. Zileuton has a short half-life and is given four times a day. Both drugs are for adults and children older than 12 years of age. Montelukast (Singulair) is a new leukotriene receptor antagonist. It has a short

half-life of 2.5 to 5.5 hours and is considered safe for use in children 6 years and older.

This category of drugs is the latest available used to control asthma. Again, they should not be used during an acute asthmatic attack. They are used for prophylactic and maintenance drug therapy for chronic asthma.

GLUCOCORTICOIDS (STEROIDS)

Glucocorticoids, members of the corticosteroid family are used in the treatment of respiratory disorders, particularly asthma. These drugs have an antiinflammatory action and are indicated if the asthma is unresponsive to bronchodilator therapy or if the client has an asthma attack while on maximum doses of a theophylline or an adrenergic drug.

Side effects are significant with long-term oral use and include fluid retention, hyperglycemia, and impaired immune response. It is thought that glucocorticoids have a synergistic effect when given with a beta$_2$ agonist.

Glucocorticoids can be given by (1) aerosol inhaler: beclomethasone (Vanceril, Beclovent); (2) tablet: triamcinolone (Amcort, Aristocort, Azmacort), dexamethasone (Decadron), prednisone, prednisolone, and methylprednisolone; and (3) injection: dexamethasone (Decadron), hydrocortisone. Inhaled glucocorticoids are *not* helpful in treatment of a severe asthmatic attack. It may take 1 to 4 weeks for an inhaled steroid to reach its full effect.

Glucocorticoid preparations are discussed in detail in Chapter 45.

These drugs can be irritating to the gastric mucosa and should be taken with food to avoid ulceration. When discontinuing glucocorticoids, the dosage should be tapered slowly to prevent adrenal insufficiency. A single dose usually does not cause adrenal suppression. The use of an oral inhaler minimizes the risk of adrenal suppression that is associated with oral systemic glucocorticoid therapy. Inhaled glucocorticoids are preferred to the oral preparations unless they fail to control the asthma.

SIDE EFFECTS AND ADVERSE REACTIONS

Side effects associated with the oral inhalers generally are local rather than systemic (e.g., throat irritation, hoarseness, dry mouth, and coughing). Oral, laryngeal, and pharyngeal fungal infections have occurred but are reversible with discontinuation and antifungal treatment. Using a spacer for the inhaler may prevent these effects.

Oral and injectable glucocorticoids have many side effects. Occasionally, short-term use does not cause significant side effects. Most adverse reactions are seen within 2 weeks of glucocorticoid therapy.

Table 36-5
Antiinflammatory Drugs for Chronic Obstructive Pulmonary Disease

GENERIC (BRAND)	ROUTE AND DOSAGE	USES AND CONSIDERATIONS
LEUKOTRIENE MODIFIERS (DO *NOT* ADMINISTER FOR ACUTE ASTHMATIC ATTACK)		
Leukotriene receptor antagonists		
Zafirlukast (Accolate)	A: PO: 20 mg, b.i.d. 1 h before or 2 h after meals C >12 y: PO: same as adults	For prophylaxis and maintenance therapy for chronic asthma. Reduces inflammation within the bronchial tubes and airways. *Pregnancy category:* B; PB: >99%, t½: 10 h
Montelukast (Singulair)	A: PO: 10 mg daily in evening without food C >6 y: PO: 5 mg daily in evening without food	Newest leukotriene antagonist. Effective for mild-moderate persistent asthma. Reduces inflammation in airways. Better tolerated than zafirlukast and zileuton. *Pregnancy category:* UK; PB: UK; t½: 2.5-5.5 h
Leukotriene synthesis inhibitors		
Zileuton (Leutrol, Zyflo)	A: PO: 600 mg q.i.d. C >12 y: PO: 600 mg q.i.d.	For prophylaxis and maintenance therapy for chronic asthma. Reduces inflammation in the airways and decreases bronchoconstriction. Hepatotoxicity may result; liver enzymes should be closely monitored. *Pregnancy category:* C; PB: 93%; t½: 2.5 h

GLUCOCORTICOIDS (CORTICOSTEROIDS)

Intranasal spray (see Chapter 35, Table 35-3)
  Beclomethasone (Beconase, Vanconase)
  Budesonide (Pulmicort, Rhinocort)
  Dexamethasone (Decadron)
  Flunisolide (AeroBid, Nasalide)
  Fluticonsone (Flonase, Flovent)
  Mometasone furoate (Elocon)
  Triamcinolone (Nasacort)

Aerosol inhalation (see Chapter 45, Table 45-5)
  Beclomethasone (Beconase, Vanceril)
  Dexamethasone (Decadron)
  Flunisolide (AeroBid, Nasalid)
  Triamcinolone (Azmacort, Kenalog, Nasacort)

Oral, intramuscular, and intravenous (see Chapter 45, Table 45-5)
  Betamethasone (Celestone)
  Cortisone acetate (Cortone acetate, Cortistan)
  Dexamethasone (Decadron)
  Flurocortisone acetate (Florinef acetate)
  Hydrocortisone (Cortef, Hydrocortone)
  Methylprednisolone (Medrol, Solu-Medrol, Depo-Medrol)
  Paramethasone acetate (Haldone)
  Prednisolone (Delta-Cortef, Hydeltrasol)
  Prednisone
  Triamcinolone (Aristocort, Kenacort, Azmacort)

Cromolyn and nedocromil (do *NOT* use for an acute asthmatic attack)		
Cromolyn sodium (Intal)	A: C >6 y: Inhalation: 1 puff q.i.d.; available: oral solution and powder, intranasal	For chronic asthma and prophylactic use. Suppresses inflammation in the bronchial tube; does not have bronchodilating effects. Prevents the release of histamine. *Pregnancy category:* B; PB: UK; t½: 80 min
Nedocromil sodium (Tilade)	A: C >6 y: Inhalation: 2 puffs, q.i.d.; may decrease to b.i.d. to t.i.d.	For maintenance therapy for mild-moderate asthma. Has antiinflammatory effect. Suppresses the release of histamine. *Pregnancy category:* B; PB: UK; t½: 1.5-3 h

KEY: A: adult; C: child; PO: by mouth; PB: protein-binding; UK: unknown; t½: half-life; >: greater than.

BRONCHODILATOR

Assessment

- Obtain a medical and drug history; report probable drug-drug interaction.
- Obtain baseline vital signs (VS) for identifying abnormalities and for future comparisons.
- Assess for wheezing, decreased breath sounds, cough, and sputum production.
- Assess sensorium levels for confusion and restlessness due to hypoxia and hypercapnia.
- Assess theophylline blood levels. Toxicity occurs at a higher frequency with levels of >20 μg/mL.
- Assess hydration; diuresis may result in dehydration in the elderly and children.

Potential Nursing Diagnosis

- Airway clearance, ineffective
- Activity intolerance
- Knowledge deficit related to over-the-counter (OTC) drugs

Planning

- Client will be free of wheezing or significantly improved and lung fields will be clear within 2 to 5 d.
- Client is taking oral drugs and using inhaler as prescribed.

Nursing Interventions

- Monitor VS. Blood pressure may decrease and heart rate may increase. Check for cardiac dysrhythmias.
- Provide adequate hydration. Fluids aid in loosening secretions. Monitor drug therapy. Observe for side effects.
- Check serum plasma theophylline levels (normal level is 10 to 20 μg/mL).
- Administer medication at regular intervals around the clock to have a sustained therapeutic level.
- Administer medication after meals to decrease GI distress.
- Do *not* crush enteric-coated or sustained-release (SR) tablets or capsules.
- Provide pulmonary therapy by chest clapping and postural drainage, as appropriate.

Client Teaching

General
- Advise the client that if allergic reaction occurs (rash, urticaria), drug should be discontinued and health care provider notified.
- Advise the client not to take OTC preparations without first checking with the health care provider. Some OTC products may have an additive effect.
- Encourage the client to stop smoking under medical supervision. Avoid marked sudden changes in smoking amounts, which could affect theophylline blood levels. Smoking increases drug elimination, which may require an increase of drug dose.
- Discuss ways to alleviate anxiety such as relaxation techniques and music.
- Advise the client having frequent or severe asthma attacks to wear an ID bracelet or tags.
- Encourage the client contemplating pregnancy to seek medical advice before taking a theophylline preparation.
- Advise the client to keep drug stored out of reach of small children; request child safety caps.

Self-Administration
- Instruct the client to correctly use the nebulizer in conjunction with theophylline.
- Teach the client to monitor pulse rate and report any irregularities in comparison to baseline to health care provider.

Diet
- Advise the client that a high-protein, low-carbohydrate diet increases theophylline elimination. Conversely, a low-protein, high-carbohydrate diet prolongs the half-life; dosage may need adjustment.

Nursing Process continued on following page

Evaluation

- Evaluate the effectiveness of the bronchodilators. The client is breathing without wheezing and without side effects of the drug:
- Evaluate serum theophylline levels to make sure they are within the accepted range.
- Evaluate tolerance to activity.

When steroids are used over a prolonged time, fluid retention (puffy eyelids, edema in the lower extremities, moon face, and weight gain), thinning of the skin, purpura, abnormal subcutaneous (fat) distribution, increased blood sugar, and impaired immune response are likely to occur.

CROMOLYN AND NEDOCROMIL

Cromolyn sodium (Intal) is used for prophylactic treatment of bronchial asthma and therefore must be taken on a daily basis. It is *not* used for acute asthmatic attacks. Cromolyn does not have bronchodilator or antiinflammatory properties, but acts by inhibiting the release of histamine, which can cause an asthma reaction. The most common side effects are cough and a bad taste in the mouth. These effects can be decreased by drinking a few sips of water before and after the inhalation.

The method of administration of cromolyn is by inhalation. It can be used with beta adrenergics and xanthine derivatives. Rebound bronchospasm is a serious side effect of cromolyn. The drug should not be discontinued abruptly because a rebound asthmatic attack can result.

Action and uses of nedocromil sodium are similar to those of cromolyn sodium. It has an antiinflammatory effect and suppresses the release of histamine, leukotrienes, and other mediators from the mast cells. Like cromolyn, it should not be used for an acute asthmatic attack but it is used to prevent incidence of bronchospasm and an acute asthmatic attack. The inhalation may cause an unpleasant taste. It is thought that nedocromil may be more effective than cromolyn. Table 36–5 lists the antiinflammatory drugs for COPD, which include leukotriene receptor antago-

nists, leukotriene synthesis inhibitors, glucocorticoids (intranasal spray, aerosol, inhalation, oral, intramuscular, and intravenous, and cromolyn sodium and nedocromil sodium).

MUCOLYTICS

Mucolytics act like detergents by liquefying and loosening thick mucous secretions so they can be expectorated. Acetylcysteine (Mucomyst) is administered by nebulization. The drug should not be mixed together with other drugs. The medication should be administered with a bronchodilator for clients with asthma or hyperactive airways disease because the increased secretions may obstruct the bronchial airways. The bronchodilator should be given 5 minutes before the mucolytic. Side effects include nausea and vomiting, stomatitis (oral ulcers), and "runny nose."

Acetylcysteine (Mucomyst) can be used as an antidote for acetaminophen overdose if given within 12 to 24 hours after the overdose ingestion. Acetylcysteine can be given orally diluted in juice or soft drink.

Dornase alfa (Pulmozyme) is an enzyme that digests the DNA in thick sputum secretions of cystic fibrosis (CF) clients. This agent helps to reduce respiratory infections and improves pulmonary function. With the use of dornase alfa, the improvement usually occurs in 3 to 7 days. Side effects include chest pain, sore throat, laryngitis, and hoarseness.

ANTIMICROBIALS

Antibiotics are used only if an infection results from retained mucous secretions.

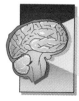

Critical Thinking in Action

M. A., age 55 years, was recently diagnosed as having bronchial asthma. She has a family history of asthma: her mother and three brothers also have asthma. In the past year, M. A. has had three asthmatic attacks that were treated with prednisone and albuterol (Proventil) inhaler. Prednisone 10 mg was prescribed for 5 days as follows: day 1, one tablet four times that day; day 2, one tablet three times that day; day 3, one tablet two times that day; day 4, one tablet in the morning; day 5, one-half tablet in the morning.

1. Explain the purpose for the use of prednisone during an asthmatic attack. Explain why the dosage is decreased (tapered) over a period of 5 days.
2. May cromolyn sodium be substituted for prednisone during an asthmatic attack? Explain.
3. M. A. is prescribed albuterol. What effect does albuterol have on controlling asthma?
4. Albuterol is administered by an inhaler. For each drug dose, M. A. is to receive two puffs. What instructions would you give her concerning the use of the inhaler?

To minimize the frequency of asthmatic attacks, the health care provider prescribed TheoDur 200 mg, b.i.d., for M. A. The albuterol inhalation is to be taken as needed. Nursing interventions include client history of asthmatic attacks and physical assessment.

5. What should the nurse include when taking the client's history concerning asthmatic attacks? What physical assessment would suggest an asthmatic attack?
6. What type of drug is TheoDur? Why should the nurse ask M. A. whether she smokes?
7. What are the side effects and adverse reactions and drug interactions related to TheoDur?
8. What nonpharmacologic measures can the nurse suggest that may decrease the frequency of asthmatic attacks?

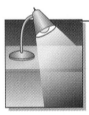

Study Questions

1. Your client is using an albuterol aerosol inhaler four times a day to prevent an asthmatic attack. What type of drug is albuterol? What is its action? What client teaching would you include concerning dose administration and side effects?

2. Theophylline drugs are administered by tablets for preventing asthmatic attacks and in intravenous fluids for an acute asthmatic attack. What is the effect of theophylline? What is its serum therapeutic range? Why is the serum level monitored?

3. When is cromolyn sodium used for treating asthma? Why should cromolyn not be discontinued abruptly?

4. S. D. is to use two aerosol inhalers, one a bronchodilator (Proventil) and the second a glucocorticoid (Vanceril). What client teaching would you include on administering these drugs together?

5. E. W. was having a mild asthmatic attack. The health care provider ordered methylprednisolone 4 mg for 6 days with decreasing dosages over the 6 days (six tablets the first day, five tablets the second day, four tablets the third day, and so forth). The questions the client asks include the following: What is the purpose of this drug for treating my asthma? Why am I taking fewer tablets each day? Why do I take it with food or after a meal? What are appropriate responses?

6. What are mucolytics? When are they used?

Unit IX

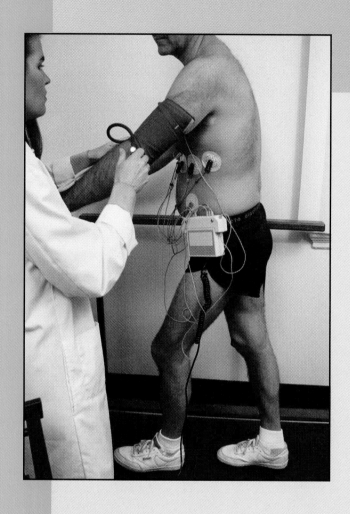

Cardiovascular Agents

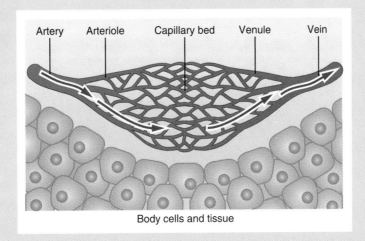

Figure IX–1
Basic structures of the vascular system.

Artery   Arteriole   Capillary bed   Venule   Vein

Body cells and tissue

The cardiovascular system includes the heart, blood vessels (arteries and veins), and blood. Blood rich in oxygen, nutrients, and hormones moves through vessels called arteries, which narrow to arterioles. Capillaries transport rich nourished blood to body cells and absorb waste products such as carbon dioxide (CO_2), urea, creatinine, and ammonia. The deoxygenated blood is returned to the circulation by the venules and veins for elimination with waste products by the lungs and kidneys (Fig. IX–1).

The pumping action of the heart is the energy source for circulation of blood to body cells. Blockage of vessels can inhibit blood flow.

HEART

The heart is composed of four chambers: the right and left atria and the right and left ventricles (Fig. IX–2). The right atrium receives deoxygenated blood from the circulation, and the right ventricle pumps blood to the pulmonary artery to the lungs for gas exchange (CO_2 for O_2). The left atrium receives oxygenated blood, and the left ventricle pumps the blood into the aorta for systemic circulation.

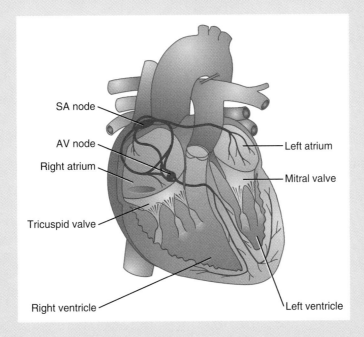

SA node
AV node
Right atrium
Tricuspid valve
Right ventricle
Left atrium
Mitral valve
Left ventricle

Figure IX–2
Anatomy of the heart. (SA node: sinoatrial node; AV node: atrioventricular node.)

653

The heart muscle is called the **myocardium** and surrounds the atria and ventricles. The ventricles are thick walled, especially the left ventricle, to achieve the muscular force needed to pump blood to the pulmonary and systemic circulations. The atrium is thin walled, because it serves as a receptacle for blood from the circulation and from the lungs and has no pumping action.

The heart has a fibrous covering called the **pericardium** that protects it from injury and infection. The **endocardium** is a three-layered membrane that lines the inner part of the heart chambers. Four valves—two atrioventricular (tricuspid and mitral) and two semilunar (pulmonic and aortic)—control blood flow between the atria and ventricles and between the ventricles and the pulmonary artery and the aorta. Three major coronary arteries (right, left, and circumflex) provide nutrients to the myocardium. Blockage in one or more of these arteries can result in a myocardial infarction, or heart attack.

CONDUCTION OF ELECTRICAL IMPULSES

The myocardium is capable of generating and conducting its own electrical impulses. The cardiac impulse usually originates in the **sinoatrial (SA) node** located in the posterior wall of the right atrium. The SA node is frequently referred to as the *pacemaker*, because it regulates the heartbeat (firing of cardiac impulses), which is approximately 60 to 80 beats a minute. The **atrioventricular (AV) node,** located in the posterior right side of the interatrial septum, has a continuous tract of fibers called the bundle of His, or the AV bundle. These two conducting systems (SA node and AV node) can act independently of each other. The ventricle can contract independently 30 to 40 times per minute.

Drugs that affect cardiac contraction include calcium, digitalis preparations, and quinidine and related preparations. The autonomic nervous system (ANS) and the drugs that stimulate or inhibit it influence heart contractions. The sympathetic nervous system and drugs that stimulate it increase heart rate; the parasympathetic nervous system and drugs that stimulate it decrease heart rate.

REGULATION OF HEART RATE AND BLOOD FLOW

The heart beats approximately 60 to 80 times a minute in an adult, pumping blood into the systemic circulation. As blood travels, resistance to blood flow develops and arterial pressure increases. The average systemic arterial pressure, known as blood pressure, is 120/80 mmHg. Arterial blood pressure is determined by peripheral resistance and **cardiac output,** the volume of blood expelled from the heart in 1 minute, which is calculated by multiplying the heart rate by the stroke volume. The average cardiac output is 4 to 8 L/min. **Stroke volume,** the amount of blood ejected from the left ventricle with each heart beat, is approximately 70 mL/beat.

Three factors, preload, contractility, and afterload, determine the stroke volume (Fig. IX–3). **Preload** refers to the blood flow force that stretches the ventricle. **Contractility** is the force of ventricular contraction, and **afterload** is the resistance to ventricular ejection of blood caused by opposing pressures in the aorta and systemic circulation.

Specific drugs can increase or decrease preload and afterload, affecting both stroke volume and cardiac output. Most vasodilators decrease preload and afterload, thus decreasing arterial pressure and cardiac output.

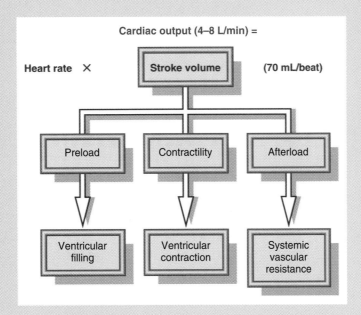

Cardiac output (4–8 L/min) =

Heart rate ✕   **Stroke volume**   (70 mL/beat)

Preload   Contractility   Afterload

Ventricular filling   Ventricular contraction   Systemic vascular resistance

Figure IX–3
Cardiac output and stroke volume.

CIRCULATION

There are two types of circulation—systemic, or peripheral, and pulmonary. With pulmonary circulation, the heart pumps deoxygenated blood from the right ventricle through the pulmonary artery to the lungs. In this situation, the artery is carrying blood that has a high concentration of CO_2. Oxygenated blood is returned to the left atrium by the pulmonary vein.

With systemic or peripheral circulation, the heart pumps blood from the left ventricle to the aorta into the general circulation. The blood is carried by arteries and arterioles to capillary beds. Nutrients in the capillary blood are transferred to cells in exchange for waste products. Blood returns to the heart through venules and veins.

BLOOD

Blood is composed of plasma, red blood cells (erythrocytes), white blood cells (leukocytes), and platelets. Plasma, made up of 90% water and 10% solutes, constitutes 55% of the total blood volume. The solutes in plasma include glucose, protein, lipids, amino acids, electrolytes, minerals, lactic and pyruvic acids, hormones, enzymes, oxygen, and carbon dioxide.

The major function of blood is to provide nutrients, including oxygen, to body cells. Most of the oxygen is carried in the hemoglobin of red blood cells (RBCs). The white blood cells (WBCs) are the major defense mechanism of the body and act by engulfing microorganisms. They also produce antibodies. The platelets are large cells that cause blood to coagulate. RBCs have a life span of approximately 120 days, where as the WBCs' life span is only 2 to 24 hours.

Unit IX, Cardiovascular Agents, is composed of four chapters dealing with drugs for cardiac disorders, diuretics and antihypertensive drugs, and drugs for circulatory disorders. Cardiac glycosides, antianginals, and antidysrhythmics are described in Chapter 37. Five categories of diuretics are included in Chapter 38. Five major categories of antihypertensive agents are presented in Chapter 39. Anticoagulants, thrombolytics, antilipidemics, and peripheral vasodilators are the four drug groups discussed in Chapter 40. Two Critical Thinking in Action and four groups of Study Questions are presented in this unit.

37 **Drugs for Cardiac Disorders**

Outline

Objectives

- Explain the actions of cardiac glycosides, antianginal drugs, and antidysrhythmics.
- Describe the signs and symptoms of digitalis toxicity.
- Identify the side effects and adverse reactions of nitrates, beta blockers, calcium channel blockers, quinidine, and procainamide.
- Explain the nursing process, including client teaching, related to cardiac glycosides, antianginal drugs, and antidysrhythmic drugs.

Terms

afterload	calcium channel blockers	hypokalemia
angina pectoris	cardiac dysrhythmias	hypoxia
antianginal drugs	cardiac glycosides	inotropic
antiarrhythmics	chronotropic	myocardial ischemia
antidysrhythmics	congestive heart failure	nitrates
atrial fibrillation	depolarization	preload
atrial flutter	dromotropic	repolarization
bradycardia	heart failure	tachycardia
beta blockers	hypercapnia	therapeutic serum level

INTRODUCTION

Three groups of drugs, the cardiac glycosides, the antianginals, and the antidysrhythmics, are discussed in this chapter. Drugs in these groups regulate heart contraction, heart rate and rhythm, and blood flow to the myocardium (heart muscle).

CARDIAC GLYCOSIDES

Digitalis, one of the oldest drugs, used as early as A.D. 1200, is still used in a purified form. Obtained from the purple and white foxglove plant, it can be poisonous. In 1785, William Withering of England used digitalis for alleviating "dropsy," edema of the extremities caused by kidney and cardiac insufficiency. Digitalis preparations are effective in treating congestive heart failure (CHF). (Withering did not realize that "dropsy" was the result of heart failure.) When the heart muscle (myocardium) weakens and enlarges; it loses its ability to pump blood through the heart and into the systemic circulation. This is called **heart failure,** or pump failure. When compensatory mechanisms fail and the peripheral and lung tissues are congested, the condition is **congestive heart failure.** Heart failure can be left sided or right sided. The client is in left-sided heart failure when the left ventricle does not contract sufficiently to pump the blood returned from the left atrium and lungs into the aorta, causing excessive amounts of blood to remain in the lung tissue. Right-sided heart failure occurs when the heart does not pump sufficiently for the amount of blood returning from the systemic circulation, and the blood and its constituents are pushed into peripheral tissues. One type of heart failure can lead to the other.

With heart failure, there is an increase in preload and afterload. An increase in preload is an increase in blood in the ventricle after diastole. With an increased afterload, there is an increased pressure or force in the ventricular wall caused by increased resistance in the aorta that must be overcome to open the aortic valve to eject blood into the circulation.

Cardiac glycosides are also called digitalis glycosides. This group of drugs inhibits the sodium-potassium pump; thus, they increase intracellular calcium, which causes the cardiac muscle fibers to contract more efficiently. Digitalis preparations have three effects on the heart muscle: (1) a positive **inotropic** action (increases myocardial contraction), (2) a negative **chronotropic** action (decreases heart rate), and (3) a negative **dromotropic** action (decreases conduction of the heart cells). The increase in myocardial contractility increases cardiac, peripheral, and kidney function by increasing cardiac output, decreasing preload, improving blood flow to the periphery and kidneys, decreasing edema, and increasing fluid excretion. As a result, fluid retention in the lung and extremities is decreased.

Digitalis preparations are also used to correct **atrial fibrillation** (cardiac dysrhythmia with rapid uncoordinated contractions of atrial myocardium) and **atrial flutter** (cardiac dysrhythmia with rapid contractions of 200 to 300 beats per minute [bpm]).

Nonpharmacologic Measures for Treating Heart Failure

Nondrug therapy is an integral part of the regimen for controlling heart failure. The client should limit the salt intake to 2 grams daily, which is approximately 1 teaspoon of salt. Alcohol intake should be decreased to one drink per day or completely avoided. Excess alcohol use can lead to cardiomyopathy. Smoking should be avoided because it deprives the heart of oxygen. Obesity increases cardiovascular problems; thus, obese clients should decrease fat and caloric intake. Mild exercise is recommended, such as walking or bicycling.

The nondrug component should be tailored to meet the needs of each client. Heart failure control requires the combined approach of nondrug and pharmacologic therapies.

Digoxin

Chart 37–1 gives the pharmacologic data for digoxin, a cardiac glycoside.

PHARMACOKINETICS

The absorption rate of digoxin in oral tablet form is >70%, and with the liquid preparation is 90%. The protein-binding power for digoxin is low; however, its half-life is 36 h; thus drug accumulation can occur. Side effects and serum digoxin level should be closely monitored to detect digitalis toxicity.

Thirty percent of digoxin is metabolized by the liver and 65% is excreted by the kidneys mostly unchanged. Kidney dysfunction can affect the excretion of digoxin. Thyroid dysfunction can alter metabolism of cardiac glycosides. For clients with hypothyroidism, the dose of digoxin should be decreased; in hyperthyroidism, the dose may need to be increased.

Digitoxin is a potent cardiac glycoside that has a very long half-life and is highly protein-bound. This drug is seldom prescribed. The names of *digoxin* and *digitoxin* are very similar, and the nurse must be extremely careful to administer the correct drug. The client should consistently take the same brand-name digoxin to avoid unnecessary side effects or adverse reactions.

Chart 37–1.   Cardiac Glycosides (Inotropic Agents, Cardiotonics)

CARDIAC GLYCOSIDE

Drug Name

Digoxin (Lanoxin), 🍁 Novodigoxin
   Pregnancy Category: C

Dosage

A: PO: 0.5–1 mg initially in 2 divided doses
(digitalization); *maint:* 0.125–0.5 mg/d;
elderly: 0.125 mg/d. IV: Same as PO dose given
over 5 min
C: PO: 1 mo–2 y: 0.01–0.02 mg/kg in 3 divided
doses; 2–10 y: 0.012–0.04 mg/kg in divided
doses; maint: 0.012 mg/kg/d in 2 divided
doses.
Pediatric doses are usually ordered in μg (mcg)
in elixir form. IV: Dosage varies

Contraindications

Ventricular dysrhythmias, 2nd- or 3rd-degree
heart block
Caution: AMI, renal disease, hypothyroidism,
hypokalemia

Drug-Lab-Food Interactions

Drug: *Increase* digoxin serum level with quinidine, flecainide, verapamil; *decrease* digoxin absorption with antacids, colestipol; *increase* risk
for digoxin toxicity with thiazide diuretics, loop
diuretics
Lab: hypokalemia, hypomagnesemia, hypercalcemia

Pharmacokinetics

Absorption: PO: 60%–76%; liq PO: 90%
Distribution: PB: 25%
Metabolism: t½: 30–45 h
Excretion: 70% in urine; 30% by liver metabo-
lism

Pharmacodynamics

PO: Onset: 1–5 h
     Peak: 6–8 h
     Duration: 2–4 d
IV: Onset: 5–30 min
     Peak: 1–5 h
     Duration: 2–4 d

Therapeutic Effects/Uses

To treat CHF, atrial tachycardia, flutter, or fibrillation.

Mode of Action: It inhibits the sodium-potassium ATPase, thus promoting increased force of cardiac
contraction, cardiac output, and tissue perfusion; decreases ventricular rate.

Side Effects

Anorexia, nausea, vomiting, headache, blurred
vision (yellow-green halos), diplopia, photophobia, drowsiness, fatigue, confusion

Adverse Reactions

Bradycardia, visual disturbances
Life-threatening: Atrioventricular block, cardiac
dysrhythmias

Assessment and Planning

Interventions

Evaluation

NURSING PROCESS

KEY: A: adult; C: child; PO: by mouth; IV: intravenous; AMI: acute myocardial infarction; CHF: congestive heart failure; PB: protein-
binding; t½: half-life; 🍁: Canadian drug name.

PHARMACODYNAMICS

In clients with a failing heart, cardiac glycosides increase myocardial contraction, which increases cardiac
output and improves circulation and tissue perfusion.
Because these drugs decrease conduction through the
atrioventricular node, the heart rate is decreased.

The onset and peak actions of oral and intraven-

ous digoxin vary. The **therapeutic serum level** is
0.5 to 2.0 ng/mL for digoxin and 10 to 35 ng/mL for
digitoxin. To treat CHF, the lower serum therapeutic
levels should be obtained, and for atrial flutter or
fibrillation, the higher therapeutic serum levels are
required.

Of these two drugs, digoxin is more frequently

Table 37-1
Cardiac Glycosides

GENERIC (BRAND)	ROUTE AND DOSAGE	USES AND CONSIDERATIONS
RAPID-ACTING DIGITALIS		
Digoxin (Lanoxin)	See Chart 37-1	For CHF atrial flutter, or atrial fibrillation. Low pulse rate may indicate digitalis toxicity. Serum therapeutic level is 0.5–2. *Pregnancy category:* C; PB: 25%; t½: 30–45 h
LONG-ACTING DIGITALIS		
Digitoxin (Crystodigin)	A: PO/IV: LD: 0.8–1.2 mg; *maint:* PO: 0.05–3 mg/d	For CHF. Serum therapeutic level is 15–30 ng/mL. Due to its long half-life, this drug is seldom given. *Pregnancy category:* C; PB: 97%; t½: 1–3 wk
POSITIVE INOTROPIC BIPYRIDINES		
Amrinone lactate (Inocor)	A: IV: LD: 0.75 mg/kg within 2–3 min; *maint:* 5–10 µg/kg/min; *max:* 10 mg/kg/d	For CHF, amrinone may be prescribed when digoxin and diuretics have not been effective. It may be used in conjunction with diuretic. Drug is for short-term use. *Pregnancy category:* C; PB: 10%–50%; t½: 3.5–7 h
Milrinone lactate (Primacor)	A: IV: Initially: 50 µg/kg/over 10 min *Continuous infusion:* 0.375–0.75 µg/kg/min with 0.45%–0.9% saline	For short-term treatment of CHF. May be given before heart transplantation. Heart rate and blood pressure should be monitored. *Pregnancy category:* C; PB: 70%; t½: 1.5–2.5 h
ANTIDOTE FOR DIGITALIS TOXICITY		
Digoxin immune Fab (ovine, Digibind)	Dose varies. Use manufacturer's dosing guidelines. Approx 760 mg, IV diluted in 50 mL of NSS. Infuse over 30 min.	To correct serious digitalis toxicity. This agent binds with digoxin to form complex molecules. A serum digoxin level >2.0 ng is indicative of digitalis toxicity. Onset of action is 30 min and duration of action can be 3–4 d. *Pregnancy category:* C; PB: UK; t½: 15–20 h

KEY: A: adult; PO: by mouth; IV: intravenous; LD: loading dose; PB: protein-binding; t½: half-life; CHF: congestive heart failure; NSS: normal saline solution.

used. It can be administered orally or intravenously. Table 37-1 lists the drug data for digitalis preparations.

DIGITALIS TOXICITY

Overdose or accumulation of digoxin causes digitalis toxicity. Signs and symptoms include anorexia, diarrhea, nausea and vomiting, **bradycardia** (pulse rate below 60 beats per minute [bpm]), premature ventricular contractions, cardiac dysrhythmias, headaches, malaise, blurred vision, visual illusions (white, green, yellow halos around objects), confusion, and delirium. Older adults are more prone to toxicity.

Cardiotoxicity is a serious adverse reaction to digoxin; ventricular dysrhythmias result. There are three cardiac-altered functions that contribute to digoxin-induced ventricular dysrhythmias: (1) suppression of atrioventricular (AV) conduction, (2) increased automaticity, and (3) decreased refractory period in ventricular muscle. The antidysrhythmics phenytoin and lidocaine are effective in treating digoxin-induced ventricular dysrhythmias.

ANTIDOTE FOR CARDIAC/DIGITALIS GLYCOSIDES

Digoxin immune Fab (ovine, Digibind) may be given to treat severe digitalis toxicity. This agent binds with digoxin to form complex molecules that can be excreted in the urine; thus, digoxin is unable to bind at the cellular site of action. Signs and symptoms of digoxin toxicity should be reported promptly to the health care provider. Serum digoxin levels should be closely monitored. Digitalis toxicity may result in first-degree, second-degree, or complete heart block.

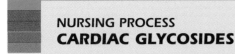

NURSING PROCESS
CARDIAC GLYCOSIDES

Assessment

- Obtain a drug history. Report if a drug-drug interaction is probable. If the client is taking digoxin and a potassium-wasting diuretic or cortisone drug, hypokalemia might result, causing digitalis toxicity. A low serum potassium level enhances the action of digoxin. A client taking a thiazide and/or cortisone along with digoxin should be taking a potassium supplement.
- Obtain a baseline pulse rate for future comparisons. Apical pulse should be taken for a full minute and should be >60 bpm.
- Assess for signs and symptoms of digitalis toxicity. Common symptoms include anorexia, nausea, vomiting, bradycardia, cardiac dysrhythmias, and visual disturbances. Report symptoms immediately to the health care provider.

Potential Nursing Diagnoses

- Decreased cardiac output
- Altered tissue perfusion (cardiopulmonary, cerebral)
- Anxiety related to cardiac problem

Planning

- Client checks pulse rate daily before taking digoxin. Client will report pulse rate of <60 bpm or a marked decline in pulse rate.
- Client eats foods rich in potassium to maintain a desired serum potassium level (see Client Teaching, Diet).

Nursing Interventions

- Do *not* confuse **digoxin** with **digitoxin.** Read the drug labels carefully. Digoxin has a long half-life but has a shorter half-life than digitoxin.
- Check the apical pulse rate before administering digoxin. Do *not* administer if pulse rate is <60 bpm.
- Check the signs of peripheral and pulmonary edema, which indicate CHF.
- Check the serum digoxin level. The normal therapeutic drug range for digoxin is 0.5 to 2.0 ng/mL. A serum digoxin level of >2.0 ng/mL is indicative of digitalis toxicity. Check serum potassium level (normal range, 3.5 to 5.3 mEq/L) and report if hypokalemia (<3.5 mEq/L) is present.

Nursing Process continued on following page

DRUG INTERACTIONS

Drug interaction with digitalis preparations can cause digitalis toxicity. Many of the potent diuretics such as furosemide (Lasix) and hydrochlorothiazide (Hydro-DIURIL) promote the loss of potassium from the body. The resultant **hypokalemia** (low serum potassium level) increases the effect of the digitalis preparation, and digitalis toxicity results. Cortisone preparations taken systemically promote sodium retention and potassium excretion or loss, and can also cause hypokalemia. Clients taking digoxin along with a potassium-wasting diuretic or a cortisone drug should consume foods rich in potassium or take potassium supplements to avoid hypokalemia and digitalis toxicity. Antacids can decrease digitalis absorption if taken at the same time. Staggering doses prevents this problem.

OTHER AGENTS USED TO TREAT HEART FAILURE

Vasodilators may be used for treating heart failure. The venodilators decrease venous blood return to the heart, thus there is a decrease in cardiac filling, ventricular stretching, and oxygen demand on the heart. The arteriolar dilators act in three ways: (1) reduce cardiac afterload, which increases cardiac output, (2) dilate the arterioles of the kidneys, which improves renal perfusion and increases fluid loss, and (3) improve circulation to the skeletal muscles.

Angiotensin-converting enzyme (ACE) inhibitors are usually prescribed for heart failure. ACE inhibitors dilate venules and arterioles, which improves renal blood flow and decreases blood fluid volume. It moderately decreases the release of aldosterone; thus, sodium retention is reduced as is fluid retention.

Client Teaching

General

- Explain to the client the importance of compliance with the drug therapy. A visiting nurse may ensure that the medications are properly taken.
- Advise the client not to take over-the-counter (OTC) drugs without first consulting the health care provider to avoid adverse drug interactions.
- Keep drugs out of reach of small children. Request child safety cap bottle.
- Instruct the parent to check child's pulse rate before administering the drug.

Self-Administration

- Instruct the client how to check the pulse rate before taking digoxin and to call the health care provider for pulse rate <60 bpm or irregular pulse.

Diet

- Advise the client to eat foods rich in potassium such as fresh and dried fruits, fruit juices, and vegetables, including potatoes.

Side Effects

- Instruct the client to report side effects such as a pulse rate of <60 bpm, nausea, vomiting, headache, and visual disturbances, including diplopia.

Cultural Considerations

- It is essential that clients from various cultural backgrounds taking digoxin, diuretics, and potassium supplements for heart failure do not miss drug doses of their medication. The client should be fully aware of adverse effects and readily report them to the health care provider.

Evaluation

- Evaluate the effectiveness of digoxin by noting the client's response to the drug (decreased heart rate, decreased chest rales), and the absence of side effects. Continue monitoring the pulse rate.

Diuretics are the first-line drug treatment for reducing fluid volume and are frequently prescribed with digoxin or other agents.

Spironolactone (Aldactone), a potassium-sparing diuretic, is effective in treating moderate to severe CHF, more so than the ACE inhibitors. Aldosterone secretions are increased in CHF; this promotes body loss of potassium and magnesium needed by the heart and increases sodium and water retention. Spironolactone blocks the production of aldosterone.

Beta blockers had been contraindicated for clients in heart failure. This drug class reduces cardiac contractility. In some cases, this therapy can improve cardiac performance, for example, the beta blocker carvedilol (Coreg).

ANTIANGINAL DRUGS

Antianginal drugs are used to treat **angina pectoris** (acute cardiac pain caused by inadequate blood flow resulting from plaque occlusion in the coronary arteries of the myocardium or from spasms of the coronary arteries). With decreased blood flow, there is a decrease in oxygen to the myocardium that causes pain. Anginal pain is frequently described by the client as tightness, pressure in the center of the chest, and pain radiating down the left arm. Referred pain felt in the neck and left arm commonly occurs with severe angina pectoris. Anginal attacks may lead to myocardial infarction (heart attack). Anginal pain usually lasts for only a few minutes.

Types of Angina Pectoris

The frequency of anginal pain depends on many factors, including the type of angina, which includes (1) classic (stable)—occurs with stress or exertion, (2) unstable (preinfarction)—occurs frequently over the course of a day with progressive severity, and (3) variant (Prinzmetal, vasospastic)—occurs during rest. The first two types are caused by a narrowing or partial occlusion of the coronary arteries; variant angina is due to vessel spasm (vasospasm). It is not uncommon for the client to have both classic and variant angina. Unstable angina often indicates an impending myocardial infarction (MI). This is an emergency and needs immediate medical intervention.

Types of Antianginal Drugs

Antianginal drugs increase blood flow either by increasing oxygen supply or by decreasing oxygen demand by the myocardium. Three types of antianginals are the (1) nitrates, (2) beta blockers, and (3) calcium channel blockers. The major systemic effect of nitrates is a reduction of venous tone, which decreases the workload of the heart and promotes vasodilation. Beta blockers and calcium channel blockers decrease the workload of the heart and decrease oxygen demands.

Nitrates and calcium channel blockers are effective in treating variant or vasospastic angina pectoris. Beta blockers are not effective for this type of angina. With stable angina, beta blockers are effective in preventing angina attacks. Table 37–2 lists the effects of antianginal drug groups on angina.

There are various types of organic nitrates. Isosorbide dinitrate (Isordil, Sorbitrate) can be administered sublingually (SL) by tablets and orally by chewable tablets, immediate-release tablets, and sustained-release tablets and capsules. Isosorbide mononitrate (Monoket, Imdur) can be given orally by immediate-release and sustained-release tablets.

Stress tests, cardiac profile laboratory tests, and cardiac catheterization may be needed to determine the degree of blockage in the coronary arteries. A combination of pharmacologic and nonpharmacologic measures is usually necessary to control and prevent anginal attacks.

Nonpharmacologic Measures to Control Angina

Nonpharmacologic ways of decreasing anginal attacks are to avoid heavy meals, smoking, extremes in weather changes, strenuous exercise, and emotional upset. Proper nutrition, moderate exercise (only after consulting with a health care provider if the client already has angina), adequate rest, and relaxation techniques should be employed as preventive measures.

Nitrates

Nitrates, developed in the 1840s, were the first agents used to relieve angina. Nitroglycerin is not swallowed because it undergoes first-pass metabolism by the liver, which decreases its effectiveness; instead it is given sublingually (under the tongue) and is absorbed readily into the circulation through the sublingual vessels. The sublingual tablet comes in various dosages, but the average dose prescribed is 0.4 mg or gr 1/150 following cardiac pain, repeated every 5 min for a total of three doses. The client may experience dizziness, faintness, or headache as a result of the peripheral vasodilation. If pain persists, the client should immediately call for medical assistance. Nitroglycerin is also available in topical (ointment, transdermal patch) and intravenous forms. Chart 37–2 summarizes the action of the nitroglycerin (nitrates).

PHARMACOKINETICS

Nitroglycerin, taken sublingually, is absorbed rapidly and directly into the internal jugular vein and the right atrium. Approximately 40% to 50% of nitrates absorbed through the gastrointestinal (GI) tract are inactivated by liver metabolism (first-pass metabolism

Table 37–2
Effects of Antianginal Drug Groups on Angina

DRUG GROUP	VARIANT (VASOSPASTIC) ANGINA	CLASSIC (STABLE) ANGINA
Nitrates	Relaxation of coronary arteries, which decreases vasospasms and increases oxygen supply	Dilation of veins, which decreases preload and decreases oxygen demands
Beta blockers	Not effective	Decreases heart rate and contractility, which decreases oxygen demand
Calcium channel blockers	Relaxation of coronary arteries, which decreases vasospasms and increases oxygen supply	Dilation of arterioles, which decreases afterload and decreases oxygen demand. Verapamil and diltiazem decrease heart rate and contractility.

Adapted from Lehne, R. A.: Pharmacology for Nursing Care. Philadelphia: WB Saunders, p. 464, 1998.

Chart 37–2.   Antianginals: Nitroglycerin

NITRATE

Drug Name

Nitroglycerin
(Nitrostat, Nitro-Bid, Transderm-Nitro patch,
NTG), ❁ Nitrogard SR, Nitrol
Nitrate
Pregnancy Category: C

Contraindications

Marked hypotension, AMI, increased intracra-
nial pressure (ICP), severe anemia
Caution: Severe renal or hepatic disease, early
MI

Dosage

A: PO/SL: 0.3, 0.4, 0.6 mg; repeat q5min × 3 as
needed. SR: 2.5 mg q8–12 h
IV: Initially: 5 μg/min; dose may be increased
Oint: 2% 1–2 inch to chest or thigh area
Patch: 2.5–15 mg/d to chest or thigh area

Drug-Lab-Food Interactions

Drug: *Increase* effect with alcohol, beta blockers,
calcium blockers, antihypertensives; *decrease* effects of heparin

Assessment and Planning

Pharmacokinetics

Absorption: SL: >75% absorbed; oint and
patch: slow absorption
Distribution: PB: 60%
Metabolism: t½: 1–4 min
Excretion: Liver and urine

Pharmacodynamics

SL:	Onset: 1–3 min
	Peak: 4 min
	Duration: 20–30 min
SR: Cap:	Onset: 20–45 min
	Duration: 3–8 h
Oint:	Onset: 20–60 min
	Peak: 1–2 h
	Duration: 3–8 h
Patch:	Onset: 30–60 min
	Peak: 1–2 h
	Duration: 20–24 h
IV:	Onset: 1–3 min
	Duration: 0.5–2 h

Interventions

NURSING PROCESS

Therapeutic Effects/Uses

To control angina pectoris (anginal pain).

Mode of Action: Decrease myocardial demand for oxygen; decrease preload by dilating veins, thus
indirectly decreasing afterload.

Side Effects

Nausea, vomiting, headache, dizziness, syncope,
weakness, flushing, confusion, pallor, rash, dry
mouth

Adverse Reactions

Hypotension, reflex tachycardia, paradoxical
bradycardia
Life-threatening: Circulatory collapse

Evaluation

KEY: A: adult; C: child; PO: by mouth; SL: sublingual; SR: sustained-release; IV: intravenous; PB: protein-binding; t½: half-life; NTG:
nitroglycerin; AMI: acute myocardial infarction; MI: myocardial infarction; ❁: Canadian drug names.

---

of the liver). The nitroglycerin in Nitro-Bid ointment
and in the Transderm-Nitro patch is absorbed slowly
through the skin. It is excreted primarily in the urine.

PHARMACODYNAMICS

Nitroglycerin acts directly on the smooth muscle of
blood vessels, causing relaxation and dilation. It decreases cardiac **preload** (the amount of blood in the

ventricle at the end of diastole) and **afterload** (peripheral vascular resistance) and reduces myocardial oxygen demand. With dilation of the veins, there is less
blood return to the heart, and with dilation of the
arteries, there is less vasoconstriction and resistance.

The onset of action of nitroglycerin depends on the
method of administration. With sublingual and intravenous use, the onset of action is rapid (1 to 3 min);

Table 37–3
Antianginals

GENERIC (BRAND)	ROUTE AND DOSAGE	USES AND CONSIDERATIONS
NITRATES		
Amyl nitrite	A: Inhal: 0.18–0.3 mL amp PRN	For acute anginal attack. Rarely used. *Pregnancy category:* C; PB: UK; $t_{\frac{1}{2}}$: 1–4 min
Isosorbide dinitrate (Isordil, Sorbitrate)	A: SL: 2.5–10 mg q.i.d. Chewable: 5–10 mg PRN PO: 2.5–30 mg q.i.d. a.c. and h.s. SR: 40 mg q6–12h	To prevent anginal attacks. Drug can lower blood pressure. Tolerance builds up over time. Headaches, dizziness, lightheadedness, and flushing may occur. *Pregnancy category:* C; PB: UK; $t_{\frac{1}{2}}$: 1–4 h
Isosorbide mononitrate (Imdur)	A: PO: SR: 30–60 mg q morning: *max:* 240 mg/d	To prevent anginal attacks. Sustained-release form provides controlled delivery and a 6-h drug-free period. By allowing a drug-free period, tolerance to nitrates is reduced; effectiveness is increased. *Pregnancy category:* C; PB: 5%; $t_{\frac{1}{2}}$: 6.6 h
Nitroglycerin (Nitrostat, Nitro-Bid, Transderm-Nitro)	See Chart 37–2	To control angina pectoris. IV used for treating severe angina and hypertension. Headaches occur approximately 50% when first used. *Pregnancy category:* C; PB: 60%; $t_{\frac{1}{2}}$: 1–4 min (IV)
BETA-ADRENERGIC BLOCKERS		
Atenolol (Tenormin) (Beta$_1$)	A: PO: 50–100 mg/d; *max:* 200 mg/d	To control angina pectoris. Also effective in managing hypertension. Blood pressure and heart rate should be monitored. Cardioselective drug, blocking beta$_1$. Can be used by asthmatic clients. *Pregnancy category:* C; PB: 5%–15%; $t_{\frac{1}{2}}$: 6–7 h
Metoprolol tartrate (Lopressor) (Beta$_1$)	A: PO: Initially: 50–100 mg/d in 1–2 divided doses; *maint:* 100–400 mg/d SR: 100 mg, daily; *max:* 400 mg/d	Same as atenolol. Monitor heart rate and blood pressure. *Pregnancy category:* C; PB: 12%; $t_{\frac{1}{2}}$: 3–7 h
Nadolol (Corgard) (Beta$_1$ and beta$_2$)	A: PO: 40 mg daily; dose may be increased	To treat angina pectoris and hypertension. *Pregnancy category:* C; PB: 28%; $t_{\frac{1}{2}}$: 10–24 h (renal disease: 45 h)
Propranolol HCl (Inderal) (Beta$_1$ and beta$_2$)	A: PO: Initially: 10–20 mg t.i.d.–q.i.d.; *maint:* 20–60 mg t.i.d.–q.i.d.; *max:* 320 mg/d SR: 80–160 mg/d	First beta blocker, blocking beta$_1$ and beta$_2$. It is no longer the drug of choice to prevent angina because of the risk of bronchospasm. Heart rate, blood pressure, and respiratory status should be monitored. *Pregnancy category:* C; PB: 90%; $t_{\frac{1}{2}}$: 3–6 h
CALCIUM CHANNEL BLOCKERS		
Amlodipine (Norvasc)	A: PO: Initially: 10 mg; maint: 2.5–10 mg/d Elderly: Initially: 2.5 mg/d	Management of angina pectoris and hypertension. May be given with another antianginal or antihypertensive drug. *Pregnancy category:* C; PB: 95%; $t_{\frac{1}{2}}$: 30–50 h
Bepridil HCl (Vascor)	A: PO: Initially 200 mg/d × 10 d; *maint:* 300 mg/d; *max:* 400 mg/d	Treatment of angina pectoris. May be used as single drug or in combination with nitrates. Given as a single dose. *Pregnancy category:* C; PB: 99%; $t_{\frac{1}{2}}$: 2–24 h
Diltiazem HCl (Cardizem)	A: PO: 30–60 mg q.i.d.; may increase to 360 mg/d in 4 divided doses SR: 60 mg q12h; *max:* 360 mg/d CD: 120–180 mg/d; *max:* 360 mg/d	For angina pectoris. Hypotensive effect is not as severe as with nifedipine. Kidney function should be monitored. *Pregnancy category:* C; PB: 70%–85%; $t_{\frac{1}{2}}$: 3.5–9 h

Table 37–3 *Continued*
Antianginals

GENERIC (BRAND)	ROUTE AND DOSAGE	USES AND CONSIDERATIONS
Felodipine (Plendil)	A: PO: Initially: 5 mg/d single dose; *maint:* 2.5–10 mg/d Elderly: Initially: 2.5 mg/d	To treat chronic angina pectoris and manage hypertension. Reduces oxygen demand by the heart. A potent peripheral vasodilator, thus increasing heart rate and myocardial contractility. *Pregnancy category:* C; PB: >99%; $t_{\frac{1}{2}}$: 10–16 h
Isradipine (DynaCirc)	A: PO: 2.5–7.5 mg t.i.d.	Primary use is to treat hypertension. Also can be given for angina pectoris. *Pregnancy category:* C; PB: 99%; $t_{\frac{1}{2}}$: 5–11 h
Nicardipine HCl (Cardene, Cardene SR)	A: PO: 20 mg t.i.d.; maint: 20–40 mg t.i.d. SR: 30 mg b.i.d.; maint: 30–60 mg b.i.d.	Used for angina pectoris. May be used alone or in combination with other antianginals. Used also for hypertension. Peripheral edema, headache, dizziness, and lightheadedness may occur. *Pregnancy category:* C; PB: 95%; $t_{\frac{1}{2}}$: 5 h
Nifedipine (Procardia, Adalat)	A: PO: 10–30 mg q6–8h; *max:* 180 mg/d	For angina pectoris. Blood pressure should be closely monitored, especially if client is taking nitrates or beta blockers. Is a potent calcium blocker. *Pregnancy category:* C; PB: 92%–98%; $t_{\frac{1}{2}}$: 2–5 h
Nisoldipine (Sular, Nisocor)	A: PO: Initially: 20 mg/d; *maint:* 20–40 mg/d Elderly: A: PO: 10–20 mg/d	To treat angina pectoris and hypertension. Suppresses contraction of cardiac and vascular smooth muscle. Increases heart rate and cardiac output. Decreases blood pressure. *Caution:* Clients with heart disease are prone to MI and CHF. *Pregnancy category:* C; PB: >99%; $t_{\frac{1}{2}}$: 7–12 h
Verapamil HCl (Calan, Isoptin, Verelan)	A: PO: 40–120 mg t.i.d.; *max:* 480 mg/d IV: 5–10 mg over 2 min	Treatment of angina pectoris, cardiac dysrhythmias, and hypertension. Peripheral edema, constipation, dizziness, headache, and hypotension may occur. *Pregnancy category:* C; PB: 90%; $t_{\frac{1}{2}}$: 3–8 h

KEY: A: adult; PO: by mouth; IV: intravenous; SL: sublingual; SR: sustained-release; CD: controlled delivery; a.c.: before meals; PB: protein-binding; $t_{\frac{1}{2}}$: half-life; PRN: as necessary; UK: unknown; MI: myocardial infarction; CHF: congestive heart failure.

it is slower with the transdermal method (30 to 60 min). The duration of action of the Transderm-Nitro patch is approximately 24 h. Because Nitro-Bid ointment is effective for only 6 to 8 h, it must be reapplied three to four times a day. The use of Nitro-Bid ointment has declined since the advent of the Transderm-Nitro patch, which needs to be applied only once a day. Table 37–3 lists drug data for the nitrates.

SIDE EFFECTS AND ADVERSE REACTIONS

Headaches are one of the most common side effects of nitroglycerin, but they may become less frequent with continued use. Otherwise, acetaminophen may provide some relief. Other side effects include hypotension, dizziness, weakness, and faintness. When nitroglycerin ointment or transdermal patches are dis-

continued, the dose should be tapered over several weeks to prevent the rebound effect of severe pain caused by **myocardial ischemia** (lack of blood supply to the heart muscle). Nitrate tolerance can occur with a continual increase in dosage or with prolonged use.

Beta Blockers

Beta-adrenergic blockers block the beta$_1$ receptor site. Beta blockers decrease the effects of the sympathetic nervous system by blocking the release of the catecholamines epinephrine and norepinephrine, thereby decreasing the heart rate and blood pressure. They are used as antianginal, antidysrhythmic, and antihypertensive drugs. Beta blockers are effective as antianginals because, by decreasing the heart rate and myocardial contractility, they reduce the need for oxygen consumption and, consequently, the pain of angina. These drugs are more useful for classic (stable) angina.

Beta blockers, which are discussed in detail in Chapter 21, are subdivided into nonselective beta blockers (blocking beta$_1$ and beta$_2$) and selective (cardiac) beta blockers (blocking beta$_1$). Examples of nonselective beta blockers are propranolol (Inderal), nadolol (Corgard), and pindolol (Visken). These drugs decrease the pulse rate and can cause bronchoconstriction. The selective (cardioselective) beta blockers act more strongly on the beta$_1$ receptor, thus decreasing the pulse rate. Examples are atenolol (Tenormin) and metoprolol (Lopressor). This latter group is the choice for controlling angina pectoris. Table 37–3 lists the beta blockers most frequently used for angina.

PHARMACOKINETICS

Orally, the beta blockers are well absorbed. Absorption of sustained-release capsules is slow. The half-life of propranolol (Inderal) is 3 to 6 h. Of the selective beta blockers, atenolol (Tenormin) has a half-life of 6 to 7 h, and metoprolol (Lopressor), 3 to 7 h. Propranolol and metoprolol are metabolized and excreted by the liver. Fifty percent of atenolol is excreted unchanged by the kidneys, and 50% is excreted unabsorbed in the feces.

PHARMACODYNAMICS

Because beta blockers decrease the force of myocardial contraction, the oxygen demand by the myocardium is reduced, and the client can tolerate increased exercise with less oxygen need. Beta blockers tend to be more effective for classic (stable) angina than for variant (vasospastic) angina.

The onset of action of the nonselective beta blocker propranolol is 30 min, its peak action is reached in 1 to 1.5 h, and its duration is 4 to 12 h. For the selective beta blockers, the onset of action of atenolol is 60 min, the peak action occurs in 2 to 4 h, and the duration of action is 24 h; the onset of action of metoprolol is reached in 15 min and the duration of action is 6 to 12 h.

SIDE EFFECTS AND ADVERSE REACTIONS

Both nonselective and selective beta blockers cause a decrease in pulse rate and blood pressure. For the nonselective beta blockers, bronchospasm, behavioral or psychotic response, and impotence (with use of Inderal) are potential adverse reactions.

The vital signs need to be closely monitored in the early stages of beta blocker therapy. With discontinuation of use, the dosage should be tapered for a week or two to prevent a rebound effect (reflex tachycardia and vasoconstriction).

Calcium Channel Blockers

Calcium channel blockers, also known as calcium blockers, are the newest group of drugs to be marketed (1982) for the treatment of angina pectoris, certain dysrhythmias, and hypertension. Calcium activates myocardial contraction, increasing the workload of the heart and the need for more oxygen. Calcium blockers decrease cardiac contractility (negative inotropic effect by relaxing smooth muscle) and the workload of the heart, thus decreasing the need for oxygen. They are effective in controlling variant (vasospastic) angina by relaxing coronary arteries and for classic (stable) angina by decreasing oxygen demand.

PHARMACOKINETICS

Three calcium blockers, verapamil (Calan), nifedipine (Procardia), and diltiazem (Cardizem), have been effectively used in long-term treatment of angina. Eighty to ninety percent of calcium channel blockers are absorbed through the GI mucosa. However, the first-pass metabolism by the liver decreases the availability of free circulating drug, and only 20% of verapamil, 45% to 65% of diltiazem, and 35% to 40% of nifedipine are bioavailable. All three drugs are highly protein-bound (80%–90%) and their half-life is 2 to 6 h.

Several other calcium blockers are available: nicardipine HCl (Cardene), amlodipine (Norvasc), bepridal HCl (Vascor), felodipine (Plendil), and nislodipine (Sular). All five of these drugs are highly protein-bound (>95%). Nicardipine has the shortest half-life.

PHARMACODYNAMICS

Bradycardia is a common problem with verapamil, the first calcium blocker. Nifedipine, the most potent of the calcium blockers, promotes vasodilation of the coronary and peripheral vessels, and hypotension can result. The onset of action is 10 min for verapamil and 30 min for nifedipine and diltiazem. Duration of action is 3 to 7 h (PO) and 2 h (IV) for verapamil and 6 to 8 h for nifedipine and diltiazem.

Table 37–3 presents the drug data for the calcium blockers used in treating angina.

SIDE EFFECTS AND ADVERSE REACTIONS

The side effects of calcium blockers include headache, hypotension (more common with nifedipine and less common with diltiazem), dizziness, and flushing of the skin. Reflex tachycardia can occur as a result of hypotension. Calcium blockers can cause changes in liver and kidney function, and serum liver enzymes should be checked periodically. Calcium blockers are frequently given with other antianginal drugs such as nitrates to prevent angina.

NURSING PROCESS
ANTIANGINALS: NITROGLYCERIN, BETA AND CALCIUM BLOCKERS

Assessment

- Obtain baseline vital signs (VS) for future comparisons.
- Obtain health and drug histories. Nitroglycerin is contraindicated for marked hypotension or acute myocardial infarction (AMI).

Potential Nursing Diagnoses

- Decreased cardiac output
- Anxiety related to cardiac problems
- Acute pain
- Activity intolerance

Planning

- Client takes nitroglycerin or other antianginals and angina pain is controlled.

Nursing Interventions

- Monitor VS. Hypotension is associated with most antianginal drugs.
- Have the client sit or lie down when taking a nitrate for the first time. After administration, check the VS while the client is lying down and then sitting up. Have the client rise slowly to a standing position.
- Offer sips of water before giving sublingual (SL) nitrates; dryness may inhibit drug absorption.
- Monitor effects of IV nitroglycerin. Report angina that persists.
- Apply Nitro-Bid ointment to the designated mark on paper. Do *not* use fingers because the drug can be absorbed; use a tongue blade or gloves. For the Transderm-Nitro patch, do not touch the medication portion.
- Do *not* apply the Nitro-Bid ointment or the Transderm-Nitro patch in any area on the chest in the vicinity of defibrillator-cardioverter paddle placement. Explosion and skin burns may result.

Client Teaching

General
- A nitroglycerin SL tablet is used if chest pain occurs. Repeat in 5 min if the pain has not subsided and again in another 5 min if it persists. Do *not* give more than three tablets. If the chest pain persists >15 min, immediate medical help is necessary.
- Instruct the client not to ingest alcohol while taking nitroglycerin to avoid hypotension, weakness, and faintness.
- Tolerance to nitroglycerin can occur. If the client's chest pain is not completely alleviated, the client should notify the health care provider.

Beta Blockers and Calcium Blockers
- Instruct the client not to discontinue these drugs without the health care provider's approval. Withdrawal symptoms, such as reflex tachycardia and pain, may be severe.

Self-Administration
- Instruct the client about SL nitroglycerin tablets. The tablet is placed under the tongue for quick absorption. A stinging or biting sensation may indicate the tablet is fresh. With the newer SL nitroglycerin, the biting sensation may not be present. The bottle is stored away from light and kept dry.
- Instruct the client about the Transderm-Nitro patch. Apply once a day, usually in the morning. Rotation of skin sites is necessary. Usually the patch is applied to the chest wall; however, the thighs and arms are used. Avoid hairy areas.

Nursing Process continued on following page

Side Effects
- Headaches commonly occur when first taking nitroglycerin products and last about 30 min. Acetaminophen is suggested for relief.
- If hypotension results from SL nitroglycerin, place the client in supine position with legs elevated.

Beta Blockers and Calcium Blockers
- Instruct the client how to take a pulse rate. Advise the client to call the care provider if dizziness or faintness occurs; this may indicate hypotension.

Cultural Considerations

- Ascertain from the African-American, Hispanic, and obese clients their understanding of foods common to people from their culture that may contribute to cardiac conditions.
- Discuss with clients from various cultures the importance of the drug regimen. An interpreter may be necessary to ensure the client's compliance with drug and diet regimens.

Evaluation

- Evaluate the client's response to nitrate product for relieving anginal pain. Note headache, dizziness, or faintness.

ANTIDYSRHYTHMICS

Cardiac Dysrhythmias

A **cardiac dysrhythmia (arrhythmia)** is defined as any deviation from the normal rate or pattern of the heartbeat; this includes heart rates that are too slow (bradycardia), too fast **(tachycardia)**, or irregular. The terms *dysrhythmia* (disturbed heart rhythm) and *arrhythmia* (absence of rhythm) are used interchangeably, despite the slight difference in meaning.

The electrocardiogram (ECG) identifies the type of dysrhythmia. The P wave of the ECG reflects atrial activation, the QRS complex indicates the ventricular depolarization, and the T wave reflects ventricular **repolarization** (return of cell membrane potential to resting after depolarization). The PR interval indicates atrioventricular conduction time, and the QT interval reflects the ventricular action potential duration. Atrial dysrhythmias prevent proper filling of the ventricles and decrease the cardiac output by one third. Ventricular dysrhythmias are life-threatening because ineffective filling of the ventricle results in decreased or absent cardiac output. With ventricular tachycardia, ventricular fibrillation is likely to occur, followed by death. Cardiopulmonary resuscitation (CPR) is a necessity in treating these clients.

Cardiac dysrhythmias frequently follow a myocardial infarction (heart attack) or can result from **hypoxia** (lack of oxygen to body tissues), **hypercapnia** (increased carbon dioxide in the blood), excess catecholamines, or electrolyte imbalance.

Cardiac Action Potentials

When sodium and calcium enter a cardiac cell, **depolarization** (myocardial contraction) occurs. Sodium enters rapidly to start the depolarization, and calcium enters later to maintain it. These electrolytes irritate the cell and cause contraction. In the presence of myocardial ischemia, the contraction can be irregular.

Cardiac action potentials are frequent depolarization followed by repolarization of myocardial cells. Figure 37–1 illustrates the action potential of a five cardiac cell to conduct impulses. There are five phases. Phase 0 is the depolarization caused by an influx of sodium ions. Phase 1 is rapid repolarization. Phase 2 is the influx of calcium ion, which prolongs the action potential and promotes atrial and ventricular muscle contraction. Phase 3 is rapid repolarization caused by the potassium ion. Phase 4 is the spontane-

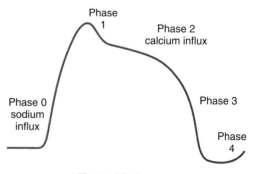

Figure 37–1
Cardiac action potential.

ous depolarization, or automaticity, which initiates the action potential cycle.

Types of Antidysrhythmic Drugs

The desired action of antidysrhythmics is restoration of normal cardiac rhythm, which is accomplished by various mechanisms (Table 37–4).

The antidysrhythmics are grouped into four classes: (1) fast (sodium) channel blockers IA (I), IB (II), and IC (III); (2) beta blockers; (3) those that prolong repolarization; and (4) slow (calcium) channel blockers. Table 37–5 lists the classes and actions of antidysrhythmic drugs.

CLASS I: FAST (SODIUM) CHANNEL BLOCKERS

Fast (sodium) channel blockers decrease the fast sodium influx to the cardiac cells. The drug response is decreased conduction velocity in the cardiac tissues, suppression of the automaticity that decreases the likelihood of ectopic foci, and increased recovery time (repolarization or refractory period). There are three subgroups of fast channel blockers: IA (I) slows conduction and prolongs repolarization (quinidine, procainamide, disopyramide), IB (II) slows conduction and shortens repolarization (lidocaine, mexiletine HCl), and IC (III) prolongs conduction with little to no effect on repolarization (encainide, flecainide). Chart 37–3 summarizes the action of the fast (sodium) channel blocker procainamide HCl.

CLASS II: BETA BLOCKERS

The drugs in the second class, beta blockers, decrease conduction velocity, automaticity, and recovery time (refractory period). Examples are propranolol (Inderal) and acebutolol (Sectral).

CLASS III: PROLONG REPOLARIZATION

Drugs in the third class prolong repolarization and are used in emergency treatment of ventricular dys-

Table 37–4
Pharmacodynamics of Antidysrhythmics

MECHANISMS OF ACTION
Block adrenergic stimulation of the heart
Depress myocardial excitability and contractility
Decrease conduction velocity in cardiac tissue
Increase recovery time (repolarization) of the myocardium
Suppress automaticity (spontaneous depolarization to initiate beats)

Table 37–5
Classes and Actions of Antidysrhythmic Drugs

CLASSES	ACTIONS
CLASS I	
Sodium channel blockers	
IA	Slows conduction; prolongs repolarization
IB	Slows conduction and shortens repolarization
IC	Prolongs conduction with little to no effect on repolarization
CLASS II	
Beta blockers	Reduces calcium entry; decreases conduction velocity, automaticity, and recovery time (refractory period)
CLASS III	
Prolong repolarization	Prolongs repolarization during ventricular dysrhythmias. Prolongs action potential duration
CLASS IV	
Calcium channel blockers	Blocks calcium influx; slows conduction velocity, decreases myocardial contractility (negative inotropic), and increases refraction in the AV node

rhythmias when other antidysrhythmics are not effective. These drugs, bretylium (Bretylol) and amiodarone (Cordarone), increase the refractory period (recovery time) and prolong the action potential duration (cardiac cell activity).

CLASS IV: CALCIUM CHANNEL BLOCKERS

The fourth class, the calcium channel blocker verapamil (Calan, Isoptin), a slow (calcium) channel blocker, blocks calcium influx, thus decreasing the excitability and contractility (negative inotropic) of the myocardium. It increases the refractory period of the AV node, which decreases ventricular response. Verapamil is contraindicated for clients with AV block or congestive heart failure.

Pharmacokinetics

The IA or fast (sodium) channel blockers I, quinidine (Cardioquin, Quinidex), procainamide (Pronestyl, Procan), and disopyramide (Norpace), are absorbed rapidly from the GI mucosa. Food and pH change the absorption rate. The salt content of quinidine affects absorption: quinidine sulfate is absorbed more readily

Chart 37–3.   Antidysrhythmics: Fast Channel Blocker (IA)

FAST CHANNEL BLOCKER I (IA)

Drug Name

Procainamide HCl (Procan, Pronestyl)
Fast channel (sodium) blocker I
Pregnancy Category: C

Dosage

A: PO: 250–500 mg q3–4h. SR: 250 mg–1 g q6h
or 50 mg/kg/d in 4 divided doses. IV: 20–30
mg/min; *maint:* 1–4 mg/min; *max:* 17 mg/kg
C: PO: 40–60 mg/kg/d in 4 divided doses. IV:
3–6 mg/kg q10–30 min; *max:* 100 mg/dose
TDM: 4–8 μg/mL

Contraindications

Hypersensitivity to procaine, blood dyscrasias,
heart block, cardiogenic shock, myasthenia
gravis
Caution: Hypotension, CHF, MI, renal or hepatic insufficiency

Drug-Lab-Food Interactions

Drug: *Increase* effects with histamine$_2$ blockers;
increase hypotensive effects with antihypertensives, nitrates; *decrease* effects with barbiturates
Lab: May *increase* ALP, AST, LDH, bilirubin

Pharmacokinetics

Absorption: PO: 75%–95%
Distribution: PB: 20%
Metabolism: t½: 3–4 h
Excretion: 60% unchanged in urine (half as an
active metabolite)

Pharmacodynamics

PO: Onset: 30 min
      Peak: 1–1.5 h
      Duration: 3–4 h (SR: 8 h)
IV: Onset: Minutes
      Peak: 25–60 min
      Duration: 3–4 h

Assessment and Planning

Interventions

Evaluation

NURSING PROCESS

Therapeutic Effects/Uses

To control cardiac dysrhythmias (premature ventricular contractions [PVCs], ventricular tachycardia.

Mode of Action: Depression of myocardial excitability by slowing conduction of cardiac tissue
through the atrium, bundle of His, and ventricle to decrease cardiac dysrhythmias.

Side Effects

Anorexia, nausea, vomiting, diarrhea, headache,
dizziness, weakness, flushing, rash, pruritus,
lupus-like syndrome with rash

Adverse Reactions

Life-threatening: Atrioventricular block, pleural
effusion, ventricular tachycardia/fibrillation,
thrombocytopenia, agranulocytosis, cardiovascular collapse, torsades de pointes

KEY: A: adult; C: child; PO: by mouth; IV: intravenous; TDM: therapeutic drug monitoring; SR: sustained-release; PB: protein-binding;
t½: half-life; CHF: congestive heart failure; MI: myocardial infarction; ALP: alkaline phosphatase; ALT: alanine aminotransferase; AST:
aspartate aminotransferase; LDH: lactic dehydrogenase.

than quinidine gluconate or quinidine polygalact-
uronate.

Quinidine is highly protein-bound, whereas procainamide is 20% protein-bound, and disopyramide is
moderately protein-bound. All of these antidysrhythmics are excreted by the kidneys unchanged.
Procainamide has a shorter half-life than quinidine or
disopyramide.

Pharmacodynamics

Quinidine, procainamide, and disopyramide have
similar onset-of-action times. The peak action is
longer with disopyramide and the duration is shorter
with procainamide.

Table 37–6 lists the drug data for the commonly
administered antidysrhythmics.

Table 37–6
Antidysrhythmics

GENERIC (BRAND)	ROUTE AND DOSAGE	USES AND CONSIDERATIONS
CLASS I		
Fast (sodium) channel blockers I		
Disopyramide phosphate (Norpace, Napamide)	A: PO: 100–200 mg q6h CR: 300 mg q12h C 4–12 y: PO: 10–15 mg/kg/d in divided doses 13–18 y: PO: 6–15 mg/kg/d in divided doses	Prevention and suppression of unifocal and multifocal premature ventricular contractions (PVCs). For ventricular dysrhythmias. May cause anticholinergic symptoms. Serum therapeutic level: 3–8 μg/mL. *Pregnancy category:* C; PB: 50%–66%; $t\frac{1}{2}$: 4–10 h
Procainamide (Pronestyl, Procan)	See Chart 37–3	For atrial and ventricular dysrhythmias. Has less hypotensive effect than quinidine. Serum therapeutic level: 4–8 μg/mL. *Pregnancy category:* C; PB: 20%; $t\frac{1}{2}$: 3–4 h
Quinidine sulfate, polygalactorate, gluconate (Quinidex, Cardioquin)	A: PO: 200–400 mg t.i.d.–q.i.d. C: PO: 30 mg/kg or 900 mg/m² in 5 divided doses	For atrial, ventricular, and supraventricular dysrhythmias. Nausea, vomiting, diarrhea, abdominal pain, or cramps are common side effects. If given with digoxin, it can increase digoxin concentration. Serum therapeutic level: 2–6 μg/mL. *Pregnancy category:* C; PB: 80%; $t\frac{1}{2}$: 6–7 h
Fast (sodium) channel blockers II		
Lidocaine (Xylocaine)	A: IV: 50–100 mg bolus in 2–3 min; then 20–50 μg/kg/min	For acute ventricular dysrhythmias following MI and cardiac surgery. Serum therapeutic range: 1.5–6 μg/mL. *Pregnancy category:* B; PB: 60%–80%; $t\frac{1}{2}$: 1.5–2 h
Mexiletine HCl (Mexitil)	A: PO: 200–400 mg q8h	Analogue of lidocaine. Treatment for acute and chronic ventricular dysrhythmias. Take with food to decrease GI distress. Common side effects include nausea, vomiting, heartburn, tremor, dizziness, nervousness, lightheadedness. Serum therapeutic range: 0.5–2 μg/mL. *Pregnancy category:* C; PB: 50%–60%; $t\frac{1}{2}$: 10–12 h
Fast (sodium) channel blockers III		
Encainide HCL **Available for compassionate use only**	A: PO: 25 mg q8h; may increase to 50–75 mg q8h	For ventricular dysrhythmia, but may cause new ventricular dysrhythmia. FDA approved for life-threatening situations. *Pregnancy category:* B; PB: 75%–85%; $t\frac{1}{2}$: 3–12 h
Flecainide (Tambocor)	A: PO: Initial: 50–100 mg q12h, increase by 50 mg q12h q4d; *maint:* 150 mg q12h; *max:* 300 mg/d	For life-threatening ventricular dysrhythmias; prevention of paroxysmal supraventricular tachycardia (PSVT) and paroxysmal atrial fibrillation or flutter (PAF). Avoid use in cardiogenic shock, second- or third-degree heart block, or right bundle branch block. *Pregnancy category:* C; PB: UK; $t\frac{1}{2}$: 12–27 h
Propafenone HCl (Rythmol)	A: PO: 150–300 mg q8h; *max:* 900 mg/d	Treatment of life-threatening ventricular dysrhythmias. Avoid use if cardiogenic shock, uncontrolled CHF, heart block, severe hypotension, bradycardia, and bronchospasms occur. *Pregnancy category:* C; PB: 97%; $t\frac{1}{2}$: 5–8 h
Tocainide HCl (Tonocard)	A: PO: LD: 600 mg PO: 400 mg q8h; *max:* 2.4 g/d	For ventricular dysrhythmias, especially PVC. Similar to lidocaine except in oral form. Serum therapeutic level: 4–10 μg/mL. *Pregnancy category:* C; PB: 70%–80%; $t\frac{1}{2}$: 10–17 h

Table continued on following page

Table 37–6 *Continued*
Antidysrhythmics

GENERIC (BRAND)	ROUTE AND DOSAGE	USES AND CONSIDERATIONS
OTHER CLASS I		
Moricizine (Ethmozine)	A: PO: Initially: 200 mg q8h; *maint:* 300 mg q8h	To treat life-threatening ventricular dysrhythmias. Blocks sodium channels, decreases conduction velocity in atria and ventricles, and prolongs refractory period in the AV node. May cause bradycardia, heart block, and CHF in high doses. *Pregnancy category* B; PB: UK; $t\frac{1}{2}$: 1.5–3.5 h
CLASS II		
Beta-adrenergic blockers		
Acebutolol HCl (Sectral) Beta₁ blocker	A: PO: 200 mg b.i.d.; may increase dose	Management of ventricular dysrhythmias. Also used for angina pectoris and hypertension. Primarily for PVC. New beta blocker that affects the beta₁ receptor in the heart. Can cause bradycardia and decrease cardiac output. *Pregnancy category:* B; PB: 26%; $t\frac{1}{2}$: 3–13 h
Esmolol (Brevibloc) Beta₁ blocker	A: IV: LD: 500 µg; kg/over 1 min; *maint:* 100 µg/kg/min *max:* 200 µg/kg/min	To control atrial flutter and fibrillation. For short-term use only. Mainly for clients having dysrhythmias during surgery. May cause bradycardia, heart block, CHF. *Pregnancy category:* UK; PB: UK; $t\frac{1}{2}$: 9 min
Propranolol HCl (Inderal) Beta₁ and beta₂ blocker	A: PO: 10–30 mg t.i.d.–q.i.d. A: IV bolus: 0.5–3 mg at 1 mg/min	For ventricular dysrhythmias, PAT, and atrial and ventricular ectopic beats. Asthmatic clients should not use drug. *Pregnancy category:* C; PB: 90%; $t\frac{1}{2}$: 3–6 h
Sotalol HCl (Betapace) Beta₁ and beta₂ blocker (also Class III)	A: PO: 80 mg b.i.d.; *max:* 240–320 mg/d in divided doses Increase dose interval with renal dysfunction	For ventricular dysrhythmias. Avoid if bronchial asthma or heart block is present. *Pregnancy category:* B; PB: 0%; $t\frac{1}{2}$: 12 h
CLASS III		
Prolong repolarization		
Adenosine (Adenocard)	A: IV: 6 mg (bolus: 1–2 sec); repeat if necessary, 12 mg bolus	Treatment of paroxysmal supraventricular tachycardia (PSVT), Wolff-Parkinson-White syndrome. Avoid if second- or third-degree AV block, or atrial flutter or fibrillation is present. *Pregnancy category:* C; PB: UK; $t\frac{1}{2}$: <10 sec
Amiodarone HCl (Cordarone)	A: PO: LD: 400–1600 mg/d in divided doses; *maint:* 200–600 mg/d	For life-threatening ventricular dysrhythmias. Initially dosage is greater and then decreases over time. Therapeutic serum level: 1–2.5 µg/mL. *Pregnancy category:* C; PB: 96%; $t\frac{1}{2}$: 5–100 d
Bretylium tosylate (Bretylol)	A: IM: 5–10 mg/kg q6–8h IV: 5–10 mg/kg; repeat in 15–30 min, IV drip or IV bolus	For ventricular tachycardia and fibrillation (to convert to a normal sinus rhythm). Used when lidocaine and procainamide are ineffective. *Pregnancy category:* C; PB: UK; $t\frac{1}{2}$: 4–17 h
Sotalol (Betapace)	A: PO: Same as class II *(See sotalol in class II)*	Beta blocker. Can be classified as class II or class III. To treat life-threatening ventricular dysrhythmias (ventricular tachycardia). Slows heart rate, decreases AV conduction, increases AV refractory period, and decreases systolic and diastolic BP. *Caution:* second- and third-degree heart block. *(See sotalol in class II.)*

Table continued on following page

Table 37–6 *Continued*
Antidysrhythmics

GENERIC (BRAND)	ROUTE AND DOSAGE	USES AND CONSIDERATIONS
CLASS IV		
Calcium channel blockers		
Verapamil HCl (Calan)	A: PO: 240–480 mg/d in 3–4 divided doses IV: 5–10 mg IV push	For supraventricular tachydysrhythmias, prevention of PSVT. Also used for angina pectoris and hypertension. Avoid use if cardiogenic shock, second- or third-degree AV block, severe hypotension, severe CHF occur. Serum therapeutic level 80–300 ng/mL or 0.08–0.3 μg/mL. *Pregnancy category:* C; PB: 90%; $t\frac{1}{2}$: 3–8 h
Diltiazem (Cardizem)	A: IV: 0.25 mg/kg IV bolus over 2 min, or 5–10 mg/h in IV infusion	For PSVT and atrial flutter or fibrillation. Avoid use if second- or third-degree AV block or hypotension occurs. *Pregnancy category:* C; PB: 70%–80%; $t\frac{1}{2}$: 3–8 h
OTHERS		
Phenytoin (Dilantin)	A: IV: 100 mg q5–10 min until dysrhythmia ceases; *max:* 1000 mg	Treatment of digitalis-induced dysrhythmias. Not approved as dysrhythmic drug by FDA. Serum level <20 μg/mL. *Pregnancy category:* D; PB: 95%; $t\frac{1}{2}$: 22 h
Digoxin (Lanoxin)	A: IV: LD: 0.6–1 mg/d in 24 h C >10 y: IV: LD: 8–12 μg/kg	For atrial flutter or fibrillation; to prevent recurrence of paroxysmal atrial tachycardia. *Pregnancy category:* A; PB: 20%–25%; $t\frac{1}{2}$: >36 h
Ibutilide fumarate (Corvert)	A >60 kg: IV infusion: 1 mg (10 mL), may repeat in 10 min	To treat atrial flutter and fibrillation. Prolongs cardiac action potential and increases atrial and ventricular refractories. *Pregnancy category:* C; PB: UK; $t\frac{1}{2}$: 6 h

KEY: A: adult; PO: by mouth; IV: intravenous; UK: unknown; PB: protein-binding; $t\frac{1}{2}$: half-life; m^2: square meter of body surface area; LD: loading dose; MI: myocardial infarction; CHF: congestive heart failure; AV: atrioventricular; BP: blood pressure; >: greater than; <: less than; PAT: paroxysmal atrial tachycardia.

Lidocaine, a IB or fast (sodium) channel blocker II, was used in the 1940s as a local anesthetic and is still used for that purpose. Later, it was determined that lidocaine had antidysrhythmic properties and was and still is most effective for treating acute ventricular dysrhythmias. It slows conduction velocity and decreases action potential amplitude. Onset of action (intravenously) is rapid.

Side Effects and Adverse Reactions

Quinidine, the first drug used to treat cardiac dysrhythmias, has many side effects, such as nausea, vomiting, diarrhea, confusion, and hypotension. It can also cause heart block and neurologic and psychiatric symptoms. Procainamide causes less cardiac depression than quinidine.

High doses of lidocaine can cause cardiovascular depression, bradycardia, and hypotension. Side effects may include dizziness, lightheadedness, and confusion.

Side effects of beta blockers are bradycardia and hypotension. Bretylium and amiodarone can cause nausea, vomiting, hypotension, and neurologic problems. Side effects of calcium blockers include nausea, vomiting, hypotension, and bradycardia.

NURSING PROCESS
ANTIDYSRHYTHMICS

Assessment

- Obtain health and drug histories. The history may include shortness of breath (SOB), heart palpitations, coughing, chest pain (type, duration, and severity), previous angina or cardiac dysrhythmias, and drugs that the client is currently taking.
- Obtain baseline vital signs (VS) and ECG for future comparisons.
- Check early cardiac enzyme results (AST, LDH, CPK) to compare with future laboratory results.

Potential Nursing Diagnoses

- Decreased cardiac output
- Anxiety related to irregular heartbeat
- Risk for activity intolerance

Planning

- Client will no longer experience abnormal sinus rhythm.
- Client will comply with the antidysrhythmic drug regimen.

Nursing Interventions

- Monitor VS. Hypotension can occur.
- When the drug is ordered IV push or bolus, administer it over a period of 2 to 3 min or as prescribed.
- Monitor ECG for abnormal patterns and report findings, such as PVCs, increased PR and QT intervals, and/or widening of the QRS complex. Increased QT interval is a risk factor for torsades des pointes.

Client Teaching

General
- Instruct the client to take the prescribed drug as ordered. Drug compliance is essential.
- Provide specific instructions for each drug, such as photosensitivity for amiodarone.

Side Effects
- Instruct the client to report side effects and adverse reactions to the health care provider. These can include dizziness, faintness, nausea, and vomiting.
- Advise the client to avoid alcohol, caffeine, and cigarettes. Alcohol can intensify the hypotensive reaction; caffeine increases the catecholamine level; and cigarette smoking promotes vasoconstriction.

Cultural Considerations

- Same as for antianginal drugs.

Evaluation

- Evaluate the effectiveness of the prescribed antidysrhythmic by comparing heart rates with the baseline heart rate and assessing the client's response to the drug. Report side effects and adverse reactions. The drug regimen may need to be adjusted. A proarrhythmic effect may occur, which may require discontinuation of the drug.

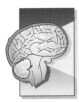

Critical Thinking in Action

S. T., age 64 years, has congestive heart failure (CHF), which has been controlled with digoxin, furosemide (Lasix), and a low-sodium diet. She is taking potassium chloride (KCl), 20 mEq orally per day. Three days ago, S. T. had flu-like symptoms of anorexia, lethargy, and diarrhea. Her fluid and food intake were diminished. She refused to take the KCl, stating that the drug makes her "sick." She has taken the daily digoxin and furosemide.

The nurse's assessment during the home visit includes poor skin turgor, poor muscle tone, irregular pulse rate, and decreased bowel sounds. The nurse obtained a blood sample for serum electrolytes; results indicated potassium (K) 2.9 mEq/L, sodium (Na) 137 mEq/L, and chloride (Cl) 96 mEq/L.

1. What are the reference values for serum potassium (K), serum sodium (Na), and serum chloride (Cl)? Are S. T.'s electrolytes within normal range? Explain.
2. What physical findings are indicative of which electrolyte imbalance?
3. What are the reasons for the electrolyte imbalance?
4. S. T. said she was not taking KCl because the drug makes her "sick." What information can you give her concerning the administration of potassium?
5. What is the affect of furosemide on digoxin when there is a potassium deficit? Explain.
6. The nurse should be assessing S. T. for digitalis toxicity. Why? List the signs and symptoms of digitalis toxicity.

S. T. was referred to the health care provider because of the serum potassium deficit and its effect on digoxin. A repeat serum potassium determination was taken and the result was 2.8 mEq/L. A liter of dextrose 5% in water with KCl 40 mEq/L was administered over a 4-h period.

7. How many milliequivalents of KCl per hour would S. T. receive? Does this amount constitute an acceptable dosage?
8. Why is it important that the nurse check the rate of intravenous fluids containing potassium, the hourly urine output, and vital signs?
9. Because of the low serum potassium level, what other electrolyte value should be checked and why?

After S. T.'s serum electrolytes returned to normal, the health care provider instructed her to continue to take the prescribed KCl dosage daily with her other medications.

10. S. T. asked why she has to continue taking these drugs. What should your response be?
11. The nurse instructs S. T. to eat foods rich in potassium. Which foods are the richest sources of potassium?

D. K., 72 years old, had a myocardial infarction (MI) 5 years ago. He has been having angina attacks at night and at rest when watching TV. He complains of stabbing pain in the chest that last 5 minutes. Pain does not radiate to the arm. D. K., is prescribed propranolol (Inderal), 20 mg q.i.d. His vital signs are blood pressure, 108/58; pulse, 56 (at times irregular); respirations, 28. His clinical history indicates that he has mild asthma.

1. What other clinical information would you need in regard to D. K.'s health problem and drug?
2. Of the various types of angina, D. K.'s angina occurrence may indicate which type of angina? Give your rationale.
3. What are the assessments that the nurse should make while D. K. is taking propranolol? Is propranolol an appropriate anginal drug for D. K.? Explain.

4. What should be included in client teaching for D. K. in regard to his health history and drug?

D. K. notified the health care provider that he was having "dizzy spells." His blood pressure was 86/50, pulse 46, and respirations 30. His propranolol was stopped and diltiazem (Cardizem), 30 mg q.i.d., was ordered. He is experiencing an increasing amount of wheezing.

5. What are the correlations between D. K.'s dizziness, wheezing, vital signs, and propranolol?
6. Is the diltiazem ordered for D. K. within the therapeutic dosage range? In what ways would this drug benefit D. K.?
7. List the side effects of diltiazem that should be included in client teaching. What other pertinent information should the nurse include in the teaching data for D. K.?
8. What other drug regimen might be helpful to D. K.?

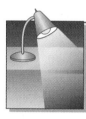

Study Questions

1. Your client is taking digoxin 0.25 mg/d. What are the nursing responsibilities for client teaching in regard to pulse monitoring and side effects? What is the serum therapeutic range?
2. Drug interactions are associated with digitalis drugs. What are the effects of potassium-wasting diuretics and cortisone with digitalis?
3. What effects do electrolytes have on digitalis toxicity?
4. How are nitroglycerin products administered? Explain. What is a common side effect (temporary) of nitrates that occurs early in the course of administration? How is this side effect treated?
5. Beta blockers are administered from which drug groups for cardiac conditions? What are two side effects of beta blockers?
6. Calcium blockers are given from what drug groups for cardiac conditions? Which calcium blockers are used for dysrhythmias?
7. How do the fast sodium channel blockers affect the heart?

Diuretics

38

Outline

Objectives

- Explain the action and uses of diuretics.
- Identify the various groups of diuretics.
- Describe several side effects and adverse reactions related to thiazide, loop, and potassium-sparing diuretics.
- Explain the nursing interventions, including client teaching, related to diuretics, especially thiazide, loop, and potassium-sparing diuretics.

Terms

antihypertensives

diuresis

diuretics

hypercalcemia

hyperglycemia

hyperkalemia

hypertension (essential or secondary)

hyperuricemia

hypokalemia

natriuresis

oliguria

osmolality

potassium-sparing diuretics

potassium-wasting diuretics

saluretic

INTRODUCTION

Hypertension is an elevated blood pressure. Diuretics are used for two main purposes: to decrease hypertension (lower blood pressure), and to decrease edema (peripheral and pulmonary) in congestive heart failure (CHF) and renal or liver disorders. Diuretics discussed in this chapter are used either singly or in combination to decrease blood pressure and reduce edema.

Diuretics produce increased urine flow (**diuresis**) by inhibiting sodium and water reabsorption from the kidney tubules. Most sodium and water reabsorption occurs throughout the renal tubular segments (proximal, loop of Henle [descending loop and ascending loop], and collecting tubule). Diuretics can affect one or more segments of the renal tubules. Figure 38-1

illustrates the renal tubule along with the normal process of water and electrolyte reabsorption and diuretic effects on the tubules.

Every 1½ h, the total volume of the body's extracellular fluid (ECF) goes through the kidneys (glomeruli) for cleansing; this is the first process for urine formation. Small particles such as electrolytes, drugs, glucose, and waste products from protein metabolism are filtered in the glomeruli. Larger products such as protein and blood are not filtered with normal renal function and they remain in the circulation. Sodium and water are the largest filtrate substances.

Normally, 99% of the filtered sodium that passes through the glomeruli is reabsorbed. From 50% to 55% of sodium reabsorption occurs in the proximal tubules, 35% to 40% in the loop of Henle, 5% to 10% in the distal tubules, and <3% in the collecting tu-

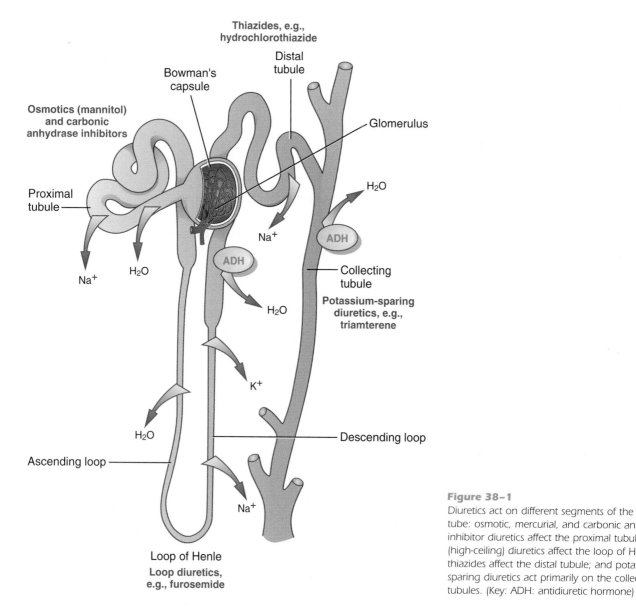

Figure 38-1

Diuretics act on different segments of the renal tube: osmotic, mercurial, and carbonic anhydrase inhibitor diuretics affect the proximal tubule; loop (high-ceiling) diuretics affect the loop of Henle; thiazides affect the distal tubule; and potassium-sparing diuretics act primarily on the collecting tubules. (Key: ADH: antidiuretic hormone)

Table 38-1
Diuretics: Thiazides

GENERIC (BRAND)	ROUTE AND DOSAGE	USES AND CONSIDERATIONS
SHORT-ACTING		
Chlorothiazide (Diuril, Diachlor)	*Hypertension:* A: PO: 250–500 mg daily or b.i.d. *Edema:* A: PO: 500–2000 mg daily or b.i.d. C >1 y: PO: 20 mg/kg/d C <6 mon: PO: 10–30 mg/kg/d in divided doses	For hypertension and peripheral edema. Adults may be given IV chlorothiazide, but it is not recommended for infants and children. *Pregnancy category:* D; PB: 20%–80%; $t_{\frac{1}{2}}$: 1–2 h
Hydrochlorothiazide (HydroDIURIL, HCTZ)	See Chart 38–1	For hypertension and edema. Hydrochlorothiazide (HCTZ) is inexpensive and is usually well tolerated by most clients. Usually HCTZ is the first thiazide prescribed. HCTZ may be used as a single antihypertensive drug or in combination with other antihypertensives. It is used in edema associated with CHF, cirrhosis of the liver, and steroids (glucocorticoids). Electrolyte imbalance can occur. *Pregnancy category:* B; PB: 65%; $t_{\frac{1}{2}}$: 6–15 h
INTERMEDIATE ACTING		
Bendroflumethiazide (Naturetin)	A: PO: 2.5–20 mg/d C: PO: maint: 0.05–0.1 mg/kg/d or 1.5–3 mg/m² daily or in divided doses	Treatment of hypertension and edema associated with CHF and cirrhosis. Has similar effects as the prototype drug HCTZ. Hypokalemia, hyperglycemia, and hyperuricemia may occur. *Pregnancy category:* UK; PB: 94%; $t_{\frac{1}{2}}$: 3–4 h
Benzthiazide (Aquatag, Hydrex)	*Hypertension:* A: PO: 25–100 mg/daily or 25–100 mg in divided doses *Edema:* A: PO: 25–200 mg daily C: PO: 1–4 mg/kg/d in 3 divided doses	Similar to hydrochlorothiazide. *Pregnancy category:* D; PB: UK; $t_{\frac{1}{2}}$: UK
Hydroflumethiazide (Saluron, Diucardin)	*Hypertension:* A: PO: 50–100 mg/d *Edema:* A: PO: 25–200 mg/d C: PO: 1 mg/kg/d	Similar to hydrochlorothiazide, its effects, side effects, adverse reactions, and abnormal laboratory results. *Pregnancy category:* C; PB: 74%; $t_{\frac{1}{2}}$: 17 h
LONG ACTING		
Methyclothiazide (Aquatensen, Enduron)	*Hypertension/edema:* A: PO: 2.5–10 mg/d C: PO: 0.05–0.1 mg/kg/d	For hypertension and edema associated with CHF, renal and liver dysfunction. Side effects and drug interactions are similar to those of HCTZ. It has a long duration of action. *Pregnancy category:* C; PB: UK; $t_{\frac{1}{2}}$: UK
Polythiazide (Renese-R)	*Hypertension:* A: PO: 2–4 mg/d *Edema:* A: PO: 1–4 mg/d C: PO: 0.02–0.08 mg/kg/d	Similar to hydrochlorothiazide. *Pregnancy category:* D; PB: 84%; $t_{\frac{1}{2}}$: 25 h
Trichlormethiazide (Metahydrin, Naqua)	*Hypertension:* A: PO: 2–4 mg *Edema:* A: PO: 1–4 mg/daily or b.i.d. C: PO: 0.07 mg/kg/d in divided doses	Similar to HCTZ. It has a long duration of action (24 h). *Pregnancy category:* B; PB: UK; $t_{\frac{1}{2}}$: 2.5–7 h
THIAZIDE-LIKE DIURETICS (This group has similar effects to but not exactly like HCTZ)		
Chlorthalidone (Hygroton)	*Hypertension:* A: PO: 12.5–50 mg/d *Edema:* A: PO: 25–100 mg/d C: PO: 2 mg/kg/3 × wk	For hypertension and edema associated with CHF, renal and liver dysfunction. It has a very long duration of action (24–72 h). *Pregnancy category:* C; PB: 75%; $t_{\frac{1}{2}}$: 40–54 h

Table continued on following page

Table 38–1 *Continued*
Diuretics: Thiazides

GENERIC (BRAND)	ROUTE AND DOSAGE	USES AND CONSIDERATIONS
Indapamide (Lozol)	*Hypertension and edema:* A: PO: 2.5 mg/d; may increase to 5 mg/d	For hypertension and edema. A long-acting diuretic. May be classified as a loop diuretic. *Pregnancy category:* B; PB: 75%; $t_{\frac{1}{2}}$: 14–18 h
Metolazone (Zaroxolyn)	*Hypertension:* A: PO: 2.5–5.0 mg/d *Edema:* A: PO: 5–20 mg/d	For hypertension and edema. Intermediate-acting diuretic. More effective than thiazides in clients with decreased renal function. *Pregnancy category:* D; PB: 33%; $t_{\frac{1}{2}}$: 8–14 h
Quinethazone (Hydromox)	A: PO: 50–100 mg/d; *max:* 200 mg/d in divided doses	For edema. Intermediate-acting diuretic. *Pregnancy category:* D; PB: UK; $t_{\frac{1}{2}}$: UK

KEY: *A: adult; C: child; PO: by mouth; m²: body surface area; >: greater than; <: less than; PB: protein-binding; $t_{\frac{1}{2}}$: half-life; CHF: congestive heart failure.*

bules. Diuretics that act on the tubules closest to the glomeruli have the greatest effect in causing **natriuresis** (sodium loss in the urine). A classic example is the osmotic diuretic mannitol. The diuretic effect is dependent on the drug reaching the kidneys and its concentration in the renal tubules.

Diuretics have an antihypertensive effect by promoting sodium and water loss by blocking sodium and chloride reabsorption. This causes a decrease in fluid volume and lowering of blood pressure. Also with fluid loss, edema (fluid retention in body tissues) should decrease. When sodium is retained, water is also retained in the body and the blood pressure increases.

Many diuretics cause loss of other electrolytes, including potassium, magnesium, chloride, and bicarbonate. The diuretics that promote potassium excretion are classified as **potassium-wasting diuretics,** and those that promote potassium retention are called **potassium-sparing diuretics.** Combination diuretics have been marketed that have both potassium-wasting and potassium-sparing action.

The five categories of diuretics effective in removing water and sodium are:

- thiazide and thiazide-like
- loop or high-ceiling
- osmotic
- carbonic anhydrase inhibitor
- potassium-sparing

The thiazide, loop or high-ceiling, and potassium-sparing diuretics are the most frequently prescribed types for hypertension and edema associated with CHF. All of these diuretics are potassium wasting, except those in the potassium-sparing group.

THIAZIDES AND THIAZIDE-LIKE DIURETICS

The first thiazide marketed was chlorothiazide (1957), followed 1 year later by hydrochlorothiazide. There are numerous thiazide and thiazide-like preparations (Table 38–1). Thiazides act on the distal convoluted renal tubule, beyond the loop of Henle, to promote sodium, chloride, and water excretion. Thiazides are used in the treatment of hypertension and peripheral edema. They are not effective for immediate diuresis.

This diuretic group is primarily used for clients with normal renal function. If the client has a renal disorder and his or her creatinine clearance is less than 30 mL/min, the effectiveness of the thiazide diuretic is greatly decreased. Thiazides cause a loss of sodium, potassium, and magnesium, but they promote calcium reabsorption. **Hypercalcemia** (calcium excess) may result, which can be a hazard to the client if he or she is digitalized or has cancer that is causing hypercalcemia. Thiazides affect glucose tolerance; thus, hyperglycemia can occur. Thiazides should be used with caution in clients with diabetes mellitus. Laboratory test (electrolytes and glucose) results need to be monitored. The pharmacologic data for the prototype thiazide diuretic hydrochlorothiazide are presented in Chart 38–1.

Pharmacokinetics

Thiazides are well absorbed from the gastrointestinal (GI) tract. Hydrochlorothiazide has a moderate protein-binding power, and the half-life of the thiazide drugs is longer than that of the loop diuretics. For

Chart 38–1. Diuretic: Thiazides

THIAZIDE DIURETIC

Drug Name

Hydrochlorothiazide (HydroDIURIL, HCTZ, Esidrix, Oretic); ♣ Apo-Hydro, Urozide
Pregnancy Category: B

Dosage

A: PO: Hypertension: 12.5–100 mg/d
Edema: Initially: 25–200 mg in divided doses; maint: 25–100 mg/d
C: PO: 1–2 mg/kg/d in divided doses
C: <6 mo: PO: 1–3 mg/kg/d in divided doses

Contraindications

Renal failure with anuria, electrolyte depletion
Caution: Hepatic cirrhosis, renal dysfunction, diabetes mellitus, gout, systemic lupus erythematosus (SLE)

Drug-Lab-Food Interactions

Drug: *Increase* digitalis toxicity with digitalis and hypokalemia; *increase* potassium loss with steroids; potassium loss; *decrease* antidiabetic effect; *decrease* thiazide effect with cholestyramine and colestipol
Lab: *Increase* serum calcium, glucose, uric acid; *decrease* serum potassium, sodium, magnesium

Pharmacokinetics

Absorption: Readily absorbed from the GI tract
Distribution: PB: 65%
Metabolism: t½: 6–15 h
Excretion: In urine

Pharmacodynamics

PO: Onset: 2 h
Peak: 3–6 h
Duration: 6–12 h

Therapeutic Effects/Uses

To increase urine output. To treat hypertension, edema from CHF, hepatic cirrhosis, renal dysfunction

Mode of Action: Action is on the renal distal tubules by promoting sodium, potassium, and water excretion, decreasing preload and cardiac output; also edema. Acts on arterioles, causing vasodilation, thus decreasing blood pressure.

Side Effects

Dizziness, vertigo, weakness, nausea, vomiting, diarrhea, hyperglycemia, constipation, rash, photosensitivity

Adverse Reactions

Severe dehydration, hypotension
Life-threatening: Severe potassium depletion, marked hypotension, uremia, aplastic anemia, hemolytic anemia, thrombocytopenia, agranulocytosis

Assessment and Planning
Interventions
Evaluation
NURSING PROCESS

KEY: A: adult; C: child; PO: by mouth; <: less than; PB: protein-binding; t½: half-life; CHF: congestive heart failure; ♣: Canadian drug names.

this reason, thiazides should be administered in the morning to avoid nocturia (nighttime urination) and sleep interruption.

Pharmacodynamics

Thiazides act directly on arterioles, causing vasodilation, which can lower blood pressure. Other action is the excretion of sodium chloride and water, causing a decrease in vascular fluid and thus decreasing cardiac output and blood pressure. The onset of action of hydrochlorothiazide occurs within 2 h. The peak concentration times are long, 3–6 h. Thiazides are divided into three groups according to their duration of action: the short-acting thiazides with a duration time of less than 12 h; intermediate-acting, with a duration

NURSING PROCESS
DIURETICS: THIAZIDES

Assessment

- Assess vital signs (VS), weight, urine output, and serum chemistry values (electrolytes, glucose, uric acid) for baseline levels.
- Check peripheral extremities for presence of edema. Note pitting edema.
- Obtain a history of drugs that are taken daily. Review for drugs that may cause drug interaction, including digoxin, corticosteroids, antidiabetics.

Potential Nursing Diagnoses

- Risk for fluid volume deficit
- Altered patterns of urinary elimination

Planning

- Client's blood pressure will be decreased and/or return to normal value.
- Client's edema will be decreased.
- Client's serum chemistry levels remain within normal ranges.

Nursing Interventions

- Monitor VS and serum electrolytes, especially potassium, glucose, uric acid, and cholesterol levels. Report changes. If client is taking digoxin and hypokalemia occurs, digitalis toxicity frequently results.
- Observe for signs and symptoms of hypokalemia, such as muscle weakness, leg cramps, and cardiac dysrhythmias.
- Check the client's weight daily at a specified time. A weight gain of 2.2 to 2.5 lb is equivalent to an excess liter of body fluids.
- Monitor urine output to determine fluid loss or retention.

Client Teaching

General
- Emphasize the need for compliance. Client may not "feel better" for some time or may not "feel worse" if treatment is missed or discontinued.

Nursing Process continued on following page

Table 38-2
Serum Chemistry Abnormalities Associated with Thiazides

SERUM CHEMISTRY PARAMETER	ABNORMAL RESULTS
ELECTROLYTES	
Potassium	Hypokalemia (low serum potassium) is excreted from the distal renal tubule.
Magnesium	Hypomagnesemia (low serum magnesium). Potassium and sodium loss prompt magnesium loss.
Calcium	Hypercalcemia (elevated serum calcium). Thiazides may block calcium excretion.
Chloride	Hypochloremia (low serum chloride). Sodium and potassium losses produce chloride loss.
Bicarbonate	Minimal bicarbonate loss from proximal tubule.
Uric acid	Hyperuricemia (elevated uric acid). Thiazides can block uric acid excretion.
Blood sugar	Hyperglycemia (increased blood sugar). Thiazides increase fasting blood sugar levels and those of prediabetic state.
Blood lipids	Cholesterol, low-density lipoproteins, and triglycerides can be elevated.

- Suggest that the client take hydrochlorothiazide in early morning to avoid sleep disturbance resulting from nocturia.
- Keep drugs out of reach of small children. Request child safety cap bottle.

Self-Administration
- Instruct the client or family member how to take and record his or her blood pressure. Record daily results.

Diet
- Instruct the client to eat foods rich in potassium, such as fruits, fruit juices, and vegetables. Potassium supplements may be ordered.
- Advise the client to take drugs with food to avoid GI upset.

Side Effects
- Instruct the client to change positions from lying to standing slowly because dizziness may occur as a result of orthostatic (postural) hypotension.
- Advise the client who may be prediabetic to have blood sugar checked periodically because large doses of hydrochlorothiazide increase blood glucose levels.
- Advise the client to use sunscreen when in direct sunlight.

Cultural Considerations

- Respect cultural beliefs and values. If the client from a foreign background tells the health care provider that she or he only eats pasta and does not eat fruits and vegetables, the nurse may have two options: to encourage the client to eat fruits and vegetables or to contact the health care provider so that an adequate potassium supplement would be prescribed to overcome potassium loss. An interpreter may be necessary.
- Emphasize the importance of the client taking a potassium supplement with the potassium-wasting diuretic. Also advise the client of consequences and dangers of not taking potassium supplements or lack of appropriate diet with potassium-wasting diuretics.

Evaluation

- Evaluate the effectiveness of drug therapy. Client's blood pressure and edema will be reduced and blood chemistry will remain within normal range.
- Determine the absence of side effects and adverse reactions to therapy.

---

time of 12 to 24 h; and long-acting, with a duration time of greater than 24 h.

Table 38–1 lists the drugs, dosages, and uses and considerations for the thiazide and thiazide-like diuretics. Drug dosages for hypertension and edema are similar.

Side Effects and Adverse Reactions

Side effects and adverse reactions of thiazides include electrolyte imbalances (hypokalemia, hypercalcemia, hypomagnesemia, and bicarbonate loss), **hyperglycemia** (elevated blood sugar), **hyperuricemia** (elevated serum uric acid level), and hyperlipidemia (elevated blood lipid level). Signs and symptoms of hypokalemia should be assessed, and serum potassium levels must be closely monitored. Potassium supplements are frequently needed. Serum calcium and uric acid levels should be checked because thiazides block calcium and uric acid excretion; hypercalcemia (elevated blood calcium levels) and hyperuricemia may result. Thiazides affect the metabolism of carbohydrates, and hyperglycemia can result, especially in clients with

high to high-normal blood sugar levels. Thiazides can increase serum cholesterol, low-density lipoprotein, and triglyceride levels. A drug to lower blood lipids may be ordered. Other side effects include dizziness, headaches, nausea, vomiting, constipation, urticaria (hives) (rare), and blood dyscrasias (rare).

Table 38–2 summarizes the serum chemistry abnormalities that can occur with the use of thiazides.

Contraindications

Thiazides are contraindicated for use in renal failure. Symptoms of severe kidney impairment or shutdown include **oliguria** (marked decrease in urine output), elevated blood urea nitrogen (BUN), and elevated serum creatinine.

Drug Interactions

Of the numerous drug interactions, the most serious occurs with digoxin. Thiazides can cause hypokalemia, which enhances the action of digoxin, and digitalis toxicity can occur. Potassium supplements are

Chart 38–2.   Diuretic: Loop (High-Ceiling)

HIGH-CEILING (LOOP) DIURETIC

Drug Name

Furosemide (Lasix, Furodide); ❀ fumide, furomide
Pregnancy Category: C

Dosage

A: PO: 20–80 mg single dose; repeat in 6–8 h; *max:* 600 mg/d
IM/IV: 20–80 mg single dose; over 1–2 min IV; repeat 20 mg in 2 h
C: PO: 2 mg/kg single dose; repeat in 6–8 h; *max:* 6 mg/kg/d
IM/IV: 1 mg/kg single dose; repeat 1 mg/kg in 2 h

Contraindications

Presence of severe electrolyte imbalances, hypovolemia, anuria, hypersensitivity to sulfonamides, hepatic coma

Drug-Lab-Food Interactions

Drug: *Increase* orthostatic hypotension with alcohol; *increase* ototoxicity with aminoglycosides; *increase* bleeding with anticoagulants; *increase* potassium loss with steroids; *increase* digitalis toxicity and cardiac dysrhythmias with digitalis and hypokalemia; *increase* lithium toxicity; *increase* amphotericin B ototoxicity and nephrotoxicity
Lab: *Increase* BUN, blood/urine glucose, serum uric acid, ammonia; *decrease* potassium, sodium, calcium, magnesium, chloride serum levels

Pharmacokinetics

Absorption: PO: Readily absorbed from the GI tract
Distribution: PB: 95%
Metabolism: $t\frac{1}{2}$: 30–50 min
Excretion: In urine, some in feces; crosses placenta

Pharmacodynamics

PO: Onset: <60 min
    Peak: 1–4 h
    Duration: 6–8 h
IV: Onset: 5 min
    Peak: 20–30 min
    Duration: 2 h

Therapeutic Effects/Uses

To treat fluid retention/fluid overload due to CHF, renal dysfunction, cirrhosis; hypertension; acute pulmonary edema.

Mode of Action: Inhibition of sodium and water reabsorption from the loop of Henle and distal renal tubules. Potassium, magnesium, and calcium also may be excreted.

Side Effects

Nausea, diarrhea, electrolyte imbalances, vertigo, cramping, rash, headache, weakness, ECG changes, blurred vision, photosensitivity

Adverse Reactions

Severe dehydration; marked hypotension
Life-threatening: Renal failure, thrombocytopenia, agranulocytosis

(Right margin, vertical text:) Assessment and Planning | Interventions | Evaluation | **NURSING PROCESS**

KEY: A: adult; C: child; PO: by mouth; IM: intramuscular; IV: intravenous; PB: protein-binding; BUN: blood urea nitrogen; ECG: electrocardiogram; GI: gastrointestinal; <: less than; $t\frac{1}{2}$: half-life; CHF: congestive heart failure; ❀: Canadian drug names.

frequently prescribed and serum potassium levels are monitored. Thiazides also induce hypercalcemia, which enhances the action of digoxin that may cause digitalis toxicity. Signs and symptoms of digitalis toxicity (bradycardia, nausea, vomiting, visual changes) should be reported. Thiazides also enhance the action of lithium, and lithium toxicity can occur. Thiazides potentiate the action of other antihypertensive drugs, which may be used in combination drug therapy for hypertension.

LOOP (HIGH-CEILING) DIURETICS

The loop, or high-ceiling, diuretics act on the ascending loop of Henle by inhibiting chloride transport of sodium into the circulation (inhibits passive reabsorption of sodium). Sodium and water are lost, together with potassium, calcium, and magnesium. They have little effect on the blood sugar; however, the uric acid level increases. The drugs in this group are potent and cause marked depletion of water and electrolytes. The effects of loop diuretics are dose related; that is, increasing the dose increases the effect and response of the drug. This response is referred to as high-ceiling diuretics. Loop diuretics are more potent than thiazides as diuretics, inhibiting reabsorption of sodium two to three times more effec-

tively, but they are less effective as **antihypertensive agents.**

Loop diuretics can increase renal blood flow up to 40%. It is a common choice of diuretic for clients whose creatinine clearance is less than 30 mL/min and for those with end-stage renal disease. This group of diuretics causes excretion of calcium, unlike thiazides, which inhibit calcium loss.

Ethacrynic acid (Edecrin) (late 1950s) and furosemide (Lasix) (1960) were the first loop diuretics marketed. Bumetanide (Bumex) is more potent than furosemide on a per milligram-for-milligram basis. Furosemide and bumetanide are derivatives of sulfonamides. Ethacrynic acid, a phenoxyacetic acid derivative, is a seldom-chosen loop diuretic, usually reserved for a client who is allergic to sulfa drugs.

Table 38–3
Physiologic and Laboratory Changes Associated with High-Ceiling (Loop) Diuretics

PHYSIOLOGIC/LAB CHANGES	POSSIBLE EFFECTS OF HIGH-CEILING (LOOP) DIURETICS
PHYSIOLOGIC CHANGES	
Hypotension	Postural (orthostatic) hypotension can result because of extracellular fluid volume (ECFV) deficit.
Ototoxicity	Hearing impairment, although rare, may occur. It is more common with use of ethacrynic acid. Diuretics in other categories are not considered to be ototoxic. *Caution:* Avoid taking a loop diuretic with a drug that can be ototoxic, such as aminoglycoside.
Skin disturbances	Pruritus, urticaria, exfoliative dermatitis, and purpura may occur in some persons allergic to the drug or when taking the loop diuretic in high doses over a long period of time.
Photosensitivity	When exposed to sun or sunlamp for a prolonged time, severe sunburn could result. The client should use sunscreen and avoid long sun exposure.
Hypovolemia	Excess extracellular fluid is lost through increased urine excretion.
LABORATORY CHANGES	
Hypokalemia, hypomagnesemia, hyponatremia, hypocalcemia, hypochloremia	Potassium, magnesium, sodium, calcium, and chloride are lost from the body from increased urine excretion. Chloride, an anion, is attached to the cations potassium and sodium; thus, chloride is lost along with potassium and sodium.
Hyperglycemia	Increased glycogenolysis may contribute to an elevated blood sugar level. Diabetics should closely monitor their blood glucose levels when taking a loop diuretic.
Hyperuricemia	Elevated uric acid levels are common in clients susceptible to gout.
Elevated BUN and creatinine	These elevations may result from ECFV loss. Hemoconcentration can cause elevated BUN and creatinine levels, which are reversible when fluid volume returns to normal levels.
Thrombocytopenia, leukopenia	A decrease in platelet and white blood cell counts is rare, but they should be closely monitored.
Elevated lipids	Loop diuretics can decrease high-density lipoproteins (HDL) and increase low-density lipoproteins (LDL). Clients with elevated cholesterol levels should have their levels of HDL and LDL checked. Regardless of the lipid effects, loop diuretics are useful for clients with serious fluid retention caused by a cardiac condition such as CHF.

KEY: BUN: blood urea nitrogen; CHF: congestive heart failure.

Table 38–4
Diuretics: Loop (High-Ceiling) Osmotics, Carbonic Anhydrase Inhibitors

GENERIC (BRAND)	ROUTE AND DOSAGE	USES AND CONSIDERATIONS
LOOP (HIGH-CEILING)		
Bumetanide (Bumex)	A: PO: 0.5–2.0 mg/d; *max:* 10 mg/d IV: 0.5–1.0 mg/dose; repeat in 2–4 h C: PO: 0.015 mg/kg/d	Treatment of hypertension and edema associated with CHF, and renal disease. Similar effects as furosemide. *Pregnancy category:* C; PB: 95%; $t_{\frac{1}{2}}$: 1–1.5 h
Ethacrynic acid (Edecrin)	A: PO: 50–200 mg/d IV: 0.5–1.0 mg/kg/dose C: PO: 25 mg/d	For severe edema (pulmonary and peripheral). It is a potent diuretic and has rapid action. Also used for mild–moderate hypertension, and for hypercalcemia. *Pregnancy category:* B; PB: 95%; $t_{\frac{1}{2}}$: 1–1.5 h
Furosemide (Lasix)	See Chart 38–2	For pulmonary and peripheral edema caused by CHF, hypertension, renal failure *without* anuria, and hypercalcemia. Furosemide promotes calcium excretion. Hypokalemia may result. *Pregnancy category:* C; PB: 95%; $t_{\frac{1}{2}}$: 0.5–1 h
Torsemide (Demadox)	*Hypertension:* A: PO/IV: Initially: 5 mg/d; *maint:* PO: 5–10 mg/d IV: in 2 min *CHF:* A: PO/IV: 10–20 mg/d	Similar to furosemide. *Pregnancy category:* C; PB: >97%; $t_{\frac{1}{2}}$: 2–4 h
OSMOTICS		
Mannitol	*ICP, IOP:* A: IV: 1.5–2.0 g/kg; 15%–25% sol infused over 30–60 min *Edema, ascites, or oliguria:* A: IV: 50–100 g; 10%–20% sol infused over 90 min to 6 h	For decreasing ICP (increased intracranial pressure) and for oliguria. To prevent acute renal failure. Used in narrow-angle glaucoma for reducing intraocular pressure. Client should have effective renal function. It is a potent diuretic. *Pregnancy category:* C; PB: UK; $t_{\frac{1}{2}}$: 1.5 h
Urea (Ureaphil)	A: IV: 1.0–1.5 g/kg of 30% sol C (>2 y): IV: 0.5–1.5 g/kg of 30% sol	Same uses as mannitol. Not the drug of choice. Used during prolonged surgery to prevent acute renal failure. *Pregnancy category:* C; PB: UK; $t_{\frac{1}{2}}$: 1 h
CARBONIC ANHYDRASE INHIBITORS		
Acetazolamide (Diamox)	A: PO/IV: 250 mg q12h; dose may vary C: PO: 10–15 mg/kg/d in divided doses C: IV: 5–10 mg/kg q6h	For edema, treating absence (petit mal) seizures, and open-angle glaucoma. May cause hyperglycemia, hyperuricemia, and hypercalcemia. Metabolic acidosis can result. *Pregnancy category:* C; PB: 90%; $t_{\frac{1}{2}}$: 2.5–5.5 h
Dichlorphenamide (Daranide, Oratrol)	A: PO: 100 mg q12h; *maint:* 25–50 mg daily-t.i.d.	Treatment of open-angle glaucoma by reducing the IOP and for narrow-angle glaucoma prior to surgery. *Pregnancy category:* C; PB: UK; $t_{\frac{1}{2}}$: UK
Methazolamide (Neptazane)	A: PO: 50–100 mg b.i.d.–t.i.d.	Similar to dichlorphenamide. *Pregnancy category:* C; PB: 50%–60%; $t_{\frac{1}{2}}$: 14 h

KEY: A: adult; C: child; PO: by mouth; IV: intravenous; ICP: intracranial pressure; IOP: intraocular pressure; CHF: congestive heart failure; maint: maintenance dose; >: greater than; PB: protein-binding; $t_{\frac{1}{2}}$: half-life; sol: solution.

Chart 38–2 lists the drug data for the loop diuretic furosemide.

Pharmacokinetics

Loop diuretics are rapidly absorbed by the GI tract. These drugs are highly protein-bound with half-lives (t½) that vary from 30 min to 1.5 h. Loop diuretics compete for protein-binding sites with other highly protein-bound drugs.

Pharmacodynamics

Loop diuretics have a great **saluretic** (sodium-losing) effect and can cause rapid diuresis, thus decreasing vascular fluid volume and causing a decrease in cardiac output and blood pressure. Furosemide is a more potent diuretic than thiazide diuretics. It causes a vasodilatory effect, thus increasing renal blood flow before diuresis. It is used when other conservative measures fail, such as sodium restriction and use of less potent diuretics. The oral dose of furosemide is usually twice that of an intravenous dose.

The onset of action of loop diuretics occurs within 30 to 60 min. The onset of action for intravenous (IV) furosemide is 5 min. Duration of action is shorter than that of the thiazides.

Side Effects and Adverse Reactions

The most common side effects are fluid and electrolyte imbalances, such as hypokalemia, hyponatremia, hypocalcemia, hypomagnesemia, and hypochloremia. Hypochloremic metabolic alkalosis may result, which can worsen the hypokalemia. Orthostatic hypotension can occur. Thrombocytopenia, skin disturbances, and transient deafness are seen rarely. Prolonged use of loop diuretics could cause thiamine deficiency. Table 38–3 lists the physiologic and laboratory changes associated with loop diuretics.

Drug Interaction

The major drug interaction is with digitalis preparations. If the client takes digoxin with a loop diuretic, digitalis toxicity can result. The client needs potassium replacement with food or supplements. Hypokalemia enhances the action of digoxin and increases the risk of digitalis toxicity. Table 38–4 lists the data for the four loop (high-ceiling) diuretics.

OSMOTIC DIURETICS

Osmotic diuretics increase the **osmolality** (concentration) of the plasma and fluid in the renal tubules. Sodium, chloride, potassium (to a lesser degree), and water are excreted. This group of drugs is used to prevent kidney failure, to decrease intracranial pressure (ICP) (e.g., cerebral edema), and to decrease intraocular pressure (IOP) (e.g., glaucoma). Mannitol is a potent potassium-wasting diuretic that is used frequently in emergency situations such as for ICP and IOP. Also, mannitol can be used with cisplatin and carboplatin in cancer chemotherapy to induce a frank diuresis with decreased side effects of treatment.

Mannitol is the most frequently prescribed osmotic diuretic, followed by urea. Diuresis occurs within 1 to 3 h after intravenous administration. Table 38–4 describes the two osmotic diuretics.

Side Effects and Adverse Reactions

The side effects and adverse reactions of mannitol include fluid and electrolyte imbalance, pulmonary edema from rapid shift of fluids, nausea, vomiting, tachycardia from rapid fluid loss, and acidosis. Crystallization of mannitol in the vial may occur when the drug is exposed to a low temperature. The vial should be warmed to dissolve the crystals. The mannitol solution should *not* be used for intravenous infusion if the crystals are present and have not been dissolved.

CARBONIC ANHYDRASE INHIBITORS

The carbonic anhydrase inhibitors acetazolamide, dichlorphenamide, ethoxzolamide, and methazolamide block the action of the enzyme carbonic anhydrase needed to maintain the acid–base balance (hydrogen and bicarbonate ion balance). Inhibition of this enzyme causes increased sodium, potassium, and bicarbonate excretion. With prolonged use, metabolic acidosis can occur.

This group of drugs is used primarily to decrease intraocular pressure in clients with open-angle (chronic) glaucoma. These drugs are not used in narrow-angle or acute glaucoma. Other uses include diuresis, management of epilepsy, and treatment of high-altitude or acute mountain sickness. Table 38–4 presents the drug data for carbonic anhydrase inhibitor diuretics. The drug may also be used for a client in metabolic alkalosis who needs a diuretic. Carbonic anhydrase inhibitors may be alternated with a loop diuretic.

Side Effects and Adverse Reactions

Acetazolamide can cause fluid and electrolyte imbalance, metabolic acidosis, nausea, vomiting, anorexia, confusion, orthostatic hypotension, and crystalluria. Hemolytic anemia and renal calculi can also occur. These drugs are contraindicated during the first trimester of pregnancy.

NURSING PROCESS
DIURETICS: LOOP (HIGH-CEILING)

Assessment

- Obtain a history of drugs that are taken daily. Note whether client is taking a drug that may cause an interaction, such as alcohol, aminoglycosides, anticoagulants, corticosteroids, lithium, amphotericin B, or digitalis. Recognize that furosemide is highly protein-bound and can displace other protein-bound drugs such as Coumadin.
- Assess vital signs (VS), serum electrolytes, weight, and urine output for baseline levels.
- Compare client's drug dose with recommended dose and report discrepancy.
- Note whether client is hypersensitive to sulfonamides.

Potential Nursing Diagnosis

- Risk for fluid volume deficit

Planning

- Client's edema and/or hypertension will be decreased.
- Client's serum chemistry levels will remain within normal ranges.

Nursing Interventions

- Check the half-life of furosemide. With a short half-life, the drug can be repeated or given more than once a day.
- Check onset of action for furosemide, orally and intravenously. If the drug is given intravenously, the urine output should increase in 5 to 20 min. If urine output does not increase, notify the health care provider. Severe renal disorder may be present.
- Monitor urinary output to determine body fluid gain or loss. Urinary output should be at least 25 mL/h or 600 mL/24 h.
- Check the client's weight to determine fluid loss or gain. A loss of 2.2 to 2.5 lb is equivalent to a fluid loss of 1 liter.
- Monitor VS. Be alert for marked decrease in blood pressure.
- Administer IV furosemide slowly; hearing loss may occur if rapidly injected.
- Observe for signs and symptoms of hypokalemia (<3.5 mEq/L), such as muscle weakness, abdominal distention, leg cramps, and/or cardiac dysrhythmias.
- Check serum potassium levels, especially when a client is taking digoxin. Hypokalemia enhances the action of digitalis, causing digitalis toxicity.

Client Teaching

General
- Instruct the client to take furosemide early in the morning and *not* in the evening, to prevent sleep disturbance and nocturia.

Diet
- Suggest taking furosemide at mealtime or with food to avoid nausea.

Side Effects
- Instruct the client to arise slowly to prevent dizziness resulting from fluid loss.

Cultural Considerations

- These are the same as for thiazide.

Evaluation

- Evaluate the effectiveness of drug action: decreased fluid retention or fluid overload, decreased respiratory distress, and increased cardiac output.
- Check for side effects and increase in urine output.

Chart 38–3.   Diuretic: Potassium-Sparing

POTASSIUM-SPARING DIURETIC

Drug Name

Triamterene (Dyrenium)
Pregnancy Category: B

Dosage

A: PO: Edema: 100 mg q.d., b.i.d.; not to exceed
300 mg/d
C: PO: 2–4 mg/kg/d in divided doses

Contraindications

Severe kidney or hepatic disease, severe hyperkalemia
Caution: Renal or hepatic dysfunction, diabetes
mellitus

Drug-Lab-Food Interactions

Drug: *Increase* serum potassium level with potassium supplements; *increase* effects of antihypertensives and lithium; life-threatening hyperkalemia if given with ACE inhibitor
Lab: *Increase* serum potassium level; may *increase* BUN, AST, alkaline phosphatase levels;
decrease serum sodium, chloride

Pharmacokinetics

Absorption: PO: Rapidly absorbed from GI tract
Distribution: PB: 67%
Metabolism: $t\frac{1}{2}$: 1.5–2.5 h
Excretion: In urine, mostly as metabolites and
bile

Pharmacodynamics

PO: Onset: 2–4 h
    Peak: 6–8 h
    Duration: 12–16 h

Therapeutic Effects/Uses

To increase urine output; to treat fluid retention/overload associated with CHF, hepatic cirrhosis, or
nephrotic syndrome.

Mode of Action: Action on the distal renal tubules to promote sodium and water excretion and
potassium retention.

Side Effects

Nausea, vomiting, diarrhea, rash, dizziness,
headache, weakness, dry mouth, photosensitivity

Adverse Reactions

Life-threatening: Severe hyperkalemia, thrombocytopenia, megaloblastic anemia

Assessment and Planning — Interventions — Evaluation — NURSING PROCESS

KEY: A: adult; C: child; PO: by mouth; PB: protein-binding; CHF: congestive heart failure; $t\frac{1}{2}$: half-life; ACE: angiotensin-converting enzyme;
BUN: blood urea nitrogen; GI: gastrointestinal; AST: asparate aminotransferase.

POTASSIUM-SPARING DIURETICS

Potassium-sparing diuretics, weaker than thiazides and loop diuretics, are used as mild diuretics or in combination with antihypertensive drugs. Continuous use of potassium-wasting diuretics requires a daily oral potassium supplement because potassium, sodium, and body water are excreted through the kidneys. However, potassium supplements are not used when the client takes a potassium-sparing diuretic; in fact, serum potassium excess, **hyperkalemia**, results when a potassium supplement is taken with a potassium-sparing diuretic. Potassium-sparing diuretics act primarily in the collecting distal duct renal tubules to promote sodium and water excretion and potassium retention. The drugs interfere with the sodium-potassium pump that is controlled by the mineralocorticoid hormone aldosterone (sodium retained and potassium excreted). Potassium is reabsorbed and sodium is excreted.

Spironolactone (Aldactone), an aldosterone antagonist discovered in 1958, was the first potassium-sparing diuretic. Aldosterone is a mineralocorticoid hormone that promotes sodium retention and potassium excretion. Aldosterone antagonists inhibit the sodium-potassium pump (i.e., potassium is retained and so-

Table 38–5
Diuretics: Potassium-Sparing

GENERIC (BRAND)	ROUTE AND DOSAGE	USES AND CONSIDERATIONS
SINGLE AGENTS		
Amiloride HCl (Midamor)	A: PO: 5 mg/d; may increase to 10–20 mg/d in 1–2 divided doses	For diuretic-induced hypokalemia; used for hypertension, CHF, and cirrhosis of the liver. Serum potassium level should be monitored to detect hyperkalemia. *Pregnancy category:* B; PB: 23%; $t\frac{1}{2}$: 6–9 h
Spironolactone (Aldactone)	*Hypertension:* A: PO: 25–100 mg/d *Edema:* A: PO: 25–200 mg/d in divided doses C: PO: 3.3 mg/kg/d in divided doses	For edema and hypertension. Dosage for hypertension is usually slightly lower than for edema. Has a long duration of action. *Pregnancy category:* C; PB: 98%; $t\frac{1}{2}$: 1.5–2 h
Triamterene (Dyrenium)	See Chart 38–3	It blocks the luminal sodium channels. For edema due to CHF, cirrhosis, nephrosis, and steroid-induced edema. Should be taken with meals. Intermediate-acting diuretic. *Pregnancy category:* B; PB: 67%; $t\frac{1}{2}$: 1.5–2.5 h
COMBINATIONS		
Amiloride HCl and hydrochlorothiazide (Moduretic)	A: PO: 1–2 tab (amiloride 5 mg/hydrochlorothiazide 50 mg)	Combinations contain potassium-wasting and potassium-sparing diuretics. Drugs are to control hypertension and edema. They are used to prevent the occurrence of hypokalemia.
Spironolactone and hydrochlorothiazide (Aldactazide)	A: PO: 25/25 and 50/50 mg tab	Same as Moduretic
Triamterene and hydrochlorothiazide (Dyazide, Maxzide)	A: PO: 1–2 cap b.i.d., p.c. (Dyazide: triamterene 50 mg/hydrochlorothiazide 25 mg)	Dyazide: each tablet contains triamterene 50 mg and hydrochlorothiazide 25 mg. Maxzide comes in two strengths: triamterene 37.5 mg or 75 mg and hydrochlorothiazide 50 mg or 75 mg. *Pregnanacy category:* B; PB: UK; $t\frac{1}{2}$: UK

KEY: A: adult; C: child; cap: capsule; PO: by mouth; CHF: congestive heart failure; p.c.: after meals; UK: unknown; PB: protein-binding; $t\frac{1}{2}$: half-life.

dium is excreted). The effects of spironolactone may take 48 hours. Amiloride and triamterene are two additional potassium-sparing diuretics commonly prescribed. Amiloride (Midamor) is effective as an antihypertensive agent. Triamterene is useful in the treatment of edema caused by CHF or cirrhosis of the liver. Spironolactone (Aldactone), amiloride (Midamor), and triamterene (Dyrenium) should not be taken with angiotensin-converting enzyme (ACE) inhibitors because they can also increase serum potassium levels. Chart 38–3 provides the pharmacologic data of triamterene.

When potassium-sparing diuretics are used alone, they are less effective than when used in combination in reducing body fluid and sodium. These drugs are usually combined with a potassium-wasting diuretic, such as a thiazide, primarily hydrochlorothiazide, or a loop diuretic. The combination of potassium-sparing and potassium-wasting diuretics intensifies the diuretic effect and prevents potassium loss. The com-

mon combination diuretics are spironolactone and hydrochlorothiazide (Aldactazide), amiloride and hydrochlorothiazide (Moduretic), and triamterene and hydrochlorothiazide (Dyazide, Maxzide).

When diuretic combinations are used, either combined in one tablet or as separate tablets, the dose of each is usually less than the dose of any single drug. Table 38–5 lists the potassium-sparing diuretics and the combination potassium-wasting and potassium-sparing diuretics.

Side Effects and Adverse Reactions

The main side effect of these drugs is hyperkalemia. Caution must be used when giving potassium-sparing diuretics to a client with poor renal function, because 80% to 90% of the potassium is excreted by the kidneys. Urine output should be at least 600 mL per day. Clients should *not* use potassium supplements while

NURSING PROCESS
DIURETIC: POTASSIUM-SPARING

Assessment

- Obtain a history of drugs that are taken daily. Note whether the client is taking a potassium supplement or using a salt substitute.
- Assess vital signs (VS), serum electrolytes, weight, and urinary output for baseline levels.
- Compare the client's drug dose with the recommended dose and report any discrepancy.

Potential Nursing Diagnosis

- Risk for fluid volume deficit

Planning

- Client's fluid retention and blood pressure will be decreased.
- Client's serum electrolytes remain within their normal values.

Nursing Interventions

- Check the half-life of triamterene. With a long half-life, drug dose is usually administered once a day and sometimes twice a day.
- Monitor urinary output. Urine output should increase. Report if urine output is <30 mL/h or 600 mL/day.
- Monitor VS. Report abnormal changes.
- Observe for signs and symptoms of hyperkalemia (increased serum potassium level: >5.3 mEq/L), such as nausea, diarrhea, abdominal cramps, tachycardia and later bradycardia, peaked narrow T wave on electrocardiogram, or oliguria.
- Administer triamterene in the early morning and not in the evening, to avoid nocturia.

Client Teaching

General
- Instruct the client to take triamterene with or after meals to avoid nausea.
- Do not discontinue drug without consulting the health care provider.

Diet
- Advise clients with high average serum potassium levels to avoid foods rich in potassium when taking potassium-sparing diuretics.

Side Effects
- Instruct the client to avoid exposure to direct sunlight because the drug can cause photosensitivity.
- Advise the client to report possible side effects of the drug, such as rash, dizziness, or weakness.

Evaluation

- Evaluate the effectiveness of the potassium-sparing diuretic such as triamterene. The presence of fluid retention (edema) is decreased or absent.
- Determine whether urine output has increased and the serum potassium level is within normal range.

taking potassium-sparing diuretics unless the serum potassium level is low. If a potassium-sparing diuretic is given with the antihypertensive drug angiotensin-converting enzyme (ACE) inhibitor, hyperkalemia could become severe or life-threatening because both drugs retain potassium. Monitoring serum potassium levels is necessary. GI disturbances (anorexia, nausea, vomiting, diarrhea) can occur.

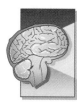

Critical Thinking in Action

J. Q., 58 years old, has recently been diagnosed as having minor hypertension. His blood pressure is 158/92. He has been prescribed hydrochlorothiazide (HydroDIURIL), 50 mg, q.d. He has been told to eat foods rich in potassium.

1. How does hydrochlorothiazide differ from furosemide? What are their similarities and differences?
2. Why is it necessary for J. Q. to eat foods rich in potassium when taking hydrochlorothiazide? Explain.
3. What are the nursing interventions that should be considered while J. Q. is taking HydroDIURIL?

J. Q. became weak and complained of nausea and vomiting. His muscles were "soft." His serum potassium level was 3.3 mEq/L. J. Q.'s diuretic was changed to triamterene/hydrochlorothiazide (Dyazide). Again he is advised to eat foods rich in potassium. Refer to Chapter 13 as needed.

4. Explain the rationale for changing J. Q.'s diuretic.
5. Should J. Q. receive a potassium supplement? Explain.
6. What nursing interventions should be followed for J. Q.?
7. What care plan should the nurse develop for J. Q. in relation to client teaching?
8. What medical follow-up care is needed for J. Q.?

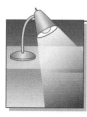

Study Questions

1. The client is receiving hydrochlorothiazide (HydroDIURIL) 50 mg daily and digoxin 0.25 mg daily. Is hydrochlorothiazide a potassium-wasting or potassium-sparing diuretic? What types of electrolyte imbalances can occur? Explain.
2. Client teaching is essential when caring for a client receiving the two drugs in question 1. How would you instruct the client regarding diet and vital signs? What are the signs and symptoms of digitalis toxicity?
3. What electrolyte imbalances may occur when taking hydrochlorothiazide over a prolonged period of time?
4. Your client has diabetes mellitus and is taking hydrochlorothiazide. Why should the client's blood glucose level be closely monitored?
5. Furosemide (Lasix) is what type of diuretic? What electrolyte imbalances can be caused by this drug?
6. Your client is taking triamterene. What type of diuretic is triamterene? What effect may this have on the potassium level?
7. Why would a combination diuretic (triamterene and hydrochlorothiazide) be prescribed?
8. The client's blood pressure is 142/92. What nonpharmacologic measures would you suggest to lower the blood pressure?

Antihypertensive Drugs

Outline

Objectives

- Identify the categories of antihypertensive drugs, and the stepped-care approach and the modified pharmacologic approach to antihypertensive drugs.

- Explain the pharmacologic action of the individual groups of antihypertensive drugs.

- Describe the side effects and adverse reactions to sympatholytics (beta blockers, centrally acting and peripherally acting alpha blockers, alpha and beta blockers), direct-acting vasodilators, and angiotensin antagonists.

- Explain the nursing interventions, including client teaching, related to antihypertensives.

Terms

antihypertensives

hypertension (essential and secondary)

stepped-care hypertensive approach

sympatholytics

HYPERTENSION

Hypertension is an increase in blood pressure such that the systolic pressure is greater than 140 mmHg and the diastolic pressure is greater than 90 mmHg. **Essential hypertension** is the most common type, affecting 90% of persons with high blood pressure. The exact origin of essential hypertension is unknown; however, contributing factors include (1) a family history of hypertension, (2) hyperlipidemia, (3) African-American background, (4) diabetes, (5) obesity, (6) aging, (7) stress, and (8) excessive smoking and alcohol ingestion. Ten percent of hypertension is related to renal and endocrine disorders and is classified as **secondary hypertension.**

Selected Regulators of Blood Pressure

The kidneys and the blood vessels strive to regulate and maintain a "normal" blood pressure. The kidneys regulate blood pressure via the renin-angiotensin system. The process is illustrated in Figure 39–1. Renin (from the renal cells) stimulates production of angiotensin II (a potent vasoconstrictor), which causes the release of aldosterone (adrenal hormone that promotes sodium retention and thereby water retention). Retention of sodium and water causes fluid volume to increase, thus elevating blood pressure. The baroreceptors in the aorta and carotid sinus and the vasomotor center in the medulla assist in the regulation of blood pressure. Norepinephrine, an adrenal hormone of the sympathetic nervous system, increases blood pressure.

Physiologic Risk Factors

Certain physiologic risk factors contribute to hypertension. Diet with excess fat and carbohydrate can increase blood pressure. Carbohydrate intake can affect sympathetic nervous activity. Mild to moderate sodium restriction can decrease blood pressure. Alcohol increases renin secretions, thus causing the production of angiotensin II. Obesity affects the sympathetic and cardiovascular systems by increasing cardiac output, stroke volume, and left ventricular filling. Two-thirds of hypertensive persons are obese. Normally, weight loss can decrease hypertension.

NONPHARMACOLOGIC CONTROL OF HYPERTENSION

A sufficient decrease in blood pressure may be accomplished by nonpharmacologic methods. There are many nonpharmacologic ways to decrease blood

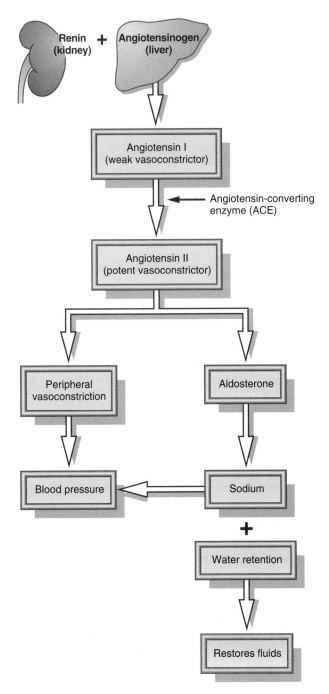

Figure 39–1
Renin-angiotensin system. Renin, an enzyme located in the juxtaglomerular cells of the kidney, is released when blood pressure decreases. This diagram shows how the renin-angiotensin system restores fluid balance and stabilizes blood pressure.

pressure; however, if the systolic pressure is greater than 140 mmHg, **antihypertensive** drugs are generally ordered. Nondrug methods to decrease blood pressure include (1) stress reduction techniques, (2) exercise (increases high-density lipoproteins [HDL]), (3) salt restriction, (4) decreased alcohol ingestion, and (5) weight reduction (Fig. 39–2).

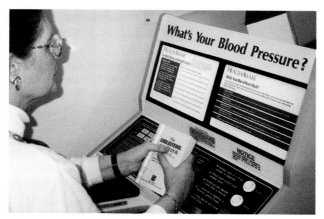

Figure 39–2
Blood pressure should be charted at specific intervals, especially if the client has an elevated cholesterol level or has borderline hypertension.

Table 39–1
Four Stages of Hypertension According to Blood Pressure

| STAGES | BLOOD PRESSURE RANGE (mmHg) | |
	Systolic	Diastolic
Normal	<130	<85
Stage 1	140–159	90–99
Stage 2	160–179	100–109
Stage 3	180–209	110–119
Stage 4	>210	>120

When hypertension *cannot* be controlled by nonpharmacologic means, antihypertensive drugs are prescribed. However, nonpharmacologic methods should be combined with antihypertensive drugs to control hypertension.

PHARMACOLOGIC CONTROL OF HYPERTENSION

An individualized approach to the treatment of hypertension is used by many health care providers, and all drugs when first prescribed for hypertension are considered as initial agents. Reduction of other cardiovascular risk factors and the use of fewer drugs (substituting instead of adding drugs) at the lowest effective doses are emphasized. It has been suggested that, after a client has taken an antihypertensive drug for a year, the drug dose might be decreased to determine whether the client needs less drug dosage.

Several years ago, the American Heart Association's Joint National Committee on Detection, Evaluation, and Treatment of High Blood Pressure recommended a **stepped-care hypertensive approach** to pharmacologic treatment of hypertension. Severity of hypertension is classified within four stages of blood pressure range (Table 39–1). According to their approach, step I drugs are used to control stage I hypertension. If the blood pressure is not controlled, then step II drugs are prescribed. Adverse effects are more prevalent with each increasing step. By using less potent drugs and combination therapy (lower dosages) for controlling high blood pressure, side effects are decreased.

The stepped-care approach by the American Heart Association is still used by some health care providers; however, many of them individualize their pharmacologic approach for treating hypertension.

Figure 39–3 illustrates the stepped-care approach and a modified pharmacologic approach in the management of hypertension.

It has been estimated that some 20% to 30% of clients receiving antihypertensive drugs are not truly hypertensive when hypertension is determined by 24-h ambulatory blood pressure measurement. Another large percentage are being overtreated because of a perceived inefficacy of antihypertensive drugs and the subsequent increase in dosage or numbers of antihypertensive drugs.

Antihypertensive drugs, used either singly or in combination with other drugs, are classified into five categories: (1) diuretics, (2) sympathetic depressants (sympatholytics), (3) direct arteriolar vasodilators, (4) angiotensin antagonists, and (5) calcium channel blockers.

Diuretics

Diuretics promote sodium depletion, which decreases extracellular fluid volume (ECFV). Diuretics are effective as first-line drug for treating mild hypertension. Hydrochlorothiazide (HydroDIURIL), a thiazide, is the most frequently prescribed diuretic to control mild hypertension. Hydrochlorothiazide can be used alone for recently diagnosed or mild hypertension or with other antihypertensive drugs. Many antihypertensive drugs can cause fluid retention; therefore, diuretics are often administered with antihypertensive agents. The various types of diuretics are discussed in Chapter 38.

Thiazides should not be used for clients with renal insufficiency (creatinine clearance level <30 mL/min). The loop (high-ceiling) diuretics such as furosemide (Lasix) are usually recommended because they do not depress renal blood flow. Diuretics are not used if hypertension is the result of renal-angiotensin-aldosterone involvement because they tend to elevate the serum renin level.

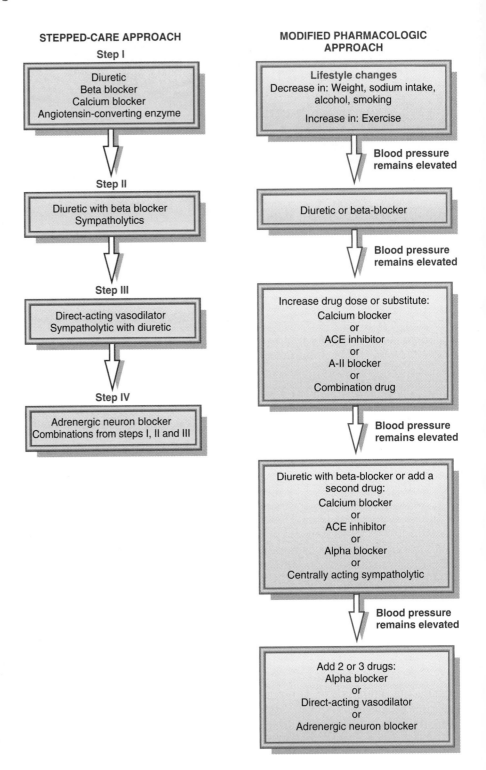

STEPPED-CARE APPROACH

Step I

Diuretic
Beta blocker
Calcium blocker
Angiotensin-converting enzyme

Step II

Diuretic with beta blocker
Sympatholytics

Step III

Direct-acting vasodilator
Sympatholytic with diuretic

Step IV

Adrenergic neuron blocker
Combinations from steps I, II and III

MODIFIED PHARMACOLOGIC APPROACH

Lifestyle changes
Decrease in: Weight, sodium intake, alcohol, smoking

Increase in: Exercise

Blood pressure remains elevated

Diuretic or beta-blocker

Blood pressure remains elevated

Increase drug dose or substitute:
Calcium blocker
or
ACE inhibitor
or
A-II blocker
or
Combination drug

Blood pressure remains elevated

Diuretic with beta-blocker or add a second drug:
Calcium blocker
or
ACE inhibitor
or
Alpha blocker
or
Centrally acting sympatholytic

Blood pressure remains elevated

Add 2 or 3 drugs:
Alpha blocker
or
Direct-acting vasodilator
or
Adrenergic neuron blocker

Figure 39–3
Stepped-care and modified pharmacologic approaches to drug management of hypertension.

The combination of potassium-wasting and potassium-sparing diuretics may be useful instead of a single thiazide drug; less potassium excretion would occur. Also, thiazides can be combined with other antihypertensive drugs to increase their effectiveness. Table 39–2 lists the combinations of thiazides with other drugs. Hydrochlorothiazides are combined with beta blockers and angiotensin-converting enzyme (ACE) inhibitors. ACE inhibitors tend to increase the serum potassium (K) level so when they are combined with the thiazide diuretic, serum potassium loss is minimized.

Table 39–2
Combination of Thiazides with Antihypertensive Drugs

THIAZIDE WITH POTASSIUM-SPARING DIURETICS

Hydrochlorothiazide with spironolactone (Aldactazide)

Hydrochlorothiazide with amiloride (Moduretic)

Hydrochlorothiazide with triamterene (Dyazide, Maxzide)

THIAZIDE WITH BETA BLOCKERS

Hydrochlorothiazide with bisoprolol fumarate (Ziac)

Hydrochlorothiazide with metoprolol (Lopressor HCT)

Hydrochlorothiazide with propranolol (Inderide)

Hydrochlorothiazide with timolol (Timolide)

Chlorthalidone (thiazide-like diuretic) with atenolol (Tenoretic)

THIAZIDE WITH ACE INHIBITORS

Hydrochlorothiazide with benazepril (Lotensin HCT)

Hydrochlorothiazide with captopril (Capozide)

Hydrochlorothiazide with enalapril maleate (Vaseretic)

Hydrochlorothiazide with lisinopril (Prinzide, Zestoretic)

Hydrochlorothiazide with moexipril (Uniretic)

THIAZIDE WITH ANGIOTENSIN II ANTAGONISTS

Hydrochlorothiazide with losartan potassium (Hyzaar)

Sympatholytics (Sympathetic Depressants)

The sympatholytics comprise five groups of drugs: (1) beta-adrenergic blockers, (2) centrally acting sympatholytics (adrenergic blockers), (3) alpha-adrenergic blockers, (4) adrenergic neuron blockers (peripherally acting sympatholytics), and (5) alpha- and beta-adrenergic blockers. The beta-adrenergic blockers block the beta receptors. The alpha-adrenergic blockers block the alpha receptors.

BETA-ADRENERGIC BLOCKERS

Beta-adrenergic blockers, frequently referred to as *beta blockers,* are used as step I antihypertensive drugs or in combination with a diuretic in the step II approach to treating hypertension. Beta blockers are also used as antianginals and antidysrhythmics (see Chapter 37).

Beta (B_1 and B_2)-adrenergic blockers reduce cardiac output by diminishing the sympathetic nervous system response. With continued use of beta blockers, vascular resistance is diminished and blood pressure is lowered. They reduce heart rate and contractility. Beta blockers also reduce renin release. There is a greater hypotensive response by clients who have higher renin levels.

Hypertensive clients who are African-American do not respond well to beta blockers for control of hypertension. However, in this group, hypertension can be controlled by combining beta blockers with diuretics.

There are numerous types of beta blockers. The nonselective beta blockers such as propranolol (Inderal) inhibit beta$_1$ (heart) and beta$_2$ (bronchial) receptors. Heart rate slows (blood pressure decreases secondary to the decrease in heart rate), and bronchoconstriction occurs. Cardioselective beta blockers are preferred because they act mainly on the beta$_1$ rather than the beta$_2$ receptors; as a result, bronchoconstriction is less likely to occur. Acebutolol (Sectral), atenolol (Tenormin), betaxolol (Kerlone), bisoprolol (Zebeta), and metoprolol (Lopressor) are cardioselective beta blockers, blocking beta$_1$ receptors.

Cardioselectivity does not confer absolute protection from bronchoconstriction. In tests measuring forced expiratory volume in 1 sec (FEV_1), as a measure of B_2 reactivity, only atenolol demonstrated true protection. Other cardioselective beta blockers were only partially effective. Studies also show that, at the upper end of the dosage range, cardioselectivity is less effective. In clients with preexisting bronchospasms or other pulmonary disease, beta blockers, even those considered cardioselective, should be used with caution. Some experts regard this as a relative contraindication. The real value of beta selectivity is in maintaining renal blood flow and minimizing the hypoglycemic effects of beta blockade.

The combination of beta blockers with hydrochlorothiazides is packaged together in tablet form (see Table 39–2). Usually, the hydrochlorothiazide dose is 25 mg, approximately one-half of the average dose.

Again, beta blockers tend to be more effective in lowering blood pressure in clients who have an elevated serum renin level. The cardioselective prototype drug metoprolol (Lopressor) is presented in Chart 39–1.

Beta blockers should not be used by clients with second- or third-degree atrioventricular (AV) block, sinus bradycardia, or congestive heart failure (CHF). A noncardioselective beta blocker such as propranolol (Inderal) should not be given to a client with chronic obstructive pulmonary disease (COPD).

Pharmacokinetics

Metoprolol is well absorbed from the gastrointestinal (GI) tract. Its half-life is short. Metoprolol is highly

Chart 39–1. Antihypertensives: Beta Blocker

BETA BLOCKER

Drug Name

Metoprolol tartrate
♦ Betaloc, Apo-Metoprolol, Toprol SR
Adrenergic blocker, sympatholytic, beta$_2$ blocker
Pregnancy Category: C

Dosage

Hypertension:
A: PO: 50–100 mg/d in 1–2 divided doses;
maint: 100–450 mg in divided doses; *max:* 450
mg/d in divided doses
SR: 50–100 mg/d; max: 450 mg/d
Myocardial infarction:
A: PO: 100 mg b.i.d.
IV: 5 mg q2min × 3 doses

Contraindications

Second- and third-degree heart block, cardiogenic shock, CHF, sinus bradycardia
Caution: Hepatic, renal, or thyroid dysfunction; asthma; peripheral vascular disease, IDDM

Drug-Lab-Food Interactions

Drug: *Increase* bradycardia with digitalis; *increase* hypotensive effect with other antihypertensives, alcohol, anesthetics

Pharmacokinetics

Absorption: PO: 95%
Distribution: PB: 12%
Metabolism: t½: 3–4 h
Excretion: In urine

Pharmacodynamics

PO: Onset: 15 min
    Peak: 1.5 h
    Duration: 10–19 h
IV: Onset: Immediate
    Peak: 20 min
    Duration: 5–10 h

Therapeutic Effects/Uses

To control hypertension.

Mode of Action: Promotion of blood pressure reduction via beta$_1$-blocking effect.

Side Effects

Fatigue, weakness, dizziness, nausea, vomiting, diarrhea, mental changes, nasal stuffiness, impotence, decreased libido, depression

Adverse Reactions

Bradycardia, thrombocytopenia
Life-threatening: Complete heart block, bronchospasm, agranulocytosis

Assessment and Planning
Interventions
Evaluation
NURSING PROCESS

KEY: A: adult; PO: by mouth; IV: intravenous; PB: protein-binding; t½: half-life; IDDM: insulin-dependent diabetes mellitus; CHF: congestive heart failure; ♦: Canadian drug names.

protein-bound and competes with other highly protein-bound drugs. Free drug is released from the protein-binding site and can have adverse effects.

Pharmacodynamics

Beta-adrenergic blockers block sympathetic stimulation, thus decreasing heart rate and blood pressure. The nonselective beta blockers block beta$_2$ receptors, which can result in bronchial constriction. Beta blockers cross the placental barrier and can enter breast milk.

The onset of action of oral beta blockers is usually 30 min or less, and the duration of action is 6 to 12 h. When beta blockers are administered intravenously, the onset of action is immediate, peak time is 20 min intravenously (compared to 1½ h orally), and duration of action is 4 to 10 h.

Side Effects and Adverse Reactions

Side effects and adverse reactions include decreased pulse rate, markedly decreased blood pressure, and bronchospasm (nonselective beta$_2$ blockers). Beta blockers should not be abruptly discontinued because

Table 39-3
Antihypertensives: Beta Blockers and Central Alpha₂ Agonists

GENERIC (BRAND)	ROUTE AND DOSAGE	USES AND CONSIDERATIONS
BETA-ADRENERGIC BLOCKERS		
Acebutolol HCl (Sectral) Cardioselective beta$_1$	A: PO: 400–800 mg/d in 1 or 2 divided doses; *max:* 1200 mg/d	For hypertension and cardiac dysrhythmia. It may be used alone or in combination with a diuretic. Side effects include dizziness, fatigue, hypotension, bradycardia, constipation/diarrhea. Vital signs should be closely monitored. *Pregnancy category:* B; PB: 26%; t$\frac{1}{2}$: 3–13 h
Atenolol (Tenormin) Cardioselective beta$_1$	A: PO: 25–100 mg/d	For hypertension and angina. Similar side effects as acebutolol. *Pregnancy category:* C; PB: 6%–16%; t$\frac{1}{2}$: 6–7 h
Betaxolol HCl (Kerlone) Cardioselective beta$_1$	A: PO: 10–20 mg/d Also for ophthalmic use: glaucoma	For hypertension and glaucoma. Ophthalmic preparation is used to decrease intraocular pressure (IOP). *Pregnancy category:* C; PB: UK; t$\frac{1}{2}$: 14–22 h
Bisoprolol fumarate (Zebeta) Beta$_1$ blocker	A: PO: Initially: 5 mg/d; maint: 2.5–20 mg/d	For hypertension and angina pectoris. Long-acting beta$_1$ blocker. Heart rate and blood pressure may be decreased. *Pregnancy category:* C; PB: <30%; t$\frac{1}{2}$: 9–12 h
Carteolol HCl (Cartrol) Nonselective beta$_1$ and beta$_2$	A: PO: 2.5–5.0 mg/d	For hypertension and glaucoma. It should be avoided for clients who have asthma because of its beta$_2$ effect. It may be used in combination with a thiazide diuretic. *Pregnancy category:* C; PB: 23%–30%; t$\frac{1}{2}$: 4–6 h
Metoprolol (Lopressor) Cardioselective beta$_1$	See Chart 39–1	For hypertension and angina pectoris. A commonly used drug to decrease blood pressure. *Pregnancy category:* C; PB: 12%; t$\frac{1}{2}$: 3–4 h
Nadolol (Corgard) Nonselective beta$_1$ and beta$_2$	A: PO: 40–80 mg/d; *max:* 320 mg/d	For hypertension and angina pectoris. Similar to carteolol HCl. *Pregnancy category:* C; PB: 30%; t$\frac{1}{2}$: 10–24 h
Penbutolol SO$_4$ (Levatol) Nonselective beta$_1$ and beta$_2$	A: PO: 10–20 mg/d; *max:* 80 mg/d	Treatment of stage 1 and 2 hypertension. Clients with asthma should avoid taking drug. *Pregnancy category:* C; PB: 80%–98%; t$\frac{1}{2}$: 5 h
Pindolol (Visken) Nonselective beta$_1$ and beta$_2$	A: PO: 5 mg b.i.d.–t.i.d.; maint: 10–30 mg in divided doses; *max:* 60 mg/d in divided doses	For hypertension. May be used alone or in combination with thiazide diuretic. Also may be used for angina pectoris. *Pregnancy category:* B; PB: 50%; t$\frac{1}{2}$: 3–4 h
Propranolol (Inderal) Nonselective beta$_1$ and beta$_2$	A: PO: Initially: 40 mg b.i.d. SR: 80 mg/d; maint: 120–240 mg/d in divided doses C: PO: Initially 1 mg/kg/d in 2 divided doses; maint: 2 mg/kg/d	For hypertension, angina, and cardiac dysrhythmias. The first beta blocker. May cause bronchospasm, decrease in heart rate and blood pressure. *Pregnancy category:* C; PB: 90%; t$\frac{1}{2}$: 3–6 h
Timolol maleate (Blocadren) Nonselective beta$_1$ and beta$_2$	A: PO: Initially 10 mg b.i.d.; maint: 20–40 mg/d in 2 divided doses; *max:* 60 mg/d Also for ophthalmic use: glaucoma	For hypertension, angina pectoris, and glaucoma. It is used as step 1 antihypertensive, like most of the beta blockers. Similar to propranolol. *Pregnancy category:* C; PB: 60%; t$\frac{1}{2}$: 3–4 h
CENTRAL ALPHA$_2$ AGONISTS		
Clonidine HCl (Catapres)	A: PO: Initially: 0.1 mg b.i.d.; maint: 0.2–1.2 mg/d in divided doses; *max:* 2.4 mg/d A: Transdermal patch: 100 μg (0.1 mg)/d 200 μg (0.2 mg)/d 300 μg (0.3 mg)/d	For hypertension. Long-acting. Well absorbed from GI tract. Can be taken with a diuretic. Step 2 antihypertensive drug. Decreases sympathetic effect. Drowsiness, dizziness, and dry mouth may occur. *Pregnancy category:* C; PB: 20%–40%; t$\frac{1}{2}$: 6–20 h

Table continued on following page

Table 39–3 *Continued*
Antihypertensives: Beta Blockers and Central Alpha$_2$ Agonists

GENERIC (BRAND)	ROUTE AND DOSAGE	USES AND CONSIDERATIONS
Guanabenz acetate (Wytensin)	A: PO: 4 mg b.i.d.; may increase to 4–8 mg/d; *max:* 32 mg b.i.d.	For hypertension and tachycardia. Can be taken with a thiazide diuretic. Intermediate-acting. May cause drowsiness, dizziness, headache, fatigue, and dry mouth. If GI distress occurs, take with food. *Pregnancy category:* C; PB: 90%; t$\frac{1}{2}$: 4–14 h
Guanfacine HCl (Tenex)	A: PO: 1 mg h.s.; may increase to 2–3 mg/d	For hypertension. Long-acting. May be taken alone or with a thiazide diuretic. *Pregnancy category:* B; PB: 70%; t$\frac{1}{2}$: >17 h
Methyldopa (Aldomet)	A: PO: 250–500 mg b.i.d.; *max:* 3 g/d IV: 250 mg–1 g q6h C: PO: 10 mg/kg/d in 2–4 divided doses	For stage 1 to 3 hypertension. May be used alone or in combination with a diuretic. Long-acting. Can be given intravenously. If GI upset occurs, take with food. *Pregnancy category:* C; PB: <15%; t$\frac{1}{2}$: 1.7 h

KEY: A: adult; C: child; PO: by mouth; IV: intravenous; PB: protein-binding; GI: gastrointestinal; t$\frac{1}{2}$: half-life; >: greater than; <: less than; UK: unknown.

rebound hypertension, angina, dysrhythmias, and myocardial infarction can result. Beta blockers can cause insomnia, depression, nightmares, and sexual dysfunction. Other side effects are discussed in Chapter 37. Table 39–3 presents the drug data for beta blockers that are commonly used in treating hypertension.

Noncardioselective beta blockers inhibit the liver's ability to convert glycogen to glucose in response to hypoglycemia. Because of this side effect, beta blockers should be used with caution in clients with diabetes mellitus. In addition, the depression of heart rate masks the symptom (tachycardia) of hypotension.

CENTRALLY ACTING SYMPATHOLYTICS (ADRENERGIC BLOCKERS)

Centrally acting sympatholytics decrease the sympathetic response from the brain stem to the peripheral vessels. Centrally acting sympatholytics stimulate the alpha$_2$ receptors, which in turn decrease sympathetic activity, increase vagus activity, and decrease serum epinephrine, norepinephrine, and renin release; thus, peripheral vascular resistance is reduced.

This group of drugs has minimal effects on cardiac output and blood flow to the kidneys. Drugs in this group include methyldopa, clonidine, guanabenz, and guanfacine. Methyldopa (Aldomet) was one of the first drugs widely used in controlling hypertension. In high doses, methyldopa and clonidine can cause sodium and water retention. Frequently, these drugs are administered with diuretics, vasodilators, calcium blockers, or ACE inhibitors. Beta blockers are not given with centrally acting sympatholytics that can

interfere with the antihypertensive effect. Guanabenz and guanfacine are new centrally acting sympatholytics with effects similar to clonidine.

Clonidine is available in a transdermal preparation that provides a 7-day duration of action. New transdermal patches are replaced every 7 days. Skin irritations have occurred in approximately 20% of the clients. Guanfacine has a long half-life and usually is taken once a day. Table 39–3 lists the centrally acting sympatholytics along with the beta blockers.

Side Effects and Adverse Reactions

The side effects and adverse reactions include drowsiness, dry mouth, dizziness, and slow heart rate (bradycardia). Methyldopa should not be used in clients with impaired liver function, and serum liver enzymes should be monitored periodically in all clients. This group of drugs must not be abruptly discontinued because a hypertensive crisis can result. If the drug needs to be stopped immediately, another antihypertensive drug is usually prescribed to avoid rebound hypertensive symptoms such as restlessness, tachycardia, tremors, headache, and increased blood pressure. Rebound hypertension is less likely to occur with guanabenz and guanfacine. The nurse should emphasize the need to take the medication as prescribed. This group of drugs can cause sodium and water retention, resulting in peripheral edema. A diuretic may be ordered with methyldopa or clonidine to decrease water and sodium retention (edema). Clients who are pregnant or contemplating pregnancy should avoid clonidine. Methyldopa is frequently used to treat chronic or pregnancy-induced hypertension; however, it crosses the placental barrier, and

NURSING PROCESS
ANTIHYPERTENSIVES: BETA BLOCKERS

Assessment

- Obtain a medication history from the client. Report if a drug-drug interaction is probable.
- Obtain vital signs (VS). Report abnormal blood pressure. Compare VS with baseline finding.
- Check laboratory values related to renal and liver function. An elevated blood urea nitrogen (BUN) and serum creatinine may be caused by metoprolol or cardiac disorder. Elevated cardiac enzymes, such as aspartate transaminase (AST) and lactate dehydrogenase (LDH), could result from use of metoprolol or from a cardiac disorder.

Potential Nursing Diagnoses

- Decreased cardiac output
- Noncompliance with drug regimen
- Altered sexual dysfunction

Planning

- Client's blood pressure will be decreased and/or return to normal value.
- Client takes the medication as prescribed.

Nursing Interventions

- Monitor VS, especially blood pressure and pulse.
- Monitor laboratory results, especially BUN, serum creatinine, AST, and LDH.

Client Teaching

General
- Instruct the client to comply with drug regimen: *abrupt discontinuation of the antihypertensive drug may cause rebound hypertension.*
- Suggest that the client avoid over-the-counter drugs without first checking with the health care provider. Many OTC drugs carry warnings against use in the presence of hypertension.
- Suggest that the client wear a Medic Alert bracelet or carry a card indicating the health problem and prescribed drugs.
- Instruct the client in a trauma situation to inform the health care provider of drugs taken daily, such as a beta blocker. Beta blockers block the compensatory effects of the body to the shock state. Glucagon may be needed to reverse the effects so that the client can be resuscitated.

Self-Administration
- Instruct the client or family member how to take a radial pulse and blood pressure. Advise the client to report abnormal findings to the health care provider.

Diet
- Teach the client and family members nonpharmacologic methods to decrease blood pressure, such as a low-fat and low-salt diet, weight control, relaxation techniques, exercise, smoking cessation, and decreased alcohol ingestion (1 to 2 oz/d).
- Advise the client to report constipation. Foods high in fiber, a stool softener, and increased water intake (except in clients with CHF) are usually indicated.

Side Effects
- Advise the client that antihypertensives may cause dizziness resulting from orthostatic hypotension and possible sexual dysfunction caused by impotence. Instruct the client to remain in a sitting position for several minutes before standing.
- Instruct the client to report dizziness, slow pulse rate, changes in blood pressure, heart palpitation, confusion, or GI upset to the health care provider.
- Caution client with diabetes mellitus of possible hypoglycemic symptoms.

Nursing Process continued on following page

NURSING PROCESS *Continued*
ANTIHYPERTENSIVES: BETA BLOCKERS

Cultural Considerations

- African-American clients who are hypertensive should avoid taking beta blockers because these agents are not generally effective in controlling their hypertension. Taking a diuretic with a beta blocker increases the effectiveness of the drug for controlling hypertension for the African-American client.

Evaluation

- Evaluate the effectiveness of the drug therapy, that is, decreased blood pressure and the absence of side effects.
- Determine that the client is adhering to the drug regimen.

---

small amounts may enter breast milk in a lactating client.

ALPHA-ADRENERGIC BLOCKERS

This group of drugs blocks the alpha-adrenergic receptors, resulting in vasodilation and decreased blood pressure. They help to maintain the renal blood flow rate. The alpha blockers are useful in treating hypertension in clients with lipid abnormalities. They decrease the very low-density lipoproteins (VLDL) and the low-density lipoproteins (LDL) that are responsible for the buildup of fatty plaques in the arteries (atherosclerosis). Also, they increase high-density lipoprotein (HDL) levels ("friendly" lipoprotein). Alpha blockers are safe for diabetics because they do not affect glucose metabolism. They do not affect respiratory function.

Prazosin, terazosin, and doxazosin (selective alpha$_1$ adrenergic blockers) are used mainly for reducing blood pressure and can be used in treatment of benign prostatic hypertrophy (BPH). Prazosin is a commonly prescribed drug. Doxazosin and terazosin have longer half-lives than prazosin, and they are normally given once a day. When prazosin is taken with alcohol or other antihypertensives, the hypotensive state can be intensified.

These drugs, like the centrally acting sympatholytics, cause sodium and water retention with edema, and diuretics are frequently given with them to decrease fluid accumulation in the extremities.

The more potent alpha blockers, phentolamine, phenoxybenzamine, and tolazoline, are used primarily for hypertensive crisis and severe hypertension resulting from tumors of the adrenal medulla (pheochromocytomas).

Side Effects and Adverse Reactions

Side effects of phentolamine include hypotension, reflex tachycardia due to the severe decrease in blood pressure, nasal congestion because of the vasodilating effect, and GI disturbances.

The side effects of prazosin, doxazosin, and terazosin include orthostatic hypotension (dizziness, faintness, lightheadedness, increased heart rate), which may occur with first dose, nausea, drowsiness, nasal congestion due to vasodilation, edema, and weight gain.

Drug Interactions

Drug interactions occur when alpha-adrenergic blockers are taken with antiinflammatory drugs and nitrates (nitroglycerin) for angina. Peripheral edema is intensified when prazosin and an antiinflammatory drug are taken daily. Nitroglycerin taken for angina lowers the blood pressure. If prazosin is taken with nitroglycerin, syncope (faintness) caused by a decrease in blood pressure can occur. The selective alpha-adrenergic blocker prazosin is shown in Chart 39–2.

Pharmacokinetics

Prazosin is absorbed through the GI tract; however, a large portion of prazosin is lost during hepatic first-pass metabolism. The half-life is short, so the drug should be administered twice a day. Prazosin is highly protein-bound, and when it is given with other highly protein-bound drugs, the client should be assessed for adverse reactions.

Pharmacodynamics

The selective alpha-adrenergic blockers dilate the arterioles and venules, decreasing peripheral resistance and lowering the blood pressure. With prazosin, the heart rate is only slightly increased, whereas with alpha blockers such as phentolamine and tolazoline, the blood pressure is greatly reduced and reflex tachycardia can occur. Alpha blockers are more effective for acute hypertension; selective alpha blockers are more useful for long-term essential hypertension.

The onset of action of prazosin occurs between 30 min and 2 h. The duration of action of prazosin is 10 h. Table 39–4 presents the drug data for selective and nonselective alpha blockers.

Chart 39-2.   Antihypertensives: Alpha-Adrenergic Blocker

ALPHA-ADRENERGIC BLOCKER

Drug Name

Prazosin HCl
  (Minipress)
Sympatholytic, selective alpha-adrenergic
blocker
Pregnancy Category: C

Dosage

A: PO: 1 mg b.i.d.–t.i.d.; maint: 3–15 mg/d;
max: 20 mg/d in divided doses

Contraindications

Renal disease

Drug-Lab-Food Interactions

Drug: *Increase* hypotensive effect with other antihypertensives, nitrates, alcohol

Pharmacokinetics

Absorption: GI: 60% (5% to circulation)
Distribution: PB: 95%
Metabolism: t½: 3 h
Excretion: 10% in urine; in bile and feces

Pharmacodynamics

IV: Onset: 0.5–2 h
  Peak: 2–4 h
  Duration: 10 h

Therapeutic Effects/Uses

To control hypertension, refractory CHF, treatment of benign prostatic hypertrophy (BPH).

Mode of Action: Dilation of peripheral blood vessels via blocking the alpha-adrenergic receptors.

Side Effects

Dizziness, drowsiness, headache, nausea, vomiting, diarrhea, impotence, vertigo, urinary frequency, tinnitus, dry mouth, incontinence, abdominal discomfort

Adverse Reactions

Orthostatic hypotension, palpitations, tachycardia, pancreatitis

Assessment and Planning

Interventions

NURSING PROCESS

Evaluation

KEY: A: adult; PO: by mouth; PB: protein-binding; CHF: congestive heart failure; t½: half-life.

ADRENERGIC NEURON BLOCKERS (PERIPHERALLY ACTING SYMPATHOLYTICS)

Adrenergic neuron blockers are potent antihypertensive drugs that block norepinephrine from the sympathetic nerve endings, causing a decrease in norepinephrine release that results in a lowering of blood
pressure. There is a decrease in both cardiac output
and peripheral vascular resistance. Reserpine and
guanethidine (the two most potent drugs) are used to
control severe hypertension. Orthostatic hypotension
is a common side effect: the client should be advised
to rise slowly from a reclining or sitting position. The
drugs in this group can cause sodium and water retention. Use of reserpine may cause vivid dreams,
nightmares, and suicidal intention. This group is classified as step IV drugs and these drugs can be taken
alone or with a diuretic to decrease peripheral edema.

ALPHA₁ AND BETA₁ ADRENERGIC BLOCKERS

This group of drugs blocks both the alpha$_1$ and beta$_1$
receptors. Labetalol (Normodyne) and carteolol (Car-
trol) are examples of alpha/beta blockers. By blocking
the alpha$_1$ receptor, dilation of the arterioles and
veins occurs. The effect on the alpha receptor is
stronger than the effect on the beta receptor; therefore, blood pressure is lowered and pulse rate is
moderately decreased. With blocking the cardiac
beta$_1$, the heart rate and AV contractility are decreased. Large doses of alpha/beta blockers could
block beta$_2$ adrenergic receptors, thus increasing airway resistance. Clients who are severe asthmatics
should not take large doses of carteolol or labetalol.
Table 39–4 lists the two alpha/beta blockers.

Common side effects of these drugs include orthostatic (postural) hypotension, GI disturbances, nerv-

Table 39–4
Antihypertensives: Sympatholytics: Alpha-Adrenergic and Peripherally Acting Blockers and Direct-Acting Vasodilators

GENERIC (BRAND)	ROUTE AND DOSAGE	USES AND CONSIDERATIONS
SELECTIVE ALPHA-ADRENERGIC BLOCKERS		
Doxazosin mesylate (Cardura)	A: PO: Initially: 1 mg/d; maint: 2–4 mg/d; *max:* 16 mg/d	For stage 1 or 2 hypertension. May be used alone or with another antihypertensive. May cause orthostatic hypotension, headache, dizziness, and GI upset. *Pregnancy category:* C; PB: 98%; $t\frac{1}{2}$: 22 h
Prazosin HCl (Minipress)	See Chart 39–2	For hypertension. Intermediate-acting. May be taken with a diuretic. Commonly used antihypertensive. *Pregnancy category:* C; PB: 95%; $t\frac{1}{2}$: 3 h
Terazosin HCl (Hytrin)	A: PO: Initially 1 mg h.s.; maint: 1–5 mg/d; *max:* 20 mg/d	For stage 1 or 2 hypertension. May be used alone or with another antihypertensive drug. Dizziness and headache may occur. *Pregnancy category:* C; PB: 95%; $t\frac{1}{2}$: 9–12 h
ALPHA-ADRENERGIC BLOCKERS		
Phenoxybenzamine HCl (Dibenzyline)	A: PO: Initially: 10 mg/d; maint: 20–40 mg/d C: PO: 0.2 mg/kg/d in 1–2 divided doses; may increase dose by 0.2 mg	For hypertension related to adrenergic excess, pheochromocytoma. It lowers peripheral resistance. Has a long action. *Pregnancy category:* C; PB: UK; $t\frac{1}{2}$: 24 h
Phentolamine (Regitine)	A: IM/IV: 2.5–5 mg; repeat q5min until controlled; then q2–3h PRN C: IM/IV: 0.05–0.1 mg/kg; repeat if needed	For hypertensive crisis due to pheochromocytoma, MAO inhibitors, or clonidine withdrawal. It is a potent antihypertensive drug. In heart failure, it decreases afterload and increases cardiac output. For hypertension, it antagonizes the effects of epinephrine and norepinephrine causing vasodilation. *Pregnancy category:* C; PB: UK; $t\frac{1}{2}$: 20 min
Tolazoline HCl (Priscoline HCl)	NB: IV: Initially: 1–2 mg/kg; followed by 1–2 mg/kg/h for 24–48 h; expected effect within 30 min of initial dose A: IM/IV: 10–50 mg q.i.d.	For pulmonary hypertension of newborn, and for peripheral vasospastic disorders. *Pregnancy category:* C; PB: UK; $t\frac{1}{2}$: 3–10 h
ADRENERGIC NEURON BLOCKERS (PERIPHERALLY ACTING SYMPATHOLYTICS)		
Guanadrel sulfate (Hylorel)	A: PO: Initially: 5 mg b.i.d.; maint; 20–75 mg/d in divided doses	For moderate to severe hypertension. Intermediate-acting duration. Rapid onset: *Pregnancy category:* B; PB: 20%; $t\frac{1}{2}$: 10–12 h
Guanethidine monosulfate (Ismelin)	A: PO: Initially: 10 mg/d; maint: 25–50 mg/d; *max:* 300 mg/d C: PO: 0.2 mg/kg/d; *max:* 1–1.6 mg/kg/d	For severe hypertension. Long-acting. Can be taken with a diuretic. Potent antihypertensive drug. May cause marked orthostatic hypotension, edema, weight gain, diarrhea, bradycardia. *Pregnancy category:* C; PB: UK; $t\frac{1}{2}$: 5 d
Reserpine (Serpasil, Serpalan)	A: PO: Initially: 0.25–5.0 mg daily for 1–2 wk; maint: 0.1–0.25 mg/d	One of the early antihypertensives. For hypertension. Currently, not frequently used. May cause nightmares, vivid dreams. *Pregnancy category:* D; PB: UK; $t\frac{1}{2}$: 4.5–11 h
ALPHA₁ AND BETA₁ ADRENERGIC BLOCKER		
Carteolol HCl (Cartrol, Ocupress)	A: PO: Initially: 2.5 mg, q.d.; maint: 2.5–5 mg q.d.; *max:* 10 mg q.d.	To treat hypertension. It may be used alone or in combination with other antihypertensive agents. Not for hypertensive crisis or client with open-angle glaucoma. *Pregnancy category:* C; PB: UK; $t\frac{1}{2}$: 4–6 h

Table continued on following page

Table 39–4 *Continued*

Antihypertensives: Sympatholytics: Alpha-Adrenergic and Peripherally Acting Blockers and Direct-Acting Vasodilators

GENERIC (BRAND)	ROUTE AND DOSAGE	USES AND CONSIDERATIONS
Labetalol HCl (Trandate, Normodyne)	A: PO: Initially: 100 mg b.i.d.; maint: 200–800 mg/d in 2 divided doses A: IV: 2 mg/min in infusion; *max:* 300 mg as total dose	For stage 1 or 2 hypertension. May be used alone or with a thiazide diuretic. May cause orthostatic hypotension, palpitation, syncope. *Pregnancy category:* C; PB: 50%; t½: 4–8 h
DIRECT-ACTING VASODILATORS		
Diazoxide (Hyperstat, Proglycem)	A & C: IV: 1–3 mg/kg in bolus (30 sec); repeat in 5–15 min as needed; *max:* 150 mg	For hypertensive emergency. Dose may be repeated in 5–15 min until adequate decrease in blood pressure is achieved. Oral antihypertensive drugs may follow. *Pregnancy category:* C; PB: 90%; t½: 20–45 h
Hydralazine HCl (Apresoline HCl)	A: PO: Initially: 10 mg q.i.d.; maint: 25–50 mg q.i.d. Severe hypertension IM–IV: 10–40 mg: repeat as needed C: PO: 3–7.5 mg/kg/d in 4 divided doses	For hypertension. Short-acting duration. Can be taken with diuretic to decrease edema and beta blocker to prevent tachycardia. Dizziness, tremors, headaches, tachycardia, and palpitation may occur. Vital signs should be closely monitored. *Pregnancy category:* C; PB: 87%; t½: 2–6 h
Minoxidil (Loniten, Rogaine, Minodyl)	A: PO: Initially: 5 mg/d; maint: 10–40 mg/d in single or divided doses; *max:* 100 mg/d C: PO: Initially: 0.2 mg/kg/d; *max:* 5 mg/d; maint: 0.25–1 mg/kg/d in divided doses; *max:* 50 mg/d *Topical for alopecia:* 2% sol b.i.d.	For hypertension. Can be taken with a diuretic to reduce edema and with a beta blocker to prevent tachycardia. Long-acting effect. When discontinuing drug, it should be slowly decreased to avoid rebound hypertension; should not be abruptly withdrawn. Vital signs should be closely monitored. *Pregnancy category:* C; PB: 0%; t½: 3.5–4 h
Sodium nitroprusside (Nipride, Nitropress)	A: IV: 1–3 µg/kg/min in D₅W; *max:* 10 µg/kg/min	For hypertensive crisis. A potent antihypertensive drug. Drug decomposes in light; container must be wrapped in aluminum foil. Good for 24 hours. Drug should be discarded if red or blue. Can cause cyanide toxicity. Measure cyanide and thiocyanate levels. May cause profound hypotension. *Pregnancy category:* C; PB: UK; t½: 2–7 d

KEY: *A: adult; C: child; PO: by mouth; IM: intramuscular; IV: intravenous; UK: unknown; PB: protein-binding; t½: half-life; MAO: monoamine oxidase.*

ousness, dry mouth, and fatigue. Large doses of these agents may cause AV heart block.

Direct-Acting Arteriolar Vasodilators

Vasodilators are potent antihypertensive drugs. Direct-acting vasodilators are step III drugs that act by relaxing the smooth muscles of the blood vessels, mainly the arteries, causing vasodilation. Vasodilators promote an increase in blood flow to the brain and kidneys. With vasodilation, the blood pressure decreases and sodium and water are retained, resulting in peripheral edema. Diuretics can be given with a direct-acting vasodilator to decrease the edema. Reflex tachycardia is caused by the vasodilation and decrease in blood pressure. Beta blockers are frequently prescribed with arteriolar vasodilators to decrease the heart rate; this counteracts the effect of reflex tachycardia. Two of the direct-acting vasodilators, hydralazine and minoxidil, are used for moderate to severe hypertension; nitroprusside and diazoxide are prescribed for acute hypertensive emergency. The latter two drugs are very potent vasodilators that rapidly decrease the blood pressure. Nitroprusside

NURSING PROCESS
ANTIHYPERTENSIVES: ALPHA-ADRENERGIC BLOCKERS

Assessment

- Obtain a medication history from the client, including current drugs. Report if a drug-drug interaction is probable. Prazosin is highly protein-bound and can displace other highly protein-bound drugs.
- Obtain baseline vital signs (VS) and weight for future comparisons.
- Check urinary output. Report if it is decreased (< 600 mL/d), because drug is contraindicated if renal disease is present.

Potential Nursing Diagnoses

- Risk for activity intolerance
- Knowledge deficit related to drug regimen
- Altered sexuality patterns

Planning

- Client's blood pressure will decrease.
- Client will follow proper drug regimen.

Nursing Interventions

- Monitor VS. The desired therapeutic effect of prazosin may not fully occur for 4 wk. A sudden marked decrease in blood pressure should be reported.
- Check daily for fluid retention in the extremities. Prazosin may cause sodium and water retention.

Client Teaching

General
- Instruct the client to comply with drug regimen. *Abrupt discontinuation of the antihypertensive drug may cause rebound hypertension.*
- Inform the client that orthostatic hypotension may occur. Explain that before rising, the client should sit and dangle his or her feet.

Self-Administration
- Instruct the client or family member how to take a blood pressure reading. A record for daily blood pressures should be kept.

Diet
- Encourage the client to decrease salt intake unless otherwise indicated by the health care provider.

Side Effects
- Caution the client that dizziness, lightheadedness, and drowsiness may occur, especially when the drug is first prescribed. If these symptoms occur, the health care provider should be notified.
- Inform the male client that impotence may occur if high doses of the drug are prescribed. This problem should be reported to the health care provider.
- Instruct the client to report if edema is present in the morning.
- Instruct the client not to take cold, cough, or allergy over-the-counter (OTC) medications without first contacting the health care provider.

Cultural Considerations
- Same as for beta blockers.

Evaluation

- Evaluate the effectiveness of the drug in controlling blood pressure and the absence of side effects.
- Evaluate the client's adherence to medication schedule.

Chart 39–3. Antihypertensives: Angiotensin Antagonist

ANGIOTENSIN-CONVERTING ENZYME (ACE) INHIBITOR

NURSING PROCESS

Assessment and Planning

Drug Name

Captopril
   (Capoten), Apo-Captopril, Novo-Capto
Pregnancy Category: C

Dosage

A: PO: Initially: 12.5–25 mg b.i.d.–t.i.d.; *max:* 450 mg/d; maint: 25–50 mg t.i.d.

Contraindications

Heart block
Caution: Leukemia, chronic obstructive pulmonary disease (COPD), renal or thyroid disease

Drug-Lab-Food Interactions

Drug: *Increase* hypotensive effect with nitrates, diuretics, adrenergic blockers, vasodilators, other antihypertensives; *increase* serum potassium with potassium-sparing diuretics or with potassium supplements

Interventions

Pharmacokinetics

Absorption: PO: 65% (food decreases absorption)
Distribution: PB: 25%–30%
Metabolism: t½: normal kidney function: 2–3 h
Excretion: In urine

Pharmacodynamics

PO: Onset: 15 min
      Peak: 1 h
      Duration: 6–12 h

Evaluation

Therapeutic Effects/Uses

To reduce blood pressure; to control CHF.

Mode of Action: Suppression of the ACE; inhibits angiotensin I conversion to angiotensin II.

Side Effects

Dizziness, cough, nocturia, impotence, rash, polyuria, hyperkalemia, taste disturbance

Adverse Reactions

Oliguria, urticaria, severe hypotension
Life-threatening: Acute renal failure, bronchospasm, angioedema, agranulocytosis

KEY: A: adult; PO: by mouth; PB: protein-binding; t½: half-life; CHF: congestive heart failure; ACE: angiotensin-converting enzyme; : Canadian drug names.

acts on the arterial and venous vessels, and diazoxide acts on the arterial vessels. Table 39–4 lists direct-acting vasodilators.

SIDE EFFECTS AND ADVERSE REACTIONS

The effects of hydralazine are numerous and include tachycardia, palpitations, edema, nasal congestion, headache, dizziness, GI bleeding, lupus-like symptoms, and neurologic symptoms (tingling, numbness). Minoxidil has similar side effects, along with tachycardia, edema, and excess hair growth. It can precipitate an anginal attack.

Nitroprusside and diazoxide can cause reflex tachycardia, palpitations, restlessness, agitation, nausea, and confusion. Hyperglycemia can occur with diazoxide because the drug inhibits insulin release from the beta cells of the pancreas. Nitroprusside and diazoxide are discussed in greater detail in Chapter 52.

Angiotensin Antagonists (Angiotensin-Converting Enzyme Inhibitors)

Drugs in this group inhibit angiotensin-converting enzyme (ACE), which in turn inhibits the formation of angiotensin II (vasoconstrictor) and blocks the release of aldosterone. Aldosterone promotes sodium retention and potassium excretion. When aldosterone is blocked, sodium is excreted along with water and potassium is retained. ACE inhibitors cause little

Table 39-5
Antihypertensives: ACE Inhibitors and Angiotensin II Antagonists

GENERIC (BRAND)	ROUTE AND DOSAGE	USES AND CONSIDERATIONS
ANGIOTENSIN ANTAGONISTS (ACE INHIBITORS)		
Benazepril HCl (Lotensin)	A: PO: Initially: 10 mg/d; maint: 20–40 mg/d in 2 divided doses	Management of stage 1 and 2 hypertension. Headache, dizziness, hypotension, nausea, diarrhea, or constipation may occur. *Pregnancy category:* D; PB: 97%; $t\frac{1}{2}$: 10 h
Captopril (Capoten)	See Chart 39–3	For stage 1 or 2 hypertension and CHF. Can be taken alone or with a diuretic. Duration of action is moderate. Food can decrease absorption time. Commonly prescribed drug. Should *not* be taken with potassium-sparing diuretics to avoid hyperkalemia (potassium excess). *Pregnancy category:* C; PB: 25%–30%; $t\frac{1}{2}$: 2–3 h
Enalapril maleate (Vasotec)	A: PO: Initially: 5 mg/d; maint: 10–40 mg/d in 1–2 divided doses IV: 1.25 mg q6h infuse in 5 min	For hypertension and CHF. Similar to captopril and benazepril. Has a long duration of action (orally). *Pregnancy category:* D; PB: 50%–60%; $t\frac{1}{2}$: 1.5–2 h
Enalaprilat (Vasotec IV)	A: IV: 1.25 mg q6h	A potent ACE inhibitor for control of hypertension. Similar to enalapril (Vasotec)
Fosinopril (Monopril)	A: PO: 5–40 mg/d; *max:* 80 mg/d	To treat hypertension and heart failure. Reduces peripheral resistance (afterload) and improves cardiac output. Dose does not have to be reduced because of renal insufficiency. *Pregnancy category:* C (first trimester), D (second and third trimester); PB: 90%; $t\frac{1}{2}$: 3–4 h
Lisinopril (Prinivil, Zestril)	A: PO: Initially: 10 mg/d; maint: 20–40 mg/d; *max:* 80 mg/d	For hypertension and CHF. Usually given in combination with a diuretic. Has a long duration of action (24 h). Monitor vital signs. *Pregnancy category:* D; PB: 0%; $t\frac{1}{2}$: 12 h
Moexipril (Univasc)	A: PO: 7.5 mg/d; *max:* 30 mg/d in divided doses	For the treatment of hypertension. Reduce dose with renal insufficiency; creatinine clearance <40 mL/min. May increase serum lithium levels and cause toxicity. *Pregnancy category:* C and D (see fosinopril) PB: 50%; $t\frac{1}{2}$: 2–9 h
Quinapril HCl (Accupril)	A: PO: 10–20 mg/d; *max:* 80 mg/d in divided doses Elderly: A: PO: 2.5–5 mg/d	To treat hypertension and heart failure. A potent, long-acting second-generation ACE inhibitor. Reduces systemic vascular resistance and increases cardiac output. *Pregnancy category:* D; PB: 97%; $t\frac{1}{2}$: 2 h
Ramipril (Altace)	A: PO: 2.5–5 mg/d; *max:* 20 mg/d	Treatment of stage 1 and 2 hypertension and CHF. Similar to captopril. Has a long duration of action (24 h). *Pregnancy category:* D; PB: 97%; $t\frac{1}{2}$: 2–3 h
Trandolapril (Mavik)	A: PO: 1 mg/d; may increase weekly to 2–4 mg/d; *max:* 8 mg/d	To treat hypertension. May be used alone or combined with other antihypertensives. Diuretics should be discontinued 2 to 3 days before taking trandolapril. Reduce dose if client has renal (creatinine clearance <30 mL/min) or hepatic insufficiency. African-Americans respond to trandolapril including those with low-renin hypertension. *Pregnancy category:* C and D. PB: 80%; $t\frac{1}{2}$: 6 h
COMBINATIONS WITH CALCIUM BLOCKERS		
Benazepril with amlodipine (Lotrel) Enalapril with diltiazem (Teczem) Enalapril with felodipine (Lexxel) Trandolapril with verapamil (Tarka)		

Table continued on following page

Table 39–5 *Continued*
Antihypertensives: ACE Inhibitors and Angiotensin II Antagonists

GENERIC (BRAND)	ROUTE AND DOSAGE	USES AND CONSIDERATIONS
ANGIOTENSIN II RECEPTOR ANTAGONISTS		
Candesartan (Atacand)	A: PO: 16 mg/d.; maint: 8–32 mg/d.	For treating hypertension. It may be used when the client does not respond or cannot tolerate ACE inhibitors. It may be combined with the calcium blocker, amlodipine, for a more effective response in decreasing high blood pressure. *Pregnancy category:* C (first trimester) and D (second and third trimester); PB: >99%; t½: 9 h
Irbesartan (Avapro)	A: PO: 150 mg/d.; maint: 150–300 mg/d.	For treating hypertension. It may be used alone or in combination with other antihypertensive drugs. *Pregnancy category:* C and D (see candesartan); PB: 90%; t½: 11–15 h
Losartan potassium (Cozaar)	A: PO: 25–50 mg/d., in single dose or in 2 divided doses; *max:* 100 mg/d	For treating hypertension. It may be used alone or in combination with other antihypertensive drugs. *Pregnancy category:* C and D (see candesartan); PB: 95%; t½: 1.5–2 h
Valsartan (Diovan)	A: PO: 80 mg/d.; *max:* 320 mg/d.	For treating hypertension. Similar action to candesartan, irbesartan, losartan. *Pregnancy category:* C and D (see candesartan); PB: 99%; t½: 6 h

KEY: A: adult; PO: by mouth; SR: sustained-release; PB: protein-binding; t½: half-life; CHF: congestive heart failure; maint: maintenance.

change in cardiac output or heart rate, and they lower peripheral resistance. Figure 39–1 illustrates the renin-angiotensin system. These drugs can be used in clients who have elevated serum renin levels.

ACE inhibitors are used primarily to treat hypertension; some of the agents are also effective in treating heart failure. The first ACE inhibitor, captopril (Capoten), became available in the early 1970s. By the mid 1990s, there were five ACE inhibitors, and in the late 1990s, there were 10. These 10 ACE inhibitors include benazepril (Lotensin), captopril (Capoten), enalapril maleate (Vasotec), enalaprilat (Vasotec IV), fosinopril (Monopril), lisinopril (Prinivil, Zestril), moexipril (Univasc), quinapril (Accupril), ramipril (Altace), and trandolapril (Mavik), which are presented in Table 39–5. These drugs are not intended for first-line antihypertensive therapy. Chart 39–3 gives the pharmacologic data related to captopril.

African-Americans and the elderly do not respond with effective reduction in blood pressure to ACE inhibitors, but when taken with a diuretic, the blood pressure usually will be lowered. ACE inhibitors should not be given during pregnancy because they reduce placental blood flow. The major adverse effects are first-dose hypotension and hyperkalemia. Hypotension results because of the vasodilating effect. First-dose hypotension is more common in clients also taking diuretics.

Except for moexipril (Univasc), which should be taken on an empty stomach for maximum effectiveness, ACE inhibitors can be administered with food. It is necessary to reduce the drug dose, except for fosinopril (Monopril), for clients with renal insufficiency.

SIDE EFFECTS AND ADVERSE REACTIONS
The side effects of these drugs include nausea, vomiting, diarrhea, headache, dizziness, fatigue, insomnia, serum potassium excess (hyperkalemia), and tachycardia. Because of the risk of hyperkalemia, these drugs should not be taken with potassium-sparing diuretics or salt substitutes that contain potassium.

Angiotensin II Receptor Antagonists (Blockers)

Angiotensin II receptor antagonists (A-II blockers) are a new group of antihypertensive drugs. This group is similar to ACE inhibitors in that they prevent the release of aldosterone (sodium-retaining hormone). They act on the renin-angiotensin system. The difference between A-II blockers and ACE inhibitors is that A-II blockers block the angiotensin II from the AT_1 receptors found in many tissues, and ACE inhibitors prevent the angiotensin-converting enzyme in the formation of angiotensin II. A-II blockers cause vasodilation and decrease peripheral resistance.

NURSING PROCESS
ANTIHYPERTENSIVES: ANGIOTENSIN ANTAGONIST (ACE) INHIBITORS

Assessment

- Obtain a drug history from the client of current drugs that are being taken. Report if a drug-drug interaction is probable.
- Obtain baseline vital signs (VS) for future comparisons.
- Check the laboratory values for serum protein, albumin, BUN, creatinine, and white blood cell (WBC) count, and compare with future serum levels.

Potential Nursing Diagnoses

- Knowledge deficit related to drug regimen
- Anxiety related to hypertensive state

Planning

- Client's blood pressure will be within desired range.
- Client is free of moderate to severe side effects.

Nursing Interventions

- Monitor laboratory tests related to renal function (BUN, creatinine, protein) and blood glucose levels. *Caution:* Watch for hypoglycemic reaction in a client with diabetes mellitus. Urine protein may be checked in the morning using a dipstick.
- Report to the health care provider occurrences of bruising, petechiae, and/or bleeding. These may indicate a severe adverse reaction to an angiotensin antagonist such as captopril.

Client Teaching

General
- Instruct the client not to abruptly discontinue use of captopril without notifying the health care provider. *Rebound hypertension could result.*
- Inform the client not to take over-the-counter (OTC) drugs (cold, allergy medications) without first contacting the health care provider.

Self-Administration
- Teach the client how to take and record his or her blood pressure. Blood pressure chart should be established, and blood pressure changes should be reported.

Diet
- Instruct the client to take captopril 20 min to 1 h before a meal. Food decreases 35% of captopril absorption.
- Inform the client that the taste of food may be diminished during the first month of drug therapy.

Side Effects
- Explain to the client that dizziness and/or light-headedness may occur during the first week of captopril therapy. If dizziness persists, the health care provider should be notified.
- Instruct the client to report any occurrence of bleeding.

Cultural Considerations

- African-Americans do not respond well to ACE inhibitors.

Evaluation

- Evaluate the effectiveness of the drug therapy: the absence of severe side effects and blood pressure return to desired range.

Table 39–6
Antihypertensives: Calcium Channel Blockers

GENERIC (BRAND)	ROUTE AND DOSAGE	USES AND CONSIDERATIONS
PHENYLALKYLAMINES		
Verapamil (Calan SR, Is-optin SR)	A: PO SR: 120–240 mg/d in 2 divided doses; *max:* 480 mg/d	For hypertension (sustained release form). One of the first calcium blockers. Also used for variant angina and cardiac dysrhythmias. Common side effects: dizziness, headache, hypotension, bradycardia, and constipation. *Pregnancy category:* C; PB: 90%; t½: 3–8 h
BENZOTHIAZEPINES		
Diltiazem HCl (Cardizem, Cardizem CD or SR)	A: PO SR: Initially: 60–120 mg b.i.d.; *max:* 240–360 mg/d	For hypertension (sustained-release form). Also for angina pectoris; IV form for cardiac dysrhythmias (atrial fibrillation). Headache, bradycardia, and hypotension may occur. *Pregnancy category:* C; PB: 70%–80%; t½: 3.5–9 h
DIHYDROPYRIDINES		
Amlodipine (Norvasc)	A: PO: 5–10 mg/d. Elderly: 2.5–5.0 mg/d	To treat mild and moderate hypertension and angina pectoris. Decreases peripheral vascular resistance (vasodilation). May be used alone or with other antihypertensives. *Pregnancy category:* C; PB: >95%; t½: 30–50 h (elderly with hepatic insufficiency: 50–100 h)
Felodipine (Plendil)	A: PO: Initially: 5 mg; maint: 5–10 mg/d; *max:* 20 mg/d	Treatment for stage 1 and 2 hypertension, CHF, and angina. Potent calcium blocker. Flushing, peripheral edema, palpitations, dizziness, headache may occur. Long duration of action. *Pregnancy category:* C; PB: 99%; t½: 10–16 h
Isradipine (DynaCirc)	*Hypertension:* A: PO: 1.25–10 mg b.i.d.; *max:* 20 mg/d	Management of hypertension, CHF, and angina pectoris. For hypertension, drug may be used alone or with a diuretic. *Pregnancy category:* C; PB: 99%; t½: 5–11 h
Nicardipine HCl (Cardene, Cardene SR)	A: PO: 20–40 mg t.i.d. SR: 30–60 mg b.i.d. A: IV: initially: 5 mg/h; increase dose as needed; *max:* 15 mg/h C: IV: 1–3 µg/kg/min	To treat essential hypertension and vasospastic angina. IV therapy for short-term therapy for hypertension. Decreases systemic resistance; heart rate and cardiac output are increased. *Pregnancy category:* C; PB: 95%; t½: 8.5 h
Nifedipine (Procardia)	A: PO: 10–20 mg t.i.d. A: PO SR: 30–90 mg/d; *max:* 120 mg/d	For hypertension and angina pectoris. Potent calcium channel blocker. Common side effects include dizziness, lightheadedness, headache, flushing, peripheral edema, and nausea. Drug may be taken alone or with a diuretic. *Pregnancy category:* C; PB: 92%–98%; t½: 2–5 h
Nisoldipine (Sular, Nisocor)	A: PO: 10–20 mg/d in 2 divided doses; *max:* 40 mg/d	To treat hypertension and angina. It can be used alone or combined with another antihypertensive drug. It is similar to nifedipine, causing vasodilation and is 10 times more potent than nifedipine. It is considered a potent coronary vasodilator. *Pregnancy category:* C; PB: 99%; t½: 2–14 h

KEY: *A: adult; C: child; PO: by mouth; IV: intravenous; UK: unknown; PB: protein-binding; t½: half-life; SR: sustained release.*

Losartan (Cozaar), valsartan (Diovan), irbesartan (Avapro), and candesartan cilexetil (Atacand) are examples of A-II blockers. These agents block the vasoconstrictor effects of angiotensin II at the receptor site. They are approved by the Food and Drug Administration (FDA) for the treatment of hypertension. Candesartan cilexetil (Atacand) is the fourth A-II blocker to be approved for treating high blood pressure. The combination of losartan potassium and hydrochlorothiazide tablet is also available and should not cause serum potassium excess or loss.

Like ACE inhibitors, the angiotensin II receptor antagonists (A-II blockers) are less effective for treating hypertension in African-American persons. Also, A-II blockers, like ACE inhibitors, may cause angioedema. These agents can be taken with or without food, and are suitable for clients with mild hepatic and renal insufficiency.

Calcium Channel Blockers

Slow calcium channels are found in the myocardium (heart muscle) and smooth muscle cells. Free calcium increases muscle contractility, peripheral resistance, and blood pressure. Calcium channel blockers, also known as calcium antagonists and calcium blockers, decrease calcium levels and promote vasodilation. The large arteries are not as sensitive to calcium blockers as the coronary and cerebral arteries and the peripheral resistance vessels. Calcium blockers are highly protein-bound but have a short half-life. Slow-release preparations decrease the frequency of administering calcium blockers. Calcium blockers are also discussed in Chapter 37.

Verapamil (Calan) is used for treating chronic hypertension, angina pectoris, and cardiac dysrhythmias. Verapamil and diltiazem act on the arterioles and the heart. The dihydropyridines are the largest family group of calcium channel blockers and are composed of seven drugs; six drugs are used to control hypertension. The calcium blocker, nimodipine, is used to treat subarachnoid hemorrhage.

Nifedipine (Procardia) was the first drug in this group. Nifedipine decreases blood pressure in those with low serum renin values and in the elderly. Nifedipine and verapamil are potent calcium blockers. Normally, beta blockers are not prescribed with calcium blockers because both drugs decrease myocardium contractility. Calcium blockers lower blood pressure better in African-Americans than with other drug categories. Table 39–6 lists the calcium blockers.

SIDE EFFECTS AND ADVERSE REACTIONS
The side effects and adverse reactions of calcium blockers include flushing, headache, dizziness, ankle edema, bradycardia, and atrioventricular block.

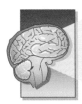

Critical Thinking in Action

G. G., a 72-year-old African-American, has congestive heart failure (CHF). She is a diabetic. Her vital signs are BP: 176/94; P: 92; R: 30. Her medications include hydrochlorothiazide 50 mg/d, atenolol 50 mg/d, and digoxin 0.25 mg/d.

1. Why was hydrochlorothiazide prescribed for G. G.? Explain the effects of hydrochlorothiazide on the blood pressure (refer to Chapter 38 if necessary).
2. Abnormal electrolytes and other laboratory test results may occur when taking hydrochlorothiazide. Indicate if the serum electrolyte and laboratory values are expected to *increase* or *decrease*.
    a. Sodium _____   d. Magnesium _____
    b. Potassium _____   e. Glucose _____
    c. Calcium _____   f. Uric acid _____
3. Why should G. G.'s blood glucose level be monitored when taking hydrochlorothiazide?
4. What effect may result when G. G. takes digoxin and hydrochlorothiazide? Explain.
5. Atenolol is what type of antihypertensive? Would atenolol be effective in lowering G. G.'s blood pressure if given as the only antihypertensive drug? Explain.
6. How effective is the combination of hydrochlorothiazide and atenolol for controlling G. G.'s blood pressure? Explain.
7. When using a combination drug therapy to correct hypertension, would the dosage for each drug be the same? Explain.
8. When abruptly discontinuing beta blockers for hypertension without the client taking another antihypertensive, what could occur? Explain how adverse effects can be avoided.

G. G.'s blood glucose is 229. Her drugs for controlling hypertension are changed to prazosin 10 mg, t.i.d. Her cholesterol and low-density lipoprotein are elevated. Her serum potassium level was low, 3.2 mEq/L.

9. Why were G. G.'s drugs, hydrochlorothiazide and atenolol, discontinued? Explain.
10. What type of antihypertensive is prazosin? What is the physiologic action of prazosin for lowering the blood pressure?
11. What effect does prazosin have on the blood glucose level? What effect could prazosin have on G. G.'s abnormal lipid levels? Explain.

G. G.'s ankles have become edematous. Hydrochlorothiazide was prescribed.

12. Why was hydrochlorothiazide added to the drug regimen? Give at least two reasons.
13. Is the prazosin daily dose within the safe therapeutic prescribed range? See prototype drug chart for prazosin (Chart 39–2). Explain.
14. What groups of antihypertensive drugs can cause sodium and water retention?

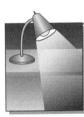

Study Questions

1. What nonpharmacologic methods can be practiced to decrease blood pressure?
2. What is the purpose of the stepped-care approach or modified pharmacologic approach in the treatment of hypertension? Explain the function of diuretics in controlling hypertension.
3. A major side effect of sympatholytic drugs and direct-acting vasodilators is sodium and water retention. How would you assess this problem? What drug is given with the antihypertensives to decrease this side effect? What electrolyte imbalances might occur with the use of the additional drug?
4. What are the similarities and differences between ACE inhibitors and A-II blockers?
5. What antihypertensive drug might be given for a hypertensive crisis? How would it be administered?
6. Describe the nursing process as it relates to administering beta-adrenergic blockers, alpha-adrenergic blockers, angiotensin antagonists, and calcium blockers.

40 Drugs for Circulatory Disorders

Outline

Objectives

- Describe the action of each of the four main drug groups: anticoagulants, thrombolytics, antilipemics, and peripheral vasodilators.
- Identify the side effects and adverse reactions of anticoagulants, thrombolytics, antilipemics, and peripheral vasodilators.
- Describe the nursing process, including client teaching, of anticoagulants, thrombolytics, antilipemics, and peripheral vasodilators.

Terms

aggregation

activated partial thromboplastin time (aPTT)

anticoagulants

antilipemics

chylomicrons

fibrinolysis

high-density lipoproteins (HDL)

hyperlipidemia

international normalized ratio (INR)

ischemia

lipoproteins

low-density lipoproteins (LDL)

myocardial infarction

necrosis

partial thromboplastin time (PTT)

peripheral vasodilators

prothrombin time (PT)

thromboembolism

thrombolytics

thrombosis

very low-density lipoproteins (VLDL)

INTRODUCTION

Various drugs are used to maintain, preserve, or restore circulation. The four major groups are (1) anticoagulants and antiplatelets (antithrombotics), (2) thrombolytics, (3) antilipemics, and (4) peripheral vasodilators. Anticoagulants prevent the formation of clots that inhibit circulation. The antiplatelets prevent platelet aggregation (clumping together of platelets to form a clot). The thrombolytics, popularly referred to as *clot busters*, attack and dissolve blood clots that have already formed.

Antilipemics, also called *hypolipemics* or *antihyperlipemics*, decrease blood lipid concentrations. The peripheral vasodilators promote dilation of vessels narrowed by vasospasm. Each of these four drug groups are discussed separately.

Thrombus Formation

A clot is a thrombus that has formed in an arterial or venous vessel. The formation of an arterial thrombus could be due to blood stasis (because of decreased circulation), platelet aggregation on the blood vessel wall, and blood coagulation. Arterial thrombus begins with platelet adhesion to the vessel wall. Adenosine diphosphate (ADP) is released from platelets, which in turn causes more platelet aggregation. As the thrombus inhibits blood flow, fibrin, platelets, and red blood cells (erythrocytes) surround the clot, building the clot's size and structure. As the clot occludes the blood vessel, tissue ischemia occurs.

The venous thrombus usually develops because of slow blood flow. The venous clot can occur rapidly. Small pieces of the venous clot can detach and travel to the pulmonary artery and then to the lung. Inadequate oxygenation and gas exchange in the lungs result.

Oral and parenteral anticoagulants (warfarin and heparin) primarily act by preventing venous thrombosis, whereas antiplatelet drugs act primarily by preventing arterial thrombosis. However, both groups of drugs suppress thrombosis.

ANTICOAGULANTS

Anticoagulants are used to inhibit clot formation. Unlike thrombolytics, they do *not* dissolve clots that have already formed but rather act prophylactically to prevent new clots. Anticoagulants are used in clients with venous and arterial vessel disorders that put them at high risk for clot formation. The venous problems include deep vein thrombosis and pulmonary embolism (ultimately an arterial problem), and the arterial problems include coronary thrombosis

(myocardial infarction), presence of artificial heart valves, and cerebrovascular accidents (CVA, or stroke). Antiplatelet drugs such as aspirin, dipyridamole (Persantine), and sulfinpyrazone (Anturane) are prescribed for the prevention of platelet aggregation.

Heparin

Anticoagulants are administered orally or parenterally (subcutaneously and intravenously). Heparin, introduced in 1938, is a natural substance in the liver that prevents clot formation. It was first used in blood transfusions to prevent clotting. Heparin is used in open heart surgery to prevent blood from clotting and in the critically ill client with disseminated intravascular coagulation (DIC). Its primary use is to prevent venous thrombosis that can lead to pulmonary embolism or stroke.

Heparin combines with antithrombin III, thus inactivating thrombin and other clotting factors. By inhibiting the action of thrombin, conversion of fibrinogen to fibrin does not occur and the formation of a fibrin clot is prevented (Fig. 40–1).

Heparin is poorly absorbed through the gastrointestinal (GI) mucosa, and much is destroyed by heparinase, a liver enzyme. Because heparin is poorly absorbed orally, it is given subcutaneously for prophylaxis or intravenously to treat acute thrombosis. It can be administered as an intravenous (IV) bolus or in IV fluid for continuous infusion. Heparin prolongs clotting time, and **partial thromboplastin time (PTT)** and **activated partial thromboplastin time (aPTT)** are monitored during therapy. Heparin can decrease the

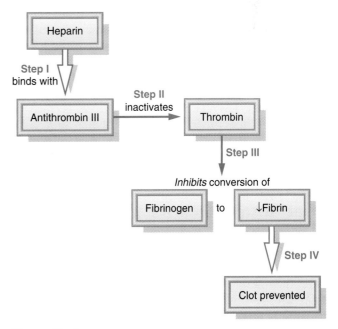

Figure 40–1
Action of the parenteral anticoagulant heparin.

platelet count, causing thrombocytopenia. If hemorrhage occurs, the anticoagulant antagonist protamine sulfate is given intravenously. Protamine can be an anticoagulant, but in the presence of heparin, it is an antagonist. Before discontinuing heparin, oral therapy with warfarin therapy is begun.

LOW MOLECULAR WEIGHT HEPARINS (LMWHs)

These derivatives of standard heparin were recently introduced for the prevention of venous thromboembolism. By extracting only the low molecular weight fractions of standard heparin through depolymerization; studies have shown the equivalent of anticoagulation with a lower risk of bleeding. LMWHs produce more stable responses at recommended doses. As a result, frequent laboratory monitoring is not required. LMW heparins bind to antithrombin III, which inhibits the synthesis of factor Xa and the formation of thrombin.

At present, there are two (LMWHs)—enoxaparin sodium (Lovenox) and dalteparin sodium (Fragmin). These agents have been approved for prevention of deep venous thrombosis (DVT) following hip and knee replacement surgery (enoxaparin) and abdominal surgery (dalteparin). They can be administered at home because aPTT monitoring is not necessary; heparin is given in the hospital. The LMWH is administered subcutaneously twice a day. The drugs are available in prefilled syringes with attached needles. The client or family member is taught how to administer the subcutaneous injection, which is usually given in the abdomen. The average treatment is for 7 to 14 days. The LMWH is usually started in the hospital within 24 hours following surgery.

The half-life of LMWH is two to four times longer than that of heparin. Clients should be instructed not to take antiplatelet drugs such as aspirin while taking LMWHs or heparin.

Bleeding as result of LMWH is less likely to occur than when heparin is given. Heparin has a shorter half-life than LMWH. LMWH overdose is rare; if bleeding occurs, protamine sulfate is the anticoagulant antagonist used. The dosage for protamine sulfate is 1 mg of protamine for every 1 mg of LMWH given.

Oral Anticoagulants

The coumarin group of oral anticoagulants consists of warfarin (Coumadin) and dicumarol. Warfarin is the most widely used coumarin. Warfarin is synthesized from dicumarol. Before warfarin was available for human use, it was used in rodenticides to kill rats by causing hemorrhage.

Oral anticoagulants inhibit hepatic synthesis of vitamin K, thus affecting the clotting factors II, VII, IX, and X. These drugs are used mainly to prevent thromboembolic conditions, such as thrombophlebitis, pulmonary embolism, and embolism formation caused by atrial fibrillation. Oral anticoagulants prolong clotting time and are monitored by the **prothrombin time (PT)**. This laboratory test is usually performed before administering the next drug dose until the therapeutic level has been reached. **International normalized ratio (INR)** is a new laboratory test, introduced to account for the variability in reported PTs from different laboratories. Reagents used in the PT test are compared to an international reference standard and reported as the INR. The normal INR is 1.3 to 2.0. Clients on warfarin therapy are maintained at an INR of 2.0 to 3.0.

Monitoring at regular intervals is required for the duration of drug therapy. The coumarins have long half-lives and very long durations of action (dicumarol has a longer action than warfarin); therefore, drug accumulation can occur, which may cause internal bleeding. The nurse must observe for petechiae, ecchymosis, tarry stools, and hematemesis.

Parenteral and oral anticoagulants (heparin and warfarin) are presented in Chart 40–1.

PHARMACOKINETICS

Heparin is poorly absorbed through the GI mucosa, and much is destroyed by heparinase, a liver enzyme. Heparin is given parenterally, either subcutaneously for prophylactic anticoagulant therapy or intravenously (bolus or continuous infusion) for an immediate response. Warfarin, an oral anticoagulant, is well absorbed through the GI mucosa; however, food will delay but not inhibit absorption.

The half-life of heparin is dose-related; high doses prolong the half-life. The half-life of warfarin is 0.5 to 3 days, in contrast to 1 to 2 h for heparin. Because warfarin has a long half-life and is highly protein-bound, the drug can have cumulative effects. Bleeding can occur, especially if another highly protein-bound drug is administered with warfarin. Kidney and liver disease prolong the half-life of both heparin and warfarin. Warfarin is metabolized to inactive metabolites that are excreted by the kidneys and in bile.

PHARMACODYNAMICS

Heparin, administered for acute thromboembolic disorders, prevents thrombus formation and embolism. It has been effectively used in disseminated intravascular coagulation (DIC), which causes multiple thrombi in small blood vessels. Warfarin is effective for long-term anticoagulant therapy. The PT level should be 1.5 to 2 times the reference value to be therapeutic, or INR should be 2.0 to 3.0. INR has effectively replaced the use of PT, because PT can vary from laboratory to laboratory, plus reagent to reagent. Higher INR levels are usually required for

Chart 40–1.   Anticoagulants

ANTICOAGULANTS

Drug Name

Heparin (H)
   (Lipo-Hepin, Calciparine), 🍁 Hepalean,
   Calcilean
Pregnancy Category: C

Warfarin sodium (W)
   (Coumadin), 🍁 Warfilone
Pregnancy Category: D

Dosage

H:
A: SC: 5000–7500 units, q6h or 8000–10,000
units q8h IV: Bolus: 5000 units; inf: 20,000–
40,000 units over 24 h
C: IV: 50 units/kg bolus; 50–100 units/kg q4h
or 20,000 units m²/24 h
W:
A: PO: LD: 10 mg/d for 2–3 d; maint: 2–10
mg/d
Elderly: PO: 2.5 mg/d IV: Dose is usually titrated according to INR

Contraindications

H and W:
Bleeding disorder, peptic ulcer, severe hepatic
or renal disease, hemophilia, CVA
W:
Blood dyscrasias, eclampsia

Drug-Lab-Food Interactions

H:
Drug: Increase effect with aspirin, NSAIDs,
thrombolytics, probenecid; decrease effect with
nitroglycerin, protamine

W:
Drug: Increase effect with amiodarone, aspirin,
NSAIDs, sulfonamides, thyroid drugs, allopurinol, histamine₂ blockers, oral hypoglycemics,
metronidazole, miconazole, methyldopa, diuretics, oral antibiotics, vitamin E; decrease effect
with barbiturates, laxatives, phenytoin, estrogens, vitamins C and K, oral contraceptives,
rifampin
Lab: May increase AST, ALT
Food: Decrease diet rich in vitamin K

Pharmacokinetics

Absorption: (H): SC or IV; (W): PO: well ab-
sorbed
Distribution: PB: (H): >80%; (W): 99%
Metabolism: t½: (H): 1–2 h; (W): 0.5–3 d
Excretion: (H): slowly in urine and reticuloen-
dothelial system; (W): in urine and bile

Pharmacodynamics

(H):
SC: Onset: 20–60 min
     Peak: 2 h
     Duration: 8–12 h
IV: Onset: immediate
     Peak: 5–10 min
     Duration: 2–6 h
(W):
PO: Onset: >2 d
     Peak: 1–3 d
     Duration: 2.5–5 d

Therapeutic Effects/Uses

(H and W): To prevent blood clotting.

Mode of Action: (H): Inhibits thrombin, which prevents the conversion of fibrinogen to fibrin.
(W): Depression of hepatic synthesis of vitamin K clotting factors (II [prothrombin], VII, IX, and X).

Side Effects

(H): Itching, burning
(W): Anorexia, nausea, vomiting, diarrhea, abdominal cramps, rash, fever

Adverse Reactions

(H and W): Bleeding, ecchymoses
(W): stomatitis
Life threatening: (H and W): hemorrhage

Assessment and Planning · **Interventions** · **Evaluation** · **NURSING PROCESS**

KEY: A: adult; C: child; PO: by mouth; SC: subcutaneous; IV: intravenous; PB: protein-binding; NSAIDs: nonsteroidal antiinflammatory drugs; t½: half-life; INR: international normalized ratio; >: greater than; 🍁: Canadian drug names; ALT: alanine aminotransferase; AST: aspartate aminotransferase.

Table 40-1
Comparison of Oral and Parenteral Anticoagulants

FACTORS TO CONSIDER	HEPARIN	WARFARIN (COUMADIN)
Methods of administration	Subcutaneously Intravenously	Primarily orally
Drug action	Binds with antithrombin III, which inactivates thrombin and clotting factors, thus inhibiting fibrin formation	Inhibits hepatic synthesis of vitamin K, which decreases prothrombin and the clotting factors VII, IX, X
Uses	Treatment of venous thrombosis, pulmonary embolism, thromboembolic complications; e.g., heart surgery, disseminated intravascular coagulation (DIC)	Treatment of deep venous thrombosis, pulmonary embolism, transient ischemic attack (TIA), prophylactic for cardiac valves
Contraindication/caution	Hemophilia, peptic ulcer, severe (stage 3 or 4) hypertension, severe liver or renal disease, dissecting aneurysm	Hemophilia, peptic bleeding ulcer, blood dyscrasias, severe liver or kidney disease, acute myocardial infarction (AMI), alcoholism
Laboratory tests	PTT (partial thromboplastin time): 60–70 sec Anticoagulant: 1.5–2 × control in seconds aPTT (activated partial thromboplastin time): 40 sec Anticoagulant: PTT: 60–80 sec	PT (prothrombin time): 11–15 sec Anticoagulant: 1.25–2.5 × control in seconds INR (international normalized ratio): 1.3–2.0 Anticoagulant: INR 2.0–3.0
Side/adverse effects	Bleeding, hemorrhage, hematoma, severe hypotension	Bleeding, hemorrhage, gastrointestinal (GI) bleeding, ecchymoses, hematuria
Antidote	Protamine sulfate, 1 mg per 100 units of heparin; see Table 40–2	Vitamin K_1 PO/SC//IM/IV: 2.5–10 mg, C: SC/IM: 5–10 mg Infant: 1 mg Vitamin K_4: A: PO/IM/IV: 5–15 mg/d; see Table 40–2

KEY: A: adult; C: child; IV: intravenous; IM: intramuscular; SC: subcutaneous.

clients with prosthetic heart valves, cardiac valvular disease, and recurrent emboli. Heparin does not cross the placental barrier, unlike warfarin; therefore, warfarin use is not suggested during pregnancy.

Intravenous heparin has a rapid onset, its peak time of action is reached in minutes, and its duration of action is short. After an IV heparin dose, the client's clotting time will return to normal in 2 to 6 h. Subcutaneous heparin is more slowly absorbed through the blood vessels in fatty tissue. The coumarins (warfarin and dicumarol) have long onset of action, peak concentration, and duration of action times; thus, drug accumulation may occur. Dicumarol has a longer action time than warfarin. Vitamin K counteracts the effect of warfarin, but it can take up to 24 h for it to be effective.

Table 40–1 gives the comparison summary between oral and parenteral anticoagulants, according to methods of administration, drug action, uses, contraindications, laboratory tests, side/adverse effects, and antidotes.

SIDE EFFECTS AND ADVERSE REACTIONS

Bleeding (hemorrhaging) is the major adverse effect of warfarin. Clients should be monitored closely for signs of bleeding, that is, petechiae, ecchymosis, hematemesis. PT or INR testing should be scheduled at recommended intervals.

DRUG INTERACTIONS

Because warfarin and dicumarol are highly protein-bound, they are affected by drug interactions. Aspirin, nonsteroidal antiinflammatory drugs (NSAIDs), antiinflammatory drugs, sulfonamides, phenytoin, cimetidine (Tagamet), allopurinol, and oral hypoglycemic drugs for diabetes can displace warfarin or dicumarol from the protein-bound site, causing more free circulating anticoagulant. Numerous drugs increase the action of warfarin, and bleeding is apt to occur. Acetaminophen (Tylenol) should be used instead of aspirin for clients taking warfarin or dicumarol. For frank bleeding resulting from excess free drug, parenteral vitamin K is given as a coagulant to decrease

Table 40–2
Anticoagulants, Antiplatelets, and Anticoagulant Antagonists

GENERIC (BRAND)	ROUTE AND DOSAGE	USES AND CONSIDERATIONS
ANTICOAGULANT: LMWHS		
Dalteparin sodium (Fragmin)	A: SC: 2500 IU/d for 5–10 d starting 1–2 h before surgery	For prevention of DVT prior to surgery and for those who are at risk of thromboembolism. Similar to enoxaparin. *Pregnancy category:* B; PB: UK; $t_{\frac{1}{2}}$: UK
Enoxaparin sodium (Lovenox)	A: SC: 30 mg b.i.d.	For thromboembolism. Prevents and treats DVT and pulmonary embolism. Bleeding is an adverse reaction. Monitor CBC. *Pregnancy category:* B; PB: UK; $t_{\frac{1}{2}}$: 4.5 h
HEPARINS		
Heparin sodium (Lipo-Hepin)	A: SC: 5000–7500 units q6h or 8000–10,000 units q8h A: IV: Bolus: 5000 units Inf: 20,000–40,000 units over 24 h; dose varies according to aPTT level C: IV: units/kg bolus, 50–100 units/kg q4h or 20,000 units/m²/24 h	For thromboembolism as a prophylaxis against clotting. Is not given IM because of pain and hematoma. Drugs that inactivate heparin: digitalis, tetracycline, IV penicillin, phenothiazine, and quinidine, aPTT should be monitored. Protamine sulfate is the antidote for bleeding control. Dose is 1–1.5 mg for every 100 units of heparin SC. *Pregnancy category:* C, PB: 95%; $t_{\frac{1}{2}}$: 1–1.5 h
ANTICOAGULANTS: COUMARINS		
Dicumarol (Bishydroxycoumarin)	A: PO: LD: 200–300 mg/24 h; maint: 25–200 mg/d based on PT	For thromboembolism as long-term prophylaxis. Has a longer duration than warfarin. INR should be monitored. Oral absorption may be erratic. *Pregnancy category:* D; PB: 99%; $t_{\frac{1}{2}}$: 1–2 d
Warfarin (Coumadin)	See Chart 40–1	Used in thromboembolism for long-term prophylaxis after heparin is discontinued. Monitor PT or INR. PT should be 1.25–2.5 times the control. INR should be 2.0–3.0. Drug has many drug interactions; see text. Has a long half-life. Check for bleeding. *Pregnancy category:* D; PB: 99%; $t_{\frac{1}{2}}$: 0.5–3 d
ANTIPLATELETS		
Aspirin	A: PO: 325 mg/d or q.o.d.	For prevention of thrombosis prior to or after CVA or MI. Client should check with health care provider before taking aspirin for antiplatelet therapy. Aspirin should be avoided with peptic ulcer or liver dysfunction. Enteric-coated preparation decreases GI upset. *Pregnancy category:* D; PB: 55%; $t_{\frac{1}{2}}$: 10–12 h
Dipyridamole (Persantine)	A: PO: 50–100 mg t.i.d.–q.i.d.	For prevention of thromboembolism post-MI and associated with prosthetic devices (heart valves and hip replacement); prevention of TIA. Monitor blood pressure. *Pregnancy category:* C; PB: >91%; $t_{\frac{1}{2}}$: 10–12 h
Sulfinpyrazone (Anturane)	A: PO: 200–400 mg b.i.d.; *max:* 800 mg/d	Used for treating gout. Has antiplatelet function. May be used in AV shunts for hemodialysis to prevent clotting. *Pregnancy category:* C; PB: 95%–99%; $t_{\frac{1}{2}}$: 3 h
Ticlopidine (Ticlid)	A: PO: 250 mg b.i.d.	To prevent the risk of strokes and thrombin formation. To treat intermittent claudication and sickle cell disease. Avoid if client has a hematopoietic disorder such as thrombocytopenia or bleeding peptic ulcer. *Pregnancy category:* B; PB: UK; $t_{\frac{1}{2}}$: 8–12 h

Table continued on following page

Table 40–2 *Continued*
Anticoagulants, Antiplatelets, and Anticoagulant Antagonists

GENERIC (BRAND)	ROUTE AND DOSAGE	USES AND CONSIDERATIONS
ANTIPLATELETS FOR ANGIOPLASTY AND ACUTE CORONARY SYNDROMES		
Abciximab (ReoPro)	A: IV bolus: 0.25 mg/kg given 10–60 min before PTCA. Inject 4.5 mL abciximab into 250 mL of NSS or D_5W. Follow with a continuous infusion of 10 μg/min (17 mL/h) for 12 h	To prevent acute cardiac ischemic prior to and following PTCA and for unstable angina. *Pregnancy category:* C; PB: UK; $t\frac{1}{2}$: 30 min
Eptifibatide (Integrilin)	A: IV bolus: 180 μg/kg, then 2 μg/kg/min for up to 72 h	For acute cardiac syndromes (unstable angina and non–Q-wave MI). Can be used with angioplasty. *Pregnancy category:* UK; PB: UK; $t\frac{1}{2}$: UK
Tirofiban (Aggrastat)	A: IV: 0.4 μg/kg/min for 30 min, then 0.1 μg/kg/min for 48–108 h	New agent. For acute cardiac syndromes (unstable angina and non–Q-wave MI). Also may be used with angioplasty. *Pregnancy category:* UK; PB: UK; $t\frac{1}{2}$: UK
ANTICOAGULANT ANTAGONISTS		
Protamine SO_4	A: IV: Initially: 1 mg/100 units heparin administered; 10–50 mg in 3–10 min slow push; *max:* 50 mg in any 10-min period	Used to stop bleeding during heparin therapy. Binds and neutralizes heparin. *Pregnancy category:* C; PB: UK; $t\frac{1}{2}$: UK
Vitamin K_1, phytonadione (AquaMEPHYTON, Mephyton, Konakion)	A: PO/IM/IV: 2–10 mg q12–24 h as needed C: SC/IM: 5–10 mg	For control of bleeding due to warfarin or dicumarol. If frank bleeding occurs, fresh or frozen plasma or plasmanate may be needed. Depending on form and route, vitamin K takes effect in 1–24 h. Hemorrhage is usually controlled in 3–6 h. *Pregnancy category:* C; PB: UK; $t\frac{1}{2}$: UK
Vitamin K_4, menadiol sodium diphosphate	A: PO/SC/IM/IV: 5–10 mg/d C: PO: 50–100 μg/d	For control of bleeding caused by warfarin or dicumarol. Not effective to control bleeding caused by heparin. *Pregnancy category:* C; PB: UK; $t\frac{1}{2}$: UK

KEY: *A: adult; C: child; PO: oral; IM: intramuscular; IV: intravenous; SC: subcutaneous; I: initially; PT: prothrombin time; aPTT: activated partial thromboplastin time; CVA: cerebrovascular accident; MI: myocardial infarction; AV: arteriovenous; UK: unknown; PB: protein-binding; $t\frac{1}{2}$: half-life; TIA: transient ischemic attack; DVT: deep vein thrombosis; LMWHs: low molecular weight heparins; INR: international normalized ratio; LD: loading dose; PTCA: percutaneous transluminal coronary angioplasty; NSS: normal saline solution.*

bleeding and promote clotting. However, caution must be used with this approach because the prothrombin can remain depressed for prolonged periods.

Table 40–2 lists the drug data for the anticoagulants, the antiplatelets, and the anticoagulant antagonists.

ORAL ANTICOAGULANT ANTAGONISTS

Vitamin K_1 (phytonadione), antagonist of warfarin, is used for warfarin overdose or uncontrollable bleeding. Usually 1 to 10 mg of vitamin K_1 is given at once if bleeding occurs. Bleeding occurs in about 10% of clients taking oral anticoagulants. If vitamin K_1 fails to control bleeding, fresh whole blood or fresh-frozen platelets are then generally given.

Antiplatelet Drugs

Antiplatelet drugs are used to prevent thrombosis in the arteries by suppressing platelet aggregation. Heparin and warfarin prevent thrombosis in the veins.

Antiplatelet drug therapy is mainly for prophylactic use such as: (1) prevention of myocardial infarction or stroke for clients with familial history, (2) prevention of a repeat myocardial infarction, and (3) prevention of a stroke for clients having transient ischemic attacks (TIAs). Recommended dose for clients with familial history of stroke and/or myocardial infarction is 81 to 325 mg per day. Aspirin should be discontinued 7 days before surgery.

Other oral antiplatelet drugs include dipyridamole

ANTICOAGULANTS: WARFARIN (COUMADIN) AND HEPARIN

Assessment

- Obtain a history of abnormal clotting or health problems that affect clotting, such as severe alcoholism or severe liver or renal disease. Warfarin is contraindicated for clients with blood dyscrasias, peptic ulcer, cerebral vascular accident (CVA), hemophilia, or severe hypertension. Caution its use in a client with acute traumatic injury.
- Obtain a drug history of current drugs the client is taking. Report if a drug-drug interaction is probable. Warfarin is highly protein-bound and can displace other highly protein-bound drugs, or warfarin could be displaced, which may result in bleeding.
- Develop a flow chart that lists PT or INR and warfarin dosages. A baseline PT or INR should be obtained before warfarin is administered.

Potential Nursing Diagnoses

- Risk for injury (bleeding)
- Knowledge deficit

Planning

- Client's PT will be 1.25 to 2.5 times the control level or INR will be 2.0 to 3.0. For a client receiving heparin, the aPTT should be checked.
- Abnormal bleeding will be rapidly addressed while the client is taking an anticoagulant. The PT, INR, PTT, or aPTT level(s) will be closely monitored.

Nursing Interventions

- Monitor vital signs (VS). An increased pulse rate followed by a decreased systolic pressure can indicate a fluid volume deficit resulting from external or internal bleeding.
- Check PT or INR for warfarin (Coumadin) and aPTT for heparin before administering the anticoagulant. The PT should be 1.25 to 2.5 times the control level or INR 2.0 to 3.0. The platelet count should be monitored, because anticoagulants can decrease platelet count.
- Check for bleeding from the mouth, nose (epistaxis), urine (hematuria), and skin (petechiae, purpura).
- Check stools periodically for occult blood.
- In elderly clients, monitor closely for bleeding. Their skin is thin and capillary beds are fragile.
- Keep anticoagulant antagonists (protamine for heparin and vitamin K for warfarin) available when drug dose is increased or there are indications of frank bleeding. Fresh or frozen plasma may be needed for transfusion.

Client Teaching

General
- Instruct the client to inform the dentist when taking an anticoagulant. Contacting the health care provider may be necessary.
- Instruct the client to use a soft toothbrush to avoid causing the gums to bleed.
- Instruct the client to shave with an electric razor. Bleeding from shaving cuts may be difficult to control.
- Advise the client to have laboratory tests such as PT performed as ordered by the health care provider. Warfarin dose is regulated according to the INR derived from the PT.
- Instruct the client to carry or wear a medical identification card or jewelry (Medic-Alert) listing the person's name, telephone number, and drug name.
- Encourage the client *not* to smoke. Smoking increases drug metabolism; thus, the warfarin dose may need to be increased. If the person insists on smoking, notify the health care provider.
- Instruct the client to check with the health care provider before taking over-the-counter (OTC) drugs. Aspirin should *not* be taken with warfarin because aspirin intensifies its action and bleeding is apt to occur. Suggest that the client use acetaminophen.

Nursing Process continued on following page

NURSING PROCESS *Continued*
ANTICOAGULANTS: WARFARIN (COUMADIN) AND HEPARIN

- Teach the client to control external hemorrhage (bleeding) from accidents or injuries by applying firm, direct pressure for at least 5 to 10 min with a clean, dry absorbent material.

Diet
- Advise the client to avoid alcohol, which could contribute to increased bleeding, and large amounts of green leafy vegetables, fish, liver, coffee, or tea (caffeine), which are rich in vitamin K.

Side Effects
- Advise the client to report bleeding, such as petechiae, ecchymosis, purpura, tarry stools, bleeding gums, epistaxis, or expectoration of blood.

Cultural Considerations

- Certain cultural groups may lack understanding related to health problems, drug therapy, adverse effects, and follow-up care concerning thrombophlebitis or other conditions that cause a thrombus formation.
- Respect the cultural beliefs of a client regarding his or her method for treating a vascular problem. If the method may be harmful, explanations along with nursing plan should be initiated.

Evaluation

- Evaluate the effectiveness of drug therapy. Client's PT or INR values are within the desired range, and client is free of significant side effects.

(Persantine), ticlopidine (Ticlid), abciximab (ReoPro), eptifibatide (Integrilin), and tirofiban (Aggrastat). Dipyridamiole and ticlopidine have similar effects as aspirin and are more expensive than aspirin. Abciximab, eptifibatide, and tirofiban (the latter two drugs are the newest antiplatelet agents) are primarily used for acute coronary syndromes (unstable angina or non–Q-wave myocardial infarction) and for preventing reocclusion of coronary arteries following percutaneous transluminal coronary angioplasty (PTCA). These drugs are usually given before and after PTCA. The drug of choice for angioplasty is abciximab. These three agents block the binding of fibrinogen to the glycoprotein IIb/IIIa receptor on the platelet surface. They are referred to as platelet glycoprotein (GP) IIb/IIIa receptor antagonists. Following IV infusion, the antiplatelet effects for abciximab perisist for 24 to 48 hours, and for eptifibatide and tirofiban, the antiplatelet effects last for 4 hours.

THROMBOLYTICS

Thromboembolism (occlusion of an artery or vein caused by a thrombus or embolus) results in ischemia (deficient blood flow) that causes **necrosis** (death) of the tissue distal to the obstructed area. It takes ap-

proximately 1 to 2 weeks for the blood clot to disintegrate by natural fibrinolytic mechanisms. If a new thrombus or embolus could be dissolved more quickly, the necrosis would be minimized and blood flow would be reestablished faster. This is the basis for thrombolytic therapy.

Thrombolytics have been used since the early 1980s to promote the fibrinolytic mechanism (converting plasminogen to plasmin, which destroys the fibrin in the blood clot). The thrombus, or blood clot, disintegrates when a thrombolytic drug is administered within 4 h following an **acute myocardial infarction** (AMI); necrosis resulting from the blocked artery is prevented or minimized and hospitalization time may be decreased. The need for cardiac bypass or coronary angioplasty can be evaluated soon after thrombolytic treatment. These drugs are also used for pulmonary embolism, deep vein thrombosis, and noncoronary arterial occlusion from an acute thromboembolism.

Five commonly used thrombolytics are streptokinase, urokinase, tissue plasminogen activator (t-PA, alteplase), anisoylated plasminogen streptokinase activator complex (APSAC, anistreplase), and reteplase (Retavase). Streptokinase and urokinase are enzymes that act systemically and promote the conversion of plasminogen to plasmin. t-PA and APSAC activate plasminogen by acting specifically on the clot. They

Chart 40–2. Thrombolytics

THROMBOLYTIC ENZYME

Drug Name

Streptokinase
  (Streptase, Kabikinase)
Pregnancy Category: C

Dosage

Myocardial Infarction:
A: IV: 1,500,000 IU diluted in 45 mL; infuse over 60 min
Pulmonary Embolism (PE) and Deep Vein Thrombosis (DVT):
A: IV: LD: 250,000 IU Inf: 100,000 IU/h for 24–72 h (24 h for PE; 72 h for DVT)

Contraindications

Recent CVA, cerebral neoplasm, active bleeding, severe hypertension, ulcerative colitis, anticoagulant therapy

Drug-Lab-Food Interactions

Drug: *Increase* risk of bleeding with heparin, oral anticoagulants, aspirin, antiplatelets, NSAIDs

Pharmacokinetics

Absorption: IV: Directly administered
Distribution: PB: UK
Metabolism: t½: 20–80 min
Excretion: In urine and bile

Pharmacodynamics

IV: Onset: Immediate
  Peak: Rapid
  Duration: 4–12 h

Therapeutic Effects/Uses

To dissolve blood clots due to coronary artery thrombi, deep vein thrombosis, pulmonary embolism.

Mode of Action: Conversion of plasminogen to plasmin (fibrinolysin) for dissolving fibrin deposits.

Side Effects

Headache, nausea, flushing, rash, fever

Adverse Reactions

Bleeding, urticaria, unstable blood pressure
Life-threatening: Hemorrhage, bronchospasm, cardiac dysrhythmias, anaphylaxis

KEY: A: adult; C: child; IV: intravenous; LD: loading dose; Inf: infusion; NSAIDs: nonsteroidal antiinflammatory drugs; UK: unknown; PB: protein-binding; t½: half-life.

also promote the conversion of plasminogen to plasmin. Plasmin, an enzyme, digests the fibrin in the clot. Plasmin also degrades fibrinogen, prothrombin, and other clotting factors. These five drugs induce fibrinolysis (fibrin breakdown). Chart 40–2 gives the pharmacologic data for streptokinase.

Streptokinase may cause hypotension when first administered. Drug dosage may need to be adjusted. Reteplase (Retavase), a derivative t-PA, is the newest thrombolytic drug. Anticoagulants and antiplatelet drugs increase the risk of hemorrhage; these types of drugs should be avoided until the thrombolytic effect has passed. The health care provider needs to determine whether the client has taken any of these drugs before seeking treatment.

Pharmacokinetics

Streptokinase has a short half-life (20 min), but can persist up to 82 min. It is administered intravenously and absorbed immediately.

Pharmacodynamics

Streptokinase stimulates the fibrinolytic mechanism to dissolve blood clots. Streptokinase is derived from bacterial species so that antibody formation can occur. In rare cases, anaphylaxis has been reported. Initially, a large loading dose is needed to prevent antibody resistance and to induce lysis. The onset of action and peak time are immediate and rapid. Duration of

Table 40-3
Thrombolytics

GENERIC (BRAND)	ROUTE AND DOSAGE	USES AND CONSIDERATIONS
THROMBOLYTICS		
Anistreplase (APSAC, Eminase)	A: IV: 30 units over 2–5 min	Treatment following an AMI, causing lysis of the thrombi. Decreases the infarction size. *Pregnancy category:* C; PB: UK; $t\frac{1}{2}$: 1.5–2 h
Reteplase (Retavase)	A: IV bolus: 10 units over 2 min, then repeat 10 units in 30 min (total of 20 units)	To treat coronary thrombosis by causing lysis of the thrombi; inhibits the fibrin aspect of the thrombus. A derivative of t-PA (Alteplase). Considered more effective than t-PA with less risk of hemorrhage. *Pregnancy category:* C; PB: UK; $t\frac{1}{2}$: 13–16 min
Streptokinase (Streptase, Kabikinase)	See Chart 40-2	For DVT, PE, coronary thrombosis, AV cannula occlusion. Least expensive of the three drugs. May be associated with anaphylactic reactions. Anistreplase and streptokinase should not be administered for more than 5 days or within 6 months of last dose because of possible formation of antistreptokinase antibodies, which decrease effectiveness and increase the likelihood of allergic reaction. If thrombin time is not significantly different from the normal after 4 h, discontinue because of streptokinase resistance. *Pregnancy category:* C; PB: UK; $t\frac{1}{2}$: 20–80 min
Tissue-type plasminogen activator (t-PA, alteplase, Activase)	*AMI* A: IV: Total: 100 mg over 1.5 h Bolus: 15 mg (over 2 min); then 0.75 mg/kg (not to exceed 50 mg) over 30 min; then 0.5 mg/kg (not to exceed 35 mg) over 60 min	For coronary thrombosis. A clot-specific drug. Very expensive drug. Not associated with anaphylactic reactions. Also used for pulmonary thromboembolism. Adverse reactions include internal and superficial bleeding. *Pregnancy category:* C; PB: UK; $t\frac{1}{2}$: 30 min
Urokinase (Abbokinase)	A: IV: LD: 4400 IU/kg diluted over 10 min Inf: 4400 IU/kg over 12–24 h *Occluded coronary artery:* Dose may be increased	Same uses as streptokinase. Causes less allergic reaction and is more expensive than streptokinase. Not susceptible to antistreptokinase antibodies. May also be used for peripheral artery occlusion. *Pregnancy category:* B; PB: UK; $t\frac{1}{2}$: 10–20 min
PLASMINOGEN INACTIVATOR		
Aminocaproic acid (Amicar)	A: PO/IV: LD: 5 g first hour Inf: 1–1.25 g/h for 8 h; *max:* 30 g/d	Treatment for excessive bleeding that may result from heart surgery, severe trauma, abruptio placentae, and thrombolytic drugs such as streptokinase, t-PA, urokinase. Side effects include dizziness, headache, orthostatic, hypotension, thrombophlebitis. *Pregnancy category:* C; PB: 0%; $t\frac{1}{2}$: 1–2 h

KEY: A: adult; IV: intravenous; LD: loading dose; DVT: deep vein thrombosis; AMI: acute myocardial infarction; PE: pulmonary embolism; AV: arteriovenous; IU: international units; UK: unknown; PB: protein-binding; $t\frac{1}{2}$: half-life.

action can be extended to 12 h. After drug therapy is discontinued, the risk of bleeding can persist for 24 h.

The most expensive thrombolytic is t-PA, which costs approximately $2500 per treatment. It changes the plasminogen to plasmin in breaking down and destroying the fibrin in the clot. It has the advantage of a short half-life (5 to 7 min) and is not associated with anaphylactic reactions.

Side Effects and Adverse Reactions

Allergic reactions can complicate thrombolytic therapy. Anaphylaxis (vascular collapse) occurs more frequently with streptokinase than with the other thrombolytics. If the drugs are administered through an intracoronary catheter after myocardial infarction, reperfusion dysrhythmia or hemorrhagic infarction at

NURSING PROCESS
THROMBOLYTICS

Assessment

- Assess baseline vital signs (VS) and compare with future values.
- Check baseline CBC, PT, or INR values before administration of streptokinase.
- Obtain a medical and drug history. Contraindications for use of streptokinase include a recent CVA, active bleeding, severe hypertension, and anticoagulant therapy. It should be reported if the client is taking aspirin or NSAIDs. Thrombolytics are contraindicated for the client with a recent history of traumatic injury, especially head injury.

Potential Nursing Diagnoses

- Decreased cardiac output
- Anxiety related to severe health problem
- Impaired tissue integrity
- Risk for injury

Planning

- The blood clot will be dissolved, and the client will be closely monitored for active bleeding.
- Client's VS will be monitored for stability during and after thrombolytic therapy.
- Thrombolytic drug should be administered 4 to 6 h after MI.

Nursing Interventions

- Monitor VS. Increased pulse rate followed by decreased blood pressure usually indicates blood loss and impending shock. Record VS and report changes.
- Observe for signs and symptoms of active bleeding from the mouth or rectum. Hemorrhage is a serious complication of thrombolytic treatment. Aminocaproic acid can be given as an intervention to stop the bleeding.
- Check for active bleeding for 24 h after thrombolytic therapy has been discontinued: q15min for the first hour, q30min until the eighth hour, and then hourly.
- Observe for signs of allergic reaction to streptokinase, such as itching, hives, flushing, fever, dyspnea, bronchospasm, hypotension, and/or cardiovascular collapse.
- Avoid administering aspirin or NSAIDs for pain or discomfort when the client is receiving a thrombolytic.
- Monitor the electrocardiogram (ECG) for the presence of reperfusion dysrhythmias as the blood clot is dissolving; antidysrhythmic therapy may be indicated.
- Avoid venipuncture/arterial sticks.

Client Teaching

General
- Explain the thrombolytic treatment to the client and family. Be supportive.

Side Effects
- Instruct the client to report any side effects, such as lightheadedness, dizziness, palpitations, nausea, pruritus, or urticaria.

Evaluation

- Determine the effectiveness of drug therapy. The client's clot has dissolved; VS are stable; there are no signs and symptoms of active bleeding; and the client is pain free.

the myocardial necrotic area can result. The major complication of thrombolytic drugs is hemorrhage. The antithrombolytic drug aminocaproic acid (Amicar) is used to stop bleeding by inhibiting plasminogen activation, which inhibits thrombolysis.

Table 40–3 lists the drug data for the thrombolytic drugs.

Table 40-4
Lipoprotein Groups

| LIPOPROTEIN SUBGROUPS | Protein (%) | COMPOSITION OF THE LIPOPROTEINS | | |
		Cholesterol (%)	Triglycerides (%)	Phospholipids (%)
Chylomicrons	1–2	1–3	80–95	3–6
Very low density (VLDL)	6–10	8–20	45–65	15–20
Low density (LDL)	18–22	45–50	4–8	18–24
High density (HDL)	45–55	15–20	2–7	26–32

Adapted from Henry: Clinical Diagnosis and Management by Laboratory Methods, *18/E. Philadelphia, WB Saunders, p. 189, 1991.*

ANTILIPEMICS

Antilipemics lower abnormal blood lipid levels. Lipids composed of cholesterol, triglycerides, and phospholipids are transported in the body bound to protein in various amounts. These lipoproteins are classified as **chylomicrons, very low-density lipoproteins (VLDL), low-density lipoproteins (LDL),** and **high-density lipoproteins (HDL).** The HDL (friendly or "good" lipoproteins) have a higher percentage of protein and less lipids. Their function is to remove cholesterol from the bloodstream and deliver it to the liver. The other three lipoproteins are composed mainly of cholesterol and triglycerides and contribute to atherosclerotic plaque in the blood vessels; they are "bad" lipoproteins. Table 40–4 presents the composition of the lipoproteins.

Serum cholesterol and triglyceride measurements are frequently part of a regular physical examination or readmission evaluation and are used as baseline test results. If the levels are high, a 14-hour fasting lipid profile may be ordered. When cholesterol, tri-

glycerides, and LDL are elevated, the client is at increased risk for coronary artery disease. Table 40–5 lists the various serum lipids and their reference values (normal serum levels) according to a risk classification.

Nonpharmacologic Methods for Cholesterol Reduction

Before antilipemics are prescribed, nondrug therapy should be initiated for decreasing blood pressure. The saturated fats and cholesterol in the diet should be reduced. Total fat intake should be 30% or less of caloric intake and cholesterol intake should be 300 mg or less. The client needs to read labels on containers and buy appropriate foods. Clients should choose lean meats, especially chicken and fish.

In many cases, diet alone will not lower blood lipid levels. Because 75% to 85% of serum cholesterol is endogenously (internally) derived, dietary modification alone will typically lower total cholesterol levels by only 10% to 30%. This, and the fact that adher-

Table 40-5
Serum Lipid Values

| LIPIDS | NORMAL VALUE (mg/dL) | Low Risk (mg/dL) | LEVEL OF RISK FOR CAD | |
			Moderate Risk (mg/dL)	High Risk (mg/dL)
Cholesterol	150–240	<200	200–240	>240
Triglycerides	40–190	Values vary with age		>190
Lipoproteins:				
LDL	60–160	<130	130–159	>160
HDL	29–77	>60	35–50	<35

KEY: LDL: low-density lipoproteins; HDL: high-density lipoproteins; CAD: coronary artery disease; <: less than; >: greater than.

ence to dietary restrictions is often short lived, explains why many clients do not respond to diet modification alone.

Exercise is an important aspect of the nonpharmacologic method to reduce cholesterol. For the hypertensive elderly person, exercise can be walking and bicycling. If the client is obese, body weight reduction decreases cholesterol levels and the risk of coronary artery disease (CAD). Another risk factor that should be eliminated is smoking. Smoking increases LDL-cholesterol and decreases the HDL.

If nonpharmacologic methods are ineffective for reducing cholesterol and the lipoproteins LDL and VLDL and hyperlipemia remains, antilipemic drugs are prescribed. It must be emphasized to the client that dietary changes need to be made and an exercise program followed even after drug therapy has been initiated. The type of antilipemics ordered depends on the lipoprotein phenotype (Table 40–6).

Types of Antilipemics

One of the first antilipemics was cholestyramine (Questran), introduced in 1959. It is a resin that binds with bile acids in the intestine and is effective against hyperlipidemia type II. The drug comes in a gritty powder, which is mixed thoroughly in water or juice.

Colestipol (Colestid) is a new resin antilipemic similar to cholestyramine. Both of these drugs are effective in lowering cholesterol. Bile acid sequestrants should not be used as the only therapy in clients with elevated triglycerides, because they typically raise triglyceride levels.

Table 40–6
Hyperlipidemia: Lipoprotein Phenotype

TYPE	MAJOR LIPIDS
I	Increased chylomicrons and increased triglycerides. Uncommon.
IIA	Increased low-density lipoprotein (LDL) and increased cholesterol
IIB	Increased very low-density lipoprotein (VLDL), increased LDL, increased cholesterol and triglycerides. Very common.
III	Moderately increased cholesterol and triglycerides. Uncommon.
IV	Increased VLDL and markedly increased triglycerides. Very common.
V	Increased chylomicrons, VLDL, and triglycerides. Uncommon.

Types II and IV are commonly associated with coronary artery disease.

Clofibrate (Atromid-S) and gemfibrozil (Lopid) are fibric acid derivatives that are effective in reducing triglyceride and VLDL levels. They are used primarily to reduce hyperlipidemia type IV but can also be used for type II hyperlipidemia. These drugs are highly protein-bound and should not be taken with anticoagulants because they compete for protein sites. The anticoagulant dose should be reduced during antilipemic therapy, and the INR should be closely monitored. Clofibrate, once a popular antilipemic, is not suggested for long-term use due to its many side effects, such as cardiac dysrhythmias, angina, thromboembolism, and gallstones.

Nicotinic acid, or niacin (vitamin B_2), reduces VLDL and LDL. Nicotinic acid is actually very effective at lowering cholesterol levels, and its effect on the lipid profile is highly desirable. Because it has numerous side effects and large doses are required, as few as 20% of clients can tolerate niacin initially; however, with proper client counseling, careful drug titration, and concomitant use of aspirin, this number can be increased to as high as 60% to 70%.

Probucol, a bisphenol, is poorly absorbed after oral dosage. It lowers the LDL and cholesterol levels in type II hyperlipidemia, but it is not as effective as other antilipemic drugs. It is highly lipid soluble and is stored in body fat; thus it is slow to be eliminated from the body. Diarrhea may result from use. Probucol is contraindicated for clients with cardiac dysrhythmias.

VASTATINS OR STATINS

The statin drugs inhibit the enzyme HMG CoA reductase in cholesterol biosynthesis; thus the statins are referred to as HMG CoA reductase inhibitors. By inhibiting cholesterol synthesis in the liver, this group of antilipemics decreases the concentration of cholesterol and decreases the LDL and slightly increases the HDL cholesterol. Reduction of LDL cholesterol may be seen in as early as 2 weeks.

Numerous statins have been approved in the past few years. The present group of statins include atorvastatin calcium (Lipitor), cerivastatin (Baycol), fluvastatin (Lescol), lovastatin (Mevacor), pravastatin sodium (Pravachol), and simvastatin (Zocor). Lovastatin was the first statin used to decrease cholesterol. It is effective in lowering LDL (hyperlipidemia type II) within several weeks; GI disturbances, headaches, muscle cramps, and tiredness are early complaints. Serum liver enzymes should be monitored and an annual eye examination done because cataract formation may result from lovastatin therapy. The other five statins have actions that are similar to lovastatin in decreasing serum cholesterol, LDL, VLDL, and triglycerides, and they slightly elevate HDL. The statin group has been useful in decreasing coronary artery disease (CAD) and reducing mortality rates.

Chart 40–3.   Antilipemic

ANTILIPEMIC, ANTIHYPERLIPIDEMIC

	NURSING PROCESS
Drug Name	**Assessment and Planning**

Drug Name

Lovastatin
   (Mevacor)
Pregnancy Category: X

Dosage

A: PO: 20–80 mg/d in 1–2 divided doses with meals

Contraindications

Hepatic disease, pregnancy
Caution: Increase with alcohol consumption, seizure disorder, trauma

Drug-Lab-Food Interactions

Drug: *Increase* effect with other antilipemics; *increase* effect of Coumadin
Lab: May *increase* CPK, AST, ALT

Pharmacokinetics

Absorption: PO: 30%
Distribution: PB: 95%
Metabolism: $t_{\frac{1}{2}}$: 1–2 h
Excretion: 10% in urine, 80% in feces, bile

Pharmacodynamics

PO: Onset: 2–3 d
    Peak: UK
    Duration: UK

Therapeutic Effects/Uses

To control hypercholesterolemia; to decrease low-density lipoprotein (LDL); and to slightly increase high-density lipoprotein (HDL).

Mode of Action: Reduction of HMG-CoA reductase (enzyme), which inhibits cholesterol synthesis.

Side Effects

Nausea, diarrhea or constipation, abdominal pain or cramps, flatulence, dizziness, headache, blurred vision, rash, pruritus

Adverse Reactions

Hepatic dysfunction (elevated serum liver enzymes), myositis

Side margin labels: Interventions; Evaluation

KEY: A: adult; C: child; UK: unknown; PO: by mouth; PB: protein-binding; $t_{\frac{1}{2}}$: half-life; CPK: creatine phosphokinase; ALT: alanine aminotransferase; AST: aspartate aminotransferase.

If antilipemic therapy is withdrawn, cholesterol and LDL levels return to pretreatment levels. The client taking an antilipemic should understand that antilipemic drug therapy is a lifetime commitment for maintaining a decrease in serum lipid levels.

PHARMACOKINETICS

Thirty percent of lovastatin is absorbed, and much of the drug is lost as a result of extensive first-pass metabolism by the liver. When taken with food, 50% of lovastatin is absorbed. Lovastatin is highly protein-bound, and other highly protein-bound drugs such as warfarin should be avoided when taking

antilipemics. Chart 40–3 gives the drug data for lovastatin.

PHARMACODYNAMICS

Lovastatin inhibits hepatic synthesis of cholesterol, thus lowering the serum cholesterol level. If the drug has not been effective in lowering the serum lipid levels after 3 months, it should be discontinued and another antilipemic started. Lovastatin should not be administered with gemfibrozil.

The onset and peak time of action of lovastatin occurs in hours; however, it takes several days for the drug to have a therapeutic effect. Duration of action may be up to 3 weeks.

Table 40–7 lists the drug data for the antilipemics.

Table 40–7
Antilipemics

GENERIC (BRAND)	ROUTE AND DOSAGE	USES AND CONSIDERATIONS
Cholestyramine resin (Questran)	A: PO: 4 g t.i.d. a.c. and hs; mix powder in 120–240 mL of fluid; *max:* 24 g/d	Cholestyramine resin was the first antilipemic produced. For type II hyperlipoproteinemia (LDL). Decrease in LDL is apparent in a week. Drug powder should be mixed well in fluid. It does not have any effect on VLDL and HDL, but could increase triglyceride levels. GI upset and constipation can occur. Vitamin A, D, K deficiency may occur due to decreased GI absorption. *Pregnancy category:* C; PB: UK; t½: UK
Clofibrate (Atromid-S)	A: PO: 500 mg q.i.d.	For lowering cholesterol, VLDL, and triglyceride; and for types IIB (VLDL), IV, V hyperlipidemia. Drug is more effective for higher cholesterol levels. Therapeutic effect occurs in 2–5 d. Drug should not be taken during pregnancy. Gallstones can occur with long-term use. *Pregnancy category:* C; PB: 90%–95%; t½: 12–25 h
Colestipol HCl (Colestid)	A: PO: 10–30 g/d in divided doses before meals	To reduce cholesterol and LDL levels. Same as cholestyramine. *Pregnancy category:* C; PB: UK; t½: UK
Fenofibrate (Lipidil)	A: PO: 100 mg/d	Treatment of type IV and V hyperlipidemia. Specified diet should be part of the drug therapy. *Pregnancy category:* UK; PB: UK; t½: UK
Gemfibrozil (Lopid)	A: PO: 600 mg b.i.d. before meals; *max:* 1500 mg/d	For VLDL and elevated triglycerides; LDL may decrease and HDL may increase. For types II (VLDL, LDL), III, IV, V hyperlipidemia. Do not use in combination with lovastatin due to increase in CPK. *Pregnancy category:* B; PB: >90%; t½: 1.5 h
Nicotinic acid (Niacin)	A: PO: Initially: 100 mg t.i.d.; maint; 1–3 g/d p.c. in 3 divided doses; *max:* 6 g/d	For VLDL and LDL: types II, III, IV, V hyperlipidemia. Doses are 100 times higher than for RDA to lower VLDL. See text. *Pregnancy category:* C; PB: UK; t½: 45 min
Probucol (Lorelco)	A: PO: 500 mg b.i.d. with meals	For LDL and elevated cholesterol (type II hyperlipidemia). Contraindicated in clients with cardiac dysrhythmias. *Pregnancy category:* B; PB: UK; t½: 20 d
VASTATINS AND STATINS (HMG-CoA REDUCTASE INHIBITORS)		
Atorvastatin calcium (Lipitor)	A: PO: 10 mg/d.; *max:* 80 mg/d	To reduce hyperlipidemia (LDL, cholesterol, and triglycerides). May increase digoxin levels. *Caution* in clients with history of liver disease. *Pregnancy category:* X; PB: 98%; 14 h
Cerivastatin (Baycol)	A: PO: 0.3 mg/d. in evening; *max:* 0.3 mg/d. *Renal insufficiency:* 0.2 mg/d	To reduce hyperlipidemia. Decreases LDL, VLDL, cholesterol, triglycerides, and slightly increases HDL. Similar to other statins. The newest statin and least expensive. *Pregnancy category:* UK; PB: UK; t½: UK
Fluvastatin (Lescol)	A: PO: Initially: 20 mg h.s.; maint: 20–40 mg/d in 1 or 2 divided doses	A recently approved antilipemic drug. Treatment of types IIA and IIB hyperlipidemia, total cholesterol, and elevated triglycerides. HDL is slightly increased. Monitor liver function (liver enzymes). *Pregnancy category:* B; PB: UK; t½: UK
Lovastatin (Mevacor)	See Chart 40–3	For LDL and elevated cholesterol (type II hyperlipidemia), and to increase HDL. Dose dependent on serum cholesterol level. Monitor liver function. Do not exceed 20 mg/d in clients on immunosuppressive drugs. Do not use in combination with gemfibrozil. *Pregnancy category:* X; PB: 95%; t½: 1–2 h

Table continued on following page

Table 40–7 *Continued*
Antilipemics

GENERIC (BRAND)	ROUTE AND DOSAGE	USES AND CONSIDERATIONS
Pravastatin sodium (Pravachol)	A: PO: 10–40 mg/d	A recently approved antilipemic drug. Decreases serum cholesterol, LDL, VLDL, and triglycerides. HDL is slightly increased. Monitor liver enzymes. *Pregnancy category:* X; PB: 55%; t½: 1.5–2.5 h
Simvastatin (Zocor)	A: PO: Initially: 5–10 mg/d in evening; maint: 20–40 mg/d in 1 or 2 divided doses; *max:* 40 mg/d	Similar to lovastatin. Monitor liver enzymes. *Pregnancy category:* X; PB: 95%; t½: UK

KEY: A: adult; PO: by mouth; LDL: low-density lipoprotein; VLDL; very low-density lipoprotein; HDL: high-density lipoprotein; CPK: creatine phosphokinase; RDA: recommended daily allowance; UK: unknown; PB: protein-binding; t½: half-life; GI: gastrointestinal.

SIDE EFFECTS AND ADVERSE REACTIONS

Side effects and adverse reactions of **cholestyramine** include constipation and peptic ulcer. Constipation can be decreased or alleviated by increasing intake of fluids and foods high in fiber. Early signs of peptic ulcer are nausea and abdominal discomfort, followed later by abdominal pain and distention. To avoid GI discomfort, the drug must be taken with and followed by sufficient fluids.

The many side effects of nicotinic acid, including GI disturbances, flushing of the skin, abnormal liver function (elevated serum liver enzymes), hyperglycemia, and hyperuricemia, decrease its usefulness. However, as mentioned, aspirin and careful drug titration can reduce side effects to a manageable level in most clients.

PERIPHERAL VASODILATORS

A common problem in the elderly is peripheral vascular disease. It is characterized by numbness and coolness of the extremities, intermittent claudication (pain and weakness of limb when walking and symptoms are absent at rest), and possible leg ulcers. The primary cause is hyperlipemia resulting in atherosclerosis, and arteriosclerosis. The arteries become occluded.

Peripheral vasodilators increase blood flow to the extremities. They are used in peripheral vascular disorders of venous and arterial vessels. They are more effective for disorders resulting from vasospasm (Raynaud's disease) than from vessel occlusion or arteriosclerosis (arteriosclerosis obliterans, thromboangiitis obliterans [Buerger's disease]). In Raynaud's disease, cold exposure or emotional upset can trigger vasospasm of the toes and fingers; these clients have benefited from vasodilators.

Although the following drugs have different actions, they all promote vasodilation: tolazoline (Priscoline), an alpha-adrenergic blocker; isoxsuprine (Vasodilan) and nylidrin (Arlidin), beta-adrenergic agonists; and cyclandelate (Cyclan), nicotinyl alcohol, and papaverine (Cerespan, Genabid), direct-acting peripheral vasodilators. The alpha blocker prazosin (Minipress), and the calcium channel blocker nifedipine (Procardia) have also been used.

Isoxsuprine hydrochloride (Vasodilan) is effective for relaxing the arterial walls within skeletal muscles. Chart 40–4 gives the drug data for isoxsuprine.

Isoxsuprine

PHARMACOKINETICS

Isoxsuprine is readily absorbed from the GI tract. It has a short half-life of 1.25 to 1.5 h. Because of its half-life, the drug can be taken three to four times a day.

PHARMACODYNAMICS

Isoxsuprine is a beta$_2$-adrenergic agonist. It causes vasodilation on arteries within the skeletal muscles. Bronchodilation also may occur. This drug has a short onset of action, peak time, and duration of action.

SIDE EFFECTS AND ADVERSE REACTIONS

Lightheadedness, dizziness, orthostatic hypotension, tachycardia, palpitation, flushing, and GI distress may occur.

The effectiveness of these drugs in increasing blood flow by vasodilation is questionable in the presence of arteriosclerosis. These drugs may decrease some of the symptoms of cerebrovascular insufficiency. The drug data for the peripheral vasodilators are given in Table 40–8.

A new drug, pentoxifylline (Trental), classified as

NURSING PROCESS
ANTILIPEMICS: LOVASTATIN (MEVACOR) AND OTHERS

Assessment

- Assess vital signs (VS) and serum chemistry values (cholesterol, triglycerides, AST, ALT, CPK) for baseline values.
- Obtain a medical history. Lovastatin is contraindicated for clients with a liver disorder. Pregnancy category is X.

Potential Nursing Diagnoses

- Impaired tissue integrity
- Anxiety related to elevated cholesterol level

Planning

- Client's cholesterol level will be <200 mg/dL in 6 to 8 wk.
- Client will be taught to choose foods low in fat, cholesterol, and complex sugars.

Nursing Interventions

- Monitor the client's blood lipid levels (cholesterol, triglycerides, low-density lipoprotein [LDL], and high-density lipoprotein [HDL] every 6 to 8 wk for the first 6 mo after lovastatin therapy and then every 3 to 6 mo. For lipid level profile, the client should fast for 12 to 14 h. Desired cholesterol value is <200 mg/dL; triglyceride value is <150 mg/dL (can vary); LDL is <130 mg/dL; and HDL is >60 mg/dL. Cholesterol levels of >240 mg/dL, LDL levels of >160 mg/dL, and HDL levels of <35 mg/dL can lead to severe cardiovascular or cerebral vascular accident.
- Monitor laboratory tests for liver function, such as ALT, ALP, and GGTP. Antilipemic drugs may cause liver disorder.
- Observe for signs and symptoms of GI upset. Taking the drug with sufficient water or with meals may alleviate some of the GI discomfort.

Client Teaching

General
- Advise the client that if there is a family history of hyperlipidemia, his or her children should have a baseline blood lipid level obtained and monitored. Instruct the client that children should decrease fatty foods in the diet.
- Emphasize the need to comply with the drug regimen to lower the blood lipids. Side effects should be reported to the health care provider.
- Inform the client that it may take several weeks before blood lipid levels decline. Explain that laboratory tests for blood lipids (cholesterol, triglycerides, LDL, and HDL) are usually ordered every 3 to 6 mo.
- Advise the client to have serum liver enzymes monitored as indicated by the health care provider. Lovastatin, pravastatin, and simvastatin are contraindicated in acute hepatic disease and pregnancy.
- Instruct the client to have an annual eye examination and to report changes in visual acuity.

Clofibrate, Gemfibrozil, Probucol
- Advise the client taking clofibrate and probucol that decreased libido and impotence may occur and should be reported. Drug dosage can be changed or another antilipemic may be ordered.
- Instruct diabetic or prediabetic clients to monitor blood glucose levels if they are taking gemfibrozil. Dietary changes or insulin adjustment may be necessary.
- Advise the client with cardiac dysrhythmias to tell the health care provider before starting probucol. Cardiac dysrhythmias should be monitored and reported.

Nursing Process continued on following page

NURSING PROCESS *Continued*
ANTILIPEMICS: LOVASTATIN (MEVACOR) AND OTHERS

Self-Administration
- For cholestyramine and cholestipol, instruct the client to mix the powder well in water or juice.

Diet
- Explain to the client that GI discomfort is a common problem with most antilipemics. Suggest increasing fluid intake when taking the medication.
- Instruct the client to maintain a low-fat diet by eating foods that are low in animal fat, cholesterol, and complex sugars. Lovastatin and other antilipemics are not a substitute for a diet that is low in fat.

Nicotinic Acid
- Advise the client to take the drug with meals to decrease GI discomfort.

Side Effects—Cholestyramine, Cholestipol, and Nicotinic Acid (Niacin)
- Advise the client that constipation may occur with cholestyramine and cholestipol. Increasing fluid intake and food bulk should help in alleviating the problem.
- Explain to the client that flushing is common and should decrease with continued use of the drug. Usually, the drug is started at a low dose.
- Advise the client that large doses of nicotinic acid can cause vasodilation, producing dizziness, and faintness (syncope).

Cultural Considerations

- Respect the client's belief of how to control his or her cholesterol level. Explanations and modification to plan of care may be necessary if the method the client is using is not effective or is unsafe.

Evaluation

- Evaluate the effectiveness of the antilipemic drug. The client's cholesterol level is within desired range.
- Determine that the client is on a low-fat, low-cholesterol diet.

Table 40–8
Vasodilators (Peripheral)

GENERIC (BRAND)	ROUTE AND DOSAGE	USES AND CONSIDERATIONS
ALPHA-ADRENERGIC BLOCKER		
Tolazoline HCl (Priscoline HCl)	A: SC/IM/IV: 10–50 mg q.i.d. NB: IV: Initially: 1–2 mg/kg, followed by 1–2 mg/kg/h for 24–48 h; initial dose effect: 30 min	For neonatal pulmonary hypertension and in vascular occlusive diseases in adults. Causes vasodilation and decreases peripheral resistance. Improves circulation in thromboangiitis obliterans, Raynaud's disease, frostbite, and peripheral vasospastic disorders. *Pregnancy category:* C; PB: UK; t½: A: 10 h, NB: 3–10 h
BETA₂-ADRENERGIC AGONISTS		
Isoxsuprine HCl (Vasodilan)	See Chart 40–4	For symptoms of TIA and peripheral vascular diseases (e.g., Raynaud's and Buerger's diseases). May cause hypotension and tachycardia. May take several weeks for therapeutic effects. *Pregnancy category:* C; PB: UK; t½: 1.25–1.5 h

Table continued on following page

Table 40–8 *Continued*
Vasodilators (Peripheral)

GENERIC (BRAND)	ROUTE AND DOSAGE	USES AND CONSIDERATIONS
Nylindrin HCl (Arlidin)	A: PO: 3–12 mg t.i.d.–q.i.d.	For peripheral vascular disorders. May cause tachycardia and heart palpitations. *Pregnancy category:* C; PB: UK; $t\frac{1}{2}$: UK
DIRECT-ACTING PERIPHERAL VASODILATORS		
Cyclandelate (Cyclospasmol)	A: PO: 20 mg q.i.d.; maint: 400–800 mg/d in 2–4 divided doses; dose may be reduced; *max:* 1600 mg/d	For peripheral vascular disorders. Acts on vascular smooth muscle. Has greater vasodilating effect than papaverine. Skin flushing and tachycardia can occur. Short-term use rarely of benefit; long-term treatment usually needed. *Pregnancy category:* C; PB: UK; $t\frac{1}{2}$: UK
Ergoloid mesylates (Hydergine)	A: PO/SL: 1 mg t.i.d.; dose may increase to 4–12 mg/d	For cerebrovascular insufficiency. To improve cognitive skills, self-care, and mood, especially in the older adult. SL tablets should be placed under the tongue. May cause GI distress, orthostatic hypotension. *Pregnancy category:* C; PB: UK; $t\frac{1}{2}$: 3–12 h
Nicotinyl alcohol (Ronigen [Canada only])	A: PO: 150–300 mg b.i.d.	Acts as vasodilator. Can cause flushing and orthostatic hypotension. *Pregnancy category:* UK; PB: UK; $t\frac{1}{2}$: UK
Papaverine (Pavabid)	A: PO: 100–300 mg, 3–5 × d SR: 150 mg q12h; *max:* 300 mg q12h IV: 30–120 mg q3h PRN	For arterial spasms. Reduces ischemia of the brain, heart, and peripheral vessels. One of the oldest vasodilators. Side effects: flushing, GI upset, headaches, increased heart rate and respiration. *Pregnancy category:* C; PB: 90%; $t\frac{1}{2}$: 1.5 h
HEMORRHEOLOGIC		
Pentoxifylline (Trental)	A: PO: 400 mg t.i.d. with meals	For peripheral vascular disorders. Alleviates intermittent claudication. Also improves cerebral function for those with cerebrovascular insufficiency and may decrease stroke incidence for those having recurrent TIA. *Pregnancy category:* C; PB: UK; $t\frac{1}{2}$: 0.5–1 h

KEY: A: adult; NB: newborn; PO: by mouth; SR: sustained-release tablet; SL: sublingual; TIA: transient ischemic attack; GI: gastrointestinal; PRN: as necessary; UK: unknown; PB: protein-binding; $t\frac{1}{2}$: half-life.

an antihemorrheologic agent, improves microcirculation and tissue perfusion, thus increasing tissue oxygenation. It is not a vasodilator, although it dilates rigid arteriosclerotic blood vessels including arterioles, capillaries, and venules. It is a derivative from the xanthine group. Pentoxifylline is used for clients having intermittent claudication, and in Buerger's disease resulting from arterial occulsions.

Reactions to an overdose of pentoxifylline include flushing of the skin, faintness, sedation, and GI disturbances. The drug should be taken with food. The client should avoid smoking because nicotine increases vasoconstriction. Clients taking an antihypertensive drug along with pentoxifylline may need to have the antihypertensive dosage decreased to avoid side effects.

Chart 40–4.   Vasodilators

PERIPHERAL VASODILATOR

Drug Name

Isoxsuprine HCl
  (Vasodilan, Voxsuprine)
Beta-adrenergic agonist
Pregnancy Category: C

Dosage

A: PO: 10–20 mg t.i.d.–q.i.d.

Contraindications

Arterial bleeding, severe hypotension, postpartum, tachycardia
Caution: Bleeding disorders, tachycardia

Drug-Lab-Food Interactions

Drug: *Decrease* blood pressure with antihypertensives

Pharmacokinetics
Absorption: PO: Readily absorbed
Distribution: PB: UK
Metabolism: $t\frac{1}{2}$: 1.25–1.5 h
Excretion: In urine

Pharmacodynamics

PO: Onset: 0.5 h
      Peak: 1 h
      Duration: 3 h

Therapeutic Effects/Uses

To increase circulation due to peripheral vascular disease (Raynaud's disease, arteriosclerosis obliterans) and cerebrovascular insufficiency.

Mode of Action: Action is directly on vascular smooth muscle.

Side Effects

Nausea, vomiting, dizziness, syncope, weakness, tremors, rash, flushing, abdominal distention, chest pain

Adverse Reactions

Hypotension, tachycardia, palpitations

Assessment and Planning

Interventions

NURSING PROCESS

Evaluation

KEY: A: adult; PO: by mouth; PB: protein-binding; $t\frac{1}{2}$: half-life; UK: unknown.

NURSING PROCESS
VASODILATORS: ISOXSUPRINE (VASODILAN)

Assessment

- Obtain baseline vital signs (VS) for future comparison.
- Assess for signs of inadequate blood flow to the extremities: pallor, coldness of extremity, and pain.

Potential Nursing Diagnoses

- Impaired tissue integrity
- Pain related to inadequate blood flow to extremity

Planning

- Client's blood flow to the extremities will improve, and the client's pain will be controlled.

Nursing Interventions

- Monitor VS, especially blood pressure and heart rate. Tachycardia and orthostatic hypotension can be problematic with peripheral vasodilators.

Client Teaching

General
- Inform the client that a desired therapeutic response may take 1.5 to 3 mo.
- Advise the client not to smoke; smoking increases vasospasm.
- Instruct the client to use aspirin or aspirin-like compounds only with the health care provider approval. Salicylates help in preventing platelet aggregation.

Diet
- Advise the client with GI disturbances to take isoxsuprine with meals.
- Advise the client not to ingest alcohol with a vasodilator because it may cause a hypotensive reaction.

Side Effects
- Encourage the client to change position slowly but frequently to avoid orthostatic hypotension. Orthostatic hypotension is common when taking high doses of a vasodilator.
- Instruct the client to report side effects of isoxsuprine, such as flushing, headaches, and dizziness.

Evaluation

- Evaluate the effectiveness of the isoxsuprine therapy; blood flow is increased in the extremities and pain has subsided.
- Client is experiencing no side effects from the prescribed drug.

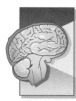

Critical Thinking in Action

T. M., 57 years old, has thrombophlebitis in the right lower leg. IV heparin, 5000 units by bolus, was given. Following the IV bolus, heparin 5000 units, SC, q6h was prescribed. Other therapeutic means to decrease pain and alleviate swelling and redness were also prescribed. An aPTT test was ordered.

1. Was T. M.'s heparin order per day within the safe daily range?
2. What are the various methods for administering heparin?
3. Why was an aPTT test ordered? How would you determine whether T. M. is within the desired range? Explain.

After 5 days of heparin therapy, T. M. was prescribed warfarin (Coumadin) 5 mg PO daily. PT and INR tests were ordered.

4. What is the pharmacologic action of warfarin? Is the warfarin dose within the daily dosage range? Explain.
5. What is the half-life and protein-binding for warfarin? If a client is taking a drug that is highly protein-bound, would there be a drug interaction? Explain.
6. Why would PT or INR be ordered for T. M.? What is the desired range?
7. What serious adverse reactions could result with prolonged use and/or large doses of warfarin?
8. What client teaching interventions should the nurse include? Give three client teaching interventions.
9. Months later, T. M. had hematemesis. What nursing action should be taken?

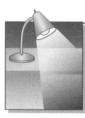

Study Questions

1. In what routes can heparin be administered? When? Why? Give rationale for your explanations.
2. What drugs can enhance the action of Coumadin (drug interaction)? How is Coumadin therapy monitored? Explain.
3. Explain how protamine is used. What is its action?
4. Plan a nursing plan of care for a client with thrombocytopenia.
5. The client has had an AMI within the last 3 hours. A thrombolytic drug is given. What type of nursing assessment should be performed and for how long?
6. Name at least three client situations that would contradict the use of thrombolytic therapy.
7. Explain the difference between an anticoagulant and a thrombolytic.
8. The client has a serum cholesterol level of 265 mg/dL, a triglyceride level of 235 mg/dL, and an LDL level of 180 mg/dL. Do these serum levels indicate hypolipidemia, normolipidemia, or hyperlipidemia? What nonpharmacologic measure should the nurse suggest that can aid in decreasing blood lipids?
9. Name the "friendly" lipoprotein. Which antilipemics tend to elevate this lipoprotein?
10. What are the uses of peripheral vasodilators? What two common side effects can occur?

Unit X

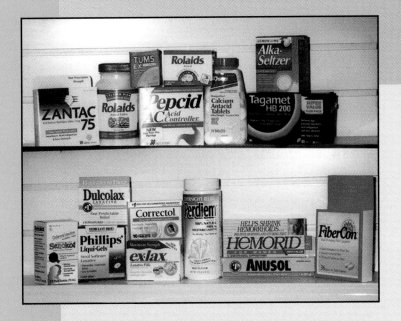

Gastrointestinal Agents

INTRODUCTION

The gastrointestinal (GI) system (tract), comprising the alimentary canal and the digestive tract, begins at the oral cavity of the mouth and ends at the anus. Major structures of the GI system are (1) the oral cavity (mouth, tongue, and pharynx), (2) the esophagus, (3) the stomach, (4) the small intestine (duodenum, jejunum, and ileum), (5) the large intestine (cecum, colon, and rectum), and (6) the anus. The accessory organs and glands that contribute to the digestive process are (1) the salivary glands, (2) the pancreas, (3) the gallbladder, and (4) the liver (Fig. X–1). The main functions of the GI system are digestion of food particles and absorption of the digestive contents (nutrients, electrolytes, minerals, and fluids) into the circulatory system for cellular use. Absorption and digestion take place in the small intestine and, to a lesser extent, in the stomach. Undigested material passes through the lower intestinal tract with the aid of peristalsis to the rectum and anus, where it is excreted as feces, or stool.

ORAL CAVITY

The oral cavity, or mouth, starts the digestive process by (1) breaking up food into smaller particles; (2) adding saliva, which contains the enzyme amylase for digesting starch (the beginning of the digestive process); and (3) swallowing, a voluntary movement of food that becomes involuntary (peristalsis) in the esophagus, stomach,

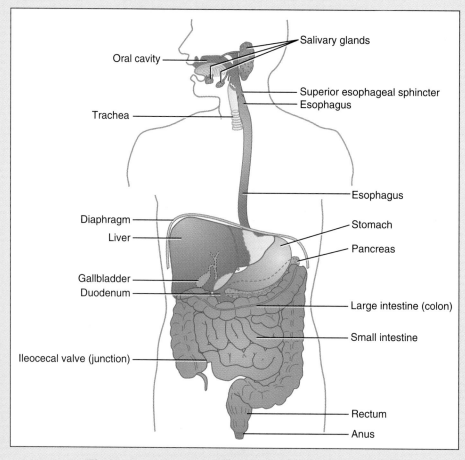

Figure X–1
The gastrointestinal system and alimentary canal.

and intestines. Swallowing occurs in the pharynx (throat), which connects the mouth and esophagus.

ESOPHAGUS

The esophagus, a tube that extends from the pharynx to the stomach, is composed of striated muscle in its upper portion and smooth muscle in its lower portion. The inner lining of the esophagus is a mucous membrane that secretes mucus. The peristaltic process of contraction begins in the esophagus and ends in the lower large intestine. There are two sphincters: the superior esophageal (hyperpharyngeal) sphincter and the lower esophageal sphincter. The lower esophageal sphincter prevents gastric reflux into the esophagus, a condition called *reflux esophagitis.*

STOMACH

The stomach is a hollow organ that lies between the esophagus and the intestine. The body of the stomach has lesser and greater curvatures. It can hold 1000 to 2000 mL of gastric contents, and empties in 2 to 6 h (average, 3 to 4 h), depending on gastric content and motility. Two sphincters, the cardiac sphincter, which lies at the upper opening of the stomach, and the pyloric sphincter, located at the lower portion of the stomach or the head of the duodenum, regulate the entrance of food into the stomach.

The interior lining of the stomach has mucosal folds that contain glands that secrete gastric juices. The four types of cells in the stomach mucosa that secrete these juices are (1) the chief cells, which secrete the proenzyme pepsinogen (pepsin), (2) the parietal cells, which secrete hydrochloric acid (HCl), (3) the gastrin-producing cells, which secrete gastrin, a hormone that regulates enzyme release during digestion, and (4) mucus-producing cells that release mucus to protect the stomach lining, which extends into the duodenum.

SMALL INTESTINE

The small intestine begins at the pyloric sphincter of the stomach and extends to the ileocecal valve at the cecum. Most drug absorption occurs in the duodenum, but lipid-soluble drugs and alcohol are absorbed from the stomach. The digestive process begins in the stomach, but most of the digestive contents are absorbed from the small intestine. The duodenum releases the hormone secretin, which suppresses gastric acid secretion, causing the intestinal juices to have a higher pH than the gastric juices. The intestinal cells also release the hormone cholecystokinin, which in turn stimulates the release of pancreatic enzymes and contraction of the gallbladder to release bile into the duodenum. Hormones, bile, and pancreatic enzymes (trypsin, chymotrypsin, lipase, and amylase) complete the digestion of carbohydrates, protein, and fat in preparation for absorption.

LARGE INTESTINE

The large intestine accepts undigested material from the small intestine, absorbs water, secretes mucus, and with peristaltic contractions moves the remaining intestinal contents to the rectum for elimination. Defecation completes the process.

Vomiting, diarrhea, and constipation are gastrointestinal problems that frequently require drug intervention. Chapter 41 describes the antiemetics used to control vomiting. Antiemetic groups include antihistamines, anticholinergics, selected phenothiazines, cannabinoids, and nonclassified antiemetics. Also discussed in the chapter are drugs that induce vomiting for elimination of ingested toxins and drugs. The antidiarrheal drugs include opiates, opiate-related drugs, and adsorbent drugs. Osmotic, contact-stimulant, bulk-forming, and emollient laxatives are discussed. The nursing process is considered in relation to each of the drug groups.

Drugs used to prevent and treat peptic ulcers (gastric and duodenal) are discussed in Chapter 42. Predisposing factors for peptic ulcers are described. Drug groups used for treating peptic ulcers include (1) selected tranquilizers, (2) anticholinergics, (3) antacids, (4) histamine$_2$ (H$_2$) blockers, (5) pepsin inhibitor (also known as mucosal protective drug), (6) gastric acid secretion inhibitor, (7) prostaglandin E$_1$ analog, and (8) GI stimulants. The nursing process is discussed in relation to these drugs.

Drugs for Gastrointestinal Tract Disorders

41

Outline

Objectives

* Identify causes of vomiting, diarrhea, and constipation.
* Explain the action and side effects of antiemetics, emetics, antidiarrheals, and laxatives.
* Describe the nursing process, including client teaching, of antiemetics, emetics, antidiarrheals, and laxatives.
* Identify contraindications to use of antiemetics, emetics, antidiarrheals, and laxatives.

Terms

adsorbents

antidiarrheals

antiemetics

cannabinoids

cathartics

chemoreceptor trigger zone (CTZ)

constipation

diarrhea

emetics

emollients

laxatives

opiates

osmotics

purgatives

vomiting center

INTRODUCTION

Drug groups used to correct or control vomiting, diarrhea, and constipation are antiemetics, emetics, antidiarrheals, and laxatives. Each of these drug groups is discussed separately. Drugs used to treat peptic ulcers are discussed in Chapter 42.

VOMITING

Vomiting (emesis), the expulsion of gastric contents, has a multitude of causes, such as motion sickness, viral and bacterial infection, food intolerance, surgery, pregnancy, pain, shock, effects of selected drugs, including antineoplastics, radiation, and disturbances of the middle ear affecting equilibrium. The cause of the vomiting needs to be identified. Nausea, a queasy sensation, may or may not precede the act of vomiting. Antiemetics can mask the underlying cause of vomiting and should not be used until the cause has been determined, unless the vomiting is so severe as to cause dehydration and electrolyte imbalance.

Two major cerebral centers—the **chemoreceptor trigger zone (CTZ),** which lies near the medulla, and the **vomiting center** in the medulla—cause vomiting when stimulated (Fig. 41–1). The CTZ receives most of the impulses from drugs, toxins, and the vestibular center in the ear and transmits them to the vomiting center. The neurotransmitter dopamine stimulates the CTZ, which in turn stimulates the vomiting center. Levodopa, a drug with dopamine-like properties, can

cause vomiting by stimulating the CTZ. Some sensory impulses such as odor, smell, taste, and gastric mucosal irritation are transmitted directly to the vomiting center. The neurotransmitter acetylcholine is also a vomiting stimulant. When the vomiting center is stimulated, the motor neuron responds by causing contraction of the diaphragm, the anterior abdominal muscles, and the stomach. The glottis closes, the abdominal wall moves upward, and vomiting occurs.

Nonpharmacologic measures should be used first when nausea and vomiting occur. If the nonpharmacologic measures are not effective, then antiemetics are combined with nonpharmacologic measures. There are two major groups of antiemetics: nonprescription (antihistamines, bismuth subsalicylate, phosphorated carbohydrate solution) and prescription (antihistamines, dopamine antagonists, benzodiazepines, serotonin antagonists, glucocorticoids, cannabinoids, and miscellaneous antiemetics).

Nonpharmacologic Measures

The nonpharmacologic methods of decreasing nausea and vomiting include administration of weak tea, flattened carbonated beverage, gelatin, Gatorade, and Pedialyte (children). Crackers and dry toast may be helpful. When dehydration becomes severe, intravenous fluids are needed to restore body fluid balance.

Nonprescription Antiemetics

Nonprescription **antiemetics** (antivomiting agents) can be purchased as over-the-counter (OTC) drugs. These drugs are frequently used to prevent motion sickness and have minimal effect on controlling severe vomiting resulting from anticancer agents (antineoplastics), radiation, and toxins. To prevent motion sickness, the antiemetic should be taken 30 min before travel. These drugs are not effective in relieving motion sickness if taken after vomiting has occurred.

Selected antihistamine antiemetics such as dimenhydrinate (Dramamine), cyclizine hydrochloride (Marezine), meclizine hydrochloride (Antivert), and diphenhydramine hydrochloride (Benadryl) can be purchased OTC to prevent nausea, vomiting, and dizziness (vertigo) caused by motion by inhibiting vestibular stimulation in the middle ear. Benadryl is also used to prevent or alleviate allergic reactions to drugs, insects, and food by acting as an antagonist to the histamine$_1$ (H$_1$) receptors.

The side effects of these drugs are similar to those of anticholinergics: drowsiness, dryness of the mouth, and constipation. Table 41–1 lists the nonprescription antihistamines used for vomiting associated with motion sickness.

Several nonprescription drugs such as bismuth subsalicylate (Pepto-Bismol) act directly on the gastric

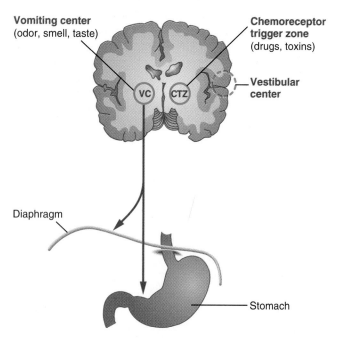

Figure 41–1
The chemoreceptor trigger zone and vomiting center.

Vomiting center (odor, smell, taste)

Chemoreceptor trigger zone (drugs, toxins)

Vestibular center

VC   CTZ

Diaphragm

Stomach

Table 41–1
Nonprescription Antiemetics: Antihistamine

GENERIC (BRAND)	ROUTE AND DOSAGE	USES AND CONSIDERATIONS
MOTION SICKNESS		
Buclizine HCl (Bucla-din-S [Softab])	*Prophylaxis:* A: PO: 50 mg 0.5 h before travel; may repeat in 4–6 h	Prevention of motion sickness that may cause nausea and vomiting. Drowsiness and dry mouth can occur. Avoid taking alcohol and central nervous system (CNS) depressants. *Pregnancy category:* C; PB: UK; t½: UK
Cyclizine HCl (Mare-zine)	A: PO: 50 mg 0.5 h before travel; may repeat in 4–6 h; *max:* 200 mg/d IM: 50 mg q4–6h PRN C 6–12 y: PO: 25 mg q.d./t.i.d. *Postoperative vomiting:* A: IM: 50 mg 0.5 h before surgery ends; may repeat q4–6h PRN	Similar to buclizine. Has been used for post-operative nausea and vomiting. *Pregnancy category:* B; PB: UK; t½: UK
Dimenhydrinate (Calm-X, Dimetabs, Dramamine)	A: PO: 50–100 mg q4–6h; *max:* 400 mg/d; IM/IV: 50 mg PRN C 6–12 y: PO: 25–50 mg q6–8h; *max:* 150 mg/d C < 2 y: Not recommended	Primarily used to prevent motion sickness. Drowsiness, dizziness, dry mouth, and hypotension may occur. *Pregnancy category:* B; PB: UK; t½: UK
Meclizine HCl (Anti-vert, Antrizine, Bon-ine)	A & C > 12 y: PO: 25–50 mg 1 h before travel, after meal; may repeat q24h *Vertigo:* A: PO: 25–100 mg/d in divided doses	Prevention of nausea, vomiting, and dizziness. Drowsiness and dry mouth may occur. *Pregnancy category:* B; PB: UK; t½: UK

KEY: *A: adult; C: child; PO: by mouth; >: greater than; <: less than; UK: unknown; PB: protein-binding; t½: half-life; max: maximum; PRN: as necessary.*

mucosa to suppress vomiting. They are marketed in liquid and chewable tablet forms and can be taken for gastric discomfort or diarrhea. Phosphorated carbohydrate solution (Emetrol), a hyperosmolar carbohydrate, decreases nausea and vomiting by changing the gastric pH; it may also decrease smooth muscle contraction of the stomach. Its effectiveness as an antiemetic has not been verified. Clients with diabetes mellitus should avoid this drug owing to its high sugar content.

Antiemetics were once used frequently for the treatment of nausea and vomiting during the first trimester of pregnancy, but they are no longer recommended because of possible harm to the fetus. Non-pharmacologic methods should be used to alleviate nausea and vomiting and OTC antiemetics should be avoided. If the vomiting becomes severe and threatens the well-being of the mother and fetus, an antiemetic such as trimethobenzamide (Tigan) has been administered although the drug is classified as pregnancy category C.

Prescription Antiemetics

Prescription antiemetics are classified into eight groups: (1) antihistamines, (2) anticholinergics, (3) do-pamine antagonists, (4) benzodiazepines, (5) serotonin antagonists, (6) glucocorticoids, (7) cannabinoids (for cancer clients), and (8) miscellaneous. Many of these drugs act as antagonists to dopamine, histamine, serotonin, and acetylcholine, which are associated with vomiting. Antihistamines and anticholinergics act primarily on the vomiting center; they also act by decreasing stimulation of the CTZ and vestibular pathways. Phenothiazines and the miscellaneous antiemetics such as benzquinamide, diphenidol, metoclopramide, and trimethobenzamide act on the CTZ center. The cannabinoids act on the cerebral cortex.

ANTIHISTAMINES AND ANTICHOLINERGICS

Only a few prescription antihistamines and anticholinergics are used in the treatment of nausea and vomiting; Table 41–2 lists these drugs, dosages, and uses and considerations.

Side Effects and Adverse Reactions

Side effects include drowsiness, which can be a major problem, dry mouth, blurred vision caused by pupillary dilation, tachycardia (with use of anticholinergics), and constipation. These drugs should *not* be used in clients with glaucoma because they dilate the pupils (mydriasis).

Table 41–2
Prescription Antiemetics

DRUG	DOSAGE	USES AND CONSIDERATIONS
PRESCRIPTION ANTIHISTAMINES		
Hydroxyzine (Vistaril, Atarax)	A: PO/IM: 25–100 mg t.i.d. or q.i.d. PRN	For postoperative nausea and vomiting, vertigo (dizziness). Given preoperatively with narcotics to decrease nausea. Give hydroxyzine deep IM. Drowsiness and dry mouth usually occur. *Pregnancy category:* C; PB: UK; $t_{\frac{1}{2}}$: 3 h
Promethazine (Phenergan)	A: PO: 12.5–25 mg q4–6h PRN C: PO: 0.25–0.5 mg/kg PRN Also suppository	Drug is a phenothiazine but has antihistamine effects. For postoperative nausea and vomiting, vertigo, motion sickness. *Pregnancy category:* C; PB: 60%–90%; $t_{\frac{1}{2}}$: UK
ANTICHOLINERGIC		
Scopolamine (Transderm Scop)	A: transdermal patch Deliver: 0.5 mg in 3 d	For motion sickness. Has numerous anticholinergic side effects. One patch behind ear at least 4 h before antiemetic effect is required. Patch is effective for 3 d. Alternate ears if using for longer than 3 d. Wash hands after applying patch disc. Wear no more than one disc/patch at a time. *Pregnancy category:* C; PB: <25%; $t_{\frac{1}{2}}$: 8 h
PHENOTHIAZINES		
Chlorpromazine (Thorazine)	A: PO/IM: 10–25 mg q4–6h PRN	Primarily used for psychosis but may be used to treat nausea and vomiting. Drowsiness, dizziness, EPS, and blurred vision may occur. *Pregnancy category:* C; PB: >90%; $t_{\frac{1}{2}}$: biphasic: 2–30 h
Perphenazine (Trilafon)	See Chart 41–1	For nausea and vomiting, especially as a result of chemotherapy (anticancer drug). Give before and after each cancer treatment. Side effects may include EPS, dry mouth and eyes, drowsiness, hypotension, dizziness, and syncope. *Pregnancy category:* C; PB: >90%; $t_{\frac{1}{2}}$: 8 h
Prochlorperazine maleate (Compazine)	A: PO/IM: 5–10 mg t.i.d.–q.i.d., PRN (give deep IM) SR: 10 mg q12h Rect: 5–25 mg PRN C: PO/Rect: 2.5 mg b.i.d.–t.i.d.	Primary use is for severe nausea and vomiting. Secondary use is to reduce anxiety and tension and for psychosis. Drowsiness, dizziness, EPS, dry mouth may occur. *Pregnancy category:* C; PB: >90%; $t_{\frac{1}{2}}$: 23 h
Thiethylperazine (Torecan, Norzine)	A: PO/IM/PR: 10 mg q.d./t.i.d.	To control nausea and vomiting by acting on CTZ and vomiting center. Same side effects as prochlorperazine. *Pregnancy category:* UK (X); PB: UK; $t_{\frac{1}{2}}$: UK
Triflupromazine (Vesprin)	A: PO: 20–30 mg/d A: IM: 5–15 mg q4–6 h C: PO/IM: 0.2 mg/kg/d; *max:* 10 mg/d	For severe nausea and vomiting. Secondary use is for psychosis without depression. Similar to prochlorperazine. *Pregnancy category:* C; PB: >90%; $t_{\frac{1}{2}}$: UK
BENZODIAZEPINE		
Lorazepam (Ativan)	A: PO: 2–6 mg/d in 2–3 divided doses; *max:* 10 mg/d	For prevention of nausea and vomiting resulting from cancer chemotherapy. It is usually administered with an antiemetic such as metoclopramide. *Pregnancy category:* D; PB: 85%; $t_{\frac{1}{2}}$: 10–20 h

Table continued on following page

Table 41–2 *Continued*
Prescription Antiemetics

DRUG	DOSAGE	USES AND CONSIDERATIONS
CANNABINOIDS		
Dronabinol (Marinol) CSS II	*Chemotherapy-induced nausea:* A: PO: 5 mg/m² 1–3 h before chemotherapy; then q2–4h after; *max:* 15 mg/m²/dose	For nausea and vomiting due to cancer chemotherapy. Taken before and for 24 h after chemotherapy. It can be an appetite stimulant for clients with AIDS. Common side effects include drowsiness, dizziness, dry mouth, impaired thinking, and euphoria. *Pregnancy category:* B; PB: 98%; t½: 20–24 h
Nabilone (Cesamet) CSS II	*Chemotherapy-induced nausea:* A: PO: 1–2 mg b.i.d. 1–3 h before chemotherapy, continue for 48 h after	For chemotherapy-induced nausea and vomiting, especially for cisplatin chemotherapy. May be used when other antiemetics are ineffective. It is a synthetic derivative of marijuana. Alcohol and CNS depressants should be avoided. *Pregnancy category:* B; PB: UK; t½: 2 h
MISCELLANEOUS		
Benzoquinamide HCl (Emete-con)	A & C > 12 y: IM: 50 mg q3–4h PRN IV: 25 mg or 0.2–0.4 mg/kg diluted in D₅W as one dose; give remainder of dose as IM	Treatment of nausea and vomiting due to anesthesia and postoperative surgery. It depresses the CTZ. It has anticholinergic, antihistamine, and sedative properties. Can cause drowsiness. *Pregnancy category:* C; PB: 60%; t½: 30–45 min
Diphenidol HCl (Vontrol)	*Nausea, vomiting, vertigo:* A: PO: 25–50 mg q4h C > 6 y: PO: 0.9 mg/kg; *max:* 5.5 mg/kg/d	For nausea, vomiting, and vertigo due to Ménière's disease and surgery of the middle ear. *Pregnancy category:* C; PB: UK; t½: 4 h
Droperidol (Inapsine)	A: IM/IV: 2.5–10 mg, 0.5–1 h before surgery C 2–12 y: IM/IV: 0.088–0.165 mg/kg, 0.5–1 h prior to surgery C < 2 y: Not recommended	Prevention of nausea and vomiting during surgical and diagnostic procedures. May cause hypotension, tachycardia, and EPS. *Pregnancy category:* C; PB: UK: t½: 2.5 h
Granisetron (Kytril)	A: PO: 1 mg b.i.d. (1 h before and 12 h after chemotherapy) A: IV: 10 μg/kg/30 min before chemotherapy	Prevention of nausea and vomiting due to cancer chemotherapy. Acts on the CTZ and vomiting center. Headache may occur. *Pregnancy category:* B; PB: 65%; t½: 4–10 h
Metoclopramide monohydrochloride monohydrate (Reglan)	A: PO: 10 mg a.c. and h.s. IV: 1–2 mg/kg 30 min before chemotherapy; then repeat q2h for 2 doses; then q3h for 3 doses; infuse diluted solution over not less than 15 min	For nausea and vomiting related to cancer chemotherapy treatment. It increases gastric and intestinal emptying. Avoid alcohol and CNS depressants. EPS may occur. *Pregnancy category:* B; PB: 30%; t½: 4–7 h
Ondansetron HCl (Zofran)	A: PO: 8 mg b.i.d. (1st dose 30 min before and 8 h after chemotherapy) A: IV: 0.15 mg/kg 30 min before chemotherapy; then 4 and 8 h after (total, 3 doses)	For nausea and vomiting related to cancer chemotherapy, especially cisplatin. *Pregnancy category:* B; PB: 70%–75%; t½: 4 h
Trimethobenzamide HCl (Tigan, Arrestin, Ticon)	A: PO: 250 mg t.i.d.–q.i.d.; IM/PR: 200 mg t.i.d.–q.i.d. C: 15–40 kg; PO/PR: 15–20 mg/kg/d divided in 3–4 doses or 100–200 mg, t.i.d.–q.i.d.	For postoperative nausea and vomiting, motion sickness, and vertigo. Avoid if sensitive to benzocaine or similar local anesthetics, and with CNS depressants. *Pregnancy category:* C; PB: UK; t½: UK

KEY: *A: adult; C: child; PO: by mouth; IM: intramuscular; IV: intravenous; PRN: whenever necessary; Rect: rectally; a.c.: before meals; h.s.: hour of sleep; EPS: extrapyramidal symptoms; CTZ: chemoreceptor trigger zone; UK: unknown; PB: protein-binding; t½: half-life; >: greater than; <: less than; CNS: central nervous system; CSS: Controlled Substance Schedule; AIDS: acquired immunodeficiency syndrome.*

DOPAMINE ANTAGONISTS

These agents suppress emesis by blocking dopamine$_2$ receptors in the CTZ. The categories of dopamine antagonists include phenothiazines, butyrophenones, and metoclopramide. Common side effects of the dopamine antagonists are extrapyramidal symptoms (EPS), which are caused by blocking the dopamine receptors, and hypotension.

PHENOTHIAZINE ANTIEMETICS

The largest group of drugs used for nausea and vomiting are the phenothiazines, primarily the piperazine phenothiazines which are also discussed in Chapter 19. These drugs are used to treat severe nausea and vomiting resulting from surgery, anesthetics, chemotherapy, and radiation sickness. They act by inhibiting the CTZ. When used in cancer clients, these drugs are commonly given the night before treatment, the day of the treatment, and for 24 h after treatment. Not all phenothiazines are effective antiemetic agents. When prescribed for vomiting, the drug dosage is usually smaller than when used for psychiatric disorders. Promethazine (Phenergan), a phenothiazine introduced as an antihistamine in the 1940s, has a sedative effect and can be used for motion sickness.

Chlorpromazine (Thorazine) and prochlorperazine edisylate (Compazine) were the first tranquilizers used for both psychosis and vomiting. Prochlorperazine, a piperazine phenothiazine, is the most frequently prescribed antiemetic drug. It is administered orally, intramuscularly, and rectally. Among the newer phenothiazines are perphenazine (Trilafon), fluphenazine (Prolixin), thiethylperazine (Torecan), and triflupromazine (Vesprin).

Chart 41–1 describes the action and effects of perphenazine (Trilafon), a phenothiazine antiemetic that is frequently used with anticancer therapy.

Pharmacokinetics

Absorption of the oral solid form of perphenazine is erratic; however, the liquid form is more stable with a faster absorption rate. It has a long protein-binding power and its half-life is moderate. Perphenazine is metabolized by the liver and gastrointestinal (GI) mucosa, and most of the drug is excreted in the urine.

Pharmacodynamics

Perphenazine inhibits dopamine in the CTZ, thus decreasing CTZ stimulation of the vomiting center. This drug is also used as an antipsychotic. The onset of action of oral perphenazine varies from 2 to 6 h, and the duration of action from 6 to 12 h. The onset of action of intramuscular and intravenous perphenazine is rapid, and the duration of action is the same as for the oral preparation.

Drug Interactions

Perphenazine interacts with numerous drugs. When perphenazine is taken with alcohol, antihypertensive agents, and nitrates, hypotension can result. There is an increase in central nervous system (CNS) depression when it is taken with alcohol, narcotics, sedative-hypnotics, and general anesthetics. Anticholinergic effects are increased when perphenazine is combined with antihistamines, anticholinergics such as atropine, and other phenothiazines. Laboratory test results may reveal increased levels of serum liver and cardiac enzymes, cholesterol, and blood glucose.

Side Effects and Adverse Reactions

Phenothiazines have antihistamine and anticholinergic properties. The side effects of phenothiazine antiemetics are moderate sedation, hypotension, extrapyramidal symptoms, which are those of parkinsonism, CNS effects (restlessness, weakness, dystonic reactions, agitation), and mild anticholinergic symptoms (dry mouth, urinary retention, constipation). Because the dose is lower for vomiting than for psychosis, the side effects are not as severe.

Table 41–2 lists the drug data for the phenothiazines along with other prescription antiemetics.

BUTYROPHENONES

Haloperidol (Haldol) and droperidol (Inapsine), like phenothiazines, block the dopamine$_2$ receptors in the CTZ. They are used for treatment of postoperative nausea and vomiting and the emesis associated with toxins, cancer chemotherapy, and radiation therapy. Also as with phenothiazines, EPS are likely to occur if these drugs are used over an extended time. Hypotension may result; blood pressure should be monitored.

METOCLOPRAMIDE

Metoclopramide (Reglan) suppresses emesis by blocking the dopamine and the serotonin receptors in the CTZ. It is used in the treatment of postoperative emesis, cancer chemotherapy, and radiation therapy. High doses can cause sedation and diarrhea. With this agent, the occurrence of EPS is more prevalent in children than in adults. Metoclopramide should not be given if the client has GI obstruction, hemorrhage, or perforation.

BENZODIAZEPINES

Selected benzodiazepines indirectly control nausea and vomiting that may occur with cancer chemotherapy. Lorazepam is the choice drug. Previously, diazepam (Valium) was the desired benzodiazepine. Lorazepam may be given with an antiemetic such as metoclopramide.

Chart 41–1. Antiemetics: Phenothiazine

PHENOTHIAZINE ANTIEMETIC

Drug Name

Perphenazine
   (Trilafon)
Pregnancy Category: C

Dosage

A: PO: 8–16 mg/d in divided doses; *max:*
24 mg
IV: *Max:* 5 mg, diluted or slow IV drip
A & C > 12 y: IM: 5–10 mg PRN: *max:* 15 mg
ambulatory care; *max:* 30 mg acute care

Contraindications

Narrow-angle glaucoma, severe liver disease, intestinal obstruction, blood dyscrasias, bone marrow depression
Caution: Children <12 y, seizures, cardiovascular disease

Drug-Lab-Food Interactions

Drug: *Increase* effects of alcohol, sedative-
hypnotics, beta-adrenergic blockers; *decrease*
levodopa, lithium, other phenothiazines;
Toxicity with epinephrine
Lab: *Increase* liver and cardiac enzymes, cholesterol, blood sugar; *decrease* hormones; false pregnancy test

Pharmacokinetics

Absorption: PO: Erratic absorption; liquid: ab-
sorption is increased
Distribution: PB: >90%
Metabolism: $t\frac{1}{2}$: 8 h
Excretion: In urine and feces

Pharmacodynamics

PO: Onset: 2–6 h
    Peak: 2–4 h
    Duration: 6–12 h
IM: Onset: 10 min
    Peak: 1–2 h
    Duration: 6–12 h
IV: Onset: Rapid
    Peak: UK
    Duration: UK

Therapeutic Effects/Uses

To treat and prevent vomiting, especially from anticancer drug; to treat alcoholism.

Mode of Action: Effects of dopamine changed in CNS; inhibits medullary chemoreceptor trigger
zone as antiemetic; anticholinergic blocking agent.

Side Effects

Anorexia, dry mouth and eyes, constipation,
blurred vision, extrapyramidal symptoms, rash,
photosensitivity, orthostatic hypotension, impotence, weight gain, amenorrhea, gynecomastia,
transient leukopenia, pain at IM injection site.

Adverse Reactions

Extrapyramidal syndrome (tardive dyskinesia,
akathesia), tachycardia
Life-threatening: Agranulocytosis, respiratory
depression, laryngospasm, allergic reactions,
cardiac arrest

Assessment and Planning
Interventions
Evaluation
NURSING PROCESS

KEY: A: adult; C: child; PO: by mouth; IM: intramuscular; PB: protein-binding; $t\frac{1}{2}$: half-life; IV: intravenous; >: greater than; UK: unknown.

SEROTONIN ANTAGONISTS

Serotonin antagonists suppress nausea and vomiting by blocking the serotonin receptors ($5\text{-}HT_3$) in the CTZ and the afferent vagal nerve terminals in the upper GI tract. It reacts to the serotonergic initiation of the reflex.

Two serotonin antagonists—ondansetron (Zofran) and granisetron (Kytril)—are effective in suppressing cancer chemotherapy–induced emesis. Ondansetron, the first serotonin antagonist, and granisetron do not block the dopamine receptors; therefore, they do not cause extrapyramidal symptoms as do the phenothiazine antiemetics. Both drugs can be administered orally and intravenously. Common side effects include headache, diarrhea, dizziness, and fatigue.

GLUCOCORTICOIDS (CORTICOSTEROIDS)

Dexamethasone (Decadron) and methylprednisolone (Solu-Medrol) are two agents that are effective in suppressing emesis associated with cancer chemotherapy. These drugs are administered intravenously. Because of the intravenous (IV) route and with short-term use of the drug, the side effects caused by glucocorticoids may be diminished. Glucocorticoids are discussed in Chapter 45.

CANNABINOIDS

Cannabinoids, the active ingredients in marijuana, had been appoved for clinical use in 1985 to alleviate nausea and vomiting resulting from cancer treatment. These agents may be prescribed for clients receiving chemotherapy who do not respond to or are unable to take other antiemetics. They are contraindicated for clients with psychiatric disorders. Cannabinoids can be used as an appetite stimulant for clients with acquired immunodeficiency syndrome (AIDS). The two cannabinoids, dronabinol (Marinol) and nabilone (Cesamet), are described in Table 41–2.

Side Effects and Adverse Reactions

Side effects occurring as the result of cannabinoid use include mood changes, euphoria, drowsiness, dizziness, headaches, depersonalization, nightmares, confusion, incoordination, memory lapse, dry mouth, orthostatic hypotension or hypertension, and tachycardia. Less common symptoms are depression, anxiety, and manic psychosis.

MISCELLANEOUS ANTIEMETICS

Benzquinamide hydrochloride (Emete-Con), diphenidol (Vontrol), and trimethobenzamide (Tigan) are several miscellaneous antiemetics because they do not act strictly as antihistamines, anticholinergics, or phenothiazides. These drugs suppress the impulses to the CTZ. Diphenidol also prevents vertigo by inhibiting impulses to the vestibular area.

Benzquinamide appears to have antiemetic, antihistaminic, and anticholinergic effects. It inhibits stimulation to the CTZ center and decreases activity in the vomiting center. This drug can also increase cardiac output and elevate blood pressure.

Side Effects and Adverse Reactions

The side effects and adverse reactions of the miscellaneous antiemetics are drowsiness and anticholinergic symptoms (dry mouth, increased heart rate, urine retention, constipation, blurred vision). Benzquinamide should be used cautiously in clients with cardiac problems such as dysrhythmias. Benzquinamide can cause CNS stimulation, including nervousness, excitement, and insomnia. Trimethobenzamide can cause hypotension, diarrhea, and extrapyramidal symptoms (abnormal involuntary movements, postural disturbances, and alteration in muscle tone). Metoclopramide can also cause extrapyramidal effects.

Table 41–2 lists the drug data for the miscellaneous antiemetics along with other prescription antiemetics.

EMETICS

When an individual has consumed certain toxic substances, induced vomiting (emesis) may be indicated to expel the substance before absorption occurs. There are many ways to induce vomiting without using drugs, such as putting the finger in the back part of the throat.

Vomiting should not be induced if caustic substances have been ingested, such as ammonia, chlorine bleach, lye, toilet cleaners, or battery acid. Regurgitating these substances can cause additional injury to the esophagus. To prevent aspiration, vomiting should also be avoided if petroleum distillates are ingested; these include gasoline, kerosene, paint thinners, and lighter fluid. Activated charcoal is given when emesis is contraindicated.

Ipecac

Ipecac is an OTC drug. Most health care providers instruct parents to keep ipecac in the household; however, it should be kept out of reach of children. When the client is purchasing ipecac, instruct the client to get ipecac syrup and *not* ipecac fluid extract, which is more potent. Ipecac syrup induces vomiting by stimulating the CTZ in the medulla and acting directly on the gastric mucosa. Ipecac should be taken with a glass of water or other fluid (do not give milk or carbonated beverages). If vomiting does not occur in 20 to 30 minutes, the dose could be repeated. Ipecac can be toxic if it does not induce vomiting and is absorbed; treat with activated charcoal and/or gastric lavage and give cardiovascular support if necessary. Chart 41–2 gives the drug data for ipecac.

PHARMACOKINETICS

Following a dose of ipecac, eight or more ounces of tepid water or juice should be given. The absorption of ipecac is minimal. The protein-binding is unknown, and the half-life is short.

PHARMACODYNAMICS

Ipecac acts on the chemotherapeutic trigger zone (CTZ) in the medulla and on the gastric mucosa to induce vomiting. The onset of action for ipecac is 15

NURSING PROCESS
ANTIEMETICS

Assessment

- Obtain a history of the onset, frequency, and amount of vomiting and contents of the vomitus. If appropriate, elicit from the client possible causative factors such as food (seafood, mayonnaise).
- Obtain a history of present health problems. Clients with glaucoma should avoid many of the antiemetics.
- Assess vital signs (VS) for abnormalities and for future comparison.
- Assess urinalysis before and during therapy.

Potential Nursing Diagnoses

- Altered nutrition: less than body requirements
- Risk for fluid volume deficit related to vomiting

Planning

- Client will adhere to nonpharmacologic methods and/or drug regimen for alleviating vomiting.
- The underlying cause of vomiting is determined and corrected.

Nursing Interventions

- Monitor VS. If vomiting is severe, dehydration may occur, and shock-like symptoms may be present.
- Monitor bowel sounds for hypoactivity or hyperactivity.
- Provide mouth care after vomiting. Encourage the client to maintain oral hygiene.

Client Teaching

General
- Instruct the client to store drug in tight, light-resistant container if required.
- Instruct the client to avoid over-the-counter (OTC) preparations.
- Instruct the client not to consume alcohol while taking antiemetics. Alcohol can intensify the sedative effect.
- Advise pregnant women to avoid antiemetics during the first trimester due to possible teratogenic effect on the fetus. Encourage them to seek medical advice about OTC or prescription antiemetics.

Side Effects
- Advise the client to report sore throat, fever, and mouth sores; notify health care provider and have blood drawn for a complete blood count (CBC).
- Instruct the client to avoid driving a motor vehicle or engaging in dangerous activities because drowsiness is common with antiemetics. If drowsiness becomes a problem, a decrease in dosage may be indicated.
- Advise the client with a hepatic disorder to seek medical advice before taking phenothiazines. Instruct the client to report dizziness.
- Suggest to the client nonpharmacologic methods of alleviating nausea and vomiting such as flattened carbonated beverages, weak tea, crackers, and dry toast.

Cultural Considerations

- Respect clients' cultural beliefs and alternative methods for treating nausea and vomiting. Discuss with clients the safety of their methods, other nondrug methods, and the purpose of an antiemetic if prescribed.
- An interpreter may be needed to assist non–English-speaking clients to understand the drug schedule for prescribed antiemetics and their side effects.

Evaluation

- Evaluate the effectiveness of the nonpharmacologic methods or antiemetic by noting the absence of vomiting. Identify any side effects that may result from drug.

Chart 41–2.   Emetics

EMETIC

Drug Name

Ipecac Syrup
Pregnancy Category: C

Dosage

A: PO: 15–30 mL, followed by 200–300 mL tepid water
C: >1–12 y: PO: 15 mL, followed by 200–300 mL tepid water
C: <1 y: PO: 5–10 mL, followed by 100–200 mL tepid water
Repeat initial dose if vomiting does not occur within 30 min only if the child is older than 1 yr

Contraindications

Hypersensitivity, depressed gag reflex, unconsciousness or semiconsciousness, poisoning with caustic or petroleum products, convulsions

Drug-Lab-Food Interactions

Drug: *Decrease* effect with activated charcoal, carbonated beverages, or milk

Pharmacokinetics

Absorption: Minimal
Distribution: PB: UK
Metabolism: t½: 2 h
Excretion: GI

Pharmacodynamics

PO: Onset: 15–30 min
      Peak: UK
      Duration: 20–25 min

Therapeutic Effects/Uses

To induce vomiting after poisoning

Mode of Action: Acts on chemoreceptor trigger zone (induces vomiting) and irritates gastric mucosa.

Side Effects

Diarrhea, sedation, lethargy; protracted vomiting

Adverse Reactions

Life-threatening: Cardiotoxicity if ipecac is not vomited (hypotension, tachycardia, chest pain)

Assessment and Planning / Interventions / Evaluation — NURSING PROCESS

KEY: A: adult; C: child; >: greater than; <: less than; PO: by mouth; GI: gastrointestinal; UK: unknown; PB: protein-binding; t½: half-life.

to 30 minutes and the duration of action is 20 to 25 minutes.

Apomorphine

Apomorphine is a morphine-derived emetic that can be administered subcutaneously or intramuscularly. Fluids are given before the injection, and vomiting should occur within 15 min. The drug is classified as a narcotic and can depress the respiratory center and decrease blood pressure; therefore, it is not used for narcosis due to CNS depressants, such as opiates, barbiturates, and alcohol. Side effects of apomorphine include restlessness, tremors, euphoria, tachycardia, hypotension, nausea, increased salivation, perspira-

tion, and lacrimation. Table 41–3 presents the drug data for ipecac syrup and apomorphine.

DIARRHEA

Diarrhea (frequent liquid stool) is a symptom of an intestinal disorder. Causes include (1) foods (spicy, spoiled), (2) fecal impaction, (3) bacteria (*Escherichia coli, Salmonella*) or virus (parvovirus, rotavirus), (4) toxins, (5) drug reaction, (6) laxative abuse, (7) malabsorption syndrome caused by lack of digestive enzymes, (8) stress and anxiety, (9) bowel tumor, and (10) inflammatory bowel disease, such as ulcerative colitis or Crohn's disease. Diarrhea can be mild to

Table 41-3
Emetics and Adsorbent

GENERIC (BRAND)	ROUTE AND DOSAGE	USES AND CONSIDERATIONS
EMETICS		
Apomorphine CSS II	A: SC: 4–10 mg C: SC: 0.07–0.1 mg/kg; 100–200 mL of water or evaporated milk before injection; do not repeat	To induce vomiting. Dose should *not* be repeated if vomiting does not occur. Schedule II drug. Fluids should be given before injection. Large doses could cause CNS depression (bradycardia and decreased respirations). *Pregnancy category:* C; PB: UK; t½: UK
Ipecac syrup (OTC preparation)	See Chart 41-2	To induce vomiting; contraindicated when caustic or petroleum substances have been ingested. Give with water (at least 200 mL). If vomiting does not occur, give activated charcoal to absorb ipecac and substance, or gastric lavage. *Pregnancy category:* C; PB: UK; t½: UK
ADSORBENT		
Charcoal (Charcoaid, CharcoCaps)	*For Poisoning:* *Charcoaid:* A: PO: 30–100 g dose in 6–8 oz of water *For Flatus:* *CharcoCaps:* A: PO: 520 mg, after meals; repeat PRN; *max:* 4 g/d	Promotes absorption of poison/toxic substances. Promotes absorption of intestinal gas. Both drugs are not systemically absorbed. *Pregnancy category:* C; PB: NA; t½: NA

KEY: A: adult; C: child; PO: by mouth; SC: subcutaneous; UK: unknown; NA: not applicable; PB: protein-binding; t½: half-life; PRN: as necessary; OTC: over-the-counter; CNS: central nervous system; CSS: Controlled Substance Schedule.

severe. Antidiarrheals are not to be used longer than 2 days and should not be used if fever is present.

Because intestinal fluids are rich in water, sodium, potassium, and bicarbonate, diarrhea can cause minor or severe dehydration and electrolyte imbalances. The loss of bicarbonate places the client at risk for developing metabolic acidosis. Clients with diarrhea should avoid foods rich in fat and milk products. Diarrhea can develop very quickly and can be life-threatening to the young and elderly, who may not be able to compensate for the fluid and electrolyte losses.

Nonpharmacologic Measures

The cause of diarrhea should be identified. Nonpharmacologic treatment for diarrhea is recommended until the underlying cause can be determined. This includes use of clear liquids and oral solutions (Gatorade, Pedialyte or Ricolyte [children]) and intravenous electrolyte solutions. Antidiarrheal drugs are frequently used in combination with nonpharmacologic treatment.

Traveler's Diarrhea

Traveler's diarrhea, also known as acute diarrhea and Montezuma's revenge, is usually caused by *E. coli.* It ordinarily lasts less than 2 days; however, if it becomes severe, fluoroquinolone antibiotics are generally prescribed. Loperamide may be used to slow peristalsis and decrease the frequency of defecation, but it may slow the exit of the organism from the GI tract. Traveler's diarrhea can be reduced by using bottled water, washing fruit, and eating cooked vegetables. Meats should be cooked until well done.

Antidiarrheals

There are various antidiarrheals for treating diarrhea and decreasing hypermotility (increased peristalsis). Usually there is an underlying cause of the diarrhea that needs to be corrected as well. The antidiarrheals are classified as (1) **opiates,** (2) opiate-related agents, (3) **adsorbents,** and (4) antidiarrheal combinations.

NURSING PROCESS
EMETIC: IPECAC SYRUP

Assessment

- Determine the toxic substance ingested. Do *not* induce vomiting if caustics or petroleum products have been ingested.
- Determine the time elapsed since the ingestion; lavage may be indicated.
- Check the client's vital signs (VS). Report abnormal findings.

Potential Nursing Diagnoses

- Potential risk for absorption of toxic substance
- Potential risk for infection

Planning

- Toxic substance will be expelled before absorption. There will be no bodily harm due to the toxic substance.
- Client will be closely monitored for adverse effects of the toxic substance for 24 to 48 h depending on the substance.

Nursing Interventions

- Call the poison control center to report the toxic ingestion and for instructions.
- Monitor VS. Report changes.
- Offer sufficient fluids with ipecac syrup; warm clear liquids are best: *no* milk or milk products. Have client in high Fowler's position. Fluids dilute the toxic substance and are vehicles for expelling the substance; avoid carbonated beverages as they cause abdominal distention. If emetic is unsuccessful, gastric lavage may be performed or activated charcoal given to adsorb the toxic substance.
- Do not offer ipecac syrup or fluids to a semiconscious or unconscious person because of the danger of aspiration. Gastric lavage is usually performed in such cases.
- Do not induce vomiting if the toxic substance is a caustic or a petroleum distillate.
- Prepare for forceful vomiting; have large basin ready, and move clothing to protected area.

Client Teaching

General

- Instruct the parent or other family member to have ipecac syrup on hand. Explain that ipecac syrup is an OTC drug.
- Explain to the parent that ipecac should be given with sufficient fluids. Advise that ipecac syrup is *not* given if the toxic substance is a caustic or petroleum product.
- Advise the client or parents to *never* remove toxic substances from original labeled containers. Instruct parents on the use of child safety caps for future prevention.
- Advise the parent to keep readily available the telephone numbers of the poison control center and all emergency services.

Cultural Considerations

- Recognize that clients from various cultural groups may need additional guidance in regard to storing drugs and chemical agents out of reach of children, giving first aid related to the substance the child ingested, and knowing how to contact a poison center. A written information sheet in the client's language may be beneficial.

Evaluation

- Evaluate the effectiveness of ipecac syrup for inducing vomiting.
- Continue monitoring VS.
- Continue monitoring for signs and symptoms related to effect of ingested substance.

Chart 41–3. Antidiarrheals

DIPHENOXYLATE WITH ATROPINE

Drug Name

Diphenoxylate with atropine
  (Lomotil)
Pregnancy Category: C
CSS V

Dosage

A: PO: 2.5–5 mg b.i.d.–q.i.d.
C: >2 y: PO: 0.3–0.4 mg/kg daily in 4 divided
doses or 2 mg 3–5 ×/d (use liquid form only)

Contraindications

Severe hepatic or renal disease, glaucoma, severe electrolyte imbalance, child <2 y

Drug-Lab-Food Interactions

Drug: *Increase* CNS depression with alcohol, an-
tihistamines, narcotics, sedative-hypnotics.
MAOIs may *enhance* hypertensive crisis
Lab: *Increase* serum liver enzymes, amylase

Pharmacokinetics

Absorption: PO: Well absorbed
Distribution: PB: UK
Metabolism: t½: 2.5 h
Excretion: In feces and urine

Pharmacodynamics

PO: Onset: 45–60 min
    Peak: 2 h
    Duration: 3–4 h

Therapeutic Effects/Uses

To treat diarrhea by slowing intestinal motility.

Mode of Action: Inhibition of gastric motility.

Side Effects

Drowsiness, dizziness, constipation, dry mouth,
weakness, flushing, rash, blurred vision, mydriasis, urine retention

Adverse Reactions

Angioneurotic edema
Life-threatening: Paralytic ileus, toxic mega-
colon, severe allergic reaction

Assessment and Planning

Interventions

NURSING PROCESS

Evaluation

KEY: A: adult; C: child; PO: by mouth; >: greater than; <: less than; UK: unknown; PB: protein-binding; t½: half-life; MAOIs: monoamine oxidase inhibitors.

OPIATES

Opiates decrease intestinal motility, thus decreasing peristalsis. Constipation is a common side effect of opium preparations. Examples are tincture of opium, paregoric (camphorated opium tincture), and codeine. Opiates are frequently combined with other antidiarrheal agents. Opium antidiarrheals can cause CNS depression when taken with alcohol, sedatives, or tranquilizers. Duration of action of opiates is approximately 2 h.

OPIATE-RELATED AGENTS

Diphenoxylate (Lomotil, Reasec [in Europe]), and loperamide (Imodium) are synthetic drugs that are chemically related to the narcotic meperidine (Demerol). They decrease intestinal motility (peristalsis) and are taken for "traveler's diarrhea." Loperamide causes less CNS depression than diphenoxylate and can be purchased as an OTC drug. Loperamide hydrochloric acid (Imodium) protects against diarrhea longer than a similar dose of diphenoxylate HCl with atropine sulfate (Lomotil), reduces fecal volume, and decreases intestinal fluid and electrolyte losses. Difenoxin (with atropine [Motofen]) is an active metabolite derived from diphenoxylate. This agent is prescribed to treat nonspecific and chronic diarrhea.

These drugs can cause nausea, vomiting, drowsiness, and abdominal distention. Tachycardia, paralytic ileus, urinary retention, decreased secretions, and physical dependence can occur with prolonged use.

Anticholinergic drugs decrease cramping, intestinal motility, and hypersecretion. They can be used in combination with opiates. Diphenoxylate product is approximately 50% atropine. (Atropine is added to

Table 41–4
Antidiarrheals: Opiates, Opiate Related, Adsorbents, and Miscellaneous

GENERIC (BRAND)	ROUTE AND DOSAGE	USES AND CONSIDERATIONS
OPIATES		
Deodorized opium tincture CSS II	A: PO: 0.6 mL or 10 gtt q.i.d. mixed with water; *max:* 6 mL/d C: PO: 0.005–0.01 mL/kg/dose q3–4 h; *max:* 6 doses/d	For acute, nonspecific diarrhea. To treat withdrawal symptoms in neonates of mothers who are addicted to opiates. Not to be used for diarrhea caused by poison. Avoid taking alcohol and CNS depressants. *Pregnancy category:* B (D at term); PB: UK; $t\frac{1}{2}$: 2–3 h
Camphorated opium tincture (paregoric) CSS III	Camphorated: 5–10 mL b.i.d.–q.i.d. C: PO: 0.25–0.5 mL/kg daily–q.i.d.	To decrease incidence of diarrhea. Decreases GI peristalsis. *Pregnancy category:* B (D at term); PB: UK; $t\frac{1}{2}$: 2–3 h
OPIATE RELATED		
Diphenoxylate with atropine (Lomotil) CSS V	A: PO: 2.5–5 mg b.i.d.–q.i.d. C > 2 y: 0.3–0.4 mg/kg daily in 4 divided doses or 2 mg 3–5 × d	For acute, nonspecific diarrhea. Inhibits GI motility. Diphenoxylate is a synthetic narcotic; atropine prevents possible narcotic abuse and decreases GI motility. Contraindicated in glaucoma, ulcerative colitis. *Pregnancy category:* C; PB: UK; $t\frac{1}{2}$: 2.5 h
Loperamide HCl (Imodium)	A: PO: Initially: 4 mg; then 2 mg after each loose stool; *max:* 16 mg/d C 2–5 y: PO: 1 mg t.i.d.; 6–8 y: 2 mg b.i.d.; 9–12 y: 2 mg t.i.d.	For diarrhea. Newest OTC drug. Does not affect the CNS. Less than 1% reaches systemic circulation. *Pregnancy category:* B; PB: 98%; $t\frac{1}{2}$: 7–12 h
ADSORBENTS		
Bismuth salts (Pepto-Bismol)	*Prevention of traveler's diarrhea:* A: PO: 2 tab q.i.d. a.c. and h.s. *Treatment:* A: PO: 2 tab or 30 mL q30–60 min PRN	For diarrhea, gastric distress. OTC liquid and tablet form. *Pregnancy category:* UK; PB: UK; $t\frac{1}{2}$: UK
Kaolin-pectin (Kapectolin, Kaopectate)	A: 60–120 mL after each loose stool C 6–12 y: 30–60 mL after each loose stool	For diarrhea. Administered after each loose stool. OTC drug. *Pregnancy category:* B; PB: 97%; $t\frac{1}{2}$: 7–14 h
MISCELLANEOUS		
Furazolidone (Furoxone)	A: PO: 100 mg q.i.d.; *max:* 400 mg/d C > 1 mo: PO: 5–8 mg/kg/d in 4 divided doses	Management of diarrhea and enteritis due to bacteria or protozoa. Common side effects include nausea and vomiting. *Pregnancy category:* C; PB: UK; $t\frac{1}{2}$: UK
Lactobacillus acidophilus and *Lactobacillus bulgaricus* (one or both) (Bacid [plus carboxymethylcellulose sodium], Lactinix, More-Dophilus)	A & C > 3 y: PO: 2 cap 2–9×/d Granules: 1 pkg with cereal, food, water t.i.d.–q.i.d. Powder: 1 tsp daily with fluid C < 3 y: Not recommended	Management of diarrhea due to bacteria. *Pregnancy category:* UK; PB: UK; $t\frac{1}{2}$: UK
Octreotide acetate (Sandostatin)	*Diarrhea related to carcinoid tumors:* A: SC: Initially 0.05 mg/d in divided doses for 2 wk; then increase according to response; *max:* 0.75 mg/d	For severe diarrhea resulting from metastatic carcinoid tumors. It suppresses secretion of serotonin, gastrin, and pancreatic peptides. *Pregnancy category:* B; PB: 65%; $t\frac{1}{2}$: 1.5 h

Table continued on following page

Table 41-4 *Continued*
Antidiarrheals: Opiates, Opiate Related, Adsorbents, and Miscellaneous

GENERIC (BRAND)	ROUTE AND DOSAGE	USES AND CONSIDERATIONS
COMBINATIONS		
Difenoxin and atropine (Motofen) CSS IV	A: PO: Initially: 2 mg; then 1 mg after each loose stool; *max:* 8 mg/d for 2 d C < 2 y: Not recommended	For acute nonspecific and chronic diarrhea. Combination of a synthetic narcotic and atropine. Avoid use in narrow-angle glaucoma. Dry mouth, flushing, and tachycardia may occur. *Pregnancy category:* C; PB: UK; t½: 12–24 h
Diphenoxylate with atropine (Lomotil)	See Chart 41-3	Similar to difenoxin and atropine
Parepectolin CSS V	A & C > 12 y: 15–30 mL after each loose stool; *max:* 120 mL/d C 6–12 y: 5–10 mL after each loose stool; *max:* 40 mL/d	Contains paregoric (an opiate) and kaopectate. OTC drug; however, must be signed for at pharmacy because it contains opium. *Pregnancy category:* D; PB: UK; t½: UK

KEY: *A: adult; C: child; PO: by mouth; OTC: over-the-counter; <: less than; >: greater than; PB: protein-binding; t½: half-life; CNS: central nervous system; UK: unknown; CSS: Controlled Substance Schedule.*

discourage abuse; the amount of atropine is subtherapeutic.) Clients with hepatic impairment should be cautioned about taking diphenoxylate because it may precipitate hepatic coma. Pediatric and geriatric clients taking diphenoxylate are more susceptible to respiratory depression than other age groups. The action and effects of diphenoxylate with atropine are listed in Chart 41-3.

Pharmacokinetics

Diphenoxylate with atropine is well-absorbed from the GI tract. The diphenoxylate is metabolized by the liver mainly as metabolites. There are two half-lives: 2½ h for diphenoxylate and 3 to 20 h for the diphenoxylate metabolites. The drug is excreted in the feces and urine.

Pharmacodynamics

Diphenoxylate with atropine is an opium agonist with anticholinergic properties (atropine) that decreases GI motility (peristalsis). It has a moderate onset of action time of 45 to 60 min, and the duration of action is 3 to 4 h. Many side effects are due to the anticholinergic atropine. Clients with severe glaucoma should take another antidiarrheal that does not have an anticholinergic effect. If this drug is taken with alcohol, narcotics, or sedative-hypnotics, CNS depression can occur.

ADSORBENTS

Adsorbents act by coating the wall of the GI tract and adsorbing the bacteria or toxins that are causing the diarrhea. Adsorbent antidiarrheals include kaolin and pectin. These agents are combined in Kaopectate, a

mild or moderate antidiarrheal that can be purchased OTC and used in combination with other antidiarrheals. An example is Parepectolin, which contains paregoric (an opiate) and Kaopectate (an adsorbent). Bismuth salts (Pepto-Bismol) is considered an adsorbent because it adsorbs bacterial toxins. Bismuth salts can also be used for gastric discomfort. It is an OTC drug that is used for traveler's diarrhea. Colestipol and cholestyramine (Questran) are presciptive drugs that have been used to treat diarrhea, although they have not been approved by the Food and Drug Administration for that purpose. Table 41-4 lists the drug data for the commonly used antidiarrheals.

MISCELLANEOUS ANTIDIARRHEALS

There are various miscellaneous antidiarrheals that are prescribed to control diarrhea. These drugs are colistin sulfate, furazolidone, loperamide (Imodium), lactobacillus, and octreotide acetate. Combination drugs with brand names are used to alleviate diarrhea and these include Lomotil (diphenoxylate HCl with atropine sulfate) and Parepectolin (paregoric, kaolin, pectin, alcohol). Most of these combination drugs contain a synthetic narcotic ingredient. Table 41-4 includes these drugs.

CONSTIPATION

Constipation (accumulation of hard fecal material in the large intestine) is a relatively common complaint and a major problem of the elderly. Insufficient water intake and poor dietary habits are contributing factors. Other causes include (1) fecal impaction, (2)

NURSING PROCESS
ANTIDIARRHEALS

Assessment

- Obtain a history of any viral or bacterial infection, drugs taken, and foods ingested that could be contributing factors to diarrhea. Many of the antidiarrheals are contraindicated if the client has liver disease, narcotic dependence, ulcerative colitis, or glaucoma.
- Check vital signs (VS) to provide baseline for future comparison and to determine body fluid and electrolyte losses.
- Assess frequency and consistency of bowel movements.
- Assess bowel sounds. Hyperactive sounds can indicate increased intestinal motility.
- Report if the client has a narcotic drug history. If opiate or opiate-related antidiarrheals are given, drug misuse or abuse may occur.

Potential Nursing Diagnoses

- Diarrhea
- Altered nutrition
- Alteration in fluid volume

Planning

- Client's bowel movements will no longer be diarrhea.
- Client's body fluids will be restored.

Nursing Interventions

- Monitor VS. Report tachycardia or a systolic blood pressure decrease of 10 to 15 mmHg. Monitor respirations. Opiates and opiate-related drugs can cause CNS depression.
- Monitor the frequency of bowel movements and bowel sounds. Notify the health care provider if intestinal hypoactivity occurs when taking drug.
- Check for signs and symptoms of dehydration resulting from persistent diarrhea. Fluid replacement may be necessary. With prolonged diarrhea, check serum electrolytes.
- Administer antidiarrheals cautiously to clients with glaucoma, liver disorders, or ulcerative colitis or who are pregnant.
- Recognize that drug may need to be withheld if diarrhea continues for more than 48 h or acute abdominal pain develops.

Client Teaching

General
- Instruct the client not to take sedatives, tranquilizers, or other narcotics with drug. CNS depression may occur.
- Advise the client to avoid over-the-counter (OTC) preparations; they may contain alcohol.
- Instruct the client to take the drug only as prescribed. Drug may be habit forming; do not exceed recommended dose.
- Encourage the client to drink clear liquids. Advise the client not to ingest fried foods or milk products until after the diarrhea has stopped.
- Advise the client that constipation can result from the overuse of this drug.

Evaluation

- Evaluate the effectiveness of the drug; diarrhea has stopped.
- Monitor long-term use of opiates and opiate-related drugs for possible abuse and physical dependence.
- Continue to monitor VS. Report abnormal changes.

bowel obstruction, (3) chronic laxative use, (4) neurologic disorders (paraplegia), (5) ignoring the urge to have a bowel movement, (6) lack of exercise, and (7) selected drugs, such as anticholinergics, narcotics, and certain antacids.

Nonpharmacologic Measures

Nonpharmacologic management includes a diet that contains bulk (fiber) and water, exercise, and routine bowel habits. A "normal" number of bowel movements is one to three a day to three a week. What is normal varies from person to person; the nurse should determine what "normal" bowel habits are for the client. At times, a laxative may be needed, but the client should also use nonpharmacologic measures to prevent constipation.

Laxatives

Laxatives and **cathartics** are used to eliminate fecal matter. Laxatives promote a soft stool and cathartics result in a soft to watery stool with some cramping. Frequently, the dosage determines whether the drug acts as a laxative or cathartic.* A **purgative** is a "harsh" cathartic, causing a watery stool with abdominal cramping. There are four types of laxatives: (1) osmotics (saline), (2) stimulants (contact or irritants), (3) bulk-forming, and (4) emollients.

Laxatives should be avoided if there is any question that the client has an intestinal obstruction, severe abdominal pain, or symptoms of appendicitis, ulcerative colitis, or diverticulitis. Most laxatives stimulate peristalsis. Laxative abuse from chronic use of laxatives is a common problem, especially with the elderly. Laxative dependence can be a problem, so client teaching is an important nursing responsibility.

OSMOTIC LAXATIVES

Osmotics (hyperosmolar laxatives) include salts or saline products, lactulose, and glycerin. The saline products are composed of sodium or magnesium, and a small amount is systemically absorbed. Serum electrolytes should be monitored to avoid electrolyte imbalance. The hyperosmolar salts pull water into the colon and increase water in the feces to increase bulk, which stimulates peristalsis. Saline cathartics cause a semiformed to watery stool according to low or high doses. Good renal function is needed to excrete any excess salts. Saline cathartics are contraindicated for clients with congestive heart failure.

Osmotic laxatives contain three types of electrolyte salts, including the sodium salts (sodium phosphate

or phospho-soda, sodium biphosphate), magnesium salts (magnesium hydroxide [milk of magnesia], magnesium citrate, magnesium sulfate [Epsom salts]), and potassium salts (potassium bitartrate, potassium phosphate). High doses of salt laxatives are used for bowel preparation for diagnostic and surgical procedures. Another laxative used for bowel preparation is polyethylene glycol (PEG) with electrolytes, commonly referred to as Colyte or GoLYTELY. With PEG, however, a large volume of solutions, approximately 3 to 4 liters over 3 hours, is used. Clients may be advised to keep GoLYTELY refrigerated to make it more palatable. The positive aspect is that the solution is an isotonic, nonabsorbable osmotic substance that contains sodium salts and potassium chloride, thus can be used by clients with renal impairment or cardiac disorder.

Lactulose, another saline laxative that is not absorbed, draws water into the intestines and promotes water and electrolyte retention. It decreases the serum ammonia level and is useful in liver diseases, such as cirrhosis. Glycerin acts like lactulose, increasing water in the feces in the large intestine. The bulk that results from the increased water in the feces stimulates peristalsis and defecation.

Side Effects and Adverse Reactions

Adequate renal function is needed to excrete excess magnesium. Clients who have renal insufficiency should avoid magnesium salts. Hypermagnesemia can result from continuous use of magnesium salts, causing symptoms such as drowsiness, weakness, paralysis, complete heart block, hypotension, flushing, and respiratory depression.

The side effects of lactulose from excess use include flatulence, diarrhea, abdominal cramps, nausea, and vomiting. Clients who have diabetes mellitus should avoid lactulose because it contains glucose and fructose.

STIMULANT (CONTACT) LAXATIVES

Stimulant (contact or irritant) laxatives increase peristalsis by irritating sensory nerve endings in the intestinal mucosa. Types include those containing phenolphthalein (Ex-Lax, Feen-A-Mint, Correctol), bisacodyl (Dulcolax), cascara sagrada, senna (Senokot), and castor oil (purgative). Bisacodyl and phenolphthalein are two of the most frequently used and abused laxatives. They can be purchased OTC. The results of the use of these agents usually occur in 6 to 12 hours. Bisacodyl and several other of these drugs are used to empty the bowel before diagnostic tests (barium enema). Chart 41–4 gives the pharmacologic data for the contact/stimulant laxative bisacodyl.

Castor oil is a harsh laxative (purgative) that acts on the small bowel and produces a watery stool. The action is quick, within 2 to 6 hours, and the laxative

---

*These terms are often used interchangeably: "laxative" refers to both terms in this chapter.

Chart 41–4.   Laxatives: Stimulant (Contact)

STIMULANT LAXATIVE

Drug Name

Bisacodyl
    (Dulcolax); ❧ Apo-Bisacodyl, Bisco-Lax
Pregnancy Category: C

Dosage

A: PO: 10–15 mg in a.m./p.m.; *max:* 30 mg
C: >3 y: PO: 5–10 mg; 0.3 mg/kg/d
A & C: >2 y: Rectal supp: 5–10 mg/d
C < 2 y & infants: 5 mg

Contraindications

Hypersensitivity, fecal impaction, intestinal/biliary obstruction, appendicitis, abdominal pain, nausea, vomiting, rectal fissures

Drug-Lab-Food Interactions

Drug: *Decrease* effect with antacids, histamine$_2$ blockers, milk

Pharmacokinetics

Absorption: Minimal absorption (5%–15%)
Distribution: PB: UK
Metabolism: t$\frac{1}{2}$: UK
Excretion: In bile and urine

Pharmacodynamics

PO: Onset: 10–15 min; act: 6–12 h
      Peak: UK
      Duration: UK
Rect: Onset: 15–60 min
      Peak: UK
      Duration: UK

Therapeutic Effects/Uses

Short-term treatment for constipation: bowel preparation for diagnostic tests.

Mode of Action: Increases peristalsis by direct effect on smooth muscle of intestine.

Side Effects

Anorexia, nausea, vomiting, cramps, diarrhea

Adverse Reactions

Dependence, hypokalemia
Life-threatening: Tetany

KEY: A: adult; C: child; PO: by mouth; >: greater than; <: less than; UK: unknown; PB: protein-binding; t$\frac{1}{2}$: half-life; Rect: rectally; ❧: Canadian drug names.

Assessment and Planning · *Interventions* · *Evaluation* — **NURSING PROCESS**

should not be taken at bedtime. Castor oil is seldom used for correction of constipation. It is used mainly for bowel preparation.

Pharmacokinetics

The contact laxative bisacodyl is minimally absorbed from the GI tract. It is excreted in the feces, but due to the small amount of bisacodyl absorption, a portion is excreted in the urine.

Pharmacodynamics

Bisacodyl promotes defecation. Bisacodyl irritates the colon, causing defecation, and psyllium compounds increase fecal bulk and peristalsis. The onset of action of oral bisacodyl occurs within 6 to 12 h and within 15 to 60 min with the suppository (rectal administration).

Side Effects and Adverse Reactions

Side effects include nausea, abdominal cramps, weakness, and reddish-brown urine due to excretion of phenolphthalein, senna, or cascara.

With excessive and chronic use of bisacodyl, fluid and electrolyte (especially potassium and calcium) imbalances are likely to occur. Systemic effects occur infrequently because of minimal absorption of bisaco-

Table 41–5
Laxatives: Osmotic and Stimulant

GENERIC (BRAND)	ROUTE AND DOSAGE	USES AND CONSIDERATIONS
OSMOTICS: SALINE		
Glycerin	A: Supp: 3 g C < 6 y: Supp: 1–1.5 g	To relieve constipation. Use with caution for clients with cardiac, renal, or liver disease and for the elderly or for those who are dehydrated. *Pregnancy category:* C; PB: UK; $t\frac{1}{2}$: 30–45 min
Lactulose (Cephulac, Cholac, Constilec, Enulose)	*Chronic Constipation:* A: PO: 30–60 mL/d PRN C: PO: 7.5 mL/d after breakfast	For constipation. Also used in liver disease for ammonia elimination. May be used for constipation after barium studies. Poorly absorbed. *Pregnancy category:* C; PB: UK; $t\frac{1}{2}$: UK
Magnesium citrate (Citroma, Evac-Q-Mag)	A: PO: 120–240 mL C: PO: 4 mL/kg/dose or $\frac{1}{2}$ adult dose	For constipation or to complete bowel elimination prior to diagnostic procedures and surgery. *Pregnancy category:* UK; PB: UK; $t\frac{1}{2}$: UK
Magnesium hydroxide (milk of magnesia)	A: PO: 20–60 mL/d C: PO: 0.5 mL/kg/dose	For constipation. Take with a glass of water in morning or evening. With frequent use, good renal function is necessary. *Pregnancy category:* B; PB: UK; $t\frac{1}{2}$: UK
Magnesium oxide (Maox, Mag-Ox)	A: PO: 2–4 g h.s. with 8 oz water Do not use in client with renal failure	Similar to magnesium hydroxide. *Pregnancy category:* B; PB: UK; $t\frac{1}{2}$: UK
Magnesium SO$_4$ (Epsom salts)	A: PO: 10–15 g in 8 oz water C: PO: 5–10 mg in water	For complete bowel elimination before surgery. Hypermagnesemia can occur if used frequently. Also used in pregnancy to control seizures with severe toxemia of pregnancy (given IV). Caution for use in renal dysfunction. *Pregnancy category:* B; PB: UK; $t\frac{1}{2}$: UK
Sodium biphosphate (Fleet Phospho-Soda)	A: PO: 15–30 mL mixed in water	For constipation or bowel preparation. Contraindicated with CHF. *Pregnancy category:* UK; PB: UK; $t\frac{1}{2}$: UK
Sodium phosphate with sodium biphosphate (Fleet Enema)	*Enema:* A: 60–120 mL C: 30–60 mL	For constipation or bowel preparation for diagnostic procedures. Frequent Fleet Enema may cause fluid imbalance in the elderly. *Pregnancy category:* UK; PB: UK; $t\frac{1}{2}$: UK
STIMULANTS		
Bisacodyl (Dulcolax)	See Chart 41–4	For constipation or bowel preparation for diagnostic procedures. Onset: 6–8 h for oral and 15–30 min for suppository. Used for clients with decreased colon (motor) response due to spinal cord damage. *Pregnancy category:* C; PB: UK; $t\frac{1}{2}$: UK
Cascara sagrada	A: PO: Tab: 325 mg/d Fluid extract: 1 mL/d Aromatic fluid extract: 5 mL/d	For acute constipation or bowel preparation. Can be mixed with milk of magnesia. Onset: 6–12 h. *Pregnancy category:* C; PB: UK; $t\frac{1}{2}$: UK
Castor oil (Emulsoil, Neoloid, Purge)	A: PO: 15–60 mL C 6–12 y: 5–15 mL	For bowel preparation for diagnostic tests. Harsh cathartic or purgative. Not commonly used for constipation. *Pregnancy category:* X; PB: UK; $t\frac{1}{2}$: UK
Phenolphthalein (Ex-Lax, Feen-A-Mint, Correctol)	A & C > 12 y: 60–240 mg/d C 6–12 y: 30–60 mg	For acute constipation. Onset: 6–10 h. Urine is reddish color. *Pregnancy category:* C; PB: UK; $t\frac{1}{2}$: UK
Senna (Senokot)	A: PO: 2 tab or 1–4 tsp (granules) diluted in water; *max:* 8 tab/d	For constipation. Available in granules, syrup, and suppository. Prolonged use may cause fluid and electrolyte imbalances. Flatus and abdominal cramps may occur. *Pregnancy category:* C; PB: UK; $t\frac{1}{2}$: UK

KEY: *A: adult; C: child; PO: by mouth; >: greater than; <: less than; UK: unknown; PB: protein-binding; $t\frac{1}{2}$: half-life; CHF: congestive heart failure.*

LAXATIVES: STIMULANT

Assessment

- Obtain a history of constipation and possible causes such as insufficient water/fluid intake, diet deficient in bulk or fiber, or inactivity; a history of the frequency and consistency of stools; and the general health status.
- Obtain baseline vital signs (VS) for identification of abnormalities and for future comparisons.
- Assess renal function.
- Assess electrolyte balance of clients with frequent laxative use.

Potential Nursing Diagnoses

- Constipation
- Altered nutrition
- Risk for fluid deficit
- Knowledge deficit related to overuse of laxatives
- Altered health maintenance

Planning

- Client will be free of constipation.
- Client will exercise, eat foods high in fiber, and have adequate fluid intake to avoid constipation.

Nursing Interventions

- Monitor fluid intake and output. Note signs and symptoms of fluid and electrolyte imbalances that may result from watery stools. Habitual use of laxatives can cause fluid volume deficit and electrolyte losses. Also, it can cause a loss of urge for defecation.

Client Teaching

General
- Instruct the client to increase water intake, if not contraindicated, which will decrease hard, dry stools.
- Advise the client to avoid overuse of laxatives, which can lead to fluid and electrolyte imbalances and drug dependence. Suggest exercise to help increase peristalsis.
- Instruct the client not to chew the tablets; swallow them whole.
- Advise the client to store suppositories at <86°F.
- Advise the client to take the drug only with water to increase absorption.
- Instruct the client not to take drug within 1 h of any other drug.
- Remind the client that drug is not for long-term use; tone of bowel may be lost.
- Instruct the client to time administration of drug so as not to interfere with activities or sleep.

Diet
- Advise the client to increase foods rich in fiber such as bran, grains, and fruits.

Side Effects
- Instruct the client to discontinue use if rectal bleeding, nausea, vomiting, or cramping occurs.

Cultural Considerations
- Provide explanation and written information as needed to clients from various cultural groups related to the use and abuse of stimulant laxatives.

Evaluation

- Evaluate the effectiveness of nonpharmacologic methods for alleviating constipation.
- Evaluate the client's use of laxatives in managing constipation; constipation will be alleviated. Identify laxative abuse.

Chart 41-5. Laxatives: Bulk Forming

BULK-FORMING LAXATIVE

Drug Name

Psyllium hydrophilic muciloid
  (Metamucil, Naturacil); ❦ Karasil
Pregnancy Category: C

Dosage

A: PO: 1–2 tsp in 8 oz water/d followed by
8 oz water
C: >6 y: PO: 0.5–1 tsp in 4 oz water, followed
by ≥4 oz water

Contraindications

Hypersensitivity, fecal impaction, intestinal obstruction, abdominal pain

Drug-Lab-Food Interactions

Drug: *Decrease* absorption of oral anticoagulants,
aspirin, digoxin, nitrofurantoin

Pharmacokinetics

Absorption: Not absorbed
Distribution: PB: UK
Metabolism: $t_{\frac{1}{2}}$: UK
Excretion: In feces

Pharmacodynamics

PO: Onset: 10–24 h
      Peak: 1–3 d
      Duration: UK

Therapeutic Effects/Uses

To control chronic constipation.

Mode of Action: Bulk-forming laxative by drawing water into the intestine.

Side Effects

Anorexia, nausea, vomiting, cramps,
diarrhea

Adverse Reactions

Esophageal and/or intestinal obstruction if not
taken with adequate water
Life-threatening: Bronchospasm, anaphylaxis

KEY: A: adult; C: child; PO: by mouth; >: greater than; UK: unknown; PB: protein-binding; $t_{\frac{1}{2}}$: half-life; ❦: Canadian drug name.

---

dyl. Mild cramping and diarrhea are side effects of bisacodyl.

Castor oil should not be used in early pregnancy because it stimulates uterine contraction. Spontaneous abortion may result. Prolonged use of senna can damage nerves, which may result in loss of intestinal muscular tone. Table 41–5 lists the osmotic and contact laxatives.

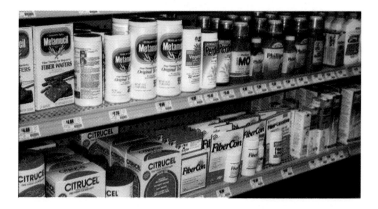

Figure 41-2
Various over-the-counter laxatives are available. The bulk-forming laxatives, such as Metamucil, Perdiem, Citrucel, and FiberCon, do not cause laxative dependence.

NURSING PROCESS
LAXATIVE: BULK FORMING

Assessment

- Obtain a history of constipation and possible causes such as insufficient water/fluid intake, diet deficient in bulk or fiber, or inactivity; a history of the frequency and consistency of stools; and the general health status.
- Obtain baseline vital signs (VS) for identification of abnormalities and for future comparisons.
- Assess renal function, urine output, blood urea nitrogen (BUN), and serum creatinine.

Potential Nursing Diagnoses

- Constipation
- Risk for fluid deficit

Planning

- Client will be free of constipation.
- Client will exercise, eat foods high in fiber, and have adequate fluid intake to avoid constipation.

Nursing Interventions

- Monitor fluid intake and output. Note signs and symptoms of fluid and electrolyte imbalances that may result from watery stools. Habitual use of laxatives can cause fluid volume deficit and electrolyte losses.
- Monitor bowel sounds.
- Identify the cause of constipation.
- Avoid inhalation of psyllium dust.

Client Teaching

General
- Instruct the client to mix drug with water immediately before use.
- Instruct the client to *not* swallow the drug in dry form.

Nursing Process continued on following page

BULK-FORMING LAXATIVES

Bulk-forming laxatives are natural fibrous substances that promote large, soft stools by absorbing water into the intestine, increasing fecal bulk and peristalsis. These agents are nonabsorbable. Defecation usually occurs within 8 to 24 h; however, it may take up to 3 d after drug therapy is started for the stool to be soft and well formed. Powdered bulk-forming laxatives, which sometimes come in flavored and sugar-free forms, should be mixed in a glass of water or juice, stirred, and drunk immediately, followed by a half to a full glass of water. Insufficient fluid intake can cause the drug to solidify in the GI tract, which can result in intestinal obstruction. This group of laxatives does not cause laxative dependence and may be used by clients with diverticulosis, irritable

bowel syndrome, and ileostomy and colostomy (Fig. 41–2).

Calcium polycarbophil (FiberCon), methylcellulose (Citrucel), fiber granules (Perdiem), and psyllium hydrophilic mucilloid (Metamucil) are examples of bulk-forming laxatives. Clients with hypercalcemia should avoid calcium polycarbophil because of the calcium in the drug. Chart 41–5 presents the bulk-forming laxative psyllium (Metamucil).

Pharmacokinetics

The bulk-forming laxative Metamucil is a nondigestible and nonabsorbent substance that, when mixed with water, becomes a viscous solution. Because it is not absorbed, there is no protein-binding or half-life for the drug. Metamucil is excreted in the feces.

NURSING PROCESS *Continued*
LAXATIVE: BULK FORMING

- Advise the client to avoid overuse of laxatives, which can lead to fluid and electrolyte imbalances and drug dependence. Suggest exercise to help increase peristalsis.
- Advise the client to avoid inhaling psyllium dust; it may cause watery eyes, runny nose, and wheezing.

Diet
- Instruct the client to increase water intake, which will decrease hard, dry stools. Drink at least eight 8-oz glasses of fluids per day.
- Instruct the client to mix the drug in 8 to 10 oz of water, stir, and drink immediately. At least one glass of extra water should follow. Insufficient water can cause the drug to solidify and lead to fecal impaction.
- Advise the client to increase foods rich in fiber such as bran, grains, and fruits.

Side Effects
- Instruct client to discontinue use if nausea, vomiting, cramping, or rectal bleeding occurs.

Cultural Considerations

- Respect the client's cultural beliefs and alternative methods for treating constipation. Give nonpharmacologic methods that might benefit the client.
- Provide additional explanation and written information as needed to clients from various cultural groups related to the use and abuse of laxatives.

Evaluation

- Evaluate the effectiveness of nonpharmacologic methods for alleviating constipation.
- Evaluate the client's use of laxatives in managing constipation. Identify laxative abuse.

Pharmacodynamics
The onset of action for Metamucil is 10 to 24 h. Peak action is 1 to 3 d. The duration of action is unknown.

Side Effects and Adverse Reactions
Bulk-forming laxatives are not systemically absorbed; therefore, there is no systemic effect. If bulk-forming laxatives are excessively used, nausea, vomiting, flatus, or diarrhea may occur. Abdominal cramps may occur if the drug is used in dry form.

EMOLLIENTS (SURFACTANTS)
Emollients are stool softeners (surface-acting drugs) and lubricants used to prevent constipation. These drugs decrease straining during defecation. Stool softeners work by lowering surface tension and promoting water accumulation in the intestine and stool. They are frequently prescribed for clients following myocardial infarction or surgery. They are also given prior to administration of other laxatives in treating fecal impaction. Docusate calcium (Surfak), docusate potassium (Dialose), docusate sodium (Colace), and docusate sodium with casanthranol (Peri-Colace) are examples of stool softeners.

Lubricants such as mineral oil increase water retention in the stool. Mineral oil absorbs essential fat-soluble vitamins A, D, E, and K. Some of the minerals can be absorbed into the lymphatic system.

Side Effects and Adverse Reactions
Side effects include nausea, vomiting, diarrhea, and abdominal cramping. This drug is not indicated for children, the elderly, or clients with debilitating diseases because they might aspirate the mineral oil, resulting in lipid pneumonia.

The docusate group of drugs may cause mild cramping.

Contraindications
Contraindications to the use of laxatives include inflammatory disorders of the GI tract, such as appendicitis, ulcerative colitis, undiagnosed severe pain that could be due to an inflammation of the intestine (diverticulitis, appendicitis), pregnancy, spastic colon, or bowel obstruction. Laxatives are contraindicated when any of these conditions is suspected.

Table 41–6 presents the drug data for the laxatives.

Table 41–6
Laxatives: Bulk Forming, Emollients, and Evacuants

GENERIC (BRAND)	ROUTE AND DOSAGE	USES AND CONSIDERATIONS
BULK FORMING		
Calcium polycarbophil (FiberCon, Fiberall, Mitrolan)	A: PO: 1 g, qid *max:* 6 g/d C 6–12 y: PO: 500 mg/d t.i.d.; *max:* 3 g C 2–5 y: PO: 500 mg/d b.i.d.; *max:* 1.5 g/d	Prevention of constipation. Also used to treat acute nonspecific diarrhea or diarrhea associated with irritable bowel syndrome. For diarrhea, it absorbs water and produces a formed stool. For constipation, chew tablet and follow with a full glass of water. *Pregnancy category:* C; PB: NA; $t\frac{1}{2}$: NA
Methylcellulose (Cologel, Citrucel)	A: PO: 5–20 mL t.i.d. in 8–10 oz water C: 5–10 mL b.i.d. with 8 oz water	For constipation. Effects are similar to Metamucil. Mix in at least 8 oz of water and take immediately. *Pregnancy category:* UK; PB: NA; $t\frac{1}{2}$: NA
Psyllium hydrophilic mucilloid (Metamucil)	See Chart 41–5	For preventing constipation. Dry fiber should be diluted in full glass of water and taken immediately to prevent solidification; follow with extra water. Insufficient water may cause bowel obstruction. Available as OTC with sugar or sugar-free. *Pregnancy category:* C; PB: UK; $t\frac{1}{2}$: UK
EMOLLIENT: STOOL SOFTENERS		
Docusate calcium (Surfak)	A: PO: 240 mg/d C: PO: 60–120 mg/d	Prevention of constipation. Softens the stool. Acts on the small and large intestines and has little absorption. When first used it may take 1–5 d for effectiveness. Available with calcium, potassium, or sodium. Drug should not be taken if CHF is present because of the sodium content. *Pregnancy category:* C; PB: NA; $t\frac{1}{2}$: NA
Docusate potassium (Dialose)	A: PO: 100–300 mg/d	
Docustate sodium (Colace)	A: PO: 50–300 mg/d C > 6 y: 40–120 mg/d	
Docusate sodium with casanthranol (Peri-Colace)	A: PO: 1–2 cap/d C: PO: 1 cap/d	For preventing constipation. Combination drug: docusate sodium 100 mg with casanthranol 30 mg. *Pregnancy category:* C; PB: NA; $t\frac{1}{2}$: NA
EMOLLIENT: LUBRICANT		
Mineral oil	A: PO: 15–45 mL/h.s. C 6–12 y: PO: 5–20 mL	Relief of constipation and fecal impaction. May be useful for those with cardiac disorder and following anorectal surgery. Avoid prolonged use because vitamins A, D, E, and K may be lost. *Pregnancy category:* UK; PB: NA; $t\frac{1}{2}$: NA
EVACUANT/BOWEL PREP		
Polyethylene glycol-electrolyte solution (Colyte, GoLYTELY)	Prep for GI exam requires 4 h; fasting for 3–4 h A: PO: 240 mL q10–15 min for total of 4 L C: PO: 25–40 mL/kg/h for 4–10 h Administer via NGT to those unable or unwilling to drink solution (prepared with tap water and refrigerated)	For bowel preparation before GI examination. *Pregnancy category:* C; PB: NA; $t\frac{1}{2}$: NA

KEY: *A: adult; C: child; PO: by mouth; UK: unknown; NA: not applicable; >: greater than; NGT: nasogastric tube; $t\frac{1}{2}$: half-life; OTC: over-the-counter; CHF: congestive heart failure; PB: protein-binding.*

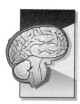

Critical Thinking in Action

C. S., 34 years old, has been vomiting for 48 hours. In the last 12 hours, C. S. has had diarrhea. Prochlorperazine (Compazine) 10 mg was administered intramuscularly.

1. What nonpharmacologic measures should the nurse suggest when vomiting occurs?
2. Why was C. S. given prochlorperazine intramuscularly and not orally or rectally? Prochlorperazine should be given deep intramuscularly. Why?
3. What electrolyte imbalances may occur as a result of vomiting and diarrhea? Explain how they can be replaced.
4. What are the side effects of prochlorperazine? May this occur to C. S.? Explain.
5. Could a serotonin antagonist be given to C. S. instead of prochlorperazine? Explain.

C. S. was prescribed diphenoxylate with atropine (Lomotil), 2.5 mg, t.i.d.

6. Is the Lomotil dosage for C. S. within the normal prescribed range? Explain.
7. What clinical conditions are contraindicated for the use of Lomotil?
8. What are some of the combination drugs that may be prescribed to control diarrhea? Give their advantages and disadvantages.
9. Name at least two over-the-counter (OTC) antidiarrheals and explain how frequently they should be administered.
10. Give an example of an adsorbent. Do you think C. S. should receive an adsorbent? Explain.

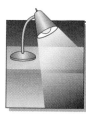

Study Questions

1. The client complains of motion sickness. What types of drugs might be suggested? What are the side effects?
2. Certain phenothiazines are prescribed for vomiting. What are the pharmacodynamics (actions)? Give examples of phenothiazine antiemetics.
3. What is ipecac syrup? How is it administered? For what conditions is ipecac contraindicated?
4. The client is taking paregoric for diarrhea. How does this drug differ from opium tincture? What type of antidiarrheal is paregoric?
5. Diphenoxylate (Lomotil) is what type of drug? What are the side effects?
6. What is the difference between laxatives and cathartics? What is the action of contact (irritant) laxatives? What are the side effects?
7. The client is taking a bulk-forming laxative. What instructions should you give?

42 Antiulcer Drugs

Outline

Objectives

- Identify the predisposing factors for peptic ulcers.
- Define peptic ulcer, gastric ulcer, and duodenal ulcer.
- Describe the actions of five groups of antiulcer drugs used in the treatment of peptic ulcer: tranquilizers, anticholinergics, antacids, histamine₂ blockers, proton pump inhibitors, and pepsin inhibitor.
- Identify at least two drugs from each of the following drug groups: anticholinergics, antacids, and H₂ blockers.
- Describe the side effects of anticholinergics and systemic and nonsystemic antacids.
- Describe the nursing process, with client teaching, related to antiulcer drugs.

Terms

antacids

duodenal ulcer

esophageal ulcer

gastric mucosal barrier (GMB)

gastric ulcer

histamine₂ receptor antagonists

hydrochloric acid

pepsin

peptic ulcer

stress ulcer

INTRODUCTION

Peptic ulcer is a broad term for an ulcer occurring in the esophagus, stomach, or duodenum within the upper gastrointestinal (GI) tract. The ulcers are more specifically named according to the site of involvement: esophageal, gastric, and duodenal ulcers. Duodenal ulcers occur 10 times more frequently than gastric and esophageal ulcers. The release of **hydrochloric acid** (HCl) from the parietal cells of the stomach is influenced by histamine, gastrin, and acetylcholine. Peptic ulcers are caused by hypersecretion of hydrochloric acid and pepsin, which erode the GI mucosal lining.

The gastric secretions in the stomach strive to maintain a pH of 2 to 5. **Pepsin,** a digestive enzyme, is activated at a pH of 2, and the acid-pepsin complex of gastric secretions can cause mucosal damage. If the pH of gastric secretion increases to pH 5, the activity of pepsin declines. The **gastric mucosal barrier** (GMB) is a thick, viscous, mucous material that provides a barrier between the mucosal lining and the acidic gastric secretions. The GMB maintains the integrity of the gastric mucosal lining and is a defense against corrosive substances. The two sphincter muscles—the cardiac, located at the upper portion of the stomach, and the pyloric, located at the lower portion of the stomach—act as barriers to prevent reflux of acid into the esophagus and the duodenum. Figure 42-1 illustrates common sites of peptic ulcers.

Esophageal ulcers result from reflux of acidic gastric secretion into the esophagus as a result of a defective or incompetent cardiac sphincter. **Duodenal**

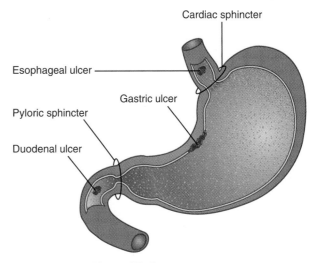

Figure 42-1
Common sites of peptic ulcers.

ulcers are caused by hypersecretion of acid from the stomach that passes to the duodenum because of (1) insufficient buffers to neutralize the gastric acid in the stomach, (2) a defective or incompetent pyloric sphincter, or (3) hypermotility of the stomach. **Gastric ulcers** frequently occur because of a breakdown of the GMB.

PREDISPOSING FACTORS IN PEPTIC ULCER DISEASE

The nurse needs to assist the client in identifying possible causes of the ulcer and to teach ways to

Table 42-1
Predisposing Factors in Peptic Ulcer Disease

PREDISPOSING FACTORS	EFFECTS
Mechanical disturbances	Hypersecretion of acid and pepsin. Inadequate GMB mucus secretion. Impaired GMB resistance. Hypermotility of the stomach. Incompetent (defective) cardiac or pyloric sphincter.
Genetic influences	Increased number of parietal cells in the stomach. Susceptibility of mucosal lining to acid penetration. Susceptibility to excess acetylcholine and histamine. Excess hydrochloric acid caused by external stimuli.
Environmental influences	Foods and liquids containing caffeine; fatty, fried, and highly spiced foods; alcohol. Nicotine products, including cigarettes. Stressful situations. Pregnancy, massive trauma, major surgery.
Helicobacter pylori (H. pylori)	A gram-negative bacterium, *H. pylori* infects the gastric mucosa and can cause gastritis, gastric ulcer, and duodenal ulcer. If the *H. pylori* is not eradicated, peptic ulcer may return as frequently as every year. *H. pylori* can lead to atropic gastritis in some clients. Serology and special breath tests can detect the presence of *H. pylori*.
Drugs	NSAIDs, including aspirin and aspirin compounds, ibuprofen (Motrin, Advil, Nuprin), and indomethacin (Indocin); corticosteroids (cortisone, prednisone); potassium salts; antineoplastic drugs.

KEY: GMB: gastric-mucosal barrier; NSAIDs: nonsteroidal antiinflammatory drugs.

alleviate them. Predisposing factors include mechanical disturbances, genetic influences, bacterial organisms, environmental factors, and certain drugs. Healing of an ulcer takes 4 to 8 weeks. Complications can occur as the result of scar tissue. Table 42–1 lists the predisposing factors for peptic ulcers and their effects.

The classic symptom of peptic ulcers is gnawing, aching pain. With a gastric ulcer, pain occurs 30 min to 1½ h after eating, and with a duodenal ulcer, 2 to 3 h after eating. Small, frequent meals of nonirritating foods decrease the pain. With treatment, pain usually subsides in 10 days; however, the healing process takes 1 to 2 months.

A **stress ulcer** usually follows a critical situation such as extensive trauma or major surgery (e.g., burns, cardiac surgery). Prophylactic use of antiulcer drugs decreases the incidence of stress ulcers.

Helicobacter pylori

Helicobacter pylori (H. pylori), a gram-negative bacillus, is linked with the development of peptic ulcer. *H.*

pylori is known to cause gastritis, gastric ulcer, and duodenal ulcer. When a peptic ulcer recurs after antiulcer therapy, and the ulcer is not caused by nonsteroidal antiinflammatory drugs (NSAIDs) such as aspirin or ibuprofen, the client should be tested for the presence of the bacterium *H. pylori,* which may have infected the gastric mucosa. In the past, endoscopy and a biopsy of the gastric antrum would be needed to check for *H. pylori.* Currently, a noninvasive breath test, the Meretek UBT, can detect *H. pylori.* This test consists of drinking a liquid containing ^{13}C urea and breathing into a container. If *H. pylori* is present, the bacterial urease hydrolyzes the urea, releasing $^{13}CO_2$, which is detected by a spectrometer. This test is 90% to 95% effective for detecting *H. pylori.* Also, a serology test may be performed to check for antibodies of *H. pylori.*

There are various protocols for treating *H. pylori* infection. Antibacterial agents are the choice for treating *H. pylori.* One antibacterial agent is not effective for eradicating *H. pylori,* because the bacterium can readily become resistent to the drug. Treatment to

Table 42–2
Various Regimens Used for the Eradication of *Helicobacter pylori*

TYPE OF THERAPY	DRUGS	TREATMENT DURATION	ERADICATION RATE
Dual therapy	Ranitidine bismuth citrate, 400 mg b.i.d. Clarithromycin, 500 mg t.i.d.	2–4 wk	82%
	Omeprazole, 40 mg/d. Clarithromycin, 500 mg t.i.d.	2–4 wk	64–82%
	Lansoprazole, 30 mg b.i.d. Clarithromycin, 400 mg b.i.d.	14 d	72%
Triple therapy	Colloidal bismuth subcitrate, 120 mg q.i.d. Metronidazole, 250 mg q.i.d. Tetracycline, 250 mg q.i.d. OR tetracycline, 500 mg q.i.d.	14 d 7 d	96% 83%
	Bismuth subsalicylate, 300 mg q.i.d. Metronidazole, 500 mg t.i.d. Amoxicillin, 500 mg t.i.d. OR Bismuth with clarithromycin, 500 mg t.i.d. Tetracycline, 500 mg q.i.d.	14 d 14 d	84% 93%
	Metronidazole, 500 mg b.i.d. OR amoxicillin, 1 g b.i.d. Omeprazole, 20 mg b.i.d. OR lansoprazole, 30 mg b.i.d. Clarithromycin, 500 mg b.i.d. Combinations of: Metronidazole, omeprazole, clarithromycin Metronidazole, omeprazole, amoxicillin Lansoprazole, clarithromycin, and metronidazole Lansoprazole, amoxicillin, and clarithromycin Omeprazole, amoxicillin, clarithromycin	7–14 d	>90%
Quadruple therapy	Colloidal bismuth subcitrate, 120 mg q.i.d. Tetracycline, 500 mg q.i.d. Metronidazole, 500 mg t.i.d. Omeprazole, 20 mg b.i.d. Other combinations may be used	7 d	98%

eradicate this bacterial infection includes using a dual, triple, or quadruple drug therapy program in a variety of combination of drugs such as amoxicillin, tetracycline, clarithromycin (Biaxin), omeprazole (Prilosec), lansoprazole (Prevacid), metronidazole (Flagyl), bismuth subsalicylate (Pepto-Bismol), and ranitidine bismuth citrate (Tritec) on a 7- to 14-day treatment plan. The combination of drugs differs for each client according to the client's drug tolerance. A common treatment protocol is the triple therapy of metronidazole (or amoxicillin), omeprazole (or lansoprazole), and clarithromycin (MOC). The drug regimen eradicates more than 90% of peptic ulcer caused by *H. pylori.*

One of the proton pump inhibitors (PPIs), omeprazole or lansoprazole, is frequently used as one of the combination drugs because each suppresses the acid secretion by inhibiting the enzyme hydrogen/potassium ATPase, which makes gastric acid. These agents block the final steps of acid production. If triple therapy fails to eradicate *H. pylori*, then the quadruple therapy using two antibiotics, a proton pump inhibitor, and a bismuth or H_2 blocker is recommended. After completion of the treatment regimen, 6 weeks of standard acid suppression, such as histamine$_2$ blocker therapy, has been recommended. Table 42–2 lists various combinations of treatment regimens for

eradicating *H. pylori* and Table 42–3 lists data for the drugs used in treating *H. pylori.*

Gastroesophageal Reflux Disease

In the United States, 40% to 44% of adults have heartburn, which in many cases is due to gastroesophageal reflux disease (GERD).

GERD, also called reflux esophagitis, is inflammation of the esophageal mucosa caused by a reflux of gastric acid content into the esophagus. Its main cause is an incompetent lower esophageal sphincter. Smoking and obesity tend to accelerate the disease process.

The medical treatment for GERD is similar to the treatment for peptic ulcers, which includes the use of the common antiulcer drugs to neutralize gastric contents and to reduce gastric acid secretion, such as proton pump inhibitors (PPIs) including omeprazole (Prilosec) and lansoprazole (Prevacid), and histamine$_2$ (H_2) blocker, such as ranitidine (Zantac). The proton pump inhibitor relieves symptoms faster and maintains healing better than does the H_2 blocker. Once the strictures are relieved by dilation, they are less likely to recur if the the client was taking PPIs rather than receiving an H_2 blocker.

GERD is a chronic disorder that requires continu-

Table 42–3
Pharmacologic Agents for Treatment of *Helicobacter pylori*

GENERIC (BRAND)	ROUTE AND DOSAGE	USES AND CONSIDERATIONS
ANTIINFECTIVE AGENTS		
Metronidazole HCl (Flagyl, Protostat)	A: PO: 250–500 mg b.i.d., t.i.d., q.i.d.	To treat numerous organisms including *H. pylori.* It is used in combination with other drugs for the treatment of *H. pylori*
Amoxicillin (Amoxil)	A: PO: 500 mg t.i.d.	Used in the triple or quadruple therapy for *H. pylori*
Clarithromycin (Biaxin)	A: PO: 500 mg b.i.d.–t.i.d.	Used in the dual and triple therapy for *H. pylori*
Tetracycline	A: PO: 500 mg q.i.d.	Used in the triple and quadruple therapy for *H. pylori*
PROTON PUMP INHIBITORS (PPIs)		
Omeprazole (Prilosec)	A: PO: 20 mg/d. or 40 mg/d.	Used in dual, triple, and quadruple therapy for *H. pylori*
Lansoprazole (Prevacid)	A: PO: 30 mg b.i.d.	Used in dual and triple therapy for *H. pylori*
ANTACIDS		
Bismuth subsalicylate	A: PO: 300 mg q.i.d.	Used in combination with other drugs for the treatment of *H. pylori*
Colloidal bismuth sub-citrate	A: PO: 120 mg q.i.d.	Used in combination with other drugs for the treatment of *H. pylori*
Ranitidine bismuth citrate (Tritec)	A: PO: 400 mg b.i.d.	Used in combination with other drugs for the treatment of *H. pylori*

ous management. The purpose is to keep the esophageal mucosa healed and the client free of symptoms.

NONPHARMACOLOGIC MEASURES FOR MANAGING PEPTIC ULCER AND GASTROESOPHAGEAL REFLUX DISEASE

With a GI disorder, nonpharmacologic measures, along with drug therapy, are an important part of the treatment. Once the GI problem is resolved, the client should continue to follow nonpharmacologic measures in order to avoid recurrence of the GI disorder.

Avoiding smoking and alcohol can decrease gastric secretions. With GERD, nicotine relaxes the lower esophageal sphincter, thus permitting gastric acid reflux. Obesity enhances the problem of GERD. Weight loss is helpful in decreasing symptoms. The client should avoid hot, spicy, and greasy foods, which could aggravate the gastric problem. Nonsteroidal antiinflammatory drugs (NSAIDs), which include aspirin, should be taken with food or in a decreased dosage. Glucocorticoids can cause gastric ulceration, and food should be taken with these drugs.

To relieve symptoms of GERD, the client should raise the head of his or her bed, not eat before bedtime, and wear loose-fitting clothing.

ANTIULCER DRUGS

There are eight groups of antiulcer agents: (1) tranquilizers, which decrease vagal activity; (2) anticholinergic drugs, which decrease acetylcholine by blocking the cholinergic receptors; (3) antacids, which neutralize gastric acid; (4) histamine$_2$ (H$_2$) blockers, which block the histamine$_2$ receptor; (5) the proton pump inhibitors, which inhibit gastric acid secretion regardless of acetylcholine or histamine release; (6) the pepsin inhibitor sucralfate; (7) the prostaglandin E$_1$ analogue misoprostol, which inhibits gastric acid secretion and protects the mucosa; and (8) GI stimulants such as cisapride (Propulsid), which increase the lower esophagus sphincter pressure and lower esophagus peristalsis. Figure 42–2 illustrates the action of the eight antiulcer drug groups, each of which is discussed separately.

Tranquilizers

Tranquilizers have minimal effect in preventing and treating ulcers; they reduce vagal stimulation and decrease anxiety. Librax, a combination of the anxiolytic

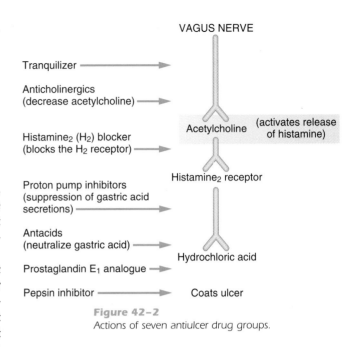

Figure 42–2
Actions of seven antiulcer drug groups.

chlordiazepoxide (Librium) and the anticholinergic clidinium (Quarzan), is used in the treatment of ulcers.

Anticholinergics

Anticholinergics (antimuscarinics, parasympatholytics) and antacids were for many years the drugs of choice for peptic ulcers. However, with the introduction of histamine$_2$ blockers in 1975, anticholinergic use has declined. These drugs relieve pain by decreasing GI motility and secretion; they act by inhibiting acetylcholine and blocking histamine and hydrochloric acid. Anticholinergics delay gastric emptying time, so they are used more frequently for duodenal ulcers than for gastric ulcers. An anticholinergic, pirenzepine (Gastrozepine), available in Canada, inhibits gastric secretions and does not cause tachycardia or decrease GI motility. Its action is selective for gastric acid secretory cells.

Anticholinergics should be taken before meals to decrease the acid secretion that occurs with eating. Antacids can slow the absorption of anticholinergics and should therefore be taken 2 h after anticholinergic administration.

Table 42–4 lists selected anticholinergic drugs that are used in the treatment of peptic ulcer. Anticholinergics should be used as adjunctive therapy and not as the only antiulcer drug. Anticholinergics are discussed in more detail in Chapter 22.

SIDE EFFECTS AND ADVERSE REACTIONS

Anticholinergics have many side effects, including dry mouth, decreased secretions, tachycardia, urinary

Table 42–4
Antiulcer: Anticholinergics

GENERIC (BRAND)	ROUTE AND DOSAGE	USES AND CONSIDERATIONS
Belladonna tincture	A: PO: 0.3–1 mL t.i.d.–q.i.d.	For peptic ulcers; decreases gastric secretions. Contraindicated in narrow-angle glaucoma, myasthenia gravis, paralytic ileus, urinary retention. Dry mouth and constipation can occur. *Pregnancy category:* C; PB: UK; $t_{\frac{1}{2}}$: 18–36 h
Clidinium bromide and chlordiazepoxide HCl (Librax)	A: PO: 1–2 cap t.i.d.–q.i.d. a.c., h.s.	Decreases anxiety and GI distress. Contains a benzodiazepine. *Pregnancy category:* C; PB: UK; $t_{\frac{1}{2}}$: UK
Glycopyrrolate (Robinul)	A: PO: 1 mg b.i.d.–t.i.d. IM/IV: 0.1–0.2 mg (100–200 μg) t.i.d.–q.i.d.	For peptic ulcers and gastric disorder due to hyperacidity. Used as one of the preanesthetic drugs. Same contraindications as belladonna. *Pregnancy category:* B; PB: UK; $t_{\frac{1}{2}}$: UK
Pirenzepine (Gastrozepine)	A: PO: 50 mg b.i.d.–t.i.d.	For peptic ulcers. It blocks the muscarinic receptors that regulate gastric acid secretion without causing severe anticholinergic side effects. *Pregnancy category:* UK; PB: UK; $t_{\frac{1}{2}}$: 10 h
Propantheline bromine (Pro-Banthine)	A: PO: 15 mg t.i.d. 30 min a.c. and 30 mg h.s.	For peptic ulcers; decreases gastric secretions, irritable bowel syndrome, pancreatitis, and urinary bladder spasm. Standard anticholinergic side effects. *Pregnancy category:* C; PB: UK; $t_{\frac{1}{2}}$: 9 h
Tridihexethyl chloride (Pathilon)	A: PO: 25–50 mg t.i.d.–q.i.d. a.c. and h.s.	For peptic ulcers; decreases gastric secretions. *Pregnancy category:* C; PB: UK; $t_{\frac{1}{2}}$: UK

KEY: A: adult; PO: by mouth; a.c.: before meals; h.s.: hour of sleep; UK: unknown; PB: protein-binding; $t_{\frac{1}{2}}$: half-life.

retention, and constipation. Because anticholinergics decrease GI motility, the gastric emptying time is delayed, which can stimulate gastric secretions and aggravate the ulceration.

Antacids

Antacids promote ulcer healing by neutralizing hydrochloric acid and reducing pepsin activity; they do not coat the ulcer. There are two types of antacids: those that have a systemic effect and those that have a nonsystemic effect.

Sodium bicarbonate, a systemically absorbed antacid, was one of the first antiulcer drugs. Because it has many side effects (sodium excess, causing hypernatremia and water retention; metabolic alkalosis caused by the excess bicarbonate; and acid rebound [excess acid secretion]), sodium bicarbonate is seldom used for treating peptic ulcers. Examples of sodium bicarbonate compounds are Bromo-Seltzer and Alka-Seltzer.

Calcium carbonate is most effective in neutralizing acid; however, 1/3 to 1/2 of the drug can be systemically absorbed and cause acid rebound. Hypercalcemia and "milk-alkali syndrome" can result from ex-

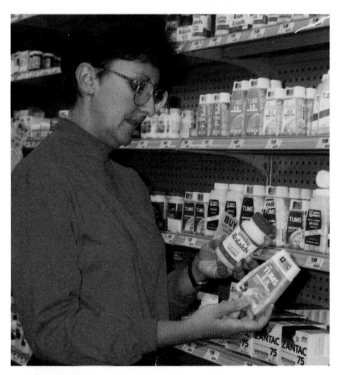

Figure 42–3
Numerous over-the-counter antacids are available. This client is deciding which of these antacids would best help her "upset stomach."

Chart 42-1. Antiulcer: Antacids

ANTACID

Drug Name	**Dosage**
Aluminum hydroxide (Amphojel, ALternaGEL, Alu-Tab) *Pregnancy Category:* C	*Antacid:* A: PO: 600 mg 1 h p.c. and h.s.; chewed with water or milk Susp: 5–10 mL 1 h p.c. and h.s. *Hyperphosphatemia:* A: PO: 2 cap or 12.5 mL t.i.d.–q.i.d. with meals
Contraindications	**Drug-Lab-Food Interactions**
Hypersensitivity to aluminum products, hypophosphatemia **Caution:** In elderly	**Drug:** *Decrease* effects with tetracycline, phenothiazine, isoniazid, phenytoin, digitalis, quinidine, amphetamines; may *increase* effect of benzodiazepines **Lab:** *Increase* urine pH
Pharmacokinetics	**Pharmacodynamics**

Absorption: PO: Small amount absorbed
Distribution: PB: UK
Metabolism: t½: UK
Excretion: In feces; small amount in urine
	PO: Onset: 15–30 min
	      Peak: 0.5 h
	      Duration: 1–3 h

Therapeutic Effects/Uses

To treat hyperacidity, peptic ulcer, and reflux esophagitis; to reduce hyperphosphatemia.

Mode of Action: Neutralization of gastric acidity.

Side Effects	**Adverse Reactions**
Constipation	Hypophosphatemia; long term: GI obstruction

Nursing Process labels (right margin): Assessment and Planning; Interventions; Evaluation; NURSING PROCESS

KEY: A: adult; PO: by mouth; UK: unknown; PB: protein-binding; t½: half-life; p.c.: after meals; h.s.: at bedtime.

cessive use of calcium carbonate. Milk-alkali syndrome is intensified if milk products are ingested with calcium carbonate. It is identified by the presence of alkalosis, hypercalcemia, and, in severe cases, crystalluria and renal failure.

The nonsystemic antacids are composed of alkaline salts such as aluminum (aluminum hydroxide, aluminum carbonate) and magnesium (magnesium hydroxide, magnesium carbonate, magnesium trisilicate, and magnesium phosphate). There is a small degree of systemic absorption with these drugs, mainly of aluminum. Magnesium hydroxide has greater neutralizing power than aluminum hydroxide. Magnesium compounds can cause diarrhea, and aluminum and calcium compounds can cause constipation with long-term use. A combination of magnesium and aluminum salts neutralizes gastric acid without causing constipation or severe diarrhea. Simethicone (an anti-gas agent) is found in many antacids, including Mylanta II, Maalox Plus, and Gelusil II (Fig 42–3).

Chart 42–1 gives the drug data for the aluminum hydroxide antacid (Amphojel).

PHARMACOKINETICS

Aluminum hydroxide (Amphojel) was one of the first antacids used for neutralizing hydrochloric acid. Aluminum products are frequently used to lower high serum phosphate (hyperphosphatemia). Because aluminum hydroxide alone can cause constipation and magnesium products alone can cause diarrhea, combination drugs, such as aluminum hydroxide and magnesium hydroxide (Maalox), have become popular.

Only a very small amount of Amphojel is absorbed from the GI tract. It is primarily bound to phosphate and excreted in the feces. The small portion that is absorbed is excreted in the urine.

Table 42–5
Antiulcers: Antacids

GENERIC (BRAND)	ROUTE AND DOSAGE	USES AND CONSIDERATIONS
Aluminum carbonate (Basaljel)	A: PO: 10–30 mL or 2 tab/cap q2h Extra strength 5–15 mL	To alleviate gastric hyperacidity related to gastritis, gastric and duodenal ulcers, esophageal reflux, and hiatal hernia. Increases gastric pH and inhibits pepsin activity. Also is used to decrease hyperphosphatemia for clients with renal dysfunction. Duration of action is 2 to 3 h when taken 1 h after meals. *Pregnancy category:* C; PB: UK; $t_{\frac{1}{2}}$: UK
Aluminum hydroxide (Amphojel, ALternaGEL)	A: PO: 30 mL, 1–3 h p.c. and h.s. *Peptic ulcer disease:* A: PO: 15–45 mL, 1–3 h p.c. and h.s. C: PO: 5–15 mL, 1–3 h p.c. and h.s. *Prophylaxis GI bleeding:* A: PO: 30–60 mL, qh C: PO: 5–15 mL, q1–2h; maintain gastric pH >5	Same as aluminum carbonate. Constipation can occur. *Pregnancy category:* C; PB: UK; $t_{\frac{1}{2}}$: UK
Calcium carbonate (Tums, Dicarbosil)	A: PO: 2 tab or 10 mL q2h; *max:* 12 doses/d	To alleviate heartburn, acid indigestion, esophagitis, and hiatal hernia due to hyperacidity. Also to treat hyperphosphatemia for clients with renal disorders. OTC drug. One-third of the drug dose is absorbed from GI tract. Constipation can be a problem. *Pregnancy category:* C; PB: UK; $t_{\frac{1}{2}}$: UK
Dihydroxyaluminum sodium carbonate (Rolaids Antacid)	A: PO: Chew 1–2 tab PRN	Similar to calcium carbonate except it contains sodium instead of calcium. *Pregnancy category:* C; PB: UK; $t_{\frac{1}{2}}$: UK
Magaldrate (Riopan, Lowsium [plus simethicone])	A: PO: 5–15 mL, PRN; *max:* 100 mL/d; or 1–2 tab PRN; *max:* 20 tab/d	To alleviate heartburn, gastritis, esophagitis, peptic ulcers due to hyperacidity. Contains aluminum and magnesium hydroxide. Low sodium content. Simethicone decreases flatus. Drug is minimally absorbed. *Pregnancy category:* C; PB: UK; $t_{\frac{1}{2}}$: UK
Magnesium hydroxide and aluminum hydroxide (Maalox)	A: PO: 2–4 tab PRN; *max:* 16 tab/d or 10–30 mL, 1–3 h p.c. and h.s.	Same as magaldrate. Caution for clients with renal disorder due to the magnesium content. OTC drug. *Pregnancy category:* UK; PB: UK; $t_{\frac{1}{2}}$: UK
Magnesium hydroxide, aluminum hydroxide, and calcium carbonate (Camalox)	A: PO: 10–20 mL, PRN; *max:* 80 mL/d; or 2–4 tab PRN; *max:* 16 tab	Same as magaldrate except it also contains calcium. *Pregnancy category:* UK; PB: UK; $t_{\frac{1}{2}}$: UK
Magnesium hydroxide and aluminum hydroxide with simethicone (Aludrox, Mylanta, Mylanta III, Maalox Plus, Gelusil-I, Gelusil-II, Gelusil-M, Di-Gel)	A: PO: 10–20 mL, PRN; *max:* 120 mL/d; or 2–4 tab PRN; *max:* 24 tab	Same as magaldrate. It also contains simethicone, which decreases flatus. OTC drug. *Pregnancy category:* UK; PB: UK; $t_{\frac{1}{2}}$: UK
Magnesium trisilicate (Gaviscon)	A: PO: 1–2 tab PRN; *max:* 8 tab/d	To relieve gastric disorders due to hyperacidity. OTC drug. Contains magnesium trisilicate and aluminum hydroxide. *Pregnancy category:* UK; PB: UK; $t_{\frac{1}{2}}$: UK
Sodium bicarbonate	A: PO: 0.5 tsp of powder in 8 oz water	Previously used for gastric hyperacidity. It is a short-acting, potent antacid that is systemically absorbed. Acid-base imbalance could occur. *Pregnancy category:* C; PB: UK; $t_{\frac{1}{2}}$: UK

KEY: *A: adult; C: child; PO: by mouth; PB: protein-binding; $t_{\frac{1}{2}}$: half-life; PRN: as necessary; >: greater than; OTC: over-the-counter; UK: unknown.*

NURSING PROCESS
ANTIULCER: ANTACIDS

Assessment

- Assess the client's pain, including the type, duration, severity, and frequency.
- Assess the client's renal function.
- Assess for fluid and electrolyte imbalances, especially serum phosphate and calcium levels.
- Obtain drug history; report probable drug-drug interactions.

Potential Nursing Diagnoses

- Pain
- Knowledge deficit related to (mis)use of antacids

Planning

- Client will be free of abdominal pain after 1 to 2 wk of antiulcer drug management.

Nursing Interventions

- Avoid administering antacids with other oral drugs, because antacids can delay their absorption. An antacid should definitely not be given with tetracycline, digoxin, or quinidine because it binds with and inactivates most of the drug. Antacids are given 1 to 2 h after other medications.
- Shake suspension well before administering: follow with water.
- Monitor urinary pH, calcium, and phosphate levels, and electrolytes.

Client Teaching

General
- Instruct the client to report pain, coughing, or vomiting of blood.
- Encourage client to drink 1 oz of water after antacid to ensure that the drug reaches the stomach.
- Advise the client to take the antacid 1 to 3 h after meals and at bedtime. Do not take antacids at mealtime; they slow gastric emptying time, causing increased GI activity and gastric secretions.

Nursing Process continued on following page

PHARMACODYNAMICS

Amphojel neutralizes gastric acid, including hydrochloric acid, and increases the pH of gastric secretions (an elevated pH inactivates pepsin). The onset of action is fairly rapid, but the duration of action varies depending on whether the antacid is taken with or without food. If the antacid is taken after a meal, the duration of action may be up to 3 h because food delays gastric emptying time. Frequent dosing may be necessary if the antacid is given during a fasting state or early in the course of treatment.

The ideal dosing interval for antacids is 1 and 3 h after meals (maximum acid secretion occurs after eating) and at bedtime. Antacids taken on an empty stomach are effective for 30 to 60 min before passing into the duodenum. Chewable tablets should be followed by water. Liquid antacids should also be taken with water (2 to 4 oz) to ensure that the drug reaches the stomach; however, no more than 4 oz of water should be taken, because water quickens gastric emptying time.

The dosage for antacids is determined according to the health care provider's order or the directions on the drug label (1 to 2 tsp or 5 to 10 mL). Overuse or overdosing can result in side effects and some systemic absorption. Table 42–5 lists the drug data for antacids.

Antacids containing magnesium salts are contraindicated in clients with impaired renal function because of the risk of hypermagnesemia. Prolonged use of aluminum hydroxides can cause hypophosphatemia (low serum phosphate). If hyperphosphatemia

ANTIULCER: ANTACIDS

- Advise the client to notify the health care provider if constipation or diarrhea occurs; the antacid may have to be changed. Self-treatment should be avoided.
- Stress that antacids are not candy and that an unlimited amount is contraindicated.
- Advise the client to avoid taking acids with milk or foods high in vitamin D.
- Instruct the client to avoid taking antacids within 1 to 2 h of other oral medications because there may be interference with absorption.
- Advise the client to check antacid labels for sodium content if on a sodium-restricted diet.
- Alert the client to consult with the health care provider before taking self-prescribed antacids for longer than 2 wk.
- Instruct the client on the use of relaxation techniques.

Self-Administration
- Instruct the client how to take antacids correctly. Chewable tablets should be thoroughly chewed and followed with water. With liquid antacid, 2 to 4 oz of water should follow the antacid.

Side Effects
- Advise the client to avoid foods and liquids that can cause gastric irritation, such as caffeine-containing beverages, alcohol, and spices.
- Advise the client that stools may become speckled or white.

Cultural Considerations

- Respect the client's cultural beliefs and alternative methods for treating gastrointestinal discomfort. Discuss with the client the safety of his or her methods and the use of drugs prescribed to heal and lessen the symptoms.
- Recognize that clients of various cultural backgrounds may need guidance in understanding the disease process of their GI disturbance. Use of a written plan of care with modification should be considered.

Evaluation

- Determine the effectiveness of the antiulcer treatment and the presence of side effects. The client should be free of pain, and healing should be progressing.

occurs because of poor renal function, aluminum hydroxide can be given to decrease the phosphate level. In clients with renal insufficiency, aluminum salt ingestion can cause encephalopathy from accumulation of aluminum in the brain.

Histamine₂ Blockers

The **histamine₂** (H₂) blockers (histamine₂ receptor antagonists) are the most popular drugs used in the treatment of gastric and duodenal ulcers. H₂ blockers prevent acid reflux in the esophagus (reflux esophagitis). These drugs block the H₂ receptors of the parietal cells in the stomach, thus reducing gastric acid secretion and concentration. Antihistamines, used to treat allergic conditions, act against histamine₁ (H₁); they are not the same as H₂ blockers.

The first H₂ blocker was cimetidine (Tagamet), introduced in 1975. Cimetidine, which has a short half-life and a short duration of action, blocks about 70% of acid secretion for 4 h. Good kidney function is necessary, because approximately 50% to 80% of the drug is excreted unchanged in the urine. If renal insufficiency is present, cimetidine dose and frequency may need to be reduced. Antacids can be given an hour before or after cimetidine as part of the antiulcer drug regimen; however, if they are given at the same time, they decrease the effectiveness of the H₂ blocker.

Three H₂ blockers, ranitidine (Zantac, 1983), famotidine (Pepcid, 1986), and nizatidine (Axid, 1988), are more potent than cimetidine. In addition to blocking gastric acid secretions, they also promote healing of the ulcer by eliminating its cause. Their duration of action is longer, thus decreasing the frequency of dosing, and they have fewer side effects and fewer drug interactions than cimetidine. Chart 42–2 gives the pharmacologic data for ranitidine (Zantac), the most popular H₂ blocker.

Chart 42–2. Antiulcer: Histamine₂ Blockers

HISTAMINE₂ BLOCKER

Drug Name	**Dosage**
Ranitidine (Zantac) *Pregnancy Category:* B	A: PO: 150 mg q12h or 300 mg h.s.; maint: 300 mg h.s. IM: 500 mg q6–8h IV: 50 mg q6–8h diluted C: PO: 2–4 mg/kg/d divided q12h IV: 1–2 mg/kg/d divided q6–8h

Contraindications

Hypersensitivity, severe renal or liver disease
Caution: Pregnancy, lactation

Drug-Lab-Food Interactions

Drug: *Decrease* absorption with antacids; *decrease* absorption of ketoconazole; *toxicity* with metoprolol
Lab: *Increase* serum alkaline phosphatase

Pharmacokinetics

Absorption: PO: Well absorbed, 50%
Distribution: PB: 15%
Metabolism: $t\frac{1}{2}$: 2–3 h
Excretion: In urine and feces

Pharmacodynamics

PO: Onset: 15 min
      Peak: 1–3 h
      Duration: 8–12 h

IM/IV: Onset: 10–15 min
      Peak: 15 min
      Duration: 8–12 h

Therapeutic Effects/Uses

To prevent and treat peptic ulcers, gastroesophageal reflux, and stress ulcers.

Mode of Action: Inhibition of gastric acid secretion by inhibiting histamine at histamine₂ receptors in parietal cells.

Side Effects

Headache, confusion, nausea, vertigo, diarrhea or constipation, depression, rash, blurred vision, malaise

Adverse Reactions

Life-threatening: Hepatotoxicity, cardiac dysrhythmias, blood dyscrasias

Assessment and Planning · *Interventions* · *Evaluation* — **NURSING PROCESS**

KEY: A: adult; C: child; PO: by mouth; IM: intramuscular; IV: intravenous; PB: protein-binding; $t\frac{1}{2}$: half-life; h.s.: at bedtime.

PHARMACOKINETICS

Ranitidine is 5 to 12 times more potent than cimetidine; however, it is less potent than famotidine. It is rapidly absorbed and reaches its peak concentration after a single dose in 1 to 3 h. Ranitidine has a low protein-binding power and a short half-life. With liver disease, the half-life of ranitidine is prolonged. About 50% of the absorbed drug is excreted unchanged in the urine.

Ulcer healing occurs in 4 weeks for 70% of clients and in 8 weeks for 90% of clients taking ranitidine. Large doses of ranitidine are effective for controlling Zollinger-Ellison syndrome, whereas cimetidine is not effective in controlling the symptoms of this disorder.

PHARMACODYNAMICS

Ranitidine inhibits histamine at the H₂ receptor site. The drug is effective in treating gastric and duodenal ulcers and can be used prophylactically. It is also useful in relieving symptoms of reflux esophagitis, preventing stress ulcers that can occur following major surgery, and preventing aspiration pneumonitis that can result from aspiration of gastric acid secretions.

Table 42–6
Antiulcers: Histamine₂ Blockers

GENERIC (BRAND)	ROUTE AND DOSAGE	USES AND CONSIDERATIONS
Cimetidine (Tagamet)	A: PO: 300 mg q.i.d. with meals and h.s. or 800 mg h.s.; maint: 300 mg h.s. IV: 300 mg q6–8h diluted in 50 mL (administered over 15–30 min) IV: continuous infusion: 37.5 mg/h over 24 h; *max:* 900 mg/d C: PO/IV: 10–40 mg/kg/d divided q6h	For peptic ulcers (gastric and duodenal). The first H_2 blocker marketed. Has many drug interaction and side effects. Duration of action is 4–6 h. *Pregnancy category:* B; PB: 20%; $t_{\frac{1}{2}}$: 2 h
Famotidine (Pepcid)	A: PO: 20 mg q12h or 40 mg h.s.; maint: 20 mg h.s. IV: 20 mg q12h diluted C: PO: 1 mg/kg/d divided q8–12h C: IV: 0.6–0.8 mg/kg/d divided q8–12h	For treatment of active duodenal ulcer. Inhibits gastric secretion. More potent than cimetidine. *Pregnancy category:* B; PB: 15%–20%; $t_{\frac{1}{2}}$: 2.5–4 h
Nizatidine (Axid)	A: PO: 150 mg q12h or 300 mg h.s.; maint: 150 mg h.s.	Same as famotidine. Also to treat gastroesophageal reflux. Give drug after meals or at bedtime. Do not give within 1 h of antacids. *Pregnancy category:* B; PB: 35%; $t_{\frac{1}{2}}$: 1–2 h
Ranitidine (Zantac)	See Chart 42–2	Commonly prescribed H_2 blocker. To treat peptic ulcers (gastric and duodenal) and gastroesophageal reflux disease (GERD). Administer after meals or at bedtime. Do not give within 1 h of antacids. If creatinine clearance is <50 mL/min, dose should be decreased. Drug is more potent than cimetidine. *Pregnancy category:* B; PB: 15%; $t_{\frac{1}{2}}$: 2–3 h

KEY: A: adult; C: child; h.s.: hour of sleep; IV: intravenous; PB: protein-binding; PO: by mouth; $t_{\frac{1}{2}}$: half-life; <: less than.

Ranitidine has a longer onset of action and duration of action (up to 12 h) than cimetidine. Because cimetidine has a duration of action of only 4 to 5 h, it is frequently given three to four times a day.

Cimetidine increases the effects of theophylline, beta blockers, oral anticoagulants, anticonvulsants (phenytoin), diazepam (Valium), and the antidysrhythmics. Cimetidine can cause an increase in blood urea nitrogen (BUN), serum creatinine, and serum alkaline phosphatase. Neither cimetidine nor ranitidine should be taken with antacids because their H_2 blocking action could be decreased. Ranitidine can increase the effect of oral anticoagulants.

Famotidine is 50% to 80% more potent than cimetidine and is five to eight times more potent than ranitidine. It is indicated for short-term use (4 to 8 weeks) for duodenal ulcer and for Zollinger-Ellison syndrome.

Nizatidine (Axid) is the latest H_2 blocker. It can relieve noctural gastric acid secretion for 12 hours. This drug is similar to famotidine and ranitidine, and neither of these agents suppress the metabolism of other drugs. The dosage for prevention of recurrence of duodenal uclers for nizatidine is 150 mg per day at bedtime and for famotidine is 20 mg per day at bedtime. Both nizatidine and famotidine have similar protein-binding times and half-life. Table 42–6 lists the H_2 blockers, their dosages, and uses and considerations.

SIDE EFFECTS AND ADVERSE REACTIONS

Side effects and adverse reactions of H_2 blockers include headaches, dizziness, constipation, pruritus, skin rash, gynecomastia, decreased libido, and impotence.

DRUG INTERACTIONS

Cimetidine interacts with many drugs. By inhibiting hepatic drug metabolism, it enhances the effects of oral anticoagulants, theophylline, caffeine, phenytoin (Dilantin), diazepam (Valium), propranolol (Inderal), phenobarbital, and calcium channel blockers. Ranitidine and famotidine have fewer side effects than cimetidine. Table 42–6 lists the drug data for the H_2 blockers.

NURSING PROCESS
ANTIULCER: HISTAMINE₂ BLOCKER

Assessment

- Assess the client's pain, including the type, duration, severity, frequency, and location.
- Assess GI complaints.
- Assess mental status.
- Assess fluid and electrolyte imbalances, including intake and output.
- Assess gastric pH (>5 is desired), BUN, and creatinine.
- Assess drug history; report probable drug-drug interactions.

Potential Nursing Diagnoses

- Pain related to gastric dysfunction

Planning

- Client will no longer experience abdominal pain after 1 to 2 wk of drug therapy.

Nursing Interventions

- Do not confuse drug with alprazolam (Xanax).
- Administer drug just before meals to decrease food-induced acid secretion or at bedtime.
- Be alert that reduced doses of drug are needed by the elderly, who have less gastric acid; need to prevent metabolic acidosis.
- Administer drug intravenously in 20 to 100 mL of IV solution.

Client Teaching

General
- Instruct the client to report pain, coughing, or vomiting of blood.
- Advise the client to avoid smoking because it can hamper the effectiveness of the drug.
- Remind the client that the drug must be taken exactly as prescribed to be effective.
- Instruct the client to separate ranitidine and antacid dosage by at least 1 h, if possible.
- Instruct the client not to drive a motor vehicle or engage in dangerous activities until stabilized on the drug.
- Tell the client that drug-induced impotence and gynecomastia are reversible.
- Instruct the client on the use of relaxation techniques to decrease anxiety.

Diet
- Advise the client to eat foods rich in vitamin B₁₂ to avoid deficiency as a result of drug therapy.
- Advise the client to avoid foods and liquids that can cause gastric irritation, such as caffeine-containing beverages, alcohol, and spices.

Cultural Considerations

- Same as for Antacids.

Evaluation

- Determine the effectiveness of the drug therapy and the presence of any side effects or adverse reactions. The client should be free of pain, and healing should be progressing.

Chart 42–3. Antiulcer: Pepsin Inhibitor

PEPSIN INHIBITOR

Drug Name

Sucralfate
    (Carafate), 🍁: Sulcrate
Pregnancy Category: B

Dosage

Active Disease:
A: PO: 1 g q.i.d. 1 h a.c. and h.s.
Maintenance:
A: PO: 1 g b.i.d.

Contraindications

Hypersensitivity
Caution: Renal failure

Drug-Lab-Food Interactions

Drug: *Decrease* effects with tetracycline, phenytoin, fat-soluble vitamins, digoxin; *altered absorption* with ciprofloxacin, norfloxacin, antacids

Pharmacokinetics

Absorption: PO: Minimal absorption (<5%)
Distribution: PB: UK
Metabolism: t½: 6–20 h
Excretion: In urine

Pharmacodynamics

PO: Onset: 30 min
    Peak: UK
    Duration: 5 h

Therapeutic Effects/Uses

To prevent gastric mucosal injury from drug-induced ulcers (aspirin, NSAIDs); to manage ulcers.

Mode of Action: In combination with gastric acid forms a protective covering on the ulcer surface.

Side Effects

Dizziness, nausea, constipation, dry mouth,
rash, pruritus, back pain, sleepiness

Adverse Reactions

None significant

Assessment and Planning

Interventions

Evaluation

NURSING PROCESS

KEY: A: adult; PO: by mouth; UK: unknown; PB: protein-binding; t½: half-life; a.c.: before meal; NSAIDs: nonsteroidal antiinflammatory drugs; h.s.: at bedtime; 🍁: Canadian drug names.

Proton Pump Inhibitors (Gastric Acid Secretion Inhibitors, Gastric Acid Pump Inhibitors)

Proton pump inhibitors (PPIs) suppress gastric acid secretion by inhibiting the hydrogen/potassium ATP-ase enzyme system located in the gastric parietal cells. They tend to inhibit gastric acid secretion up to 90% greater than the H₂ blockers (histamine antagonists). These agents block the final step of acid production.

Omeprazole (Prilosec) was the first PPI marketed. Eight years ago, lansoprazole (Prevacid) became available. Both agents are extremely effective in suppressing gastric acid secretions and are used for treatment of peptic ulcers and GERD. These drugs have a 24-hour duration and a short half-life, and are highly protein-bound (97%). Caution should be taken for clients with hepatic impairment; liver enzymes should be monitored. Possible side effects include headache, dizziness, diarrhea, abdominal pain, and rash.

Pepsin Inhibitor

Sucralfate (Carafate), a complex of sulfated sucrose and aluminum hydroxide, is classified as a pepsin inhibitor, or mucosal protective drug. It is nonabsorbable and combines with protein to form a viscous substance that covers the ulcer and protects it from acid and pepsin. This drug does not neutralize acid or decrease acid secretions.

NURSING PROCESS
ANTIULCER: PEPSIN INHIBITOR

Assessment

- Assess the client's pain, including the type, duration, severity, and frequency. Ulcer pain usually occurs after meals and during the night.
- Assess the client's renal function. Report urine output of <600 mL/d or <25 mL/h.
- Assess for fluid and electrolyte imbalances.
- Assess gastric pH (>5 is desired).

Potential Nursing Diagnoses

- Pain related to GI dysfunction

Planning

- Client will be free of abdominal pain after 1 to 2 wk of antiulcer drug management.

Nursing Interventions

- Administer drug on empty stomach.
- Administer an antacid 30 min before or after sucralfate. Allow 1 to 2 h to elapse between sucralfate and other prescribed drugs; sucralfate binds with certain drugs such as tetracycline, phenytoin, thus reducing the effect of the other drugs.

Client Teaching

General
- Advise client to take drug exactly as ordered. Therapy usually requires 4 to 8 wk for optimal ulcer healing. Advise the client to continue to take drug even if feeling better.
- Increase fluids, dietary bulk, and exercise to relieve constipation.
- Instruct the client on the use of relaxation techniques.
- Monitor for severe, persistent constipation.
- Stress need for follow-up medical care.
- Emphasize cessation of smoking, as indicated.

Diet
- Advise the client to avoid foods and liquids that can cause gastric irritation, such as caffeine-containing beverages, alcohol, and spices.

Side Effects
- Instruct the client to report pain, coughing, or vomiting of blood.

Evaluation

- Determine the effectiveness of the antiulcer treatment and the presence of any side effects. The client should be free of pain, and healing should be progressing.

The dosage of sucralfate is 1 g, usually four times a day before meals and at bedtime. If antacids are added to decrease pain, they should be given either 30 min before or after the administration of sucralfate. Because sucralfate is not systemically absorbed, side effects are few; however, it can cause constipation. If the drug is stored at room temperature in a tight container, it will remain stable for up to 2 years.

The action and effects of sucralfate are shown in Chart 42-3.

PHARMACOKINETICS
Less than 5% of sucralfate is absorbed by the GI tract. It has a half-life of 6 to 20 h. Ninety percent of the drug is excreted in the feces.

PHARMACODYNAMICS

Sucralfate promotes healing by adhering to the ulcer surface. The onset of action occurs within 30 min, and the duration of action is short. Sucralfate decreases the absorption of tetracycline, phenytoin, fat-soluble vitamins, and the antibacterial agents ciprofloxacin and norfloxacin. Antacids decrease the effects of sucralfate.

Prostaglandin Analogue Antiulcer Drug

Misoprostol, a synthetic prostaglandin analogue, is a new drug for prevention and treatment of peptic ulcer. It appears to suppress gastric acid secretion and increases cytoprotective mucus in the GI tract. It causes a moderate decrease in pepsin secretion. Misoprostol is considered to be as effective as cimetidine. Clients having complaints of gastric distress from taking NSAIDs, such as aspirin or indomethacin prescribed for long-term therapy, can benefit from use of misoprostol. When the client is taking high doses of NSAIDs, misoprostol is frequently recommended for the duration of the NSAID therapy. Misoprostol is contraindicated during pregnancy and for women of child-bearing age. Table 42–7 lists drug data for pepsin inhibitors, proton pump inhibitors, prostaglandin analogues, and GI stimulants.

Table 42–7

Antiulcers: Pepsin Inhibitor, Gastric Acid Secretion Inhibitor, Prostaglandin Analogue, and GI Stimulant

GENERIC (BRAND)	ROUTE AND DOSAGE	USES AND CONSIDERATIONS
PEPSIN INHIBITOR		
Sucralfate (Carafate)	See Chart 42–3	Management of duodenal ulcer. May be used for aspirin-induced gastric ulcer. Produces a pasty substance to protect the damaged mucosa. May cause nausea and constipation. *Pregnancy category:* B; PB: UK; $t_{\frac{1}{2}}$: 6–20 h
PROTON PUMP INHIBITORS (GASTRIC ACID SECRETION INHIBITORS)		
Lansoprazole (Prevacid)	*Duodenal ulcer:* A: PO: 15 mg/d a.c. for 4 wk *Erosive esophagitis:* A: PO: 30 mg/d a.c. for 8 wk	Short-term treatment for duodenal ulcer and erosive esophagitis. Used in drug combination for treatment of *H. pylori*. Also effective for treating Zollinger-Ellison syndrome. Swallow capsule whole (do not chew or crush). *Pregnancy category:* B; PB: UK; $t_{\frac{1}{2}}$: UK
Omeprazole (Prilosec)	*Gastroesophageal reflux disease (GERD):* A: PO: 20 mg/d for 4–8 wk *Hypersecretory:* A: PO: Initially: 60 mg daily; may increase to 120 mg t.i.d. in divided doses	Treatment of gastroesophageal reflux disease, including esophagitis, Zollinger-Ellison syndrome and *H. pylori*. Poorly absorbed with only 35%–40% in circulation. Antacids can be taken with drug. *Pregnancy category:* C; PB: 95%; $t_{\frac{1}{2}}$: 0.5–1.5 h
PROSTAGLANDIN ANALOGUE		
Misoprostol (Cytotec)	A: PO: 100–200 μg q.i.d. with food C <18 y: PO: Safety and efficacy not established	Prevention of NSAID-induced gastric ulcer. May be taken during NSAID therapy, including with aspirin. Side effects include diarrhea, abdominal pain, flatulence, nausea and vomiting, constipation, menstrual spotting. Has a short duration of action. *Pregnancy category:* X; PB: 85%; $t_{\frac{1}{2}}$: 1.5 h
GI STIMULANTS		
Cisapride (Propulsid)	*Heartburn and GERD:* A: PO: 10 mg, 15 min a.c. and h.s.	For nocturnal heartburn and gastroesophageal reflux disease (GERD). Avoid alcohol intake with drug. *Pregnancy category:* C; PB: 98%; $t_{\frac{1}{2}}$: 8–10 h

KEY: A: adult; C: child; h.s.: hour of sleep; PB: protein-binding; PO: by mouth; $t_{\frac{1}{2}}$: half-life; <: less than; NSAID: nonsteroidal antiinflammatory drug.

Gastrointestinal Stimulants

GI stimulants have been useful for treating noctural heartburn caused by GERD. This group acts by increasing gastric emptying time, thus preventing acid reflux into the esophagus. It enhances the release of acetylcholine at the myenteric plexus and also can be classified as a parasympathomimetic (direct-acting cholinergic). Although GERD may lead to ulcer formation, this type of drug, helpful for GERD, would not be used for peptic ulcers.

Cisapride (Propulsid) is an example of the GI stimulant. Cisapride should *not* be used for clients having cardiac dysrhythmias, especially ventricular tachycardia, ventricular flutter, or fibrillation. This agent is contraindicated for clients with ischemic heart disease, congestive heart failure, uncorrected electrolyte disorders (hypokalemia, hypomagnesemia), and renal or respiratory failure. An electrocardiogram should be done before and during drug therapy. Cisapride is primarily prescribed for clients who do not respond adequately to other drug or nondrug therapy. If the client has hepatic insufficiency, the daily dose should be halved.

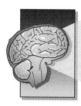

Critical Thinking in Action

J. H., 48 years old, complained of a gnawing, aching pain in the abdominal area that usually occurs several hours after eating. He said that Tums helped some, but the pain has recently intensified. Diagnostic tests indicated that the client has a duodenal ulcer.

1. Differentiate between peptic ulcer, gastric ulcer, and duodenal ulcer. Explain.
2. What are the predisposing factors related to peptic ulcers? What additional information do you need from J. H.?
3. What nonpharmacologic measures can you suggest for alleviating symptoms related to peptic ulcer?

The health care provider prescribed Mylanta 2 tsp to be taken 2 h after meals, and ranitidine (Zantac) 150 mg, b.i.d. Mylanta is to be taken either 1 h before or 1 h after the ranitidine.

4. J. H. asks the nurse the purposes for Mylanta and ranitidine. What would your response be?
5. The health care provider may suggest that the client take ranitidine with meals. Why? Why should Mylanta and ranitidine not be taken at the same time?
6. In what ways are ranitidine and cimetidine the same and how do they differ? Explain.
7. As part of client teaching, the nurse discusses side effects of ranitidine with J. H. What might be the most effective way to present this information? Develop a plan.

The client states he drinks beer at lunch and has two gin and tonics in the midafternoon. He states that these drinks help him to relax.

8. What nursing intervention should be taken in regard to his alcoholic intake?
9. What foods should he avoid?

A week later the client states that he discontinued the prescribed medications because he "felt better." However, the pain recurred and he asked if he should resume taking the medications.

10. What would your response be? What client teaching should be included?

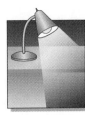

Study Questions

1. What is the action of antacids used in the treatment and control of peptic ulcers?

2. Your client is taking Maalox 15 mL four times a day. At what times should the drug be taken? What would the duration of action be if the drug were taken with food and without food? How should it be taken?

3. What is a major side effect of antacids containing aluminum salts and magnesium salts?

4. Your client is taking ranitidine (Zantac). What type of drug is ranitidine?

5. What is sucralfate (Carafate)? What is its action in treating peptic ulcer?

6. What are the actions of omeprazole and misoprostol?

Unit XI

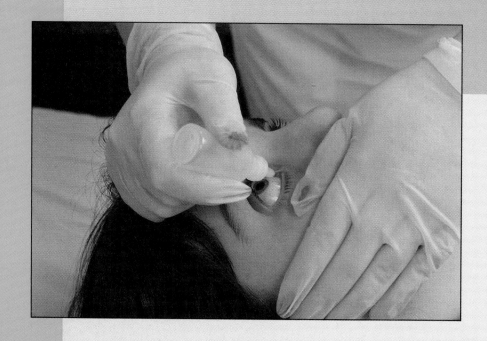

Eye, Ear, and Skin Agents

Many of the drugs used in the treatment of eye and ear disorders are discussed in other chapters of this text, for example, antibiotics in Chapters 25, 26, and 27. Of particular interest and importance in Chapter 43 are drugs used in the treatment of glaucoma and ocular infections.

OVERVIEW OF THE EYE

The eyeballs, protected within the orbits of the skull, are controlled by the third, fourth, and sixth cranial nerves, connected to six extraocular muscles. The eye has three layers: (1) the cornea and sclera, (2) the choroid, iris, and ciliary body, and (3) the retina. Figure XI–1 illustrates the basic structures of the eye.

The cornea, the anterior covering of the eye, is transparent, enabling the light to enter the eye. The cornea, which has no blood vessels, receives nutrition from the aqueous humor. An abraded cornea is susceptible to infection. Loss of corneal transparency is generally caused by increased intraocular pressure.

The sclera is the opaque, white fibrous envelope of the eye. Within the sclera are the posterior chamber and the anterior chamber. The posterior chamber has a blind spot (not sensitive to light) around the optic nerve. The lens, held in place by ligaments, separates these two chambers. The normally transparent lens focuses light on the retina by changing its shape through a process called accommodation.

The anterior chamber, filled with aqueous humor secreted by the ciliary body, lies in front of the lens. The fluid flows into the anterior chamber through a space between the lens and iris. The excess fluid drains into the canal of Schlemm. A rise in intraocular pressure, resulting in glaucoma, occurs with increased production or decreased drainage of aqueous humor.

The choroid, iris, and ciliary body (thickened part of vascular covering of the eye; provides attachment to ligaments and support to lens) constitute the second layer. The choroid absorbs light. The iris, which surrounds the pupil and gives the eye its color, controls the quantity of light reaching the lens through dilation and constriction.

The retina, the third layer, is composed of nerves, rods, and cones that serve as visual sensory receptors. The retina is connected to the brain via the optic nerve.

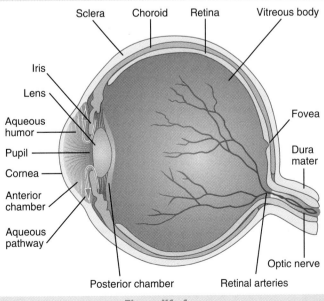

Figure X1–1

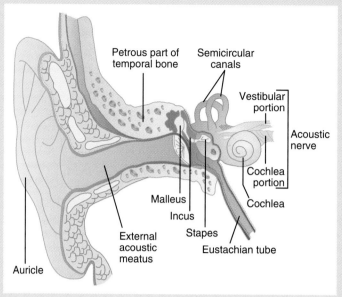

The eyebrows, eyelashes, eyelids, tears, and corneal and conjunctival reflexes all serve to protect the eye. Bilateral blinking occurs every few seconds during waking hours to keep the eye moist and free of foreign material.

OVERVIEW OF THE EAR

The ear is divided into the external, middle, and inner ear. Figure XI–2 illustrates the basic structures of the ear.

The **external ear** consists of the pinna and the external auditory canal. The external auditory canal transmits sound to the tympanic membrane (eardrum), a transparent partition between the external and middle ear. The eardrum in turn transmits sound to the bones of the middle ear and also serves a protective function.

The three auditory ossicles (malleus, incus, and stapes) transmit sound waves to the inner ear and are located in the **middle ear,** an air-filled cavity. The tip of the malleus is attached to the eardrum; its head is attached to the incus, which is attached to the stapes. The eustachian tube provides a direct connection to the nasopharynx and equalizes air pressure on both sides of the eardrum to prevent it from rupturing. Swallowing, yawning, and chewing gum help the eustachian tube to relieve pressure changes on airplane flights.

The **inner ear,** a series of labyrinths (canals), consists of a bony section and a membranous section. The vestibule, cochlea, and semicircular canals make up the bony labyrinth. The vestibular area is responsible for maintaining equilibrium and balance. The cochlea is the principal hearing organ.

Professional evaluation of ear problems is essential because hearing loss can result from untreated disorders. Middle ear problems require prescription medications and are not treated with over-the-counter preparations.

SKIN

Skin, the largest organ of the body, is composed of two major layers: the epidermis, which is the outer layer of the skin; and the dermis, which is the layer of skin beneath the epidermis. The functions of the skin include (1) body protection from the environment, (2) aiding in body temperature control, and (3) preventing body fluid loss.

The epidermis has four layers (1) the basal layer (stratum germinativum), the deepest layer lying over the dermis, (2) the spinous layer (stratum spinosum), (3) the granular layer (stratum granulosum), and (4) the cornified layer (stratum corneum), the outer layer of the epidermis. As the epidermal cells migrate to the surface, they die and their cytoplasm is converted to keratin (hard and rough texture), forming keratinocytes. Eventually the keratinocytes slough off as new layers of epidermal cells migrate upward.

The dermis has two layers: the papillary layer, next to the epidermis; and the reticular layer, which is the deeper layer of the dermis. The dermal layers consist of fibroblasts, collagen fibers, and elastic fibers. The collagen and elastic fibers give the skin its strength and elasticity. Within the dermal layer, there are sweat glands, hair follicles, sebaceous glands, blood vessels, and sensory nerve terminals. Figure XI–3 shows the layers of the skin.

The subcutaneous tissue, primarily fatty tissue, lies under the dermis. Besides fatty cells, subcutaneous tissue contains blood and lymphatic vessels, nerve fibers, and elastic fibers. It supports and protects the dermis. Chapter 44 discusses the drugs for dermatologic disorders.

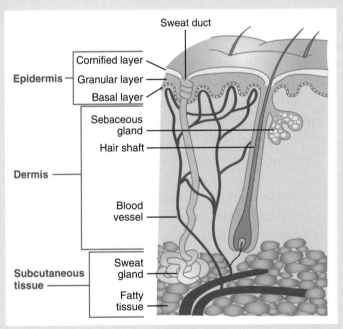

Figure X1–3

43 Drugs for Disorders of the Eye and the Ear

Outline

Objectives

- Identify medication groups commonly used for disorders of the eye and the ear.
- List mechanisms of action, route, side effects and adverse reactions, and contraindications for selected drugs in each group.
- Describe content of teaching plans for groups of drugs presented.
- Describe the nursing process, including client teaching, related to disorders of the eye and ear.

Terms

carbonic anhydrase inhibitors
cerumen
ceruminolytic
conjunctivitis

cycloplegics
lacrimal duct
miosis
miotics
mydriatics

ophthalmic
optic
osmotics
otic

INTRODUCTION

This chapter describes the most commonly used drugs for eye and ear disorders. Many of these drugs have other uses and are discussed in greater detail in other chapters.

The nurse must be alert to the fact that a variety of systemic diseases have ocular findings that are characteristic. Examples of these systemic disorders are acquired immunodeficiency syndrome (AIDS), coronary vascular disease, muscular and endocrine disorders, and hematologic and neurologic diseases.

DRUGS FOR DISORDERS OF THE EYE

Diagnostic Aids

Diagnostic aids are used frequently to locate lesions or foreign objects and to provide local anesthesia to the area. Drugs commonly used as diagnostic aids are presented in Table 43–1.

Topical Anesthetics

Topical anesthetics are used in selected aspects of a comprehensive eye examination and in the removal of foreign bodies from the eye. The two most common topical anesthetics are proparacaine HCl (Ophthaine, Ophthetic) and tetracaine HCl (Pontocaine).

Corneal anesthesia is achieved within 1 min and generally lasts about 15 min. The blink reflex is temporarily lost; therefore, the corneal epithelium is not kept moist. To protect the eye, a patch is usually

Normal flow of aqueous humor

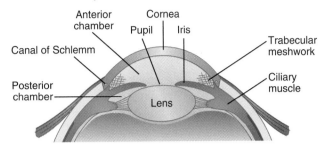

Impeded flow of aqueous humor, resulting in intraocular pressure

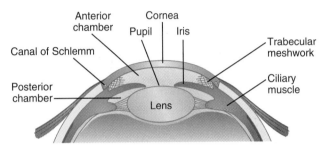

Obstructive flow to canal of Schlemm

Figure 43–1
Increased intraocular pressure (see p. 794).

worn over the eye until the effects of the drug are gone. These drugs are not to be self-administered by the client. Repeated doses are given only under strict medical supervision.

Antiinfectives

Antiinfectives are frequently used for eye infections. **Conjunctivitis** (inflammation of the delicate membrane covering the eyeball and lining the eyelid) and local skin and eye irritation are possible side effects of topical **ophthalmic** antiinfective drugs. Screen for previous allergic reactions. Conjunctivitis is also one type of eye infection that can be bacterial or viral in origin. For more comprehensive information on antiinfectives, see Chapters 25, 26, and 27. The drug data for optic antiinfectives are presented in Table 43–2; antiinflammatory drug data are presented in Table 43–3.

Lubricants

Both healthy and ill persons may need to use eye lubricants. Healthy clients who complain of "dryness of the eyes" use lubricants as artificial tears; lubricants are also used to moisten contact lenses or artificial eyes. Lubricants are used to alleviate discomfort associated with dryness and to maintain integrity of the epithelial surface. Lubricants are also used during

Table 43–1	
Diagnostic Aids for Eye Disorders	
DIAGNOSTIC AIDS	PURPOSE
Fluorescein sodium	A dye used to demonstrate defects in corneal epithelium. Corneal scratches turn bright green; foreign bodies are surrounded by green ring. Loss of conjunctiva shows orange yellow. Dye appears in nasal secretions if lacrimal duct patent.
Fluress (fluorescein sodium and benoxinate HCl)	Used for short corneal and conjunctival procedures, including removal of foreign bodies. Dye and local anesthetic.

Table 43-2
Ophthalmic: Antiinfectives

GENERIC (BRAND)	ROUTE AND DOSAGE*	USES AND CONSIDERATIONS
ANTIBACTERIALS		
Chloramphenicol (AK-Chlor, Chloromycetin Ophthalmic)	A&C: Ophthalmic: Instill 1–2 gtt or $\frac{1}{2}$ inch oint q3–4 h for 48 h; increase interval to b.i.d./t.i.d.	Effective against both gram-negative and gram-positive bacteria. For treatment of severe infections or when other antibacterials not effective. Continue treatment for at least 48 h after eye appears normal. *Pregnancy category:* C; PB: NA; t½: NA
Ciprofloxacin (Cipro)	Day 1: 2 qtt q15min for 6 h then 2 gtt q30min for the rest of the day Day 2: 2 gtt qh Days 3–14: 2 gtt q4h	Effective against bacterial conjunctivitis. To treat corneal ulceration. Minimal absorption through cornea or conjunctiva. *Pregnancy category:* C; PB: NA; t½: NA
Erythromycin (Ilotycin)	Oint 0.5%: 0.5–1 cm q.d./q.i.d.	Most commonly used antibacterial; for superficial ocular infections and prevention of ophthalmia neonatorum. *Pregnancy category:* B; PB: NA; t½: NA
Gentamicin sulfate (Garamycin Ophthalmic)	A&C: Sol 0.3%: 1–2 gtt q4h; may increase to 2 gtt qh for severe infections Oint 0.3%: $\frac{1}{2}$ inch ribbon b.i.d./t.i.d.	For infections of the external eye: *Pregnancy category:* C; PB: NA; t½: NA
Norfloxacin (Chibroxin)	A&C > 1 y: Sol 3%: instill 1–2 gtt in affected eye(s) q.i.d. for ≤ 7 d	For treatment of conjunctivitis. *Pregnancy category:* C; PB: NA; t½: NA
Tobramycin (Nebcin, Tobrex)	0.3% Oint: $\frac{1}{2}$ inch b.i.d./t.i.d. 0.3% Sol: 1–2 gtt q4h *For severe infections:* Oint: $\frac{1}{2}$ inch q 3–4 h Sol: 2 gtt q 30–60 min until improvement, then decrease frequency	*Pregnancy category:* D; PB: NA; t½: NA
Silver nitrate 1% (Dey-Drop)	Neonate: Instill 2 gtt in each eye within 1 h of birth	For prevention and treatment of ophthalmia neonatorum. *Pregnancy category:* C; PB: NA; t½: NA
Tetracycline HCl (Achromycin Ophthalmic)	A: Instill 1–2 gtt b.i.d./q.i.d. A: Instill $\frac{1}{2}$ inch q2–12h	Bacteriostatic action; alternative to silver nitrate for prevention of ophthalmia neonatorum. *Pregnancy category:* D; PB: NA; t½: NA
ANTIFUNGAL		
Natamycin (Natacyn Ophthalmic)	A&C: Sol 5%: 1 gt q2h for 3–4 d; then 1 gt q3h for 14–21 d	May cause transient stinging or temporary blurring of vision. *Pregnancy category:* C; PB: NA; t½: NA
ANTIVIRAL		
Idoxuridine (IDU, Herplex Liquifilm)	A&C: Sol (1%): Initially: 1 gt q1h during the day and q2h at night; when definite improvement occurs, use 1 gt q2h during the day and q4h at night; continue 3–7 d after healing occurs 0.5% Oint: Place $\frac{1}{2}$ inch q4h while awake	To treat cytomegalovirus or herpes simplex keratitis. Store in refrigerator; do not mix with boric acid. If no response in 1 week, discontinue. *Pregnancy category:* C; PB: NA; t½: NA
Trifluridine (Viroptic)	A: 1% sol: Instill 1 gt into infected eye q2h while awake; max: 9 gtt/d until corneal ulcer reepithelialized; then 1 gt q4h for 7 d; max: 21 d of treatment	For treatment of keratoconjunctivitis caused by herpes simplex virus types 1 and 2; herpetic ophthalmic infections. *Pregnancy category:* C; PB: NA; t½: NA
Vidarabine monohydrate (Vira-A)	A&C: Oint 3%: $\frac{1}{2}$ inch 5 × d at 3-h intervals	For treatment of keratoconjunctivitis and herpes simplex keratitis. *Pregnancy category:* C; PB: NA; t½: NA

To minimize systemic absorption, apply gentle pressure on inner canthus.
KEY: A: adult; C: child; gt: drop; gtt: drops; oint: ointment; PB: protein-binding; sol: solution; t½: half-life; UK: unknown.

Table 43-3
Ophthalmic: Antiinflammatories

GENERIC (BRAND)	ROUTE AND DOSAGE*	USES AND CONSIDERATIONS
Dexamethasone (AK-Dex Ophthalmic)	A&C: Oint: Apply into conjunctival sac t.i.d./q.i.d.; gradually decrease to discontinue Susp: Instill 2 gtt qh while awake and q2h during night; taper to q3–4h; then t.i.d./q.i.d.	For uveitis, allergic conditions, and inflammation of conjunctiva, cornea, and lids. Should not be used for minor abrasions and wounds. *Pregnancy category:* C; PB: NA; $t\frac{1}{2}$: NA
Diclofenac Na (Voltaren)	A: 1 gt to affected eye q.i.d. for 2 wk; start 24 h after cataract surgery	*Pregnancy category:* B; PB: NA; $t\frac{1}{2}$: NA
Flurbiprofen Na (Ocufen)	A: Instill 1 gt q30 min 2 h before surgery, total dose is 4 gtt	To decrease corneal edema; miosis. *Pregnancy category:* C; PB: NA; $t\frac{1}{2}$: NA
Suprofen (Profenal)	*Preoperative:* A: Instill 2 gtt in sac q4h while awake on day preceding surgery; instill 2 gtt in conjunctival sac at 3, 2, and 1 h before surgery	Used to prevent intraoperative miosis. *Pregnancy category:* C; PB: NA; $t\frac{1}{2}$: NA
Ketorolac tromethamine (Acular)	A: 0.5% sol: Instill 1 gt q.i.d.	Nonsteroidal. Efficacy has not been established beyond 1 wk of therapy. Used for the relief of itching associated with seasonal allergic conjunctivitis. *Pregnancy category:* C; PB: NA; $t\frac{1}{2}$: NA
Olopatadine HCl Ophthalmic solution (Patanol)	A: 1 gt b.i.d. C: >3y: 1 gt b.i.d.	For temporary prevention of itching of eye caused by allergic conjunctivitis. Convenient twice daily dosing. Topical use only. Combines antihistamines and mast cell stabilizing action. Persons wearing contact lenses should wait at least 10 min after instillation before reinserting lenses. *Pregnancy category:* C; PB: NA; $t\frac{1}{2}$: NA
Medrysone (HMS Liquifilm)	A&C: Susp. Initially: Instill 1 gt in conjunctival sac q1–2h (1–2 d); then 1 gt b.i.d./q.i.d.	To treat allergic conditions, burns, inflammation of conjunctiva, cornea, and lids. *Pregnancy category:* C; PB: NA; $t\frac{1}{2}$: NA
Prednisolone acetate (Econopred)	A: Initially: Instill 1–2 gtt in conjunctival sac qh while awake, q2h during night until desired effect; maint: 1 gt q4h Susp: 0.125% and 1%	Steroidal. To treat uveitis, allergic conditions, burns, inflammation of conjunctiva, cornea, and lids. *Pregnancy category:* C; PB: NA; $t\frac{1}{2}$: NA
Prednisolone Na phosphate (AK-Pred, Inflamase)	A&E Elderly: Sol: 0.125% & 1%: 1–2 gtt q1h during day; q2h during night; with response give 1 gt q4h, then 1 gt t.i.d./q.i.d. Oint: thin coat t.i.d./q.i.d.; with response Decrease to b.i.d., then daily.	To prevent or decrease tissue response to inflammatory process
Combination: TobraDex (tobramycin 0.3% and dexamethasone 0.1%)	A: 1–2 gtt q2–6 h 1st 24–48h; then q4–6h or less until symptoms decrease. Max: 20 mL for 1st treatment C: not recommended Oint: A: Apply to conjunctival sac up to t.i.d./q.i.d. Max: 8g for initial treatment Oint: C: not recommended.	Combines antiinflammatory power of dexamethasone with antibiotic. Increased tolerability and comfortable pH. For treatment of fungal, mycobacterial, or viral infection of eye.

*To minimize systemic absorption, apply gentle pressure to inner canthus.
KEY: A: adult; C: child; gt: drop; gtt: drops; oint: ointment; PB: protein-binding: sol: solution; susp: suspension; $t\frac{1}{2}$: half-life; NA: not applicable.

Table 43–4
Miotics: Cholinergics and Beta-Adrenergic Blockers

GENERIC (BRAND)	ROUTE AND DOSAGE	USES AND CONSIDERATIONS
DIRECT-ACTING CHOLINERGICS		
Acetylcholine Cl (Miochol)	A: Intraocular: 0.5–2 mL of 1% sol injected in anterior chamber before or after suturing	To achieve miosis in cataract and other anterior segment surgery. *Pregnancy category:* C; PB: NA; t½: NA
Carbachol intraocular (Miostat)	A: Ophthalmic: 1–2 gtt daily/q.i.d. A: IO: 0.5 mL into anterior chamber before or after suturing	For miosis during eye surgery. To reduce intraocular pressure, especially when pilocarpine is ineffective. *Pregnancy category:* C; PB: NA; t½: NA
Pilocarpine HCl (Isopto Carpine)	See Chart 43–1	
Pilocarpine nitrate (Ocusert Pilo-20, Pilo-40)	See Chart 43–1	
Echothiophate iodide (Phospholine Iodide)	A: 0.03%–0.25% sol: 1 gt daily/b.i.d.	Used to treat chronic open-angle glaucoma and glaucoma following cataract surgery. *Pregnancy category:* C; PB: NA; t½: NA
INDIRECT-ACTING CHOLINESTERASE INHIBITORS: SHORT ACTING		
Physostigmine salicylate (Isopto Eserine)	A&C: Oint 0.25%: ¼ inch up to daily/t.i.d. Sol 0.25–0.5%: 1–2 gtt daily/q.i.d.	For wide-angle glaucoma. *Pregnancy category:* C; PB: NA; t½: NA
LONG-ACTING		
Demecarium bromide (Humorsol)	A: Sol 0.125–0.25%: 1–2 gtt 2 × wk or 1–2 gtt b.i.d.	Used for open-angle glaucoma when shorter-acting agents have been unsuccessful, conditions affecting aqueous outflow, accommodative strabismus. *Pregnancy category:* C; PB: NA; t½: NA
BETA-ADRENERGIC BLOCKERS		
Betaxolol HCl (Betoptic)	0.25% Susp or 0.5% sol: Usual dose: 1 gt b.i.d.	Beta blockers. Used to decrease elevated intraocular pressure in chronic open-angle glaucoma and ocular hypertension. Contraindicated in clients with asthma due to increased airway resistance from systemic absorption. Use caution in clients receiving oral beta blockers. *Pregnancy category:* C; PB: NA; t½: NA
Levobunolol HCl (Betagan Liquifilm, AKBeta)	0.25%–0.5% Sol: 1–2 gtt daily/b.i.d.	Lowers intraocular pressure. *Pregnancy category:* C; PB: NA; t½: NA
Timolol maleate (Timoptic)	A: Sol 0.25%–0.5% initially: 1 gt b.i.d.; maint: 1 drop daily once response occurs with initial dosage	Reduces production of aqueous humor. Monitor vital signs during initial therapy. Concurrent use of similar drugs must be individualized. Blurred vision decreases with use. *Pregnancy category:* C; PB: NA; t½: NA

KEY: *A: adult; C: child; NA: not applicable; oint: ointment; PB: protein-binding; sol: solution; susp: suspension; t½: half-life; gt: drop; gtt: drops; IO: intraocular.*

Chart 43–1.   Direct-Acting Miotic

Drug Name

Pilocarpine
   (Isopto Carpine, Pilopine HS, Ocusert Pilo-20
   and -40)
Pregnancy Category: C

Dosage

A&C: sol: 1–2%, 1–2 gtt, t.i.d./q.i.d.
Gel: Apply 0.5-in ribbon in lower eyelid at bedtime
Ocusert: Replaced q7d

Contraindications

Retinal detachment, adhesions between iris and lens, acute ocular inflammation; must avoid systemic absorption of drug with coronary artery disease, obstruction of GI/GU tract, epilepsy, asthma

Drug-Lab-Food Interactions

Avoid use with carbachol and echothiophate
Decrease antiglaucoma effects with belladonna alkaloids, *decrease* dilation with phenylephrine

Pharmacokinetics

Absorption: PO: Some systemic absorption
Distribution: PB: UK
Metabolism: t½: UK; binds to ocular tissue
Excretion: UK

Pharmacodynamics

Miosis:
Ophthalmic: Onset:10–30 min
                     Peak: 20 min
                     Duration: 4–8 h
Reduce IOP:
Ophthalmic: Onset: 45–60 min
                     Peak: 75 min
                     Duration: 4–14 h
Ocusert: Onset: 1 h
                     Peak: 1.5–2 h
                     Duration: 7 d
Gel: Onset: 1 h
                     Peak: 3–12 h
                     Duration: 18–24 h

Therapeutic Effects/Uses

To induce miosis; to decrease IOP in glaucoma.
Mode of Action: Stimulation of pupillary and ciliary sphincter muscles.

Side Effects

Blurred vision, eye pain, headache, eye irritation, brow ache, stinging and burning, nausea, vomiting, diarrhea, increased salivation and sweating, muscle tremors, contact allergy
Conjunctival irritation with Ocusert

Adverse Reactions

Dyspnea, hypertension, tachycardia, retinal detachment; long term: bronchospasm
Corneal abrasion and visual impairment potential with Ocusert

KEY: A: adult; C: child; IOP: intraocular pressure; PB: protein-binding; sol: solution; t½: half-life; UK: unknown; G2: gastrointestinal; GU: genitourinary.

anesthesia and in acute or chronic central nervous system (CNS) disorders that result in unconsciousness or decreased blinking.

Most lubricants are available over-the-counter (OTC) in both liquid and ointment form. Popular lubricants are Isopto Tears, Tearisol, Ultra Tears, Tears Naturale, Tears Plus, Lens Mate, and Lacri-Lube. Be alert to allergic response to preservatives in lubricants.

Miotics

In open-angle glaucoma, **miotics** are used to lower the intraocular pressure, thereby increasing blood flow to the retina and decreasing retinal damage and loss of vision. Direct-acting cholinergics and cholinesterase inhibitors, the two types of miotics, differ in their mechanism of action. Miotics cause a contraction of the ciliary muscle and widening of trabecular meshwork. Figure 43–1 illustrates increased intraocular pressure resulting in glaucoma. Table 43–4 presents the drug data for miotics.

PHARMACOKINETICS

Systemic absorption is possible but not common with the use of miotics. Pilocarpine binds to the ocular tissues; its half-life is unknown. The metabolism and elimination of this drug are also currently unknown.

PHARMACODYNAMICS

Pilocarpine produces **miosis** and decreases intraocular pressure. The onset of action, peak, and duration of action vary with the dose, desired effect, and form. The onset of action of pilocarpine given to produce miosis is 10 to 30 min, the time of peak action is unknown, and the duration of action is 4 to 8 h. When used to reduce intraocular pressure, ophthalmic pilocarpine has an unknown onset of action, peak time of 75 min, and duration of action of 4 to 14 h. With the ocular therapeutic system Ocusert, the onset of action is unknown, the peak is 1.5 to 2 h, and the duration of action is 7 d.

Ocusert is a wafer-thin disk impregnated with time-release pilocarpine. The disk is replaced every 7 d. Clients should check for presence of the Ocusert disk in the conjunctival sac daily at bedtime and on arising.

The drug data for pilocarpine are shown in Chart 43–1.

CONTRAINDICATIONS

Contraindications to pilocarpine include retinal detachment, adhesions between the iris and lens, and acute ocular infections. Caution is advised for clients with the following conditions: asthma, hypertension, corneal abrasion, hyperthyroidism, coronary vascular disease, urinary tract obstruction, gastrointestinal (GI) obstruction, ulcer disease, parkinsonism, and bradycardia.

DRUG INTERACTIONS

Ophthalmic epinephrine, timolol, levobunolol, betaxolol, and systemic carbonic anhydrase inhibitors have the added effect of lowering intraocular pressure. Cyclopentolate, ophthalmic belladonna alkaloids, and antidepressants antagonize the therapeutic effects.

Use of beta-adrenergic blockers, such as betaxolol

Table 43–5
Carbonic Anhydrase Inhibitors

DRUG	DOSAGE	USES AND CONSIDERATIONS
Acetazolamide (Diamox)	A: PO: 250–1000 mg daily given in divided doses for amounts >250 mg; doses >1000 mg show no increased benefit	To reduce aqueous humor formation, thus lowering intraocular (IO) pressure. Monitor for dehydration and postural hypotension. Monitor electrolytes. Avoid hazardous activities due to drowsiness. Most frequently prescribed. *Pregnancy category:* C; PB: UK; $t_{\frac{1}{2}}$: 2–6 h
Brinzolamide ophthalmic susp 1% (Azopt)	A: 1gt t.i.d. C: not recommended	*Topical:* Treatment of elevated IO pressure in clients with ocular hypertension or open-angle glaucoma by suppressing production of aqueous humor. *Pregnancy category:* UK; PB: UK; $t_{\frac{1}{2}}$: UK
Dichlorphenamide (Daranide)	A: PO: Initially: 100–200 mg followed by 100 mg q12h until desired response is obtained	As above. Can cause confusion, especially in elderly. *Pregnancy category:* C; PB: UK; $t_{\frac{1}{2}}$: UK
Dorzolamide (Trusopt)	A: 2% sol: 1 gt t.i.d.	Do not use with oral carbonic anhydrase inhibitors. Side effects include burning, stinging, bitter taste. *Pregnancy category:* UK; PB: UK; $t_{\frac{1}{2}}$: UK
Methazolamide (Neptazane)	A: 50–100 mg, b.i.d. or t.i.d.	Similar to Diamox and Daranide. Increases action of amphetamines. Increases effects of salicylates, lithium, and barbiturates. *Pregnancy category:* C; PB: UK; $t_{\frac{1}{2}}$: 14 h

KEY: A: adult; C: child; gt: drop; PB: protein-binding; PO: by mouth; $t_{\frac{1}{2}}$: half-life; UK: unknown.

NURSING PROCESS
MIOTICS

Assessment

- Obtain medical and drug history. Miotics are contraindicated in clients with narrow-angle glaucoma, acute inflammation of the eye, heart block, coronary artery disease, obstruction of the GI or urinary tract, and asthma.
- Check vital signs (VS). Baseline VS can be compared with future findings.
- Assess the client's level of anxiety. The possibility of diminished vision or blindness increases anxiety.
- Assess the client's eye pigment; clients with dark, heavily pigmented eyes may benefit from a pilocarpine concentration greater than 4%.

Potential Nursing Diagnoses

- Altered visual perception
- High risk for injury

Planning

- Client will take miotics as prescribed.
- Client's intraocular pressure will decrease and be within the accepted range.

Nursing Interventions

- When administering eye drops, apply gentle pressure to the inner canthus to prevent or minimize systemic absorption.
- Monitor VS. Heart rate and blood pressure may decrease with large doses of cholinergics.
- Monitor for side effects such as headache, eye pain, and decreased vision.
- Monitor for postural hypotension. Instruct client to rise slowly from a recumbent position.
- Check breath sounds for rales and rhonchi; cholinergic drugs can cause bronchospasms and increase bronchial secretions.
- Maintain oral hygiene with excessive salivation.
- Have atropine available as antidote for pilocarpine.

Nursing Process continued on following page

HCl, levobunolol HCl, and timolol maleate, represents the most recent approach to the treatment of open-angle glaucoma. Refer to Chapter 21 for a comprehensive discussion of adrenergic blockers. The commonly prescribed miotics are listed in Table 43–4. Chart 43–1 presents the actions and effects of pilocarpine.

SIDE EFFECTS AND ADVERSE REACTIONS

Miotic side effects include headache, eye pain, decreased vision, brow pain, and, less frequently, hyperemia of the conjunctiva. Systemic absorption can cause nausea, vomiting, diarrhea, frequent urination, precipitation of attacks in asthma clients, increased salivation, diaphoresis, muscle weakness, and respiratory difficulty. Manifestations of toxicity include vertigo, bradycardia, tremors, hypotension, syncope, cardiac dysrhythmias, and seizures. Atropine sulfate must be available in case of systemic toxicity.

Carbonic Anhydrase Inhibitors

Carbonic anhydrase inhibitors interfere with production of carbonic acid, which leads to decreased aqueous humor formation and decreased intraocular pressure. These drugs, which were developed as diuretics, have come to be used for the long-term treatment of open-angle glaucoma. It is recommended that they be used only when pilocarpine, beta blockers, epinephrine, and cholinesterase inhibitors have not been effective. Table 43–5 presents the drug data for carbonic anhydrase inhibitors.

SIDE EFFECTS AND ADVERSE REACTIONS

Side effects include lethargy, anorexia, drowsiness, paresthesia, depression, polyuria, nausea, vomiting, hypokalemia, and renal calculi. Clients frequently discontinue medications because of the side effects. These drugs are contraindicated during the first trimester of pregnancy. Do not use in persons allergic to

Client Teaching

General
- Instruct the client or family on correct administration of eye drops and ointment; include return demonstration. See Figures 3–9 and 3–10.
- Instruct client on need for regular and ongoing medical supervision.
- Instruct the client not to stop medication suddenly without prior approval of the health care provider.
- Advise client to avoid driving or operating machinery while vision is impaired.
- Instruct the client on the use of relaxation techniques for decreasing anxiety, if appropriate.
- Instruct the client with glaucoma to avoid atropine-like drugs, which increase intraocular pressure. Clients should check labels on OTC drugs or check with a pharmacist.

Ocular Therapeutic Systems (Ocusert)
- Store drug in refrigerator.
- Discard damaged or contaminated disks.
- Explain that the myopia is minimized by bedtime insertion in the upper conjunctival sac.
- For self-administration, advise clients to follow instructions related to insertion and removal.
- Instruct client to check for presence of disk in conjunctival sac at bedtime and when arising.
- Explain that temporary stinging is expected; notify health care provider if blurred vision or brow pain occurs.

Cholinesterase Inhibitors
- First dose should be administered by health care provider and followed by tonometry reading.
- Instruct client to tightly cap tube because ointment is inactivated by water.

Evaluation

- Evaluate the effectiveness of drug therapy and the presence of side effects. Intraocular pressure will be within desired range or reduced.

Table 43–6
Osmotics

DRUG	DOSAGE	USES AND CONSIDERATIONS
Glycerin	A: PO: 1–1.5 g/kg given 1–1.5 h prior to surgery	Decreases volume of intraocular fluid, thus lowering ocular tension. Carbohydrate; use with caution in diabetics. *Pregnancy category:* C; PB: UK; $t_{\frac{1}{2}}$: 30–45 min
Isosorbide (Ismotic)	A: 45% sol, 1.5–3 g/kg, b.i.d./q.i.d.	Monitor I&O and electrolytes. *Pregnancy category:* C; PB: UK; $t_{\frac{1}{2}}$: 5–9.5 h
Mannitol (Osmitrol)	A: IV: 15–20% sol, 1.5–2 g/kg over 0.5–1 h	Monitor I&O; weigh daily. Contraindicated in severe pulmonary congestion, anuria, and dehydration. Use with caution in clients with CHF. *Pregnancy category:* C; PB: UK; $t_{\frac{1}{2}}$: 15–100 min
Urea (Ureaphil)	A: IV: 30% sol, 1–1.5 g/kg over 1–3 h; max: 4 mL/min C > 2 y: IV: 0.5–1.5 g/kg up to 4 mL/min C < 2 y: IV: 0.1 g/kg up to 4 mL/min	Monitor I&O; weigh daily. Do *not* mix with any other medication or blood. Contraindicated with intracranial bleeding and dehydration. *Pregnancy category:* C; PB: UK; $t_{\frac{1}{2}}$: <60 min

KEY: A: adult; C: child; sol: solution; IV: intravenous; I&O: intake and output; PB: protein-binding; $t_{\frac{1}{2}}$: half-life; UK: unknown; PO: by mouth; CHF: congestive heart failure.

NURSING PROCESS
CARBONIC ANHYDRASE INHIBITORS

Assessment

- Obtain medical and drug history. Use is contraindicated during first trimester of pregnancy.
- Check vital signs (VS). Baseline VS can be compared with future readings.
- Assess level of anxiety. Eye disorders carrying the possibility of blindness promote high anxiety state in clients.

Potential Nursing Diagnoses

- Altered visual perception
- High risk for injury

Planning

- Client will take carbonic anhydrase inhibitors as prescribed.
- Client's intraocular pressure will decrease to within the desired range.

Nursing Interventions

- Monitor for side effects such as lethargy, anorexia, drowsiness, polyuria, nausea, and vomiting.
- Monitor electrolytes because drug can cause hypokalemia.

- Increase fluid intake, unless contraindicated. Record intake and output; weigh daily.
- Maintain oral hygiene.

Client Teaching

General
- Encourage use of artificial tears for "dry eyes."
- Encourage client to maintain oral hygiene if mouth is dry; ice chips and sugarless gum are recommended.
- Instruct client not to abruptly discontinue medication. Clients frequently discontinue drug because of side effects.
- Instruct client on need for regular and ongoing medical supervision.
- Advise client to avoid driving or operating hazardous machinery while vision is impaired.

Self-Administration
- Instruct client or family on the correct administration of eye drops and ointment. Include return demonstration. See Figures 3–9 and 3–10.

Side Effects
- Advise client to avoid prolonged exposure to sunlight because of the potential for photosensitivity.

Evaluation

- Determine effectiveness of drug therapy and presence of side effects. Intraocular pressure will be within desired range.

NURSING PROCESS
OSMOTICS

Assessment
- Obtain medical and drug history.
- Check vital signs (VS). Obtain baseline data to compare with future findings.
- Assess level of anxiety. Possibility of blindness increases anxiety.

Potential Nursing Diagnoses
- Altered visual perception
- High risk for injury

Planning
- Client's intraocular pressure will be lowered.

Nursing Interventions
- Monitor for side effects.
- Monitor for potassium depletion and electrolyte imbalances.
- Increase fluid intake, unless contraindicated.
- Record input and output and weigh daily.
- Monitor changes in level of orientation, especially in the elderly.

Client Teaching

General
- Instruct client regarding side effects of drugs.
- Osmotics are usually administered intravenously in a health care setting.

Evaluation
- Determine the effectiveness of drug therapy and presence of side effects. Intraocular pressure will be within desired range.

---

sulfonamides; carbonic anhydrase inhibitors can also cause photosensitivity.

Osmotics

Osmotics are generally used preoperatively and postoperatively to decrease vitreous humor volume, thereby reducing intraocular pressure. These drugs are used primarily in the emergency treatment of acute closed-angle glaucoma because of their ability to rapidly reduce intraocular pressure. Commonly prescribed osmotic drugs are presented in Table 43–6.

SIDE EFFECTS AND ADVERSE REACTIONS
Osmotic medications can cause headache, nausea, vomiting, and diarrhea. Especially in the elderly, disorientation resulting from electrolyte imbalances can result from use of mannitol and urea.

Anticholinergic Mydriatics and Cycloplegics

Mydriatics dilate the pupils; **cycloplegics** paralyze the muscles of accommodation. Both are used in diagnostic procedures and ophthalmic surgery. (Refer to Chapters 20 and 22 for a review of the autonomic nervous system and comprehensive discussion of anticholinergics.) Anticholinergics cause both dilation of the pupils and paralysis of the muscles of accommodation by relaxing the ciliary and dilator muscles of the iris by blocking acetylcholine. Commonly prescribed anticholinergic mydriatics and cycloplegics are presented in Table 43–7.

SIDE EFFECTS AND ADVERSE REACTIONS
Cycloplegics
Cycloplegics can cause tachycardia, photophobia, dryness of the mouth, edema, conjunctivitis, and derma-

Table 43-7

Mydriatics and Cycloplegics

GENERIC (BRAND)	ROUTE AND DOSAGE*	USES AND CONSIDERATIONS
Atropine sulfate (Atropisol, Isopto Atropine)	A: Sol 1%: 1–2 gtt up to q.i.d. C: Sol 0.5%: 1–2 gtt up to t.i.d. 1% Oint: Apply in lower eyelid sac up to t.i.d.	Most potent cycloplegic. For refraction, especially in children; for iritis and uveitis. *Not* for use with glaucoma or tachycardia. Wait 5 min before using other drugs. *Pregnancy category:* C; PB: NA; t½: NA
Cyclopentolate HCl (AK-Pentolate, Cyclogyl, Pentolair)	A: Sol 0.5%–2%: 1–2 gtt; then 1 gt in 5 min C: 1–2 gtt × 1; may repeat × 1 in 5–10 min with 0.5% or 1% sol	Mydriasis and cycloplegia for eye examination. *Pregnancy category:* C; PB: NA; t½: NA
Dipivefrin HCl (Propine)	A: Sol 0.1%; 1 gt q12h	Control of intraocular pressure in chronic open-angle glaucoma. *Pregnancy category:* B; PB: NA; t½: NA
Epinephrine HCl (Epifrin, Glaucon)	A&C: Sol 0.1%–2%: 1–2 gtt daily/b.i.d.	For open-angle glaucoma and during eye surgery. Discard brown or precipitate solution. *Pregnancy category:* C; PB: NA; t½: NA
Epinephrine borate (Epinal)	*Surgery:* A: 0.5–1% sol: Instill 1–2 gtt ≤ 3 × *Open-angle glaucoma:* A: 0.5% or 1.0% sol: Instill 1 gt in eye b.i.d.	For treatment of open-angle glaucoma and during ocular surgery. Contraindicated in narrow-angle glaucoma. Monitor tonometer readings with long-term use. Increased pressor effects. *Pregnancy category:* C; PB: UK; t½: UK
Homatropine hydrobromide (Isopto Homatropine)	A&C: Sol 2% and 5%: 1–2 gtt q3–4h Cy: Use only 2%	Similar to atropine, but faster onset and shorter duration. Mydriasis and cycloplegia for eye examination. *Pregnancy category:* C; PB: NA; t½: NA
Phenylephrine HCl (AK-Dilate)	*Mydriasis:* A&C: 2.5% or 10% sol: Instill 1 gt in eye before examination *Mydriasis with vasoconstriction:* A&C > 12 y: Instill 1 gt in eye; repeat × 1 in 1 h PRN Cy: 2.5% sol: Instill 1 gt in eye; repeat × 1 in 1 h PRN	For eye examination or surgery; treatment of wide-angle glaucoma and uveitis. *Pregnancy category:* C; PB: UK; t½: UK
Scopolamine hydrobromide (Isopto Hyoscine)	A: Sol: 0.25% 1–2 gtt 1 h before exam; 1–2 gtt for treatment up to q.i.d.	Used for clients sensitive to atropine sulfate. More rapid onset and shorter duration than atropine. *Pregnancy category:* C; PB: NA; t½: NA
Tropicamide (Mydriacyl Ophthalmic, Tropicacyl, Opticyl)	*Refraction:* 1%: 1–2 gtt; repeat in 5 min *Fundus exam:* 0.5%: 1–2 gtt 15–20 min before exam	Mydriasis and cycloplegia for eye exam. *Pregnancy category:* C; PB: NA; t½: NA

*To minimize systemic absorption, apply gentle pressure to lacrimal duct.
KEY: Cy: cycloplegic; A: adult; C: child; gt: drop; gtt: drops; oint: ointment; sol: solution; PB: protein-binding; t½: half-life; NA: not applicable; UK: unknown; PRN: as necessary.

titis. Symptoms of atropine toxicity include dry mouth, blurred vision, photophobia, constipation, fever, tachycardia, confusion, hallucinations, delirium, and coma. Toxicity is treated with physostigmine. Cycloplegics are contraindicated in clients with glaucoma because of their increased intraocular pressure.

Adrenergic Mydriatics

Side effects include headache, brow pain, allergic reaction, and worsening of narrow-angle glaucoma. Adrenergic mydriatics are contraindicated in cardiac dysrhythmias and cerebral atherosclerosis and should be used with caution in the elderly and clients with prostatic hypertrophy, diabetes mellitus, or parkinsonism. The health care provider should be notified of blurring of vision or loss of sight, difficulty in breathing, sweating, or flushing.

Administration of Eye Drops and Ointments

The techniques for administering eye drops and ointments are described in Tables 3–5 and 3–6 and illustrated in Figures 3–9 and 3–10. Individuals who wear contact lenses need to be knowledgeable about the products associated with some of the lenses. (See Figure 43–2.)

Clients with Eye Disorders: General Suggestions for Client Teaching

• Eye disorders carrying the possibility of blindness promote a high anxiety state in clients. Provide time, instructions, and return demonstration in all teaching plans.
• Use caution with confused or forgetful clients in order to prevent overdose.
• Instruct client or family in proper administration of eye drops or ointment. Maintain sterile technique and prevent dropper contamination. Expect some blurriness from ointments. Apply at bedtime, if possible, to avoid safety problems from diminished vision.
• Instruct client to report changes in vision, blurring, loss of vision, difficulty in breathing, or flushing.
• Instruct client to store drug in light-resistant container away from heat.

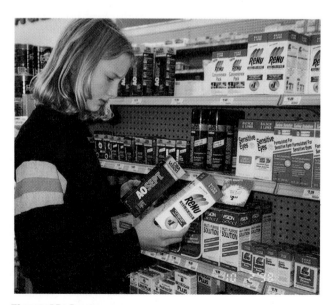

Figure 43–2
Teenager selecting products to meet her contact lens care needs.

• Instruct client not to suddenly stop medication without *prior* approval from the prescribing health care provider.
• Instruct client to record medications administered. Prepare a chart so the client can record when eye medications were given.
• Instruct client with glaucoma to avoid atropine-like drugs, which increase intraocular pressure. Some drugs for glaucoma are long acting and require only daily dosing if the client is forgetful or needs another person to administer the medicine.
• Clients should be alerted to check labels on OTC drugs with pharmacist.
• Instruct client to carry a medical alert identification card or bracelet at all times if he or she is allergic to any medications.
• Encourage the client to keep health care appointments.
• Individuals who wear contact lenses need to be knowledgeable about the products associated with the care of the lenses.

DRUGS FOR DISORDERS OF THE EAR

The medications most often used to treat **otic** disorders are the same preparations used to treat similar problems in other areas of the body; e.g., antiinfectives. Refer to the appropriate chapter in the text for a comprehensive discussion of the specific drug group.

Antibacterials

Several antibacterials are commonly prescribed for external use for otic disorders. Refer to Chapters 25, 26, and 27 on antibiotics. Table 43–8 presents the drug data for selected antibacterial medications.

SIDE EFFECTS AND ADVERSE REACTIONS
Side effects include overgrowth of nonsusceptible organisms. Prior hypersensitivity is a contraindication.

Antihistamine-Decongestants

Antihistamine-decongestants are thought to reduce nasal and middle ear congestion in acute otitis media. (Refer to Chapter 35 for a comprehensive discussion of upper respiratory agents.) Reduction of the edema around the orifice of the eustachian tube promotes drainage from the middle ear. There are numerous antihistamine-decongestant medications on the market, including Actifed, Allerest, Dimetapp, Drixoral, Novafed, Ornade, Phenergan, and Triaminic. Com-

Table 43–8
Otic: Antiinfectives

GENERIC (BRAND)	ROUTE AND DOSAGE	USES AND CONSIDERATIONS
EXTERNAL		
Acetic acid and aluminum acetate (Otic Domeboro)	A&C: Sol 2%: Insert saturated wick, keep moist × 24 h; instill 4–6 gtt q2–3h	Provides an acid medium; has antibacterial activity. Low cost. *Pregnancy category:* UK; PB: NA; t½: NA
Boric acid (Ear-Dry), Carbamide peroxide (Debrox)	A&C > 12 y: Instill 5–10 gtt b.i.d.; tilt head to unaffected side to keep gtt in ear or put cotton plug in outer ear	OTC preparations to dry the ear canal and to loosen and remove impacted wax (cerumen) from the ear canal. Debrox—instill for up to 4 d. If no improvement, call health care provider. *Pregnancy category:* C; PB: NA; t½: NA
Chloramphenicol (Chloromycetin Otic)	A&C: 0.5% otic sol: Instill 2–3 gtt into ear t.i.d.	Topically for infections of ear canal. *Pregnancy category:* C; PB: NA; t½: NA
Polymyxin B	A&C: 3–4 gtt t.i.d./q.i.d. for 7–10 d	Usually given in combination with neomycin and hydrocortisone. For disorders of external ear. Discontinue after 10 d to prevent fungal overgrowth. *Pregnancy category:* B; PB: NA; t½: NA
Tetracycline (Achromycin)	A&C: 1–2 gtt b.i.d./q.i.d.	Similar to polymyxin B. *Pregnancy category:* D; PB: NA; t½: NA
Trolamine polypeptide oleate-condensate (Cerumenex)	A&C: Fill ear canal and insert cotton plug for 15–30 min; flush ear with lukewarm water; repeat × 1 if needed.	To loosen and remove impacted wax (cerumen) from the ear canal. *Pregnancy category:* C; PB: NA; t½: NA
INTERNAL		
Amoxicillin (Amoxil, Augmentin)	A: PO: 250–500 mg q8h C: PO: 20–40 mg/kg/d in 3 divided doses	For treatment of otitis media. Eighty percent absorbed by mouth; food does not prevent absorption. Long duration of action. *Pregnancy category:* B; PB: 20%; t½: 1–1.5 h
Ampicillin trihydrate (Polycillin)	A: PO: 250–500 mg q6h IM/IV: 2–8 g/d in divided doses C: PO: 50–200 mg/kg/d in divided doses IM/IV: 50–200 mg/kg/d in divided doses	First broad-spectrum penicillin. Fifty percent of drug absorbed by GI tract. Effective against gram-negative and gram-positive bacteria. Individuals allergic to penicillin may also be allergic to ampicillin. *Pregnancy category:* B; PB: 15%–28%; t½: 1–2 h
Cefaclor (Ceclor)	A: PO: 250–500 mg q8h; *max,* 4 g/d C: PO: 20–40 mg/kg/d in 3 divided doses; *max:* 1 g/d	Second-generation cephalosporin. To treat ampicillin-resistant and gram-negative strains. Third-line drug for otitis media. Not for infants < 1 mo. Monitor electrolytes in long-term therapy. *Pregnancy category:* B; PB: 25%; t½: 0.5–1 h

Table continued on following page

mon side effects are drowsiness, blurred vision, and dry mucous membranes.

Combination Products

Combination products such as Cortisporin Otic are not held in high regard by most health care providers who believe that only what is needed should be used. These drugs combine local anesthetics or antiinflammatory drugs with antiinfectives.

Ceruminolytics

Cerumen (earwax), produced by glands in the outer half of the ear canal, usually moves to the external os by itself and is washed away. However, **ceruminolytics** are sometimes needed to loosen and remove impacted cerumen from the ear canal. Irrigation with hydrogen peroxide solution (3% diluted to half strength with water) can be done to flush cerumen deposits out of the ear canal. For chronic impaction, 1

Table 43–8 *Continued*
Otic: Antiinfectives

GENERIC (BRAND)	ROUTE AND DOSAGE	USES AND CONSIDERATIONS
Erythromycin (E-Mycin)	A: PO: 250–500 mg q6h 　IV: 1–4 g/d in 4 divided doses C: PO: 30–50 mg/kg/d in 4 divided doses 　IV: 20–50 mg/kg/d in 4 divided doses	To treat gram-positive and gram-negative bacterial infections in clients allergic to penicillin. Enteric-coated tablet to prevent gastric acid from destroying drug. *Pregnancy category:* B; PB: 65%; $t_{\frac{1}{2}}$: PO, 1–2 h; IV, 3–5 h
Penicillin (Pentids, Pen-V)	*Penicillin G potassium (Pentids):* A: PO: 200,000–50,000 U q6h 　IM: 500,000–5 million U/d in divided doses 　IV: 4–20 million U/d in divided doses diluted in IV solution C: PO: 25,000–90,000 U/d in divided doses 　IV: 50,000–100,000 U/kg/d in divided doses *Penicillin V potassium (Pen-V):* A: PO: 125–500 mg q6h C: PO: 15–50 mg/kg/d in 3–4 divided doses	For otitis media and mastoiditis. Take before or after meals. Penicillin G: electrolytes should be monitored; injectable solution is clear. Penicillin V: not recommended in renal failure. *Pregnancy category:* B; PB: (G) 60%, (V) 80%; $t_{\frac{1}{2}}$ (G) 0.5–1 h, (V) 0.5 h
Sulfonamides (Azulfidine [sulfasalazine], Bactrim [trimethoprim and sulfamethoxazole])	Dose and route vary See Chapter 27	Most are highly protein-bound. Increase fluid intake to decrease crystalluria. Side effects include allergic response. Blood disorders may result from long-term use and high doses. Avoid in third trimester of pregnancy. *Pregnancy category:* B, D; PB: 50–95%; $t_{\frac{1}{2}}$: 4.5–12 h
Clarithromycin (Biaxin)	A: PO: 250–500 mg q12h C: PO: 7.5 mg/kg q12h	For otitis media. Cautious use in renal impairment. Efficacy not established in children < 12 y. *Pregnancy category:* C; PB: UK; $t_{\frac{1}{2}}$: 3–5 h
Amoxicillin and potassium clavulanate (Augmentin)	A: PO: 250 mg q8h C: PO: 40 mg/kg/d divided q8h	For otitis media. Clavulanate inhibits beta lactamase degradation of amoxicillin. *Pregnancy category:* B; PB: UK; $t_{\frac{1}{2}}$: 1–3 h
Loracarbef (Lorabid)	A: PO: 200 mg q12h C: PO: 30 mg/kg/d q12h	For otitis media. Second-generation cephalosporin. Cautious use in renal impairment and seizures. *Pregnancy category:* B; PB: UK; $t_{\frac{1}{2}}$: 45–60 min

KEY: A: adult; C: child; PO: by mouth; IM: intramuscular; IV: intravenous; gtt: drops; sol: solution; PB: protein-binding; $t_{\frac{1}{2}}$: half-life; NA: not applicable; UK: unknown; OTC: over-the-counter; GI: gastrointestinal.

to 2 drops of olive oil or mineral oil softens the wax. Cerumenex (prescription) and Debrox (OTC) cost more and are no more effective than hydrogen peroxide solution.

Administration of Ear Medications

Ear medications are generally contained in a liquid vehicle for ease of administration. Guidelines for the administration of ear drops are given in Table 3–7 and Figure 3-11*A* and *B*.

IRRIGATION

Irrigations of the ear may also be ordered. Irrigation is best accomplished when there is direct visualization of the tympanic membrane (eardrum). It must be done *gently* to avoid damage to the eardrum. Frequently used irrigating solutions include Burow's solution, hydrogen peroxide 3% (with water), hypertonic sodium chloride solution 3%, and acetic acid (vinegar) solution. Contraindications include perforation of the eardrum and prior hypersensitivity.

NURSING PROCESS
ANTIINFECTIVES FOR EAR DISORDERS

Assessment

- Obtain a medical and drug history including any allergies.
- Check vital signs (VS). Obtain baseline data that can be compared with future findings.

Potential Nursing Diagnoses

- Altered auditory perception
- Pain

Planning

- Client will be free of ear infection after completion of drug regimen.

Nursing Interventions

- Complete culture and sensitivity before starting drug.
- Monitor input and output.
- Report hematuria or oliguria. High doses of antibacterials are nephrotoxic.
- Relief of associated pain, if present.
- Monitor renal function, liver studies, and blood studies (white cell count, red cell count, hemoglobin and hematocrit, bleeding time).
- Store medication in airtight container.
- Report dizziness to health care provider.
- Report fatigue, fever, or sore throat, any of which could indicate superimposed infection.

Client Teaching

- Instruct client to complete entire course of medication (10 to 14 d) and *not* to stop medication when he or she "feels better."
- Encourage client to eat yogurt or buttermilk to maintain intestinal flora.
- If client is prone to otitis after swimming or in warm weather, instruct him or her to keep ear canals dry; instillation of drops of alcohol into the ear canal may be helpful. Check with the health care provider.
- Instruct client to have medical alert identification with him or her at all times if allergic to medications.

Evaluation

- Determine the effectiveness of drug therapy and the presence of side effects.

Clients with Ear Disorders: General Suggestions for Client Teaching

- Instruct client not to insert any foreign objects into the ear canal.
- Instruct client to take drug as prescribed.
- Instruct client to keep drug in light-resistant container.
- Instruct client about expected effect of drug, dosage, and side effects, and when to notify health care provider.
- Encourage client to keep follow-up appointments.

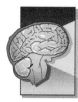

Critical Thinking in Action

Mrs. H. has been on pilocarpine for several days; a 2% solution, 4 gtt q.i.d. She tells you that she must need new glasses because newsprint and the TV picture are a bit "fuzzy."

1. Is any action indicated? If so, what?
2. What additional advice would be appropriate if the client had coronary vascular disease and bradycardia?
3. Are there any expected effects on Mrs. H's vital signs? If so, what?
4. What suggestions would you give Mrs. H. to avoid systemic absorption of the medication?

Mrs. Z. brings 7-year-old Chris to the HMO practice because he has been complaining of "pain in my ear" for 2 days. Following an assessment, the health care provider determines that Chris has an infection in the external right ear canal. Polymyxin B is prescribed to be administered 3 to 4 gtt t.i.d. for 14 days.

1. Is the drug regimen appropriate for Chris? What is the nurse's responsibility?
2. What is a consequence of long-term use of this drug?
3. What drug may be used in combination to decrease edema, itching, and redness?

Client teaching is an integral part of the therapeutic drug regimen. Explain the role of the nurse in relation to the following:

4. What position should Chris be in to receive the drugs?
5. What instructions would you give Mrs. Z. regarding the administration of ear drops, including the actual positioning of the ear prior to administering the drops? In what way would you modify these instructions if the child were 2 years old?
6. What advice do you give Chris about putting things in his ear?

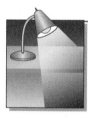

Study Questions

1. Miotics are used in the treatment of what disorders? What is the mechanism of action of miotics?

2. What information would be required in a teaching plan for a client receiving pilocarpine?

3. What drug is the most potent cycloplegic? What are the nursing implications of the use of this medication?

4. The client E.H., aged 85 years, was just started on acetazolamide. What category of drug is this? What is the brand name? What are the nursing interventions associated with clients receiving this drug?

5. Mannitol is a commonly used osmotic. What are the contraindications for use of this drug?

6. Your client is being prepared for an eye examination. In taking the health history, you discover she is sensitive to atropine sulfate. What drug might be used instead for the examination?

7. Describe appropriate general teaching strategies for clients with eye disorders.

8. What is a disadvantage to the use of combination products such as Cortisporin Otic?

9. What product is recommended for the treatment and prevention of chronic impaction of cerumen?

10. What is included in the nursing assessment of the client before the start of an antibacterial drug for the treatment of an ear infection?

Drugs for Dermatologic Disorders

44

Outline

Objectives

* Define acne vulgaris, psoriasis, drug-induced dermatitis, and contact dermatitis.
* Describe nonpharmacologic measures for treating mild acne vulgaris.
* List three drugs that can cause drug-induced dermatitis and their characteristic symptoms.
* Identify the topical antibacterial agents used in prevention and treatment of burn tissue infection.
* Describe the nursing process, including client teaching, related to commonly used drugs for acne vulgaris, psoriasis, and burns.

Terms

acne vulgaris	papule	tinea capitis
contact dermatitis	plaques	tinea pedis
macule	psoriasis	vesicle

INTRODUCTION

There are numerous skin lesions and eruptions requiring mild to aggressive drug therapy. Some of the skin disorders include acne vulgaris, psoriasis, eczema dermatitis, contact dermatitis, drug-induced dermatitis, and burn infection. Skin eruptions may result from viral infections (e.g., herpes simplex, herpes zoster) and from fungal infections (e.g., **tinea pedis** [athlete's foot], **tinea capitis** [ringworm]), as well as from bacterial infections. These skin eruptions may be treated with over-the-counter (OTC) drugs and are not discussed in this chapter. Antiviral drugs are presented in Chapter 29.

Most of the treatments for skin eruptions include topical creams, ointments, pastes, lotions, and solutions. Skin lesions may appear as **macules** (flat with varying colors), **papules** (raised, palpable, and less than 1 cm in diameter), **vesicles** (raised, filled with fluid, and less than 1 cm in diameter), or **plaques** (hard, rough raised, and flat on top). Selected skin disorders and their drug therapy regimens are discussed separately.

ACNE VULGARIS

Acne vulgaris is the formation of papules, nodules, and cysts on the face, neck, shoulders, and back resulting from keratin plugs at the base of the pilosebaceous oil glands near the hair follicles. Ninety percent of persons with acne are adolescents. The increase in androgen production that occurs during adolescence increases the production of sebum, an oily skin lubricant. The sebum combines with keratin to form a plug.

Nonpharmacologic Approach

Nonpharmacologic measures should be tried before drug therapy is initiated. A prescribed or suggested cleansing agent is necessary with all types of acne. Skin should be gently cleansed several times a day. Vigorous scrubbing should be avoided. Well-balanced diet is indicated. Megadoses of vitamin A were once used for treating acne. Vitamin A is fat-soluble and is retained in tissues, especially the liver, for long periods; excessive doses of vitamin A, therefore, can be highly toxic, so megadosing with vitamin A is no longer a valid therapy for treating acne. High doses of vitamin A may also cause teratogenic effects to a fetus. Decreasing emotional stress and increasing emotional support are suggested. If drug therapy is necessary, the nonpharmacologic measures should be maintained.

Topical Antiacne Drugs

Mild acne may require gentle cleansing and the use of keratolytics (keratin dissolvers, such as benzoyl peroxide, resorcinol, salicylic acid). Benzoyl peroxide is applied as a cream, lotion, or gel once or twice a day. This agent loosens the outer, horny layer of the epidermis.

Tretinoin (Retin-A, Renova), a derivative of vitamin A, is a topical drug for treating mild to moderate acne by altering keratinization. There are two new antiacne agents, adapalene (Differin) and azelaic acid (Azelex), used for mild to moderate acne. Adapalene is similar in action to tretinoin. It has antiinflammatory and comedolytic (eliminating blackheads) properties, and tends to be more effective in reducing the number of acne lesions than is tretinoin. Adapalene should not be used before or after extended sun exposure or sunburn. It can increase the risk of sunburn and intensify the existing sunburn. Azelaic acid appears to be as effective as benzoyl peroxide and tretinoin. Adapalene and azelaic acid can cause burning, pruritus, and erythema after several applications; however, with azelaic acid, it is not as common as it is with adapalene.

Moderate acne requires a stronger concentration of benzoyl peroxide (10%), and topical antibiotics, such as tetracycline, erythromycin, clindamycin, or meclocycline, may be used. Erythromycin and clindomycin are most frequently prescribed with fewest side effects.

Systemic Antiacne Drugs

For severe acne, oral antibiotics (tetracycline [drug of choice] or erythromycin), and topical glucocorticoids may be prescribed. Tetracycline inhibits bacterial protein synthesis. It is used in the treatment of acne with a lower maintenance dose over a period of months. Tetracycline should not be taken with antacids or milk products, because these bind the tetracycline into an insoluble compound, thus decreasing its absorption. A major side effect of tetracycline is photosensitivity. Exposure to the sun can result in a severe sunburn. Pregnant women should not take tetracycline because of the possible teratogenic effects on the fetus.

Isotretinoin (Accutane), a derivative of vitamin A, is used for severe cystic acne. It can be administered orally or topically. It decreases sebum formation and secretion, and it has antiinflammatory and antikeratinizing (keratolytic) effects. It can cause adverse reactions such as nosebleeds, pruritus, and inflammation of the eyes and lips. Isotretinoin should not be used during pregnancy because of teratogenic effects. Also, it can elevate triglyceride levels. Table 44–1 lists the drugs used for controlling acne vulgaris.

Table 44–1
Drugs for Acne Vulgaris and Psoriasis

DRUG	DOSAGE	USES AND CONSIDERATIONS
ACNE VULGARIS		
Systemic Preparations		
Tetracycline (Sumycin)	A: PO: 250–500 mg b.i.d.	For moderate to severe acne. Inexpensive. Should not be taken during pregnancy. Should not be taken with milk products or antacids. *Pregnancy category:* D; PB: 65%; t½: 6–12 h
Erythromycin (E-Mycin)	A: PO: 250–500 mg, b.i.d.	For moderate to severe acne. A substitute for tetracycline. *Pregnancy category:* B; PB: 75%–90%; t½: 1.5–2 h
Isotretinoin (Accutane)	A: PO: 0.5–2 mg/kg/d, in 2 divided doses, for 15 wk	For severe acne. Decreases sebum secretion. Used when oral antibiotics have failed. Avoid use with tetracycline and vitamin A to reduce toxic effects. *Pregnancy category:* X; PB: 99%; t½: 10–20 h
TOPICAL PREPARATIONS		
Keratolytic Agents		
Adapalene (Differin)	A: C >12 y: topical: 0.1% gel; apply daily h.s. after washing	To treat mild to moderate acne. Do not use before or after extended sun exposure. It intensifies sunburn. Pruritus may occur. *Pregnancy category:* C; PB: UK; t½: UK
Azelaic acid (Azelex)	A: C >12 y: Topical: cream 20%; apply b.i.d.	To treat mild to moderate acne. Inhibits hyperactivity of normal melanocytes. Mild pruritus, erythema, dryness, and peeling of skin might result. *Pregnancy category:* B; PB: UK; t½: 12 h
Benzoyl-peroxide (Benzac, Persa-Gel)	2.5%–10%, once to four times/d (cream, gel, or lotion)	For mild to moderate acne. Promotes keratolysis (removal of horny layer of the epidermis). May cause skin irritation (burning, blistering, or swelling)
Salicylic acid (Sebulex)	*Antiacne/antiseborrheic:* 2%–10%, cream, gel, shampoo; use as directed	For mild to moderate acne; promotes desquamation
Resorcinol (Bicozene)	1%–10% cream, ointment, lotion, and shampoo	For mild to moderate acne
Resorcinol and sulfur	2% resorcinol + 5% sulfur 2% resorcinol + 8% sulfur Use as directed	For mild to moderate acne
Antibiotics		
Tetracycline	Ointment: 3%; sol: 2.2 mg/mL	For moderate acne. *Pregnancy category:* B
Erythromycin	Ointment: 2%; gel: 1.5%–2%	
Clindamycin (Cleocin)	Gel: ⅕; lotion: 1%; sol: 1%	
Meclocycline (Meclan)	Ointment, b.i.d.	
Tretinoin (Retin-A)	Cream: 0.05%–0.1% Gel: 0.025%–0.1% Liquid: 0.05% daily h.s.	For mild to moderate acne. Vitamin A derivative. May be used with benzoyl peroxide or topical antibiotic. Should not be applied to open wounds. Area should be cleansed first. *Pregnancy category:* B
PSORIASIS		
Methoxsalen (Oxsoralen)	A: PO: 10–20 mg, 2 h before exposure to therapeutic ultraviolet rays. Topical application before exposure to ultraviolet rays	For severe psoriasis. Systemic antimetabolite drug. Avoid during pregnancy. Avoid sunlight during drug therapy; sunlight could cause burning and blistering. *Pregnancy category:* C; PB: 80%–90%; t½: >2 h
Etretinate (Tegison)	A: PO: 0.5–0.75 mg/kg/d, in divided doses, not to exceed 1.5 mg/kg/d	For recalcitrant psoriasis. Related to vitamin A. It may take up to 1–6 mo for a response to treatment. *Pregnancy category:* X; PB: 99%; t½: 4–8 d

Table continued on following page

Table 44–1 *Continued*
Drugs for Acne Vulgaris and Psoriasis

DRUG	DOSAGE	USES AND CONSIDERATIONS
Topical Preparations		
Calcipotriene (Dovonex)	A: Topical: cream, ointment, and scalp; sol: 0.005%, q.d., or b.i.d.	To treat mild to moderate plaque psoriasis. Burning, stinging, erythema may occur. Excess use may increase serum calcium level. *Pregnancy category:* C; PB: UK; t$\frac{1}{2}$: UK
Coal tar (Estar, Psorigel)	Shampoo, cream, gel, paste, soap, ointment, lotion, solution	For mild to moderate psoriasis. Suppresses DNA synthesis, decreasing mitotic activity. May stain clothing, skin, and hair
Anthralin (Anthra-Derm)	0.1%–1.0% ointment and cream	For moderate-type psoriasis. It inhibits DNA synthesis, thus suppressing proliferation of the epidermal cells. It can stain clothing, skin, and hair
Keratolytic Drugs		
Salicyclic acid, sulfur, resorcinol		See acne vulgaris

KEY: A: adult; PO: by mouth; PB: protein-binding; sol: solution; t$\frac{1}{2}$: half-life; >: greater than.

PSORIASIS

Psoriasis is a chronic skin disorder that affects 1% to 2% of the U.S. population. It is more common in whites than blacks. Onset of psoriasis may be as early as at age 10 years but usually appears before the age of 30 years. Psoriasis is characterized by erythematous papules and plaques covered with silvery scales. It appears on the scalp, elbows, palms of the hands, knees, and soles of the feet. With psoriasis, epidermal cell growth and epidermal turnover is accelerated to approximately five times the normal expected epidermal growth. Antipsoriatic drug therapy uses preparations such as coal tar products and anthralin to keep the psoriasis in check; however, there are usually periods of remission and exacerbation.

Topical and Systemic Preparations for Psoriasis

The psoriatic scales may be loosened with keratolytics (salicylic acid, sulfur). Topical glucocorticoids are used at times for mild psoriasis. Other topical preparations for psoriasis include anthralin (Anthra-Derm, Lasan) and coal tar (Estar, PsoriGel). Applications of 1% anthralin may cause erythema to occur. This agent can stain clothing, skin, and hair. Coal tar products are available in shampoos, lotions, and creams. They have an unpleasant odor and can cause burning and stinging. Systemic toxicity does not occur with anthralin and coal tar. A new topical product for mild to moderate psoriasis is calcipotriene (Dovonex), a synthetic vitamin D_3 derivative. It is useful for suppressing cell proliferation. This drug may cause local irritation, but the serious adverse effects are hypercalciuria and hypercalcemia (increased urine and serum calcium levels).

The anticancer drug methotrexate slows high growth fraction. It is prescribed to decrease the acceleration of epidermal cell growth in severe psoriasis. Etretinate (Tegison) is used for severe pustular psoriasis, more so than the plaque-type psoriasis. It is used when other agents have failed to control psoriasis. Etretinate has an antiinflammatory effect and inhibits keratinization and proliferation of the epithelial cells. Ultraviolet A (UVA) may be used to suppress mitotic (cell division) activity. Photochemotherapy, a combination of ultraviolet radiation with a psoralen derivative, methoxsalen (photosensitive drug), is used to decrease proliferation of epidermal cells. This type of therapy is called psoralen and ultraviolet A (PUVA). The use of PUVA permits lower doses of drug and ultraviolet A to be given. Table 44–1 lists the drugs used for controlling psoriasis.

SIDE EFFECTS AND ADVERSE REACTIONS

Acne Vulgaris

TETRACYCLINE

Nausea, vomiting, diarrhea, rash, urticaria, photosensitivity. **Adverse reactions:** Oral candidiasis, superinfection, blood dyscrasias, hepatotoxicity, and nephrotoxicity.

ISOTRETINOIN

Nosebleeds; dryness of the nose, mouth, especially in corners of mouth, and skin; inflamed eyes; pruritus; photosensitivity; anorexia, nausea, vomiting; elevated liver enzymes. **Adverse reactions:** Thrombocytopenia, hematuria.

BENZOYL PEROXIDE

Dry and irritated skin with burning, scaling, and swelling.

TRETINOIN

Skin irritation, such as burning, swelling, blistering, and peeling.

ADAPALENE

Burning, pruritus, erythema, dryness, and scaling, usually occurring during the second to fourth weeks of treatment, but subsiding later in treatment. Severe sunburn can occur during extended exposure to the sun.

Psoriasis

COAL TAR

Skin irritation, such as burning; photosensitivity; and staining effect.

ANTHRALIN

Erythema (redness) to normal skin, inflamed eyes, and staining effect.

METHOXSALEN

Nausea, headache, vertigo, rash, pruritus, burning and peeling of skin. **Adverse reactions:** Anemia, leukopenia, thrombocytopenia, ulcerative stomatitis, bleeding; alopecia, cystitis.

ETRETINATE

Anorexia, vomiting, dry skin and nasal mucosa, rash, pruritus, fatigue, bone or joint pain, peeling of skin, photosensitivity. **Adverse reactions:** Alopecia, cardiac dysrhythmias, hepatitis, hematuria.

VERRUCA VULGARIS (WARTS)

The common wart is a hard, horny nodule that may appear anywhere on the body, but particularly on the hands and feet. Warts are benign lesions. They may be removed by freezing, electrodesiccation, or surgical excision. Drugs used include salicylic acid, podophyllum resin, and cantharidin. Salicylic acid promotes desquamation. It can be absorbed through the skin, and salicylism (toxicity) might occur. Podophyllum resin is indicated mainly for venereal warts and is not as effective against the common wart. This drug also can be absorbed through the skin, so toxic symptoms such as peripheral neuropathy, blood dyscrasias, and kidney impairment could result if a large area is treated. Podophyllum can cause teratogenic effects and should not be used during pregnancy. Cantharidin (Cantharone, Verr-Canth) is used to remove the common wart; however, it can be harmful to the normal skin. For treating the common wart, cantharidin is applied to the wart, the topical agent is allowed to dry, and then it is covered with a nonporous tape for 24 hours. The procedure can be repeated in a week or two.

There are many over-the-counter (OTC) agents used to remove warts. The efficiency of some of the OTC agents is questionable; however, some that contain chemical compounds such as salicylic acid may be effective.

DRUG-INDUCED DERMATITIS

An adverse reaction to drug therapy may result in skin lesions, which may vary from a rash, urticaria, papules, and vesicles, to life-threatening skin eruptions, such as erythema multiforme (red blisters over a large portion of the body) or Stevens-Johnson syndrome (large blisters in the oral and anogenital mucosa, pharynx, eyes, and viscera). The hypersensitive reaction to a drug is caused by the formation of sensitizing lymphocytes. If multiple drug therapy is used, the last drug given may be the cause of the hypersensitivity and skin eruptions. The usual skin reactions are a rash that may take several hours or a day to appear and urticarias (hives), which usually take a few minutes to appear. Certain drugs, such as penicillin, are known to cause hypersensitivity.

Other drug-induced dermatitides include discoid lupus erythematosus (DLE) and exfoliative dermatitis. Hydralazine hydrochloride (Apresoline), isoniazid (INH), phenothiazines, anticonvulsants, and antidysrhythmics, such as procainamide (Pronestyl), may cause lupus-like symptoms. If lupus symptoms occur, the drug should be discontinued. Certain antibacterials and anticonvulsants may cause exfoliative dermatitis, resulting in erythema of the skin, itching, scaling, and loss of body hair.

CONTACT DERMATITIS

Contact dermatitis, also called exogenous dermatitis, is caused by chemical or plant irritation. It is characterized by a skin rash with itching, swelling, blistering, oozing, or scaling at the affected skin sites. The

NURSING PROCESS
ACNE VULGARIS AND PSORIASIS

Assessment

- Obtain a history from the client of the onset of skin lesions. Note whether there is a familial history of the skin disorder.
- Assess the client's skin eruptions. Describe the lesions, location, and drainage, if present.
- Assess the psychological effects of skin lesions and changes in body image.
- Obtain a culture of a purulent draining skin lesion.
- Obtain baseline vital signs (VS). Report any elevation in temperature.

Potential Nursing Diagnoses

- Risk for impaired skin integrity
- Risk for infection
- Body image disturbance related to skin lesions

Planning

- The client's skin lesions will be decreased in size or will be absent after drug therapy and skin care.

Nursing Interventions

- Apply topical medications to the skin lesions using aseptic technique.
- Monitor VS and report abnormal findings.
- Check the lesion sites during drug therapy for improvement or adverse reactions to the drug therapy, such as blistering, swelling, or scaling.

Client Teaching

- Instruct the client not to use harsh cleansers on the skin. Tell the client to clean the skin several times a day.
- Teach the client how to apply topical ointments and creams using a clean technique.
- Teach the client about the side effects and adverse reactions associated with the drugs being taken.
- Tell the client to report abnormal findings immediately. Inform the client not to take milk or antacids with tetracycline.
- Inform the client to alert the health care provider if pregnant or if there is a possibility of pregnancy. Many agents for treating acne can cause teratogenic effects on the fetus.
- Instruct the client to keep health care appointments and have laboratory tests performed as prescribed.

Cultural Considerations

- Respect the client's cultural beliefs and alternative methods for treating acne vulgaris or psoriasis. Plan may need modification to include pharmacologic treatment for the acne or psoriasis.

Evaluation

- Evaluate the effectiveness of the drug therapy on the skin lesions. If improvement is not apparent, the drug therapy and skin care regimen may need to be changed.

chemical contact may include cosmetics, cleansing products (such as soaps and detergents), perfume, clothing, dyes, and topical drugs. Plant contacts include poison ivy, oak, or sumac.

Nonpharmacologic measures include avoiding direct contact with the causative irritant. Protective gloves or clothing may be necessary if the chemical is associated with work. Cleanse the skin area that has been in contact with the irritant immediately. Patch testing may be needed to determine the causal factor.

Treatment may consist of wet dressings containing Burow's solution (aluminum acetate); lotions, such as calamine, that contain zinc oxide; calcium hydroxide solution; and glycerin. Calamine lotion may contain the antihistamine diphenhydramine and is used primarily for plant irritations. If itching persists, antipruritics (topical or systemic diphenhydramine [Benadryl]) may be used. Topical antipruritics should not be applied to open wounds or near the eyes or genital area. Other agents used as antipruritics are

- Systemic drugs, such as cyproheptadine hydrochloride (Periactin) and trimeprazine tartrate (Temaril)
- Antipruritic baths of oatmeal or Alpha-Keri
- Solutions of potassium permanganate, aluminum subacetate, or normal saline
- Glucocorticoid ointments, creams, or gels

Dexamethasone (Decadron) cream, hydrocortisone ointment or cream, methylprednisolone acetate (Medrol) ointment, triamcinolone acetonide (Aristocort), and flurandrenolide (Cordran) are examples of topical glucocorticoids that aid in alleviating dermatitis. Table 44–2 lists selected topical glucocorticoids according to their potency for relieving the itching and inflammation associated with dermatitis.

A portion of topical glucocorticoids can be systemically absorbed into the circulation, the amount and rate of absorption depending on the vehicle (cream, lotion), drug concentration, drug composition, and skin area to which the glucocorticoid is applied. Absorption is greater where the skin is more permeable: at the face, scalp, eyelids, neck, axilla, and genital area. Side effects and adverse reactions may occur with prolonged use of the topical drug and if the drug is continuously covered with a dressing. Prolonged use of topical glucocorticoids can cause thinning of the skin with atrophy of the epidermis and dermis, and purpura from small-vessel eruptions.

HAIR LOSS AND BALDNESS

When the hair shaft is lost and the hair follicle cannot regenerate, male pattern baldness, or alopecia, occurs. Permanent hair loss is associated with a familial history and occurs during the aging process, earlier in some individuals than others. Drugs and health conditions that are also known to cause alopecia include the anticancer (antineoplastic) agents, gold salts, sulfonamides, anticonvulsants, aminoglycosides, and some of the nonsteroidal antiflammatory drugs (NSAIDs), such as indomethacin. Severe febrile illnesses, pregnancy, myxedema (condition resulting from hypothyroidism), and cancer therapies are some of the conditions contributing to temporary hair loss.

A 2% minoxidil (Rogaine) solution has been approved by the Food and Drug Administration (FDA) for treating male pattern baldness. Minoxidil causes vasodilation, thus increasing cutaneous blood flow. The increased blood flow tends to stimulate hair folli-

Table 44–2
Topical Glucocorticoids

POTENCY	DRUG NAME	DRUG FORM
High	Amcinonide 0.1% (Cyclocort)	Cream, ointment
	Betamethasone dipropionate 0.05% (Diprosone)	Cream, ointment, lotion
	Desoximetasone 0.25% (Topicort)	Cream, ointment
	Desoximetasone 0.05%	Gel
	Diflorasone diacetate 0.05% (Florone)	Cream, ointment
	Halcinonide 0.1% (Halog)	Cream, ointment
	Triamcinolone acetonide 0.5% (Aristocort A, Kenalog)	Cream, ointment
Moderate	Betamethasone benzoate 0.025% (Benisone)	Cream, ointment
	Betamethasone valerate 0.1% (Valisone)	Cream, ointment, lotion
	Desoximetasone 0.05% (Topicort LP)	Cream, gel
	Fluocinolone acetonide 0.025% (Fluonid)	Cream, ointment
	Flurandrenolide 0.025% (Cordran, Cordran SP)	Cream, ointment, lotion
	Halcinonide 0.025% (Halog)	Cream, ointment
	Hydrocortisone valerate 0.2% (Westcort)	Cream, ointment
	Mometasone furoate 0.1% (Elocon)	Cream, ointment, lotion
	Triamcinolone acetonide 0.025%–0.1% (Aristocort A, Kenalog)	Cream, ointment, lotion
Low	Dexamethasone 0.1% (Decadron)	Cream
	Desonide 0.05% (Tridesilon)	Cream
	Fluocinolone acetonide 0.01% (Fluonid)	Solution
	Hydrocortisone 0.25%, 0.5%, 1.0%, 2.5% (Cortef, Hytone)	Cream, ointment
	Methylprednisolone acetate 0.25%, 1.0% (Medrol)	Ointment

Table 44–3
Degree and Tissue Depth of Burns

TYPE	DEGREE	DEPTH	CHARACTERISTICS
Superficial epidermal	First	Epidermis	Erythema (redness), painful
Partial thickness superficial	First-second	Epidermis, upper dermis	Blistering, very painful
Deep thickness	Second	Epidermis, lower dermis	Mottled, blistering, intense pain
Full thickness	Third	Epidermis, dermis, nerve ending involvement, subcutaneous tissue	Pearly white skin, charred, no pain

cle growth. When the drug is discontinued, however, hair loss occurs within 3 to 4 months. Systemic absorption of minoxidil is minimal, so adverse reactions seldom occur. Occasionally, there may be headaches and a slight decrease in systolic blood pressure.

BURNS AND BURN PREPARATIONS

Burns from heat (thermal burns), electricity (electrical burns), and chemical agents (chemical burns) can cause skin lesions. Burns are classified according to degree and tissue depth of burns and are described in Table 44–3.

A moderately severe sunburn is an example of a first-degree burn. A severe sunburn can result in a second-degree burn. A burn needs immediate attention regardless of the degree and tissue depth of the burn.

For first-degree and minor burns, a cold wet compress should be applied to the burned area to constrict blood vessels and decrease swelling. This treatment also decreases the amount of pain. The quicker the burn area is cooled, the less tissue damage occurs.

Table 44–4
Topical Antiinfectives: Burns

GENERIC (BRAND)	ROUTE AND DOSAGE	USES AND CONSIDERATIONS
Nitrofurazone (Furacin)	0.2% cream, ointment, sol *Adjunctive therapy:* Apply directly or to dressing daily for 2°–3° burns; q4–5d for 2° burns with scant exudate	For second- and third-degree burns. Can cause photosensitivity, so avoid sunlight. May cause contact dermatitis. *Pregnancy category:* C; PB: NA; t$\frac{1}{2}$: NA
Mafenide acetate (Sulfamylon)	See Chart 44–1	For prevention and treatment of sepsis caused by 2°–3° burns. Pain and burning on application are common side effects. Allergic reaction (itching, rash, edema) may occur 10–14 d after use of mafenide. *Pregnancy category:* C; PB: UK; t$\frac{1}{2}$: UK
Silver nitrate	0.5 sol; 10%, 25% sticks; apply only to affected area 2–3×/wk for 2–3 wk	For second- and third-degree burns. Dressings are soaked in 0.5% silver nitrate solution and the dressings are removed before they dry. Effective against some gram-negative organisms. May cause electrolyte imbalance (hypokalemia) if used extensively. *Pregnancy category:* C; PB: NA; t$\frac{1}{2}$: NA
Silver sulfadiazine (Silvadene, SSD)	1% cream, apply daily–b.i.d. in $\frac{1}{16}$-inch layer	Prevent and treat infection of second- and third-degree burns. Ten percent of the drug is absorbed. Excessive use or extensive application area may cause sulfa crystals (crystalluria). *Pregnancy category:* C; PB: NA; t$\frac{1}{2}$: NA

KEY: NA: nonapplicable; UK: unknown; <: less than; PB: protein-binding; t$\frac{1}{2}$: half-life; sol: solution.

Chart 44-1. Antiinfectives: Burns

ANTIINFECTIVE: SULFONAMIDE

Drug Name

Mafenide acetate (Sulfamylon)
Pregnancy Category: C

Dosage

A & C: Topical: Apply $\frac{1}{16}$-inch layer evenly to affected area daily/b.i.d.; reapply as necessary

Contraindications

Hypersensitivity, inhalation injury

Drug-Lab-Food Interactions

None known

Pharmacokinetics

Absorption: Some absorbed
Distribution: PB: UK
Metabolism: t½: UK
Excretion: In urine

Pharmacodynamics

PO: Onset: On contact
     Peak: 2–4 h
     Duration: As long as applied

Therapeutic Effects/Uses

To treat second- and third-degree burns; to prevent organism invasion of burned tissue areas; to treat burn infections.

Mode of Action: Inhibits bacterial cell wall synthesis.

Side Effects

Rash, burning sensation, urticaria, pruritus, swelling

Adverse Reactions

Metabolic acidosis, respiratory alkalosis, blistering, superinfection
Life-threatening: Bone marrow suppression, fatal hemolytic anemia

Assessment and Planning

Interventions

Evaluation

NURSING PROCESS

KEY: A: Adult; C: child; UK: unknown; PB: protein-binding; t½: half-life.

No greasy ointment, butter, or greasy dressing should be applied, because they can inhibit heat loss from the burn and increase the damage to the tissues. A nonprescription antibiotic, such as bacitracin with polymyxin B (Polysporin), may be used for minor burns. Polymyxin B and neomycin, used separately, are not drugs of choice because they do not have a broad-spectrum effect. With chemical burns, the clothing should be removed immediately and the skin thoroughly flushed with water.

Persons with second- and third-degree burns that involve dermis and subcutaneous tissue should undergo treatment in a burn center or other hospital setting. Intravenous therapy is started immediately and a nonnarcotic or narcotic analgesic is given for pain. Burn areas are cleansed with sterile saline solution and an antiseptic, such as povidone-iodine (Betadine). If a povidone-iodine solution is used, it should be determined that the client is not allergic to iodine or seafood. Broad-spectrum topical antibacterials, usually effective against many gram-positive and gram-negative as well as yeast infections, are applied to burn areas to prevent infection. Examples of these antibacterials include mafenide acetate (Sulfamylon), silver sulfadiazine (Silvadene), silver nitrate 0.5% solution, and nitrofurazone (Furacin). Chart 44–1 lists the drug data for the antibacterial agent mafenide acetate (Sulfamylon).

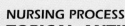

NURSING PROCESS
TOPICAL ANTIINFECTIVES: BURNS

Assessment

- Assess burned tissue for infection. Culture an oozing wound.
- Check client's vital signs (VS). Report abnormal findings such as an elevated temperature.
- Assess fluid status. Report signs and symptoms of hypovolemia or hypervolemia.

Potential Nursing Diagnoses

- Risk for infection related to loss of skin integrity
- Pain related to thermal injury
- Body image disturbance

Planning

- Aseptic technique will be enforced when caring for burned tissue, and tissue will be free from infection.

Nursing Interventions

- Administer prescribed analgesia before application, if needed.
- Cleanse burned tissue sites using aseptic technique.
- Apply topical antibacterial drug and dressing with sterile technique.
- Monitor client's fluid balance and renal function.
- Monitor client for side effects of and adverse reactions to topical drug.
- Monitor client's VS and be alert for signs of infection. Use with caution in client with acute renal failure.
- Closely monitor client's acid–base balance, especially in the presence of pulmonary or renal dysfunction.
- Store drug in dry place at room temperature.

Client Teaching

General
- Instruct client and family about changes in respiratory status.

Self-Administration
- Explain to client and family the care given to the burned tissue areas, using aseptic technique.
- Instruct client and family to apply topical agent and dressings to the burned areas.

Evaluation

- Evaluate effectiveness of treatment interventions to burned tissue areas by determining whether healing is proceeding and sites are free from infection.

Mafenide Acetate

PHARMACOKINETICS
Mafenide acetate is absorbed through the skin and is metabolized by the liver to a metabolite. The drug is excreted in the urine. The drug and its metabolite are strong carbonic anhydrase inhibitors, which may lead to acid–base imbalances, such as metabolic acidosis and respiratory alkalosis, and fluid loss from the mild diuretic effect. If respiration becomes rapid, labored, or shallow, the cream should be discontin-ued for a few days until the acid–base balance is restored.

PHARMACODYNAMICS
Mafenide, a sulfonamide derivative, interferes with bacterial cell wall synthesis and metabolism and is bacteriostatic. It is used as a topical water-soluble antibacterial agent to prevent or combat a burn infection. After the burn is cleansed and debrided, 1/16 inch of mafenide cream is applied to the affected area daily or twice a day and is covered lightly with a

dressing. The client may complain of a burning sensation when the drug is applied.

Aseptic technique should be used when caring for the burn site and applying the topical antibacterial agent. Table 44–4 lists the topical medications for burns, their strengths, uses, and considerations.

Silver Sulfadiazine

Silver sulfadiazine (Silvadene, SSD) is becoming more popular for the prevention and treatment of sepsis in second- and third-degree burns than other antibacterial agents. It acts on the cell membrane and cell wall to produce bactericidal effects. Unlike mafenide, it is *not* a carbonic anhydrase inhibitor. It is contraindicated at or near term pregnancy.

One percent or less of the silver is absorbed and up to 10% of sulfadiazine is absorbed. Side and adverse effects may include skin discoloration, burning sensation, rashes, erythema multiforme, skin necrosis, and possible leukopenia.

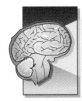

Critical Thinking in Action

M. G., 15 years old, complains about numerous blackheads and large raised pimples on her face. She seeks help from a health care provider.

1. To assist in identifying her skin problem, the health history and assessment should include _____?
2. Which nonpharmacologic measures might you discuss with M. G. in caring for her facial skin condition?

M. G.'s skin disorder does not improve. Her health care provider said she has acne vulgaris and has prescribed benzoyl peroxide and oral tetracycline.

3. M. G. asks the nurse how to use benzoyl peroxide. How would you explain the method and frequency for use of benzoyl peroxide?
4. What would you include in client teaching related to the use of oral tetracycline?
5. What other agents for acne might be used for M. G.? Explain their uses and side effects.
6. M. G. asked if she would have to remain on benzoyl peroxide and oral tetracycline for the rest of her life. What would be your answer or course of action? Explain.

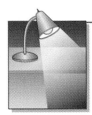

Study Questions

1. What are the actions of keratolytics? Give examples of these agents and their actions.
2. What are the similarities and differences of the topical antiacne drugs: tretinoin, adapalene, and azelaic acid?
3. What are the advantages and disadvantages for use of the oral antiacne drugs, isotretinoin, and tetracycline?
4. T. H. has psoriasis. A coal tar preparation has been suggested and anthralin has been prescribed by the health care provider. T. H. wants to know how these agents will help him. How would you respond?
5. R. Q. has poison ivy. Poison ivy is classified as what type of skin disorder? What nondrug and drug regimens may be used to alleviate the poison ivy?
6. What drug is used to treat male pattern baldness? How is it administered and how does it achieve hair follicle growth?
7. B. R. has second- and third-degree burns over 25% of his body. Mafenide acetate has been ordered. How is it administered? What care is taken before its administration? What acid–base imbalance can result from its use?

Unit XII

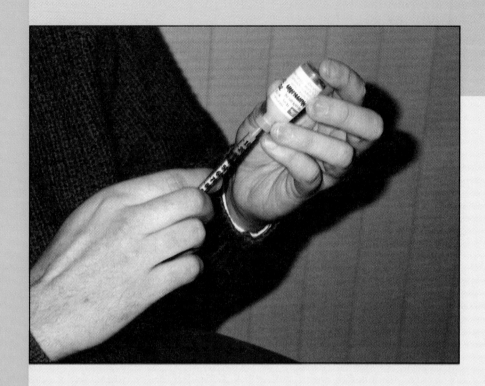

Endocrine Agents

INTRODUCTION

The endocrine system is composed of ductless glands that secrete hormones into the bloodstream. **Hormones** are chemical substances synthesized from amino acids and cholesterol that act on body tissues and organs and affect cellular activity. Hormones can be divided into two categories: (1) proteins or small peptides, and (2) steroids. Hormones from the adrenal glands and the gonads are steroid hormones; the others are protein hormones. The **endocrine glands** include the pituitary (hypophysis), thyroid, parathyroid, adrenal, gonads, and pancreas. Figure XII–1 illustrates the location and functions of these glands. This unit discusses the hormonal activity of the endocrine glands.

PITUITARY GLAND

The pituitary gland, or hypophysis, located at the base of the brain, has two lobes, the anterior pituitary (adenohypophysis) and the posterior pituitary (neurohypophysis). The anterior pituitary gland is called the *master gland,* because it secretes

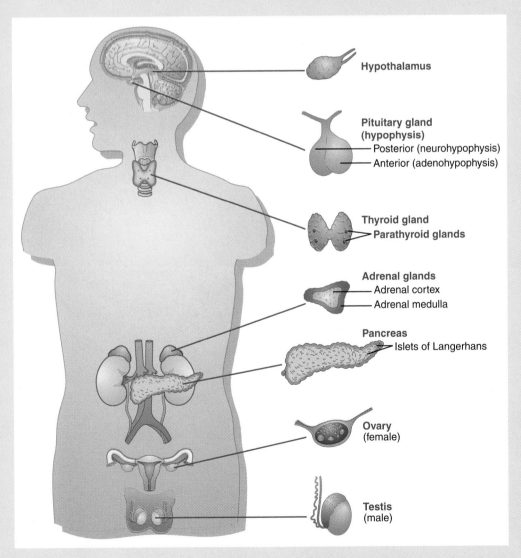

Figure XII–1
The endocrine glands.

hormones that stimulate the release of other hormones from target glands, including the thyroid, parathyroids, adrenals, and gonads. The posterior pituitary gland secretes two neurohormones, antidiuretic hormone (ADH), or vasopressin, and oxytocin. Figure XII–2 shows the anterior and posterior pituitary gland and the types of hormones that are secreted.

ANTERIOR PITUITARY GLAND

The anterior pituitary hormones are (1) thyroid-stimulating hormone (TSH), (2) adrenocorticotropic hormone (ACTH), and (3) the gonadotropins (follicle-stimulating hormone [FSH] and luteinizing hormone [LH]). They control the synthesis and release of hormones from the thyroid, adrenals, and ovaries. Other hormones secreted from the anterior pituitary (adenohypophysis) include growth hormone (GH), prolactin, and melanocyte-stimulating hormone (MSH). The amount of each hormone secreted from the anterior pituitary is regulated by a negative feedback system. If excess hormone is secreted from the target gland, hormonal release from the anterior pituitary will be suppressed. If there is a lack of hormone secretion from the target gland, there will be an increase in that particular anterior pituitary hormone.

Thyroid-Stimulating Hormone

The anterior pituitary gland secretes thyroid-stimulating hormone (TSH) in response to thyroid-releasing hormone (TRH) from the hypothalamus. TSH, or thyrotropic hormone, stimulates the release of levothyroxine (T_4) and triiodothyronine (T_3) from the thyroid gland. Hypersecretion of TSH can cause hyperthyroidism and thyroid enlargement, and hyposecretion can cause hypothyroidism. Serum TSH levels should be checked to determine whether there is a TSH deficit or excess. TSH and T_4 levels are frequently measured to differentiate pituitary from thyroid dysfunction. A decreased T_4 level and a normal or elevated TSH level can indicate a thyroid disorder.

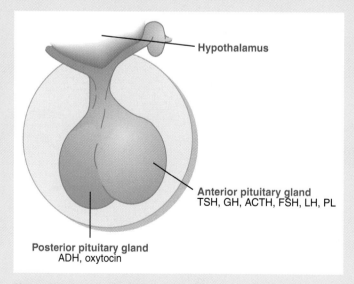

Figure XII–2
The anterior and posterior pituitary glands. (KEY: ADH: antidiuretic hormone; TSH: thyroid-stimulating hormone; GH: growth hormone; ACTH: adrenocorticotropic hormone; FSH: follicle-stimulating hormone; LH: luteinizing hormone; PL: prolactin.)

Adrenocorticotropic Hormone

Secretion of adrenocorticotropic hormone (ACTH) occurs in response to corticotropin-releasing factor (CRF) from the hypothalamus. ACTH from the anterior pituitary stimulates the release of glucocorticoids (cortisol), mineralocorticoids (aldosterone), and androgen from the adrenal cortex (adrenal glands). Elevated serum cortisol from the adrenal cortex inhibits ACTH and CRH release. When the cortisol level is low, ACTH secretion is stimulated, which in turn stimulates the adrenal cortex to release more cortisol. More ACTH is secreted in the morning than in the evening.

GONADOTROPIC HORMONES

The gonadotropic hormones regulate hormone secretion from the ovaries and testes (the gonads). Follicle-stimulating hormone (FSH), luteinizing hormone (LH), and prolactin are the gonadotropic hormones secreted from the anterior pituitary gland. FSH promotes the maturation of follicles in the ovaries and initiates sperm production in the testes. LH combines with FSH in follicle maturation and estrogen production and promotes secretion of androgens from the testes. Prolactin stimulates milk formation in the glandular breast tissue after delivery. Estrogen, progesterone, and testosterone are discussed in Chapters 47, 48, and 49, respectively.

GROWTH HORMONE

Growth hormone (GH), or somatotropic hormone (STH), acts on all body tissues, but particularly the bones and skeletal muscles. The amount of growth hormone secreted is regulated by growth hormone–releasing hormone (GHRH) and growth hormone-inhibiting hormone (GHIH, or somatostatin) from the hypothalamus. Sympathomimetics, serotonin, and glucocorticoids can inhibit the secretion of growth hormone.

Posterior Pituitary Gland

The posterior pituitary gland (neurohypophysis) secretes antidiuretic hormone (ADH, vasopressin) and oxytocin. Interconnecting nerve fibers between the hypothalamus and the posterior pituitary gland allow ADH and oxytocin to be synthesized in the hypothalamus and stored in the posterior pituitary gland. ADH increases the reabsorption of water from the renal tubules, thus returning it to the systemic circulation. Secretion of ADH is regulated by the serum osmolality (concentration of the vascular fluid). An increase in serum osmolality increases the release of ADH from the posterior pituitary; more water is then absorbed from the renal tubules to dilute the vascular fluid. Excess ADH can overload the vascular system. A decrease in serum osmolality decreases the release of ADH, promoting more water excretion from the renal tubules. Oxytocin stimulates contraction of the smooth muscles of the uterus; it is discussed in Chapters 47 and 48.

THYROID GLAND

Located anterior to the trachea, the thyroid gland has two lobes that are connected by a bridge of thyroid tissue. The thyroid gland secretes two hormones, thyroxine (T_4) and triiodothyronine (T_3 liothyronine). These hormones affect nearly every tissue and organ by controlling their metabolic rate and activity. Stimulation by the thyroid hormones results in an increase in cardiac output, oxygen consumption, carbohydrate utilization, protein synthesis, and breakdown of fat (lipolysis). Body heat regulation and the menstrual cycle are also affected by thyroid hormones. Thyroid hormone levels in the blood are regulated by negative feedback. The anterior pituitary gland secretes thyroid-stimulating hormone (TSH), which stimulates the thyroid gland to produce T_4 and T_3. An increased amount of circulating thyroid hormones suppresses the release of TSH, and a decreased amount increases the release of TSH by the adenohypophysis.

PARATHYROID GLANDS

There are four parathyroid glands (two pairs) that lie on the dorsal surface of the thyroid gland. The parathyroid gland secretes parathormone, or parathyroid hormone (PTH), which regulates calcium levels in the blood. A decrease in serum calcium stimulates the release of PTH. PTH increases calcium levels by (1) mobilizing calcium from the bone, (2) promoting calcium absorption from the intestine, and (3) promoting calcium reabsorption from the renal tubules. Calcitonin, a hormone produced primarily by the thyroid gland and to a lesser extent by the parathyroid and thymus glands, inhibits calcium reabsorption by bone and increases renal excretion of calcium. Calcitonin counteracts the action of PTH.

ADRENAL GLANDS

The adrenal glands, located at the top of each kidney, are composed of two separate sections: the adrenal medulla (the inner section) and the adrenal cortex (the section surrounding the adrenal medulla). The adrenal medulla releases the catecholamines epinephrine and norepinephrine and is linked with the sympathetic nervous system. The adrenal cortex produces two major types of hormones (corticosteroids), glucocorticoids and mineralocorticoids. The principal glucocorticoid is cortisol and the principal mineralocorticoid is aldosterone. In addition, the adrenal cortex produces small amounts of androgen, estrogen, and progestin. Glucocorticoids have a profound influence on electrolytes, and carbohydrate, protein, and fat metabolism, and deficiencies can result in serious illness and even death.

PANCREAS

The pancreas, located to the left of and behind the stomach, is both an exocrine and an endocrine gland. The exocrine section of the pancreas secretes digestive enzymes into the duodenum; these enzymes are discussed in Unit IX. The endocrine section has cell clusters called islets of Langerhans. The alpha islet cells produce glucagon, which breaks down glycogen to glucose in the liver, and the beta cells secrete insulin, which regulates glucose metabolism. Insulin, an antidiabetic agent, is used to control diabetes mellitus. Antidiabetic agents are discussed in Chapter 46.

DRUGS FOR ENDOCRINE DISORDERS

Chapters 45 and 46 discuss the drugs used in diagnosing and treating endocrine disorders. In Chapter 45 the agents for disorders involving the pituitary gland, thyroid gland, parathyroid gland, adrenal gland, and antidiuretic hormone (ADH) are discussed. The parenteral and oral antidiabetic drugs (hypoglycemic drugs) are described in Chapter 46.

Drugs discussed in Chapter 45 are used for pituitary disorders and include (1) drugs for growth hormone replacement and a drug that suppresses the release of GH and prolactin; (2) a thyroid-stimulating hormone agent for diagnosing the cause of hypothyroidism; (3) ACTH agents, used for diagnosing and treating adrenal insufficiency; and (4) drugs used to control diabetes insipidus resulting from ADH insufficiency. Hypothyroidism and hyperthyroidism are discussed in relation to their drug therapy. The use of glucocorticoids as antiinflammatory agents and in diagnosing and treating adrenocortical insufficiency is presented.

In Chapter 46, insulin and oral antidiabetic (hypoglycemic) drugs are presented. Recognition of hypoglycemia, insulin injection sites, and client teaching are emphasized. The nursing process format is applied throughout both chapters.

45

Endocrine Pharmacology: Pituitary, Thyroid, Parathyroids, and Adrenals

Outline

Objectives

* Define hormone, hypophysis, thyroxine, and glucocorticoids.
* Name the hormones secreted from the adenohypophysis and the neurohypophysis.
* Identify the actions, uses, and side effects of the pituitary hormones, T_4, T_3, PTH, and glucocorticoids.
* Describe the nursing process, including client teaching, of drug therapy related to hormonal replacement or hormonal inhibition for the pituitary, thyroid, parathyroid, and adrenal glands.

Terms

acromegaly

Addison's disease

adenohypophysis

adrenal glands

adrenocorticotropic hormone

antidiuretic hormone (ADH)

corticosteroids

cretinism

Cushing's syndrome

diabetes insipidus

endocrine

gigantism

glucocorticoids

Graves' disease

hyperthyroidism

hypophysis

hypothyroidism

mineralocorticoids

myxedema

neurohypophysis

parathyroid hormone

thyroid-stimulating hormone

thyrotoxicosis

thyroxine (T_4)

triiodothyronine (T_3)

INTRODUCTION

This chapter describes drugs used for hormonal replacement and for inhibition of hormonal secretion from the pituitary, thyroid, parathyroid, and adrenal glands. The gonadal, or sex, hormones are discussed in Chapters 47 through 51. Before reading Chapters 45 and 46, the student or nurse should review the introduction to Unit XII, which describes the locations of the endocrine glands and the hormones that they secrete. Knowledge of the various **endocrine** hormones and their functions facilitates an understanding of the drugs that act on the endocrine glands.

PITUITARY GLAND

Anterior

The pituitary gland (**hypophysis**) has an anterior and a posterior lobe. The anterior pituitary gland, called the **adenohypophysis,** secretes various hormones that target glands and tissues: (1) growth hormone (GH), which stimulates growth in tissue and bone; (2) thyroid-stimulating hormone (TSH), which acts on the thyroid gland; (3) adrenocorticotropic hormone (ACTH), which stimulates the adrenal gland; and (4) gonadotropins (follicle-stimulating hormone [FSH] and luteinizing hormone [LH]), which affect the ovaries. FSH and LH are discussed in Chapter 47. The drugs with adenohypophyseal properties used to stimulate or inhibit glandular activity are discussed according to their drug use. The negative feedback system that controls the amount of hormonal secretion from the pituitary gland and the target gland is discussed in the introduction to Unit XII.

GROWTH HORMONE

Two hypothalamic hormones regulate growth hormone (GH): (1) growth hormone releasing hormone (GHRH), and (2) growth hormone release-inhibiting hormone (somatostatin or SIH). GH does not have a specific target gland; it affects body tissues and bone. GH replacement stimulates linear growth when there is a growth hormone deficiency. Enzymes in the gastrointestinal (GI) tract inactivate GH, thus requiring subcutaneous or intramuscular administration of GH. GH drugs cannot be given orally because the drug is inactivated in the gastrointestinal tract.

If a child's height is well below the standard for a specified age, GH deficiency may be diagnosed and dwarfism can result. Because GH replacement is very expensive (cost approximately $20,000 for 1 year), various tests are performed to determine whether this therapy is essential. Because GH acts on newly forming bone, it must be administered before the epiphyses are fused. Administration of GH over a period of several years can increase height by a foot. Prolonged GH therapy can antagonize insulin secretion and eventually cause diabetes mellitus. Because of its effects on blood sugar and other side effects, athletes should be advised not to take GH to build muscle and physique.

Drug Therapy: Growth Hormone Deficiency

Somatrem (Protropin) and somatropin (Humatrope) are two growth hormones used for the treatment of growth failure in children because of pituitary growth hormone deficiency. Somatropin is a product that has the identical amino acid sequence as human growth hormone. Somatrem also has the identical sequence of pituitary growth hormone plus an additional amino acid. Development of antibodies to somatrem has occurred in 30% to 40% of clients on somatrem during the first 3 to 6 months of therapy, but in 95% of these clients, this has not decreased the effectiveness of the somatrem treatment.

Gigantism (during childhood) and **acromegaly** (after puberty) can occur with GH hypersecretion, and are frequently caused by a pituitary tumor. If the tumor cannot be destroyed by radiation, bromocriptine, a prolactin-release inhibitor, can inhibit the release of GH from the pituitary. Table 45–1 lists the drugs used to replace or to inhibit growth hormone.

Drug Therapy: Growth Hormone Excess

Octreotide (Sandostatin) is a potent synthetic somatostatin used to suppress growth hormone release. It can be used alone or with surgery or radiation. This drug is most expensive. Gastrointestinal side effects are common.

THYROID-STIMULATING HORMONE

The adenohypophysis secretes **thyroid-stimulating hormone** (TSH) in response to thyroid-releasing hormone (TRH) from the hypothalamus. TSH stimulates the thyroid gland to release levothyroxine (T_4) and triiodothyronine (liothyronine) (T_3). Excess TSH secretion can cause hyperthyroidism, and a TSH deficit can cause hypothyroidism. Hypothyroidism may be due to a thyroid gland disorder (primary cause) or a decrease in TSH secretion (secondary cause). Thyrotropin (Thytropar), a purified extract of TSH, is used as a diagnostic agent to differentiate between primary and secondary hypothyroidism (see Table 45–1).

ADRENOCORTICOTROPIC HORMONE

The hypothalamus releases corticotropin-releasing factor (CRF), which stimulates the pituitary corticotrophs to secrete **adrenocorticotropic hormone** (ACTH). ACTH secretion stimulates the release of glucocorticoids (cortisol), mineralocorticoids (aldosterone), and androgen from the adrenal cortex. Usually, ACTH and cortisol secretions follow a diurnal rhythm in

Table 45-1
Anterior and Posterior Pituitary Hormones

GENERIC (BRAND)	ROUTE AND DOSAGE	USES AND CONSIDERATIONS
ANTERIOR: GROWTH HORMONE (GH)		
Sermorelin acetate (Geref)	*Diagnostic:* A & C: IV: 0.3–1 μg/kg	Diagnostic test to determine if the pituitary gland secretes growth hormone.
Somatrem (Protropin)	*Growth hormone deficiency:* C: SC/IM: 100 μg/kg (0.1 mg/kg) 3 × wk or 0.2 U/kg 3 × wk; 48-h interval is recommended between doses	For growth hormone replacement for treating dwarfism. It affects growth of most body tissues, and promotes bone growth at epiphyseal plates of long bones. *Pregnancy category:* C; PB: UK; t½: 20–30 min
Somatropin (Humatrope)	C: SC/IM: 60 μg/kg (0.06 mg/kg) 3 × wk or 0.16 IU/kg 3 × wk; 48-h interval is recommended between doses	For treating growth hormone deficiency. Promotes bone growth at epiphyseal plates of long bones. *Pregnancy category:* D; PB: UK; t½: 15–60 min
GROWTH HORMONE EXCESS		
Octreotide acetate (Sandostatin)	A: SC: 50–100 μg t.i.d.	For treatment of acromegaly and for clients with metastatic carcinoid tumors. *Pregnancy category:* B; PB: UK; t½: 2.5 h
THYROID-STIMULATING HORMONE (TSH)		
Thyrotropin (Thytropar)	*Hypothyroidism and treatment of thyroid cancer:* A: SC/IM: 10 IU/d for 1–3 d; cancer treatment: 3–8 d	For diagnosing cause of hypothyroidism (pituitary or thyroid). Radioiodine study follows last injection. *Pregnancy category:* C; PB: UK; t½: 35 min with normal thyroid
ADRENOCORTICOTROPIC HORMONE (ACTH)		
Corticotropin (Acthar)	See Chart 45-1	For diagnostic test to evaluate adrenocortical function and ACTH replacement. For acute exacerbations of multiple sclerosis. Long-term therapy can cause side effects similar to glucocorticoids. Repository injections have long duration of action (12 to 24 h), IM. *Pregnancy category:* C; PB: UK; t½: UK
Corticotropin repository (Acthar gel)	A: SC/IM: 40–80 U/q24–72h	
Cosyntropin (Cortrosyn)	A: C > 2 y: IM: 0.25–0.75 mg IV: 0.25 mg C < 2 y: IM: 0.125 mg IV: 0.125 mg (0.04 mg/h)	For diagnostic testing to differentiate between pituitary and adrenal cause of adrenal insufficiency. Obtain a plasma cortisol level before and 30 min after cosyntropin administration. *Pregnancy category:* C; PB: UK; t½: 15 min
POSTERIOR: ANTIDIURETIC HORMONE (ADH)		
Desmopressin acetate (DDAVP)	*Diabetes insipidus:* A: Intranasal: 0.1–0.4 mL/d in divided doses C < 12 y: Intranasal: 0.05–0.3 mL/d in divided doses	For treating diabetes insipidus, hemophilia A, von Willebrand's disease. Can have a long duration of action (5 to 21 h). *Pregnancy category:* B; PB: UK; t½: 1.25 h
Desmopressin (Stimate)	A: SC/IV: 2–4 μg, in 2 divided doses C < 12 y: Inf: 0.3 μg/kg diluted in 10 mL of NSS over 15–30 min	Same as above
Lypressin (Diapid)	*Diabetes insipidus:* A & C: Intranasal: 1–2 sprays per nostril q.i.d.	Prevention or control of diabetes insipidus caused by insufficient ADH. To decrease polydipsia, polyuria, and dehydration. Duration of action is 3–8 h. *Pregnancy category:* B; PB: UK; t½: 15 min
Vasopressin (aqueous) (Pitressin)	*Diabetes insipidus:* A: SC/IM: 5–10 U, b.i.d.–q.i.d. C: SC/IM: 2.5–10 U, b.i.d.–q.i.d.	For treating diabetes insipidus. For relief of intestinal distention. Decreases GI bleeding from esophageal varices. Can also be given intranasally. Promotes reabsorption of water from the renal tubules. Duration of action is 2–8 h. *Pregnancy category:* X; PB: UK; t½: 15 min
Vasopressin tanate/oil (Pitressin Tannate)	A: IM: 1.5–5.0 U, q2–3d C: IM: 1.25–2.5 U, q2–3d	Same as for vasopressin. Action is longer due to the oil.

KEY: *A:* adult; *C:* child; *Inf:* infusion; *IM:* intramuscular; *IV:* intravenous; *SC:* subcutaneous; *PB:* protein-binding; *t½:* half-life; *UK:* unknown; *GI:* gastrointestinal.

Chart 45–1.   Pituitary: Adrenocorticotropic Hormone (ACTH)

ADRENOCORTICOTROPIC HORMONE (ACTH)

Assessment and Planning

NURSING PROCESS

Drug Name

Corticotropin
(Acthar, ACTH)
Corticotropin repository
(Acthar Gel, cortigel)
Corticotrophin-zinc hydroxide
(Cortrophin zinc)
Pregnancy Category: C

Dosage

Diagnostic testing:
A: IV: 10–25 U in 500 mL D$_5$W q8h
SC/IM: 20 U, q.i.d.
Repository injection:
A: SC/IM; 40–80 U, q24–72h
Acute multiple sclerosis
A: SC/IM: 80–120 U/d for 2–3 wk

Contraindications

Severe fungal infection, CHF, peptic ulcer
Caution: Hepatic disease, psychiatric disorders, myasthenia gravis

Drug-Lab-Food Interactions

Drug: *Increase* ulcer formation with aspirin; may *increase* effect of potassium-wasting diuretics; *decrease* effects of oral antidiabetics (hypoglycemics) or insulin

Interventions

Pharmacokinetics

Absorption: IM: Well absorbed
Distribution: PB: UK
Metabolism: t½: 15–20 min
Excretion: In urine

Pharmacodynamics

IM: Onset: <6 h
        Peak: 6–18 h
        Duration: 12–24 h
IV: Onset: UK
        Peak: 1 h
        Duration: UK

Evaluation

Therapeutic Effects/Uses

To diagnose adrenocortical disorders; acts as an antiinflammatory agent; to treat acute multiple sclerosis (MS).

Mode of Action: Stimulation of the adrenal cortex to secrete cortisol.

Side Effects

Nausea, vomiting, increased appetite, mood swing (euphoria to depression), petechiae, water and sodium retention, hypokalemia, hypocalcemia

Adverse Reactions

Edema, ecchymosis, osteoporosis, muscle atrophy, growth retardation, decreased wound healing, cataracts, glaucoma, menstrual irregularities
Life-threatening: Ulcer perforation, pancreatitis

KEY: A: adult; SC: subcutaneous; IM: intramuscular; IV: intravenous; UK: unknown; CHF: congestive heart failure; PB: protein-binding; t½: half-life.

which the ACTH and cortisol secretion is higher in the early morning and then decreases through the day. Stresses such as surgery, sepsis, and trauma override the diurnal rhythm, causing an increase in secretions of ACTH and cortisol.

The ACTH drug corticotropin (Acthar) is used in the diagnosis of adrenal gland disorders, for treating adrenal gland insufficiency, and as an antiinflammatory drug in the treatment of an allergic response. Administration of intravenous ACTH should increase the serum cortisol level in 30 to 60 minutes if the adrenal gland is functioning. If steroid deficiency is caused by pituitary insufficiency, ACTH should eventually stimulate cortisol production. ACTH decreases the symptoms of multiple sclerosis during its exacerbation phase. Chart 45–1 lists the actions and effects of corticotropin (Acthar).

Pharmacokinetics

Corticotropin stimulates the adrenal gland to secrete corticosteroids. The aqueous and gel preparations are well-absorbed into the circulation. Zinc is added to some formulations to slow the absorption rate. A portion of the drug is bound to protein; however, the

NURSING PROCESS
PITUITARY HORMONES

Assessment

- Obtain baseline vital signs (VS) for future comparison. Report abnormal results.
- Assess the client's urinary output and weight.
- Assess the client for an infectious process. Corticotropin can suppress signs and symptoms of infection.
- Assess the client's physical growth. Compare child's growth with reported standards. Report findings.

Potential Nursing Diagnoses

- Altered health maintenance
- Altered growth and development

Planning

- Client will be free of pituitary disorder with appropriate drug regimen.

Nursing Interventions

Antidiuretic Hormone (ADH)
- Monitor VS. Increased heart rate and decreased systolic pressure can indicate fluid volume loss resulting from decreased ADH production. With less ADH secretion, more water is excreted, decreasing vascular fluid (hypovolemia).
- Monitor urinary output. Increased output can indicate fluid loss caused by a decrease in ADH.

Adrenocorticotropic Hormone (ACTH), Corticotropin
- **Avoid** administering corticotropin to clients with adrenocortical hyperfunction. Corticotropin stimulates the release of cortisol from the adrenal glands.
- Monitor the growth and development of a child receiving corticotropin.
- Monitor the client's weight. If a weight gain occurs, check for edema. A side effect of corticotropin (ACTH) is sodium and water retention.
- Monitor for adverse effects when corticotropin is discontinued. Dose should be tapered and not stopped abruptly because adrenal hypofunction may result.

Nursing Process continued on following page

percent is unknown. The half-life of the drug is 15 to 20 min. It is excreted in the urine.

Pharmacodynamics

Corticotropin suppresses the inflammatory and immune responses. Also it is prescribed to treat adrenal insufficiency secondary to inadequate corticotropin secretion. The drug is administered intramuscularly and intravenously (IV). By intramuscular injection, its onset of action, peak concentration time, and duration of action are prolonged. The IV preparation is in an aqueous form; therefore, its actions are faster than those of the gel and zinc-additive preparations.

Drug Interactions

Corticotropin has numerous drug interactions. Diuretics and anti-*Pseudomonas* penicillins such as piperacillin can decrease the serum potassium level (hypokalemia). If the client is taking a digitalis preparation and hypokalemia is present, digitalis toxicity can result. Phenytoin, rifampin, and barbiturates increase the metabolic rate, which can decrease the effect of the ACTH drug. Diabetics may need increased insulin and oral antidiabetic (hypoglycemic) drugs, because ACTH stimulates cortisol secretion, which increases the blood sugar level.

POSTERIOR

The posterior pituitary gland, known as the **neurohypophysis,** secretes **antidiuretic hormone** (ADH, vasopressin) and oxytocin. (Oxytocin is discussed in Chapter 47).

NURSING PROCESS *Continued*
PITUITARY HORMONES

- Check laboratory findings, especially electrolyte levels. Electrolyte replacement may be necessary.

Growth Hormone (GH)
- Monitor blood sugar and electrolyte levels in clients receiving GH. Hyperglycemia can occur with high doses.

Client Teaching

ACTH
- Advise the client to adhere to the drug regimen. Discontinuation of certain drugs, such as corticotropin, can cause hypofunction of the gland being stimulated.
- Advise the client to decrease salt intake to decrease or avoid edema. Potassium supplement may be needed.
- Instruct the client to report side effects, such as muscle weakness, edema, petechiae, ecchymosis, decrease in growth, decreased wound healing, and menstrual irregularities.

Growth Hormone
- Advise athletes not to take GH because of its side effects. GH can be effective for children whose height is markedly below the expected norm for their age. Because GH acts on the newly forming bone, it should be administered before the epiphyses are fused.
- Inform the diabetic client to closely monitor blood sugar levels. Insulin regulation may be necessary.
- Suggest that the client or family monitor the client's growth rate.

Cultural Considerations

- There is sometimes a lack of understanding in some cultural groups such as Hispanics and African-Americans in regard to the purpose and use of growth hormones. The health care provider needs to emphasize that these are not drugs for building muscles and that they can cause many serious side effects such as diabetes mellitus when abused.

Evaluation

- Evaluate the effectiveness of the drug therapy.

ADH promotes water reabsorption from the renal tubules to maintain water balance in the body fluids. When there is a deficiency of ADH, large amounts of water are excreted by the kidneys. This condition, **diabetes insipidus** (DI), can lead to severe fluid volume deficit and electrolyte imbalances. Head injury and brain tumors resulting in trauma to the hypothalamus and pituitary gland can also cause diabetes insipidus. Fluid and electrolyte balance must be closely monitored in these clients, and ADH replacement may be needed. The ADH preparations vasopressin (Pitressin) and desmopressin acetate (DDAVP) can be administered intranasally or by injection.

Table 45–1 lists the drugs used for pituitary disorders, their dosages, and uses and considerations.

THYROID GLAND

Thyroxine (T_4) and **triiodothyronine** (T_3) are secreted by the thyroid gland. The functions of T_4 and T_3 are to regulate protein synthesis and enzyme activity and to stimulate mitochondrial oxidation. Approximately 20% of circulating T_3 is secreted from the thyroid gland and 80% of T_3 comes from the degradation of about 40% of T_4, which occurs in the periphery. T_4 and T_3 are carried in the blood by thyroxine-binding globulin (TBG) and albumin, which protects the hormones from being degraded. T_3 is more potent than T_4, and only unbound free T_3 and T_4 are active and produce a hormonal response.

T_4 and T_3 secretion from the thyroid gland is regulated by the feedback mechanisms. The hypothalamus releases thyrotropin-releasing hormone (TRH), which stimulates the release of thyroid-stimulating hormone (TSH) from the pituitary gland. TSH stimulates the synthesis and release of T_4 and T_3 from the thyroid gland. Excess free T_4 and T_3 inhibit the hypothalamus-pituitary-thyroid (HPT) axis, which results in decreased TRH and TSH secretion. Likewise, too low T_4 and T_3 increases the function of the HPT axis.

When there is a thyroid deficiency (hypothyroidism), synthetic T_4 and T_3 may be prescribed, either alone or in combination. When the thyroid gland is secreting an overabundance of thyroid hormones (hyperthyroidism), antithyroid drugs are usually indicated.

Hypothyroidism

Hypothyroidism, a decrease in thyroid hormone secretion, can have a primary (thyroid gland disorder) or a secondary cause (lack of TSH secretion). Primary hypothyroidism occurs more frequently. Decreased T_4 and elevated TSH levels indicate primary hypothyroidism, the causes of which are acute or chronic inflammation of the thyroid gland, radioiodine therapy, excess intake of antithyroid drugs, and surgery. **Myxedema** is severe hypothyroidism; symptoms include lethargy, apathy, memory impairment, emotional changes, slow speech, deep coarse voice, edema of the eyelids and face, thick dry skin, cold intolerance, slow pulse, constipation, weight gain, and abnormal menses. In children, hypothyroidism can have a congenital **(cretinism)** or prepubertal (juvenile hypothyroidism) onset. Drugs containing T_4 and T_3, alone or in combination, are used to treat hypothyroidism.

DRUG THERAPY: HYPOTHYROIDISM

Levothyroxine sodium (Levothroid, Synthroid) is the drug of choice for replacement therapy for the treatment of hypothyroidism. It increases the levels of T_3 and T_4. Levothyroxine is also used to treat simple goiter and chronic lymphocytic (Hashimoto's) thyroiditis.

Liothyronine (Cytomel) is a synthetic T_3 that has a short half-life and duration of action; it is not recommended for maintenance therapy. Liothyronine is better absorbed from the gastrointestinal tract than is levothyroxine, and because of its rapid-onset of action and short half-life, it is frequently used as the initial therapy for treating myxedema.

Liotrix (Euthroid, Thyrolar) is a mixture of levothyroxine sodium and liothyronine sodium in a 4:1 ratio. There is no significant advantage to use of liotrix for treating hypothyroidism over levothyroxine sodium used alone, because levothyroxine converts T_4 to T_3 in the peripheral tissues.

Thyroid and thyroglobulin (Proloid) are seldom used. Some clients with hypothyroidism may benefit from these agents. Chart 45–2 presents the drug data for the synthetic thyroid drug levothyroxine.

PHARMACOKINETICS

Levothyroxine (T_4) is a synthetic thyroid hormone preparation. Fifty to 75 percent of levothyroxine is absorbed by the gastrointestinal (GI) mucosa. T_4 is highly protein-bound, and when administered with other highly protein-bound drugs like oral anticoagulants, side effects can result. The half-life of levothyroxine is longer than that of liothyronine. Levothyroxine is excreted in the bile and feces.

PHARMACODYNAMICS

Levothyroxine increases metabolic rate, cardiac output, protein synthesis, and glycogen utilization. The peak concentration time and duration of action are much longer with levothyroxine than with liothyronine. Liotrix is a combination of T_4 and T_3 with a greater concentration of T_4.

DRUG INTERACTIONS

There are many drug interactions associated with T_4 and T_3 drugs. They increase the effect of oral anticoagulants because of drug displacement from the protein-binding sites. When either of these drugs is taken with an adrenergic agent, such as a decongestant or vasopressor, the cardiac and central nervous system (CNS) actions are increased. Levothyroxine and liothyronine can decrease the effectiveness of digitalis preparations. Estrogen can increase the effect of liothyronine. Insulin and oral antidiabetic drug dosages may need to be increased.

Table 45–2 lists the drug data for natural and synthetic thyroid preparations.

Hyperthyroidism

Hyperthyroidism is an increase in circulating T_4 and T_3 levels, which results from an overactive thyroid gland or excessive output of thyroid hormones from one or more thyroid nodules. Hyperthyroidism may be mild with few symptoms or severe, as in thyroid storm in which death may occur from vascular collapse. **Graves' disease,** or **thyrotoxicosis,** is the most common type of hyperthyroidism due to hyperfunction of the thyroid gland. It is characterized by a rapid pulse (tachycardia), palpitations, excessive perspiration, heat intolerance, nervousness, irritability, exophthalmos (bulging eyes), and weight loss.

Hyperthyroidism can be treated by surgical re-

Chart 45-2.   Thyroid Hormone: Replacement

THYROID SYNTHETIC HORMONE

Drug Name	**Dosage**	
Levothyroxine sodium, T$_4$, 🍁 Eltroxin (Synthroid, Levothroid) *Pregnancy Category:* A	A: PO: Initially: 50 μg/d (0.05 mg/d); maint: 50–200 μg/d (0.05–0.2 mg/d) IV: 0.2–0.5 mg initial dose C: >3 y: PO: 50–100 μg/d (0.05–0.1 mg/d)	Assessment and Planning
Contraindications	**Drug-Lab-Food Interactions**	
Thyrotoxicosis, MI, severe renal disease **Caution:** Cardiovascular disease, hypertension, angina pectoris	**Drug:** *Increase* cardiac insufficiency with epinephrine; *increase* effects of anticoagulants, tricyclic antidepressants, vasopressors, decongestants; *decrease* effects of antidiabetics (oral and insulin), digitalis products; *decrease* absorption with cholestyramine, colestipol	
Pharmacokinetics	**Pharmacodynamics**	

Absorption: PO: 50%–75%
 Distribution: PB: 99%
 Metabolism: t½: 6–7 d
 Excretion: In bile and feces
	PO: Onset: UK
	      Peak: 24 h–1 wk
	      Duration: 1–3 wk
	 IV: Onset: 6–8 h
	      Peak: 24–48 h
	      Duration: UK
		Interventions

Therapeutic Effects/Uses

To treat hypothyroidism, myxedema, and cretinism.

Mode of Action: Increase metabolic rate, oxygen consumption, and body growth.

Side Effects	**Adverse Reactions**
Nausea, vomiting, diarrhea, cramps, tremors, nervousness, insomnia, headache, weight loss	Tachycardia, hypertension, palpitations **Life-threatening:** Thyroid crisis, angina pectoris, cardiac dysrhythmias, cardiovascular collapse

NURSING PROCESS — Evaluation

KEY: A: adult; PO: by mouth; IV: intravenous; UK: unknown; PB: protein-binding; t½: half-life; 🍁: Canadian drug name.

moval of a portion of the thyroid gland (subtotal thyroidectomy), radioactive iodine therapy, or antithyroid drugs, which inhibit either the synthesis or the release of thyroid hormone. Any of these treatments can cause hypothyroidism. Propranolol (Inderal) can control the cardiac symptoms, such as palpitations and tachycardia, that result from hyperthyroidism.

DRUG THERAPY: HYPERTHYROIDISM

The purpose of antithyroid drugs is to reduce the excessive secretion of thyroid hormones (T$_4$ and T$_3$) by inhibiting thyroid secretion. The use of surgery

(subtotal thyroidectomy) and radioiodine therapy frequently leads to hypothyroidism. Thiourea derivatives (thioamides) are the drugs of choice used to decrease thyroid hormone production. This drug group interferes with the incorporation of iodide into thyroglobulin.

Propylthiouracid (PTU) and methylthiouracil (Tapazole) are effective thioamide antithyroid drugs. They are useful for treating thyrotoxic crisis and in preparation for subtotal thyroidectomy. Methimazole does not inhibit peripheral conversion of T$_4$ to T$_3$ as PTU; however, it is 10 times more potent and it has a longer half-life than PTU. Prolonged use of thioamides may cause a goiter because of the increased TSH

Table 45–2
Thyroid Hormone: Replacements and Antithyroid Drugs

GENERIC (BRAND)	ROUTE AND DOSAGE	USES AND CONSIDERATIONS
THYROID REPLACEMENTS: HYPOTHYROIDISM		
Levothyroxine Na (Synthroid)	See Chart 45–2	For primary hypothyroidism. Synthetic T_4 drug. Onset of action is very slow. Effects occur in 1–3 wk. IV use for myxedema coma. Common side effects include nervousness, tachycardia, and weight loss. *Pregnancy category:* A; PB: 99%; $t\frac{1}{2}$: 6–7 d
Liothyronine Na (Cytomel)	A: PO: Initially: 5–25 μg/d; maint: 25–100 μg/d C: PO: Initially: 5 μg/d, >3 y: 50–100 μg/d	For hypothyroidism. Synthetic T_3 drug. Onset: faster acting than other thyroid drugs; Effects in 24–72 h. Cardiac side effects. *Pregnancy category:* A; PB: 99%; $t\frac{1}{2}$: 1–1.5 h
Liotrix (Euthroid, Thyrolar)	A: PO: Initially: 15–30 μg/d, *increase* q2–3wk; maint: 60–120 μg/d C: PO: Initially: same as adult C 6–12 y: 75–150 μg/d	For hypothyroidism. Synthetic T_4 and T_3 drug; 4:1 ratio. Onset of action is immediate. Duration of action is 72 h. Common side effects include irritability, nervousness, insomnia, tachycardia, weight loss. *Pregnancy category:* A; PB: 99%; $t\frac{1}{2}$: <7 d
Thyroglobulin (Proloid)	A: PO: Initially: 32 mg/d; maint: 32–200 mg/d Elderly: Initially: 16 mg/d	For hypothyroidism. From extract of hog thyroid. T_4 and T_3: 2.5:1 ratio. Seldom used. *Pregnancy category:* A; PB: 99%; $t\frac{1}{2}$: 6–7 d
Thyroid (Armour Thyroid, Thyrar)	A: PO: Initially: 15–60 mg/d, *increase* monthly as needed; maint: 60–180 mg/d C: PO: 15 mg/d, *increase* q2wk as needed	For hypothyroidism, to reduce goiter size. Natural form obtained from animals. T_4 and T_3: 4:1 ratio. Onset of action is slow; long duration of action (weeks). Common side effects include irritability, nervousness, insomnia, tachycardia, and weight loss. *Pregnancy category:* A; PB: 99%; $t\frac{1}{2}$: <7d (T_3: 1–2 h; T_4: 6–7 h)
ANTITHYROID DRUGS: HYPERTHYROIDISM		
Methimazole (Tapazole)	A: PO: Initially: 15–60 mg/d in 3 divided doses; maint: 5–15 mg/d C: PO: Initially: 0.4 mg/kg/d in divided doses; maint: 0.2 mg/kg/d in divided doses	For treating hyperthyroidism. Inhibits thyroid hormone synthesis. Onset of action: 1 wk for effect. Rash, urticaria, headache, GI upset may occur. *Pregnancy category:* D; PB: 0%; $t\frac{1}{2}$: 5–13 h
THIOAMIDE		
Propylthiouracil (PTU)	A: PO: Initially: 300–400 mg/d in divided doses; maint: 100–300 mg/d C: 6–10 y: PO: 50–150 mg/d, > 10 y: PO: Same as adult or 150 mg/m²/d	For hyperthyroidism, Graves' disease. Inhibits conversion of T_4 and T_3. May be used prior to surgery or radioactive iodine treatment and palliative control of toxic goiter. *Pregnancy category:* D; PB: 75%–80%; $t\frac{1}{2}$: 1–2 h
IODINE		
Strong iodine solution (Lugol solution, potassium iodide solution)	A & C: PO: 0.1–0.3 mL (3–5 drops) t.i.d. *Thyroid crisis:* A & C: PO: 1 mL in water p.c. t.i.d.	For hyperthyroidism. To reduce size and vascularity of thyroid gland. Dilute drug and administer after meals; sip through straw to avoid discoloration of teeth. Maximum effect after 10–15 d. *Pregnancy category:* D; PB: UK; $t\frac{1}{2}$: UK

KEY: A: adult; C: child; PO: by mouth; PB: protein-binding; $t\frac{1}{2}$: half-life; UK: unknown.

secretion that inhibits T_4 and T_3 synthesis. Minimal doses of thioamides should be given when indicated to avoid goiter formation.

Strong iodide preparations such as Lugol's solution have been used to suppress thyroid function for cli-

ents having a subtotal thyroidectomy for Graves' disease. Sodium iodide administered intravenously is useful for the management of thyrotoxic crisis. Table 45–2 gives the drug data for the antithyroid drugs used to treat hyperthyroidism.

NURSING PROCESS
THYROID HORMONE: REPLACEMENT AND ANTITHYROID DRUGS

Assessment

- Obtain baseline vital signs (VS) to compare with future data. Report abnormal results.
- Check serum T$_3$, T$_4$, and TSH levels. Report abnormal results.

Thyroid Replacement
- Obtain a history of drugs the client is currently taking. Be aware that thyroid drugs enhance the action of oral anticoagulants, sympathomimetics, and antidepressants and decrease the action of insulin, oral hypoglycemics, and digitalis preparation. Phenytoin and aspirin can enhance the action of thyroid hormone.

Antithyroid Drugs
- Assess for signs and symptoms of a thyroid crisis (thyroid storm), which includes tachycardia, dysrhythmias, fever, heart failure, flushed skin, apathy, confusion, behavioral changes, and later hypotension and vascular collapse. Thyroid crisis can result from a thyroidectomy (excess thyroid hormones released), abrupt withdrawal of antithyroid drug, excess ingestion of thyroid hormone, or failure to give antithyroid medication before thyroid surgery.

Potential Nursing Diagnoses

- Altered health maintenance
- Altered tissue perfusion

Planning

- Client's signs and symptoms of hypothyroidism will be alleviated within 2 to 4 wk with prescribed thyroid drug replacement, and the client will not experience side effects.
- Client's signs and symptoms of hyperthyroidism will be alleviated in 1 to 3 wk with the prescribed antithyroid drug.

Nursing Interventions

- Monitor VS. With hypothyroidism, the temperature, heart rate, and blood pressure are usually decreased. With hyperthyroidism, tachycardia and palpitations usually occur.
- Monitor the client's weight. Weight gain commonly occurs in clients with hypothyroidism.

Client Teaching

Thyroid Drug Replacement for Hypothyroidism
- Instruct the client to take the drug at the same time each day, preferably before breakfast. Food will hamper absorption rate.
- Advise the client to check cautions on labels of OTC drugs. Avoid OTC drugs that caution against use by persons with heart or thyroid disease.
- Advise the client to report symptoms of hyperthyroidism (tachycardia, chest pain, palpitations, excess sweating) due to drug accumulation or overdosing.
- Suggest that the client carry a medical alert card, tag, or bracelet with health condition and thyroid drug listed.

Diet
- Instruct the client to avoid foods that can inhibit thyroid secretion, such as strawberries, peaches, pears, cabbage, turnips, spinach, kale, Brussels sprouts, cauliflower, radishes, and peas.

Antithyroid Drugs for Hyperthyroidism
- Instruct the client to take the drug with meals to decrease GI symptoms.
- Advise the client about the effects of iodine and its presence in iodized salt, shellfish, and OTC cough medicines.

Nursing Process continued on following page

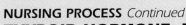

NURSING PROCESS *Continued*
THYROID HORMONE: REPLACEMENT AND ANTITHYROID DRUGS

- Emphasize the importance of drug compliance; abruptly stopping the antithyroid drug could bring on a thyroid crisis.
- Teach the client the signs and symptoms of hypothyroidism: lethargy, puffy eyelids and face, thick tongue, slow speech with hoarseness, lack of perspiration, and slow pulse. Hypothyroidism can result from treatment of hyperthyroidism.
- Advise the client to avoid antithyroid drugs if pregnant or breastfeeding. Antithyroid drugs taken during pregnancy can cause hypothyroidism in the fetus or infant.

Self-Administration
- Demonstrate to the client how to take a pulse rate. Instruct the client to monitor the pulse rate and report increases or marked decreases in pulse rate.

Side Effects
- Teach the client the side effects of antithyroid drugs, such as skin rash, hives, nausea, alopecia, loss of hair pigment, petechiae or ecchymoses, and weakness.
- Advise the client to contact the health care provider if a sore throat and fever occur while taking antithyroid drugs. A serious adverse reaction of antithyroid drugs is agranulocytosis (loss of WBCs). CBC should be monitored for leukopenia.

Cultural Considerations

- Recognize that various cultural groups may need guidance in understanding the disease process of hypothyroidism or hyperthyroidism. Support the client and family member who may be dismayed about the symptoms of either of these health problems and who lack knowledge of the prescribed drug therapy for management of the thyroid condition. Additional time in explanations and a written plan of care may be necessary for non–English-speaking persons.

Evaluation

Thyroid Replacement
- Evaluate the effectiveness of the thyroid drug and drug compliance
- Continue monitoring for side effects from drug accumulation or overdosing.

Antithyroid Drugs
- Evaluate the effectiveness of the antithyroid drug in decreasing signs and symptoms of hyperthyroidism. If signs and symptoms persist after 2 to 3 wk of therapy, other methods for correcting hyperthyroidism may be necessary.

Drug Interactions

Thyroid drugs interact with many other drugs. When used with oral anticoagulants (warfarin [Coumadin]), they can cause an increase in the anticoagulating effect. In addition, thyroid drugs decrease the effect of insulin and oral antidiabetics; digoxin and lithium increase the action of thyroid drugs; and phenytoin (Dilantin) increases serum T_3 level.

PARATHYROID GLANDS

The parathyroid glands secrete **parathyroid hormone** (PTH), which regulates calcium levels in the blood. A decrease in serum calcium stimulates the release of PTH. Calcitonin decreases serum calcium levels by promoting renal excretion of calcium. The functions of PTH and calcitonin are discussed in the introduction to Unit XII.

PTH agents treat hypoparathyroidism and synthetic calcitonin treats hyperparathyroidism. Hypocalcemia (serum calcium deficit) can be caused by PTH deficiency, vitamin D deficiency, renal impairment, or diuretic therapy. PTH replacement will help to correct the calcium deficit. PTH promotes calcium absorption from the GI tract, promotes reabsorption of calcium from the renal tubules and activates vitamin D.

Calcitriol

Calcitriol is a vitamin D analogue that promotes calcium absorption from the GI tract and secretion of calcium from bone to the bloodstream. Chart 45–3 describes the drug data related to calcitriol.

Chart 45–3. Parathyroid Hormone

VITAMIN D ANALOGUE

Drug Name	**Dosage**
Calcitriol (Rocaltrol) *Pregnancy Category:* C	A: PO: 0.25 µg/d

Contraindications

Hypersensitivity, hypercalcemia, hyperphosphatemia, hypervitaminosis D, malabsorption syndrome
Caution: Cardiovascular disease, renal calculi

Drug-Lab-Food Interactions

Drug: *Increase* cardiac dysrhythmias with digoxin, verapamil; *decrease* calcitriol absorption with cholestyramine
Lab: *Increase* serum calcium with thiazide diuretics, calcium supplements

Pharmacokinetics

Absorption: PO: Well absorbed
Distribution: PB: UK; crosses the placenta
Metabolism: t½: 3–8 h
Excretion: Mostly in feces

Pharmacodynamics

PO: Onset: 2–6 h
   Peak: 10–12 h
   Duration: 3–5 d

Therapeutic Effects/Uses

To treat hypothyroidism in chronic renal failure.

Mode of Action: Enhancement of calcium deposits in bones.

Side Effects

Anorexia, nausea, vomiting, diarrhea, cramps, drowsiness, headache, dizziness, lethargy, photophobia

Adverse Reactions

Hypercalciuria, hyperphosphatemia, hematuria

NURSING PROCESS: Assessment and Planning / Interventions / Evaluation

KEY: A: adult; PO: by mouth; UK: unknown; PB: protein-binding; t½: half-life.

PHARMACOKINETICS

Calcitriol is readily absorbed from the GI tract. Half-life is moderate (3 to 8 h). Most of the drug is excreted in the feces.

PHARMACODYNAMICS

Calcitriol is given for the management of hypocalcemia. It increases serum calcium levels by promoting calcium absorption from the intestines and from the renal tubules. Calcitriol has a long onset of action, peak action, and duration of action.

Hyperparathyroidism can be caused by malignancies of the parathyroid glands or ectopic PTH hormone secretion from lung cancer, hyperthyroidism, or prolonged immobility during which calcium is lost from bone. Table 45–3 lists the drugs used for treating hypoparathyroidism and hyperparathyroidism.

ADRENAL GLANDS

The paired **adrenal glands** are composed of the adrenal medulla and the adrenal cortex. The adrenal cortex produces two types of hormones, or corticosteroids: **glucocorticoids** (cortisol) and **mineralocorticoids** (aldosterone). Cortisol secreted by the adrenal glands is in response to the hypothalamus-pituitary-adrenal (HPA) axis as a result of the feedback mechanism. A decrease in the serum cortisol levels increases CRF and ACTH secretions, which stimulate the adrenal glands to secrete and release cortisol. An increased serum cortisol level exerts the negative feedback mechanism, which inhibits the HPA axis and less cortisol is released. Additional physiologic functions related to the hormones secreted from the adrenal medulla and adrenal cortex are described in the introduction to Unit XII.

Table 45–3
Parathyroid Hormones: Replacements and Supplements

GENERIC (BRAND)	ROUTE AND DOSAGE	USES AND CONSIDERATIONS
HYPOPARATHYROIDISM AND HYPOCALCEMIA: VITAMIN D ANALOGUES		
Calcifediol (Calderol)	A: PO: Initially: 300–350 μg/wk PO: 50–100 μg/d or 100–200 μg q.o.d.	For bone disease and hypocalcemia associated with chronic renal disease and dialysis. *Pregnancy category:* C; PB: UK; $t\frac{1}{2}$: 12–22 d
Calcitriol (Rocaltrol)	A: PO: 0.25 μmg/d; may increase 0.25 μg q4wk; *max:* 1.0 μg/d IV: 0.5 μg 3 × wk at end of dialysis C: PO: 0.014–0.041 μg/kg/d	For pseudohypoparathyroidism, hypoparathyroidism, and hypocalcemia in chronic renal disease. It is a synthetic form of vitamin D_3. It promotes calcium absorption from the GI tract and regulates calcium homeostasis. *Pregnancy category:* C; PB: UK; $t\frac{1}{2}$: 3–8 h
Dihydrotachysterol (Hytakerol)	A: PO: 0.75–2.5 mg/d for 4 d, then 0.2–1 mg/d C: PO: 1–5 mg/d for 4 d, then 0.5–1.5 mg/d	For treatment of hypoparathyroidism associated with hypocalcemia and for pseudohypoparathyroidism. Serum calcium levels should be monitored weekly during early therapy. Clients should avoid taking thiazide diuretics to prevent causing possible hypercalcemia. *Pregnancy category:* A; PB: UK; $t\frac{1}{2}$: UK
Ergocalciferol (Drisdol Drops)	A & C: PO: 50,000–200,000 IU/d or 1.25–5.0 μg/d	For hypoparathyroidism and rickets. A larger dose may be required in vitamin D–resistant rickets. It enhances calcium and phosphorus absorption. It has a long duration of action. *Pregnancy category:* C; PB: UK; $t\frac{1}{2}$: 12–24 h
HYPERPARATHYROIDISM AND HYPERCALCEMIA		
Calcitonin (human) (Cibacalcin) Calcitonin (salmon) (Calcimar)	A: SC: Initially: 0.5 mg/d; maint: 0.25 mg daily–0.5 mg b.i.d. A: SC/IM: Initially: 4 IU/kg/d; maint: 4–8 IU/kg q12h.	For treating Paget's disease of the bone (osteitis deformans), hyperparathyroidism, and hypercalcemia. Calcitonin salmon is more potent than calcitonin human. Calcitonin decreases serum calcium by binding at receptor sites on osteoclast. *Pregnancy category:* C; PB: UK; $t\frac{1}{2}$: 1–1.5 h
Etidronate (Didronel)	A: PO: 5–10 mg/kg/d; *max:* 20 mg/kg/d	For Paget's disease; for hypercalcemia due to antineoplastic therapy. *Pregnancy category:* B; PB: UK; $t\frac{1}{2}$: 6 h

KEY: A: adult; C: child; IM: intramuscular; PO: by mouth; SC: subcutaneous; PB: protein-binding; $t\frac{1}{2}$: half-life; UK: unknown.

The **corticosteroids** promote sodium retention and potassium excretion. A sodium ion is reabsorbed from the renal tubules in exchange for a potassium ion; the potassium ion is then excreted. Due to their influence on electrolytes and carbohydrate, protein, and fat metabolism, a deficiency of corticosteroids can result in serious illness or death. A decrease in corticosteroid secretion is known as adrenal hyposecretion (adrenal insufficiency, or **Addison's disease**) and an increase in corticosteroid secretion is called adrenal hypersecretion **(Cushing's syndrome)**.

Glucocorticoids

Glucocorticoids are influenced by ACTH, released from the anterior pituitary gland. They affect carbo-

hydrate, protein, and fat metabolism, as well as muscle and blood cell activity. Because of their many mineralocorticoid effects, glucocorticoids can cause sodium absorption from the kidney, resulting in water retention, potassium loss, and increased blood pressure. Cortisol, the main glucocorticoid, has antiinflammatory, antiallergic, and antistress effects. Indications for glucocorticoid therapy include trauma, surgery, infections, emotional upsets, and anxiety. Table 45–4 lists the physiologic aspects of adrenal hyposecretion (Addison's disease) and hypersecretion (Cushing's syndrome).

Most of the wide variety of glucocorticoid drugs, frequently called *cortisone* drugs, are synthetically produced. These drugs have several routes of administration: oral, parenteral (intramuscular or intravenous),

NURSING PROCESS
PARATHYROID HORMONE

Assessment

- Assess serum calcium level. Report abnormal results.
- Assess for symptoms of tetany in hypocalcemia: twitching of the mouth, tingling and numbness of the fingers, carpopedal spasm, spasmodic contractions, and laryngeal spasm.

Potential Nursing Diagnoses

- Risk for impaired tissue integrity
- Altered health maintenance

Planning

- The client's serum calcium level will be within the normal range.

Nursing Interventions

- Monitor the serum calcium level. Normal reference value is 8.5 to 10.5 mg/dL, or 4.5 to 5.5 mEq/L. A serum calcium level <8.5 mg/dL, or <4.5 mEq/L, indicates hypocalcemia, and a serum calcium level >10.5 mg/dL, or >5.5 mEq/L, indicates hypercalcemia. Serum ionized calcium levels are usually used because much of the calcium is protein-bound and is nonionized and nonactive.

Client Teaching

Hypoparathyroidism
- Advise the client to report symptoms of tetany (see Assessment).

Hyperparathyroidism
- Advise the client to report signs and symptoms of hypercalcemia: bone pain, anorexia, nausea, vomiting, thirst, constipation, lethargy, bradycardia, and polyuria.
- Instruct women to inform their health care provider about pregnancy status before taking calcitonin preparation.
- Advise the client to check OTC drugs for possible calcium content, especially if the client has an elevated serum calcium level. Some vitamins and antacids contain calcium. Tell the client to contact the health care provider before taking drugs with calcium.

Evaluation

- Monitor the effectiveness of drug therapy.
- Continue monitoring for signs and symptoms of hypocalcemia (tetany) when commercially prepared calcitonin has been given.

---

topical (creams, ointments, lotions) and aerosol (inhaler). The intramuscular form, although seldom used, should be administered deep in the muscle. The subcutaneous route is not recommended. The topical glucocorticoids are listed in Chapter 44.

Glucocorticoids are used to treat many diseases and health problems including inflammatory, allergic, and debilitating conditions. Among the inflammatory conditions that may require glucocorticoids are autoimmune disorders such as multiple sclerosis, rheumatoid arthritis, and myasthenia gravis; ulcerative colitis; glomerulonephritis; shock; ocular and vascular inflammations; head trauma with cerebral edema; polyarteritis nodosa; and hepatitis. Allergic conditions include asthma, drug reactions, contact dermatitis, and anaphylaxis. Debilitating conditions are mainly caused by malignancies. Organ transplant recipients may require glucocorticoids to prevent organ rejection.

There are many glucocorticoids, some more potent than others. Dexamethasone (Decadron) has been used for severe inflammatory response as a result of

Table 45–4
Adrenal Hyposecretion and Hypersecretion

| BODY SYSTEM | SYSTEMIC EFFECTS | |
	Hyposecretion	Hypersecretion
Metabolism		
Glucose	Hypoglycemia	Hyperglycemia
Protein	Muscle weakness	Muscle wasting; thinning of the skin; poor wound healing;
Fat		osteoporosis; fat accumulation in face, neck, and trunk (protruding abdomen, buffalo hump); hyperlipidemia; high cholesterol
Central nervous system	Apathy, depression, fatigue	Increased neural activity; mood elevation; irritability; seizures
Gastrointestinal	Nausea, vomiting, abdominal pain	Peptic ulcers
Cardiovascular	Tachycardia, hypotension, cardiovascular collapse	Hypertension; edema; heart failure
Eyes	None	Cataract formation
Fluids and electrolytes	Hypovolemia; hyponatremia; hyperkalemia	Hypervolemia; hypernatremia; hypokalemia
Blood cells	Anemia	Increased red blood cell count and neutrophils; impaired clotting

head trauma or allergic reactions. An inexpensive glucocorticoid that is frequently prescribed is prednisone. Chart 45–4 describes the pharmacologic data for prednisone.

PHARMACOKINETICS

Prednisone is readily absorbed from the GI tract. It has a short half-life of 3 to 4 h, and it has a moderately high protein-binding power. Prednisone is excreted primarily in the urine.

PHARMACODYNAMICS

The major actions of prednisone are to suppress an acute inflammatory process and for immunosuppression. It prevents cell-mediated immune reactions. Prednisone should not be confused with prednisolone. Peak action occurs in 1 to 2 h, and its duration of action is long (1 to 1.5 d).

Commonly used glucocorticoid drugs are listed in Table 45–5. Most of the glucocorticoids are pregnancy category C drugs. Agents used for adrenocortical insufficiency contain both glucocorticoids and mineralocorticoids, whereas drugs for antiinflammatory or immunosuppressive use contain mostly glucocorticoids.

SIDE EFFECTS AND ADVERSE REACTIONS

The side effects and adverse reactions of glucocorticoids that result from high doses or prolonged use include increased blood sugar, abnormal fat deposits in the face and trunk (moon face and buffalo hump), decreased extremity size, muscle wasting, edema, sodium and water retention, hypertension, euphoria or psychosis, thinned skin with purpura, increased intraocular pressure (glaucoma), peptic ulcers, and growth retardation. Long-term use of glucocorticoid drugs can cause adrenal atrophy (loss of adrenal gland function). When drug therapy is discontinued, the dose should be tapered to allow the adrenal cortex to produce cortisol and other corticosteroids. An abrupt withdrawal of the drug can result in severe adrenocortical insufficiency.

DRUG INTERACTIONS

Glucocorticoids increase the potency of drugs taken concurrently, including aspirin and nonsteroidal antiinflammatory drugs (NSAIDs), thus increasing the risk of GI bleeding and ulceration. Use of potassium-wasting diuretics (HydroDIURIL, Lasix) with glucocorticoids increases potassium loss, resulting in hypokalemia. Glucocorticoids can decrease the effect of oral anticoagulants (warfarin [Coumadin]).

Barbiturates, phenytoin, and rifampin decrease the effect of prednisone. Prolonged use of prednisone can cause severe muscle weakness.

Dexamethasone, a potent glucocorticoid, interacts with many drugs. Phenytoin, theophylline, rifampin, barbiturates, and antacids decrease the action of dexamethasone, whereas NSAIDs, including aspirin, and estrogen increase it. Dexamethasone decreases the ef-

Chart 45–4.   Adrenal Hormone

GLUCOCORTICOID

Drug Name	**Dosage**
Prednisone	A: PO: 5–60 mg/d in divided doses
(Deltasone, Meticorten, Orasone, Panasol-S), ❦	C: PO: 0.1–0.15 mg/kg/d in 2–4 divided doses
Apo-Prednisone, Winpred	or 4–5 mg/m²/d in 2 doses
Pregnancy Category: C	

Contraindications	**Drug-Lab-Food Interactions**
Hypersensitivity, psychosis, fungal infection	**Drug:** *Increase* effect with barbiturates, pheny-
Caution: Diabetes mellitus	toin, rifampin, ephedrine, theophylline; *decrease*
	effects of aspirin, anticonvulsants, isoniazid
	(INH), antidiabetics, vaccines

Pharmacokinetics	**Pharmacodynamics**
Absorption: PO: Well absorbed	PO: Onset: UK
Distribution: PB: 65%–91%; crosses the placenta	Peak: 1–2 h
Metabolism: t½: 3–4 h	Duration: 24–36 d
Excretion: In urine	

Therapeutic Effects/Uses

To decrease inflammatory occurrence; as an immunosuppressant; to treat dermatologic disorders.

Mode of Action: Suppression of inflammation and adrenal function.

Side Effects	**Adverse Reactions**
Nausea, diarrhea, abdominal distention, in-	Petechiae, ecchymosis, hypertension, tachycar-
creased appetite, sweating, headache, depres-	dia, osteoporosis, muscle wasting
sion, flushing, mood changes	**Life-threatening:** GI hemorrhage, pancreatitis,
	circulatory collapse, thrombophlebitis, embolism

(Nursing Process: Assessment and Planning / Interventions / Evaluation)

KEY: A: adult; C: child; PO: by mouth; PB: protein-binding; UK: unknown; t½: half-life; GI: gastrointestinal; ❦: Canadian drug names.

fects of oral anticoagulants and oral antidiabetics. When the drug is given with diuretics and/or anti-*Pseudomonas* penicillin preparations, the serum potassium level may decrease markedly. Glucocorticoids can increase the blood sugar levels; thus, insulin or oral antidiabetic drug dosage may need to be increased.

Glucocorticoid Inhibitors

Ketoconazole (Nizoral), an antifungal drug, and aminoglutethimide (Cytadren), an antineoplastic hormone antagonist, inhibit glucocorticoid synthesis. Ketoconazole is effective in treating clients with Cushing's syndrome and is useful as adjunct to surgery or radiation. High doses should be avoided because it can induce fatal ventricular dysrhythmias. Aminoglutethi-

mide is frequently prescribed for temporary treatment of selected clients with Cushing's syndrome, especially those clients with adrenal adenoma or carcinoma, ectopic ACTH-producing tumors, or adrenal hyperplasia.

Mineralocorticoids

Mineralocorticoids, the second type of corticosteroid, secrete aldosterone. These hormones maintain fluid balance by promoting the reabsorption of sodium from the renal tubules. Sodium attracts water, resulting in water retention. When hypovolemia (decrease in circulating fluid) occurs, more aldosterone is secreted to increase sodium and water retention and to restore fluid balance. With sodium reabsorption, potassium is lost and hypokalemia (potassium deficit)

Table 45–5
Adrenal Hormones: Glucocorticoids and Inhibitors

GENERIC (BRAND)	ROUTE AND DOSAGE	USES AND CONSIDERATIONS
GLUCOCORTICOIDS		
Beclomethasone dipropionate (Vanceril)	A: Inhal: 2 puffs b.i.d.–q.i.d	Inhalation for treating bronchial asthma and bronchial inflammation. Also to treat seasonal rhinitis. *Like all glucocorticoid inhalants, it is for prophylactic use and not for acute asthmatic attack. Pregnancy category:* C; PB: 87%; $t\frac{1}{2}$: 5–15 h
Betamethasone (Celestone, Celestone Phosphate)	A: PO: 0.6–7.2 mg/d in single or divided doses IM/IV: 1–9 mg/d; *max:* IM: 12 mg/d	Potent antiinflammatory steroid drug. It may be injected in joints. Effective for treating bronchial asthma, arthritis, severe allergic reactions, and cerebral edema. Should be taken with food. *Pregnancy category:* C; PB: 64%–90%; $t\frac{1}{2}$: 3–5 h
Cortisone acetate (Cortone Acetate, Cortistan)	A: PO/IM: 25–300 mg/d; decrease dose periodically	For adrenocortical insufficiency. Contains glucocorticoid and mineralocorticoid. Decreases inflammatory process. Oral dose is rapidly absorbed from the GI tract. Administer deep intramuscularly. With oral dose, give with food. *Pregnancy category:* C; PB: UK; $t\frac{1}{2}$: 0.5–12 h
Dexamethasone (Decadron)	*Inflammation:* A: PO: 0.25–4 mg b.i.d.–q.i.d. IM: 4–16 mg q1–3wk C: PO: 0.2 mg/kg/d in divided doses *Shock:* A: IV: 1–6 mg/kg as a single dose (IV push in IV fluids)	Potent antiinflammatory drug. For acute allergic disorders; asthmatic attack; cerebral edema; unresponsive shock. For diagnosis of Cushing's syndrome and depression. Can be administered by IV push or in IV fluids. With oral dose, give with food. *Pregnancy category:* C; PB: 80%–90%; $t\frac{1}{2}$: 3–4 h
Fludrocortisone acetate (Florinef Acetate)	A & C: PO: 0.1–0.2 mg/d	For treating adrenocortical insufficiency as in Addison's disease. Also for salt-losing adrenogenital syndrome. Used only for its mineralocorticoid effects. *Pregnancy category:* C; PB: 92%; $t\frac{1}{2}$: 3.5 h
Hydrocortisone (Cortef, Hydrocortone)	A: PO: 20–240 mg/d in 2–4 divided doses IV: 15–240 mg (phosphate q12h Rectal supp: 10–25 mg	For adrenocortical insufficiency and inflammation. Hydrocortisone sodium phosphate is parenteral form. Acetate form of drug may be injected into joints. Available in cream, ointment, lotion, and spray. *Pregnancy category:* C; PB: 79%; $t\frac{1}{2}$: 2–12 h
Methylprednisolone (Medrol, Solu-Medrol [sodium succinate] Depo-Medrol [acetate])	A: PO: 4–48 mg/d in one or more divided doses IM/IV: Succinate: 10–250 mg q6h IM: Acetate: 40–80 mg/wk	For treating inflammatory conditions such as arthritis, bronchial asthma, allergic reactions, cerebral edema. *Pregnancy category:* C; PB: UK; $t\frac{1}{2}$: 3.5 h
Paramethasone acetate (Haldrone)	A: PO: 0.5–6 mg t.i.d–q.i.d. C: PO: 58–200 μg/kg/d in 3–4 divided doses	For treating inflammatory conditions and allergic reactions. Similar to prednisone. Give with food. Do not abruptly stop dosing with long-term therapy. *Pregnancy category:* C; PB: 95%; $t\frac{1}{2}$: 3–45 h
Prednisolone (Delta-Cortef, Hydeltrasol [phosphate])	A: PO: 2.5–15 mg b.i.d.–q.i.d. IV: Phosphate: 2–30 mg q12h C: PO: 0.14–2 mg/kg/d in a single or divided doses	For antiinflammatory or immunosuppressive effect. For parenteral use. It can be injected into joints and soft tissue. Potent steroid. *Pregnancy category:* C; PB: 80%–90%; $t\frac{1}{2}$: 3.5 h (tissue: 18–36 h)
Prednisone	See Chart 45–4	For antiinflammatory or immunosuppressive effect. Inexpensive drug. This oral glucocorticoid is drug of choice. Take with food. Drug should not be abruptly stopped. *Pregnancy category:* C; PB: UK; $t\frac{1}{2}$: 3–4 h

Table continued on following page

Table 45–5 *Continued*
Adrenal Hormones: Glucocorticoids and Inhibitors

GENERIC (BRAND)	ROUTE AND DOSAGE	USES AND CONSIDERATIONS
Triamcinolone (Aristocort, Kenacort, Azmacort, Kenalog)	A: PO: 4–48 mg/d in 2–4 divided doses Inhal: 2 puffs, t.i.d.–q.i.d. Topical preparations: cream, ointment	For antiinflammatory or immunosuppressive effect. *Pregnancy category:* C; PB: UK; $t\frac{1}{2}$: 2–5 h
GLUCOCORTICOID INHIBITORS		
Aminoglutethimide (Cytadren)	*Cushing's syndrome:* A: PO: 250 mg q6h; *max:* 2 g/d	This agent is a hormonal antagonist. May be used to treat Cushing's syndrome associated with adrenal adenoma or carcinoma and ACTH-secreting tumors. It blocks the first step in steroid synthesis. *Pregnancy category:* D; PB: UK; $t\frac{1}{2}$: 13 h
Ketoconazole (Nizoral)	A: PO: 600–800 mg/d	Usually used in conjunction with surgery or radiation to inhibit glucocorticoid synthesis. Needs a higher dose to suppress steroid synthesis than for a fungal infection. *Pregnancy category:* C; PB: UK; $t\frac{1}{2}$: 8 h

KEY: A: adult; C: child; PO: by mouth; Inhal: inhalation; IV: intravenous; PB: protein-binding; $t\frac{1}{2}$: half-life; UK: unknown; GI: gastrointestinal.

can occur. Some glucocorticoid drugs also contain mineralocorticoids; these include cortisone and hydrocortisone. A severe decrease in the mineralocorticoid aldosterone leads to hypotension and vascular collapse, as seen in Addison's disease. Mineralocorticoid deficiency usually occurs with glucocorticoid deficiency, frequently called *corticosteroid deficiency.*

Fludrocortisone (Florinef) is an oral mineralocorticoid that can be given with a glucocorticoid. It can cause a negative nitrogen balance, so a high-protein diet is usually indicated. Because potassium excretion occurs with the use of mineralocorticoids and glucocorticoids, the serum potassium level should be monitored.

NURSING PROCESS
ADRENAL HORMONE: GLUCOCORTICOIDS

Assessment

- Obtain baseline vital signs (VS) for future comparison.
- Assess laboratory test results, especially serum electrolytes and blood sugar. Serum potassium level usually decreases and blood sugar level increases when a glucocorticoid such as prednisone is taken over an extensive period of time.
- Obtain the client's weight and urine output to use for future comparison.
- Assess the client's medical history. Report if the client has glaucoma, cataracts, peptic ulcer, psychiatric problems, or diabetes mellitus. Glucocorticoids can intensify these health problems.

Potential Nursing Diagnoses

- Fluid volume excess
- Risk for impaired tissue integrity

Planning

- The client's inflammatory process will abate. Side effects of glucocorticoid will be minimal.

Nursing Process continued on following page

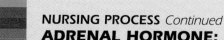

NURSING PROCESS *Continued*
ADRENAL HORMONE: GLUCOCORTICOIDS

Nursing Interventions

- Monitor VS. Glucocorticoids such as prednisone can increase blood pressure and sodium and water retention.
- Administer glucocorticoids only as ordered. Routes of administration include PO, IM (not in the deltoid muscle), IV, aerosol, and topical. Topical glucocorticoid drugs should be applied in thin layers. Rashes, infection, and purpura should be noted and reported.
- Monitor weight. Report weight gain of 5 lb in several days; this would most likely be due to water retention.
- Monitor laboratory values, especially serum electrolytes and blood sugar. Serum potassium level could decrease to <3.5 mEq/L, and blood sugar level would probably increase.
- Observe for signs and symptoms of hypokalemia, such as nausea, vomiting, muscular weakness, abdominal distention, paralytic ileus, and irregular heart rate.
- Observe for side effects from glucocorticoid drugs when therapy has lasted >10 d and the drug is taken in high dosages. The cortisone preparation should not be abruptly stopped because adrenal crisis can result.
- Monitor older adults for signs and symptoms of increased osteoporosis. Glucocorticoids promote calcium loss from the bone.
- Report changes in muscle strength. High doses of glucocorticoids promote loss of muscle tone.

Client Teaching

General
- Advise the client to take the drug as prescribed. Instruct the client *not* to abruptly stop the drug. When the drug is discontinued, the dose is tapered over 1 to 2 wk.
- For short-term use (<10 d) of glucocorticoids such as prednisone or other cortisone preparations, the drug dose still needs to be tapered. Prepare a schedule for the client to decrease the dose over a period of 4 to 5 d. For example, take 1 tab q.i.d.; the next day take 1 tab t.i.d.; the next day, take 1 tab b.i.d.; and then take 1 tab daily.
- Advise the client not to take cortisone preparations (PO or topical) during pregnancy unless necessary and prescribed by the health care provider. These drugs may be harmful to the fetus.
- Instruct the client to avoid persons with respiratory infections because these drugs suppress the immune system. This is especially important if the client is receiving a high dose of glucocorticoids.
- Advise the client receiving glucocorticoids to inform other health care providers of all drugs taken, especially before surgery.
- Advise the client to have a medical alert card, tag, or bracelet stating the glucocorticoid drug being taken.

Self-Administration
- Teach the client how to use an aerosol nebulizer. Warn the client against overuse of the aerosol to avoid possible rebound effect.

Diet
- Instruct the client to take cortisone preparations at mealtime or with food. Glucocorticoid drugs can irritate the gastric mucosa and cause a peptic ulcer.
- Advise the client to eat foods rich in potassium, such as fresh and dried fruits, vegetables, meats, and nuts. Prednisone promotes potassium loss and, thus, hypokalemia.

Side Effects
- Teach the client to report signs and symptoms of drug overdose or Cushing's syndrome, including a moon face, puffy eyelids, edema in the feet, increased bruising, dizziness, bleeding, and menstrual irregularity.

Nursing Process continued on following page

NURSING PROCESS *Continued*
ADRENAL HORMONE: GLUCOCORTICOIDS

Cultural Considerations

- Recognize that various cultural groups need guidance in understanding the disease process of Cushing's disease. Explain to the family that their family member is not "dumb or disinterested" but has an adrenal problem. Explain that the symptoms do not "go away" and may become more progressive if prescribed therapy is not followed.

Evaluation

- Evaluate the effectiveness of glucocorticoid drug therapy. If the inflammation has not improved, a change in drug therapy may be necessary.
- Continue monitoring for side effects, especially when the client is receiving high doses of glucocorticoids.

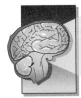

Critical Thinking in Action

M. P., age 68 years, had a severe allergic reaction to shellfish. She is taken to the emergency room. A single dose of dexamethasone 100 mg IV (direct IV over 30 seconds) was ordered. M. P. weighs 65 kg.

1. Why is M. P. receiving dexamethasone intravenously? Is the dosage of dexamethasone within safe therapeutic range? Explain.
2. Describe the various intravenous ways for administering dexamethasone. By what other routes can dexamethasone be administered?
3. What additional health information and assessment may aid the health care provider in treating M. P.'s serious health problem?

Twenty-one tablets of prednisone, 5 mg each, were prescribed to be taken over 5 days, with tapering daily doses. First day would be 10 mg four times a day; second day 10 mg three times a day; third day 10 mg two times a day; fourth day 10 mg once a day; and the fifth day 5 mg once a day.

4. Why was prednisone ordered and not oral dexamethasone? Explain.
5. What is the purpose for tapering prednisone doses? Explain.
6. Is the drug dose within safe therapeutic range? Explain.
7. Should M. P. have side effects such as peripheral edema due to water and sodium retention with tapering prednisone doses? Explain.
8. What is the difference between prednisone and prednisolone?
9. What are the adverse reactions from prolonged use of prednisone?
10. What are the nursing interventions and client teaching for M. P. and clients taking prednisone?

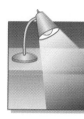

Study Questions

1. What hormones are secreted by the anterior pituitary gland (adenohypophysis) and what are their functions?

2. What is the action of ACTH? What are the nursing interventions and client teaching for clients receiving ACTH?

3. The client has diabetes insipidus. Is this the same as diabetes mellitus? Explain. What are the symptoms of diabetes insipidus? What drug is used to control this health problem?

4. What are the two hormones secreted by the thyroid gland? Differentiate between levothyroxine (Synthroid) and liothyronine (Cytomel). What are their actions?

5. For what disorders are the antithyroid drugs used? What severe side effects can result from their use?

6. What electrolyte is directly influenced by parathyroid hormone?

7. What are the physiologic effects of hypersecretion and hyposecretion of parathyroid hormone?

8. What are the subgroups of corticosteroids? What are four signs and symptoms of prolonged use of corticosteroids (cortisone)? What are the nursing implications of discontinuing a cortisone preparation? What instructions should the client receive?

9. A deficiency of the hormone cortisol leads to what health problem? What are the symptoms of this disease? What type of drug is used to control this disease?

Antidiabetic Drugs

46

Outline

Objectives

- Define diabetes mellitus, IDDM (type II), insulin, oral hypoglycemic agents, and glucagon.
- Identify the symptoms of diabetes mellitus.
- Explain a hypoglycemic reaction and describe the symptoms.
- Differentiate among rapid-acting, intermediate-acting, and long-acting insulin.
- Identify the peak concentration time for the three types of insulin action and when a hypoglycemic action is most likely to occur.
- Identify the action of oral hypoglycemic drugs and their side effects.
- Describe the nursing process including client teaching, for insulin and oral hypoglycemic agents.

Terms

diabetes mellitus
hypoglycemic reaction
IDDM
insulin

insulin shock
ketoacidosis
lipodystrophy
NIDDM

oral hypoglycemic drugs
polydipsia
polyphagia
polyuria

INTRODUCTION

Antidiabetic drugs are used primarily to control diabetes mellitus, a chronic disease that affects carbohydrate metabolism. There are two groups of antidiabetic agents: (1) insulin and (2) oral hypoglycemic drugs. Oral hypoglycemic drugs are synthetic preparations that stimulate insulin release or otherwise alter the metabolic response to hyperglycemia. **Insulin,** a protein secreted from the beta cells of the pancreas, is necessary for carbohydrate metabolism and plays an important role in protein and fat metabolism. The beta cells make up 75% of the pancreas, and the alpha cells that secrete glucagon, a hyperglycemic substance, occupy approximately 20% of the pancreas.

DIABETES MELLITUS

Diabetes mellitus, a chronic disease resulting from deficient glucose metabolism, is caused by insufficient insulin secretion from the beta cells.* This results in high blood sugar (hyperglycemia). Diabetes mellitus is characterized by the three Ps: **polyuria** (increased urine output), **polydipsia** (increased thirst), and **polyphagia** (increased hunger). The two forms of diabetes are (1) insulin-dependent diabetes mellitus **(IDDM),** or type I diabetes mellitus (also referred to as juvenile-onset diabetes with no insulin secretion), and (2) non–insulin-dependent diabetes mellitus **(NIDDM),** or type II diabetes mellitus (also known as maturity-onset or adult-onset diabetes with some insulin secretion).

How the lack of insulin causes diabetes mellitus is not fully understood. Some authorities suggest that viral infections may contribute to the onset of type I or IDDM, and heredity is a major factor in type II or NIDDM. In type II, there is some beta cell function with varying amounts of insulin secretion. Hyperglycemia may be controlled with oral antidiabetic drugs and a diet prescribed by the American Diabetic Association. However, insulin may be required during times of stress (surgery, trauma, infection, pregnancy). Persons with type II diabetes mellitus are frequently controlled by an oral antidiabetic drug, but they could become insulin-dependent years later. Approximately one third of type II diabetics receive a low dose of insulin daily.

Certain drugs increase blood sugar and can cause hyperglycemia in prediabetic persons. These include glucocorticoids (cortisone, prednisone), thiazide diuretics (hydrochlorothiazide [HydroDIURIL]), and epinephrine. Usually the blood sugar level returns to normal after the drug is discontinued.

---

*Diabetes mellitus is a disorder of the pancreas; diabetes insipidus is a disorder of the posterior pituitary gland.

Insulin

Insulin is released from the beta cells of the islets of Langerhans in response to an increase in blood glucose. Oral glucose load is more effective in raising the serum insulin level than an intravenous glucose load. This is partly due to an increase in GI hormones. Insulin promotes the uptake of glucose, amino acids, and fatty acids and converts them to substances that are stored in body cells. Glucose is converted to glycogen for future glucose needs in the liver and muscle, thereby lowering the blood glucose level. The normal range for blood glucose is 60 to 100 mg/dL and, for serum glucose, 70 to 110 mg/dL. When the blood glucose level is greater than 180 mg/dL, glycosuria (sugar in the urine) can occur. Increased blood sugar acts as an osmotic diuretic, causing polyuria. When blood sugar remains elevated (>200 mg/dL), diabetes mellitus occurs.

BETA CELL SECRETION OF INSULIN

The beta cells in the pancreas secrete approximately 0.2 to 0.5 U/kg/d. A client weighing 70 kg (154 pounds) would secrete 14 to 35 U of insulin a day. More insulin secretion may occur if the person consumes a greater caloric intake. A client with diabetes mellitus may require 0.2 to 1.0 U/kg/d. The higher range may be due to obesity, stress, or tissue insulin resistance.

COMMERCIALLY PREPARED INSULIN

Parenteral (injectable) insulin is obtained from pork and beef pancreas when the animals are slaughtered. Pork insulin is closely related to human insulin, having only one different amino acid; beef insulin has four different amino acids. Human insulin (Humulin) was introduced in 1983 and is produced by two separate methods: (1) changing the different amino acid of pork insulin or (2) using DNA technology. Pork insulin is a weaker allergen than beef insulin, and the use of human insulin has a very low incidence of allergic effects and insulin resistance. Insulin is made more pure than previously, especially the Humulin produced by DNA technology, resulting in fewer side effects. Human insulins administered subcutaneously can be absorbed faster and have a shorter duration than animal insulins. Newly diagnosed clients with insulin-dependent diabetes are usually prescribed human insulin. Also, clients in whom hyperglycemia develops during pregnancy or who are pregnant diabetics are usually prescribed human insulin. If a client has been taking animal (pork or beef) insulin without having any untoward effects, then it is not necessary to change to human insulin.

The concentration of insulin is 100 U/mL or 500 U/mL (U100/mL, U500/mL) and the insulin is packaged in a 10-mL vial (see figures on insulin in Chapter 4D). Insulin 500 U is seldom used except in emergencies and for clients with serious insulin resistance (>200 U/d). Insulin 40 U is no longer used in the United States; however, in some countries this concentration of insulin is still used. Insulin syringes are marked in units of 100 U per 1 mL for insulin U 100. Insulin syringes must be used for accurate dosing. To prevent dosage errors, the nurse must be certain that there is a match of the insulin concentration with the calibration of units on the insulin syringe. Before use, the client or nurse must roll, not shake, the bottle to ensure that the insulin and its ingredients are well mixed. Shaking a bottle of insulin can cause bubbles and an inaccurate dose. Insulin requirements vary; usually less insulin is needed with increased exercise and more insulin with infections and high fever.

ADMINISTRATION OF INSULIN

Insulin is a protein and *cannot* be administered orally because gastrointestinal (GI) secretions destroy the insulin structure. It is administered subcutaneously, at a 45- to 90-degree angle. The 90-degree angle is made by raising the skin and fatty tissue; the insulin is injected into the pocket between the fat and the muscle. In a thin person with little fatty tissue, the 45- to 60-degree angle is used. Regular insulin is the *only* type that can be administered intravenously.

The site and depth of insulin injection affect absorption. Insulin absorption is greater when given in the deltoid and abdominal areas than when given in the thighs and buttock areas. Insulin administered subcutaneously has a slower absorption rate than if administered intramuscularly. Heat and massage could increase subcutaneous absorption. Cooling the subcutaneous area can decrease absorption.

Insulin is usually given in the morning before breakfast. It can be given several times a day. Insulin injection sites should be rotated to prevent **lipodystrophy** (tissue atrophy or hypertrophy), which can interfere with insulin absorption. Lipoatrophy (tissue atrophy) is a depression under the skin surface. A frequent cause of an atrophied area is due to the use of animal insulins (beef and pork). Lipohypertrophy (tissue hypertrophy) is a raised lump or knot on the skin surface. It frequently is caused by repeated injections into the same subcutaneous site. The client needs to develop a "site rotation pattern" in order to avoid lipodystrophy and to promote insulin absorption. There are various insulin rotation programs, such as an 8-day rotation schedule (insulin is given at a different site each day). The American Diabetic Association suggests that insulin should be injected daily at a chosen site for 1 week. Injections should be 1½ inches apart (a knuckle length) at a site area each day. If a client has to take two insulin injections a day (morning and evening), one site should be cho-

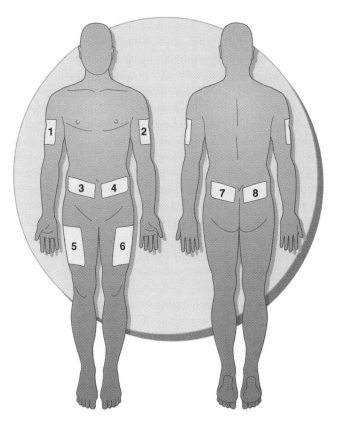

Figure 46–1
Sites for insulin injection.

sen on the right side (morning) and one site on the left side (evening). Figure 46–1 illustrates sites for insulin injections. A record of injection area sites and dates administered should be kept.

Obesity can be a causative factor of insulin resistance. Antibodies develop in persons taking animal insulin over time. This can slow the onset of insulin action and extend its duration of action. Antibody development can cause insulin resistance and insulin allergy. Skin tests with different insulin preparations may be performed to determine whether there is an allergic effect. Human and regular insulins produce fewer allergens.

Illness and stress increase the need for insulin. Insulin doses should *not* be withheld during illness, including infections and stress. Hyperglycemia and ketoacidosis may result from withholding insulin.

TYPES OF INSULIN

There are three standard types of insulin: rapid-acting, intermediate-acting, and long-acting. Rapid-acting insulin is called regular (crystalline) insulin and is a clear solution without any added substance to prolong the insulin action. The onset of action is ½ to 1 h, peak action occurs in 2 to 4 h, and the duration of action is 6 to 8 h. The onset of intermediate-acting insulin is 1 to 2 h, peak is 6 to 12 h, and the duration of action is 18 to 24 h. Long-acting insulin acts in 4 to 8 h, peaks in 14 to 20 h, and lasts for 24 to 36 h.

Rapid-acting insulins include lispro and regular insulins. **Lispro insulin (Humalog)** is a new rapid-acting insulin that was approved for use in 1996. The action of this insulin begins in 5 minutes and the duration of action is 2 to 4 hours. Lispro insulin acts faster than regular insulin; thus, lispro insulin can be administered 5 minutes before mealtime, whereas regular insulin is given 30 minutes before meals. Lispro insulin is formed by reversing two amino acids in human regular insulin (Humulin). **Regular (unmodified, crystalline) insulin** is the only type of insulin that can be administered intravenously as well as subcutaneously. Semilente insulin is no longer used as monotherapy. Insulin-dependent diabetics taking a rapid-acting insulin usually require an intermediate-acting insulin.

Intermediate-acting insulins include NPH, lente, Humulin N, and Humulin L. Neutral-protamine-Hagedorn (NPH) and Humulin N contain protamine, a protein that prolongs the action of the insulin. Lente and Humulin L contain zinc, which also prolongs the insulin action time because of the decreased solubility.

Regular insulin can be mixed with protamine or zinc insulin in the same syringe. Mixing insulin can alter absorption rate. When regular insulin is mixed with lente insulin, a portion of the effect of regular insulin is lost. Less regular insulin is decreased in effect when mixed with NPH than when mixed with lente. However, lente insulin causes less allergic response than NPH.

The **long-acting insulin** used currently is Humulin U ultralente. This insulin is absorbed slower than other insulins because of its large crystals, which dissolve slowly and prolong the duration time. PZI (protamine-zinc-insulin) has been discontinued.

Combination insulins are commercially premixed. These include Humulin 70/30, Novolin 70/30, and Humulin 50/50, and they are being widely used by diabetics. The 70/30 vials contain 70% NPH and 30% regular insulin, and the 50/50 vial contains 50% NPH and 50% regular insulin. The client does not have to mix regular and NPH insulin as long as this combination is effective. However, some clients need less than 30% regular insulin and more NPH; such a client needs to mix the the two insulins together in the prescribed proportions.

Storage of Insulin

Unopened insulin vials are refrigerated until needed. Once an insulin vial has been opened, it may be kept (1) at room temperature for 1 month or (2) in the refrigerator for 3 months. Insulin vials should not be put in the freezer. Also, insulin vials should not be placed in direct sunlight or in a high-temperature area. Prefilled syringes should be stored in the refrigerator and should be used within 1 to 2 weeks. Opened insulin vials lose their strength after approximately 3 months. Chart 46–1 compares regular insulin to NPH insulin.

Pharmacokinetics

Regular and NPH insulins are well absorbed with all routes of administration. Both insulins can be administered subcutaneously, but only regular insulin can be given intravenously. The half-life varies. Insulin is metabolized by the liver and muscle and excreted in the urine.

Pharmacodynamics

Insulin lowers blood sugar by promoting utilization of glucose by the body cells. It also stores glucose as glycogen in muscles. The onset of action of regular insulin given subcutaneously is ½ to 1 h and given intravenously, 10 to 30 min. The onset of action of NPH is 1 to 2 h. The peak action time of insulins is important because of the possibility of hypoglycemic reaction (insulin shock) occurring during that time. The peak time for regular insulin is 2 to 4 h and 6 to 12 h for NPH insulin. The nurse needs to assess for signs and symptoms of hypoglycemic reaction, such as nervousness, tremors, confusion, sweating, and increased pulse rate. Orange juice, sugar-sweetened beverages, or hard candy should be kept available and given if a reaction occurs.

Regular insulin can be given several times a day, especially during the regulation of insulin dosage. NPH insulin is usually administered once a day. Regular insulin (3 to 15 U) can be mixed with an intermediate-acting insulin (NPH or lente), especially if rapid onset of action is needed. Long-acting insulins are seldom ordered because their peak action time occurs during the night or early morning. When switching from pork to human insulin, the client may require an adjustment of insulin dose, because human insulin has a shorter duration of action.

Drug Interactions

Drugs such as thiazide diuretics, glucocorticoids (cortisone preparations), thyroid agents, and estrogen increase the blood sugar, and insulin dosage may need adjustment. Drugs that decrease insulin needs are tricyclic antidepressants, monoamine oxidase (MAO) inhibitors, aspirin products, and oral anticoagulants.

Table 46–1 lists the drug data for the rapid-acting, intermediate-acting, and long-acting insulins.

Side Effects and Adverse Reactions: Hypoglycemic Reactions and Ketoacidosis

When more insulin is administered than is needed for glucose metabolism, **a hypoglycemic (insulin) reac-**

Chart 46–1. Antidiabetic: Insulins

REGULAR AND NPH INSULIN

Drug Name

Regular Insulin
NPH Insulin
  Injectable insulins
Pregnancy Category: B

Dosage

Varies according to client's blood sugar

Contraindications

Hypersensitivity to beef, zinc, protamine insulins

Drug-Lab-Food Interactions

Drug: *Increase* hypoglycemic effect with aspirin, oral anticoagulant, alcohol, oral hypoglycemics, beta blockers, tricyclic antidepressants, MAOIs, tetracycline; *decrease* hypoglycemic effect with thiazides, glucocorticoids, oral contraceptives, thyroid drugs, smoking

Pharmacokinetics

Absorption: SC, IV (regular)
Distribution: PB: UK
Metabolism: t½: Regular IV insulin: 5–9 min; varies with type of insulin
Excretion: Mostly in urine

Pharmacodynamics

Regular Insulin:
SC: Onset: 0.5–1 h
    Peak: 2–4 h
    Duration: 4–8 h
IV: Onset: 10–20 min
    Peak: 15–30 min
    Duration: 1–2 h
NPH Insulin:
SC: Onset: 1–2 h
    Peak: 6–12 h (8–9 h average)
    Duration: 18–24 h

Therapeutic Effects/Uses

To control diabetes mellitus; to lower blood sugar.

Mode of Action: Insulin promotes utilization of glucose by body cells.

Side Effects

Hunger, tremors, weakness, headache, lethargy, fatigue, redness, irritation or swelling at insulin injection site, flushing, confusion, agitation

Adverse Reactions

Urticaria, tachycardia, palpitations, hypoglycemic reaction, rebound hyperglycemia (Somogyi effect), lipodystrophy
Life-threatening: Shock; anaphylaxis

Assessment and Planning / Interventions / Evaluation — NURSING PROCESS

KEY: SC: subcutaneous; IV: intravenous; UK: unknown; PB: protein-binding; t½: half-life; MAOIs: monoamine oxidase inhibitors.

tion, or **insulin shock,** occurs. The person may become nervous, trembling, and uncoordinated, with cold and clammy skin, and may complain of a headache. Some clients become combative and incoherent. Giving sugar orally or intravenously increases the utilization of insulin, and the symptoms disappear immediately.

With an inadequate amount of insulin, the sugar cannot be metabolized and fat catabolism occurs. The use of fatty acids (ketones) for energy causes **ketoaci-** **dosis** (diabetic acidosis or diabetic coma). Table 46–2 gives the signs and symptoms of hypoglycemic reaction and ketoacidosis.

INSULIN PUMPS

There are two types of insulin pumps: portable and implantable. The implantable insulin pump is surgically implanted in the abdomen. It delivers basal insulin infusion and bolus doses with meals, either intraperitoneally or intravenously. With the use of

Table 46-1
Antidiabetics: Insulins

GENERIC (BRAND)	ROUTE AND DOSAGE	PREGNANCY CATEGORY	HALF-LIFE	PROTEIN-BINDING	ACTION		
					Onset	Peak	Duration
RAPID-ACTING							
Lispro (Humalog)	A: SC: 5–10 U, dose individualized	B	<13 h	UK	5 min	0.5–1 h	2–4 h
Regular	A & C: SC/IV: 100 U/mL; dose is individualized according to blood sugar	B	10 min–1 h	UK	0.5–1 h	2–4 h	6–8 h
Humulin R	Same as regular insulin						
INTERMEDIATE-ACTING							
NPH insulin	See Chart 46-1	B	13 h	UK	1–2 h	6–12 h	18–24 h
Humulin N insulin	Same as NPH insulin	B	13 h	UK	1–2 h	8–12 h	18–24 h
Lente insulin	A & C: SC: 100 U/mL; dose is individualized according to blood sugar	B	13 h	UK	1–2 h	8–12 h	18–28 h
Humulin L insulin	Same as lente	B	13 h	UK	1–2 h	8–12 h	18–28 h
LONG-ACTING							
Ultralente insulin	Same as lente	B	13 h	UK	5–8 h	14–20 h	30–36 h
COMBINATIONS							
Humulin 70/30 (NPH 70%, regular 30%)	Dose individualized	B	13 h	UK	0.5 h	4–8 h	22–24 h
Humulin 50/50 (NPH 50%, regular 50%)	Dose individualized	B	13 h	UK	0.5 h	4–8 h	24 h

KEY: IV: intravenous; NPH: neutral-protamine-Hagedorn; PZI: protamine-zinc insulin; SC: subcutaneous; UK: unknown.
* Protamine and zinc suspensions are added to regular insulin.

Table 46–2
Hypoglycemic Reaction and Diabetic Ketoacidosis

REACTION	SIGNS AND SYMPTOMS
Hypoglycemic reaction (insulin shock)	Headache, lightheadedness Nervousness, apprehension Tremor Excess perspiration; cold, clammy skin Tachycardia Slurred speech Memory lapse, confusion, seizures Blood sugar level <60 mg/dL
Diabetic ketoacidosis (hyperglycemic reaction)	Extreme thirst Polyuria Fruity breath odor Kussmaul breathing (deep, rapid, labored, distressing, dyspnea) Rapid, thready pulse Dry mucous membranes, poor skin turgor Blood sugar level >250 mg/dL

implantable insulin pumps, there are fewer hypoglycemic reactions and the blood glucose levels are controlled. Long-term effectiveness of the pump is under study.

The portable or external insulin pumps have been available since 1983. The external insulin pump keeps the blood glucose levels as close to normal as possible. The insulin pump is battery-operated, connected to a small computer the size of a "call pager," and is programmed to continuously release small amounts of insulin on an hourly basis. A tubing with a small subcutaneous needle is attached to the small computer pump. Only regular insulin is used, which is similar to the body's insulin. Modified insulins (NPH and lente) are not used because of unpredictable control of blood sugars. The pump delivers exactly as much regular insulin as the client programs per hour. Insulin is delivered by bolus (the client pushing a button to deliver a bolus dose at meals), and basal rate for hourly doses. The ongoing insulin delivery helps to decrease the risk of severe hypoglycemia. Glucose levels should be monitored at least daily with or without an insulin pump.

NURSING PROCESS
ANTIDIABETICS: INSULIN

Assessment

- Assess the drugs the client is currently taking. Certain drugs, such as alcohol, aspirin, oral anticoagulants, oral hypoglycemics, beta blockers, tricyclic antidepressants, MAOIs, and tetracycline, increase the hypoglycemic effect when taken with insulin. Note that thiazides, glucocorticoids, oral contraceptives, thyroid drugs, and smoking can increase blood sugar.
- Assess the type of insulin and dosage. Note whether it is given once or twice a day.
- Check vital signs (VS) and blood sugar levels. Report abnormal findings.
- Assess the client's knowledge of diabetes mellitus and the use of insulins.
- Assess for signs and symptoms of a hypoglycemic reaction (insulin shock) and hyperglycemia or ketoacidosis.

Potential Nursing Diagnoses

- Risk for impaired tissue integrity
- Altered nutrition: more or less than body requirements
- Risk for injury

Planning

- Client's blood sugar will be within the normal values (70 to 110 mg/dL).

Nursing Interventions

- Monitor VS. Tachycardia can occur during an insulin reaction.
- Monitor blood glucose levels and report changes. The reference value is 60 to 100 mg/dL for blood glucose and 70 to 110 mg/dL for serum glucose.
- Prepare a teaching plan based on the client's knowledge of the health problem, diet, and drug therapy.

Nursing Process continued on following page

NURSING PROCESS *Continued*
ANTIDIABETICS: INSULIN

Client Teaching

General
- Instruct the client to report immediately symptoms of a hypoglycemic (insulin) reaction, such as headache, nervousness, sweating, tremors, and rapid pulse, and symptoms of a hyperglycemic reaction (diabetic acidosis), such as thirst, increased urine output, and sweet fruity breath odor.
- Advise the client that hypoglycemic reactions are more likely to occur during the peak action time. Most diabetics know whether they are having a hypoglycemic reaction; however, some have a higher tolerance to low blood sugar and can have a severe hypoglycemic reaction without realizing it.
- Explain that orange juice, sugar-containing drinks, and hard candy may be used when a hypoglycemic reaction begins.
- Instruct family members in administering glucagon by injection if the client has a hypoglycemic reaction and cannot drink sugar-containing fluid.
- Instruct the client about the necessity for compliance to prescribed insulin and diet.
- Advise the client to obtain a medical alert card, tag, and/or bracelet indicating the health problem and insulin dosage.

Self-Administration
- Instruct the client how to check the blood sugar using Chemstrip bG test.
- Instruct the client in the care of the insulin bottle and syringes. Inform the client taking NPH or lente insulin with regular insulin that the regular insulin should be drawn up before the NPH or lente insulin.

Diet
- Advise the client taking insulin to eat the prescribed diet on schedule. The diet may be from the American Diabetic Association (ADA).

Cultural Considerations

- Provide additional explanation as needed to clients from various cultural groups related to insulin action and administration, insulin reactions, and possible complications.
- Follow-up by a community nurse is needed to determine the client's compliance with insulin use, diet, and exercise regimens.

Evaluation

- Evaluate the effectiveness of the insulin therapy by noting whether blood sugar level is within the accepted range.
- Evaluate the client's knowledge of the signs and symptoms of hypoglycemic or hyperglycemic reaction.

Most insulin pumps have a memory of the last 24 boluses (time and day), 7 daily totals, 9 prime uses, and 12 alarms with time and date. An alarm is sounded when insulin is not being delivered. The pump can be disconnected from the insertion site for bathing, swimming, and the like; however, it is recommended that it not be discontinued for longer than 1 to 2 hours. Portable insulin pumps are expensive, ranging from $3000 to $5000. This method of insulin delivery is not for every diabetic. The person with IDDM may best benefit from use of an insulin pump. Figure 46–2 shows an example of an insulin pump.

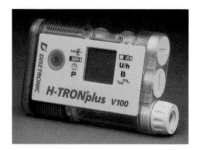

Figure 46–2

Table 46–3
Antidiabetics: Sulfonylureas

GENERIC (BRAND)	ROUTE AND DOSAGE	USES AND CONSIDERATIONS
FIRST-GENERATION: SHORT-ACTING		
Tolbutamide (Orinase)	A: PO: 500–3000 mg/d in 2–3 divided doses	For managing non–insulin-dependent diabetes mellitus (NIDDM) or type II diabetes. Drug is chemically related to sulfonamides with no antiinfective effect. Hypoglycemic reaction may occur if overdosed. *Pregnancy category:* C; PB: >90%; $t\frac{1}{2}$: 4–7 h
FIRST-GENERATION: INTERMEDIATE-ACTING		
Acetohexamide (Dymelor)	See Chart 46–2	For managing NIDDM or type II diabetes. May be given with selected type I diabetes clients. Doses >1000 mg are given twice a day. Has a diuretic effect. Duration of action is 12–24 h. *Pregnancy category:* C; PB: 90%; $t\frac{1}{2}$: 5–7 h
Tolazamide (Tolinase)	A: PO: 100–250 mg/d in 1–2 divided doses; *max:* 1 g/d	Same as acetohexamide. Diet and exercise should be a part of diabetic therapy. Duration of action is 10–20 h. *Pregnancy category:* C; PB: 90%; $t\frac{1}{2}$: 7 h
FIRST-GENERATION: LONG-ACTING		
Chlorpropamide (Diabinese)	A: PO: Initially: 100–250 mg/d; maint: 100–500 mg/d in 1–2 divided doses; *max:* 750 mg/d	For managing NIDDM or type II diabetes. May be given to selected type I diabetics for reducing insulin doses. Diet and exercise should be a part of diabetic therapy. Duration of action is 24 h. May cause water and sodium retention. *Pregnancy category:* C; PB: 95%; $t\frac{1}{2}$: 36 h
SECOND-GENERATION		
Glipizide (Glucotrol)	A: PO: Initially: 2.5–5.0 mg a.c. daily/b.i.d.; maint: 10–15 mg/d (dose should be divided if >15 mg), *max:* 40 mg/d	Same as acetohexamide and chlorpropamide. Duration of action is 10–24 h. Potent drug. *Pregnancy category:* C; PB: 90%–95%; $t\frac{1}{2}$: 2.5–5 h
Glyburide nonmicronized (DiaBeta, Micronase)	A: PO: Initially: 1.25–5 mg/d; maint: 1.25–20 mg q.d./b.i.d.; *max:* 20 mg/d	Same as chlorpropamide. Potent drug. Duration of action is 10–24 h. *Pregnancy category:* B; PB: 90%–95%; $t\frac{1}{2}$: 10 h
Glyburide micronized (Glynase)	A: PO: 1.5–3 mg/d in AM; maint: 3–4.5 mg/d; *max:* 12 mg/d in 1 or 2 divided doses	For NIDDM. Same as glyburide nonmicronized.
Glimepiride (Amaryl)	A: PO: Initially: 1–2 mg, a.c.; maint: 1–4 mg/d a.c.; *max:* 8 mg/d a.c.	To treat clients with NIDDM. May be used in combination with insulin. Can lower the 2-h postprandial glucose levels significantly. GI disturbances may occur. *Pregnancy category:* C; PB: 99.5%; $t\frac{1}{2}$: 5–9 h
NONSULFONYLUREASE		
Metformin (Glucophage)	A: PO: Initial: 500 mg daily/b.i.d.; increase dose gradually; *max:* 2500 mg/d	For NIDDM when no response to sulfonylureas. Take with meals. May be combined with sulfonylurea (dose reduction of metformin would be needed). *Pregnancy category:* B; PB: 0%; $t\frac{1}{2}$: 6.2 h
Acarbose (Precose)	A: PO: 25 mg t.i.d.; *max:* 300 mg/d	For NIDDM. Client may experience diarrhea, abdominal distention, and/or flatulence. *Pregnancy category:* C; PB: UK; $t\frac{1}{2}$: UK
Troglitazone (Rezulin)	A: PO: Initially: 200 mg/d. Dose may be increased to 200 mg; *max:* 600 mg/d	For the management of NIDDM. Taken alone, does not cause hypoglycemic reaction unless taken with insulin or a hypoglycemic drug. Decreases insulin resistance. Decreases hepatic glucose output. *Pregnancy category:* B; PB: 99%; $t\frac{1}{2}$: 16–34 h
Repaglinide (Prandin)	A: PO: 0.5–4 mg a.c. b.i.d., t.i.d., q.i.d.; *max:* 16 mg/d	To manage NIDDM. May be taken alone or in combination with metformin. Similar in action to sulfonylureas but not in structure. Increases beta cell secretion of insulin. *Pregnancy category:* UK; PB: 98%; $t\frac{1}{2}$: 1 h

KEY: A: adult; PB: protein-binding; PO: by mouth; $t\frac{1}{2}$: half-life; UK: unknown; >: greater than; a.c.: before meals.

851

INTRANASAL INSULIN

Administration of insulin intranasally is in the experimental stage. This route of insulin administration causes a rapid-onset effect and has a short duration of action. This method is primarily used to provide mealtime insulin supplements and is not used to meet basal insulin needs. Intermediate-acting insulin would still be needed. Approximately only 10% of the insulin is absorbed through the nasal membrane; thus, the intranasal insulin dose is 10 times greater than a subcutaneous dose. Also, the nasal mucous membranes can become irritated. Intranasal insulin is expensive.

INSULIN INJECTORS

Insulin jet injectors shoot insulin, without a needle, directly through the skin into the fatty tissue. Because the insulin is delivered under high pressure, stinging, pain, burning, and bruising may occur. This method of insulin insertion is not indicated for children and the elderly. This type of device is also expensive, costing approximately 2 to 10 times as much as the subcutaneous dose.

Oral Antidiabetic Drugs (Oral Hypoglycemic Drugs)

FIRST- AND SECOND-GENERATION SULFONYLUREAS

Oral antidiabetic drugs, also called **oral hypoglycemics,** were discovered in the 1950s. These drugs are used by persons with NIDDM. They should *not* be used by persons with IDDM. Persons with NIDDM have some degree of insulin secretion by the pancreas. The sulfonylureas, a group of antidiabetics that are chemically related to sulfonamides but lack antibacterial activity, stimulate the beta cells to secrete more insulin. This increases the insulin cell receptors, thus increasing the ability of the cells to bind insulin for glucose metabolism.

The sulfonylureas are classified as first- and second-generation. The first-generation sulfonylureas are divided into short-acting, intermediate-acting, and long-acting antidiabetics.

The second-generation sulfonylureas were first used in Europe, and in 1984 were approved by the Food and Drug Administration for use in the United States. The newer sulfonylureas increase the tissue response to insulin and decrease glucose production by the liver. They have a greater hypoglycemic potency than the first-generation sulfonylureas. Effective doses for the second-generation drugs are less than the dosages of the first generation. They have a longer duration and cause fewer side effects. The second-generation drugs have less displacement potential from protein-binding sites by other highly pro-

tein-bound drugs, such as salicylates and warfarin (Coumadin), than those of the first-generation drugs. The second-generation sulfonylureas should not be used when liver or kidney dysfunction is present. A hypoglycemic reaction is more likely to occur in the elderly.

The newest second-generation sulfonylurea is glimepiride (Amaryl). It directly stimulates the beta cells to secrete insulin, thus decreasing the blood glucose level. Glimepiride improves the postprandial glucose levels. It may be used in combination with insulin in persons with NIDDM. Side effects include gastrointestinal disturbances such as nausea, vomiting, diarrhea, and abdominal pain.

Table 46–3 lists the drug data for the sulfonylureas. Chart 46–2 lists the actions and effects of the first-generation, intermediate-acting sulfonylurea acetohexamide (Dymelor).

Pharmacokinetics

Acetohexamide is well absorbed from the GI tract and is highly protein-bound. Acetohexamide is metabolized by the liver with 50% converted to a metabolite. There are two half-lives: the half-life of the drug metabolite is three times as long as that of the pure drug. The kidneys excrete the drug unchanged in the urine.

Pharmacodynamics

Acetohexamide is prescribed to control NIDDM. It lowers the blood sugar by stimulating the beta cells in the pancreas to secrete insulin. Onset of action usually occurs within 1 h, and the peak action time is between 2 and 6 h. The drug is usually given once a day in the morning because of its long duration of action.

Side Effects, Adverse Reactions, and Contraindications

The side effects are similar to those of insulin. Taking antidiabetic drugs without adequate food can lead to an insulin reaction with signs and symptoms such as nervousness, tremors, and confusion. Adverse reactions are those of hematologic disorders: aplastic anemia, leukopenia, and thrombocytopenia. Sulfonylureas are contraindicated in IDDM (no functioning beta cells), pregnancy, and breastfeeding, and during stress, surgery, or severe infection.

Drug Interactions

Aspirin, anticoagulants, anticonvulsants, sulfonamides, and some NSAIDs can increase the action of sulfonylureas by binding to the plasma protein and displacing sulfonylureas. Because this causes increased free sulfonylurea, an insulin reaction can result. Sulfonylureas also enhance the action of thiazide diuretics, phenothiazines, and barbiturates. Sulfonylureas decrease the action of thyroid replacement drugs. Cli-

Chart 46–2. Antidiabetics: Sulfonylurea

SULFONYLUREA

Drug Name

Acetohexamide
  (Dymelor) 🍁 Dimelor
Oral hypoglycemic drug
Pregnancy Category: C

Contraindications

Diabetes mellitus (DM) type IDDM; severe renal, hepatic, cardiac, or thyroid disease; unstable DM

Dosage

A: PO: 250–1000 mg/d in 1 or 2 divided doses; *max:* 1.5 g/d; maint: 1000 mg/d

Drug-Lab-Food Interactions

Drug: *Increase* hypoglycemic effect with aspirin, alcohol, anticoagulants, some NSAIDs, anticonvulsants, sulfonamides, oral contraceptives, MAOIs; *decrease* hypoglycemic effect with glucocorticoids (cortisone), thiazide diuretics, estrogen, calcium channel blockers, phenytoin, thyroid drugs

Pharmacokinetics

Absorption: PO: Well absorbed
Distribution: PB: 90%
Metabolism: $t\frac{1}{2}$: Drug: 1–1.5 h metabolite; 5–7 h
Excretion: Unchanged in urine

Pharmacodynamics

PO: Onset: 1 h
    Peak: 2–6 h
    Duration: 12–24 h

Therapeutic Effects/Uses

To control DM type II (maturity-onset diabetes); to lower blood sugar.

Mode of Action: Stimulation of beta cells to secrete insulin.

Side Effects

Nausea, vomiting, diarrhea, rash, pruritus, headache, photosensitivity

Adverse Reactions

Hypoglycemic reaction
Life-threatening: Aplastic anemia, leukopenia, thrombocytopenia

NURSING PROCESS
Assessment and Planning
Interventions
Evaluation

KEY: A: adult; PO: by mouth; PB: protein-binding; $t\frac{1}{2}$: half-life; NSAIDs: nonsteroidal antiinflammatory drugs; MAOIs: monoamine oxidase inhibitors; 🍁: Canadian drug name.

ents should be alerted not to drink alcohol while taking sulfonylureas because alcohol increases the half-life and a hypoglycemic reaction can result.

There are many drug interactions associated with acetohexamide. Glucocorticoids (cortisone), thiazide diuretics, calcium channel blockers, thyroid drugs, estrogen, and phenytoin (Dilantin) can decrease the effectiveness of acetohexamide. When acetohexamide is taken with sulfonamides, aspirin, NSAIDs, MAO inhibitors, cimetidine (Tagamet), alcohol, or insulin, a hypoglycemic reaction can occur.

NONSULFONYLUREAS: NEWER DRUGS

Expanding knowledge of glucose metabolism has revealed new mechanisms for the management of NIDDM or type II diabetes. The drugs metformin and acarbose use different methods to control serum glucose levels following a meal. Unlike the sulfonylureas, which enhance insulin release and receptor interaction, these drugs affect the hepatic and gastrointestinal production of glucose. The two newest nonsulfonylureas are troglitazone and rapaglinide.

Biguanides: Metformin (Glucophage)

Metformin is a biguanide compound that acts by decreasing hepatic production of glucose from stored glycogen. This diminishes the increase in serum glucose following a meal and blunts the degree of postprandial hyperglycemia. Metformin also decreases the absorption of glucose from the small intestine. There is also evidence that it increases insulin receptor sensitivity as well as peripheral glucose uptake at the

NURSING PROCESS
ANTIDIABETICS: SULFONYLUREAS

Assessment

- Assess the drugs the client is currently taking. Aspirin, alcohol, sulfonamides, oral contraceptives, and MAOIs increase the hypoglycemic effect; decrease in oral hypoglycemic drug may be needed. Glucocorticoids (cortisone), thiazide diuretics, and estrogen increase blood sugar.
- Assess vital signs (VS) and blood sugar levels. Report abnormal findings.
- Assess the client's knowledge of diabetes mellitus and the use of oral antidiabetics (sulfonylurea).

Potential Nursing Diagnoses

- Risk for impaired tissue integrity
- Altered nutrition: more or less than body requirements

Planning

- Client's blood sugar will be within normal serum levels (70 to 100 mg/dL).
- Client will adhere to prescribed diet, blood testing, and drug.

Nursing Interventions

- Monitor VS. Sulfonylureas increase cardiac function and oxygen consumption, which can lead to cardiac dysrhythmias.
- Administer oral antidiabetics with food to minimize gastric upset.
- Monitor blood glucose levels and report changes. The reference value is 60 to 100 mg/dL for blood glucose and 70 to 110 mg/dL for serum glucose.
- Prepare a teaching plan based on the client's knowledge of health problems, diet, and drug therapy.

Client Teaching

General

- Advise the client that hypoglycemic (insulin) reaction can occur when taking an oral hypoglycemic drug. This drug stimulates the release of insulin from the beta cells of the pancreas. Oral antidiabetics are *not* insulin. Normally, clients with diabetes mellitus type I do not have functioning beta cells and should *not* take oral antidiabetics, only insulin. Sulfonylureas are prescribed for clients with diabetes mellitus type II.

Nursing Process continued on following page

cellular level. Unlike sulfonylureas, metformin does not produce hypoglycemia or hyperglycemia. It can cause GI disturbances.

Metformin is 50% to 60% bioavailable and is absorbed primarily from the small intestine. It does not undergo hepatic metabolism and is eliminated unchanged in the urine. It is not recommended for clients with renal impairment. Monotherapy with metformin is effective; however, when combined with a sulfonylurea, the drug is useful in cases resistant to oral antidiabetics (oral hypoglycemics).

Alpha-Glucosidase Inhibitor: Acarbose (Precose)

Acarbose acts by inhibiting the digestive enzyme in the small intestine responsible for the release of glu-

cose from the complex carbohydrates (CHO) in the diet. By inhibiting alpha glucosidase, the CHO cannot be absorbed and they pass into the large intestine. Acarbose has no demonstrated systemic effects and is not absorbed into the body in significant amounts. It does not cause a hypoglycemic reaction.

Acarbose is intended for use in clients who do not achieve results on diet alone. Because the dietary carbohydrates pass into the large intestine, the normal flora ferments them, producing considerable gas. The diet selected should be a standard diabetic diet with reduced complex carbohydrates.

Thiazolidinediones: Troglitazone (Rezulin)

Troglitazone (Rezulin) is unrelated to the other antidiabetic drugs. The primary action of this drug is to

NURSING PROCESS *Continued*
ANTIDIABETICS: INSULIN

- Instruct the client to recognize symptoms of hypoglycemic reaction (headache, nervousness, sweating, tremors, rapid pulse), and symptoms of hyperglycemic reaction (thirst, increased urine output, sweet fruity breath odor).
- Explain that insulin might be needed instead of an oral antidiabetic drug during stress, surgery, or serious infection. Blood sugar levels are usually elevated during stressful times.
- Instruct the client about the necessity for compliance to diet and drug.
- Advise the client to obtain a medical alert card, tag, and/or bracelet indicating the health problem and insulin dosage.

Self-Administration
- Instruct the client how to check the blood sugar level using a Chemstrip bG test. Client should record and report abnormal results.

Diet
- To avoid a hypoglycemic reaction, instruct the client not to ingest alcohol with sulfonylurea drugs. Food taken with oral antidiabetics will decrease gastric irritation.
- Advise the client taking sulfonylurea to eat the prescribed diet on schedule. Delaying or missing a meal can cause hypoglycemia.
- Explain the use of orange juice, sugar-containing drinks, and hard candy when a hypoglycemic reaction begins.

Side Effects
- Instruct the client to report side effects, such as vomiting, diarrhea, rash.

Cultural Considerations

- Respect client's cultural beliefs and alternative method for treating "sugar in the urine" and elevated blood sugar levels. Discuss with the client (the use of an interpreter may be necessary) the safety of the methods and the use of oral antidiabetic drugs to correct the "sugar problem." If the client is taking a sulfonylurea drug to decrease the blood glucose level, emphasize the importance of checking the blood sugar levels daily or as indicated. Hypoglycemic reaction can result from increased doses of sulfonylurea agent and insufficient dietary intake.

Evaluation

- Evaluate the effectiveness of drug therapy by noting whether blood sugar levels are within the accepted range.

---

decrease insulin resistance. It also helps muscle cells to respond to insulin and use glucose more effectively. It may be used in addition to sulfonylurea, metformin, or insulin for insulin-resistant clients. It may cause serious hepatic toxicity and is no longer used in England.

Rapaglinide (Prandin)
Repaglinide (classification unknown) is the newest oral antidiabetic (hypoglycemic) agent. It has been approved by the Food and Drug Administration for use alone, or in combination with metformin. It is a short-acting antidiabetic agent. The action of repaglinide is similar to that of sulfonylureas; however, it does not tend to cause a hypoglycemic reaction.

GUIDELINES FOR ORAL HYPOGLYCEMIC (ANTIDIABETIC) USE IN NIDDM
The following are criteria for the use of oral hypoglycemics:

- Onset of diabetes mellitus at age 40 years or older
- Diagnosis of diabetes for less than 5 years
- Normal weight or overweight

- Fasting blood glucose equal to or less than 200 mg/dL
- Less than 40 units of insulin required per day
- Normal renal and hepatic function

Hyperglycemic Drugs

GLUCAGON

Glucagon is a hyperglycemic hormone secreted by the alpha cells of the islets of Langerhans in the pancreas. Glucagon increases blood sugar by stimulating glycogenolysis (glycogen breakdown) in the liver. It protects the body cells, especially those in the brain and retina, by providing the nutrients and energy needed to maintain body function.

Glucagon is available for parenteral use (subcutaneous, intramuscular, and intravenous). It is used to treat insulin-induced hypoglycemia when other methods of providing glucose are not available. For example, the client may be semiconscious or unconscious and unable to ingest sugar-containing products. Diabetics who are prone to severe hypoglycemic reactions (insulin shock) should keep glucagon in the home, and family members should be taught how to administer subcutaneous or intramuscular injections during an emergency hypoglycemic reaction. The blood glucose level begins to increase within 5 to 20 min after administration. Recently, IV glucagon has been used in the acute treatment of beta blocker overdose and profound shock.

DIAZOXIDE

Oral diazoxide (Proglycem), which is chemically related to thiazide diuretics, increases blood sugar by inhibiting insulin release from the beta cells and stimulating release of epinephrine (Adrenalin) from the adrenal medulla. This drug is not indicated for hypoglycemic reactions; rather, it is used to treat chronic hypoglycemia caused by hyperinsulinism due to islet cell cancer or hyperplasia. The parenteral form of diazoxide (Hyperstat) is prescribed for malignant hypertension. Hypotension usually does not occur with oral diazoxide.

Diazoxide has a long half-life and is highly protein-bound. Its onset of action is 1 h and the duration of action is 8 h. Most of the drug is excreted unchanged in the urine.

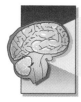

Critical Thinking in Action

T. C., 32 years old, was diagnosed as having diabetes mellitus after the birth of her first child; her blood sugar level was 180 mg/dL. Her serum glucose level has been maintained within the normal range with acetohexamide (Dymelor) 250 mg/d.

1. Why was T. C., at her age, taking an oral antidiabetic drug instead of insulin?
2. Acetohexamide is indicated for what type of diabetes mellitus? When should acetohexamide not be taken?
3. Should acetohexamide be taken with sulfonamides, aspirin, NSAIDs, cimetidine, alcohol, or insulin? Why or why not?
4. Why should T. C. monitor her blood sugar using Chemstrip bG?

Two years ago, T. C. became pregnant again. Acetohexamide was discontinued and Humulin N insulin 25 U prescribed. Since the birth of her second child, she has remained on Humulin N 25 U daily.

5. Give a possible reason why the health care provider changed the antidiabetic drug to insulin when T. C. became pregnant.
6. Humulin N is similar to what other type of insulin? How do these two types differ?
7. Give the onset, peak, and duration of action for Humulin N insulin. When is an insulin reaction most likely to occur with Humulin N?
8. What are the pros and cons for T. C. to receive Humulin 70/30 insulin?
9. What are the signs and symptoms of a hypoglycemic reaction?
10. What should be included in client teaching?

T. C. asks the nurse if she can take acetohexamide again instead of insulin because she is eating the "right foods."

11. What should your response be?

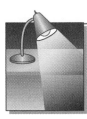

Study Questions

1. Virginia, 13 years old, has been recently diagnosed with diabetes mellitus. She is receiving 35 units of NPH insulin daily. She asks why she has to take insulin when other diabetics she knows do not. What should your response be?

2. Prepare a teaching plan for Virginia, regarding the type of insulin, sites for injections, checking the blood sugar, and recognizing the signs and symptoms of a hypoglycemic reaction.

3. Shirley is taking the sulfonylurea tolbutamide (Orinase). What generation and what type of sulfonylurea is tolbutamide?

4. Develop a nursing plan for Shirley focusing on tolbutamide. What are the side effects of this drug? How often is it usually taken? What drug interactions should she be aware of?

Unit XIII

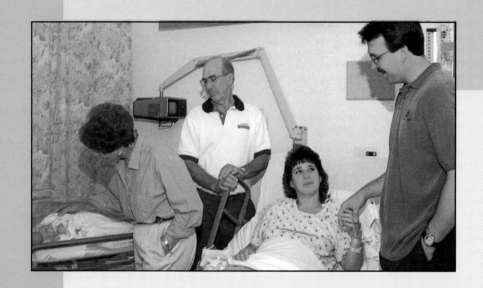

Reproductive and Gender-Related Agents

This unit comprises five chapters that focus on reproductive and gender-related drugs. Chapters 47, 48, and 49 address agents specifically associated with female health and disorders. Drugs used throughout the female reproductive cycle, including pregnancy, preterm neonate, and labor and delivery are comprehensively discussed in Chapter 47. Chapter 48 focuses on the pharmacology of the postpartum and neonatal period. Chapter 49 details the variety of oral contraceptive products and the drugs used to treat uterine dysfunction, including premenstrual syndrome, endometriosis, and menopausal discomforts. Chapter 50 describes androgens and anabolic steriods, antiandrogens, and other drugs related to male reproductive health and disorders. Chapter 51 concludes this unit with a discussion of drugs used for sexually transmitted diseases and infertility.

Each chapter uses the nursing process to illustrate the nurses' role in pharmacologic therapy. Thought-provoking study questions and Critical Thinking in Action provide the opportunity for application of the material presented.

FEMALE REPRODUCTIVE PROCESSES

The uterus is a pear-shaped, hollow, but very muscular organ located in the pelvic cavity between the rectum and the bladder; it is connected to the vagina by the cervix (Fig. XIII–1). Three distinct layers compose the uterine wall: the outer layer, the perimetrium; the muscular middle layer, the myometrium; and the inner mucosal layer, the endometrium.

The myometrium is a network of involuntary (smooth) muscles divided into three layers, with the muscles of each layer configured in different patterns. For example, the outer muscles are arranged longitudinally to assist with cervical effacement (thinning and shortening) and to expel the fetus at the time of delivery. Muscles in the middle layer are arranged in a figure-8 design. These muscles are extremely important in the control of bleeding (hemostasis). Blood vessels are threaded throughout these muscles, and when a contraction occurs the vessels are compressed, which creates a hemostatic effect. Circular muscle fibers are found in the area of the internal os and help control its sphincter. This keeps the fetus contained in the uterus for the normal gestational period. It is these muscles that stretch (dilate) the cervix to a diameter of 10 cm during labor. When all three muscle layers

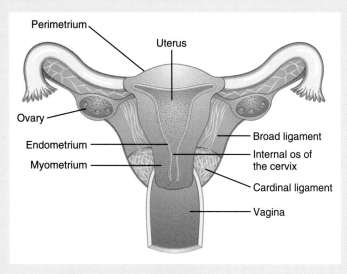

Figure XIII–1
Anatomy of the female reproductive system.

work together during labor, contractions cause cervical dilatation and descent and the delivery of the infant.

THE MENSTRUAL CYCLE

The reproductive cycle is hormonally controlled by interactions between the endocrine and reproductive systems. The hypothalamus secretes gonadotropin-releasing hormone (GnRH), which stimulates the anterior pituitary to synthesize and release follicle-stimulating hormone (FSH) and luteinizing hormone (LH). These gonadotropins stimulate the ovaries to produce estrogen and progesterone, respectively.

In most women, the menstrual cycle lasts 28 days (range, 22 to 34 days). The ovarian hormones estrogen and progesterone regulate the cycle, which has three ovarian phases, follicular, ovulatory, and luteal. Endometrial phases occur simultaneously with these ovarian phases. The **follicular phase** occurs during days 1 to 14 of the cycle. Days 1 to 6 of this period constitute the menstrual phase and days 6 to 14, the proliferative phase. During the total 14-day period, FSH increases and follicles begin to mature within the ovary. One graafian follicle from the group matures and swells by days 12 to 13, ruptures on day 14, and releases the ovum to the fallopian tube. The **ovulatory phase** occurs on day 14 when the ovum is released. The **luteal phase** occurs from days 15 to 28 and includes the secretory phase of the endometrial cycle. During this period, estrogen and progesterone are produced by the ovarian corpus luteum (the ruptured graafian follicle), reaching peak levels 8 days into the phase. Changes occur in the endometrium for optimal implantation of a fertilized ovum. FSH and LH levels decrease, mediated somewhat by dopamine, norepinephrine, and serotonin. Estrogen and progesterone are withdrawn immediately prior to menstruation and the endometrial prostaglandin level increases. The cycle begins anew with the follicular phase. In cycles that are nonovulatory, hormonal secretion of estrogen, FSH, and LH is erratic; there is also an alteration in the usual amount of progesterone. These physiologic alterations become the basis for planning and implementing pharmacologic interventions.

MALE REPRODUCTIVE PROCESSES

There are three male reproductive processes: **spermatogenesis,** or sperm production; regulation of male sexual functioning; and sexual intercourse.

Male Reproductive Anatomy and Physiology

The anatomy of the male sexual organs is depicted in Figure XIII–2. The external reproductive organs include the penis, the scrotum, and the testes. The penis is composed of three cylindrical bodies of erectile tissue: two corpora cavernosa and the corpus spongiosum. With sexual excitement, the vascular spaces fill with blood to produce an erection (Fig. XIII–3).

The scrotum has two compartments, each of which holds a testis, epididymis, and spermatic cord. The spermatic cord supports the testis and includes the vas deferens, blood vessels, nerves, and muscle fibers.

Each testis contains seminiferous tubules in which spermatogenesis occurs. The sperm then move into the epididymis. This leads into the vas deferens, the source of about 20% of ejaculate, or semen. On either side of the prostate gland, a seminal vesicle empties seminal fluid, which contains fructose to provide energy for the sperm, prostaglandins, fibrinogen, and a sperm-activating factor, into the ampulla.

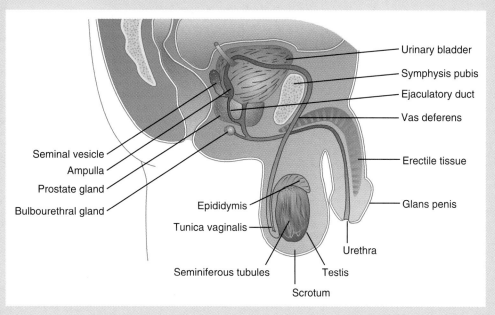

Figure XIII–2
Male reproductive anatomy.

The contents of the ampulla and the seminal vesicles empty into an ejaculatory duct that leads through the body of the prostate to empty into the urethra. Prostatic fluid, which constitutes about 20% of semen, empties from the prostate gland into the ejaculatory duct. The urethra carries semen to its distal end. The urethral glands along the length of the urethra and the bulbourethral glands near the prostatic end of the urethra supply the urethra with mucus. The bulbourethral glands secrete alkaline preejactulatory fluid to protect sperm from the acidity of the urethra.

Hormonal Regulation of Male Reproductive Functioning and Spermatogenesis

Gonadotropin-releasing hormone (GnRH) from the hypothalamus stimulates the anterior pituitary gland to secrete two major gonadotropins, follicle-stimulating hormone (FSH) and luteinizing hormone (LH), in both males and females. LH stimulates the interstitial Leydig cells of the testes to mature and produce testosterone. There is a direct relationship between the amount of circulating LH and the amount of

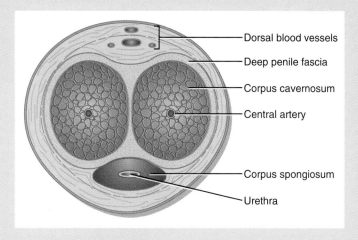

Figure XIII–3
Erectile tissue of the penis.

861

testosterone produced. Testosterone is also produced to a lesser extent in the adrenal cortex, and in the ovaries of females.

In males, FSH stimulates the Sertoli cells to begin conversion of spermatids into mature sperm. In addition, the Sertoli cells are stimulated to secrete estrogens, which may promote spermatogenesis. For spermatogenesis to be complete, testosterone must be secreted simultaneously by the Leydig cells and diffuse into the seminiferous tubules.

Testosterone is the precursor of two classes of sex steroids: 5-alpha-reduced androgens and estrogens. The net effect of endogenous androgens is the sum of the effects of the 5-alpha-reduced metabolite *dihydrotestosterone* and its estrogen derivative, *estradiol*. Most testosterone is loosely bound by plasma protein and circulates for 15 to 30 minutes before it is fixed to target tissues or metabolized. Most testosterone fixed to target cells is converted to its active form, dihydrotestosterone.

The rate of testosterone production is controlled by a negative feedback loop. With increased testosterone, the hypothalamus decreases production of GnRH (Fig. XIII–4). Also, with sperm production the Sertoli cells release a hormone called inhi-

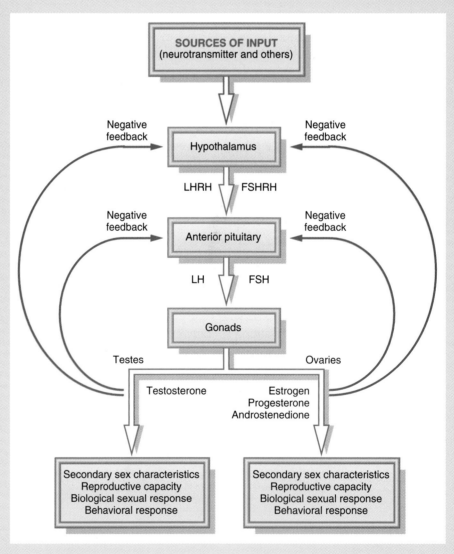

Figure XIII–4
Hypothalamic-pituitary-gonadal feedback loops. (Source: Fogel CI, Lauver D: Sexual Health Promotion. Philadelphia: WB Saunders, 1990, p. 339.)

862

bin, which suppresses FSH production by the anterior pituitary, thus maintaining a constant rate of spermatogenesis. It is not known how, before puberty, the brain stimulates the hypothalamus to begin GnRH secretion, but if the brain is not intact, this may not occur.

Sexual Function

The human sexual response cycle consists of five phases: desire, excitement, plateau, orgasm, and resolution. Sexual desire is the stimulus that causes an individual to initiate or be receptive to sexual activity. During the excitement phase, the male experiences penile erection. Males are incapable of engaging in sexual intercourse without this arousal. The plateau phase is characterized by genital enlargement, mucus secretion, generalized muscle tension, hyperventilation, tachycardia, and increased blood pressure. During the orgasmic phase, the vas deferens, seminal vesicles, ejaculatory duct, and penile urethra contract three or four times over a few seconds and the male ejaculates. During resolution, there is a refractory period in which pelvic vasocongestion declines and generalized muscle relaxation takes place.

PROCESS OF FERTILIZATION

Fertilization, or **conception,** occurs when a sperm penetrates an ovum, usually in the distal third of the fallopian tube.

In a single ejaculation, between 200 and 400 million spermatozoa are deposited in the vagina. Sperm move up the female reproductive tract by the flagellar motion of their tails. It takes an average of 4 to 6 hours for the sperm to reach the distal fallopian tube. Semen contains prostaglandins that may enhance uterine motility to facilitate sperm migration. The ciliary action of the fallopian tubes enhances migration of the ovum to the uterus and of sperm toward the ovary.

Uterine enzymes capacitate the sperm by altering their glycoprotein coat. In an acrosomal reaction, the sperm release an enzyme, hyaluronidase, that breaks through the outer layer of the ovum. The moment one sperm penetrates the ovum a chemical reaction occurs that blocks other sperm from entering. Cellular division begins immediately in what is now called the **zygote,** or fertilized egg.

After 3 days the zygote enters the uterus. It has now differentiated into an inner solid mass of cells, the **blastocyst,** and an outer layer, the **trophoblast.** Progesterone secreted by the corpus luteum of the ovary maintains a favorable uterine environment to nourish the blastocyst until **implantation** in the uterine lining occurs. The blastocyst develops into the embryo and the amniotic membrane, whereas the trophoblast develops into the chorionic membrane and the fetal side of the placenta. The maternal portion of the placenta develops under the site of the blastocyst's implantation. The **placenta** is the structure through which oxygen, nutrients, and metabolic wastes pass between the maternal and fetal circulations for the duration of pregnancy. The placenta begins to function by the fourth week of pregnancy. Within the first 8 weeks of pregnancy, organ systems are differentiated, and it is during this period that the fetus is most threatened by teratogens. Growth of the fetus throughout pregnancy depends on adequate oxygenation and nutrition, the metabolic environment, freedom from infection, and integrity of the mother's reproductive tract.

47

Drugs Associated with the Female Reproductive Cycle: Pregnancy, Preterm Neonate, Labor, and Delivery

JANE PURNELL TAYLOR and LINDA GOODWIN

Outline

Objectives

* Explain potential health-promoting and detrimental effects of substances ingested by the mother during the prenatal period.

* Describe the drugs that alter uterine muscle contractility.

* Describe drug therapy used during preterm labor to decrease the incidence or severity of neonatal respiratory dysfunction.

* Describe systemic and regional medications for pain control during labor.

* Describe the drugs used in pregnancy-induced hypertension.

* Describe the nursing process, including client teaching, associated with the drugs used during pregnancy, labor, and delivery.

Terms

ataractic drug
eclampsia
ergot alkaloids
ergotism
HELLP syndrome
labor augmentation
labor induction
L/S (lecithin/sphingomyelin) ratio

multiparous
neural tube defect
oxytocic drugs
preeclampsia
pregnancy-induced hypertension
preterm labor
primiparous
progesterone

respiratory distress syndrome
ripening
surfactant
teratogen
tocolytic therapy
uterine atony
uterine contractility
uterine inertia

INTRODUCTION

This chapter focuses on the pharmacologic aspects of pregnancy, labor, and delivery. Topics include prenatal health promotion, fetal effects of drugs, and drugs for uterine dysfunction during labor and delivery, for pain control during labor, and for pregnancy-induced hypertension.

PHYSIOLOGY OF PREGNANCY

The use of prescription and nonprescription medications raises concern throughout pregnancy and into the postpartum period. The many maternal physiologic changes that occur during pregnancy affect drug action and utilization; these include the influence of circulating steroid hormones on liver metabolism of drugs, more rapid renal excretion of drugs resulting from the increased glomerular filtration rate and increased renal perfusion, dilution of drugs by the expanded maternal circulating blood volume; and changes in the actual clearance of drugs in later pregnancy, resulting in decreases in the levels of serum and tissue concentrations of drugs. The result is that therapeutically prescribed drugs may not be ordered in lower doses with longer intervals between doses.

Medication effects are influenced by additional factors. Some drugs have shorter half-lives (e.g., antibiotics, barbiturates) during late pregnancy; events such as labor can actually increase the half-life of some drugs (e.g., analgesics, hypnotics, antibiotics), because drug clearance is believed to decrease as a result of transient reduced blood flow associated with uterine contractions and with supine maternal positioning. Increased drug accumulation is a concern in disorders with decreased renal perfusion such as diabetes and pregnancy-related hypertension.

The placenta plays an important role in drug utilization and metabolism. It allows substances to transfer quickly or slowly between mother and fetus, depending on variables such as quality of uteroplacental blood flow, the molecular weight of the substance (low-weight-substances cross more easily), the level of ionization of the drug molecules (more highly ionized substances cross less readily), and the degree to which the drug is bound to maternal plasma protein (highly bound drugs do not readily cross) versus fetal plasma protein. In addition, the placenta performs its own enzymatic activity in the biotransformation of a drug into metabolites that can affect the fetus.

Guidelines for medication administration during pregnancy must include determination that the benefits of prescribing a drug outweigh potential short- or long-term risks to the maternal-fetal system. Careful selection and monitoring for the minimum effective dose for the shortest interval in the therapeutic range with consideration given to alterations related to pregnancy physiology are required.

Drug effects may be more evident and last longer in the fetus than in the mother, because drug excretion is slower in the fetus due to the immaturity of the fetal liver. The degree of fetal exposure to a drug and its breakdown products is more important to fetal outcome than the rate at which the drug is transported to the fetus.

The mechanisms by which drugs cross the placenta are analogous to the way in which drugs infiltrate breast tissue. Lactation results in increased blood flow to the breasts, and drugs accumulate in adipose breast tissue through simple diffusion. Long-term effects on infants from drugs in breast milk are unknown.

Despite prenatal education, public service announcements, and information conveyed through the media, use of legal and illicit drugs by pregnant women continues. In addition, health care providers may prescribe drugs for maternal disorders that indirectly affect the fetus. About one-half of the medications taken by pregnant women are over-the-counter (OTC) drugs. The drugs most commonly ingested during pregnancy (other than illicit drugs) are iron and vitamins, antiemetics, antacids, nasal decongestants, mild analgesics, and antibiotics.

Drugs determined conclusively to be safe for the embryo are limited in number. Many more are possible or known **teratogens** (substances that cause developmental abnormalities). Timing, dose, and duration of exposure are of crucial importance in determining the teratogenicity of a given drug. In the human, the teratogenic period begins a few days past the first missed menstrual period and extends through the next 10 weeks—the period of organogenesis (development of major structures and organs). Examples of adverse effects of selected illicit substances commonly used during pregnancy are presented in Table 47–1.

THERAPEUTIC DRUG USE IN PREGNANCY

The most common indications for therapeutic use of drugs during pregnancy are nutritional supplementation with iron, vitamins, and minerals and treatment of nausea and vomiting, gastric acidity, and mild discomforts.

Iron

During pregnancy, approximately twice the normal amount of iron is needed to meet fetal and maternal daily requirements. Most of the required iron is needed during the last 20 weeks of pregnancy. Sup-

Table 47–1
General Adverse Effects of Selected Substances Commonly Abused During Pregnancy

SUBSTANCE	MATERNAL EFFECTS	FETAL EFFECTS*
Alcohol (high risk: 6 oz or more/d)	1 oz (2 drinks) absolute alcohol 2 ×/wk: increased risk of spontaneous abortion (2–4 times)	Fetal alcohol syndrome (FAS): mild to moderate mental retardation, altered facial features, growth retardation, low birth weight, small head circumference, hypotonia, poor motor coordination. Full FAS seen only in some children; others display only fetal alcohol effect (FAE)
Caffeine	2 cups increases epinephrine concentrations after 30 min and decreases intervillous blood flow with potential for spontaneous abortion (dosage and gestational period related)	Excess consumption (>6–8 cups/d) likely toxic to embryo. No evidence of teratogenicity
Cocaine	48-h clearance via urine Increased incidence of spontaneous abortion in first trimester. Continued use or sporadic use related to premature delivery and abruptio placentae secondary to placental vasoconstriction and hyperextension	4–5 d clearance time via urine of newborn due to liver immaturity and lack of cholinesterase. Intrauterine growth retardation, decreased head circumference, intrauterine cerebral infarction. No true withdrawal syndrome but increased irritability, hyperreflexia, tremulousness. Deficient organization and interactive abilities. By 4 month, still exhibits hypertonicity, tremulousness, and impaired motor development. By 6 month, effects may appear to be self-limited, but long-term research needed
Heroin	First trimester spontaneous abortion, premature delivery, inadequate maternal calorie and protein intake	Neonatal meconium aspiration syndrome; decreased weight and length through 9th postnatal month (weight and length catch up by 12 month); smaller head circumference (with no catch up); impaired interactive abilities (hard to console and engage); inconsistent behavioral responses; increased tremulousness and irritability
Marijuana	Heavy use (5 or more marijuana cigarettes per week). Shortened gestation (<37 wk). May hasten delivery through uterine stimulation	No higher incidence of serious birth defects due solely to marijuana. Higher incidence of meconium passage during labor
Tobacco/nicotine	Degenerative placental lesions with areas of poor O_2 exchange; higher incidence of abruptio placentae; placenta previa, vaginal bleeding during pregnancy; possible PROM; possible amnionitis; less likely to choose to breast feed	Short stature, smaller head-arm circumferences, no increase in mortality rate or congenital anomalies (some evidence of increased oral clefts); increased respiratory infections beyond the perinatal period; possibly shorter attention span beyond perinatal period
Methadone	If taken before pregnancy, will need to slow detoxification during pregnancy and decrease dose 5 mg every 2 wk. Do not detoxify prior to 14 wk gestation because of increased risk of spontaneous abortion	Smaller weight through 9 month postnatally; smaller length through 9 month postnatally (catch up on weight and length by 12 month); smaller head circumference (no catch up); withdrawal-induced fetal distress if mother detoxifies after 32-wk gestation
Barbiturates	CNS depression; lethargy; sleepiness; subtle mood alterations and impaired judgment/fine motor skills for 24 h No known inhibitory effect on uterine tone or contractility Selective anticonvulsant activity without anesthesia effects may warrant use in pregnancy for seizure disorders Active labor with imminent delivery is a contraindication since no antagonist drug is available	Rapidly cross placenta and cause CNS depression with excessive use/high doses leading to respiratory depression, hyperactivity, decreased sucking reflex

Table continued on following page

Table 47-1 *Continued*
General Adverse Effects of Selected Substances Commonly Abused During Pregnancy

SUBSTANCE	MATERNAL EFFECTS	FETAL EFFECTS*
Tranquilizers	Dose-dependent; toxic reactions include ataxia, syncope, vertigo, drowsiness; control of acute eclamptic seizures during labor	Benzodiazepine (diazepam [Valium]) use in 1st trimester not associated with oral clefts or other anomalies. Chronic 3rd trimester or labor exposure in high doses associated with hypotonia, hypothermia, hyperbilirubinemia, poor sucking reflex. Effects may be enhanced if systemic analgesics also given to mother. Fetal effects are prolonged

* Narcotic-exposed infants show downward trend in development score by age 2, suggesting that lack of environmental stimulation may be the major variable based on the Bayley Scales of Development.
KEY: PROM: premature rupture of fetal membranes; <: less than; CNS: central nervous system.

plementation is not generally necessary until the second trimester, when the fetus begins to store iron; the goal is to prevent maternal deficiency, not to supply the fetus. The fetus is adequately supplied through the placenta even though the mother is deficient; the time of greatest demand is during the third trimester.

Although normal diet generally will provide the 18 mg recommended daily allowance (RDA) for nonpregnant clients, nonanemic pregnant women usually are instructed to supplement using a dosage that provides 60 mg of elemental iron; anemic clients receive 120 mg of elemental iron. Clients are advised to continue supplements during the 6 weeks postpartum.

Pregnant women generally have a decreased hematocrit early in the third trimester; those under 30% will have their supplemental iron dosages increased and complete blood counts with platelet and ferritin measured. In those found with true iron deficiency anemia, response to iron supplementation is usually noted within 2 weeks. No teratogenic effects have been reported with physiologic doses. Numerous OTC and prescription iron products are available in varying dosages, which differ in the amount of elemental iron contained in the form of iron salt. Examples are listed in Table 47-2.

SIDE EFFECTS AND ADVERSE REACTIONS
Common side effects include nausea, constipation, black or red tarry stools, epigastric pain, vomiting, and diarrhea. In addition, liquid forms should be diluted and administered through a plastic straw to avoid temporary discoloration of the teeth.

Folic Acid

During pregnancy, folic acid (vitamin B_6, folacin) is needed in increased amounts. Folic acid deficiency early in pregnancy can result in spontaneous abortion or birth defects (e.g., **neural tube defects**), premature birth, low birth weight, and premature separation of the placenta (abruptio placentae).

The RDA for folic acid in the nonpregnant client is 180 μg. It is recommended that women trying to get pregnant should take folic acid 3 to 6 months before conception. The RDA for folic acid during pregnancy is 400 to 800 μg. Pregnancy risk factor is classified as A. (*Note:* Factor is C if dosage exceeds RDA.)

SIDE EFFECTS AND ADVERSE REACTIONS
Side effects are not common, but include allergic bronchospasm, rash, pruritus, erythema, and general malaise.

Multiple Vitamins

Prenatal vitamin preparations are routinely recommended for pregnant women. These preparations generally supply vitamins A, D, E, C, B complex (B_1, B_2, B_3, B_5, B_6), B_{12}, iron, calcium, and other minerals. Recommended daily allowances for vitamins and minerals during pregnancy are presented in Appendix D. The role of prenatal vitamins in prevention of congenital defects (e.g., cleft lip/palate, limb defects) remains undetermined.

Poor food habits cannot be rectified through supplements alone; vitamins are used most effectively by the body when taken with meals. Calories and protein are not supplied by supplements.

Megadoses of vitamins and minerals during pregnancy will not improve health and may cause harm.

Practitioners should consider *cultural* food practices and beliefs in regard to the use of prenatal vitamins. For example, in Mexico, some people view vitamins as a *hot* food that should not be ingested during pregnancy.

Table 47–2
Iron Products

DRUG	DOSAGE	USES AND CONSIDERATIONS
Ferrous sulfate (Fer-In-Sol, Feosol, Fero-Gradumet, Mol-Iron, Fer-Iron)	A: PO: 300–600 mg/d in divided doses 325 mg daily sufficient to meet needs of non–iron deficient pregnant client; with iron deficiency, should receive 325 mg 2–3 ×/d	Hematinic; for iron deficiency anemia; prophylaxis for iron deficiency in pregnancy; replaces iron stores needed for RBC development; $t_{\frac{1}{2}}$: UK; PB: UK; onset: 4 d; peak reticulocytosis: 5–10 d; hemoglobin values increase: 2–4 wk. Duration: 3–4 mo. Absorption PO is 5%–30% in intestines; therefore GI side effects; toxic reactions include pallor, hematemesis, shock, cardiovascular collapse, metabolic acidosis; contraindicated in hypersensitivity and peptic ulcer; decreased absorption of tetracycline, penicillamine, antacids; increased absorption with ascorbic acid; decreased absorption with eggs, milk, coffee, tea; can reduce availability of zinc from the diet Nursing implications. Taking iron h.s. helps to avoid GI upset. Absorption of iron is promoted when taken with orange juice or other vitamin C source. Use straw (elixir); swallow tablet/capsule whole; take with water on empty stomach, sit upright 30 min after dose to decrease reflux; increase fluids, activity, and dietary bulk; keep away from children; *Pregnancy category:* A
Ferrous gluconate (Fergon, Ferralet, Simron)	A: PO: 200–600 mg t.i.d.	Same as above
Ferrous fumarate (Fumasorb, Femiron, Feostat, Fumerin)	A: PO: 200 mg t.i.d. or q.i.d.	Same as above

KEY: *A: adult; GI: gastrointestinal; PO: by mouth; UK: unknown; RBC: red blood cell; PB: protein-binding.*

Drugs for Minor Discomforts of Pregnancy

The average prenatal client uses three drugs during pregnancy, two of which are vitamin and mineral supplements. Drug ingestion is most likely during the first and the third trimesters, the time when the minor discomforts of pregnancy tend to be most bothersome.

NAUSEA AND VOMITING

Nausea and vomiting during early pregnancy are major complaints for most (about 88%) pregnant women, possibly because of increased levels of human chorionic gonadotropin, changes in the metabolism of carbohydrates, and emotional changes. Nonpharmacologic measures to decrease nausea and vomiting to be suggested before drugs are used include (1) eating crackers, dry toast or bread, dry cereal, or other carbohydrate before rising; (2) avoiding fatty or highly seasoned foods; (3) eating small, frequent meals; (4) drinking fluids between meals rather than with meals; (5) drinking apple juice or flat carbonated beverages between meals; (6) eating a high-protein bedtime snack; (7) stopping or cutting down on smoking; and (8) taking an iron supplement at bedtime. These measures work well for most women, but if vomiting is severe, fluid replacement and pharmacologic measures may be necessary. The incidence of hyperemesis is approximately 3.5 in every 1000 pregnancies, and about 1% exhibit persistent vomiting across a variety of countries and cultures. Table 47–3 presents examples of the most commonly used drugs for management of nausea and vomiting during pregnancy. The Food and Drug Administration (FDA) has *not* given approval for any drug for use in morning sickness, nor is there consensus among health care providers who do prescribe drug therapy as to the best agents; antiemetic drug studies often find that affected individuals rate even placebo agents as "helpful."

Women who experience nausea and vomiting may experience gastric distress if they are also taking supplemental iron; temporary suspension of iron therapy may help. It is suggested that prenatal vitamins be taken at the time of day the client is least likely to vomit. Salting food to taste may help replace vomited chloride; foods rich in potassium and magnesium may also help replace lost nutrients.

Table 47–3
Examples of Drugs that Have Been Used for Management of Nausea and Vomiting During Pregnancy (Recommendation Not Implied)

DRUG	DOSAGE	USES AND CONSIDERATIONS
ANTICHOLINERGICS/ ANTIHISTAMINES		
Meclizine (Antivert, Bonine, Vertol)	PO: 20–50 mg daily	No evidence of teratogenesis; in use since 1956; considered mild; available as OTC drug; site of action is labyrinth, CNS; blocks chemoreceptor trigger zone (CTZ), which acts on vomiting center; onset of action: 1–2 h; duration of 8–24 h; metabolized in liver and excreted unchanged in feces and as metabolites in urine; $t_{\frac{1}{2}}$: 6 h; increased effect of alcohol, tranquilizers, narcotics *Pregnancy category:* B *Side effects:* Dizziness, drowsiness, dry mouth and nose, blurred vision, diplopia, urinary retention, urticaria, rash, and headache. Cardiovascular effects can include hypotension, palpitations, and tachycardia *Contraindications:* Hypersensitivity to drug or any component *Warning precautions:* Use with closed-angle glaucoma
OTHER		
Trimethobenzamide (Tigan, T-Gen)	200 mg rectally, q6–8h	Obscure action; may be mediated through CTZ; does not inhibit direct impulse to vomiting center; chemically classified as an ethanolamine derivative; precautions include use in client with cardiac dysrhythmias, narrow-angle glaucoma, asthma, and pyloroduodenal obstruction. Rectal doses of the drug are more unpredictable *Side effects:* Drowsiness, headache, blurred vision, diarrhea, depression, hypotension, muscle cramps, allergic reactions, and extrapyramidal symptoms; blood dyscrasias *Contraindications:* Benzocaine, hypersensitivity to drug; children: suppository form in neonates or preterm infants *Warning:* Avoid use in acute emesis to avoid masking of symptoms *Interactions with* phenothiazines/barbiturates, belladonna *Pregnancy category:* C; $t_{\frac{1}{2}}$: UK; onset: PO/PR: 10–40 min; IM: 15–35 min; duration: 3–4 h

KEY: *PO: by mouth; PR: by rectum; $t_{\frac{1}{2}}$: half-life; IM: intramuscular; UK: unknown; OTC: over-the-counter; CNS: central nervous system.*

Those clients whose symptoms persist and who experience severe weight loss and dehydration may require IV rehydration, including replacement of electrolytes and vitamins. Antiemetic therapy (probably with phenothiazines) may be used.

HEARTBURN

Heartburn (pyrosis) is a burning sensation perceived in the epigastric and sternal regions that occurs with reflux of acidic stomach contents. Pregnant clients experience decreased motility in the gastrointestinal (GI) tract as a result of the normal increase in the hormone **progesterone**. Progesterone also relaxes the cardiac sphincter (sphincter leading into the stomach from the esophagus), making reflux activity (reverse peristalsis) more likely. Digestion and gastric emptying are slower than in the nonpregnant state. Heartburn is common when a pregnant client sits or lies down soon after eating a normal meal, only to have her enlarged abdomen exert upward force on her stomach, causing increased reflux activity and the perception of hyperacidity. Heartburn is a disorder of the second and third trimesters of pregnancy.

Nonpharmacologic measures are preferred in the management of heartburn. These include (1) limiting the volume of food at each feeding; (2) avoiding highly seasoned, fried, or greasy foods; (3) avoiding gas-forming foods; (4) eating slowly and chewing thoroughly; (5) avoiding citrus juices; (6) drinking adequate fluids but not with meals; and (7) avoiding reclining immediately after eating. Antacids should be considered part of the therapeutic regimen only if conservative therapy is unsuccessful.

Most clients do not realize that remedies commonly used by nonpregnant individuals (e.g., baking soda [sodium bicarbonate], antacids such as Alka-Seltzer, Bromo-Seltzer, Rolaids) can be harmful during pregnancy. Selection of the wrong antacid can result in diarrhea, constipation, or electrolyte imbalance. The combination of nonpharmacologic measures plus minimal use of safe antacids should effectively meet the pregnant client's need.

The antacids of choice for the pregnant client include nonsystemic low-sodium products (those considered dietetically sodium free) containing aluminum and magnesium (in the form of hydroxide) in combination. These two ingredients can also be found in combination in the form of magaldrate (also known as hydroxymagnesium aluminate). Some products also include simethicone (an antiflatulent to decrease the surface tension of GI gas bubbles, burst them, and promote rapid gas expulsion). Calcium carbonate antacid preparations are avoided in pregnancy because of the rebound effect following acid neutralization by

Table 47–4
OTC Antacids Commonly Used in Pregnancy

DRUG	DOSAGE	USES AND CONSIDERATIONS
Aluminum hydroxide (Amphojel)	A: PO: as directed*	Contains aluminum hydroxide gel (320 mg) per 300 mg tablet or per 5 mL; ANC 8; contains saccharin and sorbitol. OTC preparation. Use: heartburn secondary to reflux; action: neutralization of gastric acidity; side effects: constipation; adverse reactions: dehydration, hypophosphatemia (long-term use), GI obstruction; *Decrease* effects with: tetracycline, phenothiazine, benzodiazepines, isoniazid, digoxin; follow dose with water *Pregnancy category:* C; t½: UK; PB: UK; Onset: 15–30 min; peak: 0.5 h; duration: 1–3 h
Magnesium hydroxide and aluminum hydroxide with Simethicone (Maalox Plus, Extra Strength Maalox Plus Suspension, Mylanta Liquid, Mylanta II)	As directed*	*Maalox Plus Tablets:* Each tablet contains magnesium hydroxide (200 mg), aluminum hydroxide (200 mg), and Simethicone (25 mg); ANC 11, 4; chewable; contains saccharin and sorbitol; OTC *Extra Strength Maalox Plus Suspension:* Each 5 mL contains magnesium hydroxide (450 mg), aluminum hydroxide (500 mg), and Simethicone (40 mg); ANC 28; contains saccharin and sorbitol; OTC *Mylanta Liquid:* Each 5 mL contains magnesium hydroxide (200 mg), aluminum hydroxide (200 mg) and Simethicone (25 mg); ANC 12.7; contains sorbitol; OTC *Mylanta II:* Each 5 mL contains magnesium hydroxide (400 mg), aluminum hydroxide (400 mg), and Simethicone (40 mg); ANC 23; OTC Use: Same as above with addition of antiflatulence action Interactions: Same, with addition of allopurinol, quinolones, ketoconazole *Pregnancy category:* C; PB: UK; t½: UK
Magaldrate with Simethicone (Riopan Plus Tablets, Riopan Plus Suspension)	As directed*	*Riopan Plus Tablets:* Each contains Magaldrate (480 mg) and Simethicone (20 mg); ANC 13.5; chewable; contains sorbitol *Riopan Plus Suspension:* Each 5 mL contains Magaldrate (540 mg) and Simethicone (20 mg); ANC 15.0; contains saccharin Use: same as above Action: same as above Side effects: same as above Adverse reactions: same as above Interaction: decreased absorption of phenothiazines, isoniazid, fluoroquinolones, tetracyclines *Pregnancy category:* C; t½: UK; PB: UK; onset: immediate; peak: UK; duration: prolonged

* Dosage recommendations for antacid preparations should be clarified by the health care provider; however, as a general rule, not more than 12 tablets or 12 tsp should be taken in a 24-h period depending on the strength of the product. Major side effects are a change in bowel habits (diarrhea or constipation), nausea, vomiting, alkalosis, and hypermagnesemia.

Antacids figure in numerous drug interactions owing to their action on gastric pH (increased) and their propensity to bind with other drugs to form poorly absorbed complexes. Antacids should not be given within 2 h of iron, digitalis products, or tetracycline. Likewise, when a client is taking a phenothiazine as an antiemetic, 2 h should elapse between administration of these drugs.

KEY: A: adult; ANC: acid-neutralizing capacity (per tablet or 5 mL); GI: gastrointestinal; OTC: over-the-counter; PB: protein-binding; PO: by mouth; t½: half-life; UK: unknown.

the antacid, in which hypersecretion of more acid occurs.

Liquid antacids are the preparations most commonly used in pregnancy owing to their even and uniform dissolution, their rapid action, and their greater activity. Tablets are also acceptable, particularly for convenience, provided these are thoroughly chewed and the client maintains an adequate fluid intake. Table 47–4 presents antacids commonly used during pregnancy.

PAIN

Headaches (up through week 26 resulting from emotional factors, hormonally induced bodily changes, sinus congestion, or eye strain), backaches, joint pains, round ligament pain resulting in mild abdominal aches and pains, and minor injuries are common in pregnancy. Nonpharmacologic pain relief measures should be tried first. These include rest, nonstimulatory environment, relaxation exercises, alteration in routine, mental imagery, ice packs, warm-moist heat, postural changes, correct body mechanics for tasks at hand, and changes in the height and style of footwear.

Acetaminophen

Acetaminophen (Tylenol, Datril), a para-aminophenol analgesic, is a pregnancy category B drug. It is the most commonly ingested nonprescription drug during pregnancy. Chapter 17 presents a drug chart for in-depth review of pharmacokinetics.

Acetaminophen is commonly used during all trimesters of pregnancy in therapeutic doses on a short-term basis, generally for its analgesic and antipyretic effects. The drug has no significant antiinflammatory effect. Acetaminophen is 20% to 50% protein-bound and crosses the placenta during pregnancy; it also is found in low concentrations in breast milk. To date, there is no concrete evidence of fetal anomalies associated with use of the drug, and no adverse effects have been noted in infants who nurse from mothers who use or did use the drug.

Use of acetaminophen during pregnancy should not exceed 12 tablets per 24 h of a 325-mg formulation (regular strength) or eight tablets per 24 h of a 500-mg (extra strength) formulation. The drug should be taken at 4- to 6-h intervals. Onset of effects following oral ingestion is within 10 to 30 min; peak action occurs at 1 to 2 h; duration of drug effects is from 3 to 5 h.

Side Effects and Adverse Reactions

Most clients *without* preexisting renal or hepatic disease tolerate acetaminophen quite well. Clients with hypersensitivity to the compound should not use it. Use cautiously in clients at risk for infection due to possibility of masked signs and symptoms. The most frequently seen side effects are skin eruptions, urticaria, unusual bruising, erythema, hypoglycemia, jaundice, hemolytic anemia, neutropenia, leukopenia, pancytopenia, and thrombocytopenia.

Aspirin

Aspirin (A.S.A., Bayer, Ecotrin, Halfprin), a salicylate, is classified as a mild analgesic. Aspirin is a pregnancy category C drug (which changes to category D if full-dose aspirin is used in the third trimester). Aspirin is presented in drug chart form in Chapter 17.

Aspirin is a prostaglandin synthetase inhibitor that has antipyretic, analgesic, and antiinflammatory properties. Teratogenic effects have not been shown conclusively, and the risk of anomalies is perceived to be small.

Aspirin can inhibit the initiation of labor and actually prolong labor through effects on uterine contractility; therefore, its use is not recommended during pregnancy. In addition, aspirin use late in pregnancy is associated with greater maternal blood loss at delivery. There may be increased risk of anemia in pregnancy and of antepartum hemorrhage as well. Hemostasis is affected in the newborn whose mother ingested aspirin during the last 2 months of pregnancy (even without use during the actual week of delivery). The platelets are unable to aggregate to form clots, and it appears that this is not a reversible effect after delivery; the baby has to wait for the bone marrow to produce new platelets.

DRUGS THAT DECREASE UTERINE MUSCLE CONTRACTILITY

Preterm Labor

Preterm labor (PTL) is labor that occurs between 20 and 37 weeks of pregnancy involving a fetus with an estimated weight between 500 and 2499 g. Regular contractions occur at less than 10-min intervals over a 30- to 60-min period that are strong enough to result in 2-cm cervical dilatation and 80% effacement. PTL occurs in approximately 5% to 10% of all births. Preterm infants who survive early delivery have significant physiologic impediments to overcome. Preterm labor that progresses to preterm delivery accounts for the majority of perinatal morbidity and mortality (excluding fetuses with anomalies) in the United States.

Although preterm labor has no single known cause, certain risk factors have been identified: maternal age of under 16 or over 35 years, low socioeconomic status, previous history of preterm delivery (PTD) (17% to 50% chance of recurrence), intrauterine infections, polyhydramnios, maternal sepsis due to re-

NURSING PROCESS
ANTEPARTUM DRUGS

Assessment

- Gather comprehensive medical and drug histories.
- Obtain baseline vital signs for comparison with future findings during the prenatal period.
- Identify clients at high risk for substance abuse and collaborate with other professionals to plan strategies to minimize risks.
- Assess drug history to determine whether there will be interference with absorption because of antacids.
- Review history of aspirin use on admission of client in labor. If aspirin has been used, alert the staff and prepare to handle possible increased bleeding.
- Obtain a medical history of alcoholism, liver disease, viral infection, and renal deficiencies. Acetaminophen should be used cautiously in these clients.

Potential Nursing Diagnoses

- Knowledge deficit related to health maintenance needs during pregnancy
- Knowledge deficit related to potential outcomes from exposure to teratogens during pregnancy

Planning

- Client will take drugs during pregnancy as advised.

Nursing Interventions

General

- Be cognizant that drug use may be part of multiple substance abuse and may also involve maternal-neonatal infections.
- Stress prenatal care and discuss fears the client may have about health care professionals and concerns about legal action in the event of substance abuse.

Specific

- Instruct on strategies to relieve common pregnancy discomforts.
- Refer to smoking or drug treatment program if appropriate.
- Instruct on nutrition/therapeutic supplements needed during pregnancy.
- Monitor hemoglobin during prenatal visits.

Iron

- Question client about nausea, constipation, and bowel habit changes if taking iron preparations.
- Give diluted liquid iron preparation through a plastic straw to prevent discoloration of teeth.
- Store iron in a light-resistant container.
- Be cognizant that client may have false-positive result of occult blood in stool if taking iron.

Client Teaching

General

- Advise pregnant woman that smoking, drinking alcohol, and heavy caffeine use may have adverse effects on the fetus.
- Stress that OTC drugs should be used sparingly: the smallest dose for the shortest time.
- Advise client not to plan to breast feed if she is using illicit drugs.

Aspirin/Acetaminophen

- Advise the client not to take aspirin during pregnancy, particularly not during the third trimester.

Nursing Process continued on following page

NURSING PROCESS *Continued*
ANTEPARTUM DRUGS

- Instruct the client not to take nonsteroidal antiinflammatory drugs (NSAIDs) with acetaminophen.

Caffeine/Alcohol/Nicotine
- Teach client to limit coffee to 1 to 2 cups per day and to limit other sources of caffeine (tea, cola, soft drinks, chocolate, certain drugs).
- Teach client to space limited caffeine intake evenly through the day because caffeine passes readily to the fetus, who cannot metabolize it. Caffeine can decrease intervillous placental blood flow.
- Suggest that client use decaffeinated products or dilute caffeinated products.
- Suggest that client use herbal teas carefully because of occasionally harmful ingredients.
- If the client plans to breast feed, tell her that 1% of the caffeine she consumes will appear in her breast milk within 15 min. Therefore, while a cup of coffee is not a problem, it is not wise to drink several cups of coffee in succession; excess caffeine will accumulate in the baby's tissues. The baby lacks enzymes to adequately clear the caffeine for 7 to 9 months after birth.
- Instruct client not to drink alcohol if she is pregnant because no safe level of alcohol has been determined and even moderate exposure has resulted in fetal alcohol effect.
- Advise client that nicotine is to be avoided.
- Advise client that smoking can cause the loss of nutrients such as vitamins A and C, folic acid, cobalamin, and calcium.

Iron
- Instruct the client about dietary sources of iron, which include organ meats (liver), nuts and seeds, wheat germ, spinach, broccoli, prunes, and cereals.
- Explain to the client that if iron is taken between meals, increased absorption (and also increased side effects) may result. Taking iron 1 h before meals is suggested. Give with juice or water, but not with milk, antacids, or eggs.

Self-Administration
- Advise the client to swallow the iron tablets whole and not to crush them. Liquid iron preparations should be taken with a plastic straw.
- Caution the client not to take antacids with iron because antacids impair absorption and are generally discouraged during pregnancy. Iron and antacids should be taken 2 h apart if both are prescribed.

Antacids
- Stress that antacids should not be taken within 1 h of taking an enteric-coated tablet because the acid-resistant coating may dissolve in the increased alkaline condition of the stomach, and the medication will not be released in the intestine as intended. Stomach upset may result.
- Advise the client to store antacid liquid suspension at room temperature, not to let it freeze, and to shake the bottle well before pouring.

Side Effects
- Advise the client to keep *iron* tablets away from children. Iron tablets look like candy, and death has been reported in small children who have ingested 2 g or less of ferrous sulfate.
- Advise the client that there may be a change in bowel habits when taking *antacids*. Aluminum products can cause constipation, whereas magnesium products can cause diarrhea. Many antacids contain both ingredients.

Evaluation

- Evaluate the effectiveness of the prescribed drug therapy. Report side effects.
- Evaluate the client's understanding of possible effects on the fetus of illegal drugs, alcohol, and smoking.

Table 47–5
Drugs Used to Decrease Uterine Contractility

DRUG	DOSAGE	USES AND CONSIDERATIONS
BETA-ADRENERGIC AGENTS		
Ritodrine (Yutopar)	See Chart 47–1	Sympathomimetic beta₂-adrenergic agonist. If long-acting corticosteroids are taken simultaneously, pulmonary edema is risk (discontinue both drugs); sufficient time must elapse before another sympathomimetic amine drug is given due to additive effect; cardiovascular effects potentiated by magnesium sulfate, meperidine, and diazoxide; beta-adrenergic blockers inhibit action of ritodrine (avoid concurrent use); IV use elevates plasma insulin and glucose and decreases plasma potassium concentrations; expect increase in maternal pulse of 20–40 bpm; expect increase in FHR of 10 bpm; more expensive than terbutaline; FDA approved; *Pregnancy category*: B; rapdily crosses placenta; absorption rate 30% (PO); PB: 32%; $t\frac{1}{2}$: 15 h (is multiphasic and varies with route); metabolized by liver; excreted by kidneys; breast feeding not contraindicated due to short half-life
Terbutaline (Brethine)	Follow agency protocols for specific directives plus individual health care provider's order; only drug that may be given SC; usually therapy is 0.25 mg SC initially (repeat as necessary); then 0.1 mg SC q4 h for maintenance; then 2.5–5 mg PO q4–6h starting with last SC dose. Some agencies begin therapy IV using 10 μg/min, increasing to 5 μg/min q10 min until contractions stop	Sympathomimetic beta₂-adrenergic agonist; action onset is within 15 min IV/SC and 30–45 min PO; peak serum levels reached in 0.5–1 h IV/SC and 1–2 h PO; *Pregnancy category*: B; partially metabolized in the liver; excreted by the kidneys; not FDA approved for labor inhibition and requires written consent; less expensive than ritodrine; 40%–50% rate of tocolytic breakthrough and recurrence of preterm labor 3 wk after start of PO therapy may require repeat therapy (may be due to desensitization of beta receptors over time); current research focused on use of low-dose continuous SC pumps that are portable and can deliver intermittent bolus doses based on data reflecting peak need periods; pumps are cost-effective with high client satisfaction; drug interactions same as for ritodrine; expected increases in maternal pulse and FHR same as for ritodrine; rapidly crosses placenta; breast feeding not contraindicated due to short half-life; duration of drug effects 4–8 h PO and 1.5–4 h SC
CALCIUM ANTAGONIST		
Magnesium sulfate	Follow agency protocols for specific directives plus individual physician orders for concentration and mL/h IV: usual LD: 4–6 g in 50–100 mL over 20–30 min Maintenance: 40 g in 1 L of IVF at 2–4 g/h. Dose based on serum magnesium levels and deep tendon reflex assessment	Calcium antagonist and CNS depressant; relaxes uterine smooth muscle through calcium displacement. Must be given by infusion pump for accurate dosage; *Pregnancy category*: B; onset: IV: immediate; duration: 30 min; freely crosses placenta; few contraindications allow for use in clients who exhibit life-threatening complications; maternal magnesium levels readily monitored through serum analyses, reflexes, respiratory rate, and urinary output (extreme care needed with decreased output); antidote: calcium gluconate; elevated levels may be evident in newborn for 7 d; observe newborn for 24–48 h for signs of toxicity if mother treated close to delivery; breast feeding not contraindicated

KEY: *bpm: beats per minute; LD: loading dose; IVF: intravenous fluid; IV: intravenous; PB: protein-binding; PO: by mouth; SC: subcutaneous; $t\frac{1}{2}$: half-life; >: greater than; FHR: fetal heart rate; FDA: Food and Drug Administration.*

lease of endotoxin with uterine irritation, multiple gestation, uterine anomalies, antepartum hemorrhage, smoking, drug use, urinary tract infections, and incompetent cervix. Attempts to arrest preterm labor are *contraindicated* in (1) pregnancy less than 20 weeks' gestation (confirmed by ultrasound); (2) bulging or premature rupture of membranes (PROM); (3) confirmed fetal death or anomalies incompatible with life; (4) maternal hemorrhage and evidence of severe fetal compromise; and (5) chorioamnionitis.

Tocolytic Therapy

When clients in true preterm labor have no contraindications, they become candidates for **tocolytic therapy** (drug therapy to decrease uterine muscle contractions) using beta-adrenergic agents (e.g., ritodrine HCl [Yutopar]; terbutaline [Brethine]) or the calcium antagonist magnesium sulfate ($MgSO_4$). The goal in tocolytic therapy is to interrupt or inhibit labor to create additional time for in utero fetal maturation.

Table 47–5 lists the drugs most commonly used to decrease uterine contractions (PTL).

RITODRINE

The beta-sympathomimetic drugs act by stimulating the $beta_2$ receptors on smooth muscle. The frequency and intensity of uterine contractions decrease as the muscle relaxes. The two beta-adrenergic agents ritodrine (Yutopar) and terbutaline (Brethine) are widely used; of these, ritodrine is the only FDA approved (1980) tocolytic drug; terbutaline is approved for medicinal use but not specifically as a tocolytic. These beta-adrenergic drugs effectively decrease uterine contractions 60% to 80%. However, the literature indicates that knowledge about the long-term cumulative effects of these drugs is still lacking.

The action and effects of ritodrine and the nursing process related to the drug are presented in Chart 47–1.

Pharmacokinetics

Ritodrine (Yutopar) has an absorption rate of 30% following oral administration. It is 32% protein-bound and has a multiphasic variable half-life. With oral administration, the half-life has two phases, 1.3 h and 12 to 20 h, and with IV administration it has three phases, 7 to 9 min, 1.5 to 2.8 h, and 15 to 17 h. Ritodrine is metabolized by the liver and excreted by the kidneys.

Clients with mild contractions may be given a subcutaneous course of terbutaline initially, followed by administration of ritodrine or terbutaline IV or a series of SC injections of terbutaline, if contraction strength is enhanced. Clients are monitored to determine whether and when contractions diminish or cease; oral therapy with ritodrine or terbutaline and/

or subcutaneous pump therapy with terbutaline may be used for long-term maintenance.

Pharmacodynamics

Oral ritodrine has an onset of action of 30 min, a peak plasma/serum concentration of 30 to 60 min, and a duration of action of 4 to 6 h. Oral administration of ritodrine is initiated 30 min before discontinuing the IV administration. The 10- to 20-mg oral dose is administered every 1 to 6 h until tocolysis is no longer needed.

Side Effects and Adverse Reactions

Side effects include tremors, malaise, weakness, dyspnea, tachycardia (maternal and fetal), increased systolic pressure and decreased diastolic pressure, chest pain, nausea, vomiting, diarrhea, constipation, erythema, sweating, hyperglycemia, and hypokalemia. More serious adverse reactions include pulmonary edema, dysrhythmias, ketoacidosis, and anaphylactic shock.

Ritodrine must be used cautiously in clients with premature rupture of the membranes, diabetes mellitus, or mild to moderate preeclampsia.

Ritodrine can cause tachycardia in the fetus and hypoglycemia in the neonate. Because the half-life is short, breast feeding is not contraindicated.

Drug Interactions

The increased effects of general anesthetics can produce additive hypotension. Pulmonary edema can occur with concurrent use of corticosteroids. Cardiovascular effects may be additive with other sympathomimetic drugs, such as epinephrine, albuterol, and isoproterenol. Ritodrine is antagonized by beta-adrenergic blocking agents such as propranolol HCl, nadolol, pindolol, timolol maleate, and metoprolol tartrate.

MAGNESIUM SULFATE

Magnesium sulfate, a calcium antagonist and central nervous system depressant, relaxes the smooth muscle of the uterus through calcium displacement. Administered intravenously, the drug has a direct depressant effect on contractility. The drug increases uterine perfusion, which has a therapeutic effect on the fetus. This drug, which is also less expensive, may be safer to use than the beta-sympathomimetics because it has fewer adverse effects; it can also be used when beta-sympathomimetics are contraindicated (e.g., in diabetes and cardiovascular disease). The drug is excreted by the kidneys and does cross the placenta. The maintenance dose must be titrated to keep uterine contractions under control, and magnesium levels are drawn based on the clinical response of the client. The effective maternal serum level range for tocolysis is 5 to 8 mg/dL. Magnesium sulfate therapy is contraindicated in clients who have

Chart 47–1.   Sympathomimetic Beta-Adrenergic Agonists: Ritodrine

RITODRINE HCl

Drug Name

Ritodrine HCl (Yutopar)
Adrenergic
Pregnancy Category: B

Dosage

IV: Mix 150 mg in 500 mL D_5W and infuse at
10–20 mL/h; increase by 10 mL/h q15 min until contractions > 15 min apart; *max:* 70 mL/h;
decrease therapy as contractions taper off
Initiate PO therapy 10–20 mg 30 min before
stopping IV drug; PO dose q1–6h until tocolysis
not needed
Refer to specific protocol.

Contraindications

Before 20th week of gestation, condition in
which maintenance of pregnancy is hazardous,
e.g., antepartal hemorrhage and intrauterine fetal death; selected preexisting maternal conditions, e.g., uncontrolled hypertension or diabetes

Drug-Lab-Food Interactions

Drug: *Increase* effects of ritodrine with diazoxide, meperidine, potent general anesthetics,
magnesium sulfate; *increase* effects of sympathomimetic amines; *decrease* effects of ritodrine with
beta blockers

Pharmacokinetics

Absorption: PO: 30%
Distribution: PB: 32%, crosses placenta; proba-
bly crosses blood–brain barrier
Metabolism: $t\frac{1}{2}$: 15 h
Excretion: In urine

Pharmacodynamics

PO: Onset: 30 min
    Peak: 30–60 min
    Duration: 4–6 h
IV: Onset: Within 5 min
    Peak: 50–60 min
    Duration: 30 min

Therapeutic Effects/Uses

To inhibit uterine contractions.
Mode of Action: Stimulation of receptors in smooth muscles of uterus, thereby decreasing intensity
and frequency of contractions.

Side Effects

Malaise, weakness, dyspnea, tachycardia (maternal and fetal), palpitations, increased chest pain,
nausea, vomiting, diarrhea, hyperglycemia, hypokalemia

Adverse Reactions

Ketoacidosis
Life-threatening: Long term: pulmonary edema,
anaphylactic shock

Assessment and Planning

Interventions

Evaluation

NURSING PROCESS

KEY: IV: intravenous; PO: by mouth; PB: protein binding; $t\frac{1}{2}$: half-life.

myasthenia gravis; impaired kidney function and recent myocardial infarction are relative contraindications; clients with renal impairment require adjusted
dosages.

Side Effects and Adverse Reactions

Dosage-related side effects in the maternal client include flushing, feelings of increased warmth, sweating, dizziness, nausea, headache, lethargy, slurred
speech, sluggishness, nasal congestion, heavy eyelids,
blurred vision, decreased GI action, increased pulse
rate, and hypotension; increased severity is evidenced
by depressed reflexes, confusion, and magnesium toxicity (respiratory depression and arrest, circulatory
collapse, cardiac arrest). Side effects in the fetus and
neonate include slight hypotonia with diminished reflexes and lethargy for 24 to 48 hours.

If maternal neurologic, respiratory, or cardiac depression is evidenced, the antidote is calcium gluconate (10 mg IV push over 3 min) or calcium chloride
(10 mL of 10% solution IV push over 10 min at a rate
of 1 mL/min).

NURSING PROCESS: BETA-ADRENERGIC AGONISTS
RITODRINE

Assessment

- Identify clients at risk for preterm labor early in pregnancy.
- Obtain a history, complete physical assessment, vital signs (VS), fetal heart rate (FHR), and urine specimen for infection screening.

Potential Nursing Diagnoses

- Risk for activity intolerance
- Altered health maintenance
- Knowledge deficit related to etiology and interventions for preterm labor
- Fear related to potential for early labor and birth

Planning

- Client's preterm contractions will be eliminated by resting in left side-lying position, increasing fluid intake, and taking tocolytic therapy as needed.
- Client has no cervical change from initial examination.

Nursing Interventions

- Monitor and assess uterine activity and FHR.
- Maintain client in left lateral position as much as possible.
- Monitor maternal and fetal VS every 15 min when the client is receiving IV dose. Report systolic blood pressure decreases, diastolic blood pressure decreases, and pulse increases.
- Report auscultated cardiac dysrhythmias. An electrocardiogram (ECG) may be ordered.
- Auscultate breath sounds every 4 h. Notify health care provider if respirations are >30/min or there is a change in quality (wheezes, rales, coughing).
- Monitor daily weight to assess fluid overload; monitor strict input and output (I & O).
- Provide passive range of motion of legs.
- Report fetal baseline heart rate >180 beats per min. or any significant contractions from pretreatment FHR baseline.
- Report persistence of contractions despite tocolytic therapy.
- Report leaking of membranes, any vaginal bleeding, or complaints of rectal pressure.
- Be alert to presence of hypoglycemia and hypoglycemia in the newborn delivered within 5 h of discontinued beta-sympathomimetic drugs.
- Administer only clear solutions of drugs if using IV route.
- Assist clients on bed rest and home tocolytic therapy to plan for assistance with self-care and family responsibilities.

Client Teaching

General

- Teach client the signs and symptoms of preterm labor (menstrual type cramps, sensation of pelvic pressure, low backache, increased vaginal discharge, and any abdominal discomfort.
- Instruct client that if she experiences preterm labor contractions at home, she should void, recline on her left side to increase uterine blood flow, and drink extra fluids. Emphasize that she should notify her health care provider if the contractions do not cease or if they increase in frequency.
- Explain the effects of beta-sympathomimetic drugs; the contractions should be arrested. Report heart palpitations or dizziness.
- Instruct client to take the drug regularly and as directed.
- Advise the client to contact the health care provider before taking any other drugs while on tocolysis.

Nursing Process continued on following page

NURSING PROCESS *Continued*
RITODRINE

Evaluation

- Evaluate the effectiveness of the tocolytic drug by noting six or fewer uterine contractions in 1 h.
- Evaluate the client's understanding of nonpharmacologic measures for decreasing preterm contractions, such as increasing oral fluid intake and resting on the left side.
- Continue monitoring the client's vital signs and fetal heart rate. Report any change immediately.

Additional Nursing Considerations

Tocolytic Therapy: Magnesium Sulfate

- Monitor VS and FHR as ordered. Respirations <12/min may indicate toxicity.
- Monitor I & O. Report urinary output less than 30 mL/h.
- Check breath and bowel sounds as ordered.
- Assess reflexes before initiation of therapy and as ordered. Notify health care provider of changes in reflexes.
- Weigh daily.
- Monitor serum magnesium levels as ordered (therapeutic level is 4 to 7 mg/dL).
- Have available calcium gluconate or calcium chloride as an antidote.
- Observe newborn for 24 to 48 h for magnesium effects if drug was given to mother before birth.

CORTICOSTEROID THERAPY IN PRETERM LABOR

The best client outcome from tocolytic therapy is prevention or cessation of preterm labor. Maternity clients (24 to 34 weeks' gestation) at risk for, or who experience, preterm labor are recommended to receive antenatal corticosteroid therapy with betamethasone or dexamethasone to accelerate lung maturation with resultant surfactant development in the fetus in utero, thereby decreasing the incidence and severity of **respiratory distress syndrome** (RDS) with increased survival of preterm infants. **Surfactant** is made up of two major phospholipids, sphingomyelin and lecithin. Sphingomyelin develops in greater quantity initially (from about the 24th week) than lecithin. However, by the 33rd to 35th weeks of gestation, lecithin production peaks, making the ratio of the two substances about 2:1 in favor of lecithin. This is referred to as the **L/S (lecithin/sphingomyelin) ratio,** measured in the amniotic fluid. The L/S ratio is a predictor of fetal lung maturity and risk of neonatal RDS.

Clients with pregnancy-induced hypertension (PIH), premature rupture of the membranes, placental insufficiency, some types of diabetes, or narcotic abuse may have amniotic fluid with higher than expected L/S ratios for gestational date because of a stress-induced increase in endogenous corticosteroid production.

Betamethasone

When preterm labor occurs before the 33rd week of gestation, corticosteroid therapy with betamethasone suspension may be prescribed. Table 47–6 provides the data for this drug.

SIDE EFFECTS AND ADVERSE REACTIONS
Side effects of betamethasone suspension are rare and include seizures, headache, vertigo, edema, hypertension, increased sweating, petechiae, ecchymoses, and facial erythema.

SURFACTANT THERAPY IN PRETERM BIRTH

Synthetic Surfactant

A second approach to addressing respiratory difficulties in the preterm infant is surfactant replacement therapy. This is done to prevent the development of respiratory distress syndrome (RDS). Clinical findings in RDS include stiff, inflexible lungs caused by

| **Table 47–6** | | |
| **Prenatal Therapy for Surfactant Development** | | |
DRUG	DOSAGE	USES AND CONSIDERATIONS
Betamethasone (Celestone, Soluspan)	IM: 12 mg q12 h × 2	Corticosteroid; given to prevent RDS in preterm infants by injecting mother prior to delivery to stimulate surfactant production in the fetal lung. Not effective in treating preterm infant after delivery. Most effective if given at least 24 h (preferably 48–72 h) but less than 7 d prior to delivery in 33rd wk or before. May be repeated if baby not delivered within 7 d. Contraindicated in severe PIH and in systemic fungal infection. Simultaneous use with terbutaline may enhance risk of pulmonary edema. Drug can mask signs of chorioamnionitis; therefore, drug not given with ruptured membranes. Metabolized in the liver and excreted by the kidneys; crosses the placenta; enters breast milk; onset of action is 1–3 h. Therapy less effective with multifetal birth and with male infants. No data available related to breast feeding. *Pregnancy category:* C; PB: 64%; $t_{\frac{1}{2}}$: 6.5 h; Peak: IV: 10–36 min

KEY: *IM: intramuscular; PB: protein binding; PIH: pregnancy-induced hypertension; RDS: respiratory distress syndrome; $t_{\frac{1}{2}}$: half-life.*

lack of surfactant, dyspnea with cyanosis, inspiratory dilatation of the nares, expiratory grunt, atelectasis with each expiration, harsh breath sounds or fine rales, significant inspiratory retractions (suprasternal, substernal, intercostal, subcostal), respiratory acidosis, and metabolic acidosis. Surfactant therapy is also used to decrease the severity of RDS following diagnosis.

The deficit in the amount of endogenous surfactant available to maintain distention of the alveolar sacs is the focus of this therapy.

Five major types of surfactant therapy have been under investigation during the past decade. Currently, the FDA has approved the use of Exosurf Pediatric, a protein-free synthetic pulmonary surfactant, which, following reconstitution, contains in 1 mL, 13.5 mg colfosceril palmitate (DPPC) (the major lipid component of natural surfactant). Beractant (Survanta) intratracheal suspension, a natural bovine lung extract, contains phospholipids, neutral lipids, fatty acids, and surfactant-associated proteins to which colfosceril palmitate (DPPC), palmitic acid, and tripalmitin are added; thus, each 1 mL of Survanta contains 25 mg of phospholipids. Survanta does not require reconstitution.

Each of these two products defines *prophylactic* and *rescue* use slightly differently (Table 47–7) and has different dosing and administration requirements.

Both products require a patent endotracheal (ET) tube for administration and special positioning of the infant with specified alterations throughout the procedure. These very precise position changes during the procedure allow gravity to assist in the distribution of

product in the lungs, particularly at the alveolar surface.

Rales and moist breath sounds may be a transient finding following administration of these products. Unless very obvious signs of airway obstruction are noted, suctioning should not be performed for 2 h following administration.

Surfactant replacement therapy has been found effective in reducing the severity of RDS; rapid improvements in lung compliance and oxygenation that may require immediate decreases in ventilator settings (to prevent lung overdistention and pulmonary air leak) may occur, requiring close monitoring; overall, mortality rate has been reduced and some studies indicate that a decrease in the incidence of bronchopulmonary dysplasia is occurring since the introduction of these products.

SIDE EFFECTS AND ADVERSE REACTIONS

Side effects during administration have included some incidents of reflux of product up the ET tube with decreases in oxygenation. Dosing is slowed or halted if the infant becomes dusky in color or agitated or experiences transient bradycardia, or oxygen saturation decreases more than 15%. Rapid improvement in underlying pathology may occur as well, requiring astute monitoring of ventilated lung function. Pulmonary hemorrhage has been seen in 2% to 4% of treated infants with Exosurf. Suctioning prior to dosing lessens the chance for endotracheal tube blockage during dosing. No long-term complications or sequelae of Exosurf Pediatric or Survanta therapy have been found.

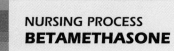

NURSING PROCESS
BETAMETHASONE

Assessment

- Assess for history of hypersensitivity.
- Assess vital signs, and report abnormal findings.
- Assess fetal heart rate (FHR).
- Assess visual status.

Potential Nursing Diagnoses

- Fear related to potential for preterm labor and birth with uncertain fetal outcome secondary to fetal immaturity
- Risk for infection

Planning

- Client will not deliver within 24 h of receiving betamethasone.

Nursing Interventions

- Observe maternal vital signs
- Maintain accurate I & O.
- Shake the suspension well. Avoid exposing it to excess heat or light.
- Inject into large muscle, not the deltoid, to avoid local atrophy.
- Check blood glucose if used for diabetic client.

Client Teaching

General
- Instruct the client to avoid exposure to infections.
- Remind diabetic client to carefully screen her glucose.

Diet
- Advise the client to avoid alcohol and to severely restrict caffeine.

Side Effects
- Instruct the client to immediately report any breathing difficulty, weakness, or dizziness.
- Instruct client to report changes in stool, easy bruising, bleeding, blurred vision, unusual weight gain, emotional changes.

Evaluation

- Continue monitoring the client's vital signs. Report changes.
- Continue monitoring FHR. Report changes.
- Monitor neonate for hypoglycemia and presence of neonatal sepsis.

FUTURE DIRECTIONS

Current research using *perfluorocarbon liquids ventilation* (PFC liquids) with respiratory-compromised infants is also being conducted as a proposed alternative approach. It is hoped that PFC liquids might distribute throughout the alveolar surface in a uniform manner and provide assistance to the area where atelectasis has occurred.

DRUGS FOR PREGNANCY-INDUCED HYPERTENSION

Pregnancy-induced hypertension (PIH), the most common serious complication of pregnancy, can have devastating maternal and fetal effects. However, with proper management, the prognosis for both mother and baby is good. Hypertensive disorders occur in

Table 47–7
Postnatal Surfactant Therapy for Prevention and Treatment of Respiratory Distress Syndrome

DRUG	DOSAGE	USES AND CONSIDERATIONS
Exosurf Pediatric	5 mL/kg per dose ET in one of two modes: *Prophylaxis:* 1 dose immediately following birth; 2 additional doses (if indicated) at 12 h and 24 h to mechanically ventilated infants *Rescue:* 1 dose as soon as RDS diagnosis is made, followed by 2nd dose 12 h later to infants who remain on mechanical ventilation After ET suctioning, administered in two 2.5-mL/kg doses via special ET tube adapter supplied with product without interrupting mechanical ventilation	FDA-approved synthetic, protein-free surfactant (artificial) given by a ventilator-experienced neonatologist as *prevention* or *rescue* in treatment of RDS; for intratracheal use only; treated infants must be on intermittent mechanical ventilation *Prophylaxis* defined as infants under 1350 g at high risk for RDS or larger infants with pulmonary immaturity. *Rescue* defined as treatment of infants with moderate to severe RDS defined in clinical trials as an arterial: alveolar oxygen tension ratio (a/A) of less than 0.22. Absorbed from alveolus into lung tissue, where extensively catabolized and reutilized for further phospholipid synthesis and secretion. Because of RDS based interruption of alveolar surface integrity, some surfactant may escape to systemic circulation; more even distribution of surfactants observed following immediate prophylaxis at birth as a result of initial availability of lung fluids. $t_{\frac{1}{2}}$: UK (however, $t_{\frac{1}{2}}$ of natural human surfactant ranges from 20–36 h; not known if generalizable to drug form). Well-tolerated in clinical trials; lesser need for ventilatory support; adverse reactions: possible reflux up ET tube during dosing (slow dosing or halt if dusky, agitated, transient bradycardia or decrease of 15% in O_2 saturation); astute monitoring of lung functioning in relation to ventilator settings required; supplied as white powder; must be reconstituted with 8 mL of supplied sterile H_2O; suspension pH 5–7; store at 15°–30°C (59°–86°F) in dry place. Stable after reconstituted for 12 h (if stored about 2°–30°C); contains no antibacterial preservatives. No known contraindications to drug use
Survanta (beractant) Intratracheal suspension	4 mL/kg per dose ET (divided into 4 aliquots) in one of two modes: *Prophylaxis:* 1 dose within 15 min of birth if possible; 3 additional doses in 1st 48 h (6 h apart) *Rescue:* Up to 4 doses in 1st 48 h of life no more frequently than q6h; 1st dose immediately following diagnosis; preferably give by 8 h of age; DO NOT SHAKE	FDA-approved natural bovine lung extract containing phospholipids, neutral lipids, fatty acids and surfactant-associated proteins to which colfosceril palmitate (DPPC), palmitic acid, and tripalmitin are added; each 1 mL contains 2.5 mg phospholipids; does not require reconstitution; must be given by a ventilator-experienced neonatologist as *prevention* or *rescue* in treatment of RDS; administered through a 5F end-hole catheter as a dosing catheter inserted into ET tube. Following administration of each quarter dose, catheter removed from ET tube and infant ventilated for 30 sec until stable. *Prophylaxis* defined as infants under 1250 g at high risk for RDS or larger infants with evidence of pulmonary immaturity. *Rescue* defined as treatment of infants with moderate to severe RDS (defined in clinical trials as need for mechanical ventilation and fractional inspired oxygen concentration [FiO_2] above 0.40). Biophysical effects occur at the alveolar surface; lowers surface tension on alveolar surfaces during respiration and stabilizes alveoli against collapse at resting pressures. Infants receiving it should be frequently monitored with arterial or transcutaneous measurement of systemic O_2 or CO_2. No known contraindications. Adverse reactions associated with dosing procedure (transient bradycardia, O_2 desaturation): less than 1% experience ET tube reflux, blockage, pallor, vasoconstriction, hypotension, hypocarbia, hypercarbia, and apnea. All reactions resolve with symptomatic treatment; drug should appear off-white to light brown; swirl vial gently; DO NOT SHAKE; foaming at surface normal; store at 2°–8°C; warm 20 min at room temperature or in hand for at least 8 min (DO NOT ARTIFICIALLY WARM); for prevention dose, begin preparation prior to infant's birth; do not warm and return drug to refrigerator more than once; protect from light

KEY: ET: endotracheal; RDS: respiratory distress syndrome; FDA: Food and Drug Administration; UK: Unknown; $t_{\frac{1}{2}}$: half-life.

EXOSURF PEDIATRIC/SURVANTA

Assessment

- Check for signed consent; need separate consents if multifetal birth.
- Check infant's vital signs (VS).

Potential Nursing Diagnosis

- Impaired gas exchange related to inadequate lung surfactant

Planning

- Infant's oxygen requirement and respiratory effort will decrease.
- Infant's need for alteration in mechanical ventilation settings will be quickly noted and accomplished.
- The infant will experience no respiratory distress after surfactant administration as evidenced by respiratory rates within normal limits (WNL), no grunting, no retractions, pink color, pulse oximetry readings ≥ 95%, within 1h of surfactant administration.

Nursing Interventions

Exosurf Pediatric
- Prepare drug within 20 min of use.
- *Reconstitute* with supplied sterile H$_2$O; draw dose from beneath the foamy layer.
- Assist with the positioning of the baby after each half-dose as detailed in the protocol.
- Store drug at 15° to 30°C in dry place; document time of reconstitution and use within 12 h.

Survanta
- Prepare drug in adequate time for drug to warm at room temperature for 20 min or in hand or at least 8 min.
- Do not artificially warm drug.
- Do not shake drug.
- Provide only off-white–light brown product for use in procedure.
- Have 5F end-hole catheter available.
- Assist with the positioning of the baby after each quarter dose as detailed in protocol.

Both Exosurf Pediatric and Survanta
- Expect the baby's lungs to sound wet after administration; do not suction through the endotracheal tube for 2 h.
- Monitor infant carefully for chest expansion, color, arterial blood gases, oxygen saturation, heart rate, facial expression, ET tube patency, blood pressure, ECG.
- Monitor ventilator pressure readings and breath sounds.

Client Teaching

General
- Explain to client what RDS is and how surfactant helps the baby.
- Explain to client the purpose of multiple monitoring devices to reduce unrealistic fears about the neonate's condition.
- Obtain consent for usage.

Side Effects
- Encourage parents to verbalize their understanding about the risks associated with the use of the drug.

Evaluation

- Evaluate preadministration breath sounds and ventilator pressure readings in comparison with postadministration findings.

Table 47-8
Predisposing Factors in Pregnancy-Induced Hypertension

African-American
Primigravida
<20 or >35 years of age (especially as primigravida)
Multifetal gestation
Family history of pregnancy-induced hypertension
Lower socioeconomic class
Gestational trophoblastic disease
Diabetes mellitus
Preexisting hypertensive, vascular, renal disease
Underweight or overweight

6% to 30% of all pregnant clients, with 5% to 7% of all pregnancies reflecting incidence of PIH. The condition is most often observed during the last 10 gestational weeks, throughout labor, and during the first 72 hours postpartum. The cause of PIH remains unknown, although numerous theories exist. The major predisposing risk factors for the development of PIH are listed in Table 47-8.

PIH is divided into two categories based on clinical manifestations: **Preeclampsia** is defined as the presence of hypertension, proteinuria, and edema in a previously normotensive prepregnant client after the 20th week of gestation. Preeclampsia is subdivided into *mild* preeclampsia and *severe* preeclampsia (see Table 47-9 for comparison).

About 5% of preeclamptic clients, notably those without adequate prenatal care, progress to the second major PIH category, **eclampsia,** in which seizure activity occurs and perinatal mortality rate is about 20%. Early diagnosis of PIH with appropriate treatment keeps most preeclamptic clients from progressing to this stage. About 25% of eclampsia occurs postpartum.

A severe sequela of PIH is known as **HELLP syndrome** (defined by *H*emolysis, *E*levated *L*iver enzymes and *L*ow *P*latelet count), which occurs in about 2% to 12% of clients with PIH. Clients who manifest severe preeclampsia are the most likely to also present with HELLP syndrome. At present, there is no effective cure for PIH except for delivery of the infant (products of conception).

Two primary treatment goals in PIH, in addition to delivery of an uncompromised fetus and psychological support for the client and her family, are prevention of seizures and reduction of vasospasm.

Thus, medically prescribed, supervised home care with nursing management or hospitalization, fetal

Table 47-9
Comparison of Mild and Severe Preeclampsia and Eclampsia

MILD PREECLAMPSIA	SEVERE PREECLAMPSIA	ECLAMPSIA
Blood pressure increase to >140 and/or >90 diastolic but <160 systolic	Blood pressure increase of more than 60 mmHg (systolic) and more than 30 mmHg (diastolic) over baseline or >160/110 on two occasions at least 6 h apart (client on bed rest)	Signs and symptoms of mild or severe PIH and ≥1 seizure
Proteinuria >500 mg in 24 h or +1 − +2; edema not generalized; noted in hands, feet	Proteinuria >5 g in 24 h or +3 or +4; edema generalized; found in face (puffy eyes, coarse features), hands, lower extremities (ankles), abdomen, and dependent areas	
Weight gain >1 lb/wk before 32 wk or >2.5 lb/wk after 34 wk	Weight gain up to 10 lb in 1 wk	
Deep tendon reflexes in arms and legs only slightly increased (0: no response; 1+: sluggish/low; 2+: normal active; 3+: brisk)	Deep tendon reflexes (DTRs) in arms and legs hyperactive (4+: hyperactive/transient clonus; 5+: brisk; clonus sustained)	
Adequate urinary output (≥1 mL/kg/h)	Oliguria present (<400 mL per 24 h)	
No major cerebral or visual symptoms May have mild frontal headache	Cerebral or visual symptoms, particularly blurred vision, spots, flashing lights, and/or persistent, severe headache in frontal area	
No epigastric pain	Epigastric pain may be present in very severe preeclampsia; pulmonary edema, cyanosis	

KEY: >: *greater than;* <: *less than;* ≥: *more than or equal to.*

well-being testing, and laboratory screening commonly are instituted until term is reached or the client's condition necessitates intervention.

Delivery of the infant (products of conception) is the only known treatment. Vaginal delivery is preferred so as not to add anesthesia or surgical risks. Those clients with HELLP syndrome may have their labor induced for a vaginal delivery at 32 or more weeks' gestation if the fetus exhibits lung maturity and well-being (based on biophysical profile score) and the client has a ripe (inducible) cervix based on a Bishop's score. For those clients with HELLP syndrome and who are at less than 32 weeks' gestation, a cesarean delivery may be considered.

If a client's disease progresses to the point of eclampsia (maternal seizure), delivery is generally postponed for 1 to 3 hours if fetal status allows. The induction or cesarean delivery is an additional stressor for the client who exhibits acidosis and hypoxia resulting from seizure. Ideally, once vital signs are stabilized with improved urinary output and decreased acidosis/hypoxia, delivery is pursued.

Table 47–10 presents the drug data for the two most commonly used drugs for treating PIH: magnesium sulfate and hydralazine.

Side Effects and Adverse Reactions

MAGNESIUM SULFATE

Early signs of increased magnesium levels in the client include flushing, feelings of increased warmth, sweating, thirst, sedation, heavy eyelids, slurred speech, hypotension, depressed reflexes, and decreased muscle tone. Adverse reactions generally oc-

Table 47–10
Drugs Used in Severe Preeclampsia

DRUG	DOSAGE	USES AND CONSIDERATION
Magnesium sulfate	Loading dose: 4–6 g in 20–30 min IV; piggyback using infusion pump/controller Maintenance dose: 1–4 g/h IV using constant infusion pump in piggyback mode	Prevention and treatment of seizures related to PIH; acts as CNS depressant; decreases acetylcholine from motor nerves, which blocks neuromuscular transmission and decreased incidence of seizures Secondarily affects peripheral vascular system with increased uterine blood flow due to vasodilation and some transient BP decrease during first hour; also inhibits uterine contractions. Depresses deep tendon reflexes and respiration; maintenance dose depends on reflexes, respiratory rate, urinary output, and magnesium level. Production of abnormally high magnesium level is main risk; therapeutic levels range from 2.5 to 6.7 mEq/L; levels of 4–7.5 mEq/L are effective in preventing seizures. Client is at risk if respiratory rate <12, output <30 mL/h, deep tendon reflex (knee jerk) is absent. *Antidote:* calcium gluconate 10 mL of 10% solution (1 g) slow IV push by physician over 3 min. Can be given IV or IM. Should not be given parenterally to clients with heart block, myocardial damage, or renal impairment. Contraindicated in myasthenia gravis. *IV:* Immediate onset; duration: 30 min; *IM:* onset 1 h; duration: 3–4 h. Absorbed magnesium is excreted by kidney; excreted in breast milk but not contraindication to breast feeding. *Pregnancy category:* B; $t_\frac{1}{2}$ UK; infusion usually stopped 24 h postpartum
Hydralazine hydrochloride (Apresoline)	IV: 100 mg in 1000 mL normal saline by infusion pump titrated at 6–12 mg/h to maintain elected BP IV Push: 5–10 mg slow IV; additional 5–10 mg doses q 20 min PRN; single dose should not be more than 20 mg IM: 5–10 mg PO: 100 mg/d in 4 divided doses IM + PO, not usually used.	Antihypertensive agent. Acts by causing arteriolar vasodilation. Usually lowers diastolic BP more than systolic BP. Objective of treatment is to maintain diastolic BP between 90 and 110 mmHg. Usually not given to pregnant PIH client with diastolic BP <105 mmHg due to risk of reduced intervillous blood flow. Clients with impaired renal function may require lower doses. *Parenteral:* onset of action 5–20 min; peak: 10–80 min; duration: 2–6 h; well-tolerated; maternal tachycardia and increased cardiac output and oxygen consumption may occur. *Oral:* onset: 20–30 min; peak: 1–2 h; duration: 2–4 h

KEY: *BP: blood pressure; IM: intramuscular; IV: intravenous; PO: by mouth; PIH: pregnancy-induced hypertension; PRN: as needed; $t_\frac{1}{2}$: half-life; UK; unknown; <: less than; CNS: central nervous system.*

PREGNANCY-INDUCED HYPERTENSION

Assessment

- Obtain baseline vital signs during early pregnancy.
- Identify client factors that may predispose to PIH.

Potential Nursing Diagnoses

- Fluid volume deficit related to shift of intravascular fluid to extravascular space as outcome of vasospasm with subsequent elevated arterial hypertension
- Knowledge deficit related to PIH, diagnosis, treatment modalities, common outcomes for mother and baby
- Potential for inadequate placental perfusion and risk to fetal well-being secondary to vasospasm
- Potential for maternal injury related to seizure activity
- Potential for maternal injury related to magnesium toxicity
- Anxiety related to possible preterm hospitalization and delivery with possible adverse fetal and/or maternal outcomes

Planning

- Client's blood pressure will be maintained within acceptable ranges.
- Client will verbalize accurate understanding of PIH-related information.
- Client will comply with planned PIH treatment regimen.
- Fetus will tolerate disease-altered intrauterine environment and subsequent delivery without injury.
- Mother will maintain therapeutic magnesium levels.
- Plan for magnesium sulfate infusion for at least 24 h postpartum and continue to check respirations and urinary output from Foley catheter hourly; assess deep tendon reflexes.

Hydralazine

- Take pulse and BP every 5 min when drug is administered or constantly by use of an electronic monitor until stabilized and then every 15 min.
- Maintain diastolic BP between 90 and 110 mmHg; or as ordered.
- Observe for change in level of consciousness.
- Monitor I & O to avoid hypotensive episodes or overload.
- Monitor fetal heart rate.
- Do not mix with any other medications in same bag.

Client Teaching

General
- Teach client information about PIH and implications for mother, fetus, and newborn.
- Provide client information about potential treatment modalities for PIH.

Safety
- Teach client how and why to rest in the left lateral recumbent position.
- Teach the client signs and symptoms of further deterioration due to progressive PIH and when and why to seek medical assistance.
- Explain to client that fetal well-being will be assessed through biophysical profile studies, a nonstress test, or contraction stress test at determined frequencies.
- Educate family regarding possibility of seizures and appropriate actions to take if seizures occur.

Diet
- Provide nutritional counseling in regard to need for additional protein intake due to protein losses, normal sodium diet, and importance of adequate fluid intake.
- Explain to client why she must be weighed daily.

Nursing Process continued on following page

Magnesium Sulfate

- Explain to the client why she will have a Foley catheter, infusion pump, continuous fetal monitoring, and routine assessment of deep tendon reflexes.
- Tell the client that therapy will extend into the postpartum period.
- Explain to the client about visitor restrictions and that she will be in a low-stimulation room.
- Tell the client that she will likely experience flushing and possibly nausea and vomiting during the loading dose.
- Tell client that evidence of magnesium levels that are within therapeutic range include decreased appetite, awkwardness when moving about, and some speech slurring.
- Tell client to report any swallowing difficulties or drooling.

Hydralazine

- Explain to client that nurses will be monitoring pulse and BP almost constantly until her BP becomes stable after administration, and then every 15 min. Explain that an electronic BP monitor may be used to obtain constant readings.
- Explain to client need for careful measuring of I & O.

Nursing Interventions

Magnesium Sulfate

- Continuous electronic fetal monitoring is indicated.
- Have available airway suction and resuscitation equipment and emergency drugs.
- Have antidote at bedside. Calcium gluconate (1 g) is usual antidote, but calcium chloride may also be used.
- Maintain client in left lateral recumbent position in low-stimulation environment. Provide constant observation.
- For IM administration, use Z-track technique and rotate sites (drug is painful and irritating).
- Monitor BP, pulse, respiratory rate per agency protocol, deep tendon reflexes, and hourly I & O with urimeter for output.
- Monitor temperature, breath sounds, and bowel sounds every 4 h.
- Check urine for protein every hour.
- Assess for epigastric pain, headache, visual symptoms, sensory changes, edema, level of consciousness, and seizure activity on ongoing basis.
- Monitor serum magnesium levels according to agency protocol for range between 4 and 7 mEq/L.
- Notify physician if following are observed:
    Respirations less than 12/min
    Absence of patellar reflexes
    Urinary output less than 30 mL/h
    Systolic BP less than or equal to 160 mmHg, unless ordered
    Magnesium level greater than 7 mEq/L
    Absent bowel sounds or altered breath sounds
    Epigastric pain, headache, visual symptoms, sensory changes, change in affect or level of consciousness, seizure activity
- Monitor laboratory reports for evidence of low platelet count, and, if present, observe for excessive bleeding.
- Monitor fetal status. FHR should remain 120 to 160.

Evaluation

- Evaluate the effectiveness of therapy to reduce BP.
- Continue monitoring of vital signs. Report changes.
- Document effect of teaching/learning opportunity upon client's knowledge deficit about PIH treatment modalities and outcomes.
- Note fetal well-being secondary to treatment with drugs as evidenced by fetal monitoring and fetal movement assessment.
- Monitor changes that occur in magnesium level per laboratory results as compared with behavioral cues.

cur with serum levels greater than 10 mEq/L. Magnesium toxicity is manifested by a rapid drop in blood pressure and respiratory paralysis. Reflexes may be absent. Heart block has been reported occasionally with levels lower than 10 mEq/L.

Decreased variability is commonly seen on the FHR tracing. If the client received magnesium sulfate close to the time of delivery, the neonate may exhibit low Apgar scores, hypotonia, lethargy, weakness, and potential respiratory distress. The fetal level of magnesium generally reaches more than 90% of maternal levels within 3 h of administration. There is no evidence linking congenital defects and maternal hypocalcemia or hypermagnesemia. The greater risk to the fetus is from maternal PIH: decreased placental blood flow and intrauterine growth retardation.

HYDRALAZINE

Observe the client for headache, nausea, vomiting, nasal congestion, dizziness, tachycardia, palpitations, and angina pectoris. In the fetus and neonate, observe for a sudden decrease in maternal blood pressure, which may cause fetal hypoxia. Hydralazine has no known adverse effects on the fetus.

DRUGS FOR PAIN CONTROL DURING LABOR

Labor and delivery, a stressful event for most clients, is divided into three stages. During the *first stage* cervical effacement and dilatation occur; the cervix becomes fully dilated at 10 cm. The *second stage* is the period during which expulsion of the fetus occurs (Fig. 47–1). During the *third stage,* the placenta separates from the uterine wall, is expelled, and initial recovery begins. As the first stage of labor progresses, uterine contractions become stronger in quality and longer in duration, the interval between them becomes shorter, and discomfort increases.

Physical causes of labor pain include uterine muscle hypoxia, cervical effacement and dilatation, referred pain, and distention of the bladder, vagina, and perineum. Possible psychological causes include past experience with pain, anticipation of pain, fear and high anxiety, knowledge deficit about what to expect, and lack of support persons.

If pharmacologic intervention is needed for pain relief, drugs should be used as an adjunct to ongoing nonpharmacologic measures. Examples of nonpharmacologic comfort and pain relief measures useful throughout labor and delivery are (1) mobility, (2) positioning supportive of the gravid uterus and promoting uterine perfusion, (3) hygiene and comfort measures, (4) presence of support persons, (5) use of

breathing and relaxation techniques, and (6) hydrotherapy (tubs and showers).

Drugs should be selected to decrease the client's pain but, at the same time, to minimize side effects for the fetus/newborn and the mother throughout the rest of her labor and delivery.

Pain relief in labor can be obtained through the use of systemic analgesics and regional anesthesia. Inhalation and general anesthesia used for delivery are not discussed in this chapter. Analgesics alter the client's perception and sensation of pain without producing unconsciousness.

Analgesia

Systemic medications (drugs that enter the circulatory system and are distributed throughout the body and to the brain) used for pain control during labor include sedative-hypnotics, narcotic agonists, and mixed narcotic agonist-antagonists.

The sedative-hypnotic drugs are generally given when an apprehensive client is in false labor or very early labor, or has ruptured membranes but no true labor. These drugs allow the mother to rest and relax and reduce her fears and anxiety. The sedative drugs most commonly used are barbiturates, generally secobarbital sodium (Seconal) and pentobarbital sodium (Nembutal). Other drugs in this category include several that can be given alone during early labor or combined with narcotic agonists and given later when the client is in active labor. Used this way, these drugs have an **ataractic** effect (potentiating the analgesic action of a low-dose narcotic) in addition to decreasing anxiety and apprehension. These drugs include promethazine (Phenergan), a sedative-antihistamine, and hydroxyzine hydrochloride (Vistaril, Atarax), a sedative-hypnotic.

The most commonly used narcotic agonist for pain relief during labor is meperidine hydrochloride (Demerol), a synthetic narcotic. Morphine sulfate may be used for pain control in labor; however, it is not commonly used in active labor and is more likely to be prescribed in prolonged latent labor for "obstetric rest." The therapeutic goal is for the woman to rest or even sleep and awaken in active labor. These drugs interfere with pain impulses at the subcortical level of the brain. Secondary effects include sedation and decreased anxiety. Narcotics received by the mother before delivery may result in neonatal respiratory depression, which may require reversal by administration of naloxone (Narcan) to the newborn. See Chapter 48 for discussion of neonatal Narcan dosing and administration.

The third group of systemic medications used for pain relief in labor is the mixed narcotic agonist-antagonists. These drugs exert effect at more than one

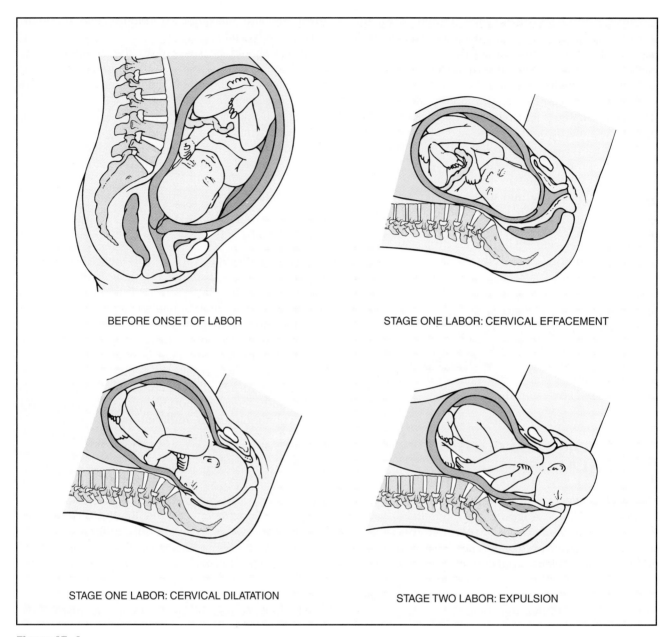

Figure 47–1
Stages one and two of labor. (From Nichols, F., and Zwelling, E. [1997]. Maternal-Newborn Nursing: Theory and Practice. Philadelphia: WB Saunders.)

site, often an agonist at one and an antagonist at another. These drugs have a not well-understood "ceiling effect," in which additional doses have no effect and do not increase the degree of respiratory depression. These drugs may be sequenced with meperidine (Demerol), but the meperidine should be given first. If an agonist-antagonist has been administered first, administration of meperidine would provide markedly diminished or no additional pain relief. If a client is addicted to narcotics, this group of drugs may cause her to exhibit extreme withdrawal symptoms. Two commonly used narcotic agonist-an-

tagonist drugs are butorphanol tartrate (Stadol) and nalbuphine (Nubain).

Table 47–11 presents additional information about these three groups of systemic medications used during labor.

SIDE EFFECTS AND ADVERSE REACTIONS
Side effects of sedative-hypnotic drugs (secobarbital, pentobarbital) for the client include paradoxically increased pain and excitability, lethargy, subdued mood, decreased sensory perception, and hypotension. Side effects include decreased heart rate variabil-

ity in the fetus and respiratory depression, sleepiness, hypotonia, delayed breast feeding with poor sucking response for up to 4 days in the neonate.

Side effects of ataractic drugs (promethazine, hydroxyzine) for the client include confusion, disorientation, excess sedation, dizziness, hypotension, tachycardia, blurred vision, headache, restlessness, weakness, and urinary retention with *promethazine;* drowsiness, dry mouth, dizziness, headache, blurred

vision, dysuria, urinary retention, and constipation with *hydroxyzine.* Decreased FHR variability can be seen, and the neonate can experience moderate CNS depression, hypotonia, lethargy, poor feeding, and hypothermia.

Side effects of narcotic agonist drugs (morphine, meperidine) for the client include orthostatic hypotension, nausea, vomiting, headache, sedation, hypotension, and confusion. Neonatal CNS depres-

Table 47–11
Common Systemic Medications Used for Pain Relief in Labor

DRUG	DOSAGE	USES AND CONSIDERATIONS
SEDATIVE-HYPNOTICS		
Secobarbital (Seconal)	IM: 50–100 mg PO: 100–200 mg	Used to decrease anxiety during latent phase of labor; onset: 10–30 min; peak: 20–30 min; duration: 4–8 h; no effects on uterine tone or contractility; rapidly crosses placenta; can cause decreased variability in FHR (pseudo-sinusoidal pattern) because of decreased CNS control over heart rate. No antagonist for barbiturates, so Seconal administered only if delivery not expected for 24–48 h. May have prolonged depressant effects on neonate. Excreted into breast milk. Compatible with breast feeding. May increase CNS depression with alcohol, narcotics, antihistamines, tranquilizers, and MAOIs. *Pregnancy category:* D; t½: 15–30 h; PB: UK
Pentobarbital (Nembutal)	PO: 20–30 mg	Short-acting barbiturate. *Pregnancy category:* D; see Chart 16–1.
ATARACTICS		
Promethazine HCl (Phenergan)	IM/IV: 12.5–25 mg q4–6h or IM: 25–50 mg with 25–75 mg meperidine or IV: 15–25 mg with 25–75 mg meperidine; repeat if needed *Max:* 100 mg in 24 h	A phenothiazine antihistamine; used as adjunct to narcotic analgesics during first stage of labor; antiemetic properties; onset: PO: 20 min; IM: 3–5 min; IV: 1–2 min; used alone to promote rest and sleep; potentiates action of narcotic agonists reducing narcotic doses; may cause decreased variability in FHR; contraindicated during lactation; at term, rapidly crosses placenta; fetal and maternal blood concentrations in equilibrium in 15 min, with infant levels persisting for 4 h; transient hypotonia, lethargy and electroencephalographic changes for 3 d in newborn; may cause maternal tachycardia; may impair newborn platelet aggregation. If given with meperidine, give slowly at beginning of contraction over several minutes to decrease amount of drug perfused immediately to the fetus via placenta. Other adverse reactions: dizziness, dry mouth, excessive sedation, weakness, blurred vision, restlessness. Do not give subcutaneous. *Pregnancy category:* C; PB: UK; t½: UK
Hydroxyzine pamoate (Vistaril, Atarax)	IM: 25–50 mg q4–6h; repeat if needed IV: not recommended	Antianxiety agent; antihistamine; antiemetic; sedative-hypnotic; used alone early in labor or later to potentiate action of narcotic agonists; can cause decreased variability in FHR; use Z-track injection for IM to reduce pain; no data available about breast feeding; onset: 15–30 min; peak: <2 h; duration: 4–6 h. Intraarterial, SC, or IV administration *not* recommended (thrombus and digital gangrene can occur); extravasation can result in sterile abscesses and marked tissue induration; use with caution in clients with chronic obstructive pulmonary disease and asthma. Adverse reactions: hypotension, drowsiness, dizziness, headache, dry mouth, pain at injection site, weakness, ataxia; may cause CNS depression with alcohol, analgesics, barbiturates, narcotics; may decrease effects of epinephrine. No effect on labor or neonatal Apgar scores. *Pregnancy category:* C; PB: UK; t½: 3 h

Table continued on following page

Table 47–11 *Continued*
Common Systemic Medications Used for Pain Relief in Labor

DRUG	DOSAGE	USES AND CONSIDERATIONS
NARCOTIC AGONISTS		
Meperidine hydro-chloride (Demerol)	IM: 50–100 mg, q3–4 h IV (slow push): 25–50 mg	Synthetic morphine-like narcotic agonist alters pain perception and depresses pain impulses by binding to opiate receptor in CNS; onset IM is 10 min with peak in 40–60 min and duration of 2–4 h; onset IV is 30 sec with peak in 5–7 min and duration of 1–2 h; crosses placenta and appears in fetus in 1–2 min after IV dose; can cause decreased variability in FHR; caution needed for use with cardiac clients due to tachycardia; well absorbed; excreted in urine as metabolites. Adverse reactions: bradycardia, severe hypotension, convulsion, respiratory depression, cardiovascular collapse, increased intracranial pressure. Respiratory depression in the newborn following use during labor is time and dose dependent; naloxone should be available; newborn may exhibit moderate CNS and mild behavioral depression. Mother may have nausea, vomiting, drowsiness, sedation, confusion. May increase or decrease uterine activity. Give drug at beginning of contraction to prevent fetal bolus of drug. *Pregnancy category:* B; PB: 60%–70%; $t\frac{1}{2}$: 3–8 h
Morphine sulfate Opioid analgesic CSS II	SC/IM: 10–15 mg	Administer drug slowly and rotate injection sites to avoid irritation of local tissue. Be alert to risk of overdose in clients with circulatory impairment; SC: onset: 5–30 min; peak: 50–90 min; duration: 4–5 h. IM: onset: 5–30 min; peak: 30–60 min; duration: 3–7 h. Crosses placenta and found in breast milk. Watch for respiratory depression in neonates of mothers who received this drug in labor. May see withdrawal symptoms in neonate if mother was regular opioid user during pregnancy. Use with extreme caution in clients with asthma, respiratory depression, anoxia, seizures, shock, and acute alcoholism. *Pregnancy category:* C; PB: UK; $t\frac{1}{2}$: 2.5–3 h
MIXED NARCOTIC AGONISTS/ ANTAGONISTS		
Butorphanol tartrate (Stadol)	IM: 2 mg, q3–4h IV: 1 mg, q3–4h	Potent nonnarcotic analgesic (2 mg dose approximately equivalent to 10–15 mg morphine); has mixed narcotic agonist-antagonist mechanism of action with central analgesic actions; binds to CNS opiate receptors and inhibits ascending pain pathways. Used for relief of moderate to severe pain, for preoperative medication, supplement to anesthesia. *Pregnancy category:* B (D, if prolonged use or high at-term dose); PB: <90%; $t\frac{1}{2}$: 2.5–4 h; onset: IM: 10–30 min; IV: 1–2 min; peak: IM: 0.5–1 h; IV: 4–5 min; duration: IM: 3–4 h; IV: 2–4 h. Additive effects with CNS depressants; may see withdrawal symptoms in narcotic-dependent clients; may cause drowsiness and respiratory depression, sedation, euphoria, hallucinations, headache, palpitations. Do not give SC; have naloxone available as antidote. Do not give if respirations <12/min. Use with caution in client having preterm baby because fetus may exhibit decreased beat-to-beat variability on FHR monitor; newborn may have moderate CNS depression, hypotonia at birth, and mild behavioral depression
Nalbuphine (Nubain)	SC/IM/IV: 10–20 mg q3–4h PRN; *Max:* 160 mg/d	Limited respiratory depression. Less analgesic effect than morphine. About 10%–15% of laboring women experience hallucinations with Nubain. Toxicity can be reversed with naloxone. *Pregnancy category:* B; PB: UK; $t\frac{1}{2}$: 5 h

KEY: FHR: fetal heart rate; IM: intramuscular; IV: intravenous; PB: protein-binding; PO: by mouth; SC: subcutaneous(ly); $t\frac{1}{2}$: half-life; UK: unknown; <: less than; CNS: central nervous system; MAOI: monoamine oxidase inhibitor.

sion and decreased FHR variability can occur with meperidine.

In the client, mixed narcotic agonist-antagonists can cause nausea, clamminess, sweating, sedation, respiratory depression, vertigo, lethargy, headache, and flushing. Side effects in the fetus and neonate include decreased FHR variability, moderate CNS depression, hypotonia at birth, and mild behavioral depression.

Anesthesia

Anesthesia in labor and delivery represents the loss of painful sensations with or without the loss of consciousness. There are two types of pain experienced in childbirth: The pain of labor arises from nociceptors in the uterine and perineal structures. *Somatic* pain caused by stretching of the perineum and vagina travels to sacral 2, 3, and 4 by way of the pudendal nerve. Visceral pain from the cervix and uterus is carried by nerves together with sympathetic fibers and enters the neuraxis at the thoracic 10, 11, 12, and lumbar 1 spinal levels.

REGIONAL ANESTHESIA
Regional anesthesia achieves pain relief during labor and delivery without loss of consciousness through temporarily blocking the conduction of painful impulses along sensory nerve pathways to the brain through the use of injected local anesthetics. The use of regional anesthesia allows an awake and aware client to experience labor and the birth of her baby with relief from discomfort in the blocked area. Regional anesthesia may inhibit the urge to push.

Local anesthetics most commonly used for regional anesthesia are chemically related to cocaine, considered to be the first natural anesthetic substance found. The chemically related drugs that have evolved since that time are much less toxic, more potent, and have longer lasting therapeutic effects. Names of frequently used local anesthetics of the amide type (metabolized in the liver) include mepivacaine (Carbocaine), lidocaine (Xylocaine), and bupivacaine (Marcaine). These potent agents have a long duration of action. They cross the placenta and, depending on the degree to which they are protein-bound, can enter the fetal circulation. The fetal effects last for 24 to 48 h after delivery. The ester type agents are rapidly metabolized by plasma pseudocholinesterase, rather than the liver. Thus, the mother's drug level is lower, and less anesthetic is placentally transferred to the fetus. Chloroprocaine (Nesacaine) is an example of an ester type agent.

Side effects from local anesthetic agents depend on their chemical properties. These include palpitations, dizziness, confusion, headache, metallic taste in the

mouth, nausea, vomiting, hypotension, seizures, and coma. IV fluids are infused to prevent hypotension.

Subarachnoid Block

Spinal Block
Indication: Need for high degree of pain relief for delivery. Preferred for cesarean delivery; seldom used for labor.

When given: Immediately before delivery; late in second stage when fetal head is on the perineum (for vaginal delivery).

Area blocked: Umbilicus to toes.

Injection site: With client side-lying, injected into subarachnoid space at L4–L5.

Considerations: Client needs to be well hydrated. Anesthetic is given immediately after a contraction to avoid impairing respiratory efforts. Client generally in curled side-lying position for administration. Contraindicated if skin over lumbar region is infected or client has severe coagulopathy, severe hypovolemia, or severe BP abnormalities.

Side effects: For client: hypotension; occasional spinal headache. For fetus or neonate: none, unless secondary to maternal hypotension. *Note:* Headache is less common because of the small size (25 gauge) of needle used; client may have nausea, backache, urinary retention.

Saddle Block
Indication: Pain relief for vaginal delivery, forceps delivery, and episiotomy repair.

When given: Same as for spinal block.

Area blocked: Perineal area, buttocks, inner area of thighs (for true saddle block); uterus and perineum (for modified saddle block).

Injection site: With client sitting, injected in S1–S5 (true saddle) or T1–S5 (modified saddle).

Advantage: Can be used for cesarean birth if injected to T4.

Considerations: Same as for spinal block.

Side effects: For client: none. For fetus and neonate: none.

Lumbar Epidural

Lumbar Epidural Block (Single Dose)
Indication: Pain relief in first and second stages of labor.

When given: Active labor.

Area blocked: T12–S5 (entire pelvis) in area of dorsal root ganglion with varying degrees of motor and sensory loss depending on dosage and agent injected.

Injection site: Epidural space (potential space between the dura mater and vertebral canal from cranium to sacrum) between L2–L3 or L3–L5 or L4–L5;

NURSING PROCESS
PAIN CONTROL DRUGS

Assessment

- Assess the laboring client's behavior for relaxation and progress of labor in relation to expected norms.
- Assess the client's verbal and nonverbal behavior for data supportive or nonsupportive of coping with labor.
- Obtain baseline vital signs, blood pressure (BP), breath sounds, quality of contractions, degree of effacement and dilatation, and fetal heart rate prior to administering the analgesic for later comparison to determine effectiveness (pain scale).
- Screen for drug history to ascertain potential for drug-drug interactions.
- Assess cultural expectations related to pain experiences.

Potential Nursing Diagnoses

- Pain related to progressive labor
- Fear of pain related to labor
- Anxiety related to uncertainty about labor experience and personal coping ability

Planning

- The client will demonstrate no severe side effects of pain control drugs during labor.
- The client will verbalize a decrease in pain on a 1 to 10 scale.

Nursing Interventions

- Offer appropriate analgesia for stage and phase of labor and the anticipated method of delivery. Encourage the client and her support persons to participate in the decision-making about analgesia.
- Document administration of the drug per agency protocol.
- Provide appropriate safety measures after administration of drugs.
- Check compatibility chart for any mixing of drugs.
- Verify that correct antidote drugs are available.
- Within agency protocols and safe obstetric practice, administer drugs before maximum intensity pain/anxiety.

Sedative-Hypnotics: Barbiturates
- Do not give if active labor is imminent.
- Observe FHR tracing; expect decreased variability.

Ataractics: Promethazine, Hydroxyzine
- *Promethazine:* If IV, give at beginning of contraction. Administer at 25 mg/min or lower rate.
- Monitor amount of promethazine the client receives in 24 h; monitor for maternal heart rate following administration.
- *Hydroxyzine:* Use IM Z-track technique only. Do not give SC, intraarterially, or IV.

Narcotic Agonists and Mixed Narcotic Agonist-Antagonists
- Consider parity of client, and likely amount of time until delivery.
- Do not give when delivery is likely within 1 to 3 h, because of greater chance of depressed fetus or neonate (i.e., birth should occur within 1 h or after 3 to 4 h following administration).
- Monitor urine output.
- Ensure that FHR tracing indicates fetal stability before drug administration.
- Observe FHR strip.

Nursing Process continued on following page

NURSING PROCESS *Continued*
PAIN CONTROL DRUGS

Meperidine
- Generally not given before active labor. Be certain a narcotic antagonist (naloxone) is available as antidote if needed.
- If drug is administered intravenously, give very slowly at beginning of a contraction over several minutes to decrease the amount of drug perfused to the fetus via the placenta.
- Check for respirations > 12 before administration.
- IM: inject deep into muscle.
- Provide restful environment as adjunctive therapy.
- Keep bed rails up when client is nonambulatory and have client solicit assistance if she does ambulate.
- Observe FHR strip.
- Have neonatal naloxone readily available.

Butorphanol Tartrate
- Observe for signs of narcotic withdrawal in narcotic-dependent clients.
- Do not administer SC.
- Observe for respiratory depression.
- Ascertain respirations > 12 before administration.
- IM: inject deep into muscle.
- Provide restful environment.
- Observe FHR strip.
- Have neonatal naloxone readily available.
- If given IV, give slowly at beginning of contraction.

Client Teaching

General
- Instruct client concerning
    Drugs ordered
    Route of administration and reason
    Expected effects of drug on labor
    Potential drug effects on fetus/newborn
- Tell the client that most drugs used for pain relief in labor and delivery are not given PO because the GI tract functions more slowly during labor. Thus, drug absorption is decreased and the route is ineffective.

Safety
- Instruct client about safety precautions that will be used while receiving the drug, including
    Positioning in bed
    Side rails
    Assistance with ambulation

Cultural Considerations

- Recognize cultural influence on client's perception of and expression of discomfort/pain.

Evaluation

- Evaluate the effectiveness of the drug in lessening or alleviating the pain.
- Evaluate fear and anxiety in regard to pain and ability to cope with the labor experience.
- Monitor respirations, heart rate, blood pressure, and FHR for alterations from baseline. Report deviations beyond those expected with a normally progressing labor.
- Document findings using agency protocols and obstetric nursing standards of care.

not into the dura. Never put in above L1. *Note:* L1–L2 is where the spinal cord ends. Nerves run off and down into the spinal canal. Nerve free-floats and can move out of the way of the epidural needle. The goal is to bathe the nerves with the dispersed local anesthetic.

Considerations: Loss of bearing-down reflex means forceps or vacuum extractor may be needed. May slow labor. Contraindicated in clients with skin infection in lumbar region or with severe coagulopathy.

Potential complications: For client: dural puncture with leak of spinal fluid, creating a true spinal block (level drug reaches determines the degree of effects); hypotension; convulsions; local anesthetic, coma, respiratory arrest. For fetus or neonate: few effects unless severe maternal hypotension occurs (late decelerations in FHR); may depend on the anesthetic agent used.

Note: Test dose (not in quantity to cause seizure) is used to confirm correct placement; if local anesthetic is injected into vein, client may experience dizziness, ringing in ears, numb mouth, toxic response.

Continuous Lumbar Epidural Block Using Indwelling Catheter in Epidural Space

Indication: Pain relief during first and second stages. Useful for prolonged labors.

When given: Progressive, active labor. This is the most widely used method for labor pain management today.

Area blocked: Same as for lumbar epidural block.

Injection site: Same as for lumbar epidural block.

Advantages: Provides continuous anesthesia from stage 1 through delivery and perineal repair. Client can feel movement and pressure but no pain. Can be used for vaginal delivery or cesarean birth. Sensory level can be altered and the density of the block can be manipulated. Can be used to deliver epidural morphine PF (Duramorph) or fentanyl (Sublimaze) into epidural space for regional analgesia (highly effective). Clients may experience itching, which may not be effectively relieved using diphenhydramine (Benadryl) or naloxone (Narcan) infusions.

Considerations: Loss of bearing-down reflex means that forceps or a vacuum extractor may be needed. Requires a large amount of local agent. Bupivacaine is used in low concentration (as low as 1/16%).

Complications: Same as for lumbar epidural block.

Side effects: Pruritus (in 2 to 3 h when drug reaches upper thoracic segments), urinary retention, and nausea and vomiting related to ineffective hydration to prevent hypotension.

Caudal (A Type of Epidural Anesthesia)

Indication: Pain in first and second stages of labor.

When given: Active labor.

Area blocked: Perineum; masks uterine contractions.

Injection site: Epidural space through sacral hiatus (S4).

Advantages: Useful for women with metabolic, lung, and heart disease. Very rapid perineal anesthesia and muscle relaxation. Can be used continuously.

Considerations: Increased need to use forceps because there is a loss of urge to push. Risk of systemic toxic reactions; level of anesthesia is more difficult to obtain.

Paracervical Block

Indication: Pain during first stage.

Time given: Active phase of first stage; may be repeated periodically until 8 cm dilated.

Area blocked: Uterus, cervix, and vagina; masks contractions.

Injection site: Transvaginally, adjacent to rim of cervix.

Advantages: Rapid onset. Lasts 60 to 90 min. Relieves pain of cervical dilatation and contractions. Does not block lower vagina or perineum.

Considerations: Rapid absorption (because injected into a very vascular area). Does not provide anesthesia for delivery or episiotomy repair. Has variable effects on labor progress.

Side effects: For client: hematomas in tissue around injection site. For fetus: mild to severe bradycardia or prolonged FHR deceleration common with decreased variability. Because of the relatively common occurrence of the prolonged FHR decelerations, use of the paracervical block has decreased significantly.

Pudendal Block

Indication: For outlet forceps, episiotomy, and repair.

When given: Immediately before birth.

Area blocked: Perineum; pudendal nerves.

Injection site: Inside birth canal deep into lower sides of vagina to bathe the pudendal nerves.

Considerations: None.

Side effects: None.

Local Infiltration

Indication: For episiotomy and repair to be done when pudendal anesthesia is not possible because of timing and position of fetal head.

When given: Just before delivery or repair.

Area blocked: Local area adjacent to injection.

Injection site: Perineal subcutaneous tissue.

Advantage: No effect on FHR or client's vital signs.

Considerations: May not obtain complete relief of pain and may need additional injections; requires large amount of agent.

Side effects: For client: mild discomfort during injection. For fetus or neonate: none.

NURSING PROCESS
REGIONAL ANESTHETICS

Assessment

- Check history for drug sensitivity to local agents.
- Assess for presence of a "labor plan" with expectations for coping with labor and beliefs about use of analgesia/anesthesia.
- Assess knowledge about regional anesthesia.
- Determine extent of cervical dilatation and labor progress.
- Review fetal status.
- Review history for presence of any contraindications to regional anesthesia; notify anesthesia provider.

Potential Nursing Diagnoses

- Pain related to progressive labor with diminished coping ability
- Knowledge deficit related to inexperience with regional anesthesia/analgesia
- Potential for impaired gas exchange to fetus if maternal hypotension occurs secondary to use of local anesthetic
- Impaired physical mobility secondary to regional anesthesia
- Potential for urinary retention secondary to regional anesthesia

Planning

- Client will verbalize pain relief during labor.
- Client will remain normotensive and maintain a normal pulse rate; FHR will remain within normal limits.
- Client will not experience bladder distention.
- Client will be able to discuss specifics of regional anesthesia.

Nursing Interventions

General
- Review hydration status before regional anesthesia is started because of the hypotensive effects. Provide IV fluids as ordered.
- Position the client on her left side or as instructed by the anesthesia provider. Place a hip roll to avoid pressure on the inferior vena cava, which would cause maternal hypotension and decreased placental perfusion.
- Monitor the progress of labor for a decrease in frequency and intensity of contractions. Monitor vital signs and fetal heart rate.
- Be certain that ephedrine, antihistamines, O₂, and resuscitation equipment are readily available.
- Be aware of signs and symptoms that might indicate postspinal headache; notify anesthesia provider.
- Be aware of how to place the client in Trendelenburg position if necessary.

Spinal
- Accurately determine when the client is having contractions, because the anesthetic agent must be given immediately after a contraction.
- Check BP for hypotensive effects per agency protocol after injection. Keep O₂ with positive pressure ventilation equipment readily available.

Epidural
- Ensure that the client has 500 to 1000 mL of an isotonic solution IV before the procedure to increase circulatory volume.
- Monitor FHR and progress of labor and recall that too much anesthetic can inhibit fetal descent.
- If hypotension occurs, maintain client on left side and increase rate of IV fluids. Notify health care provider.

Nursing Process continued on following page

NURSING PROCESS *Continued*
REGIONAL ANESTHETICS

- Check bladder status carefully. Catheterize if unable to void. Before allowing client to ambulate after delivery, be sure that adequate sensation has returned and client can support her weight when ambulating.
- Conduct ongoing pain assessment. When nature of pain changes, contact the anesthesia provider to evaluate anesthesia needs.
- Document procedure per agency protocol.

Caudal
- Place client in position requested by anesthesia provider for administration.

Paracervical Block
- Maintain continuous FHR monitoring for fetal bradycardia after administration and carefully monitor maternal BP.

Client Teaching

- Discuss technique, potential benefits, and side effects of client's particular method of anesthesia.

Side Effects
- Tell the client that regional anesthetics may slow labor and that some clients may need a drug to enhance uterine contractions.
- Explain to the client in whom a headache develops after *spinal* anesthesia that the anesthesia provider may use an epidural blood patch to seal the injection site and reduce the headache.

Skill
- Instruct client how to curl into position for *epidural* administration. Tell her that forceps or vacuum extractor may be needed for delivery (due to reduction of "urge to push" sensation).
- Instruct the client how to assume the left lateral or other position as requested by anesthesia provider for *caudal* anesthesia.

Safety
- Tell the client receiving *epidural* anesthesia that she will have an IV. Also tell her that she will have FHR monitoring to allow observation of her contractions and the effect of the anesthetic agent on the fetus.

Evaluation

- Evaluate blood pressure compared with preprocedure baseline; also evaluate FHR strips for alterations in variability and for any decelerations.
- Evaluate the effectiveness of the anesthetic in relief of discomfort; also evaluate for uniformity of anesthesia (if difference in sides of body, notify anesthesia provider).
- Evaluate urinary output and palpate for bladder distention. Catheterize if unable to void.
- Evaluate the fundus for firmness.
- Evaluate for return of sensation and mobility.

Contraindications
There are some contraindications to regional anesthesia:

- Morbid obesity
- Severe pregnancy-induced hypertension (PIH) (due to increased risk of profound hypotension, [secondary to hypovolemia] associated with underlying disease state) and risk of bleeding secondary to decreased platelets.
- Coagulation disorders (client should have a normal PTT and platelet counts)
- Generalized sepsis or local infection at needle insertion site.

DRUGS THAT ENHANCE UTERINE MUSCLE CONTRACTILITY

Oxytocic drugs enhance uterine contractility by stimulating the smooth muscle of the uterus. Oxytocin, the ergot alkaloids, and some prostaglandins make up this group of drugs.

Oxytocin is synthesized in the hypothalamus and is transported to nerve endings in the posterior pituitary. The hormone is released by the nerve endings under appropriate stimulation; capillaries absorb the substance and carry it into the general circulation where it facilitates uterine smooth muscle contraction.

In the presence of adequate estrogen levels (those normally achieved by the third trimester), intravenous oxytocin acts on the uterus to initiate labor contractions. Table 47–12 presents common medical reasons for induction.

Before a labor is induced, risks and benefits and the status of both mother and fetus must be assessed. The gestational age of the fetus must be considered together with the position of the fetus (head down and deep in the pelvis) and the size of the fetus in relation to the client's pelvis. In anticipation of a live birth, the client's cervix should be ripe (softening with progress in effacement and partial dilatation). An objective scoring system called the Bishop score is used to assess readiness for induction. The higher the score, the more likely is a positive response to induction.

Some clients are not suitable candidates for labor induction because the risks of the procedure outweigh the potential benefits. Table 47–13 presents some of the major contraindications to labor induction.

Two approaches are used to ripen, efface, and be-gin cervical dilatation in pregnant women at term (or near term) with a medical or obstetric indication for labor induction. One method is "mechanical" and involves insertion of a Foley catheter through the cervix; the bulb is then inflated. The Foley catheter bulb provides a mechanical stimulation similar to "stripping of the membranes." When the Foley "falls out," the client is started on intravenous oxytocin. The second approach uses administration of dinoprostone, the naturally occurring form of prostaglandin E_2 (PGE_2). It is thought that intracervically or intravaginally administered PGE_2 acts to create cervical effacement and softening by a combination of contraction-inducing and cervical-ripening properties, possibly secondary to collagen degradation resulting from collagenase secretion in response to PGE_2. One approach uses prefilled syringes of commercially prepared dinoprostone cervical gel 0.5 mg. (Prepidil gel); the gel is introduced just below the cervical os. A second approach is the placement in the posterior vaginal fornix of a vaginal insert (Cervidil) containing 10 mg of controlled-release dinoprostone. Table 47–14 presents the dosage, uses, and considerations for administration of dinoprostone for cervical ripening.

Intravenous oxytocin can be used to augment rather than initiate labor. It facilitates smooth muscle contraction in the uterus of a client already in labor but experiencing inadequate uterine contractility. The client with **uterine inertia** may be more responsive to oxytocin than the client who has not begun labor, and a lower starting dose will be needed.

In both labor induction and labor augmentation, oxytocin is infused at a prescribed individualized dosage rate, and this rate is increased, decreased, or maintained at fixed intervals based on uterine and fetal response. The objective is to establish an ade-

---

Table 47–13
Contraindications to Labor Induction

Disproportion between fetal head and pelvis (cephalopelvic disproportion)

Nonfavorable fetal presentation (transverse or breech)

Documented fetal distress

Prematurity

Placenta previa and/or suspected abruptio placentae

Severe pregnancy-induced hypertension

Grand multiparity

Multifetal gestation

History of uterine trauma

Previous major surgery in the area of the cervix or uterus

Excessive amniotic fluid causing overdistended uterus

Table 47–12
Indications for Labor Induction

Pregnancy-induced hypertension

Chronic hypertension

Membrane rupture >24 h

Chorioamnionitis

Postdates (>42 wk gestation)

Intrauterine growth retardation

Positive oxytocin challenge test (CST)

Maternal diabetes mellitus (classes B–F)

Maternal renal disease

Rh isoimmunization

Intrauterine fetal death

KEY: CST: contraction stress test.

Table 47–14
Dinoprostone for Cervical Ripening

DRUG	DOSAGE	USES AND CONSIDERATIONS
Dinoprostone Cervical gel, 0.5 mg (Prepidil Gel)	Endocervical: supplied in 3 g prefilled syringe applicators; 3 doses (1 dose q6h) 6 h after last dose IV oxytocin administered *Max:* 1.5 mg of drug/24 h (7.5 mL or 3 syringes)	A naturally occurring form of prostaglandin E$_2$ (PGE$_2$). Must be administered in a hospital with intensive care and acute surgical facilities. *Pregnancy category:* C. Used to ripen unfavorable cervix at or near term in pregnant women needing labor induction. Metabolized in lung, liver, and kidney; eliminated by kidney. Must be used with caution in clients with renal or hepatic dysfunction. Safety in clients with ruptured membranes has not been determined. Use with caution in asthma, glaucoma, or increased intraocular pressure. Not recommended for clients in whom oxytocic drugs are contraindicated or with prolonged uterine contractions; not recommended in clients with placenta previa or active genital herpes (vaginal delivery not indicated). Drug must *not* be placed above level of cervical os. Drug may augment other oxytocic agents; therefore, no concomitant use; sequential use 6–12 h following gel is recommended. Adverse reactions include uterine hyperstimulation, nausea, vomiting, diarrhea, back pain, fetal distress. Clients should have a reactive nonstress test before first dose. Client is to remain recumbent 1 h following each dose. Monitor uterine activity and fetal heart rate (FHR); suggest a 20 min FHR strip before doses. Must be at room temperature before administration.
Cervidil vaginal inserts	Ripening unfavorable cervix: Intravaginal: 10 mg over 12 h; remove 12 h after insertion or at onset of active labor	Administer only in setting with emergency equipment and trained personnel; use suppository at room temperature. Provider should wear gloves to decrease risk of absorption as inserted high into the vagina. After administration, client remains lying down for 10 min. Have medication available for frequent gastrointestinal side effects of abdominal cramping, diarrhea, nausea, and vomiting. Provide emotional support.

quate contraction pattern that promotes labor progress, generally represented by contractions every 2 to 3 min that last for 50 to 60 sec with moderate intensity. It is important that the client receiving oxytocin not experience uterine hyperstimulation, which causes markedly increased pain and nonreassuring fetal heart rate patterns owing to interference with placental perfusion. Continuous nursing observation during induction/augmentation is critical. The need for an accurate infusion rate requires the use of an infusion pump. Once cervical dilatation has reached 5 to 6 cm and an adequate contraction pattern is evident, the rate of oxytocin infusion can often be slowed or stopped.

Following delivery, oxytocin is usually added to an existing intravenous solution to help the uterus stay contracted and thus close the uterine sinuses at the placental site. The drug can also be given IM following the delivery of the placenta.

Oxytocin is prepared in synthetic form and marketed as Pitocin and Syntocinon. Oxytocin is an FDA-approved drug for labor induction and labor augmentation.

Chart 47–2 shows the actions and effects of oxytocin.

Oxytocin

PHARMACOKINETICS

Oxytocin (Pitocin, Syntocinon) is well absorbed from the nasal mucosa when administered intranasally for milk letdown. The protein-binding percent is low, and the half-life is 1 to 9 min. It is rapidly metabolized and excreted by the liver.

PHARMACODYNAMICS

The onset of action of intramuscularly administered oxytocin is in 3 to 5 min, the peak concentration time is unknown, and the duration of action is 2 to 3 h. The onset of action of intravenously administered oxytocin is immediate, the peak concentration time is unknown, and the duration of action is 1 h. The onset of action of intranasally administered oxytocin is a few minutes, the peak concentration time is unknown, and the duration of action is 20 min.

Chart 47-2. Oxytocic Drug: Oxytocin

OXYTOCIN

Drug Name	**Dosage**
Oxytocin (Pitocin, Syntocinon) Oxytocic *Pregnancy Category:* X	For induction or augmentation of labor, commonly A: IV: 10 units (1 amp) diluted in 1000 mL lactated Ringer's to 10 mU/mL; connect to control IV line close to the needle site of main IV line, as a piggyback line. *Post delivery* IV: 10 units added to 1 L electrolyte or dextrose solution; infuse at rate to prevent uterine atony IM: 10 units after delivery of the placenta Nasal spray: 1 spray into 1 or both nostrils 2–3 min before nursing or pumping: not for use during pregnancy
Contraindications	**Drug-Lab-Food Interactions**
Proven cephalopelvic disproportion, fetal distress, hypersensitivity, anticipated nonvaginal delivery, pregnancy (intranasal spray)	**Drug:** Hypertension with vasopressors, cyclopropane anesthetics
Pharmacokinetics	**Pharmacodynamics**

Absorption: PO: Not well absorbed
Distribution: PB: Low; widely distributed in extracellular fluid; minute amounts in fetal circulation
Metabolism: t½: 1–9 min; rapidly metabolized by liver
Excretion: In urine
	IM: Onset: 3–5 min
	    Peak: UK
	    Duration: 2–3 h
	IV: Onset: Immediate
	    Peak: UK
	    Duration: 1h
	Intranasal: Onset: Few minutes
	    Peak: UK
	    Duration: 20 min

Assessment and Planning

NURSING PROCESS

Interventions

Therapeutic Effects/Uses

To induce/augment labor contractions; to treat uterine atony; milk letdown (intranasal spray).

Mode of Action: Action of myofibrils to stimulate letdown of milk and promote uterine contractions.

Evaluation

Side Effects	**Adverse Reactions**
Maternal effects with undiluted IV use only: Hypotension, hypertension, nausea, vomiting, constipation, decreased uterine blood flow, rash, anorexia	Seizures, water intoxication with large doses **Life-threatening:** Intracranial hemorrhage, cardiac dysrhythmias asphyxia; fetus: jaundice, hypoxia

KEY: A: adult; IV: intravenous; IM: intramuscular; PO: by mouth; PB: protein-binding; t½: half-life; UK: unknown.

The medication is administered IV piggyback for induction or augmentation of labor. Pitocin is diluted in 1000 mL lactated Ringer's solution to 10 mU/mL.

DRUG INTERACTIONS

Concurrent use of vasopressors can result in severe hypertension. Hypotension can occur with concurrent use of cyclopropane anesthesia and with undiluted IV administration.

Ergot Alkaloids

The **ergot alkaloids** act by direct smooth-muscle cell receptor stimulation. These drugs are not used during labor because of their propensity to cause sustained uterine contractions (tetanic contractions), which would result in fetal hypoxia and possibly in rupture of the uterus. Following delivery, however, these sustained contractions are extremely useful for prevention or control of postpartum hemorrhage and promotion of uterine involution.

The two most commonly used ergot derivatives are ergonovine maleate (Ergotrate) and methylergonovine maleate (Methergine). These preparations can be given intramuscularly, PO, or intravenously (IV administration is recommended only for true hemorrhagic emergencies). Transient significant elevations in BP can occur, particularly after IV infusion of ei-ther drug, and clients with pregnancy-related hypertension or peripheral vascular diseases should not receive these products. Table 47–15 presents the most commonly used oxytocic drugs.

SIDE EFFECTS AND ADVERSE REACTIONS

Side effects include uterine cramping, nausea and vomiting (mostly after IV dose), dizziness, hypertension (particularly with IV administration), sweating, tinnitus, chest pain, dyspnea, itching, and sudden severe headache. Signs of ergot toxicity (ergotism) include pain in arms, legs, and lower back, numbness, cold hands and feet, muscular weakness, diarrhea, hallucinations, seizures, and blood hypercoagulability.

Table 47–15
Oxytocic Drugs Commonly Used to Enhance Uterine Motility

DRUG	DOSAGE	USES AND CONSIDERATIONS
Oxytocin (Pitocin, Syntocinon)	See Chart 47–2	
Ergonovine maleate (Ergotrate)	PO: 0.2–0.4 mg (1–2 tablets) q6–12h over 48 h IM: 0.2 mg q2–4h; *max:* 5 doses IV: 0.2 mg (only for severe bleeding) over 1 min while BP is monitored.	Oxytocic; ergot alkaloid; directly stimulates vascular smooth muscle to vasoconstrict peripheral and cerebral vessels; prevention and treatment of postpartum or postabortion hemorrhage caused by uterine atony or subinvolution. IV only for true emergencies. Limit use in clients with coronary artery disease, hypertension, PIH; contraindicated before delivery of placenta. *Pregnancy risk factor:* X. IV: Immediate onset, 45 min duration; IM: 2–5 min onset, 3 h duration; PO: 6–15 min onset, 3 h duration; $t_{\frac{1}{2}}$: 2 h. Use with caution in sepsis, hepatic or renal impairment. Adverse reactions: diaphoresis, palpitations, transient chest pain, thrombophlebitis, seizures, cerebrovascular accidents, dizziness, headache, nausea, vomiting, tinnitus, dyspnea; metabolized in liver; excreted in urine; oxytocic
Methylergonovine maleate (Methergine)	PO: 0.2–0.4 mg, q6–12h; *max:* 1 wk IM: 0.2 mg after delivery of anterior shoulder (if full obstetric supervision), after delivery of placenta, or post partum; repeat q2–4h; oral doses may follow parenteral IV: Same as for IM; but slowly over 1 min with careful monitoring of BP	Prevention and treatment of postpartum hemorrhage; subinvolution and postabortion hemorrhage; *Pregnancy risk factor:* C. IV: Immediate onset, 45 min duration; IM: 2–5 min onset; 3 h duration; PO: 5–25 min onset; 3 h duration; $t_{\frac{1}{2}}$ (biphasic): Initial: 1–5 min; terminal: 30 min–2 h. Metabolized in liver; eliminated in urine Adverse reactions: transient hypertension, diaphoresis, palpitations, dizziness, headache, nausea, vomiting, tinnitus, transient chest pain, dyspnea. Exhibits similar smooth muscle action to ergotamine but affects primarily smooth muscle, producing *sustained* contractions, and thus shortens the 3rd stage of labor. Not administered IV routinely due to possibility of sudden hypertensive and cerebrovascular accidents; limit use with clients with hypertension (especially IV); contraindicated with maternal sepsis, labor induction, threatened spontaneous abortion; do not use with vasopressors, other ergot alkaloids, or vasoconstrictors; appears in breast milk but interference with breast feeding is less than with ergonovine

KEY: BP: blood pressure; IM: intramscular; IV: intravenous; PIH: pregnancy-induced hypertension; PO: by mouth; $t_{\frac{1}{2}}$: half-life.

ENHANCEMENT OF UTERINE CONTRACTILITY: OXYTOCINS

Assessment

- For induction or augmentation of labor:
- Collect accurate baseline data before beginning infusion, including maternal pulse and blood pressure, uterine activity, and fetal heart rate (FHR).
- Interview client and review history to ascertain that there are no contraindications.

Potential Nursing Diagnosis

- Knowledge deficit related to drugs used to promote uterine contractility

Planning

- Oxytocin will enhance uterine contractions without adverse maternal or fetal effects.
- Client's vital signs (VS) will be within acceptable ranges throughout labor, delivery, and postpartum period.

Nursing Interventions

- Have magnesium sulfate and/or other tocolytic agents and oxygen readily available in case hypertonicity occurs.
- Monitor I & O.
- Monitor maternal pulse and blood pressure, uterine activity, and FHR during oxytocin infusion.
- Maintain client in lateral recumbent position or sitting to promote placental infusion.
- Be alert for signs of uterine rupture, which include FHR decelerations, sudden increased pain, loss of contractions, hemorrhage, and rapidly developing hypovolemic shock.

Client Teaching

- Explain to the client that the drug is given intravenously and the dosage adjusted in response to contraction pattern.
- For milk letdown: Teach client timing and method of nasal administration.

Evaluation

- Evaluate for effective labor progress.
- Continue monitoring VS and FHR. Report changes in VS, FHR, and vaginal bleeding.

OTHER OXYTOCICS

Assessment

Ergonovine and Methylergonovine
- Assess lochia and uterine tone before giving ergonovine or methylergonovine.
- Recognize that these two drugs have a vasoconstrictive effect, which may cause hypertension. Ergonovine is more vasoconstrictive than methylergonovine.
- Obtain baseline BP before administration.

Nursing Interventions

Ergonovine and Methylergonovine
- Monitor the client's BP as consistent with agency protocol.
- Protect drugs from light exposure.
- Observe for side effects or symptoms of ergot toxicity (ergotism). Notify physician if systolic BP increases by 25 mmHg or diastolic BP by 20 mmHg over baseline.

Nursing Process continued on following page

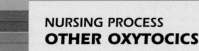

NURSING PROCESS
OTHER OXYTOCICS

Client Teaching

Ergonovine and Methylergonovine
- Explain to the client that she may feel uterine cramps after receiving the drug but may receive analgesics for pain.

Safety
- Advise the client to avoid smoking. Nicotine increases the vasoconstrictive properties of these drugs.

Side Effects
- If the client is breast feeding, explain that the drug lowers serum prolactin levels with potential to inhibit postpartum lactation; note that ergonovine is more likely to do so than methylergonovine.

Cultural Considerations

- Recognize cultural influence on client's expression or lack of expression of discomfort and/or pain.

Evaluation

- Evaluate the effectiveness of the drug.
- Continue monitoring vital signs. Report changes in vital signs or vaginal bleeding.

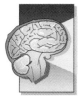

Critical Thinking In Action

Tanya, gravida 3, para 0, is at 42 weeks' gestation. At her prenatal visit, her health care provider notes signs and symptoms of pregnancy-induced hypertension and advises Tanya of the plan to induce labor after administration of prostaglandin gel. Tanya asks the nurse, "Can you help me understand all this?"

1. What objective tool (scoring system) can be used to predict the extent to which Tanya's cervix is "ripe" and therefore favorable for successful induction?

If Tanya's health care provider orders Prepidil Gel be used in her cervix, the nurse will need to be prepared to address the following aspects of the therapy for Tanya:

2. Why is the gel being used (what is to be accomplished)?
3. Who will administer the gel?
4. How often will the gel be administered?
5. How long after the last dose of gel before the intravenous oxytocic medication can be started to induce labor?
6. Why is there a period of waiting before starting the oxytocic?

It is now 16 hours since Tanya first had the gel inserted. Answering Tanya's call light, the nurse finds her in the bathroom upset that she seems to be feeling nauseous, occasionally vomiting a little bit of stomach fluid, and complaining that her stool seems "really watery." "Is something wrong?" Tanya wails.

7. Analysis of the data about Tanya's symptoms would support what conclusion about what is occurring?
8. Explain what nursing actions might be taken to support her.

9. When Tanya returns to bed and the external fetal monitor is reapplied, what data should the nurse collect, record, and report to the obstetric provider.

Twenty-four hours have elapsed since Tanya had her first gel instillation; it has been 6 hours since her last insertion. A vaginal examination reveals that Tanya's cervix is soft and 50% effaced and dilated 3 cm, the presenting part is at −2 station. Contractions are 5 minutes apart and mild. The health care provider elects to begin an oxytocin infusion.

10. Tanya asks how a medicine "running into my arm is able to make my uterus contract?" How would you explain the mode of action of oxytocin to Tanya?
11. Why is the oxytocin infusion run through a secondary line attached as a "piggyback" to the primary line? At which port along the primary line is the piggyback inserted and why at this location?
12. Why is oxytocin administered via an infusion pump?
13. What actions in regard to the IV equipment set-up should be taken as safety measures before starting the oxytocin?
14. What drugs would you want nearby in the event of an emergency with the oxytocin?
15. What information would you record during the infusion?
16. While you are setting up the oxytocin infusion, an RN orientee asks you what criteria you will use to know when to slow the rate or stop the infusion. You correctly respond that contractions would be _____ minutes apart with _____ intensity and the cervix would be at least _____ cm dilated.
17. Considering Tanya's diagnosis of pregnancy-induced hypertension, explain why you would be especially vigilant for uterine hyperstimulation during the oxytocin infusion.
18. If uterine hyperstimulation occurs explain how you would handle the situation. Address the following:
   Position Tanya _____
      Rationale _____
   IV Fluids _____
      Rationale _____
   Oxygen _____
      Rationale _____
19. Tanya asks what side effects can occur if she receives a continuous lumbar epidural. You correctly tell her that _____
_____.

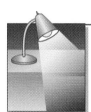

Study Questions

1. What is the main reason drug use is discouraged during pregnancy and breast feeding?
2. What are the nursing responsibilities associated with the administration of the drugs used during tocolysis?
3. What are two drugs used to protect and promote respiratory function for the premature neonate? What is the expected effect of each?
4. A client who initially planned to have "natural childbirth" has changed her mind. What information will she need about analgesics used in labor?
5. What are potential complications of an oxytocin infusion to induce labor?
6. What are the two most commonly used drugs in the treatment of pregnancy-induced hypertension?
7. What are five nursing responsibilities associated with oxytocin induction or augmentation?

48 Drugs Associated with the Postpartum and the Newborn

JANE PURNELL TAYLOR and LINDA GOODWIN

Outline

Objectives

- Identify drugs commonly administered during the postpartum period and explain their uses.
- Identify the purpose of the drugs administered to the newborn immediately after delivery.
- Describe the nursing process, including client teaching, related to drugs used during the postpartum period and for the newborn immediately after delivery.

Terms

absorption	episiotomy	prolactin
amide-type anesthetics	folliculitis	protrusion
anoderm	hydrolyzed	puerperium
anorectal	lactation	recombinant
antiflatulent	lyophilized	Rh_0 (D) immune globulin
contact dermatitis	necrosis	Rh sensitization
congenital rubella syndrome	occlusive	sensitization
denuded	percutaneous	seroconvert
dependence	perineal	titer
engorgement	permeability	urticaria

INTRODUCTION

This chapter focuses on the pharmacologic considerations for both mother and infant after delivery. Nonpharmacologic measures and pharmacologic agents related to the relief of common discomforts during the postpartum period are described. In addition, drugs commonly administered to newborns immediately after delivery are included.

DRUGS USED DURING THE POSTPARTUM PERIOD

During the **puerperium** (the period from delivery of the baby and the placenta until 6 weeks postpartum),

the maternal body physically recovers from antepartal and intrapartal stressors and returns to its prepregnant state.

Pharmacologic and nonpharmacologic measures commonly used during the postpartum period can have five main purposes: (1) prevention of uterine atony and postpartum hemorrhage (discussed in Chapter 47); (2) pain relief (from uterine contractions, perineal wounds, and hemorrhoids); (3) enhancement or suppression of lactation; (4) promotion of bowel function; and (5) enhancement of immunity.

Table 48–1 lists the nonpharmacologic measures commonly used during the postpartum period. As during pregnancy, whenever possible nonpharmacologic measures are preferred to the use of drugs or are used in conjunction with drugs.

Table 48–1
Nonpharmacologic Measures for Common Postpartum Needs

INDICATION	MEASURE
Uterine contractions	Client positioned on abdomen with pillow under abdomen periodically for 3–4 d Distraction, breathing techniques, therapeutic touch, relaxation, guided imagery, ambulation No heat to abdomen because of risk of uterine relaxation and increased bleeding
Perineal wound resulting from episiotomy or laceration	Ice covered in thin, absorbent material to protect tissue for 6–8 h after delivery Client positioned on side as much as possible with pillow between legs Early and frequent ambulation Perineal exercises Warm sitz bath 12–24 h after delivery 3–4 × per d Area cleansed front to back using perispray squeeze bottle, cleansing shower, or Surgi-Gator Client squeezes buttocks together before sitting and sits tall and flat, not rolled back onto coccyx No tampons, douche, or feminine hygiene sprays No intercourse until after bleeding has stopped or as advised by health care provider
Hemorrhoids	As above, plus most particularly: Ice Sims' position to help increase venous return Warm, moist heat; sitz bath Tucks with witch hazel
Lactation suppression	Tight bra or binder worn continuously over 5 d Normal fluid intake No manipulation or stimulation of breasts
Engorgement	As above, plus ice to axillary area of breasts if client is bottle feeding client, or apply warmth if client is breast feeding A little colostrum or milk (if breast feeding hand expressed) before putting baby to breast to ease latching-on
Sore or cracked nipples	Absorbent breast pads worn to keep moisture away from nipples No soap on nipples Air dry after feeding Only a little breast milk on nipples used as protective lubricant; lanolin no longer used because of pesticide contamination No nipple shields to prevent potential chafing Do not limit baby's time at breast to prevent nonemptying of milk ducts and increased pressure Proper positioning for feeding; nursing begun on the less sore nipple Suction broken with little finger after feeding to prevent pulling on nipple

Postpartum nursing care ideally occurs as a client-caregiver partnership. To enhance health and wellness, the nurse collaborates with the client to strengthen the new mother's self-confidence and ability to handle her own health challenges. One major challenge is management of postdelivery discomforts. An emerging trend is for postpartum mothers to be provided self-medication administration packets that contain appropriate medications (for either vaginal- or cesarean-delivered clients) with printed instructions for self-directed use in the hospital and later at home. Thus, the "well client" admitted to the hospital to deliver her baby and recover during a limited time period is not placed in a dependent "sick-role" position; instead, the mother uses her supplied medications (within instructional guidelines) when she determines the need for pain management. The nurse's role in this system is fourfold: (1) to provide astute physical and pain assessment with the client to determine healing progress within a standard and effectiveness of self-administered medications; (2) to directly administer medications for those clients unable to take their own because of nursing assessment of cognitive, psychomotor, or physiological deficits; (3) to directly administer narcotic analgesics (as prescribed) when pain control by nonnarcotic products is determined ineffective as a result of breakthrough pain episodes; and (4) to distribute the correct self-administration packet to each client on the basis of allergy/sensitivity history to contained products and to obtain signed consent forms for client participation.

Analysis of data collected from facilities employing self-medication administration programs indicates that clients use fewer narcotics overall and report satisfaction with products included in the packets for promoting comfort. Table 48–2 presents contents of a typical self-medication packet.

Table 48–2
Prototype Self-Medication Administration Packet Contents

VAGINAL DELIVERY
Witch hazel pads (Tucks)
Perineal spray (Dermoplast; Americaine)
Acetaminophen 500 mg or ibuprofen 200 mg
Docusate with casanthranol tablets

CESAREAN DELIVERY
Acetaminophen 500 mg or ibuprofen 200 mg
Docusate with casanthranol tablets
Simethicone chewable tablets

Table 48–3
Commonly Used Postpartum Systemic Analgesics

Acetaminophen (Tylenol)
Propoxyphene (Darvon)
Ibuprofen (Motrin)
Acetaminophen with codeine (Tylenol with codeine)
Codeine sulfate
Meperidine (Demerol)
Morphine sulfate (Pectoral)
Oxycodone hydrochloride (Percocet)

Pain Relief for Uterine Contractions

"Afterbirth pains" occur during the first few days postpartum when uterine tissue experiences ischemia during contractions. Table 48–3 presents a list of systemic analgesics commonly used during the postpartum period. Narcotic agents are generally reserved for more severe pain such as that experienced by the client after cesarean birth or tubal ligation. The specific drugs are described in Chapter 17.

Because some systemic analgesics (codeine, meperidine, and oxycodone) can cause decreased alertness, it is important that the nurse observe the client when she is caring for her newborn to ensure safety. Clients who receive codeine sulfate or ibuprofen need to be assessed for bowel function and gastrointestinal (GI) irritation, respectively. Clients who receive codeine or morphine need monitoring of respiratory rate.

Pain Relief for Perineal Wounds and Hemorrhoids

The process of birth places significant pressure on the perineal soft tissue. The tissue may become bruised and/or edematous. The tissue may be further stressed, with the potential for bruising, edema, and pain if episiotomy or laceration occurred as an outcome of the delivery. Clients may also have developed hemorrhoids during pregnancy, which may be exacerbated as a result of pushing during the labor process. Comfort measures and selected topical agents may be helpful.

Drugs used for relief of pain from perineal wounds and hemorrhoids are presented in Table 48–4.

SIDE EFFECTS AND ADVERSE REACTIONS
The most commonly reported side effects of local or topical agents ("caine" family drugs and witch hazel) include burning, stinging, tenderness, swelling, rash, tissue irritation, sloughing, and tissue necrosis. The

Table 48-4
Drugs Used for Pain Relief from Perineal Wounds and Hemorrhoids

AGENT	DOSAGE	USES AND CONSIDERATIONS
PERINEAL WOUNDS (EPISIOTOMY OR LACERATION)		
Benzocaine (Americaine, Dermoplast OTC)	Spray liberally t.i.d. or q.i.d. 6–12 inches from perineum following perineal cleansing Supplied as aerosol; benzocaine 20%	Local anesthetic inhibits impulses from sensory nerves as a result of alteration of cell membrane permeability to ions. Contraindicated in secondary bacterial infection of tissue and known hypersensitivity. 1-min peak effect, 30–60 min duration. Hydrolyzed in the plasma and (to lesser extent) in the liver by cholinesterase; eliminated as metabolites in urine. Well absorbed from mucous membranes and traumatized skin; apply 6–12 inches from affected area
Witch hazel pads (Tucks [50% witch hazel with glycerine, water, and methylparaben])	Apply premoistened pads t.i.d. or q.i.d. to wound site	Precipitates protein, causing tissue to contract. May be chilled/refrigerated in original container for additional comfort. If liquid, pour over ice and dip absorbent pads into solution; change when diluted. Medical intervention should be sought if rectal bleeding is present. Side effect: local irritation (discontinue use)
HEMORRHOIDS		
Hydrocortisone acetate 10 mg (Anusol HC, Anusol Ointment [Promoxine HCl 1%, mineral oil 46.7%, zinc oxide 12.5%])	One suppository b.i.d. for 3–6 d	Relieves pain and itching from irritated anorectal tissue. Contains hydrocortisone acetate. Acts as an antiinflammatory agent. Available without hydrocortisone. Contraindicated with hypersensitivity. If second infection in tissue, discontinue. Not known if excreted in breast milk; use cautiously. *Pregnancy category:* C. If anorectal symptoms do not improve in 7 d or if bleeding, protrusion, or seepage occurs, inform health care provider. Not to be used if 4th degree perineal laceration. Wear gloves. Onset: UK; peak: UK; duration: UK
Hydrocortisone acetate 1% and promazine HCl 1% topical aerosol (Proctofoam HC)	1 applicator transferred to a 2- × 2-inch pad and placed against rectum inside peripad b.i.d or t.i.d. and after bowel movements	Topical corticosteroid aerosol foam with same action and considerations as above. Also available in nonsteroidal preparation. Shake foam aerosol before use. Extent of percutaneous absorption of topical corticosteroids is determined by vehicle integrity of epidermal barrier and use of occlusive dressings (not known if any quantity detectable in breast milk). Side effects: burning, itching, irritation; dryness, infrequent folliculitis reactions. Onset: UK; peak: UK; duration: UK
Dibucaine ointment, USP 1% (Nupercaine)	Apply as above t.i.d. or q.i.d., using no more than 1 tube in 24 h	Local anesthetic ointment containing dibucaine 1%. Action same as benzocaine. Do not use if rectal bleeding is present. *Pregnancy category:* C. Onset: within 15 min; peak: UK; duration: 2–4 h. Do not use near the eyes or over denuded surfaces or blistered areas. Side effects: burning, tenderness, irritation, inflammation, contact dermatitis, urticaria, cutaneous lesions, edema. Do not use if known hypersensitivity to amide-type anesthetics

KEY: UK: unknown.

most commonly reported side effects of hydrocortisone local or topical drugs include burning, itching, irritation, dryness, folliculitis, allergic contact dermatitis, and secondary infection. These side effects are more likely to be observed if occlusive dressings are used.

Lactation Suppression

In Table 48–1, nonpharmacologic measures for **lactation** (milk formation and secretion) suppression are presented. Until recently, lactation was commonly

Text continued on page 912

NURSING PROCESS
PAIN RELIEF FROM PERINEAL WOUNDS AND HEMORRHOIDS

Assessment

- Assess the perineal area for wounds and hemorrhoids (size, color, location, pain scale).
- Check the expiration dates on topical spray cans, bottles, and ointment tubes.
- Assess for presence of infection in perineal site in order to avoid use of benzocaine on infected perineal tissue.

Potential Nursing Diagnoses

- Alteration in comfort: pain related to episiotomy, laceration, or hemorrhoids
- Knowledge deficit related to cause of discomfort and how long client may expect pain to last when products are used as directed

Planning

- Client's perineal discomfort will be alleviated by use of topical sprays, compresses, and ointment.
- Client will be free from side effects.

Nursing Interventions

- Do not use benzocaine spray when infections are present.
- Shake benzocaine spray can. Administer 6 to 12 inches from perineum with client lying on her side with top leg up and forward to provide maximum exposure. This can also be done with one foot on the toilet seat after voiding or bowel movement.
- Use witch hazel compresses (Tucks and/or witch hazel solution) with an ice pack and a peripad to provide cold in addition to the active agent.
- Store Anusol HC suppositories below 86°F, but protect from freezing. Use gloves for administration. Assess client to progress to nonhydrocortisone preparation as quickly as possible based on assessment if breast feeding.
- Check for lot numbers and expiration date.
- Use of Proctofoam HC needs to be explained carefully to the client because directions refer to placing agent inside the anus, which is not generally done with obstetric clients, who may have extensive perineal wounds extending into the anus.

Client Teaching

Perineal Wounds: Topical Spray Containing Benzocaine
- Explain expected effects.
- Tell the client that the drug is not for prolonged use (no more than 7 days) or application to a large area.
- Advise the client with bleeding hemorrhoids to use the drug carefully and to keep her health care provider informed.

Self-Administration
- Apply three to four times daily or as directed.
- Apply without touching sensitive area.
- Hold can 6 to 12 inches from affected area; side-lying in bed with upper leg lifted and spraying from behind is helpful for many clients or the client may stand with one foot on chair or toilet seat.

Safety
- Advise the client to avoid contact of the medication with eyes.
- Instruct the client not to apply anesthetic and then use a perineal heat lamp, because this could cause tissue burns.
- If condition worsens or symptoms occur again within a few days, notify the health care provider and discontinue use until directed.

Nursing Process continued on following page

NURSING PROCESS *Continued*
PAIN RELIEF FROM PERINEAL WOUNDS AND HEMORRHOIDS

- Keep out of reach of visiting children in postpartum unit and later at home. Contact poison control immediately if ingested.
- Do not store above 120°F.
- Do not puncture or incinerate can when disposing of empty can.

Witch Hazel Compresses
- Explain expected effects of product (relief of itching, burning, irritation in episiotomy site or hemorrhoid with cooling, soothing sensation).
- Notify health care provider if condition worsens or does not improve within 7 days.

Self-Administration
- If using liquid witch hazel, client may pour over chipped ice and place soft, clean absorbent squares in solution; fold and place moist square (squeezing square very slightly to eliminate excess [not all] moisture) against episiotomy/hemorrhoids.
- If using commercial medicated pads, entire container may be placed in the refrigerator.
- Instruct the client not to touch the surface of the pad that will be placed next to the perineal wound.
- Tell the client when to change the compress and show how to place an ice bag and peripad over the compress.

Safety
- Do not insert medicated pads into the rectum.
- Keep product away from children.
- Do not use if rectal bleeding is present (requires medical intervention).

Side Effects
- Discontinue use if local irritation occurs.

Hemorrhoids: Anusol Ointment and Anusol Suppositories (HC and Plain)
- Explain expected effects of product use (relief of burning, itching, discomfort from irritated anorectal tissues with soothing, lubricating, coating action of mucous membranes).
- Explain that surface analgesia lasts for several hours after use.
- Tell the client to store below 86°F so suppositories do not melt. Do not freeze.

Self-Administration
- Apply externally in postpartum period (ointment); lower portion of anal canal (suppositories) (products usually not inserted rectally with a third- or fourth-degree laceration).
- Express small quantity *ointment* into 2- × 2-inch gauze square and place against swollen anorectal tissue (approximately five times per day) inside peripad.
- If *suppository* is ordered, tell client to keep refrigerated but not to freeze; remove wrapper before inserting in rectum (hold suppository upright and peel evenly down sides); do not hold suppository for prolonged period (it will melt); if the suppository softens before use, hold in foil wrapper under cold water for 2 to 3 min.

Safety
- Tell the client to avoid contact of the medication with eyes.
- Ascertain any client hypersensitivity, to any of the components of the ointment (e.g., promazine HCl 1%, mineral oil 46.7%, zinc oxide 12.5%).

Side Effects
- Ointment may cause burning sensation occasionally in some clients—especially if anoderm is *not* intact.
- Although rare, sensitivity/allergic reactions to ingredients may develop. Discontinue use if this occurs.
- If redness, irritation, swelling, or pain develops or increases, discontinue use and consult health care provider; also notify health care provider if bleeding occurs.

Nursing Process continued on following page

NURSING PROCESS *Continued*
PAIN RELIEF FROM PERINEAL WOUNDS AND HEMORRHOIDS

Promazine and Hydrocortisone (Proctofoam HC) and Promazine Hydrochloride (Proctofoam—OTC)
- Explain expected effects of product use.
- Explain that promazine HCl is not chemically related to "caine" type local anesthetics and there is a decreased chance of cross-sensitivity reactions in clients allergic to other local anesthetics.

Self-Administration
- Tell client that product is for anal or perianal use only. In postpartum clients, product is not inserted into rectum.
- Shake foam aerosol vigorously before use.
- Do not insert any part of aerosol container into anus.
- Tell client to hold the aerosol can upright to fill applicator and to have the plunger fully extended prior to filling.
- Express contents of applicator onto a 2- × 2-inch gauze pad and place against rectum inside peripad b.i.d. or t.i.d. and after bowel movement.
- Tell the client to take the applicator apart after each use and wash with warm water.

Safety
- Keep aerosol container away from visiting children in postpartum unit and later at home.
- Store below 120°F.
- Do not puncture or burn aerosol container.

Side Effects
- Tell client it is not known whether topical administration of corticosteroids could result in sufficient systemic absorption to produce detectable quantities in breast milk.
- Infrequently, burning, itching, irritation, dryness, folliculitis reactions, especially if occlusive dressings are used, may occur as local adverse reactions.

Dibucaine Ointment 1% (Nupercainal Ointment)
- Explain that the ointment is poorly absorbed through intact skin but that it is well absorbed through mucous membrane and excoriated skin.
- Explain that effects should begin to be perceived within 15 min and last for 2 to 4 h.

Self-Administration
- Instruct the client not to place the applicator in the rectum. Instead place medication from the applicator on a tissue or 2 × 2 pad and place against the anus.

Safety
- Stress not using product near the eyes, over denuded surface or blistered areas, or if there is rectal bleeding.
- Tell the client not to use more than 1 tube (30 g size) in 24 h.
- Keep product out of the reach of children.

Side Effects
- Ask if client has any known hypersensitivity to amide-type anesthetics; if so, product is contraindicated.
- Tell client local effects may include burning, tenderness, irritation, inflammation, and contact dermatitis; client should inform her health care provider if these should occur.
- Other adverse effects may include edema, cutaneous lesions, and/or urticaria.

Evaluation

- Evaluate pain using pain scale following use of products.
- Evaluate content of client communications for need for additional pain relief.
- Reevaluate characteristics of perineal/anal tissues for integrity and healing progress within accepted standard; also evaluate for lack of side effects.

Table 48–5
Drugs Used to Promote Postpartum Bowel Function

DRUG	DOSAGE	USES AND CONSIDERATIONS
Docusate sodium (Colace) 50 mg or 100 mg capsule Docusate calcium (Sur-fak) 240 mg capsule	50–200 mg PO daily usually h.s. 50–400 mg PO daily in 1–4 divided doses	Reduces surface tension of the oil-water interface of the stool, resulting in enhanced incorporation of water and fat, allowing for stool softening: PB: NA; onset: 12–72 h; t½: NA. Docusate salts are interchangeable (amount of Na, Ca, or K per dosage is clinically insignificant). *Pregnancy category:* C. Do not use concomitantly with mineral oil. Contraindicated if intestinal obstruction, acute abdominal pain, nausea, or vomiting present. Do not use >1 wk. Prolonged, frequent, or excessive use may cause bowel dependence or electrolyte imbalance. Side effects: rash. Compatible with breast feeding
Casanthranol with docusate sodium (Peri-Co-lace); docusate sodium, 100 mg; casanthranol, 30 mg	1–2 capsules PO usually h.s.	Mild stimulant laxative. Do not use if abdominal pain, nausea, or vomiting present. Effect on stool in 8–12 h, but may require up to 24 h. *Pregnancy category:* C. Should be taken with full glass of water. Adverse reactions: rash, abdominal cramping, diarrhea, nausea. Compatible with breast feeding. PB: NA; t½: NA
Docusate potassium (Di-alose)	1 capsule PO daily/ b.i.d.	Stool softener. Sodium free. *Pregnancy category:* C. Onset 12–72 h. See docusate sodium for additional information
Casanthranol with docusate potassium (Dialose Plus)	1 capsule PO b.i.d.	Mild stimulant laxative. Sodium. *Pregnancy category:* C. Onset 8–12 h, but may require up to 24 h. See casanthranol with docusate sodium for additional information
Bisacodyl USP (Dulcolax) (suppository 10 mg or tablet 5 mg)	2–3 tablets PO or 1 suppository	Stimulant laxative. Irritates smooth muscle of the intestine, possibly the colon and intramural plexus; alters water and electrolyte secretion, increasing intestinal fluid and producing laxative effect. Onset: 6–10 h PO; 15 min–1 h rectally. Absorption: <5% absorbed systemically following oral or rectal form. Metabolized in the liver to conjugated metabolites; eliminated in breast milk, bile, and urine. Do not crush tablets (enteric coated). Do not administer within 1 h of milk or antacid because enteric coating may dissolve, resulting in abdominal cramping and vomiting. Side effects: abdominal cramps, nausea, vomiting, rectal burning, electrolyte and fluid acidosis or alkalosis, hypocalcemia. *Pregnancy category:* C
Magnesium hydroxide (Milk of Magnesia)	15–60 mL PO h.s.	Laxative. Acts by increasing and retaining water in intestinal lumen, causing distention that stimulates peristalsis and bowel elimination. Poses risk to client with renal failure because 15%–30% of magnesium is systemically absorbed. Use with caution in patients with impaired renal function because hypermagnesemia and toxicity may occur as a result of decreased renal clearance of absorbed magnesium. *Pregnancy category:* B. Contraindicated in clients with colostomy, ileostomy, abdominal pain, nausea, vomiting, fecal impaction, renal failure. Drug interactions may occur with tetracyclines, digoxin, indomethacin, or iron salts, isoniazid. Milk of Magnesia concentrate is 3 × as potent as regular-strength product. Side effects: abdominal cramps, nausea. Other adverse reactions include hypotension, hyermagnesemia, muscle weakness, and respiratory depression. Onset: 4–8 h. Excreted by kidneys (absorbed portion); unabsorbed portion excreted in feces
Magnesium hydroxide with mineral oil (Haley's M-O)	15–30 mL PO h .s.	Mild saline laxative. Acts by drawing H_2O into gut, increasing intraluminal pressure and intestinal motility. Onset: 0.5–6 h. *Pregnancy category:* B. Equivalent to magnesium hydroxide
Mineral oil (Agoral)	15–45 mL PO once daily or in divided doses	Lubricant laxative eases passages of stool by decreasing water absorption and lubricating the intestine. *Pregnancy category:* C. Onset: 6–8 h; t½: NA; PB: NA; peak; UK; duration: UK. May

Table continued on following page

Table 48–5 *Continued*
Drugs Used to Promote Postpartum Bowel Function

DRUG	DOSAGE	USES AND CONSIDERATIONS
		impair absorption of fat-soluble vitamins (A, D, E, K), oral contraceptives, coumarin, sulfonamides. Generally recommend avoidance of bedtime doses due to risk of aspiration (lipid pneumonitis). Contraindicated in clients with ileostomy, colostomy, appendicitis, ulcerative colitis, diverticulitis. Best administered on an empty stomach. Do not give with food or meals because of risk of aspiration and decreased fat-soluble vitamin absorption. Side effects: nausea, vomiting, diarrhea, abdominal cramps
Senna (Senokot)	10–15 mL syrup h.s.; 2–4 tablets PO b.i.d.	Stimulant laxative. Acts by local irritant effect on colon to promote peristalsis and bowel evacuation. Also increases moisture content of stool by accumulating fluids in intestine. Contraindicated in clients with fluid and electrolyte disturbances, abdominal pain, nausea and vomiting. Excreted in breast milk. *Pregnancy category:* C. Onset: 6–24 h; metabolized in the liver; eliminated in the feces (viable) and in urine. $t\frac{1}{2}$: NA. Drug interactions may occur with monoamine oxidase (MAO) inhibitors, disulfiram, metronidazole, procarbazine. May discolor urine or feces; liquid syrups contain 7% alcohol. May create laxative dependence and loss of bowel function with prolonged use
Simethicone (Mylicon) (chewable tablets 40 mg, 80 mg)	1 tablet q.i.d. p.c. and h.s. up to 6 × per d as needed	Antiflatulent. Acts by dispersing and preventing formation of mucus-surrounded gas pockets in GI tract; changes surface tension of gas bubbles and allows them to coalesce, making them easier to eliminate as belching and rectal flatus. *Pregnancy category:* C. Onset: UK; $t\frac{1}{2}$: UK. Excreted unchanged in the feces. May interfere with results of guaiac tests of gastric aspirates; must be chewed thoroughly before swallowing; suggest client drink a full glass of water after tablets are chewed. Double doses should not be taken to make up for missed doses. No known side effects; store below 40°C (140°F) in well-closed container

KEY: NA: not applicable; PB: protein-binding; $t\frac{1}{2}$: half-life; UK: unknown.

controlled through drug therapy by use of one of three agents: chlorotrianisene (Tace), Deladumone OB (combination of estrogen plus androgen in the form of estradiol valerate and testosterone enanthate), or bromocriptine mesylate (Parlodel). The first two agents are estrogenic substances that suppress lactation through localized inhibitory effects on the alveolar breast cells responsible for milk secretion. The third agent, a dopamine receptor agonist, is nonhormonal and acts at a systemic level on the anterior pituitary gland to inhibit the secretion of **prolactin,** which causes the milk glands to produce milk. High levels are necessary to initiate lactation. Estrogenic substances are much less popular than in the past because of the increased incidence of thrombophlebitis associated with the dosage needed to suppress lactation, as well as concerns about potential carcinogenic effects. In August 1994, the Food and Drug Administration (FDA) officially withdrew its support for the use of bromocriptine as a lactation suppressant because of the resultant severe hyperten-

sion secondary to vasospasm in some clients, ineffectiveness of the drug in some, and a rebound effect (lactation occurrence) in some. The drug is still approved for other medical conditions.

Promotion of Bowel Function

Constipation is common during the postpartum period because of the residual effects of progesterone on smooth muscle coupled with decreased peristalsis and relaxation of the abdominal muscles. Nonpharmacologic measures (high-fiber foods, early ambulation, at least 64 oz of fluids a day, prompt response to the defecation urge) are generally instituted after delivery.

Pharmacologic measures include the use of stool softeners, laxative stimulants, and, for the postcesarean client, antiflatulents. Table 48–5 presents examples of agents used to promote bowel function during the postpartum period. (See Chapter 41 for additional information about these drug groups.)

NURSING PROCESS
LAXATIVES

Assessment

- Note time of delivery, predelivery food intake, predelivery bowel emptying measures used (if any).
- Obtain history of bowel problems.
- Assess the client for bowel sounds in all four quadrants (particularly postcesarean section delivery) and abdominal distention.

Potential Nursing Diagnoses

- Potential for altered bowel elimination: high risk for constipation related to perineal discomfort, decreased peristalsis, and use of codeine
- Fear of discomfort at time of first postdelivery bowel movement (especially if extensive episiotomy or hemorrhoids present)

Planning

- Client will have a bowel movement by 2 to 4 days postpartum.
- Client will resume normal prepregnancy bowel elimination pattern within 6 weeks.

Nursing Interventions

Docusate Sodium and Casanthranol with Docusate Sodium; Docusate Potassium and Casanthranol with Docusate Potassium

- Store at room temperature.
- If a liquid preparation is ordered, give with milk or fruit juice to mask bitter taste.
- Assess client for any history of laxative dependence.
- Drug interaction may occur with mineral oil, phenolphthalein, aspirin.

Bisacodyl USP

- Store tablets and suppositories below 77°F and avoid excess humidity.
- Do not crush tablets.
- Do not administer within 1 h of milk or antacid because enteric coating may dissolve, resulting in abdominal cramping and vomiting.

Mineral Oil

- Do not give with or immediately after meals.
- Give with fruit juice or carbonated drinks to disguise taste.

Magnesium Hydroxide

- Shake container well.
- Do not give 1 to 2 h before or after PO drugs because of effects on absorption.
- Note that milk of magnesia concentrate is three times as potent as regular-strength product.
- If PO antibiotics are administered in the puerperium, avoid giving at same time; give laxative 1 h before or 1 h after antibiotic.

Senna

- Protect from light and heat.

Simethicone

- Administer after meals and at bedtime.

Nursing Process continued on following page

NURSING PROCESS *Continued*
LAXATIVES

Client Teaching

General
- Explain that oral stool softeners are not given to cause bowel evacuation, but to provide for a bowel movement without straining.
- Caution all clients against becoming laxative dependent.
- Instruct clients regarding temperature and storage requirements for particular drugs.

Docusate Sodium and Casanthranol with Docusate Sodium and Docusate Potassium and Casanthranol with Docusate Potassium
- Drink at least six 8-oz glasses of liquid daily to make stool softer. Drink one glass with each dose.
- If dosage form ordered is liquid, take with milk or fruit juice to mask bitter taste.
- Explain that many laxatives contain sodium. Tell client to check with health care provider or pharmacist before using laxative if on a low-sodium diet.
- Tell client not to take drug if she is already taking mineral oil or having acute abdominal pain, nausea, vomiting, or signs of intestinal obstruction.
- Tell client she should not use products for longer than 1 week and that prolonged, frequent, or excessive use may result in dependence on drug or electrolyte imbalance.
- Tell client to report to health care provider if skin rash occurs. If stomach or intestinal cramping occurs and does not diminish, inform health care provider.

Senna
- Tell client that drug may discolor urine or feces.
- Tell client to discontinue the drug if abdominal pain occurs.
- Tell client syrup form is 7% alcohol.

Mineral Oil
- Tell client not to take other laxatives (e.g., docusate products) if she is already taking mineral oil.
- Tell client to take mineral oil on an empty stomach; do not take with food or meals because of risk of aspiration and decreased fat-soluble vitamin absorption.
- Avoid bedtime doses because of risk of aspiration.
- Tell client to report any occurrence of nausea, vomiting, diarrhea, or abdominal cramp.

Magnesium Hydroxide
- Tell client that laxative action generally occurs in 4 to 8 h.
- Tell client to be aware of whether she is using regular strength or concentrated form of drug, because concentrate is three times as potent as regular strength.
- Tell client that drug may interact with tetracyclines, digoxin, indomethacin, iron salts, isoniazid; be certain any health care provider seen is aware of the use of this or any drug.
- Tell client to report any muscular weakness, diarrhea, or abdominal cramps.

Simethicone
- Tell client that drug will help relieve gas pains in the stomach and intestines.
- Explain the need to chew tablets thoroughly and to take after meals. Drink a full glass of water after chewing the tablets.
- Tell client that if a dose is missed, to take it as soon as possible; however, if the time is close to next scheduled dose, skip the missed dose and take the scheduled dose. Do not double doses.

Evaluation

- Evaluate the effectiveness of the drug. Return of prepregnancy regular bowel function occurs.

SIDE EFFECTS AND ADVERSE REACTIONS

The following side effects have been reported: *docusate sodium:* bitter taste, throat irritation, rash; *casanthranol and docusate sodium:* nausea, abdominal cramping, diarrhea, and rash; *bisacodyl suppositories:* proctitis and inflammation; *magnesium hydroxide:* abdominal cramps and nausea; *senna:* nausea, vomiting, diarrhea, abdominal cramps, can also result in diarrhea in breast-fed infants; *mineral oil:* nausea, vomiting, diarrhea, abdominal cramps, also lipid pneumonitis (if aspirated).

IMMUNIZATIONS
Rh₀ (D) Immune Globulin

During pregnancy, an Rh-negative client who lacks the Rh factor in her own blood may carry a fetus who is either Rh-negative or Rh-positive. The circulatory systems of client and baby do not mix during pregnancy unless an event occurs that allows some fetal blood cells to enter the maternal bloodstream. Such a situation can happen with early spontaneous or induced abortions, ectopic pregnancy, amniocentesis, chorionic villus sampling, prenatal bleeding caused by abruptio placentae, and separation of the placenta from the uterine wall at delivery. If the client and fetus are both Rh-negative, there is no difficulty. However, if the fetus is Rh-positive, the Rh-negative client is at risk for **Rh sensitization** (i.e., the development of protective antibodies against Rh-positive blood) unless preventive measures are employed. The reason why it is important to prevent formation of these antibodies is that, once created, they remain throughout life and create hemolytic difficulties for fetuses in subsequent pregnancies. Although the circulatory systems of the client and fetus do not normally mix, the protective antibodies that have been formed against Rh-positive blood are small enough to cross the placenta and cause rapid hemolysis in any Rh-positive fetus (Fig. 48–1).

The Rh sensitization process can be prevented through the administration of **Rh₀ (D) immune globulin** (RhoGAM) to nonsensitized Rh-negative clients following each actual or potential exposure to Rh-positive blood. Table 48–6 presents the drug data for Rh₀ (D) immune globulin.

SIDE EFFECTS AND ADVERSE REACTIONS

Side effects are rare, but include fever and pain at the injection site.

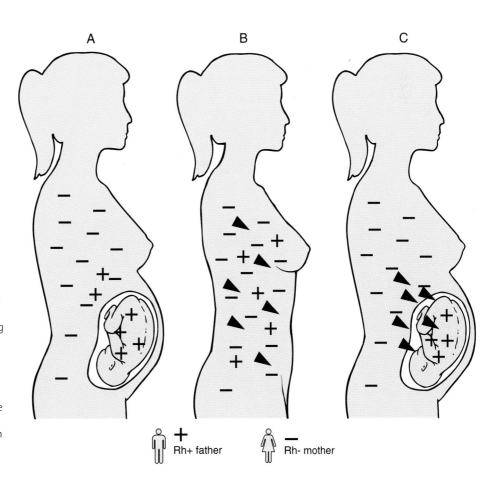

Figure 48–1

Understanding Rh isoimmunization. A, During pregnancy or delivery, a small amount of fetal blood may enter the mother's circulation. B, When the mother is Rh negative and is pregnant with an Rh-positive fetus, the mother's immune system responds by producing anti-Rh₀ (D) antibodies ▲. C, In subsequent pregnancies, these antibodies cross the placenta and enter the fetal circulation; when the fetus is Rh positive, the anti-Rh₀ (D) antibodies will attack the fetal red blood cells and cause hemolysis. (From Nichols, F., and Zwelling, E. [1997]. Maternal-Newborn Nursing: Theory and Practice. Philadelphia: W.B. Saunders.)

A   B   C

+ Rh+ father   − Rh- mother

Table 48–6
RH$_0$ (D) Immune Globulin (RhoGAM)

DOSE AND ROUTE	USES AND CONSIDERATIONS
Given IM in deltoid	A sterile concentrated solution of gamma globulin prepared from human serum containing antibodies to the Rh factor (D antigen), also expressed as anti-Rh$_0$ (D). Administered to nonsensitized Rh-negative clients. Action is to suppress active antibody response and formation of anti-Rh$_0$ (D) in Rh-negative clients exposed to RH-positive blood. Promotes destruction of Rh-positive fetal cells in maternal serum before mother can make antibodies that would cause hemolysis of RBCs in Rh-positive fetuses and newborns in subsequent pregnancies. Never give IV. *Pregnancy category:* C. Use with caution in thrombocytopenia or bleeding disorders and in IgA deficiency. Contraindicated in clients with known hypersensitivity to immune globulins or thimerosal, transfusion of Rh$_0$ (D)-positive blood in previous 3 mon or prior sensitization to Rh$_0$ (D). Adverse reactions: lethargy, splenomegaly, elevated bilirubin, myalgia, temperature elevation; most commonly (rare) fever and pain at injection site. Appears in breast milk (not absorbed by infant). $t_{\frac{1}{2}}$: 23–26 d. 1 vial (300 μg) prevents maternal sensitization if fetal red cell volume that entered maternal circulation is <15 mL. Additional vials given if more.
300 μg (1 vial) (standard dose)	Standard dose given at 28 wk gestation as prophylaxis and again after normal delivery (within 72 h) based on titer. Also given after amniocentesis. Larger than standard dose may be given if tests show large fetal-maternal blood transfusion has occurred.
50 μg (1 vial) (microdose)	Microdose given after abortion or early genetic testing (less than 12 wk gestation). Because it is a blood product, some clients may refuse because of their religious beliefs.

KEY: IM: intramuscular; IV: intravenous; $t_{\frac{1}{2}}$: half-life; RBC: red blood cell.

Rubella Vaccine

Maternal rubella is a potentially devastating infection for the fetus, depending on gestational age. If a non-immunized client contracts the virus during the first trimester, a high rate of abortion and neurologic and developmental sequelae associated with **congenital rubella syndrome** may result. Cataracts, glaucoma, deafness, heart defects, and mental retardation are seen. When infection occurs later in pregnancy, there is less risk of fetal damage because of the developmental stage of the fetus. There is no treatment for maternal or congenital rubella infection, so the goal is prevention of rubella in the childbearing population. Table 48–7 presents the drug data for rubella vaccine.

Table 48–7
Rubella Virus Vaccine, Live, MSD (Meruvax II) (Ra27/3 Strain)

DOSE AND ROUTE	USES AND CONSIDERATIONS
Given subcutaneously: 0.5 mL into outer aspect of upper arm	Live virus vaccine for immunization against German measles. Dose is the same for all persons, using either single dose or multidose vials. Do not give immune serum globulin (ISG) concurrent with vaccine. Contraindicated in pregnant women and clients with anaphylactoid reactions to neomycin, febrile respiratory illness or other febrile infection, active untreated tuberculosis, or immune deficiency conditions. Vaccinated persons can shed but not transmit the virus. Defer vaccination for 3 mo after blood or plasma transfusions; also after human ISG. Postpartum clients who received blood products may be vaccinated if repeat titer is drawn 6–8 wk later to ensure that seroconversion occurred. Excreted in breast milk; use caution. *Pregnancy category:* X. Side effects: burning, stinging at injection site; malaise; fever; headache; slight rash 2–4 wk after injection; joint pain 1–3 d within 1–10 wk of injection.

NURSING PROCESS
RH₀ (D) IMMUNE GLOBULIN

Assessment

- Determine blood type and Rh status of all prenatal clients.
- Assess the client for her understanding of her Rh status and her partner's Rh status.
- Ask the client whether she has had previous pregnancies and their outcome; ask whether she has ever received Rh₀ (D) immune globulin.
- Follow agency protocols for Rh blood work-up for client and baby at time of delivery.
- Postpartum, assess data about newborn's Rh type (if baby is Rh negative, no need for drug; if baby is Rh positive [mother negative], and mother is *not* sensitized [indirect Coombs' test negative] and the baby is direct Coombs' test negative, the mother is a candidate to receive the injection [to *prevent* antibody production, i.e., "sensitization"]).
- Obtain client's permission to receive the drug. A refusal form is required in some institutions if the drug is declined.
- Assess for history of allergy to immune globulin products.

Potential Nursing Diagnoses

- Knowledge deficit related to Rh incompatibility and sensitization
- Knowledge deficit related to Rh₀ (D) immune globulin and when and why drug is needed

Planning

- Client will receive Rh₀ (D) immune globulin as indicated within 72 h after delivery or miscarriage.
- Client will be able to explain the Rh process and actions client will need to take in subsequent pregnancies.

Nursing Interventions

- Document Rh work-up and eligibility of client to receive drug in written client record using agency protocol. Convey information in verbal report.
- Carefully check any lot numbers on vial and laboratory slip for agreement before administration; also check expiration date. Check ID band and laboratory slip for matching number. Return required slips to laboratory or blood bank.
- Give drug as soon as possible postpartum, definitely within 72 h.
- Give drug IM in deltoid.
- Drug needs to be stored at 36° to 46°F.

Client Teaching

General
- Explain to the client the purposes of the drug and review the literature with her.
- Provide the client with written documentation of date of administration for client's personal health record.

Evaluation

- Evaluate client's understanding of the need for Rh₀ (D) immune globulin.

SIDE EFFECTS AND ADVERSE REACTIONS

Side effects are generally mild and temporary. Burning or stinging at the injection site is due to the acidic pH of the vaccine. Regional lymphadenopathy, urticaria, rash, malaise, sore throat, fever, headache, polyneuritis, arthralgia, and moderate fever are also seen.

DRUGS ADMINISTERED TO THE NEWBORN IMMEDIATELY AFTER DELIVERY

Drugs routinely administered to the newborn are erythromycin ophthalmic ointment to provide pro-

NURSING PROCESS
RUBELLA VACCINE

Assessment

- Obtain a history and laboratory results indicating a need for rubella vaccine. Pregnant clients should not receive the rubella vaccine.
- Women with a rubella titer of less than 1:10 (or who are ELISA [enzyme-linked immunosorbent assay] antibody negative) are considered to be suitable postpartum recipients for the vaccine.
- Interview client and/or conduct chart review to determine whether client has
  - Received blood transfusions within past 3 mo, plasma transfusion, or human immune serum globulin.
  - Anaphylactic or anaphylactoid reactions to neomycin (dose contains 25 μg of neomycin).
  - Received other virus vaccines within 1 mo. (Do not give <1 mo before or after other virus vaccines.)
  - Active, untreated tuberculosis (TB).
  - Exhibited a primary or acquired immunodeficiency state (AIDS or other clinical manifestations of human immunodeficiency virus [HIV] infection).
  - Any febrile or respiratory illness or other active febrile infection.
- Rubella vaccine is contraindicated if any of the above exist.
- Determine whether client is also a candidate to receive Rh_0 (D) immune globulin (RhoGAM).
- Outcome may be suppression of rubella antibodies with need to recheck titer in approximately 3 mo.

Potential Nursing Diagnoses

- Knowledge deficit related to risk of rubella infection and its prevention
- Risk of injury related to rubella infection in subsequent pregnancy secondary to lack of immunity

Planning

- Client will receive the rubella vaccine to protect against rubella (also known as German measles).
- Client will state in her own words the specific plan she has to prevent pregnancy for 3 mo following injection and accurately describe how to use pregnancy prevention methods.

Nursing Interventions

- Protect vaccine from light and store it at 35.6 to 46.4°F before reconstitution.
- Use only the supplied diluent to reconstitute and use within 8 h.
- Give SC only; never inject IV.
- If tuberculin test is to be done, administer it before or simultaneously with rubella vaccine (may have temporary depression in tuberculin skin sensitivity).

Skill: Reconstitution

- Single-dose vial: withdraw entire amount of diluent into syringe.
- Inject total volume into vial of lyophilized vaccine and agitate to mix thoroughly.
- Withdraw entire contents into syringe and inject total volume of restored vaccine.
- Have epinephrine readily available in case of anaphylactic shock.
- Clearly convey in writing and verbal report that vaccination has occurred.
- Record date of administration, lot number, manufacturer, name, and title to comply with federal law.

Client Teaching

General

- Discuss the importance of immunity to rubella with client and help her understand the need to obtain titers to determine immune status.

Nursing Process continued on following page

NURSING PROCESS *Continued*
RUBELLA VACCINE

- Teach client measures to ensure adequate birth control for 3 mo after vaccine injection.
- Tell client that there is no risk to her from being near small children who received the injection even if she is pregnant and not immune.

Side Effects
- Tell client that the most common side effect is burning or stinging at site of injection; some also experience malaise, fever, headache, and slight rash about 2 to 4 wk after injection. One to 10 weeks after injection, some may experience joint pain that lasts 1 to 3 days.

Safety
- Recommend that client have titer rechecked if she also received RhoGAM.

Evaluation

- Evaluate the need for rubella vaccine.

---

phylaxis against eye infections (legally required in the United States), and vitamin K, to prevent hemorrhagic disease. In addition, a disinfectant may be applied to the cord stump during the first few hours after birth. However, recent reports in the literature support the alternative (i.e., "dry cord care") with no agents applied. Table 48–8 presents data for drugs administered to the newborn immediately after delivery.

Side Effects and Adverse Reactions

ERYTHROMYCIN OPHTHALMIC OINTMENT
Side effects include chemical conjunctivitis in about 20% of newborns, which manifests as swelling and inflammation lasting about 24 to 48 h. This may interfere slightly with eye-to-eye contact between parents and newborn.

Table 48–8
Drugs Administered to the Newborn Immediately After Delivery

DRUG	DOSAGE	USES AND CONSIDERATIONS
Erythromycin ophthalmic ointment	$\frac{1}{2}$ inch ribbon of ointment placed in lower conjunctival sac of each eye within 1 h of delivery	Prevention of gonococcal conjunctivitis (ophthalmia neonatorum), which can cause blindness. Also prevents chlamydial conjunctivitis. Source of infection is birth canal. Contains antibiotic (erythromycin) in sterile base of mineral oil and white petrolatum. Has bactericidal or bacteriostatic action based on concentration per gram and the target organisms present. Side effects: chemical conjunctivitis (swelling, inflammation 24–48 h)
Phytonadione (Vitamin K₁, Mephyton, Aqua-MEPHYTON, Konakion)	0.5–1.0 mg IM into anterior or lateral thigh within 1 h after birth	Oral anticoagulant antagonist. An aqueous colloidal solution of vitamin K₁. Newborn does not receive adequate vitamin K transplacentally and is unable to initially synthesize vitamin because of limited intestinal flora; therefore, production of clotting factors in liver is hindered and low prothrombin levels are evidenced. Phytonadione facilitates production of clotting factors equal to natural vitamin K. Newborns of mothers who received oral anticoagulants or anticonvulsants during pregnancy may need higher dosage. Dose may be repeated in 6–8 h. Side effects: pain and edema at injection site; possible allergic reactions include urticaria and rash; those who receive larger doses may exhibit hyperbilirubinemia and jaundice.

NURSING PROCESS
DRUGS ADMINISTERED TO THE NEWBORN AFTER DELIVERY

Assessment

Erythromycin Ophthalmic Ointment
• Assess baby for signs of hypersensitivity.

Phytonadione (Vitamin K₁)
• Assess newborn for bleeding from umbilical cord, circumcision site, nose, and GI tract, and for generalized ecchymoses.

Potential Nursing Diagnosis

• Potential risk of injury related to infectious process (congenital) and/or transient low prothrombin levels in the newborn

Planning

• Newborn will be free of side effects from drugs routinely received after delivery.

Nursing Interventions

Erythromycin Ophthalmic Ointment
• See procedure for administration of eye ointments (see Chapter 3).
• Delay instillation no more than 1 h; promote eye contact between parents and the baby during this period.
• Wear gloves for handling the newborn during instillations.
• Do not place tube of ointment under radiant warmer with baby before administration.
• Do not irrigate eyes following instillation.

Phytonadione (Vitamin K₁)
• Protect from light because of photosensitivity of the preparation.

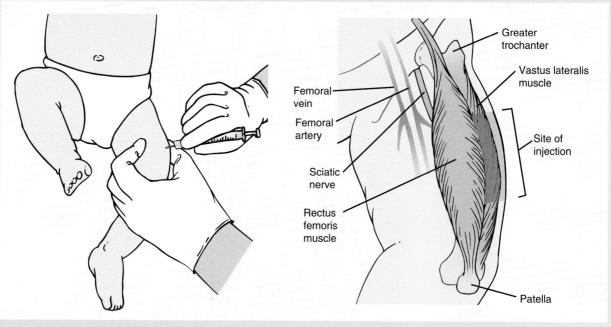

Figure 48–2
Site for giving an IM injection to a newborn shortly after birth. (From Nichols, F., and Zwelling, E. [1997]. Maternal-Newborn Nursing: Theory and Practice. Philadelphia: W.B. Saunders.)

Nursing Process continued on following page

NURSING PROCESS *Continued*
DRUGS ADMINISTERED TO THE NEWBORN AFTER DELIVERY

* Observe injection site for swelling and inflammation. (Refer to Fig. 48–2 and Chapter 3 for site.)
* The injection area should be bathed with soap and water before the injection

Client Teaching

Erythromycin Ophthalmic Ointment
* Tell parents that any swelling around eyes will usually disappear within 24 to 48 h.
* Explain that administration of eye prophylaxis is a legal requirement and that there is no harm to vision from the ointment.

Phytonadione (Vitamin K₁)
* Explain the need for the drug to parents so they do not think there is something wrong with their baby when they see an injection being given.

Evaluation

* Evaluate documentation of required drugs.

PHYTONADIONE (VITAMIN K₁)

Side effects include pain and edema at the site of the injection. Some allergic reactions, manifested by urticaria and rash, have been reported. Babies who receive larger doses may exhibit hyperbilirubinemia and jaundice resulting from competition for binding sites.

Immunization During the Newborn Period Prior to Discharge

Since 1991, the American Academy of Pediatrics and the Centers for Disease Control and Prevention (CDC) have recommended that immunization against hepatitis B virus (HBV) begin in the newborn period. The

---

Table 48–9
Hepatitis B Immunization in the Newborn Period

DRUG	DOSAGE	USES AND CONSIDERATIONS
Hepatitis B vaccine (Engerix B)	For newborns of HBsAg-*positive* mothers: 0.5 mL (10 μg) IM *within* 12 h after birth (first dose); repeated at 1 mo and 6 mo. (In addition, hepatitis B immune globulin [HBIG] is given with the first dose of hepatitis B vaccine for infants of infected mothers.) For newborns of HBsAg-*negative* mothers: 0.5 mL (10 μg) IM before discharge but no later than 2 mo of age; followed by repeat doses at 1–2 mo and 6–18 mo. (If unlikely to return for routine immunizations, may give repeat doses at 4 mo and 6–18 mo.)	Product is a recombinant hepatitis B vaccine used for immunization against infection caused by hepatitis B virus (HBV). Given to all infants regardless of HBsAg status of mother. Unvaccinated infants *younger than* 12 mo old with a mother or primary care giver with acute hepatitis B should be given HBIG because of risk of becoming an HBV carrier following infection (also start HBV vaccine series). Must be injected IM into anterolateral thigh; never inject IV. Following three doses >90% of infants and children will seroconvert. Protection in those who seroconvert will last 3–7 y with a single booster. Contraindicated if hypersensitivity to any component of vaccine (e.g., yeast)—no reports of problems published. Neonatal side effects: soreness at injection site with swelling, warmth, redness, and induration. *Pregnancy category:* C

NURSING PROCESS
HEPATITIS B VACCINE

Assessment

- Review prenatal record laboratory data for HBsAg-status of mother.
- Validate whether infant is to receive hepatitis B vaccine singly or in concert with HBIG.

Potential Nursing Diagnoses

- Injury, risk for hepatitis B infection
- Knowledge deficit related to hepatitis B and prophylaxis (maternal)

Planning

- The newborn will receive correct dosage of hepatitis B vaccine before discharge, including HBIG, if indicated.
- The newborn's caregiver will know the dates to go to primary health care provider for repeat doses.

Nursing Interventions

Skill
- Do not dilute.
- Shake well before withdrawal from vial.
- Discard if other than slightly opaque white suspension.
- Have epinephrine available for allergic reaction.
- Use full recommended dose of the vaccine.
- Monitor baby's temperature postinjection per agency protocol.

Safety
- Give IM in anterolateral thigh.
- Document site used in chart.
- Record lot number, expiration date, name, title in chart.
- Store product at 2° to 8°C.
- Do not freeze (destroys potency).

Client Teaching

General
- Inform mother of implications of her HBsAg-positive or -negative status for her newborn and recommended interventions.
- Have mother read literature and sign permission for administration of vaccine (place copy in newborn's chart).
- Inform mother when repeat doses need to be given.

Evaluation

- Evaluate mother's understanding of the need for hepatitis B vaccine for her baby.

goal is prevention of HBV infection that may result in serious long-term liver disease, cancer, and death in adulthood for the entire population through the reduction of chronic carriers of the virus.

In pregnancy, HBV transmission occurs vertically, primarily at the time of delivery. For those infants born to HBsAg-positive mothers, it is believed that infection can be prevented in 90% through postdeliv-ery screening and injection of both hepatitis B immune globulin (HBIG) and hepatitis B vaccine.

The current recommendation is that newborn infants be given three injections intramuscularly in the anterolateral thigh following a protocol based on their mother's HBsAg-positive or -negative status. Table 48–9 presents hepatitis B vaccine data for the newborn.

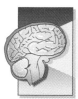

Critical Thinking In Action

Tanya, age 17 years, is the client you planned care for during labor induction in Chapter 47. Tanya was sent to the hospital for labor induction/augmentation at 42 weeks' gestation by her health care provider, because of her "post dates" pregnancy and signs and symptoms of pregnancy-induced hypertension. Tanya's mother arrived at the hospital when Tanya was dilated 8 cm, in time for the latter stages of Tanya's labor. Her mother remained as Tanya's support person throughout the delivery, which occurred at 6 AM by vacuum extraction. Tanya had a continuous epidural for her labor and delivery. An episiotomy was necessary at the time of delivery and a fourth-degree laceration occurred. A cluster of hemorrhoids is evident. Baby Jessica weighing 8 pounds and 7 ounces, had an Apgar score of 7 and 9. The baby is alert and active. Although Tanya has had three pregnancies, this is the first that has resulted in a live birth. Tanya is not married. She lives with her mother and has been going to high school and working part-time in a retail auto parts store. Tanya plans to keep this baby. She would like to breast feed "for at least 3 months." She plans on finishing school and returning to work in 6 weeks.

Immediately after the delivery, you conduct an assessment of Tanya, analyze the data, and determine and prioritize her nursing care needs. You do the same for the baby.

1. Based on the data supplied about the episiotomy, define a priority nursing diagnosis for Tanya.
2. Define an outcome-based goal for the diagnosis you stated.
3. Describe how you would intervene in regard to the episiotomy during the early postpartum period, integrating both pharmacologic and nonpharmacologic measures. Orders include benzocaine spray, witch hazel pads, Proctofoam HC, ibuprofen tablets (200 mg) at the bedside.

Baby Jessica's newborn medications must be administered within the first hour. You are also trying to promote bonding for Tanya with the baby.

4. Within the standard, how could you promote bonding, including eye contact between mother and baby, and also handle eye prophylaxis?
5. State the steps you will follow to instill the ointment into the baby's eyes, including safety aspects for yourself.
6. What would you teach Tanya about the side effects of eye prophylaxis?
7. Describe the reason for the vitamin K_1 injection for the baby in terms Tanya can understand.
8. State the steps you will follow to prepare and give the vitamin K_1 injection, including safety aspects for yourself.

Tanya is Rh negative. The baby's father's blood type is unknown. A cord blood was drawn on the baby at the time of delivery. Based on Tanya's historical data:

9. What would you be concerned about in terms of defining her as a likely or unlikely RhoGAM candidate? What information about mother and baby will be needed to aid in the decision?

Assuming Tanya is a RhoGAM candidate:

10. Define a nursing diagnosis for Tanya.
11. Define an outcome-based goal for the diagnosis you stated.
12. State the timeframe in which you would want to administer the globulin and the rationale for this timeframe.

text continued next page

13. Explain what verbal and written documentation must be addressed in regard to RhoGAM administration, both prior to administration and following administration.

14. Tanya's chart reveals that her rubella titer is 1:6. What is the implication of this titer for Tanya?

15. While reviewing Tanya's medication administration record, you notice that in the section that addresses known allergies, neomycin is listed. Considering Tanya's titer, the standing health care provider's order, and your knowledge about this vaccine, describe how you would handle the situation.

16. In a situation in which a mother is both a rubella and RhoGAM candidate, with both products being administered, what is one major piece of information the nurse should share with the client in regard to the rubella titer?

Because of her episiotomy, Tanya is concerned about having a first bowel movement. You tell her that the docusate with casanthranol product she will be supplied will help.

17. Tanya says that she does not want to take the docusate because she plans to breast feed. What nursing diagnosis could you state based on Tanya's communication?

18. Describe how you might address Tanya's concerns based on your knowledge of the product and breast feeding.

Tanya asks what can be done about the hemorrhoids. You tell her about the mode of action of the ordered pharmacologic products. She states, "So I just have to insert this syringe-type applicator up my rectum once I fill it from the big can?"

19. Analyze Tanya's communication. What is correct and incorrect in regard to the content?

20. What nursing diagnosis is appropriate for Tanya on the basis of the data supplied?

21. Describe what client teaching you need to do.

Baby Jessica is ordered to receive hepatitis B vaccine prior to discharge. Tanya is listed as being HbsAg negative.

22. Which babies are eligible to receive hepatitis B vaccine?

23. How many doses constitute the total series, and what is the time period for these?

24. What is the purpose of giving newborns this vaccine? Why is this important in today's society?

25. Tanya asks how long the baby's immunity should last provided that seroconversion occurs. How would you answer Tanya?

26. Where would you expect to find the vaccine stored at the hospital?

27. Describe the written documentation required with administration of this vaccine as a part of the permanent record.

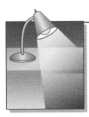

Study Questions

1. A client was supposed to chew her simethicone tablets at 8 AM, but she forgot. It is now 11:15 AM. She asks if she should chew them now or wait and take extra at the scheduled noon dose. What would you tell her? What is your rationale?

2. Describe what you would tell a newly admitted postpartum (vaginal delivery) client about the process of self-administered drugs and the specific products included. Why would you select this material?

3. What client data are required prior to postpartum administration of ergot derivatives (e.g., methergine)? (See Chapter 47.)

4. For what should the nurse assess a client prior to the client initiating laxative products?

5. Sarah is a 24-year-old woman who delivered her baby 24 h ago. She has a history of drug and alcohol abuse. Her health care provider ordered senna syrup for her as a stimulant laxative. What action would you take? Why?

6. Why are bedtime doses of mineral oil not generally recommended?

7. Your client complains during the postpartum period of "pain in my bottom where the doctor cut me." Her chart states that she has a fourth-degree laceration. What pharmacologic products are available to help this client, in addition to nonpharmacologic comfort measures? How will these help the client?

8. Mary, a postpartum client, has an order for promazine and hydrocortisone. You discover she has the product at her bedside but has not used it. When questioned, Mary said, "Oh, I forgot to tell you, I'm allergic to things like lidocaine, benzocaine." What response could you correctly make to Mary?

9. What are three aspects to evaluate concerning drugs/products for relief of pain from perineal wounds and hemorrhoids?

10. A client tells you she doesn't see any reason to use her dibucaine ointment because it "feels like nothing on my hand—not cooling or soothing—so it probably won't help my bottom." How could you correctly respond with factual information?

11. Why is a newborn given an injection of vitamin K_1 following delivery?

12. What prophylactic agent is used after delivery for newborn eye care? In what time period should it be given? How is it administered?

13. In what site would you administer hepatitis B vaccine to a newborn?

49 Drugs Related to Women's Health and Disorders

JANE PURNELL TAYLOR and LINDA GOODWIN

Outline

Objectives

- Describe the types, expected actions, and side effects of oral contraceptive products.
- Recognize new hormonal/pharmacologic products related to conception control.
- Explain the expected effects of medications used to treat uterine dysfunction, including premenstrual syndrome, endometriosis, and menopause.
- Describe nursing process, including client teaching, associated with the drugs used for women's health and disorders.

Terms

dyspareunia

endometriosis

estrogen replacement therapy (ERT)

follicular phase

hormone replacement therapy (HRT)

luteal phase

menopause

oral contraceptives

ovulatory phase

premenstrual syndrome

progestin

INTRODUCTION

Oral contraceptive products and medications for uterine dysfunction and menopause are described in this chapter. Nursing interventions and client teaching are emphasized.

ORAL CONTRACEPTIVE PRODUCTS

Among the various methods of contraception available, the **oral contraceptives** that employ hormone therapy enjoy wide popularity because of their ease of use and high degree of effectiveness with relative safety for most women. When these steroidal agents were first approved for use by the Food and Drug Administration (FDA) in 1960, little was known about the best combinations of drugs to use or optimum doses. Adverse side effects, particularly circulatory disorders, were frequent. Subsequent research has resulted in lower-dose drugs. Research continues to focus on actual and potential short- and long-term benefits and risks associated with use of low-dose oral contraceptives and new administration forms (e.g., long-acting progestin-releasing subcutaneous implants), particularly in the areas of circulatory risks and carcinogenesis. Immunologic methods of contraception are another area of current research.

There are two main types of oral contraceptives: the estrogen-progestin combination products, often referred to as "the pill," and the progestin-only products, sometimes called "the mini-pill." The combination products have the lowest pregnancy rate.

Estrogen-Progestin Combination Products

Combined estrogen-progestin oral contraceptive products prevent pregnancy by suppressing pituitary release of follicle-stimulating hormone (FSH) and luteinizing hormone (LH), which are needed to mature a graafian follicle in the ovary, thereby inhibiting ovulation. These agents also create changes in the endometrium that make it less favorable for implantation of a fertilized ovum. In addition, the quantity and viscosity of the cervical mucus is changed by progestins, making it hostile to sperm. Alterations in motility within the fallopian tube may also impede the movement of the ova.

The most commonly prescribed oral contraceptive products are the estrogen-progestin combinations. These formulations are differentiated based on the strength of the individual components and whether estrogen or progesterone effects predominate. The amount of estrogen varies among the available products. Low-dose combination products have 35 μg or less of ethinyl estradiol, or 50 μg or less of mestranol. The synthetic progesterone **progestin** incorporated in the combination products is employed to reduce the effects of estrogen. The goal of therapy is to identify the product that offers the best contraceptive protection throughout the menstrual cycle with the fewest unwanted side effects due to either the estrogen or the progestin component.

There are three types of combination products: monophasic, biphasic, and triphasic. The monophasics, the most common, provide a fixed ratio of estrogen to progestin throughout the menstrual cycle. In biphasics, the amount of estrogen is fixed throughout the cycle, but the amount of progesterone varies (reduced in the first half and increased in the second half) to provide for proliferation of the endometrium and secretory development similar to the physiologic process. Ortho-Novum 10/11-21 is an example of a biphasic. The triphasics, the newest combination products, deliver low doses of both hormones with minimal side effects, including breakthrough bleeding. With triphasics, the amount of both estrogen and progestin varies throughout the cycle in different ratios during three phases. Examples include Ortho-Novum 7/7/7, Tri-Norinyl, and Triphasil.

Progestin-Only Products

The progestin-only oral contraceptive, referred to as "the mini-pill," acts mainly by altering the cervical mucus, and secondarily by altering the endometrium to inhibit implantation. Ovulation is also inhibited in some clients through blockage of LH release. These products were designed to further decrease circulatory side effects. There is, however, a lower pregnancy prevention rate, further increased if clients miss a pill, because these drugs do not suppress activity of the hypothalamus and pituitary to the same degree as the combination products. An increase in the amount of breakthrough bleeding is also noted. Examples of progestin-only products include Ovrette, Micronor, and Nor-QD. Table 49–1 presents selected examples of the various oral contraceptive formulations.

PHARMACOKINETICS

Ethinyl estradiol is rapidly absorbed orally. It undergoes significant first-pass metabolism and elimination via the liver. Mestranol is converted in the liver to ethinyl estradiol, which is 97% to 98% bound to plasma proteins. The half-life varies from 6 to 20 h. Excretion is via bile and urine in a conjugated form. There is some enterohepatic recirculation.

Progestins are also well absorbed orally. Peak plasma levels occur from 0.5 to 4 h after ingestion, depending on the particular compound. Norethynodrel and ethynodiol diacetate are converted to noreth-

Table 49–1
Oral Contraceptives

PRODUCT	AMOUNT OF ESTROGEN (μg)	AMOUNT OF PROGESTIN (mg)	PRODUCT	AMOUNT OF ESTROGEN (μg)	AMOUNT OF PROGESTIN (mg)
COMBINATION PRODUCTS: LISTED BY DECREASING ESTROGEN CONTENT			Nelova 10/11	*Phase I:* 10 d 35 ethinyl estradiol *Phase II:* 11 d 35 ethinyl estradiol	0.5 norethindrone 1 norethindrone
MONOPHASIC PRODUCTS			Ortho-Novum 10/11	Same formulation as above but different colors for tablets	
Norinyl 1 + 50 (21 d)	50 mestranol	1 norethindrone			
Genora 1/50	50 mestranol	1 norethindrone	**TRIPHASIC PRODUCTS**		
Ovcon 50	50 ethinyl estradiol	1 norethindrone	Tri-Norinyl	*Phase I:* 7 d	
Norlestrin 1/50	50 ethinyl estradiol	1 norethindrone acetate		35 ethinyl estradiol *Phase II:* 9 d	0.5 norethindrone
Demulen 1/50	50 ethinyl estradiol	1 ethynodiol diacetate		35 ethinyl estradiol *Phase III:* 5 d	1 norethindrone
Norlestrin 21 2.5/50	50 ethinyl estradiol	2.5 norethindrone acetate		35 ethinyl estradiol	0.5 norethindrone
Ovral	50 ethinyl estradiol	0.5 norgestrel	Ortho Tri-Cyclen	*Phase I:* 7 d	
Genora 1/35	35 ethinyl estradiol	1 norethindrone		35 ethinyl estradiol *Phase II:* 7 d	0.18 norgestimate
Norcept-E 1/35	35 ethinyl estradiol	1 norethindrone		35 ethinyl estradiol *Phase III:* 7 d	0.215 norgestimate
Ortho-Novum 1/35	35 ethinyl estradiol	1 norethindrone		35 ethinyl estradiol	0.25 norgestimate
N.E.E. 1/35	35 ethinyl estradiol	1 norethindrone	Ortho-Novum 7/7/7	*Phase I:* 7 d	
Norethin 1/35 E	35 ethinyl estradiol	1 norethindrone		35 ethinyl estradiol *Phase II:* 7 d	0.5 norethindrone
Norinyl 1 + 35	35 ethinyl estradiol	1 norethindrone		35 ethinyl estradiol *Phase III:* 7 d	0.075 norethindrone
Modicon	35 ethinyl estradiol	0.5 norethindrone		35 ethinyl estradiol	1 norethindrone
Brevicon	35 ethinyl estradiol	0.5 norethindrone	Tri-Levlen	*Phase I:* 6 d	
Nelova	35 ethinyl estradiol	0.5 norethindrone		30 ethinyl estradiol *Phase II:* 5 d	0.05 levonorgestrel
Ovcon 35	35 ethinyl estradiol	0.4 norethindrone		40 ethinyl estradiol *Phase III:* 10 d	0.075 levonorgestrel
Demulen 1/35	35 ethinyl estradiol	1 ethynodiol diacetate		30 ethinyl estradiol	0.125 levonorgestrel
Desogen	30 ethinyl estradiol	0.15 desogestrel	Triphasil	Same as above	
Loestrin 21 1.5/30	30 ethinyl estradiol	1.5 norethindrone acetate	**PROGESTIN-ONLY PRODUCTS: LISTED BY DECREASING PROGESTIN CONTENT**		
Lo/Ovral	30 ethinyl estradiol	0.3 norgestrel	Micronor		0.35 norethindrone
Levlen	30 ethinyl estradiol	0.15 levonorgestrel	Nor-QD		0.35 norethindrone
Nordette	30 ethinyl estradiol	0.15 levonorgestrel	Ovrette		0.075 norgestrel
Levlite	20 ethinyl estradiol	0.10 levonorgestrel			
Loestrin 21 1/20	20 ethinyl estradiol	1 norethindrone acetate			
BIPHASIC PRODUCTS					
Jenest 28	*Phase I:* 7 d 35 ethinyl estradiol *Phase II:* 14 d 35 ethinyl estradiol	0.5 norethindrone 1.0 norethindrone			
N.E.E. 10/11	*Phase I:* 10 d 35 ethinyl estradiol	0.5 norethindrone			
N.E.E. 10/11	*Phase II:* 11 d 35 ethinyl estradiol	1.0 norethindrone			

indrone. Levonorgestrel is bioavailable and does not undergo first-pass liver metabolism; norethindrone undergoes first-pass metabolism and is 65% available. The progestins are bound to plasma proteins and to sex hormone-binding globulin. The half-life of norethindrone varies from 5 to 14 h; that of levonorgestrel from 11 to 45 h.

Dosage Schedule

COMBINATION PRODUCTS

Most monophasic products are available in 21- and 28-tablet packages. The 28-tablet packages include seven non–hormone-containing tablets (some contain iron) so that the client continues to take one tablet each day, rather than having to remember starting and stopping times. Clients are given instructions to take one tablet every day at approximately the same time each day. Many products require the client to start the tablets on the Sunday following the first day of menstruation. If menstruation actually starts on Sunday, the client starts her tablets that day. Other products instruct the client to start her tablets on day 5 of the menstrual cycle (day 1 is the day she begins her period). If the client is on a 21-day regimen, she restarts her next cycle following a 7-day break whether her bleeding has stopped or not.

The biphasic and triphasic products are taken in phases and are color-coded to assist the client. They, too, are available in 21- and 28-day regimens and are started within the guidelines previously presented. For example, the biphasic Ortho-Novum 10/11 requires 10 white tablets for 10 days, followed by 11 peach tablets for 11 days. With a 21-day regimen, the client stops for 7 days; with a 28-day regimen, the client takes seven green inert tablets during this period before beginning the next cycle. The triphasic Ortho-Novum 7/7/7 works similarly. White tablets are taken for 7 days, light peach for 7 days, darker peach for 7 days, followed by 7 days off or 7 green inert tablets. Exceptions to these guidelines include the triphasics Triphasil 21 and Tri-Levulen 21, which are started on the first day of the menstrual cycle with the designated color code followed for 6 days, 5 days, and 10 days, respectively. These, too, are available in 21- and 28-day packaging.

PROGESTIN-ONLY PRODUCTS

The progestin-only products are taken one tablet at the same time daily without interruption. The tablets are started on the first day of menstruation.

MISSED DOSES

Clients occasionally miss a tablet. If only one tablet is missed, it is unlikely that ovulation will occur. However, the risk increases with each additional missed dose. Table 49–2 presents guidelines for missed doses of oral contraceptives.

Contraindications

Not every client is a candidate for use of oral contraceptives. Table 49–3 lists contraindications to their use.

Table 49–2
Guidelines for Missed Doses of Oral Contraceptives

MISSED DOSE	RECOMMENDATIONS
COMBINATION PRODUCTS	
One tablet	Take tablet as soon as realized OR take two tablets the next day OR take one tablet and discard missed tablet and continue schedule but use secondary form of contraception until menses begin
Two tablets	Take two tablets as soon as realized with next tablet at the usual time OR take two tablets daily for the next 2 d and resume regular schedule plus use a secondary form of contraception for the rest of the cycle.
Three tablets	Start a new package of tablets 7 d after the last tablet was taken. Use another form of contraception until tablets have been taken for 7 consecutive d.
PROGESTIN-ONLY PRODUCTS	
One tablet	Take tablet as soon as realized; follow with next tablet at regular time PLUS consider secondary form of contraception
Two tablets	Take one of the missed tablets; discard the second missed tablet; follow with next scheduled tablet at regular time PLUS use secondary form of contraception until menstruation occurs or a pregnancy is tested for.
Three tablets	Discontinue use of tablets and employ another form of birth control. Observe for return of menstruation and test for pregnancy

Table 49–3
Contraindications for Oral Contraceptives

ABSOLUTE CONTRAINDICATIONS

Thromboembolic disease—history or actual

Breast cancer

Cerebrovascular disease

Myocardial infarction

Coronary artery disease

Estrogen-dependent tumors

Hepatic tumors (benign or malignant) originating during use of any estrogen product

Markedly impaired liver function

History of obstructive jaundice during pregnancy

Genital bleeding of unknown origin

Pregnancy—confirmed or suspected

Hyperlipidemia

CAUTIOUS USE

Women over age 35 who smoke

Women over age 40 who do not smoke

Women (any age) who smoke >15 cigarettes per day

Varicose veins

Diabetes or history suggesting possibility

Preexisting fibroid tumors of the uterus

Hypertension

Obesity

Anemia

Migraine headaches

Epilepsy

Elective surgery

Porphyria

Drug Interactions

The effectiveness of some drugs is impaired by oral contraceptives; other drugs impair the effectiveness of oral contraceptives. Table 49–4 lists examples of drugs for which the nurse should maintain a high index of suspicion for interactive effects with oral contraceptives. Clients receiving low-dose formulations of oral contraceptives need to be particularly cautious about potential interactions.

Side Effects and Adverse Reactions

The risk of death from the use of oral contraceptives is less than the risk from pregnancy, especially if the client does not exhibit contraindications listed in Table 49–3. Most side effects are related to differences in the estrogen-progestin ratio of the products and the client's response.

Side effects due primarily to an excess of estrogen include nausea, vomiting, dizziness, fluid retention, edema, bloating, breast enlargement, breast tenderness, chloasma (slightly more in dark-skinned clients exposed to sunlight on higher dose tablets), leg cramps, decreased tearing, corneal curvature alteration, visual changes, vascular headache, and hypertension (in about 1% to 5% of previously normotensive clients within the first few months).

Side effects due primarily to estrogen deficiency include vaginal bleeding (breakthrough bleeding) while taking the tablets (especially in the first few cycles after starting therapy) lasting several days (usually during days 1 to 14), oligomenorrhea (especially after long-term use), nervousness, and dyspareunia secondary to atrophic vaginitis.

Side effects due primarily to an excess of progestin include increased appetite, weight gain, oily skin and scalp, acne, depression, vaginitis from yeast (*Candida*), excess hair growth, and amenorrhea after cessation of use (1% to 2%), decreased breast size.

Side effects caused primarily by progestin deficiency include dysmenorrhea, bleeding late in the cycle (days 15 to 21), and heavy menstrual flow with clots, or amenorrhea.

Table 49–4
Drug Interactions with Oral Contraceptives*

Analgesics: acetaminophen, meperidine, salicylates

Antibiotics and antibacterials: ampicillin, chloramphenicol, griseofulvin, penicillins, rifampicin, sulfonamides, tetracycline

Anticoagulants (oral)

Anticonvulsants: phenytoin, phenobarbital, primidone, carbamazepine, valproic acid

Antifibrinolytic agents: aminocaproic acid

Antihistamines and decongestants

Antihypertensive agents: metoprolol

Antitubercular drugs

Benzodiazepines: lorazepam, oxazepam, temazepam

Caffeine

Cholesterol-lowering drugs: clofibrate

Corticosteroids

Mineral oil

Nonsteroidal antiinflammatory drugs (phenylbutazone, naproxon)

Theophyllines

Tricyclic antidepressants

Contraceptive effectiveness may be affected by some interactions involving one or more of these drugs. Secondary forms of contraception may be temporarily needed.

NURSING PROCESS
ORAL CONTRACEPTIVES

Assessment

- Obtain baseline blood pressure (BP) and weight. Report abnormal findings. Determine pregnancy status.
- Assess for history of smoking, hypertension, and all contraindications listed in Table 49–3.
- Recognize the need for periodic reassessment of baseline data and side effects. Most clients should be seen in 1 to 3 months after beginning regimen.

Potential Nursing Diagnoses

- Knowledge deficit related to fertility pattern
- Knowledge deficit related to oral contraceptive method(s)
- Risk for noncompliance with oral contraceptive method selected

Planning

- Client will take oral contraceptives as prescribed and will report side effects which occur.

Nursing Interventions

General

- Separate personal views from those of the client regarding contraception and use of specific products.
- Recognize that many clients on oral contraceptives abandon the method within a year; therefore, plan to provide the client with alternatives.
- Nonnursing mothers can begin combination oral contraceptives 3 to 4 weeks postpartum, regardless of whether menstruation has spontaneously occurred.

Client Teaching

- Remind client that these drugs should be used only under a health care provider's direction.
- Review with client the following aspects of oral contraceptives:

Advantages

- Easy to use and have low failure rate
- Minimal risks for teens and those in twenties
- Contraception is not linked to the sexual act
- Suppressed pain at ovulation
- Decreased dysmenorrhea
- Lighter, shorter menstrual flow
- Regular, predictable menses
- Decreased pregnancy fears may increase sexual responsivenes
- Decreased iron-deficiency anemia resulting from decreased menstrual flow.
- 80% to 90% reduced risk of functional ovarian cysts
- May provide protection against benign breast lesions and uterine and ovarian cancers
- Reduced risk of pelvic inflammatory disease
- Lower risk of ectopic pregnancy
- Decreased menstrual migraine type headache
- No concrete supportive evidence that breast cancer is caused or increased by use of oral contraceptives
- Decreased chance of endometrial cancer (possibly due to progestin) in younger women not past menopause; protection may last up to 10 years after pills have been stopped if a client has used them long-term
- Benign functional ovarian cysts are less common.

Nursing Process continued on following page

NURSING PROCESS *Continued*
ORAL CONTRACEPTIVES

- Thromboembolism risk does not appear related to duration of oral contraceptive use, rather to the dose of estrogen (lower-dose products less risky).

Disadvantages
- If nonmonogamous, increased risk of acquiring sexually transmitted diseases, because no barrier is involved
- Extremely risky for fetus if pregnancy should occur
- Bothersome side effects
- Requires medical follow-up every 6 months, which may, in addition to cost of tablets, be perceived as expensive in terms of both time and money

Side Effects
- Acquaint client with the rare but possible side effects that are considered serious, including thrombophlebitis, pulmonary embolus, myocardial infarction, cerebral vascular accident, and retinal vein thrombosis.
- As an outcome of discussion about serious side effects, teach client the acronym ACHES for dangerous side effects that must be reported to a health care provider:
  A = *A*bdominal pain (severe)
  C = *C*hest pain or shortness of breath
  H = *H*eadaches that are severe; dizziness, weakness, numbness, speech difficulties
  E = *E*ye disorders including blurring or loss of vision
  S = *S*evere leg pain or swelling in the calf or thigh

More Common Side Effects
- Inform the client that her menstrual flow may be less in amount and duration due to thinning of the endometrial lining.
- Determine whether the client wears contact lenses and discuss how to handle dry eyes caused by decreased tearing and alterations in the shape of the cornea.
- Tell the client who experiences postpill amenorrhea that 95% of women have regular periods within 12 to 18 months. Also tell her that those who participate in endurance fitness activities may have increased postpill amenorrhea.

Safety
- Counsel the client not to smoke tobacco because of the increased cardiovascular risks.
- Advise the client to use barrier method of contraception during the first month of oral contraceptive use and for 3 months after discontinuing use and before trying to conceive.
- Provide instructions about dealing with "missed pills" (see Table 49–2).
- Tell the client to report any effects from the pill to a health professional so that the therapy can be adjusted to suit her own particular needs. Encourage her not to give up and discontinue use of the pills.
- Tell the client to report breakthrough bleeding or spotting, because she may need a change in dose of oral contraceptive.
- Tell the client to always report that she takes oral contraceptives when seeing a health care provider due to possible synergistic or antagonistic responses to other therapies.
- Nursing mothers should delay use of oral contraceptives until after breast feeding is completed; another method should be selected.

Skill
- Ask the client to weigh herself regularly/weekly and observe for any edema.
- Teach the client to do a monthly breast self-examination.

Diet
- Counsel the client to moderate caffeine intake because elimination of caffeine may be decreased due to the oral contraceptives.
- Tell the client to take her pill with a snack at night or after meals to help eliminate nausea and to take the pill at the same time each day.

Nursing Process continued on following page

NURSING PROCESS *Continued*
ORAL CONTRACEPTIVES

Cultural Considerations

- Be aware of different cultures' contraception practices.
- Consider the role of each partner in the specific culture regarding decision making of contraception method.

Evaluation

- Evaluate the client's compliance with the oral contraceptive regimen.

There may also be changes in laboratory values, including thyroid and liver function, blood glucose, and triglycerides.

Adverse reactions of a more severe nature include increased risk of superficial and deep venous thrombosis, pulmonary embolism, cerebrovascular accident (thrombotic stroke), myocardial infarction, and acceleration of preexisting but nondiagnosed breast tumors.

ALTERNATIVE METHODS OF CONTRACEPTION

Alternative methods of contraception are suited to clients who select not to take a pill on a daily basis or who are usable to comply with the daily dosing.

New forms of hormone therapy that have long-lasting but reversible contraceptive effects include Norplant (approved in December, 1990), which employs low-dose levonorgestrel in six matchstick-shaped Silastic implants placed under the skin of the upper arm. Norplant is considered effective for 5 years and has the advantage of not requiring conscious daily awareness of contraception. However, the method is being requested less frequently because of side effects that include reports of rods being visible and some rods traveling up the arm, scars on the arm, breakthrough and uncontrolled bleeding, hirsutism, weight gain, increased ovarian cysts, and removal difficulties in some clients that require a minor surgical procedure.

Long-acting injectable progestin is known as medroxyprogesterone acetate (Depo-Provera), which is gaining favor because it requires only one injection every 3 months. The method is considered safe for postpartum clients to receive before discharge following delivery; clients may also breast feed. The most common side effects reported include initially irregular periods and spotting (periods may cease in about

1 year). Women who smoke may complain of headaches on Depo-Provera (usually relieved by acetaminophen). In addition, other side effects include weight gain, bloating, decreased libido, hair loss, and depression. Like oral contraceptives, there is no protection against sexually transmitted diseases. The injection, given deep IM in the gluteus, is relatively inexpensive. The site of the injection is documented in order to rotate injection sites. The client is provided with a personalized calendar for subsequent doses. The injection acts by suppressing ovulation and changing the pH of the vaginal mucosa to an environment less hospitable to sperm. In some clients, resumption of fertility may be delayed (when the injections are discontinued) for a year or more. In a rare instance, serious side effects may occur, including chest pain, hemoptysis, abdominal pain, shortness of breath, and numbness in the extremities. The drug is contraindicated in cases of undiagnosed vaginal bleeding or known or suspected pregnancy.

Inform the client about hormone-releasing intrauterine devices. Intrauterine devices (IUDs) are considered safe with use limited to those women at low risk for sexually transmitted diseases. Increased menstrual bleeding and cramps are the primary side effects. Examples of commonly used IUDs are ParaGard and Progestasert. ParaGard releases copper that interferes with sperm motility and fertilization owing to inflammation of the endometrium. ParaGard may remain in place for up to 8 years. Progestasert is thought to reduce the viability of sperm through release of progesterone. Annual replacement is required to ensure adequate release of progesterone.

Some clients may be misinformed regarding substances such as RU486 (Mefepristone), a progesterone antagonist used in France and United Kingdom (not available in the United States at this time) both as a contraceptive agent and an abortifacient (when taken within 1 month following a missed menstrual period). As debate continues about introducing RU486 in the United States, combinations of other drugs already on the market are being studied with an eye toward seeking FDA approval. Two drugs in combination currently being studied for medically induced abortion purposes are methotrexate (a chemotherapeutic agent) and misoprostol (an ulcer drug). The first agent destabilizes the uterine lining; the second agent, given a week later, triggers contractions that shed the lining within about 24 h.

EMERGENCY CONTRACEPTION

The FDA announced in February 1997 that emergency contraception (EC) pills were "safe and effective" in the prevention of pregnancy after sexual intercourse. Further, the FDA requested a pharmaceutical company to prepare an EC product with appropriate accompanying literature. The result was the Preven Emergency Contraception Kit, approved by the FDA in September 1998. The kit is Medicaid reimbursable and costs about $20, which is less than 1 month's supply of birth control pills. The kit requires a prescription and includes four tablets, each with 50 μg of ethinyl estradiol and 0.25 mg of levonorgestrel, pregnancy test, and literature. Two of the combination tablets should be taken as soon as possible and within 72 hours of unprotected intercourse; the other two tablets should be taken 12 hours later.

The mode of action of EC pills is to delay or prevent ovulation, interfere with tubal transport of the embryo, egg, or sperm, and/or change the hormones necessary for the preparation of the uterine lining. The effectiveness of EC pills is that the risk of pregnancy is decreased by 75% for each act of sexual intercourse. The major side effect is nausea; an OTC antinausea medicine (e.g., diphenhydramine, 25-50 mg) taken 1 hour before EC may be helpful. Irregular menstrual bleeding is another side effect. If a woman does not get her period within a few days of the expected time, she should have a pregnancy test done. The normal EC pill dosage should not be taken by a woman who should not take estrogen. Combined oral contraceptives used for EC are presented in Table 49–5.

If pregnancy is already established or if implantation occurred since the unprotected sexual intercourse, the pregnancy is not disrupted. EC pills do not result in an abortion and there are no reports of harm to the fetus. EC can be used when needed. EC is not as effective as taking the oral contraceptives or using condoms as directed (consistently and correctly). EC decreases the chance of pregnancy by 75% from one act of unprotected sexual intercourse; birth control pills have a much higher rate of effectiveness, almost 100%.

Other forms of EC include progestin-only pills (minipills) and a copper intrauterine device (IUD). Initiated within 48 hours of unprotected intercourse, the progestin-only pills result in less nausea but require 20 pills/dose. A copper IUD may be inserted

Table 49–5
Dosage of Some Contraceptives for Emergency Use

	ETHINYL ESTRADIOL*	PROGESTIN*	TABLETS PER DOSE†	COST‡
Preven Kit (Gynetics)	50 μg	0.25 mg levonorgestrel	2	$19.94
Ovral (Wyeth-Ayerst)	50 μg	0.50 mg norgestrel	2	44.89
Lo-Ovral (Wyeth-Ayerst)	30 μg	0.30 mg norgestrel	4	29.32
Nordette (Wyeth-Ayerst)	30 μg	0.15 mg levonorgestrel	4	28.31
Levlen (Berlex)	30 μg	0.15 mg levonorgestrel	4	28.35
Levora (Watson)	30 μg	0.15 mg levonorgestrel	4	24.07
Tri-Levlen (Berlex)§	30 μg	0.125 levonorgestrel	4	26.94
Triphasil (Wyeth-Ayerst)§	30 μg	0.125 levonorgestrel	4	27.47
Trivora (Watson)§	30 μg	0.125 levonorgestrel	4	25.82
Alesse (Wyeth-Ayerst)	20 μg	0.10 levonorgestrel	5	27.47
Ovrette (Wyeth-Ayerst)	0	0.075 norgestrel	20	56.06¶

*Content of each tablet.
†One dose is taken as soon as possible after unprotected coitus, and a second dose is taken 12 hours later.
‡Cost to the pharmacist based on wholesale price (AWP) listings in Drug Topics Red Book 1998 and October Update. Oral contraceptives are packaged in dispensers containing 21 active tablets.
§Yellow tablets only of Tri-Levlen or Triphasil, or pink tablets only of Trivora.
¶Ovrette is marketed in dispensers containing 28 active tablets.
From The Medical Letter on Drugs and Therapeutics, 40, 103, 1998.

within 5 days of unprotected intercourse and be removed after the woman's next menstrual period. The IUD may remain in place as a method of birth control for up to 10 years.

The HOTLINE for EC information is 1-888-NOT-2-LATE and the Web site is http://opr.princeton.edu/ec

DRUGS USED TO TREAT UTERINE DYSFUNCTION

Uterine dysfunction is common in premenstrual syndrome, endometriosis, and menopause. This section describes these entities and presents current pharmacologic approaches to management. The menstrual cycle is described in the unit introduction.

Premenstrual Syndrome

Premenstrual syndrome (PMS), first formally described and named in 1931, comprises a collection of varied physical, emotional, and behavioral symptoms. Table 49–6 lists commonly reported physical and

---

Table 49–6
Physical and Psychobehavioral Symptoms of Premenstrual Syndrome

---

Bloating in lower abdomen
Weight gain
Headache (migraine)
Increased appetite
Cravings for foods high in sugar or salt
Breast soreness
Fatigue
Sleep disorders
Backaches
Acne
Joint pain
Constipation
Feelings of being out of control
Emotional lability
Tension
Anxiety
Difficulty with concentration
Irritability
Agitation
Depression
Suicidal thoughts
Rage

---

psychobehavioral symptoms in PMS. More than 150 symptoms have been reported in the literature.

Premenstrual syndrome can result in decreased work effectiveness and impaired interpersonal relationships. PMS affects 40% of all adult women (4 to 5 million in the United States) to some degree, with about 5% exhibiting debilitating symptoms. There is a family history associated with the syndrome, but it is not hereditary. The syndrome is seen most commonly in women in their thirties and early forties, but it also affects adolescents. Premenstrual syndrome occurs in a repetitive regular pattern during the luteal phase (days 15 to 28) of the menstrual cycle; it decreases during the follicular phase.

There is no universal agreement about the definition, etiology, symptoms, or treatment of PMS. The most widely held theory is that PMS is linked to estrogen and progesterone levels and the relationship of these hormones to other brain chemicals. The symptoms are observed during the luteal phase when levels are high and decrease when drugs that inhibit gonadotropin-releasing hormone (GnRH) and ovulation are used. Other hypotheses center on the release of endogenous opiates (beta-endorphins), disruptions in CNS neurotransmitters (resulting in mood swings), and the role of prolactin secretion.

Diagnosis of PMS is made when the client's symptoms can be documented as consistently occurring at about the same time and in the same way over a defined number of menstrual periods. Other endocrine abnormalities need to be ruled out. One difficulty with diagnosis is that PMS is not consistent, because every cycle is not the same. Thus, measurement is problematic, particularly because every symptom that occurs associated with a menstrual cycle is not PMS.

Treatment of PMS includes nonpharmacologic and pharmacologic measures. There is not one curative therapy nor a way to know what therapy may be best for a particular client other than trial and error.

Nonpharmacologic treatment includes expression of empathy, support from family and others, correction of knowledge deficits about PMS and the menstrual cycle, exercise, and dietary changes (limiting salty foods, alcohol, caffeine, chocolate, concentrated sweets; eating four to six small high-carbohydrate, low-fat meals, which help stabilize blood sugar levels and enhance mood). Stress reduction is helpful, as is aerobic exercise, which is believed to have a regulatory effect on estrogen and progesterone secondary to hypothalamic stimulation. These measures may help the client to feel proactive in regard to her situation, give her a sense of overall well-being, and improve her general health. Also, endorphin levels are heightened, which is found to be helpful.

Pharmacologic treatment remains largely empirical because research has not consistently been done un-

NURSING PROCESS
PREMENSTRUAL SYNDROME

Assessment

- Obtain history of PMS symptoms such as bloating, weight gain, headache, and increased appetite. See Table 49–6.

Potential Nursing Diagnoses

- Knowledge deficit related to the menstrual cycle and etiology of related alterations in mood and comfort
- Individual coping ineffective
- Family processes altered

Planning

- Client will verbalize relief from PMS from nonpharmacologic and pharmacologic measures.

Nursing Interventions

- Provide quality client and family education in a supportive manner that encourages family communication.

Client Teaching

General
- Express that symptoms are real and that "crazy feelings" do not mean the client is crazy.
- Explain menstrual cycle and current knowledge about PMS verbally, in writing, and graphically.
- Share current research findings regarding PMS and known treatment modalities, with the client, her family, and community groups.
- Encourage client to include aerobic exercise in her regular activity pattern three to five times each week.
- Describe and discuss stress-reduction activities.
- Encourage family communication regarding PMS symptoms experienced by the client so that the family can understand the client's behavior.
- Suggest sources for, and potential value of, support groups.

Diet
- Encourage client to take nontoxic doses of vitamin and mineral supplements with meals.
- Encourage low-fat, low-salt, high-carbohydrate diet. Suggest four to six small meals and portable snacks (bagels, rice cakes).
- Decrease caffeine intake and increase water consumption.
- Limit alcoholic beverages; these may precipitate headaches.

Self-Administration
- Have the client keep a log of symptoms experienced during her menstrual cycle to better link events with symptoms.
- If alprazolam (Xanax) is ordered, discuss issues of dependency and withdrawal.
- If danazol (Danocrine) is ordered, see the guidelines later for use of the drug.

Evaluation

- Evaluate the effectiveness of the nonpharmacologic and pharmacologic measures for relief of PMS.

Table 49–7
Drug Therapy for Endometriosis

DRUG	DOSE	USES AND CONSIDERATIONS
Danazol (Danocrine)	PO: 400 mg b.i.d. for 4–6 mo; can extend to 9 mo; can restart if symptoms return	Pituitary gonadotropin inhibitory agent. No estrogenic or progestational action. Suppresses and atrophies intra- and extrauterine tissue; menses cease during therapy and no ovulation occurs; pain is relieved. Ovulation/menses usually recur within 90 d after treatment. Commonly used for women with infertility associated with endometriosis. Used for PMS on investigational basis. Contraindicated in pregnancy, breast feeding, abnormal genital bleeding, impaired heart, liver, or kidney function, severe hypertension. Can alter some laboratory values (e.g., decreased HDL, increased LDL). Can increase insulin requirements and, if given with warfarin, cause a prolonged PT. Therapy started during menstruation or after pregnancy. If therapy is for fibrocystic breast disease, breast carcinoma must also be ruled out before treatment. Pharmacokinetics: Absorbed well orally; 2–4 h peak action; $t\frac{1}{2}$ 4.5 h; biotransformed by the liver. Therapeutic effects occur within 3 wk of daily therapy. Excreted in the urine. *Pregnancy category:* X. Adverse effects: thrombocytopenia, hypertension, depression, headache, *hot flashes, weight gain,* androgenic effects, hemorrhagic cystitis, hematuria, hepatotoxicity, cholestatic hepatitis, acne, rashes, oily skin, hirsutism, bloating, *muscle cramps,* voice deepening (irreversible), hearing loss, mood swings, anxiety, fatigue, nausea, vomiting, diarrhea, constipation. Also produces atherogenic lipid profile. Many clients cannot tolerate side effects and discontinue drug. Alternate doses may be used for clients with hereditary angioedema and fibrocystic breast disease.
GONADOTROPIN-RELEASING HORMONE (GNRH) AGONISTS		
Leuprolide acetate for depot suspension (Lupron Depot 3.75)	IM: 3.75 mg q mo for up to 6 mo	As an agonist, initially stimulates FSH and LH, but over time, creates prolonged suppression, which causes decreased ovarian secretion of estrogen/progesterone, resulting in a hypoestrogenic state. Lack of hormonal stimulation causes regression of displaced endometrial tissue. Contains no androgen. Found as effective as danazol in reducing extent of endometriosis. Normal function returns in 4 to 12 wk after treatment discontinued. Contraindicated in actual or potential pregnancy, undiagnosed vaginal bleeding and breast feeding since is not known if excreted in breast milk. FDA classification 3B.* *Pregnancy category:* X. Pharmacokinetics: Therapeutic levels detected for at least 4 wk after injection; 85%–100% released within 4 wk with no accumulation. $t\frac{1}{2}$: 3–4.2 h; PB: 46%. Side effects: hot flashes, headaches, decreased libido, dry vagina, night sweats, mood changes, mild bone loss (usually regained within 6 mo of finishing treatment). Initial dose best given during day 1–3 of menstrual cycle to avoid affecting a pregnancy. Barrier contraceptives should be used during treatment because pregnancy is possible. Minimal changes produced in lipid profile. Retreatment not recommended because safety data beyond 6 mo are not available.

Table continued on following page

Table 49–7 *Continued*
Drug Therapy for Endometriosis

DRUG	DOSE	USES AND CONSIDERATIONS
Nafarelin acetate (Synarel Nasal Solution)	400 μg daily, administered as one spray (200 μg) into one nostril in morning and one spray (200 μg) into other nostril for up to 6 mo	Contains no androgen. Controlled studies comparing Synarel (400 μg) and danazol (600 or 800 μg/d) found higher hypoestrogenic (therapeutic state) but less androgenic side effects. Found comparable in reducing extent of endometriosis and in effect on associated client symptoms. Maintains LDL/HDL ratio. Return of normal function in 4–12 wk after treatment discontinued. Contraindicated in those sensitive to GnRH, GnRH analogs, or inert substances included in product; other contraindications include actual or potential pregnancy, undiagnosed vaginal bleeding, and breast feeding. Clients with rhinitis should have a topical decongestant prescribed by health care provider and use at least 30 min after Synarel. FDA classification 1B.† Pharmacokinetics: Maximum serum concentrations achieved in 10–40 min; serum half-life approximately 30 h (range, 0.8–10 h); 80% bound to plasma proteins; drug elimination after intranasal administration has not been studied. Side effects are those seen in a natural menopause due to a hypoestrogenic state, notably hot flashes, vaginal dryness, decreased libido, headaches, and emotional lability.

*A new formulation of a compound already on the market which offers a modest therapeutic gain over currently available agents.
†A new chemical entity that offers a modest therapeutic gain over currently available agents.
KEY: FSH: follicle-stimulating hormone; GnRH: gonadotropin-releasing hormone; HDL: high-density lipoproteins; IM: intramuscular; LDL: low-density lipoproteins; LH: luteinizing hormone; PB: protein-binding; PO: by mouth; PT: prothrombin time; t½: half-life.

der double-blind, placebo-controlled conditions. Some clients experience improvement with selected symptoms through use of vitamin B$_6$ (popular with self-help groups but not found superior to placebo) or vaginal or rectal progesterone suppositories (200 to 400 mg b.i.d.), which are commonly used but not documented as being effective and have some long-term effects; in addition, individuals who exhibit depressive symptoms tend to get worse on progesterone because of its depressant effects. Other pharmacologic trials have been diuretics (not recommended) and prostaglandin inhibitors; bromocriptine (Parlodel) (2.5 mg b.i.d. started on day 10 of cycle and taken until menstruation begins) for breast soreness; and alprazolam (Xanax) (0.25 mg t.i.d. from day 20 of cycle to day 2 of menses, followed by one tablet per day) for treatment of anxiety, irritability, and depression. Oral contraceptives have been experimentally employed as a form of anovulatory therapy but are not approved for this purpose. Breast tenderness is helped by dietary caffeine reduction more than by pharmacologic intervention. A theory under study is that stronger antiprostaglandins (NSAIDs) taken in conjunction with vitamin therapy with a product that contains magnesium, calcium, pyridoxine, vitamin E, and zinc when symptoms begin through the beginning of the menstrual period will prove useful.

A Canadian study demonstrated symptom reduction using fluoxetine (Prozac), which is thought to work through regulating serotonin use by the brain. More study is needed, and the use of Prozac may be reserved for severely affected clients with protracted symptoms.

Two other forms of experimental (not FDA approved) hormonal anovulatory treatment are danazol (Danocrine) and GnRH agonists. These formulations, which are approved for treatment of endometriosis, are presented in Table 49–7.

Endometriosis

Endometriosis is the abnormal location of endometrial tissue outside of the uterus, in the pelvic cavity; it has no single, clearly identifiable cause. Possible etiologies are retrograde menstruation (backward movement of endometrial cells through the fallopian tubes out into the abdomen) or spread through the lymphatic or vascular systems. Regardless of cause, the displaced endometrial tissue is found affixed to the ovaries, on the posterior surface of the uterus, the uterosacral ligaments, the broad ligaments, or the bowel. The displaced tissue responds to hormonal control, particularly estrogen from the ovaries in the

NURSING PROCESS
ENDOMETRIOSIS

Assessment

- Obtain a complete client history, including menstrual history.
- Identify the client's fertility plans.
- Review chart for baseline liver function studies and pregnancy test.

Leuprolide Acetate
- Review the client's history for risk factors associated with major bone loss; the drug may pose an additional risk.

Potential Nursing Diagnoses

- Discomfort (acute and chronic) related to hormonally controlled displaced endometrial tissue
- Activity limitation secondary to painful menstrual cycles
- Knowledge deficit related to menstrual cycle, displaced endometrial tissue, etiology of pain, and treatment options

Planning

- Client will be free of pain/discomfort resulting from endometriosis with the use of danazol, leuprolide acetate; or nafarelin acetate.

Nursing Interventions

Danazol
- Observe the client for signs of anxiety about potential loss of fertility and time involved in treatment.
- Recall that the drug must be started during the client's menstrual period.

Leuprolide Acetate
- Store product and diluent at room temperature.
- Must be reconstituted and used immediately (no preservatives). Reconstituted product must be shaken to create a milky suspension.

Client Teaching

Danazol
- Discuss the purpose, action, and side effects of the drug with the client. Explain that the medication is expensive. Explain length of treatment.
- Plan with the client for the use of a back-up nonhormonal form of birth control.
- Tell the client that menses will usually return in 2 to 3 months after treatment.
- Tell the client to have one menstrual cycle after treatment is completed before trying to become pregnant.

Diet
- Ask the client to keep a food history. Suggest increased exercise to help offset weight gain that is experienced by 75% (average, 4 kg); suggest caloric control plan based on history.
- Increase water consumption.

Skill
- Review breast self-examination with client.

Side Effects
- Suggest that the client wear minipads for spotting during the first month of therapy and report any bleeding to her health care provider.
- Discuss removal of unwanted hair and skin care for acne prevention. If acne occurs, consult a dermatologist.

Nursing Process continued on following page

NURSING PROCESS *Continued*
ENDOMETRIOSIS

- Suggest client wash her face and hair more often because of oily scalp and skin and use oil-free makeup and shampoo.
- If muscle cramps occur, advise client to do warm-up exercises before active workout and gradually increase exertion.

Leuprolide Acetate
- Explain to the client that the drug causes a temporary state of menopause.
- Explain that the treatment process requires one injection each month.
- Explain that the drug is palliative and temporarily effective in reducing symptoms. It does not create a change in basic physiology, metabolism, or hormone production. When treatment is complete, whatever is normal for the client will return over time.
- Advise the client that initially there may be an increase in clinical signs and symptoms of endometriosis, but these will disappear.
- Explain that 6 months is the accepted duration of therapy for GnRH agonists. Safety data are available only for 6-month use. Retreatment is not recommended.

Self-Administration
- Remind client that she must use a nonhormonal contraceptive method during treatment.

Side Effects
- If the client is concerned about potential bone loss, state that one 6-month course of treatment has been found to cause only a small loss. However, clients who are at higher risk for bone loss due to chronic alcoholism, tobacco use, strong family history of osteoporosis, or chronic use of anticonvulsants or corticosteroids should carefully discuss the decision for or against therapy with this drug. Suggest client add weight-bearing exercise and walking or low-impact aerobics to offset bone loss.
- Stress that the client must be consistent in receiving her doses of the drug, or breakthrough bleeding or ovulation can occur.
- Tell the client to inform the health care provider if menstruation persists while being treated.
- Discuss mood changes secondary to hormonal changes with drug and possible emotional lability; suggest support network and resource groups.
- If vaginal dryness occurs, suggest client use water-based lubricants and try alternate sexual positions for intercourse.
- If night sweats occur, suggest cotton bedclothes, change of clothes, resist chilling by gradually exposing body to room air from under bed covers; also, contact health care provider if sleep disturbances persist.

Diet
- Suggest increased calcium-based food products.

Nafarelin Acetate
- Explain that precise guidelines must be followed by the client if the treatment is to be effective.
- Ask the client if she is allergic to any component of the drug including nafarelin base, benzalkonium chloride, acetic acid, sodium hydroxide, hydrochloride, or sorbitol.
- Tell the client that the action of the drug, guidelines for birth control use, hypoestrogenic effects, and return of normal function are the same as for leuprolide.
- Advise the client that the medication is expensive, is provided as a 30-day supply, and needs to be continued for 6 months of therapy without interruption.

Self-Administration
- Stress that the client must use the drug twice a day (every 12 h) for the full duration of treatment.
- Tell the client to start the drug between days 2 and 4 of the menstrual period.

Nursing Process continued on following page

NURSING PROCESS Continued
ENDOMETRIOSIS

- The client must be told of the need to prime the spray pump only before the first use. The sprayer is designed to deliver the exact dose each time. A fine spray will occur after 7 to 10 pushes on the pump. If a thin stream occurs, she should call her pharmacist immediately.
- Tell the client to store the bottle upright, below 86°F, and out of light. Because she must use it every 12 h, it is suggested she put it near her toothbrush or other regularly used product (morning and night).
- Tell the client she should record each dose on the supplied chart and to refill prescription so as not to miss any doses.
- Tell the client it is permissible to use a nasal decongestant spray (with health care provider's knowledge) while on Synarel. Use the Synarel spray first and allow 30 minutes to elapse before using the decongestant spray.
- The client should blow her nose to clear both nostrils before using the drug. She should bend forward and place the spray tip in one nostril aimed at the back and outer side of her nose. She should close the other nostril with her finger and then spray one time while sniffing gently, then tilt her head back to spread the drug over the back of the nose. She must be told *not* to spray in the second nostril unless told to do so by her doctor. Alternate nostrils are used for each dose.

Side Effects
- Advise the client that she may note irregular vaginal spotting or bleeding, which should decrease and stop unless doses are missed.
- See Leuprolide—similar effects and potential remedial actions.

Diet
- See Leuprolide—same recommendations.

Evaluation

- Evaluate the effectiveness of the drug regimen. If pain or discomfort is still present, notify the health care provider. Drug dose adjustment may be necessary.

---

same way as the tissue inside the uterus. Thus, when menstruation occurs, this extrauterine tissue also bleeds. As the number of menstrual cycles increases, inflammation, scar tissue formation, and adhesions result.

Clients with endometriosis may be symptomatic (about 75%) or asymptomatic (those diagnosed during infertility work-ups). The diagnosis is based on symptoms and laparoscopic evidence of endometrial tissue. Symptoms include severe low-back and pelvic pain that increases with menstruation. Painful, sometimes bloody bowel movements during menstruation have been reported, as has painful sexual intercourse (dyspareunia). Irregular bleeding (spotting) before and after menses is common. Long term, there is an association with primary or secondary infertility; about 25% to 40% of infertile women exhibit the condition. Endometriosis may obstruct or affect the motility of the fallopian tubes. There is also a risk that nearby organs (e.g., urinary and gastrointestinal

tracts) may become obstructed by invasion by endometrial tissue.

Endometriosis is found most often in women who have delayed childbearing until their thirties, although it may occur during adolescence. There is an increased prevalence rate of 7% for siblings and daughters of affected women. Approximately 5 million women are affected in the United States. Affected women may exhibit increased ectopic pregnancy rates, and difficult pregnancies and labors.

Some success is being achieved in treating endometriosis using a laser during laparoscopy to remove or destroy endometrial growths.

Three drugs are approved for use in endometriosis: danazol (Danocrine) and two gonadotropin-releasing hormone (GnRH) agonists, leuprolide acetate (Lupron Depot) and nafarelin acetate (Synarel). Danazol has been the drug of choice, but use of the GnRH agonists is increasing. These drugs are presented in Table 49–7.

In long-term and highly painful endometriosis that has not been controlled with drug therapy or laparoscopy, hysterectomy (including ovary removal) may be elected.

Menopause

The transitional process experienced by women as they move from the reproductive into the nonreproductive stage of life is called the female climacteric, a natural event. The "change of life" experience is perceived by women in an individualized way on a continuum from no difficulty to severe difficulty. This phase of life occurs for most women somewhere between the late thirties to the late fifties. The climacteric can be divided into premenopause, menopause, and postmenopause, during which certain physiologic events occur.

Menopause is defined as the permanent end of menstruation caused by decreased ovarian function. The average age at menopause is about 50 years (range 45 to 55). Women who experience menopause before age 40 years are referred to as having premature menopause. This natural event is documented as having occurred once a woman has had no menstrual periods for 1 year. The triggering event for the onset of natural menopause is not known. Menopause can also occur abruptly as a secondary effect of surgical removal of the ovaries (oophorectomy), radiologic procedures in which ovarian function is destroyed, severe infection, ovarian tumors, or as a temporarily induced state for treatment of conditions such as endometriosis.

The premenopausal period may last for more than 5 years before true menopause occurs. During this period, menstrual variations begin to be evident. For example, menstrual periods may occur as usual, be lighter in flow, or last a shorter time. They may begin, stop, and then start again, or be of longer duration, with a heavier flow that may contain blood clots. Sudden episodes of vasodilation (hot flashes) also begin to occur in some women. Others experience vaginal dryness. These unpredictable changes may last for several years and are probably due to alterations in the hypothalamic-pituitary-ovarian feedback system.

Postmenopause is the period when the body adapts to a new hormonal environment. Although the production of estrogen and progesterone from the ovaries decreases during the late premenopausal and early postmenopausal periods, the ovary is able to secrete androgens (testosterone) in varying amounts as a result of the influence of increased LH levels. During this period, androstenedione (the main androgen secreted by the ovaries and adrenal cortex, which is present in reduced amounts postmenopause) is converted into estrone, a naturally occurring estrogen

formed in extraglandular tissue of the brain, liver, kidney, and adipose tissue. This represents the main source of available estrogen once the ovaries lose the ability to produce estradiol. Table 49–8 presents common physical effects associated with the climacteric.

HORMONE REPLACEMENT THERAPY

Hormone replacement therapy (HRT) is the most prevalent treatment for relief of vasodilation and vaginal dryness and for prevention of cardiovascular disease and osteoporosis. Oral estrogen, most commonly in the form of conjugated estrogens, is taken by the client together with the synthetic hormone progestin in one of several possible, but still controversial, treatment regimens. The progestin is added to minimize the risk of endometrial hyperplasia, endometrial cancer, and breast cancer from the use of estrogen alone. The progestin, however, has potential negative effects, including potential PMS-type symptoms, breast pathology, and alterations in lipid metabolism. Thus, progestin partially blunts the beneficial effects of estrogen and the client has much to consider when deciding on a course of action.

In the United States, the typical approach to HRT is oral estrogen in the lowest dose to control symptoms (most commonly 0.25 mg–0.625 mg/d), for days 1 to 25 of the month, with the addition of progesterone (Provera) 10 mg from days 16 to 25. In Europe, it is common for the estrogen and progesterone to be taken together every day without any days off.

Currently, there is no one absolutely correct HRT management regimen. Health care providers may prescribe either cyclic or continuous estrogen with progestin or a combined continuous approach. Other regimens are also used.

When **estrogen replacement therapy** (ERT) is selected, in conjunction with nonpharmacologic measures to prevent bone loss, it is important to start the regimen early in menopause and continue for at least 10 years following menopause. Clients who select HRT often taper off after 2 or 3 years and the menopausal symptoms, such as vaginal changes and hot flashes, return at some point.

Compliance with treatment regimens shifts with the health reports in the media that bring the latest piece of worrisome or hopeful news. For example, the two major reasons women choose not to use estrogen therapy or to decrease their compliance are fear of breast cancer and resumption of withdrawal bleeding. Women may often deemphasize the preventive health care benefits.

Dosage forms for the various types of estrogen replacement therapy include oral, transdermal, vaginal cream, injections, and pellets. The natural or biologic estrogens are composed of estrones (including conjugated equine estrogens, esterified estrogens, and piperazine estrone sulfate) and estradiols (includ-

Table 49–8
Common Physical Effects Associated with the Female Climacteric

HYPOESTROGENIC STATE	EFFECTS
Irregular menstruation	Variable frequency, duration, flow
Vasodilation	Hot flashes with transient sensations of intense heat in upper chest, neck and head; visible flushing; sweating; chills; tachycardia; sleep disruption
Vaginal alterations	Dryness; decreased lubrication during sexual stimulation; thinning. Decreased acidity and increased irritation response to stressors such as intercourse can cause increased vaginitis (itching, burning, discharge). Increased incidence of prolapse/cystocele
Decreased bone mass (osteoporosis)	Backache, reduced height, sudden fracture, particularly in thin, fair, small-boned women and those with a family history, no pregnancies, sedentary lifestyle, inadequate diet, smoking, alcohol use, or use of drugs that increase calcium loss (anticonvulsants, corticosteroids). Most rapid decrease in mass (particularly in hips, spine, and torso) occurs in first 3–5 y postmenopause and slows after age 65 years
ADDITIONAL EFFECTS DUE TO MENOPAUSE COMBINED WITH NATURAL AGING	
Urethral disorders	Loss of urethral tone, painful urination, frequency, and stress incontinence
Decreased breast size	
Decreased skin elasticity	Facial, neck, and hand wrinkling; variations in quantity and distribution of body hair
Lower HDL levels	Increased risk (3×) for cardiovascular disease as LDL levels increase
Abdominal fat development	Greater degree of central android abdominal fat accumulates due to altered peripheral resistance to insulin and increase in type II diabetes as aging progresses (lower incidence in estrogen users)
Hyperinsulinemia	Signs and symptoms of low blood sugar
Short-term memory loss	In some women estrogen may have some stabilizing effect on maintenance of short-term memory

KEY: HDL: high-density lipoproteins: LDL: low-density lipoproteins.

ing micronized estradiol and estradiol valerate or 17β-estradiol). These are preferred for use in postmenopausal clients over the synthetic estrogens (ethinyl estradiol, mestranol) used for oral contraception. Synthetic estrogens are believed to be more taxing to the renal and hepatic systems than are biologic estrogens. Conjugated estrogens, mixtures of natural estrogens isolated from the urine of pregnant mares, are the most commonly used preparations for estrogen replacement therapy. Premarin, the most frequently used conjugated estrogen product, is presented in Chart 49–1.

The goal of replacement therapy has bearing on the dosage form. For example, bone protection requires extended systemic therapy, while treatment of hot flashes may involve shorter-term therapy. Vaginal changes may be treated with local or systemic therapy, or both.

Contraindications

Contraindications to estrogen replacement therapy include pregnancy, history of endometrial or breast cancer within the last 5 years, history of thromboembolic disorders, acute liver disease or chronic impaired liver function, gallbladder or pancreatic disease, poorly controlled hypertension, undiagnosed genital bleeding, and endometriosis. Lifestyle factors, such as smoking, known to enhance risk of thromboembolism should be considered in the treatment decision. The client with a history of fibroid tumors is not started on estrogen replacement for a full year after the last period, because estrogen would likely result in tumor growth. The hypoestrogenic state associated with natural menopause usually causes existing fibroids to shrink. The presence of fibrocystic breast disease, diabetes, or obesity may require extra caution. Estrogen is not thought to cause breast cancer, but the promotion of growth in an incipient breast cancer is a possibility. Doses used in estrogen replacement therapy are generally low.

Contraindications to progestin replacement in conjunction with estrogen are the same as those for estrogen. It is extremely important to rule out the presence of known or suspected breast cancer before progestins are used.

Chart 49–1. Estrogen Replacements

CONJUGATED ESTROGENS

Drug Name

Conjugated estrogens
   (Premarin, PMB, Milprem-400)
Hormone replacement therapy (HRT)
Pregnancy Category: X

Dosage

A: PO: 0.3–1.25 mg/d cyclically (with or without progestins); most often, 0.625 mg/d

Contraindications

Breast or reproductive cancer, undiagnosed genital bleeding, pregnancy, lactation, thromboembolitic disorders, smoking
Caution: Cardiovascular disease, severe renal or hepatic disease, smoking, diabetes mellitus

Drug-Lab-Food Interactions

Drug: *Increase* effects with corticosteroids; *decrease* effects of anticoagulants, oral hypoglycemics; *decrease* effects with rifampin, anticonvulsants, barbiturates; *toxicity* with tricyclic antidepressants

Pharmacokinetics

Absorption: PO: Well absorbed
Distribution: PB: Widely distributed; crosses placenta and enters breast milk
Metabolism: $t\frac{1}{2}$: UK
Excretion: In urine and bile

Pharmacodynamics

PO/IV: Onset: Rapid
          Peak: UK
          Duration: UK
IM: Onset: Delayed
          Peak: UK
          Duration: UK

Therapeutic Effects/Uses

To relieve vasodilation, hot flashes, and vaginal dryness, to prevent cardiovascular disease and osteoporosis.

Mode of Action: Development and maintenance of female genital system, breast, and secondary sex characteristics; increased synthesis of protein.

Side Effects

Nausea, vomiting, fluid retention, breast tenderness, leg cramps and breakthrough bleeding, chloasma

Adverse Reactions

Jaundice, thromboembolic disorders, depression, hypercalcemia, gallbladder disease
Life-threatening: Thromboembolism, cerebrovascular accident, pulmonary embolism, MI, endometrial cancer

Assessment and Planning

Interventions

Evaluation

NURSING PROCESS

KEY: A: adult; PO: by mouth; tab: tablet; inj: injection; PB: protein-binding; UK: unknown; $t\frac{1}{2}$: half-life; MI: myocardial infarction.

Dosage Forms

The oral route is the most commonly used; it is well tolerated by most clients and relatively easy to use but does require daily dosing. Some clients experience GI upsets, particularly nausea and vomiting. Clients with GI disorders such as colitis, irritable bowel syndrome, peptic ulcer, or malabsorption may receive inconsistent doses with oral administration, necessitating the use of another dosage form. Oral estrogens have a particularly beneficial effect on lipids by increasing high-density lipoproteins. Although the oral route does result in complete absorption from the GI tract, there is greater impact upon liver proteins.

The transdermal skin patch (the Estraderm Transdermal System) is a convenient method because it does not require daily dosing. The patch is applied to intact skin in the prescribed dosage. Generally the lower abdomen is used, but other sites (except for the breasts) may be employed. The patch is applied twice a week for 3 weeks, with rotation of sites, followed by 1 week without use of the patch to allow for normal withdrawal bleeding. The transdermal patch

Table 49–9
Estrogens and Progestins

GENERIC (BRAND)	ROUTE AND DOSAGE	PREGNANCY CATEGORY
CONJUGATED ESTROGENS		
Premarin	See Chart 49–1	
STEROIDAL ESTROGENS		
Estradiol (Estrace, Estraderm)	*Menopausal/hypogonadism:* PO: 1–2 mg/d for 21 d; then, 7–10 d off cycle; may repeat cycle *Patch:* 10–20 cm² system 2×/wk, in above cycle *Breast cancer:* 10 mg t.i.d. *Prostate cancer:* 1–2 mg t.i.d. *Atrophic vaginitis:* Cream: 2–4 g/d for 1–2 wk; maint: 1 g 2×/wk	X
Estradiol cypionate (Depo-Estradiol Cypionate)	*Menopausal symptoms:* IM: 1–4 mg q3–4 wk *Hypogonadism:* IM: 1.5–2 mg q mo	X
Esterified estrogens (Estratab, Menest)	*Menopausal symptoms:* PO: 0.3–1.25 mg/d for 3 wk; then 7–10 d off cycle *Breast cancer:* PO: 10 mg t.i.d. *Prostate cancer:* 1.25–2.5 mg t.i.d.	X
Estrone (Theelin, Kestrone 5)	*Hypogonadism:* 0.1–2 mg/wk *Prostate cancer:* 2–4 mg 3×/wk	X
Estropipate SO₄ (Ogen, Ortho-Est)	*Hypogonadism:* 1.25–7.5 mg/d for 3 wk; then 7–10 d off cycle	X
NONSTEROIDAL ESTROGENS		
Chlorotrianisene (Tace)	*Menopausal/hypogonadism:* 12–25 mg/d for 21 d; then, 10 d off cycle; repeat cycle *Prostate cancer:* 12–25 mg/d	X
Dienestrol (DV)	*Atrophic vaginitis:* Cream: Apply q.d./b.i.d. for 1–2 wk; maint: 1–3×/wk	X
Diethylstilbestrol	*Breast cancer:* 15 mg/d *Prostate cancer:* 1–3 mg t.i.d.	X
Quinestrol (Estrovis)	*Menopausal/hypogonadism:* 100 μg daily for 7 d; then 7 d off cycle; maint: q wk	X
PROGESTINS		
Progesterone	*DUB:* IM: 5–10 mg/d for 7 d *Amenorrhea:* IM: 5–10 mg/d for 6–8 d	X
Medroxyprogesterone acetate (Amen, Curretab, Provera, Cycrin, Depo-Provera)	*DUB/amenorrhea:* 5–10 mg/d for 5–10 d *Endometriosis:* IM: 150 mg q3mo	X

Table continued on following page

Table 49–9 *Continued*
Estrogens and Progestins

Megestrol acetate (Megace)	*Breast cancer:* PO: 40 mg q.i.d. *Endometrial cancer:* 40–320 mg/d in divided doses	X
Norethindrone (Norlutin)	*DUB/amenorrhea:* 5–20 mg/d on days 5–25 of menstrual cycle	X

DUB: dysfunctional uterine bleeding.

NURSING PROCESS
ESTROGEN REPLACEMENTS

Assessment

- Assess baseline data, including height, weight, usual physical activity, diet, family history, and personal risk factors regarding osteoporosis, family and personal risk of cardiovascular disease, and the nature of the family members' climacteric experience, the client's menstrual history, and current experience with the climacteric and the drugs the client is using.
- Assess the client's perception of menopause.
- Assess the client's attitude toward resumption of menstrual periods.

Potential Nursing Diagnoses

- Sexual dysfunction
- Body image disturbance
- Health-seeking behaviors

Planning

- Client will verbalize menopausal symptoms and the nonpharmacologic and pharmacologic measures that may aid in alleviating symptoms.

Nursing Interventions

- Educate women about the nature of the climacteric, its potential effects, and nonpharmacologic as well as pharmacologic treatment. Place current educational materials in health and community sites.
- Indicate on the laboratory slip or specimen that the client is taking hormone replacement therapy (HRT).
- Administer IM route at bedtime to decrease adverse effects.

Client Teaching

General

- Review the risk-to-benefit ratio for use of estrogen replacement therapy.
- Review the contraindications to HRT.
- Advise the client to have a breast examination, pelvic examination, Pap test, and endometrial biopsy before starting HRT.
- Tell the client that warm weather and stress exacerbate vasodilation/hot flashes.
- Advise the client to use a fan, drink cool liquids, wear layered cotton clothes, decrease intake of caffeine and spicy foods, and talk with her health care provider about the use of vitamin E to cope more comfortably with vasodilation. Individuals with diabetes, hypertension, or rheumatic heart disease should use vitamin E in low doses with the health care provider's approval.

Nursing Process continued on following page

NURSING PROCESS *Continued*
ESTROGEN REPLACEMENTS

- Encourage the client on HRT to have medical follow-up every 6 to 12 mo, including blood pressure check and breast and pelvic examinations.
- Suggest that the client carry sanitary pads or tampons for breakthrough bleeding or irregular periods.
- Stress the need to use nonhormonal birth control because irregular periods may create anxiety about pregnancy. Tell the client to plan to use birth control for 2 y. If she has progesterone-induced bleeding, the only way to determine whether she is truly menopausal is by hormone assay.
- Suggest to the client that she use a water-soluble vaginal lubricant to reduce painful intercourse (dyspareunia) and prevent trauma.
- Advise the client to decrease use of antihistamines and decongestants if she is experiencing vaginal dryness.
- Advise the client to wear cotton underwear and pantyhose with a cotton liner and to avoid douche and feminine hygiene products.
- Suggest that client take Premarin after meals together with progestin to avoid nausea and vomiting.
- Tell the client to report any heavy bleeding (flooding) and to have her hematocrit and hemoglobin evaluated.
- Tell the client to report bleeding that occurs between periods or return of bleeding after cessation of menstruation.
- Advise the client starting on HRT that the withdrawal bleeding that occurs from days 25 to 30 is normal and not the same as cyclic menstrual periods. Tell her that this bleeding will usually last only 2 to 3 d and that she will not experience the same degree of premenstrual symptoms she may have had with regular periods.
- Advise the client to report if bleeding occurs other than on days 25 to 30 once she has started on HRT.
- Tell her that the withdrawal bleeding does not signify that she can become pregnant.
- Advise the client that after HRT is discontinued, there may be a recurrence of menopausal signs and symptoms such as hot flashes.

Diet
- Discuss the use of yogurt containing *Acidophilus* or *Lactobacillus* as a way of maintaining normal bacterial flora in the vagina.
- Tell the client that she may experience an occasional hot flash on days 25 to 30 when she is going through withdrawal bleeding. Instruct the client to stop treatment and contact health care provider if she has headache, visual disturbances, signs of thrombophlebitis, heaviness in legs, chest pain, or breast lumps.
- Tell the client that if she wants to stop HRT, she should do so with guidance of her health care provider.
- Suggest that the client at risk for osteoporosis have consistent exercise such as walking or bicycling, eat a well-balanced diet (low in red meat and sugar) with 1200 mg calcium/d if premenopausal or 1200 to 1500 mg/d if menopausal, and avoid smoking and alcohol.

Self-Administration
- Teach the client to perform regular breast self-examination.
- If the client is using vaginal cream, review the application procedure and suggest that she wear minipads.
- If the client is using the transdermal patch, tell her to open the package and apply it immediately, holding it in place for about 10 s; to check the edges to ensure adequate contact; to use the abdomen (except waistline) for the patch; to rotate the sites with at least 1 wk before reuse of a site; to not use the breast as a site; to not put the patch on an irritated or oily area; to reapply the patch if it loosens or put on a new one; and to follow the same cycle schedule.

Nursing Process continued on following page

NURSING PROCESS *Continued*
ESTROGEN REPLACEMENTS

Evaluation

- Evaluate the effectiveness of the nonpharmacologic or pharmacologic measures for premenopausal symptoms.
- Determine whether side effects are occurring. Plan with the client alternative measures to control menopausal symptoms.

allows for absorption of the estrogen (17β-estradiol) directly into the bloodstream through a membrane that limits the absorption rate. The advantage is that the GI tract and liver are bypassed initially, which results in less nausea and vomiting and less impact upon liver proteins.

Vaginal cream preparations are used in the treatment of vaginal atrophy, which causes painful intercourse and urinary difficulties. Vaginal cream preparations containing conjugated estrogens are rapidly absorbed into the bloodstream via the mucous membrane that lines the vagina. There is some question as to the amount of estrogen that is systemically absorbed through this route; thus, it is not usually used to provide protection against bone loss. It can be used in conjunction with another method, such as tablets or the transdermal patch.

Medroxyprogesterone acetate (Provera), the progestin most often administered in combination with the estrogen, is taken orally. Examples of progestin products are given in Table 49–9.

Pharmacokinetics

The natural estrogens are completely and rapidly absorbed from the GI tract and rapidly metabolized by the liver, necessitating daily doses when oral products that are nonesterified (a process that delays metabolism and lengthens action) are used. About 80% of estradiol is bound to sex hormone binding globulin, with 2% unbound and the rest bound to albumin. Estradiol is converted to estrone in the enterohepatic circulation, and is conjugated and excreted via the urine. Progestin (Provera) is rapidly absorbed and metabolized primarily in the liver with excretion via the kidney; distribution of the agent is not well described.

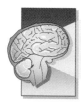

Critical Thinking in Action

Following delivery of baby Jessica, Tanya, Gr 3 P1 (gravida 3, para 1), is ready to leave the hospital. Pregnancy-induced hypertension had developed during the pregnancy but she had no prior history of hypertension. She plans to breastfeed for 3 months. She desires contraception and asks questions about hormonally controlled birth control methods.

1. Tanya asks if she can take combination birth control pills while breastfeeding. Describe a nursing diagnosis for Tanya based on her communication to you.
2. You tell her that she may breastfeed and start using combination pills in about 6 weeks once the milk flow is established. This information is:
   Correct: _____   Why? _____
   Incorrect: _____   Why? _____
3. Tanya asks if there are any advantages to the use of the oral contraceptives over using a diaphragm. List four advantages and four disadvantages that a nurse could include in her discussions.

Critical Thinking in Action continued on following page

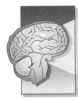

Critical Thinking in Action *Continued*

4. Tanya tells you that she smokes ¾ of a pack of cigarettes per day. Describe how this information might impact the decision for or against oral contraceptive use.

5. Tanya starts to use combination birth control pills and calls the clinic upset that she has forgotten to take one pill. What would the clinic nurse correctly tell Tanya to do? How might the nurse in the postpartum unit prepare Tanya for this situation?

6. Because milk flow needs to become established before starting on the combination birth control pills, what would you recommend to Tanya about contraception upon leaving the hospital? Consider that Tanya had a fourth-degree episiotomy and hemorrhoids.

7. Tanya states that when she has "bad allergies" she sometimes takes over-the-counter antihistamines. How would you advise Tanya?

8. How would you advise Tanya to take her birth control pills?

9. You decide to suggest injectable progestin (Depo-Provera) with Tanya as an alternative method for contraception. What advantage might this product have for Tanya over the oral products?

10. What would you advise Tanya about breastfeeding while using this product?

11. What implication does Tanya's smoking have in regard to known side effects with Depo-Provera?

12. Why should you document the site in which a Depo-Provera injection is given?

13. How would you explain to Tanya the way Depo-Provera works?

14. Tanya asks how long it will take to regain her fertility once she stops using the Depo-Provera injection. State the correct response to her question.

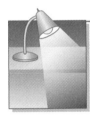

Study Questions

1. What key factors should the nurse cover in a teaching plan for oral contraceptive use? What is the degree of effectiveness of oral contraceptives? What are the advantages and disadvantages of this method?

2. What are some common symptoms associated with PMS? What are effective treatment modalities for the symptoms?

3. Explain the expected effects of drug therapy for endometriosis using danazol and gonadotropin-releasing hormone agonists.

4. A client asks you about hormonal replacement therapy. What information would you share with her in regard to (a) indications for hormone therapy, (b) routes of administration, (c) types of therapy, (d) expected duration of therapy, (e) contraindications, (f) side effects?

Drugs Related to Reproductive Health: Male Reproductive Disorders

50

Nancy C. Sharts-Hopko and Kathleen J. Jones

Outline

Objectives

- Describe the feedback loop comprising hypothalamic, anterior pituitary, and gonadal hormones.
- Describe the role of testosterone in development of primary and secondary male sex characteristics and in spermatogenesis.
- Identify common conditions for which androgen therapy and antiandrogen therapy are indicated.
- Identify clients for whom androgen therapy is particularly risky.
- Assess clients for therapeutic and adverse effects of androgen therapy.
- Identify commonly prescribed medications that can impair male sexual function.
- Explain the nursing process, including client teaching, related to drugs for male reproductive disorders.

Terms

addison's disease
anabolic steroids
androgens
antiandrogens
buccal tablet
cryptorchidism
Cushing's syndrome

delayed puberty
ejaculatory dysfunction
erectile dysfunction
gynecomastia
hirsutism
hyperthyroidism
hypogonadism

hypothyroidism
inhibited sexual desire
orchitis
priapism
spermatogenesis
testosterone
virilization

INTRODUCTION

This chapter discusses drug regimens for various alterations in male reproductive health other than the sexually transmitted diseases, which, because of their association with infertility, particularly among women, are addressed in Chapter 51.

Reproductive health requires the production of adequate quantities of various hypothalamic, pituitary, and gonadal hormones, as well as the appropriate hormone receptors. It requires normal development and patency of the reproductive tract. In addition, reproductive health implies that men and women of developmentally appropriate lifestages are fertile, that is, able to produce gametes (sperm or eggs). Finally, reproductive health entails the ability to engage in sexual intercourse with ejaculation by the male.

Alterations in reproductive health reflect a wide range of developmental, endocrine, infectious, inflammatory, hypertrophic, malignant, and psychoemotional processes. To gain a better understanding of ways in which reproductive health can be affected, reproductive processes are reviewed.

The drug family most clearly associated with male reproductive processes is the androgens. Because anabolic steroids and the antiandrogens impact male reproduction, they are also discussed.

The male reproductive processes including anatomy and physiology, sperm production, regulation of male sexual functioning, and sexual intercourse are discussed in the Unit XIII Introduction.

SUBSTANCES RELATED TO MALE REPRODUCTIVE DISORDERS

Androgens

Androgens, or male sex hormones, affect sexual processes, accessory sexual organs, cellular metabolism, and bone and muscle growth. The actions and effects of natural androgens are listed in Chart 50–1. **Testosterone,** the main androgen, is synthesized primarily in the testes and, to a lesser extent, in the adrenal cortex. In women, the ovaries synthesize small amounts of testosterone. In men, normal plasma concentrations of testosterone are 250 to 1000 mg/dL, with circadian fluctuations.

PHARMACOKINETICS

In men, about 98% of circulating testosterone is bound to protein. It is the unbound fraction that is biologically active. Estrogen elevates the production of sex hormone-binding globulin; therefore, more circulating testosterone is bound in women.

The half-life of endogenous free testosterone in the blood is 10 to 20 minutes. Exogenous testosterone is absorbed orally, but because as much as 50% is metabolized on its first pass through the hepatic circulation, high doses are needed to achieve effective plasma levels. Synthetic androgens have longer half-lives. Testosterone can be combined with esters to form esterified testosterone, in an oil base, to achieve a duration of action of up to 4 weeks.

Testosterone is excreted mainly in the urine as the metabolites androsterone and etiocholanolone. About 6% of the hormone is excreted unaltered in the feces. Synthetic androgens may be excreted as unaltered hormone or as metabolites. In some tissues, the action of testosterone depends on its reduction to 5-alpha-dihydrotestosterone, whereas in other tissues testosterone itself is the active hormone. In the central nervous system, it is the metabolite estradiol that affects hormonal action.

PHARMACODYNAMICS

Testosterone is responsible for the development of male characteristics. These include the fetal development and the maturation of the male reproductive system and the development of secondary sex characteristics such as pubic hair growth, beard and body hair growth, baldness, deepening of the male voice, thickening of the skin, sebaceous gland activity, increased musculature, bone development, and red blood cell formation.

The mechanism for these effects may be increased protein formation in the target cells. Dehydrotestosterone with its receptor acts at binding sites on the chromosomes. Increased RNA polymerase activity and increased synthesis of specific RNA and proteins result, accounting for the anabolic effects of testosterone.

The testes produce testosterone in utero. After birth until just before puberty, production is negligible. During puberty, production increases rapidly and continues until later adulthood. As men age, the number of Leydig cells decreases, sperm production declines, and luteinizing hormone (LH) and follicle-stimulating hormone FSH levels rise. Levels of unbound testosterone are reduced in elderly men to one-third to one-fifth the peak value. Although a "male menopause" does not occur, some men do experience temporary vasomotor flushing that may be alleviated by testosterone replacement therapy.

INDICATIONS FOR ANDROGEN THERAPY

Various androgens and their uses are identified in Table 50–1.

Hypogonadism

The clearest indication for androgen therapy is insufficient testosterone production by the testes, or **hypogonadism.** Hypogonadism can be primary, reflecting testicular abnormality, or secondary, reflecting hypo-

Chart 50-1. Androgens

TESTOSTERONE

Drug Name

Testosterone
　(Andro-Cyp 100, depAndro 100, Depotest 100,
　Duratest 100, DEPO-Testosterone, Testred
　Cypionate 200, Virilon, depAndrogyn, Ever-
　one)
Pregnancy Category: X
CSS III

Dosage

Androgen Replacement
PO: 10–40 mg daily
Buccal: 5–20 mg daily
SC: 150–450 mg q3–6mo
IM: 10–30 mg 2–3 times per week

Metastatic Carcinoma of the Breast:
PO: 200 mg daily
Buccal: 200 mg daily
IM: 100 mg 3 times per week

Contraindications

Pregnancy, nephrosis, hypercalcemia, pituitary
insufficiency, hepatic dysfunction, benign prostatic hypertrophy, prostatic cancer, history of
myocardial infarction, prepubertal status, non–
estrogen-dependent breast cancer

Caution: Hypertension, hypercholesterolemia,
coronary artery disease, gynecomastia, renal disease, seizure disorders, before puberty, older
adults

Drug-Lab-Food Interactions

Drug: *Increases* effects of anticoagulants;
decreases effect with barbiturates, phenytoin,
phenylbutazone; antagonizes calcitonin, parathyroid; corticosteroids exacerbate edema
Lab: *Decreases* blood glucose in diabetics; *increases* serum cholesterol, thyroid, liver function,
hematocrit

Pharmacokinetics

Absorption: IM: Well absorbed
Distribution: PB: 98%
Metabolism: t½: 10–100 min
Excretion: In urine and bile

Pharmacodynamics

IM: Onset: UK
　Peak: UK
　Duration: cypionate enanthate: 2–4 wk
　Base, propionate: 1–3 d

Therapeutic Effects/Uses

To achieve normal androgen levels; to slow progress of estrogen-dependent breast cancers.

Mode of Action: Development and maintenance of male sex organs and secondary sex characteristics.

Side Effects

Abdominal pain, nausea, diarrhea, constipation,
hives, irritation at injection site, increased salivation, mouth soreness, increased or decreased
libido, insomnia, aggressive behavior, weakness,
dizziness, pruritus

Adverse Reactions

Acne, masculinization, irregular menses, urinary
urgency, gynecomastia, priapism, red skin, jaundice, sodium and water retention, allergic reaction, depression
Life-threatening: Hepatic necrosis, hepatitis, hepatic tumors, respiratory distress

Assessment and Planning

NURSING PROCESS

Interventions

Evaluation

KEY: SC: subcutaneous; IM: intramuscular; PO: by mouth; PB: protein-binding; t½: half-life; UK: unknown.

thalamic or pituitary failure. Severely affected male
children do not experience puberty. Mild hypogonadism may result. Lack of libido or the onset of vasomotor flushing also can occur. The timing and extent
of treatment depend on the clinical manifestations.

Induction of puberty is undertaken after boys
reach 15 to 17 years of age. Hypothalamic and pituitary function is assessed. A 4- to 6-month trial of
androgen therapy is implemented, followed by a like
period of rest for reevaluation. If prolonged therapy

Table 50–1
Androgens

DRUG	DOSAGE	USES AND CONSIDERATIONS
NATURAL ANDROGENS		
Testosterone (Histerone, Tesamone, Testopel pellets, testosterone aqueous, testosterone powder)	IM: 10–25 mg 2–3 × w SC: 150–450 mg q3–6m	Androgen replacement, delayed puberty, senile or postmenopausal osteoporosis. Started at full dose and adjusted according to tolerance and therapeutic response.
	IM: 100 mg 3 × w	Carcinoma of the breast. Therapy may be life long. *Pregnancy category:* X; PB: 98%; $t_{\frac{1}{2}}$: 10–100 min
Testosterone cypionate (Andro-Cyp, Andronate, depAndro, Depotest, DEPO-Testosterone, Duratest, Testred cypionate, Virilon IM)	IM: 50–400 mg q2–6w	Androgen replacement, delayed puberty. Therapy generally lasts 3–4 yrs. *Pregnancy category:* X; PB: 98%; $t_{\frac{1}{2}}$: 10–100 min
Testosterone enanthate (Andro I.A., Andropository, Delatest, Delatestryl, Durathate, Everone, Testrin)	IM: 50–400 mg q2–6w	Androgen replacement, delayed puberty. *Pregnancy category:* X; PB: 98%; $t_{\frac{1}{2}}$: 10–100 min
Testosterone propionate (Testex, testosterone propionate powder)	IM: 50 mg 3 × w	Androgen replacement. *Pregnancy category:* X; PB: 98%; $t_{\frac{1}{2}}$: 10–100 min
SYNTHETIC ANDROGENS		
Danazol (Danocrine)	PO: 100–800 mg daily divided in 2 doses initially	Endometriosis, fibrocystic breast disease, angioedema. Initial doses are gradually reduced on an individual basis. Endometriosis therapy lasts 6–9 mo; fibrocystic breast disease therapy lasts 4–6 mo. *Pregnancy category:* X; PB: UK; $t_{\frac{1}{2}}$: 4.5 h
Fluoxymesterone (Halotestin)	PO: 10–30 mg daily divided in 1–4 doses	Androgen deficiency, carcinoma of the breast. *Pregnancy category:* X; PB: 98%; $t_{\frac{1}{2}}$: 20–100 min
Methyltestosterone (Android, Oreton Methyl, Testred, Virilon)	PO: 10–50 mg daily in divided doses initially, reduced for maintenance Buccal: 5–25 mg daily in divided doses PO: 50–200 mg daily Buccal: 2–25 mg daily in divided doses	Androgen deficiency Carcinoma of the breast. *Pregnancy category:* X; PB: UK; $t_{\frac{1}{2}}$: UK
ANABOLIC STEROIDS		
Nandrolone decanoate (Androlone-D, Deca-Durabolin, Hybolin Decanoate, Neo-Durabolic)	IM: 50–200 mg q1–4w C: IM: 25–50 mg q3–4w	Anemia of renal disease. *Pregnancy category:* X; PB: UK; $t_{\frac{1}{2}}$: UK
Nandrolone phenpropionate (Durabolin, Hybolin improved, Nandrobolic)	IM: 50–100 mg/w	Carcinoma of the breast. *Pregnancy category:* X; PB: UK; $t_{\frac{1}{2}}$: 1–9 h
Oxandrolone (Oxandrin)	PO: 5–20 mg daily, divided C: PO: 0.1 mg/kg/d	Delayed growth/puberty, osteoporotic pain, short stature, Turner's syndrome, alcoholic hepatitis. *Pregnancy category:* X; PB: UK; $t_{\frac{1}{2}}$: 1–9 h
Oxymetholone (Anadrol-50)	PO: 1–5 mg/kg/d	Anemias of deficient RBC production. *Pregnancy category:* X; PB: UK; $t_{\frac{1}{2}}$: 9 h
Stanozolol (Winstrol)	PO: 2–6 mg/d	$t_{\frac{1}{2}}$: UK

KEY: IM: intramuscular; PO: by mouth; SC: subcutaneous; C: child; PB: protein-binding; UK: unknown; $t_{\frac{1}{2}}$: half-life; RBC: red blood cell.

is required, testosterone cypionate or testosterone enanthate is given, starting with 100 mg IM every 2 weeks for 6 to 12 months, with a gradual increase to 200 mg every 2 weeks. It takes 3 or 4 years for sexual development to occur. Plasma testosterone levels should be monitored and dosages adjusted as needed to maintain normal levels.

A transdermal testosterone skin patch for daily application to the scrotum, which eliminates the need for injections, is available. This delivery system provides circadian fluctuations in dosage.

Micropenis

Neonates occasionally demonstrate inadequate penile development. Intramuscular or topical administration of low concentrations of testosterone for no longer than 3 months may promote penile growth. Treatment may be repeated later in childhood.

Constitutional Growth Delay

A height of two or more standard deviations below the mean for age and sex occurs in 2.5% of normal children. It tends to be of greater concern for boys. Delay in bone growth seems to be of little consequence by the time boys reach the age of 20 years, but in some families delayed growth causes significant emotional distress despite reassurance from health professionals. Treatment is not initiated before the age of 14 years. Therapy for 3 to 6 months or less before epiphyseal closure may result in linear growth without adverse permanent effects on hypothalamic, pituitary, or gonadal maturation. It is not known whether treatment has an effect on final adult height.

The selection of an androgen or anabolic steroid depends on the balance of growth and sexual maturation that is desired, as well as the preferred route of administration. The effectiveness of oxandrolone for this purpose has been demonstrated. Testosterone enanthate, 50 mg/month IM, has been effective, and a sublingual testosterone preparation (Andro Test-SL) is currently undergoing clinical trials.

Other Uses

Other uses of androgens include treatment of refractory anemias in men and women, the autosomal clotting disorder hereditary angioneurotic edema, tissue wasting associated with severe or chronic illness, advanced carcinoma of the breast in women, and endometriosis. The effectiveness of androgens for treatment of **cryptorchidism** and impotence has not been established. Androgens may be used in combination with estrogens for management of severe menopausal symptoms (see Chapter 49).

SIDE EFFECTS

Side effects of androgen therapy include abdominal pain, nausea, insomnia, diarrhea or constipation, hives or redness at the injection site, increased salivation, mouth soreness, and increased or decreased sexual desire. If side effects persist, worsen, or disturb the individual, the health care provider should be notified.

ADVERSE EFFECTS

Virilizing effects (the development of secondary male sex characteristics) are inappropriate when the client is not a hypogonadal adult male. Women risk such manifestations as acne and skin oiliness, the growth of facial hair, and vocal huskiness. Menstrual irregularities or amenorrhea, suppressed ovulation or lactation, baldness or increased hair growth, and hypertrophy of the clitoris may develop in women undergoing androgen therapy. Although most adverse effects slowly reverse themselves after short-term therapy is completed, vocal changes may be permanent. With long-term therapy, as in the treatment of breast cancer, adverse effects may be irreversible.

Children may experience profound virilization or feminization, as well as impaired bone growth. During pregnancy, androgens can cross the placenta and cause masculinization of the fetus.

Hypogonadal males may experience frequent or continuous erection, called **priapism; gynecomastia,** or breast swelling or soreness; and urinary urgency. Continued use of androgens by normal men can halt spermatogenesis. The sperm count may be low for 3 or more months after therapy is stopped.

Less frequent adverse effects include dizziness, weakness, changes in skin color, frequent headaches, confusion, respiratory distress, depression, pruritus, allergic skin rash, edema of the lower extremities, jaundice, bleeding, paresthesias, chills, polycythemia, muscle cramps, and sodium and water retention. Hepatic carcinoma can occur in clients who have received 17-alpha-alkyl substituted androgens over prolonged periods (i.e., 1–7 years).

Serum cholesterol may become elevated during androgen therapy. Other alterations in laboratory tests include altered thyroid and liver function tests, elevated urine 17-ketosteroids, and increased hematocrit.

Rare complications of long-term therapy include hepatic necrosis, hepatic peliosis, hepatic tumors, and leukopenia.

CONTRAINDICATIONS

Androgen therapy is contraindicated during pregnancy and in individuals with nephrosis or the nephrotic phase of nephritis, hypercalcemia, pituitary insufficiency, hepatic dysfunction, benign prostatic hypertrophy, or prostate cancer. Men with breast cancer are not treated with androgens, nor are women whose breast cancer is not estrogen dependent. A history of myocardial infarction is a contraindication.

NURSING PROCESS
ANDROGENS

Assessment

- Assess the reason for androgen therapy and the client's perception of it. If delayed puberty is the indication, the nurse will assess the client's and family's attitudes about the condition.
- Monitor the client's weight, blood pressure, liver and thyroid function, hemoglobin and hematocrit, creatinine, clotting factors, glucose tolerance, serum lipids and electrolytes, and blood count before and throughout treatment. The presence of liver or endocrine dysfunction is noted.
- Determine the pregnancy status of women of child-bearing age. Concomitant anticoagulant therapy should be noted. When a prepubertal child is treated, x-rays are obtained before, every 6 months during, and after treatment to monitor growth.
- Appraise the client's affect during therapy, particularly aggressiveness in clients taking large doses. Self-concept is an important consideration in the client on androgen therapy, particularly in children with delayed puberty and in women.

Nursing Diagnoses

- Body image disturbance
- Altered growth and development
- Self-esteem disturbance
- Sexual dysfunction
- Altered sexuality patterns
- Knowledge deficit regarding the treatment protocol

Planning

- Nursing goals for clients include adherence to the prescribed regimen for taking the medication and for monitoring.
- Long-term goals include appropriate use of the medication, avoidance of preventable adverse effects, and maintenance of a positive self-concept.

Nursing Interventions

Client Teaching

General

- The client and family need instruction on proper administration of the medications, their reasons for use, and potential undesired effects. They are informed of which effects warrant prompt medical attention (urinary problems, priapism, and respiratory distress).
- If an intermittent approach to treatment is used, the client needs to understand that this allows for monitoring of endocrine status between courses of androgen therapy. The need to return to the health care facility for monitoring is explained, and the client's ability to do so is determined. Social service referrals are made if necessary.
- Families pursuing treatment for a client with delayed puberty are instructed about the range of normal development.
- Individuals being treated for tissue wasting are urged to reduce environmental stressors and promote rest and relaxation, because stress hormones are catabolic. Muscle strength will be monitored during treatment.

Nursing Process continued on following page

Caution must be exercised in using androgen therapy in individuals with hypertension, hypercholesterolemia, coronary artery disease, gynecomastia, renal disease, or seizure disorder. It is used with caution in infants and prepubertal children because of the potential for growth disturbances and in geriatric males because of their increased risk for benign prostatic hypertrophy and prostate cancer.

DRUG INTERACTIONS

Androgens potentiate the effects of oral anticoagulants, necessitating a decrease in anticoagulant dos-

Diet

- The nutritional intake of individuals with anemia, osteoporosis, or tissue wasting is assessed and revised as needed to ensure adequate intake of calories, protein, vitamins, iron, and other minerals.
- Sodium may need to be restricted if edema develops. The client will be instructed to record body weight several times per week.
- Individuals with elevated serum calcium need 3 to 4 L of fluid per day to prevent kidney stones. Individuals on bedrest need range-of-motion exercises, whereas ambulatory clients need to engage in active weight bearing. Indicators of hypercalcemia are shown in Table 50–2. Hypercalcemia needs prompt medical attention because it can lead to cardiac arrest.

Self-Administration

- Oral androgens should be taken with food to decrease gastric distress.

Side Effects

- Women and prepubertal clients need instruction on good skin hygiene to decrease the severity of acne.
- Men undergoing androgen therapy are instructed to report priapism (painful, continuous erection) promptly. The drug dosage will be reduced to avoid subsequent erectile dysfunction. In addition, they are taught to report decreased urinary stream promptly because androgens can stimulate prostatic hypertrophy.

Evaluation

- The client's ability to adhere to the treatment regimen and response to prescribed drugs will be monitored.
- The client will be asked about therapeutic and adverse drug effects on follow-up visits. Monitoring of weight, blood pressure, and laboratory tests will continue throughout therapy, with alterations in the plan of care as needed.
- Youngsters and women who experience virilizing effects or acne will be periodically assessed for the ability to cope with these changes and maintain a positive self-concept.
- Sexual function is assessed when appropriate.
- The client's ability to adhere to the treatment plan and to discuss the treatment and its effects knowledgeably suggests that teaching has been effective and that the client accepts the treatment.

Table 50–2
Signs of Hypercalcemia

Nausea and vomiting
Lethargy
Decreased muscle tone
Polyuria
Increased urine and serum calcium

age. Androgens antagonize calcitonin and parathyroid hormones. Because androgens can decrease blood glucose in diabetics, dosages of insulin or other antidiabetic agents may need to be reduced. Concurrent use of corticosteroids exacerbates the edema that can occur with androgen therapy. Barbiturates, phenytoin, and phenylbutazone decrease the effects of androgens.

Anabolic Steroids

Anabolic steroids are testosterone derivatives developed to maximize the anabolic effects of androgens and minimize their androgenic effects. Abuse of these drugs by athletes is a growing problem. Some athletes and trainers believe these drugs enhance aerobic performance, strength, lean body mass, and muscular development. Other perceived benefits include euphoria and enhanced sexual performance. However, the dosages used may be up to 30 times the therapeutic amount, and numerous serious and sometimes irreversible adverse effects have been reported. Moreover, the adverse effects may not be recognized until several decades have passed. Because most of these drugs are obtained illegally, young people socialized to this pattern of use may be at risk for abuse of other illegal drugs. All major athletic organizations prohibit the use of anabolic steroids.

Antiandrogens

Antiandrogens, or androgen antagonists, block the synthesis or action of androgens (Table 50–3). These drugs may be useful in the management of benign prostatic hypertrophy and carcinoma of the prostate. They have been used to treat male-pattern baldness, acne, hirsutism, virilization syndrome in women, and precocious puberty in boys, although their effectiveness is not well established. The effectiveness of these drugs on the inhibition of sex drive in men who are sex offenders is controversial and not well documented.

GnRH, or an analogue such as leuprolide, is the most effective inhibitor of testosterone synthesis. When such agents are given over time, LH and testosterone levels fall. Ketoconazole is under investigation for treatment of prostatic carcinoma because of its inhibition of adrenal and gonadal steroid synthesis.

Two types of drugs have been developed to block testosterone action: androgen-receptor antagonists and agents that block conversion of testosterone to its ac-

tive form, dihydrotestosterone. Cyproterone acetate, an orally active progesterone, is a potent androgen antagonist. It also suppresses LH and FSH secretion and has progestational qualities. Cyproterone acetate competes with dihydrotestosterone for binding to the androgen receptor. Cyproterone acetate can stunt growth in youngsters. Acne and baldness have been reported.

Flutamide (Eulexin) is a nonsteroidal drug that competes with androgens at androgen receptors. Men receiving flutamide show elevations in plasma LH and testosterone levels. Flutamide is used along with GnRH blockade or estrogen in the treatment of prostate cancer. Spironolactone also competes with dihydrotestosterone at the receptor site. It is used in doses of 50 to 100 mg/d for treatment of hirsutism in women.

Finasteride, a steroid, inhibits conversion of testosterone to dihydrotestosterone. This orally active agent decreases the concentration of dihydrotestosterone in plasma and in the prostate without elevated plasma concentrations of LH or testosterone. Finasteride is used for the treatment of benign prostatic hypertrophy. Other uses are under investigation. The recommended dose (for benign prostatic hypertrophy) of 5 mg/d needs to be reevaluated at 6 months and periodically thereafter. Women of childbearing potential should not come in contact with broken or crushed tablets. Adverse reactions include impotence, decreased libido, and decreased ejaculate.

Drugs Used in Other Male Reproductive Disorders

DEVELOPMENTAL DISORDERS

Undescended testes are associated with subsequent infertility and testicular cancer. The primary treatment is orchiopexy, or surgical placement of the testicle into the scrotum, and is usually performed by the time the child is 18 months old. If subsequent hormonal therapy is indicated, the hormones testosterone and human chorionic gonadotropin (hCG) are often used. Treatment is usually initiated before the age of 6 years. The dosage of hCG in boys is 500 to 4000 IU intramuscularly two to three times per week for several weeks. Adverse reactions include headache, irritability, precocious puberty, gynecomastia, and edema.

DELAYED PUBERTY

In up to 5% of cases of delayed puberty, there is insufficient secretion of GnRH, LH, or FSH. Once the cause is determined, GnRH, LH, or FSH replacement therapy is instituted.

Table 50–3
Antiandrogens

MECHANISM	DRUGS
Elevation of GnRH level	Goserelin (Zoladex) Nafarelin (Synarel) Leuprolide acetate (Lupron, Lupron Depot)
Inhibition of testosterone synthesis	Ketoconazole (Nizoral)
Blocks conversion of testosterone to dihydrotestosterone	Finasteride (Proscar)
Receptor inhibitors	Cyproterone, cyproterone acetate (orphan drug status in the United States) Flutamide (Eulexin) Spironolactone (generic, Aldactone)

PITUITARY, THYROID, AND ADRENAL DISORDERS

Inadequate pituitary function can result in hypogonadism. In a prepubertal male, it results in lack of secondary sex characteristics and infertility; adult men may experience testicular atrophy and decreased libido, decreased potency, decreased beard growth, and decreased muscle tone. Menotropins (Pergonal), one ampule of which contains 75 IU each of LH and FSH, injected IM three times weekly over a period of years, can stimulate testosterone production. Menotropins is indicated when both LH and FSH levels are low. It is given concomitantly with hCG 2000 IU intramuscularly twice per week for at least 3 months. Adverse effects include nausea, vomiting, diarrhea, gynecomastia, and fever. Reconstituted with 1 to 2 mL sterile saline, the drug must be used immediately.

Hypothyroidism, a deficiency in thyroid hormone, can be the result of insufficient thyroid hormone production or resistance to its effects at the target organs. The problem could be congenital. It can cause inhibited sexual desire and erectile dysfunction. In **Addison's disease,** there is a deficit of both cortisol and the mineralocorticoid aldosterone. Men with Addison's disease may experience inhibited sexual desire, erectile dysfunction, or diminished fertility. Both of these conditions are highly responsive to replacement therapy with the appropriate hormones (see Chapter 45).

SEXUAL DYSFUNCTION

Sexual dysfunction is the inability to experience sexual desire, erection, ejaculation, and detumescence—the phases of the sexual response cycle. **Inhibited sexual desire** can result from androgen deficiency, an affective disorder, or discord in the sexual relationship. **Erectile dysfunction** may be due to psychoemotional problems, vascular insufficiency, neurologic disorders, androgen deficiency or resistance, or diseases of the penis. **Ejaculatory dysfunction** can be psychogenic or a result of drug therapy, androgen deficiency, or sympathetic degeneration. **Failure of detumescence** is most commonly caused by penile disease or systemic disease. Male sexual dysfunction may result from the use of various drugs, as listed in Table 50–4.

L-Dopa, used in the treatment of Parkinson's syndrome, has shown effectiveness in stimulating libido and treating erectile dysfunctions in non-Parkinson's clients. Individuals who experience premature ejaculation related to excessive anxiety about sexual intercourse may be helped by treatment with one of the monoamine oxidase (MAO) inhibitors in conjunction with psychotherapy (see Chapter 19). Erectile dysfunction caused by vascular insufficiency is occasion-

Table 50–4
Drugs Causing Sexual Dysfunction in Males

DRUG CATEGORY	DRUGS OR DRUG FAMILIES
Anticholinergics	Atropine Scopolamine Benztropine Trihexyphenidyl
Antidepressants	Tricyclic antidepressants Monoamine oxidase inhibitors
Antihistamines	Cimetidine Diphenhydramine Hydroxyzine
Antihypertensives	Central sympathetic ganglion blockers Postganglionic blockers Alpha- and beta-receptor blockers Diuretics
Antipsychotics	Phenothiazines Thioxanthenes Butyrophenone Lithium
Sedatives and social drugs	Alcohol Barbiturates Diazepam Chlordiazepoxide Cannabis Cocaine Opiates Methadone
Others	Aminocaproic acid Baclofen Steroids Ethionamide Perhexiline Digoxin Chemotherapeutic agents

ally treated on a short-term basis by local vasoactive drugs, including papaverine, phentolamine, prostaglandin E, nitroglycerin, or yohimbine (yohimbe), a systemic vasoactive drug.

A new class of drugs, the phosphodiesterase inhibitors, is available. Sildenafil citrate (Viagra) is a potent and selective reuptake inhibitor of cyclic guanosine monophosphate (cGMP) in the corpus cavernosa. This action helps to restore the erectile response. Viagra was shown to potentiate the hypotensive effects of nitrates and is contraindicated for use by any client using organic nitrates in any form. Organic nitrates include nitroglycerin, isosorbide mononitrate, isosorbide nitrate, pentaerythritol tetranitrate, erythrityl tetranitrate, isosorbide dinitrate/phenobarbital, and illicit substances (amylnitrate/nitrite, butylnitrate). Viagra is also contraindicated in clients with anatomic deformities or with a condition predisposing them to priapism.

Viagra may be taken from 30 minutes to 4 hours before sexual activity. For most clients, the recommended dose is 50 mg, taken 1 hour before sexual activity. The dosage may be different for individual clients, and clients should not take more than has been prescribed. It is necessary for the client to inform the health care provider of all other medications he is taking because Viagra can interact or interfere with their actions. For example, it is recommended not to use Viagra with other medications used in the treatment of erectile dysfunction.

Selected side effects should be reported promptly to the health care provider, including flushing, dyspepsia, nasal congestion, and diarrhea. Other rare side effects should also be discussed, including blurred vision, photosensitivity, seeing shades of color (especially blue and green) differently, and urinary tract symptoms (frequency, pain on urination, and cloudy or bloody urine).

Certain drugs are often abused by individuals seeking a heightened sexual experience. Amyl nitrate is commonly believed to be an aphrodisiac. Sudden death, myocardial infarction, and methemoglobinemia have been reported with its use. Cantharides (Spanish fly) causes bladder and urethral irritation, accounting for its use as a sexual stimulant. Permanent penile damage has been reported with its use.

NONSEXUALLY TRANSMITTED INFECTIONS

Urinary tract infections are addressed in Chapter 30. If left untreated, acute or chronic prostatitis, orchitis, or epididymitis can develop.

MALIGNANT AND BENIGN TUMORS

Prostatic cancer accounts for about 10% of all cancer deaths among American men. Most prostatic cancers are adenocarcinomas. Metastasis to lymph nodes, bone, lungs, liver, and adrenal glands is common. Prostatic cancer is often asymptomatic, but urinary obstruction is commonly the first sign. Treatment may include a combination of surgical resection, cryotherapy, antiandrogen administration, radiation therapy, chemotherapy, and pain relief.

Testicular tumors peak in early adulthood. They include malignant germinal cell tumors and benign Leydig or Sertoli cell tumors. Treatment depends on the type and stage of tumor. Surgical excision, radiation therapy, and chemotherapy are used singly or in combination.

One percent of breast cancer cases occur in men. Breast cancer in men occurs most commonly after the age of 60 years. Treatment, which is similar for men and women, entails surgery, radiation therapy, chemotherapy, and endocrine therapy. Carcinoma of the penis represents less than 1% of all malignancies among males. In situ, treatment entails local excision, radiation therapy, and local application of 5-fluorouracil cream or solution. Invasive carcinoma is treated by surgical resection of the penis and involved nodes. Radiation and chemotherapy follow as needed. Antineoplastic therapies are discussed in Unit VII.

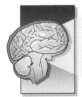

Critical Thinking In Action

Matt is a 16-year-old high school junior who is 5'3" and weighs 126 lb. He has increased feelings of discomfort about not fitting in with other students in his school because he has not yet begun sexual maturation. He is a good student and an accomplished violinist in the school orchestra. His only brother is younger than he is. His father states that he also was a "late bloomer," but he and his wife are concerned about their son's increasing social withdrawal and seem determined to seek medical intervention for him. The nurse in the clinic assesses the needs and status of Matt and his family.

1. What is the client's primary complaint? What concerns his family?
2. What information must be included in the history and physical examination?
3. What teaching should the nurse do prior to the parents making the decision to allow their son to start on androgen therapy?

The decision is made to prescribe methyltestosterone 5 mg/d by **buccal tablet** (held inside the cheek until it dissolves). Matt will be on this regimen for 4 months, during which time he is to come to the clinic at monthly intervals.

4. Matt asks why he will be treated for 4 months. What will the nurse reply?
5. About what adverse effects do Matt and his parents need to be taught?
6. What physical and psychosocial parameters will be monitored at his monthly visits?
7. What special hygiene needs does Matt have while on this regimen?
8. When should he have x-rays? Why?
9. During a clinic visit, Matt mentions that he has heard that the use of anabolic steroids might improve his chances of making the wrestling team. What should he be told about the safety and efficacy of anabolic steroid use?

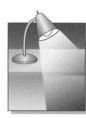

Study Questions

1. Explain the relationships among gonadotropin-releasing hormone, follicle-stimulating hormone, luteinizing hormone, and the gonadal hormones.
2. What are some desired effects of androgen therapy?
3. Why would healthy adolescents abuse androgens?
4. What is the role of androgen therapy in treatment of breast cancer?
5. What physical parameters are measured during androgen therapy?
6. In what groups must extra care be taken when androgen therapy is used?
7. What is an indication for antiandrogen therapy?
8. What are two reasons for treatment of cryptorchidism early in life?
9. What are long-term implications of infection of the male reproductive tract?
10. Identify the stages of the sexual response cycle, and identify which are most important for fertility in males and in females.
11. Identify 10 commonly used medications that can impair male sexual function.

Drugs Related to Reproductive Health: Infertility and Sexually Transmitted Diseases

NANCY C. SHARTS-HOPKO and KATHLEEN J. JONES

Outline

Objectives

- Describe male, female, and couple causes of infertility.
- Instruct couples on the relationships among ovulatory stimulation therapy, fertility awareness, and timing of coitus.
- Describe the way in which ovulatory stimulants promote fertility.
- Identify clients at risk for sexually transmitted diseases (STDs)
- Describe the relationship among STDs and infertility.
- Instruct clients in regimens for common STDs.
- Plan management for STDs for which cures do not exist.
- Counsel health care workers about management of worksite exposure to blood-borne STDs.
- Describe the nursing process, including client teaching, related to drugs for infertility and STDs.

Terms

autoimmune

blastocyst

fertilization

implantation

infertility, primary, secondary

ovulation

perinatal infection

placenta

sexually transmitted disease

trophoblast

vertical transmission

zygote

INTRODUCTION

This chapter discusses drug regimens for two broad categories of reproductive health alterations that are often interrelated: infertility and sexually transmitted diseases. Alterations in fertility reflect a wide range of developmental, endocrine, infectious, inflammatory, hypertrophic, and psychoemotional processes. As a basis for understanding infertility, the process of fertilization is reviewed. Drug therapies used in the management of female and, more briefly, male infertility are addressed, with emphasis on ovulation stimulants.

The broad category of diseases that are sexually transmitted constitutes a threat to reproductive tract integrity and functioning, as well as to neonatal health. Some, such as human immunodeficiency virus (HIV) disease, are life-threatening in and of themselves. Drug therapies for these conditions are reviewed briefly.

DRUGS RELATED TO INFERTILITY TREATMENT

Infertility is defined as the inability to conceive a child after 12 months of unprotected sexual intercourse. Women older than 35 years of age may be considered infertile after a shorter trial. Infertility is considered **primary** if a couple have never borne a live infant, and **secondary** if they have.

Assessing Infertility

Causes of infertility (Table 51–1) are numerous. In about 15% of cases, no specific cause can be found. Up to 40% of cases are the result of sexually transmitted diseases, which may result in neonatal death or altered reproductive tract integrity. Treatment of infertility depends on assessment of the cause.

General health is assessed; nutritional, reproductive, social drugs, and sexual histories are taken; and physical examinations with routine laboratory tests are conducted on both partners. Common tests to determine specific causes of infertility are listed in Table 51–2.

Induction of Ovulation

Clomiphene citrate (Serophene, Clomid), an estrogen antagonist, blocks the negative hypothalamic-pituitary-gonadal feedback loop. The precise mechanism of action is not understood, but increased gonadotropin-releasing hormone (GnRH) release increases luteinizing hormone (LH) and follicle-stimulating hormone (FSH) output. It is the most commonly used

Table 51–1
Causes of Infertility

FEMALE FACTORS	
Genetic	Chromosomal abnormalities, enzyme defects
Tubal or peritoneal	Infection, occlusion, fimbrial damage, pelvic adhesions, endometriosis
Ovarian	Anovulation/oligoovulation, inadequate luteal phase, polycystic ovaries
Cervical	Cervicitis, poor quality cervical mucus, diethylstilbestrol exposure
Uterine	Uterine fibromas, congenital malformations, adhesions, endometrial abnormalities
Endocrine	Panhypopituitarism, hypothyroidism, adrenal insufficiency, congenital adrenal hyperplasia, Cushing's disease, cirrhosis, hormone receptor defects
Other	Age, drugs, malnutrition, excess alcohol intake, smoking
MALE FACTORS	
Genetic	Klinefelter's syndrome, Reifenstein's syndrome, chromosomal abnormalities
Seminal	Failure of semen to liquefy, inadequate volume, low sperm count, decreased or erratic sperm motility, sperm dysmorphology, varicocele
Transport	Hypospadias, micropenis, retrograde ejaculation, epididymitis, impotence, ductal occlusion, ductal adhesions
Testicular	Oligospermia/azoospermia, cryptorchidism, testicular agenesis, history of high fever, postpubertal orchitis
Endocrine	Panhypopituitarism, hypothyroidism, adrenal insufficiency, congenital adrenal hyperplasia, Cushing's disease, cirrhosis, hormone receptor abnormalities
Other	Age, drugs, excess alcohol intake, smoking, pollution, malnutrition, scrotal heat exposure, autoimmunity to sperm, infectious processes
COUPLE FACTORS	Sexual technique, inappropriate timing of intercourse, immune response to sperm

Table 51-2
Common Tests for Infertility

TEST	PURPOSE
Physical examination	Assess reproductive tract function and patency by gross examination
Hematology, liver and renal function	Rule out disease processes
Hysterosalpingogram, tubal insufflation	Evaluate fallopian tube patency
Postcoital examination of cervical mucus	Assess mucus viscosity, its effect on sperm motility
Plasma progesterone	Assess function of corpus luteum
Endometrial biopsy	Assess ovulatory status or adequacy of corpus luteum
Semen analysis	Check number, structure, movement of sperm
Basal body temperature	Determine whether ovulation occurs; chart
Sperm penetration assay	Determine ability of sperm to penetrate and fertilize ovum
Laparoscopy	Visualize female pelvic organs
Hysteroscopy	Visualize uterus
Echohysteroscopy	Assess structure of woman's internal reproductive organs
Hormone assays	GnRH, FSH, LH, progesterone, estrogen, prolactin, testosterone, thyroid hormone levels
Immunologic testing	Assess cervical immunity against sperm, seminal fluid immunity against sperm, serum antisperm antibodies in either partner
Imaging	Pituitary integrity

KEY: *FSH: follicle-stimulating hormone; GnRH: gonadotropin-releasing hormone; LH: luteinizing hormone.*

Table 51-3
Ovulatory Stimulants

DRUG	DOSAGE	USE AND CONSIDERATIONS
Bromocriptine mesylate (Parlodel)	Up to 7.5 mg/d in divided doses	Normalizes prolactin levels. Possibly teratogenic. *Pregnancy category:* C; PB: 92%; $t\frac{1}{2}$: 50 h
Clomiphene citrate (Clomid, Serophene)	50–250 mg/d PO days 5–9 of cycle	Stimulates follicle growth. May be teratogenic. May impede fertilization. *Pregnancy category:* X; PB: UK; $t\frac{1}{2}$: 5–8 d
GnRH	1–10 μg/60–120 min via pump	Induces ovulation in women with hypothalamic amenorrhea. Ovarian hyperstimulation is a risk. Pregnancy loss is common. *Pregnancy category:* X; PB: UK; $t\frac{1}{2}$: 11–23 h
Human menopausal gonadotropin, menotropins and FSH, urofollitropin (Pergonal, Metrodin)	IM: 1–2 ampules/d × 5–12 d until follicle maturation; next day, hCG (5000–10,000 IU IM) administered	These contain various ratios of FSH and LH. Ovarian hyperstimulation is a risk. Ectopic pregnancy and spontaneous abortion may occur. *Pregnancy category:* X; PB: UK; $t\frac{1}{2}$: 4–70 h

KEY: *PO: by mouth; IM: intramuscular; FSH: follicle-stimulating hormone; LH: luteinizing hormone; hCG: human chorionic gonadotropin; PB: protein-binding; UK: unknown; $t\frac{1}{2}$: half-life.*

Chart 51–1.   Ovulation Stimulant: Clomiphene Citrate

CLOMIPHENE CITRATE

Drug Name

Clomiphene citrate (Clomid, Milophene, Serophene)
Ovulation stimulant
Pregnancy Category: X

Dosage

A: PO: 50–250 mg/d for days 5–9 of cycle
If ovulation does not occur with 50 mg/d, increase next course to 100 mg/d

Contraindications

Pregnancy, undiagnosed vaginal bleeding, depression, fibroids, hepatic dysfunction, thrombophlebitis, primary pituitary or ovarian failure

Drug-Lab-Food Interactions

Drug: None are significant; Danazol may inhibit response; *decrease* effects of ethinyl estradiol
Lab: *Increase* in serum thyroxine

Pharmacokinetics

Absorption: Readily absorbed from GI tract
Distribution: PB: UK
Metabolism: t½: 5–8 d
Excretion: In feces

Pharmacodynamics

PO: Onset: 5–14 d
Peak: UK
Duration: UK

Therapeutic Effects/Uses

To stimulate ovarian follicle growth.

Mode of Action: Stimulates release of follicle-stimulating hormone (FSH) and luteinizing hormone (LH).

Side Effects

Breast discomfort, fatigue, dizziness, depression, anxiety, nausea, vomiting, constipation, increased appetite, headache, flatulence, multiple gestation, hot flashes, fluid retention

Adverse Reactions

Visual disturbances, abdominal pain, weight gain, hair loss, major congenital anomalies, ovarian hyperstimulation, anxiety, ovarian cysts

Assessment and Planning

Interventions

Evaluation

NURSING PROCESS

KEY: PO: by mouth; PB: protein-binding; UK: unknown; t½: half-life.

ovulation stimulant (Chart 51–1). Some women on clomiphene citrate therapy require the addition of glucocorticoid therapy such as dexamethasone or prednisone.

Human menopausal gonadotropin (hMG) and human chorionic gonadotropin (hCG) replace or supplement FSH and LH (Table 51–3). These drugs normalize LH and FSH levels in order to stimulate follicle maturation, ovulation, and development of the corpus luteum. In a small percentage of amenorrheic women, an elevated level of prolactin is the causative factor. A portion of these women can be treated with the ergot derivative bromocriptine, 2.5 mg two or three times a day. Bromocriptine binds to dopamine receptors in the pituitary and inhibits prolactin secretion, and treatment should lead to the onset of menses in 3 to 5 weeks. Chemically, drugs in the category of ovulation stimulants are not similar.

PHARMACOKINETICS

Data on the pharmacokinetics of clomiphene citrate are limited, but clomiphene is readily absorbed from the gastrointestinal (GI) tract. It is partially metabolized in the liver and excreted in the feces via biliary elimination. Clomiphene has a half-life of about 5 days.

PHARMACODYNAMICS

The mechanism of action of clomiphene is unknown, but it is hypothesized that it competes with estrogen at receptor sites. The perception of decreased circulating estrogen by the hypothalamus and pituitary triggers the negative feedback response of increasing the secretion of FSH and LH. The result is ovarian stimulation, maturation of the ovarian follicle, and development of the corpus luteum.

SIDE EFFECTS

Side effects of clomiphene citrate include breast discomfort, fatigue, dizziness, depression, nausea, vomiting, increased appetite, weight gain, dermatitis, urticaria, anxiety, restlessness, weakness, heavier menses, vasomotor flushing, abdominal bloating or pain, and gas (Chart 51–1). Antiestrogenic effects include interference with endometrial maturation and cervical mucus production. Paradoxically, this may interfere with fertilization or implantation.

ADVERSE EFFECTS

Adverse effects include photophobia, mastalgia, diplopia, and decreased visual acuity. Ovarian hyperstimulation may result in ovarian enlargement, midcycle ovarian pain, and cysts. Reversible hair loss has been noted. Multiple gestation occurs in up to 12% of women who become pregnant. The effect of clomiphene citrate on fetal development is unclear. Neural tube defects have been reported, but have not been confirmed by controlled studies. Adverse effects of other ovulatory stimulants are listed in Table 51–4.

Table 51–4
Side Effects, Adverse Effects, and Contraindications for Selected Infertility Drugs

SIDE EFFECTS	ADVERSE EFFECTS	CONTRAINDICATIONS
HUMAN MENOPAUSAL GONADOTROPIN		
Breast pain, abdominal bloating or pain	Ovarian enlargement, ovarian hyperstimulation syndrome, fever, nausea, vomiting, diarrhea, hemoperitoneum, arterial thromboembolism, ovarian cysts, multiple births	Primary ovarian failure, pregnancy, ovarian cysts, enlargement not due to polycystic ovaries, thyroid or adrenal dysfunction, intracranial lesion, abnormal bleeding of unknown origin, infertility not caused by anovulation
UROFOLLITROPIN		
Bloating, nausea, vomiting, diarrhea, cramping, headache, breast pain, aches, fatigue, malaise, dry skin	Ovarian enlargement, ovarian hyperstimulation syndrome, hair loss, ectopic pregnancy, thromboembolism, ascites, pleural effusion, multiple births	High levels follicle-stimulating hormone, luteinizing hormone, thyroid or adrenal dysfunction, intracranial lesions, abnormal bleeding of unknown origin, ovarian cysts not due to polycystic ovary syndrome, pregnancy. Used with caution in persons with thromboembolism and nursing mothers
HUMAN CHORIONIC GONADOTROPIN		
Headache, irritability, restlessness, fatigue, depression, fluid retention, pain at injection site	Ovarian hyperstimulation syndrome, rupture of ovarian cysts, multiple births, arterial thromboembolism	Androgen-dependent neoplasms. Caution in asthma, cardiac or renal disease, epilepsy, migraine
BROMOCRIPTINE MESYLATE		
Nausea, vomiting, headache, dizziness, drowsiness, fatigue, lightheadedness, nasal congestion, diarrhea, insomnia, depression	Confusion, visual disturbances, vertigo, shortness of breath, abdominal discomfort, involuntary movements, hypotension, anxiety, dysphagia, paresthesia, blepharospasm, mottling, urinary frequency, epileptiform seizures, ergotism, transient elevations in BUN, SGOT, SGPT, creatine phosphokinase, alkaline phosphatase, serum uric acid	Ischemic heart disease, peripheral vascular disease, pregnancy, lactation, ergot nervousness, sensitivity. Caution in hypotension, epilepsy, psychoses, cardiac arrhythmia, impaired hepatic or renal function

CONTRAINDICATIONS

Contraindications for treatment with clomiphene citrate include undiagnosed vaginal bleeding, pregnancy, uterine fibroids, mental depression, history of hepatic dysfunction or thromboembolic disease, and primary pituitary or ovarian failure. If the woman has ovarian cysts, clomiphene citrate may cause them to enlarge. Contraindications to the use of other ovulatory stimulants are listed in Table 51–4.

INTERACTIONS

There are no known significant drug interactions with clomiphene citrate. Danazol may inhibit client response to clomiphene citrate, and clomiphene citrate may suppress response to ethinyl estradiol. There are no known drug interactions with hMG or hCG.

Other Drug Treatments

Other pharmacologic approaches for treatment of women with infertility include the use of pulsatile exogenous GnRH. In addition, hypothyroidism or hyperthyroidism and adrenal dysfunction must be treated. Endometriosis can be treated with a course of danazol to suppress gonadotropin output. Women with inadequate luteal-phase progesterone output are treated with progesterone 25 mg twice daily intravaginally or 12.5 mg IM.

Drug Therapy for Male Infertility

For the majority of men with infertility, no specific causal factor can be identified. They are identified as having idiopathic oligospermia and asthenospermia. There is no documented cost-effective treatment for this large group of people. Most drug regimens that have been used have never been evaluated in controlled studies. Drugs that have been tried include testosterone; hCG; GnRH; mesterolone, a synthetic androgen; antiestrogenic agents, including clomiphene citrate and tamoxifen; and testolactone, which inhibits the conversion of testosterone to estradiol. Assisted reproductive techniques currently appear to hold more promise than drug therapy.

DRUGS USED IN THE TREATMENT OF SEXUALLY TRANSMITTED DISEASES

Sexually transmitted diseases (STDs) are infections that are transmitted during sexual contact. Some pathogens are spread primarily through sexual contact. Others, such as *Shigella*, hepatitis A, or *Candida*, are transmitted primarily by other ways but can also be spread sexually. Pathogens implicated in sexually transmitted diseases are listed in Table 51–5. If not treated, STDs can result in damage to the male and female reproductive tracts that impairs fertility, in life-threatening illness and death, and in neonatal illness and death. The past 30 years have seen a dramatic increase in this problem. The emergence of STDs that are incurable or lethal in adults, such as genital herpes and HIV infection, has led to growing awareness of the seriousness of STDs, even in afflu-

Table 51–5
Pathogens Causing Sexually Transmitted Diseases

| PATHOGEN | MODE OF TRANSMISSION | | |
	Predominantly Sexual	Can be Sexual	Sexual Contact with Oral-Fecal Exposure
Bacteria	*Calymmatobacterium granulomatis* *Chlamydia trachomatis* *Haemophilus ducreyi* *Neisseria gonorrhoeae* *Treponema pallidum* *Ureaplasma urealyticum*	*Escherichia coli* *Gardnerella vaginalis* Other vaginal bacteria Group B streptococcus *Mycoplasma hominis*	*Shigella* *Campylobacter*
Viruses	Cytomegalovirus HIV-1, HIV-2 Hepatitis B Herpes simplex virus type 2 Human papillomavirus Molluscum contagiosum virus	HTLV-1 Hepatitis C, D Herpes simplex virus type 1 Epstein-Barr virus	Hepatitis A
Protozoa, fungi, ectoparasites	*Trichomonas vaginalis* *Phthirus pubis* *Sarcoptes scabei*	*Candida albicans*	*Giardia lamblia* *Entamoeba histolytica*

NURSING PROCESS
INFERTILITY

Infertility management is a highly specialized field. Nurses are most likely to encounter clients when they are in the process of trying to identify the possible causes of their infertility. Nurses need to be sensitive to the guilt, decreased self-esteem, and embarrassment that infertility may cause. Treatment of infertility requires that a couple's sexual life be directed by the health care team. Evaluation and intervention are often uncomfortable and expensive, and there is no guarantee that a viable pregnancy will result. The process is emotionally and economically draining for the couple.

Assessment

- A general health history and physical examination are required. The clients' reproductive and sexual histories are assessed, with attention to the timing and technique of coitus.
- The couple undergo an exhaustive battery of diagnostic tests to evaluate the cause of infertility. Once this is determined, conditions that contraindicate the treatment of choice are ruled out.
- It is particularly important that the couple's interpretation of their infertility be explored, along with its impact on their relationship. The nurse should help the couple discuss their feelings in a safe, supportive environment.

Potential Nursing Diagnoses

- Altered sexuality patterns
- Altered sexual functioning
- Body image disturbance
- Low self-esteem
- Knowledge deficit related to treatment regimen

Planning

- Short-term goals include the clients' adherence to the medical regimen with minimal adverse effects.
- The long-term goal is the achievement of pregnancy or the consideration of alternatives to pregnancy with the partners' self-esteem and relationship intact.

Nursing Interventions

General
- Interventions are aimed at helping clients understand the interrelationships among and timing of menses, ovulation, and coitus as they relate to conception. In addition, they need to know sexual techniques that enhance fertilization, such as the placement of a pillow under the woman's hips during coitus and her remaining supine with hips elevated for about 30 min after her partner ejaculates. In addition, clients and their partners need to understand the treatment regimen.

Specific
- The female client is taught to report adverse effects such as abdominal pain or visual disturbances to her infertility specialist at once, and to be cautious with tasks that require alertness. If she misses a dose of her medication, she should call her infertility specialist.
- Clients need to understand that treatment increases the chance of multiple births.

Client Teaching

- Couples need to be taught how to evaluate and record basal body temperature and cervical mucus changes on a chart. The first day of menses is day 1 of the cycle. Ovulation is predicted by a 0.5°F drop in basal body temperature followed by a 1°F rise. In addition, over-the-counter diagnostic kits for assessing ovulatory status can be used to time coitus. The couple is advised to engage in coitus no more frequently than every other day from 4 days before to 3 days after ovulation, to maximize the man's sperm count (Fig. 51–1).

Nursing Process continued on following page

NURSING PROCESS Continued
INFERTILITY

- The man is advised to wear boxer shorts during infertility treatment, because briefs hold the scrotum close to the body and the heat reduces the sperm count. For the same reason, if he is seated all day in his work, he is counseled to take breaks every hour or so to walk about. Some women have been helped to conceive by taking guaifenesin (Robitussin) for its effect of thinning cervical mucus.
- The woman is advised to take her medication at the same time each day to maintain steady blood levels.

Evaluation

- Successful outcomes of fertility treatment include avoidance of ovarian hyperstimulation, as well as other untoward effects. The achievement of pregnancy that results in the birth of a live infant fulfills the objectives of treatment. If pregnancy is not achieved, then intervention is aimed at helping the couple to consider alternatives to childbearing without adverse impact on their self-esteem or harm to their relationship.

---

1. Purchase a special thermometer calibrated in tenths of degrees between 96 and 100° F.
2. Place the thermometer under the tongue for at least a full 3 minutes (preferably 5 minutes) after waking in the morning and before *any* activity (e.g., lifting your head off the pillow, shaking thermometer down, intercourse, or urinating).
3. If you forget to take your temperature and have already gotten up, *do not take it.* Write *missed* on that day.
4. Take your temperature in the same manner about the same time each day.
5. Carefully record the reading on the graph by placing a dot at the proper location. Start this chart on the first day of your period.
6. Insert the month and day in the space provided.
7. The first day of menstrual flow is considered to be the start of a cycle (day 1). Each day of flow should be indicated with an M on the graph, starting at extreme left under number 1 day of cycle.
8. Record any obvious reason for temperature variation such as a cold, flu, or infection on the graph above the reading for that day.
9. If you are placed on medication, please indicate it in the space labeled medications on the days you take it.
10. If you feel you have menstrually related symptoms, such as breast tenderness or cramping, note these also.
11. If intercourse has taken place during the previous 24 hours, mark it with an (X).

Calendar for Thermal Method of Fertility Awareness

Day of Cycle: 1 2 3 4 5 6 7 8 9 10 11 12 13 14 15 16 17 18 19 20 21 22 23 24 25 26 27 28 29 30 31

Temperature
99.0
98.8
98.6
98.4
98.2
98.0
97.8
97.6
97.4
97.2
97.0

Menses (M):
Intercourse (X):

Mucus
  Color
  Consistency
  Amount

Other factors
  Medications
  Breast tenderness
  Cramps

Figure 51–1

Instructions for keeping a sympothermal record. (From Fogel, C. I., and Lauver, D. [1990]. *Sexual Health Promotion.* Philadelphia: WB Saunders, p. 253.)

Table 51-6
Risk-Reducing Behaviors for Avoidance of STDs

Sexual abstinence or sexual contact with one faithful partner

Washing and urinating before and after intercourse

Consistent use of a condom treated with nonoxynol-9

Avoiding sex with someone with genital or anal lesions

Reduction of use of alcohol or drugs, both of which impair judgment about sexual risk and immune response

Avoidance of sexual contact with HIV-infected persons, users of intravenous drugs, immigrants from high-prevalence regions, or sexual partners of all such individuals

Never sharing hypodermic needles or razors

---

ent, industrialized countries. Several infections, including those caused by HIV, human papillomavirus, human T-lymphotrophic virus, and Epstein-Barr virus, are associated with malignancies.

Transmission and Risk

Sexual transmission of pathogens can occur through breaks in the vaginal or cervical mucosa or the skin covering the shaft or glans of the penis. Recent research to better understand mechanisms of HIV transmission demonstrates that each act of coitus results in tiny, friction-induced fissures on these surfaces. This problem is exacerbated by inadequate vaginal lubrication, which may occur postmenopausally, postpartally, just following menses, or when the woman is not sufficiently aroused before penetration.

Semen, sperm cells themselves, vaginal secretions, blood, and other body fluids can carry pathogens. Skin and mucosal lesions not only can be penetrated by microorganisms but can also shed them. Sexual contact can involve skin to skin, mouth to mouth, oral-genital, oral-anal, or hand-anal transmission of pathogens through breaks in the skin or mucosal surfaces or from inoculation by infectious body fluids. Anal penetration is particularly risky because of the likelihood of tissue trauma that results in the partner's exposure to enteric microorganisms.

One practice that places individuals at high risk for the transmission of STDs, particularly HIV, is engaging in sexual activity with multiple partners. Investigators at the National Institutes of Health suggest that risk of STDs is markedly increased among individuals who have more than one sexual partner per year versus those who have fewer partners. Other high-risk practices are anal or vaginal intercourse

without a condom, hand-anal contact, blood contact during sexual activity during menses, the use of an enema before anal intercourse, and urination on broken skin or inside the body. Risk-reducing behaviors are listed in Table 51-6.

STDs are often manifested as multiple infections. Individuals undergoing treatment for one STD should be assessed for others, including HIV. This is especially true if genital or perianal ulcerations are present.

Vertical transmission, or **perinatal infection,** occurs when a fetus or neonate is infected by the mother. Microbes can travel up the reproductive tract from the vagina or cervix and enter the intrauterine environment. Transmission can occur through contact with the mother's blood at birth or through breast milk, as in the case of HIV and hepatitis B virus. Organisms that are of little consequence to healthy adults can be devastating to a fetus. Many STDs, such as syphilis, are transmitted transplacentally. Others, such as infection with herpes simplex virus type 2, require actual contact by the infant with microorganisms in the birth canal.

Common STD syndromes and their causative pathogens are listed in Table 51-7. Current guidelines from the Centers for Disease Control and Prevention (CDC) for the primary treatment of various STDs are listed in Table 51-8. All sexual contacts of an infected individual should be informed of their exposure and treated. Partners should refrain from sexual activity until each is clear of infection on follow-up evaluation or, at the very least, condoms should be used.

HIV Disease

Chapter 31 is devoted to the presentation of drugs for HIV and AIDS. These conditions involve the immune system and can be transmitted by means other than sexual contact.

SUMMARY

Reproductive health and fertility require integrity of hormonal mechanisms and reproductive anatomy. Infertility can be caused by male, female, or couple factors. Often, the use of drugs to stimulate ovulation is effective treatment. Clients need to understand the treatment regimen, and they need support in dealing with the psychological impact of this condition.

Finally, STDs can constitute a threat to reproductive health, neonatal health, fertility, and even life. Early diagnosis and treatment are crucial but less effective than prevention. HIV/AIDS is complicated by numerous opportunistic infections and autoimmune processes. For some, drug therapies may offer relief, although ultimately this disease is fatal.

Table 51–7
Common STD Syndromes and Their Causative Pathogens

SYNDROME	PATHOGENS
Acute arthritis	*Neisseria gonorrhoeae*, *Chlamydia trachomatis*, hepatitis B virus (HBV), human immunodeficiency virus (HIV)
Acquired immunodeficiency virus	HIV-1, HIV-2, and opportunistic pathogens
Cervicitis	*C. trachomatis*, *N. gonorrhoeae*, Herpes simplex virus (HSV), *Candida albicans*
Cystitis, urethritis (female)	Gram-negative bacilli, gram-positive cocci, *C. trachomatis*, *N. gonorrhoeae*
Epididymitis	*C. trachomatis*, *N. gonorrhoeae*
Genital, anal warts	Human papillomavirus (HPV)
Lymphadenopathy	Cytomegalovirus (CMV), HIV, Epstein-Barr virus (EBV)
Neoplasias Squamous cell cancers of cervix, anus, vulva, penis; Kaposi's sarcoma; lymphoid neoplasia, hepatocellular carcinoma	HPV HIV, EBV HIV, human T-lymphotrophic virus (HTLV-1)
Pelvic inflammatory disease	*Trichomonas vaginalis*, *N. gonorrhoeae*, *C. trachomatis*, *Bacteroides* spp, peptostreptococci, *Escherichia coli*, streptococci groups B and D, bacterial vaginitis-associated pathogens
Proctitis, proctocolitis or enterocolitis, enteritis	*N. gonorrhoeae*, HSV, *C. trachomatis*, *Treponema pallidum*, *Giardia lamblia*, *Campylobacter* spp, *Shigella* spp, *Entamoeba histolytica*, *Mycobacterium avium-intracellulare*, *Salmonella* spp, *Cryptosporidium*, *Isospora* (ingestion of intestinal flora)
Pubic lice	*Phthirus pubis*
Scabies	*Sarcoptes scabei*
Ulcerative lesions of the genitalia	HSV-1, HSV-2, *T. pallidum*, *C. trachomatis*, *Calymmatobacterium granulomatis*, HPV, *Haemophilus ducreyi*, molluscum contagiosum virus
Urethritis, male	*N. gonorrhoeae*, *C. trachomatis*, *T. vaginalis*, HSV, *Ureaplasma urealyticum*, *Mycoplasma hominis*, *Bacteroides urealyticum*
Vulvovaginitis	Bacterial vaginosis: *Gardnerella vaginitis* (*Haemophilus vaginalis*), *M. hominis*, *U. urealyticum*, *Mobiluncus curtisii*, *Mobiluncus mulieris*, *Bacteroides* spp, peptostreptococci, *T. vaginalis*, *C. albicans*, *Torulopsis oflabrata*

Table 51–8
Current Guidelines for Primary Therapies for Common STDs

DISEASE	PRIMARY THERAPY	NOTES
Acute urethral syndrome	Doxycycline 100 mg PO b.i.d. × 7 d *or* sulfamethoxazole 1.6 g plus trimethoprim 320 mg PO single dose	
Bacterial vaginosis	Metronidazole 500 mg PO b.i.d. × 7 d, *or* 2 g PO single dose *or* vaginal gel b.i.d. × 5 d	Avoid alcohol during therapy; contraindicated in pregnancy
Candidiasis	Fluconazole 150 mg PO × 1 dose *or* miconazole nitrate 200 mg vaginal suppository qhs × 3 d *or* miconazole nitrate 2% vaginal cream, 5 g, qhs × 3 d *or* clotrimazole 200 mg, vaginal suppository, daily × 3 d	Recurrent candidiasis may be indicative of other disease, such as diabetes or HIV infection
Chancroid	Azithromycin 1 g PO × 1 dose *or* ceftriaxone 250 mg IM × 1 *or* erythromycin base 500 mg PO q.i.d. × 7 d	Use compresses to remove necrotic material; clean ulcerative lesions t.i.d.

Table continued on following page

Table 51–8 *Continued*
Current Guidelines for Primary Therapies for Common STDs

DISEASE	PRIMARY THERAPY	NOTES
Chlamydia	Doxycycline 100 mg PO b.i.d. × 7–10 d *or* azithromycin 1 g PO × 1 *Children <45 kg:* Erythromycin 50 mg/kg/d PO divided in 4 doses, × 10–14 d *Children >45 kg:* Erythromycin base 500 mg PO q.i.d. × 7 d *or* erythromycin succinate 800 mg PO b.i.d. × 7 d *Infants:* Erythromycin 50 mg/kg/d PO divided into 4 doses × 10–14 d	A second course of therapy may be required
Epididymitis	Ceftriaxone 250 mg IM × 1 *and* doxycycline 100 mg PO b.i.d. × 10 d *or* ofloxacin 300 mg b.i.d. × 10 d	Treat for gonorrhea, then follow with treatment for nongonococcal urethritis
Genital warts	Cryotherapy *or* cryoprobe *or* podofilox 0.5% solution b.i.d. × 3 d, then 4 days off; repeat cycle × 4, *or* podophyllin 10%–25% in compound tincture of benzoin × 1/w × 6 w	Nothing eradicates HPV; podophyllin contraindicated during pregnancy
Gonorrhea	Ceftriaxone 125 mg IM × 1 *or* Norfloxicin 800 mg PO × 1 *or* trovafloxacin 100 mg PO × 1 *Children <45 kg:* Ceftriaxone 125 mg IM × 1 *or* ceftriaxone 50 mg/kg IM/IV (*max:* 1 g) daily × 7 d *Ophthalmia neonatorum:* Ceftriaxone 25–50 mg/kg IM/IV × 1 (*max:* 125 mg) *Ophthalmia neonatorum prophylaxis:* Silver nitrate (1%) aqueous × 1 *or* erythromycin (0.5%) ophthalmic ointment × 1	Treat for *Chlamydia* as well Neonate may also have scalp abscess at site of fetal monitors, rhinitis, anorectal infection
Granuloma inguinale	Doxycycline 100 mg PO b.i.d. × 7–28 d *or* erythromycin 500 mg q.i.d. PO × 14 d	
Hepatitis B	No specific therapy exists	HBV is the only STD for which a vaccine exists. The CDC recommends vaccination of all infants and adolescents. ACIP recommends vaccination of all persons with recent STD and those with more than 1 partner in the last 6 months
Herpes genitalis	*First episode, genital:* Acyclovir 200 mg PO × 5/d, × 7–10 d *Herpes proctitis, first episode:* Acyclovir 400 mg PO × 5/d, × 10 d *Recurrent:* Acyclovir 400 mg PO t.i.d. × 5 d *or* famciclovir 125 mg PO b.i.d. × 5 d *or* valacyclovir 500 mg PO b.i.d. × 5 d *Suppressive:* Acyclovir 400 mg PO b.i.d. *or* famciclovir 250 mg PO b.i.d. *or* valacyclovir 500 mg PO q.d. *Severe:* Acyclovir 5–10 mg/kg IV q8h × 5–7 d *Immunocompromised:* Acyclovir 400 mg PO × 3–5/d until resolution *Neonatal:* Acyclovir 30 mg/kg/d	Types 1 and 2 cannot be distinguished clinically. No cure is known. Systemic disease is life-threatening to neonates, and neurologic damage may result. Viral shedding is most prevalent when symptomatic; sexual relations should be avoided
Lymphogranuloma venereum	Doxycycline 100 mg PO b.i.d. × 21 d *or* erythromycin 0.5 gm PO q.i.d. × 21 d	
Molluscum contagiosum	Cryoanesthesia and curettage *or* caustic chemicals (podophyllin, trichloroacetic acid, silver nitrate) and cryotherapy	If all lesions not eradicated, may recur

Table continued on following page

Table 51–8 *Continued*

Current Guidelines for Primary Therapies for Common STDs

DISEASE	PRIMARY THERAPY	NOTES
Mucopurulent cervicitis	Doxycycline 100 mg PO b.i.d. × 7–10 d	
Nongonococcal urethritis	Doxycycline 100 mg PO b.i.d. × 7 d *or* erythromycin 500 mg PO q.i.d. × 7 d *or* azithromycin 1 gm PO × 1 dose	
Pelvic inflammatory disease (PID)	*Inpatient:* Doxycycline 100 mg IV b.i.d. *and* cefoxitin 2 g IV q.i.d. *or* defotetan 2 g IV q.i.d. *48 h after clinical improvement:* Doxycycline 100 mg PO b.i.d. for total of at least 14 d therapy *Ambulatory care:* Ofloxacin 400 mg b.i.d. *plus* metronidazole 500 mg b.i.d. × 14 d *or* ceftriaxone 250 mg IM × 1 *plus* doxycycline 100 mg PO b.i.d. × 14 d *or* trovafloxacin 200 mg PO × 14 d	Often polymicrobial. This regimen may not treat anaerobes, pelvic mass, or IUD-associated PID
Proctitis	Ceftriaxone 125 mg IM × 1 *and* doxycycline 100 mg PO b.i.d. × 7 d	
Pubic lice	Permethrin 1% creme rinse, apply for 10 min	Lindane used only if failed other therapy. Decontaminate clothes, bedding. Second treatment 7–10 d after 1st to kill newly hatched lice. If pubic lice, treat partner also
Scabies	Permethrin cream 5% applied to all affected areas from neck down, for 8–14 min *or* lindane 1% applied to all affected areas from neck down for 8 h	
Sexual assault	Ceftriaxone 125 mg IM × 1 *and* metronidazole 2 g PO × 1 *and* doxycycline 100 mg PO b.i.d. × 7 d	Tetanus-booster and gamma globulin, as well as baseline HIV testing and follow-up are recommended
Syphilis	*Primary, secondary, or <1 y duration:* Benzathine penicillin G, 2.4 million units IM *Unknown duration or >1 y:* Benzathine penicillin G, 7.2 million units divided in 2.4 million IM weekly × 3 *Allergic to penicillin:* Doxycycline 100 mg PO b.i.d. × 14–28 d	
	Penicillin-allergic pregnant women or doxycycline-intolerant: Erythromycin (stearate, ethyl succinate or base) 500 mg PO q.i.d. × 2 W *Children:* Benzathine penicillin G 50,000 units/kg IM × 1, up to 2.4 million units; repeat × 3 if unknown or >1 y duration *Infants:* Aqueous crystalline penicillin G 200,000–300,000 units/kg/d IM/IV, × 10–14 d *Congenital:* Aqueous crystalline penicillin G 100,000–150,000 units/kg/d IV, × 10–14 d *or* procaine penicillin G 50,000 units/kg/d IM × 10–14 d	Some studies indicate that pregnant women should be treated with penicillin, on an incremental basis, with an emergency set-up at the bedside, if they are allergic to penicillin. In recent years, CDC has recommended this approach
Trichomoniasis	Metronidazole 2 g PO × 1 *or* metronidazole 500 mg PO b.i.d. × 7 d	Pregnant women can be treated after the first trimester

KEY: HIV: human immunodeficiency virus; HPV: human papillomavirus; STD: sexually transmitted disease; CDC: Centers for Disease Control and Prevention; ACIP: Advisory Committee on Immunization Practices; IUD: intrauterine device; PID: pelvic inflammatory disease.

NURSING PROCESS
SEXUALLY TRANSMITTED DISEASES

Nurses need to be sensitive to clients' reasons for seeking or avoiding care for STDs. Psychosocial reactions to a diagnosis of STD may include feelings of anger, depression, shame, guilt, hurt, fear, and concern. Clients need privacy during the interview and examination, with attention to their comfort, such as warming the speculum before a pelvic examination. A second health professional should be present in the examination room during the physical examination of a female client.

Assessment

- Before physical data are gathered, a history is elicited. Less sensitive issues are addressed first so that trust can be established. The term "partners" is used in discussing sexual activity rather than value-laden terms such as "wife" or "boyfriend."
- The history includes the chief complaint, a description of the course of illness, a review of systems and general health history, a reproductive history, a sexual history, a review of lifestyle and social habits, and identification of allergies.
- Physical examination includes inspection and palpation of the genitalia and other points of inoculation.
- Laboratory tests include wet slides with microbe-specific setting agents, urinalysis, cultures, Papanicolaou smear, a complete blood count, syphilis serology, and herpes simplex virus 1 and 2 antibodies.

Potential Nursing Diagnoses

- Actual as well as potential infection
- Knowledge deficit with regard to transmission and prevention as well as treatment
- Noncompliance with known prevention strategies
- Pain
- Low self-esteem
- Altered sexuality patterns
  A medical diagnosis of HIV disease would bring with it additional nursing diagnoses:
- Fatigue
- Anxiety
- Anticipatory grieving
- Social isolation
- Self-care deficits and health maintenance needs

Planning

- Short-term goals include the client's adherence to the treatment regimen and avoidance of adverse effects.
- Long-term goals include the client's return for follow-up evaluation and adoption of risk-reducing sexual behaviors.

Nursing Interventions

- The client needs to understand procedures performed during evaluation and how to administer prescribed medications and treatments. Side effects and adverse effects that require immediate intervention are reviewed.
- Specific interventions include providing needed support as the client deals with the fact that the infection is sexually transmitted.
- The client needs to notify sexual partners so that they can be evaluated and treated.
- Ideally, sexual contact is avoided during treatment. At the least, condoms should be used until both partners are clear of infection.
- Individuals are scheduled for follow-up visits from 4 days to 4 weeks, depending on the type of infection and treatment.
- Individuals with any STD are counseled about being tested for HIV infection.

Nursing Process continued on following page

NURSING PROCESS *Continued*
SEXUALLY TRANSMITTED DISEASES

Client Teaching

- The mode of transmission of STDs, the relationship of all STDs with HIV infection, and how HIV risk is avoided should all be reviewed.
- Individuals are advised to plan periodic reproductive health check-ups.

Evaluation

- Intervention has been successful if the individual's infection is cleared up on reevaluation or, in the case of viral infections, the individual experiences quiescence of the virus.
- One important outcome to evaluate is that the infection is not transmitted to other individuals. Another is that the individual is able to avoid sexual practices that carry risk of STDs, including promiscuity, intercourse without the use of a condom, and traumatic sexual practices.

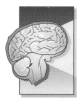

Critical Thinking in Action

Todd, a teacher, married Diane, age 32 years, 3 years ago. Diane is the only sexual partner Todd has ever had. For the last year they have been trying to conceive, without success. Diane's nurse practitioner learns when taking Diane's history that Diane had multiple sexual partners during her college years and that she was once treated for gonorrhea. Diane's menstrual history reveals an erratic pattern of unpredictable periods, about every 2 or 3 months. The nurse practitioner reviews the relationship between timing of coitus and conception, instructs Diane on taking her temperature each morning before she gets out of bed and maintaining an ovulation record, and suggests that a home test kit may be helpful in identifying when ovulation has occurred. Diane and Todd are referred to an infertility specialist.

1. What is the relevance of Diane's past sexual history to the current complaint?
2. Why would the infertility specialist consider cultures for *Chlamydia trachomatis* and *Neisseria gonorrhoeae* years after exposure?
3. What other tests would reveal damage resulting from STDs?
4. What is positive about Diane's menstrual history? What about her menstrual pattern makes conception difficult?
5. How can Diane predict when she will ovulate?
6. After a complete evaluation of Todd and Diane, a course of clomiphene citrate is prescribed. What side effects can Diane expect?
7. When should Diane take the medication?
8. When should Todd and Diane have sexual intercourse?
9. Diane experiences midcycle abdominal pain. What should she do when this occurs? How will her infertility specialist interpret this?
10. Diane becomes pregnant after four cycles on clomiphene citrate. What is one potential risk factor with this pregnancy?

Diane becomes pregnant and has a baby boy following an uneventful pregnancy. The baby has numerous upper respiratory infections during his first 4 months of life, twice requiring hospitalization, and gains weight slowly. When the family is referred to a tertiary pediatric medical center, the medical staff ask Diane if she would consider being tested for HIV.

11. What in her history puts her at risk for HIV infection?
12. Why is it possible that Diane could test positive for HIV when she has shown no sign of infection for nearly a decade after her high-risk behavior?

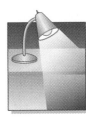

Study Questions

1. What is the relationship between STDs and infertility?
2. How should couples determine the timing of coitus when they are trying to conceive?
3. What should be the timing of coitus in relation to ovarian stimulation therapy?
4. What are some adverse effects of clomiphene citrate therapy?
5. What are some psychosocial effects of infertility therapy?
6. Which STDs cannot be cured?
7. Which STDs are associated with life-threatening illness?
8. Whenever an individual is successfully treated for an STD, what should the nurse emphasize in client teaching?
9. What reproductive tract infections may or may not be sexually transmitted? What should the client tell his or her partner when such an infection occurs?
10. Why do ulcerative STDs place an individual at risk for HIV infection?

Unit XIV

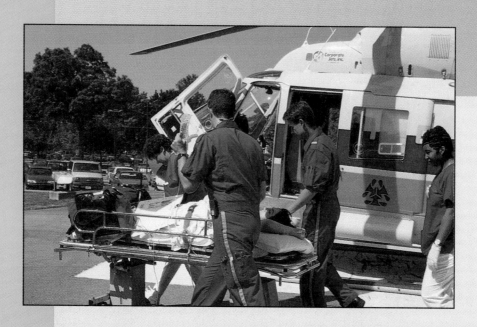

Emergency Agents

This final unit focuses on adult and pediatric emergency drugs. The chapter considers pharmacologic treatment for five categories of emergency situations: (1) cardiac, (2) neurosurgical, (3) poisoning, (4) shock, and (5) hypertensive crisis. Specific drug protocols and dosages for the pediatric client are included.

Adult and Pediatric Emergency Drugs

52

Linda Laskowski-Jones

Outline

Objectives

- Describe indications for the emergency drugs listed in this chapter.
- Define the basic mechanism of action for each emergency drug.
- List pertinent nursing considerations and actions specific for each agent.
- Explain how to administer the drugs properly.
- Describe significant adverse effects of each drug.

Terms

anaphylactic shock	emetic	hypoxemia
angina pectoris	extravasation	myocardial infarction
asthma	glycogenolysis	preload
asystole	heart block	pulse oximetry
bradycardia	hypertensive crisis	tachycardia
cathartic	hypomagnesemia	torsades de pointes
dysrhythmias	hypovolemic shock	

INTRODUCTION

The drugs described in this chapter are first-line agents commonly used to treat various medical emergencies. Nurses must have a ready knowledge of the indications and actions of these agents, because medical and surgical emergencies can occur in virtually any area of nursing practice. Learning key nursing implications before a crisis situation enables the nurse to function at the highest possible level when the client requires life-saving intervention.

At the end of each discussion on a group of emergency drugs is a summary table of the drugs, called a drug chart, their dosages, and indications. Common adult doses are listed in the tables; pediatric dosages may vary widely depending on the age and the weight of the child. The tables list only the most common indications and dosages for the emergency drugs discussed; the tables *do not* describe all possible uses and dosing regimens for the agents.

OXYGEN AS AN EMERGENCY DRUG

Oxygen can be classified as a drug because it may have both beneficial and adverse effects on the body based on the amount and manner in which it is administered. Oxygen is essential to life—without it, brain death begins within 6 minutes. Inadequate oxygenation produces hypoxemia and significant physiologic sequelae to all body systems. Therefore, oxygen is a first-line drug for all emergency situations. Depending on the circumstances, adequate oxygenation may be all that is necessary to effectively treat physiologic disturbances such as chest pain, bradycardia, and cardiac dysrhythmias.

Before the other pharmacologic agents discussed in this chapter are administered, ensure that the patient's airway and breathing are addressed to promote optimal oxygenation and ventilation. Giving a drug to treat a disorder brought on by **hypoxemia,** without effectively correcting the cause of the hypoxemia, is ineffective and, ultimately, does not produce the desired outcome. **Pulse oximetry,** which provides a digital display of oxygen saturation, is an essential monitoring tool that should be used in emergency situations to assess the adequacy of oxygenation and guide further interventions. Oxygen saturation should be kept at or above 96%.

In general, patients suffering from severe physiologic stress such as shock states, traumatic injury, acute myocardial infarction with hemodynamic instability, and cardiac arrest initially require oxygen in high concentrations (i.e., FiO_2 close to 100%). The oxygen devices of choice for these conditions include a non-rebreather mask with an oxygen reservoir (O_2 flow rate set at 10–12 L/min) for spontaneously breathing patients, and a bag-valve-mask device attached to an oxygen source at a flow rate of 12 to 15 L/min for patients who require assisted ventilation. Although caution must be exercised for patients with chronic obstructive pulmonary disease (COPD) (they may lose their hypoxic respiratory drive when given oxygen in high concentration), oxygen should never be denied to a patient who needs it. In the case of COPD, the nurse should be prepared to manually ventilate the patient with a bag-valve-mask if respiratory depression or arrest occurs. As the patient's condition stabilizes, the oxygen concentration should be decreased. An FiO_2 over 50% for a prolonged period can lead to oxygen toxicity and other detrimental effects to the pulmonary system in both adults and children.

For emergency situations that do not involve severe physiologic stress (e.g., angina, dysrhythmias, pulmonary disease), supplemental oxygen delivered by nasal cannula at 1 to 6 L/min or by simple face mask at 4 to 8 L/min may have significant physiologic benefit. Children may tolerate a face tent with a high oxygen flow of 10 to 15 L better than a nasal cannula or face mask.

EMERGENCY DRUGS FOR CARDIAC DISORDERS

Drugs described in this section are indicated for cardiac emergencies such as angina, myocardial infarction, disturbances of cardiac rate or rhythm, and cardiac arrest. These drugs often must be prepared and administered rapidly. A sound knowledge base as well as easy access to the drugs and necessary equipment is essential for the best client outcome in a cardiac emergency. These drugs are cross referenced to the specialty chapter.

Nitroglycerin

Nitroglycerin dilates coronary arteries and improves blood flow to ischemic myocardium. It is therefore the treatment of choice for **angina pectoris** (chest pain) and **myocardial infarction** (heart attack). Nitroglycerin is available in sublingual, oral, topical, and intravenous forms. Only the sublingual and intravenous preparations are discussed.

Sublingual nitroglycerin (0.3–0.4 mg) is indicated for clients experiencing an acute anginal attack. The client is taught to place one sublingual nitroglycerin tablet under the tongue and to allow it to dissolve slowly. Not all sublingual nitroglycerin preparations cause a burning sensation under the tongue, and this should not be relied on to indicate potency. If the chest pain is not relieved, sublingual nitroglycerin may be repeated at 5-min intervals until a total of three tablets has been taken. If pain persists, further interventions are necessary in an emergency or critical care setting. An ambulance should be called if the client is outside of the hospital. Blood pressure and heart rate must be monitored closely. Hypotension is a common adverse effect, especially the first time a client takes nitroglycerin. Tachycardia or, uncommonly, bradycardia also may occur.

Intravenous nitroglycerin (Tridil) is reserved for clients with unstable angina or acute myocardial infarction. A continuous infusion is usually initiated at a rate of 10 to 20 μg/min and increased by 5 to 10 μg/min every 5 to 10 min based on chest pain and blood pressure response. Continuous blood pressure and heart monitoring are required because hypotension is a common adverse effect. Hypotension usually is treated by reducing or discontinuing the nitroglycerin infusion (see Chapter 37).

Morphine Sulfate

Morphine sulfate, a narcotic analgesic, is used to treat the chest pain associated with acute myocardial infarction. It also is indicated for acute pulmonary edema. Morphine relieves pain, dilates venous vessels, and reduces the workload on the heart. The standard dosage of morphine sulfate is 1 to 3 mg intravenously (IV) over 1 to 5 min repeated until chest pain is relieved. The nurse must be aware that respiratory depression and hypotension are common adverse effects; close client monitoring is essential. The narcotic antagonist naloxone (Narcan) may be ordered to reverse the action of morphine if adverse effects pose a significant risk to the client. The dose is 0.4 to 0.8 mg every 2 to 3 min as indicated (see Chapter 17).

Atropine Sulfate

Atropine sulfate is indicated in the treatment of hemodynamically significant **bradycardia** (slow heart rate) and **heart block** (e.g., low cardiac output, hypotension), as well as asystole. Atropine acts to increase heart rate by inhibiting the action of the vagus nerve (parasympatholytic effect). Atropine sulfate is also used as an emergency drug to reverse the toxic effects of organophosphate pesticide exposure, which include bradycardia and excessive secretions. In symptomatic bradycardia, atropine is administered intravenously in 0.5- to 1.0-mg doses at 3- to 5-min intervals until the desired heart rate is achieved or until 0.03 to 0.04 mg/kg (generally not more than 3 mg) is given. In **asystole** (cardiac arrest), atropine is given as a 1.0-mg bolus dose IV, which may be repeated up to the dosing limits every 3 to 5 minutes.

The adult intravenous atropine dose should not be less than 0.5 mg or exceed 0.03 to 0.04 mg/kg (usually not more than 3 mg IV): doses below 0.5 mg can produce a paradoxical bradycardia; at doses of 0.04 mg/kg or greater, vagal activity is considered completely blocked and further atropine administration may have no benefit. Atropine sulfate can be administered through an endotracheal tube (ETT) if no venous access exists; 2 to 3 mg should be diluted in 10 mL of normal saline and instilled deep into the endotracheal tube via a feeding tube attached to a syringe. After endotracheal administration, the client should be ventilated vigorously with an Ambu bag to enhance absorption of the drug.

Continuous cardiac and blood pressure monitoring is essential for the client who receives intravenous atropine sulfate. Significant adverse effects include cardiac dysrhythmias, tachycardia, myocardial ischemia, restlessness, anxiety, mydriasis, thirst, and urinary retention.

PEDIATRIC IMPLICATIONS

Because cardiac output is dependent on heart rate in infants younger than 6 months, bradycardia (heart rate <60 beats per minute [bpm]) must be treated. Before administration of drugs, efforts should be targeted toward restoring adequate ventilation and oxygenation. If these maneuvers do not produce the desired clinical response, then atropine is indicated.

The pediatric dose of atropine is 0.02 mg/kg IV or via endotracheal tube (ETT) or intraosseous route. It is important to be cognizant that the minimum dose is 0.1 mg. The maximum total pediatric dose is 1.0 mg in a child and 2.0 mg in an adolescent. For the neonate in cardiac arrest or with a spontaneous heart rate of <80 bpm, epinephrine 0.01 to 0.03 mg/kg IV or via ETT every 3 to 5 min as indicated may be preferred to elevate the heart rate, because stressed neonates quickly deplete their own stores of catecholamines (see Chapter 22).

Isoproterenol

Isoproterenol (Isuprel) is a beta-adrenergic drug given to increase heart rate. Typically, isoproterenol is considered only after the maximum dose of atropine (3 mg), dopamine and epinephrine infusions, and a transcutaneous pacemaker have failed to produce the desired clinical response in clients with hemodynamically significant bradycardia. Thus, the client who exhibits symptomatic refractory bradycardia is a candidate for isoproterenol. Isoproterenol is administered as an IV infusion, generally 1 mg diluted in 250 mLof 5% dextrose in water, at 2 to 10 μg/min titrated to heart rate (usually 60 bpm). An electronic infusion device must be used to provide precise infusion control.

Myocardial oxygen consumption is greatly increased with isoproterenol administration; the nurse must carefully monitor the client receiving isoproterenol. Significant adverse effects include myocardial ischemia, tachycardia, and life-threatening dysrhythmias such as ventricular tachycardia and ventricular fibrillation. The nurse should alert the physician promptly if any increase in premature ventricular contractions is noted on the cardiac monitor or if the heart rate exceeds 100 bpm; the dosage may need to be decreased or the infusion stopped.

PEDIATRIC IMPLICATIONS

Epinephrine infusions may be preferable to isoproterenol infusions to increase heart rate above 60 bpm in pediatric clients. Isoproterenol can cause a large decrease in diastolic blood pressure. The typical dose is 0.1 to 1.0 μg/kg/min titrated to the desired response. As in the adult client, isoproterenol should never be used in the cardiac arrest situation (see Chapter 21).

Adenosine

Adenosine (Adenocard) is the first-line drug of choice to treat paroxysmal supraventricular tachycardia (PSVT), a sudden, uncontrolled, rapid rhythm. A natural substance found in all body cells, adenosine slows impulse conduction through the heart's atrioventricular (AV) node, interrupts dysrhythmia-producing reentry pathways, and can restore a normal rhythm in clients with PSVT. Because the half-life is less than 5 sec, adenosine is administered rapidly as a 6-mg IV bolus over 1 to 3 sec. A 12-mg bolus may be given 1 to 2 min after the initial dose if PSVT persists and can be repeated once if necessary. Dosages greater than 12 mg are not recommended.

Nursing considerations include continuous cardiac monitoring and frequent assessment of vital signs. Adenosine is inhibited by methylxanthines such as caffeine and theophylline. Although few adverse reactions have been reported, hypotension and dyspnea may occur. In addition, a short period of asystole may follow administration (up to 15 sec). Spontaneous cardiac activity resumes. Adenosine is contraindicated in clients with second- and third-degree heart block and in clients with sick sinus syndrome, except those with functioning pacemakers (see Chapter 37).

Verapamil

Verapamil (Isoptin), a calcium channel blocker, is indicated for the treatment of **tachycardia** (rapid heart rate) originating above the ventricles (paroxysmal supraventricular tachycardia [PSVT]). Such heart rates generally exceed 150 bpm. Verapamil slows conduc-tion (negative chronotropic) through the heart and has negative inotropic and vasodilating effects. In emergency situations, verapamil is administered as an intravenous bolus in variable age- and weight-dependent dosages, which should not exceed 2.5 to 5 mg given slowly over a 1- to 3-min period. Repeat doses of 5 to 10 mg may be ordered in 15 to 30 minutes. The nurse must carefully monitor heart rate and rhythm as well as blood pressure. Cardiac conduction disturbances and profound hypotension can occur. An intravenous injection of calcium may be ordered to prevent or treat calcium channel blocker–induced hypotension (see Chapters 37 and 39).

Diltiazem

Diltiazem is a calcium channel blocker like verapamil that is administered as an intravenous bolus to treat paroxysmal supraventricular tachycardia and to slow the ventricular response rate in atrial fibrillation or flutter. Diltiazem has less of a negative inotropic effect than verapamil, but it has strong negative chronotropic actions. Therefore, IV diltiazem is less likely to cause cardiac depression but is very effective in controlling heart rate.

The usual initial bolus dose of IV diltiazem is 0.25 mg/kg given over 2 min. If the supraventricular tachycardia does not convert to a normal sinus rhythm in 15 minutes, a second IV bolus of 0.35 mg/kg over 2 to 5 min. may be necessary. For ongoing control of the ventricular rate in clients with atrial fibrillation or flutter, a continuous infusion of diltiazem is indicated at a dose range of 5 to 15 mg/h, titrated according to the desired heart rate for not longer than 24 hours.

The nurse must carefully monitor blood pressure and heart rate after administering IV diltiazem. Although mild, transient hypotension is common, significant hypotension may be treated with injection of intravenous calcium to elevate blood pressure. In clients who are hypotensive before calcium channel blocker administration, intravenous calcium may be ordered as a pretreatment to prevent the hypotensive response to the drug.

Diltiazem can elevate serum digoxin levels, predisposing the client to digitalis toxicity. Simultaneous use of calcium channel blockers and beta blockers is contraindicated because their negative inotropic and negative chronotropic effects are synergistic, causing myocardial depression and bradycardia. Other contraindications include heart block or sick sinus syndrome in the client without a pacemaker and severe heart failure. The nurse should be especially careful when administering calcium channel blockers to pediatric patients, because they may have preexisting myocardial dysfunction.

Lidocaine

Lidocaine is the primary drug used to treat ventricular **dysrhythmias** (irregular heartbeats), such as premature ventricular contractions (PVCs), ventricular tachycardia, and ventricular fibrillation. Lidocaine exerts a local anesthetic effect on the heart, thus decreasing myocardial irritability. Typically, a client with ventricular dysrhythmias is given a 1- to 1.5-mg/kg bolus of lidocaine, followed by 0.5 mg/kg every 5 to 10 min until the dysrhythmia is controlled or a total dose of 3 mg/kg has been administered. A continuous lidocaine infusion is initiated at a rate of 2 to 4 mg/min to maintain a therapeutic serum level. Lidocaine may also be administered via the endotracheal route in an amount 2 to 2.5 times the IV dose.

Important nursing considerations for the client receiving lidocaine include continuous cardiac monitoring and assessment for signs and symptoms of lidocaine toxicity (confusion, drowsiness, hearing impairment, cardiac conduction defects, myocardial depression, muscle twitching, and seizures). Because lidocaine is metabolized by the liver, clients with hepatic impairment, congestive heart failure, shock, and advanced age (>70 y) are at higher risk for toxicity. In these clients, the lidocaine dose may need to be reduced by as much as 50%.

PEDIATRIC IMPLICATIONS

Ventricular ectopy is uncommon in children. Metabolic causes should be suspected if ventricular dysrhythmias occur. The pediatric dose of lidocaine is 1 mg/kg IV, ETT, or via the intraosseous route. A maintenance infusion of 20 to 50 μg/kg/min is recommended following the bolus dose (see Chapter 37). Drug data for lidocaine are presented in Chart 52–1.

Procainamide

Procainamide (Pronestyl) is an antidysrhythmic agent often prescribed when lidocaine has failed to achieve the desired clinical response. Indications include ventricular tachycardia, PVCs, and rapid supraventricular dysrhythmias. The typical intravenous loading dose of procainamide is 20 to 30 mg/min until the dysrhythmia is successfully treated. Other end points to procainamide administration include giving a total of 17 mg/kg of the drug, the development of hypotension, and specific changes on the electrocardiogram (ECG) (e.g., widening of the QRS complex by 50% or more). A continuous maintenance infusion of 1 to 4 mg/min may be ordered following the loading dose.

Procainamide administration can cause severe hypotension. Heart block, rhythm disturbances, and cardiac arrest can occur. Procainamide is contraindicated in clients with torsades de pointes. The drug is eliminated via the kidneys; therefore, clients in renal failure are at higher risk of adverse effects and often require a lower dosage (see Chapter 37).

Bretylium Tosylate

Bretylium (Bretylol) is an antidysrhythmic agent used to treat ventricular tachycardia and ventricular fibrillation when lidocaine, electric countershock, or procainamide has been ineffective. How bretylium works is not well established. For ventricular fibrillation, bretylium is administered undiluted as a rapid intravenous 5-mg/kg bolus dose. After 5 min, the dosage may be increased to 10 mg/kg if necessary. Bretylium 10 mg/kg may be repeated every 5 to 30 min until a maximum dose of 30 mg/kg is given. For ventricular tachycardia, bretylium is usually diluted in 50 mL of dextrose 5% in water or normal saline solution, and 5 to 10 mg/kg is administered slowly over 8 to 10 min; rapid infusion may cause nausea, vomiting, and low blood pressure in a conscious client. The maximum total dose of 30 mg/kg over a 24-hour period must not be exceeded. A continuous infusion of bretylium can be initiated at a rate of 1–2 mg/min. Bretylium may not take effect for up to 20 min after injection.

After bretylium administration, the nurse must monitor the client in ventricular fibrillation for return of pulses. In the client experiencing ventricular tachycardia, bretylium may cause an initial increase in blood pressure and heart rate, followed by orthostatic hypotension. Generally, placing the client in a supine position and administering IV fluids as ordered are appropriate interventions to treat the orthostatic hypotension.

PEDIATRIC IMPLICATIONS

The use of bretylium in children is not well established.

Magnesium Sulfate

Magnesium is an essential element in multiple enzymatic reactions in the body, including function of the sodium-potassium ATPase pump. Its physiologic effects can be likened to a calcium channel blocker with neuromuscular blocking properties. Hypomagnesemia is associated with the development of atrial and ventricular dysrhythmias.

The primary indications for emergency administration of magnesium sulfate are refractory ventricular tachycardia, refractory ventricular fibrillation, cardiac arrest associated with **hypomagnesemia** (low serum magnesium level), and life-threatening ventricular dysrhythmias from digitalis toxicity and tricyclic antidepressant overdose. It is also the drug of choice for the treatment of **torsades de pointes,** an unusual polymorphic ventricular tachycardia often associated with a prolonged Q-T interval. Prophylactic magne-

Chart 52–1.   Emergency Treatment of Cardiac States: Antidysrhythmic

LIDOCAINE HCl

Drug Name

Lidocaine HCl (Xylocaine)
Antidysrhythmic, class IB
Pregnancy Category: C

Dosage

A: IV: ETT*: 1–1.5 mg/kg; may repeat 0.5 mg/
kg q 5–10 min up to 3 mg/kg *(max)*
Drip: 1–4 mg/min
C: IV: ETT* or IO: Initially: 1 mg/kg; maint: 20–
50 µg/kg/min is recommended after bolus
*Note: For *endotracheal* drug administration,
dose should be 2 to 2.5 times IV dose in adults
Therapeutic Range: 1.5–5 µg/mL

Contraindications

Hypersensitivity, advanced atrioventricular
block
Caution: Liver disease, congestive heart failure,
elderly

Drug-Lab-Food Interactions

Increase effects with phenytoin, quinidine, procainamide, propranolol; *increase* risk of toxicity
with cimetidine, beta-adrenergic blockers

Pharmacokinetics

Absorption: IV
Distribution: PB: 60%–80%; concentrates in adi-
pose tissue
Metabolism: $t\frac{1}{2}$: Initial: 7–30 min; terminal: 9–
120 min
Excretion: Through the liver

Pharmacodynamics

PO: Onset: 45–60 s
       Peak: 45–60 s
       Duration: 10–20 min

Therapeutic Effects/Uses

Primary drug to treat ventricular dysrhythmias such as premature ventricular contractions (PVCs),
ventricular tachycardia, and ventricular fibrillation.

Mode of Action: Decreases automaticity; increases electrical threshold of ventricle.

Side Effects

Drowsiness, confusion, dyspnea, lethargy, hypotension, nausea, vomiting

Adverse Reactions

Life-threatening: Seizures, cardiac arrest

Assessment and Planning

Interventions

NURSING PROCESS

Evaluation

KEY: IV: intravenous; ETT: endotracheal tube; PB: protein-binding; $t\frac{1}{2}$: half-life; s: seconds.

---

sium administration may also decrease the incidence of ventricular dysrhythmias after acute myocardial infarction.

Magnesium is administered by diluting 1 to 2 g (2–4 mL of a 50% solution) in 10 mL of D_5W; in cardiac arrest, the magnesium is given by direct IV push. For patients who exhibit ventricular tachycardia with a pulse, the magnesium is administered IV over 1 to 2 minutes. Higher doses may be required to treat torsades de pointes. For patients experiencing acute myocardial infarction, a magnesium infusion of 1 to 2 g diluted in 50 to 100 mL of D_5W can be given IV over 5 to 60 minutes followed by a continuous in-

fusion of 0.5 to 1 g/h as a prophylactic agent against ventricular dysrhythmias.

Although magnesium toxicity is rare, the nurse should monitor the patient's response to magnesium administration. Hypotension is the most common adverse effect when magnesium is given by rapid IV push. Other effects include mild bradycardia, flushing, and sweating. True hypermagnesemia can cause diarrhea, respiratory depression, deep tendon reflex impairment, flaccid paralysis, and circulatory collapse. Because magnesium is eliminated via the kidneys, it should be administered with caution in patients with renal impairment.

Epinephrine

Epinephrine is a catecholamine with both alpha- and beta-adrenergic effects. Indications for administration of intravenous epinephrine include profound bradycardia, asystole, pulseless ventricular tachycardia, and ventricular fibrillation. Epinephrine is thought to improve perfusion of the heart and brain in cardiac arrest states through constriction of peripheral blood vessels. In addition, epinephrine increases the chances for successful electrical countershock (defibrillation) in ventricular fibrillation. For bradycardia, an epinephrine infusion may be ordered at 2 to 10 μg/min. For asystole, pulseless ventricular tachycardia, and ventricular fibrillation, epinephrine is administered in 1-mg doses IV every 3 to 5 min until the desired clinical response is achieved (usually, return of effective cardiac activity). High-dose epinephrine (5 mg or 0.1 mg/kg) may be considered after the initial 1.0-mg dose. Epinephrine also may be given via the ETT route, in doses of 2 to 2.5 times the IV dose.

Nursing implications for clients receiving epinephrine include constant cardiac and hemodynamic monitoring. Epinephrine can cause myocardial ischemia and cardiac dysrhythmias. Epinephrine should never be administered in the same site as an alkaline solution such as sodium bicarbonate; alkaline solutions inactivate epinephrine. In addition, the presence of metabolic or respiratory acidosis decreases the effectiveness of epinephrine. All efforts should be made to correct acid-base imbalances in the client.

PEDIATRIC IMPLICATIONS

The pediatric dose of epinephrine is 0.01 mg/kg (1:10,000 solution) given IV or via the intraosseous route for cardiac arrest (see Chapter 21). The ETT dose should be given using the 1:1000 solution.

Sodium Bicarbonate

Sodium bicarbonate is prescribed to treat the metabolic acidosis that often accompanies cardiac arrest. The current standard is to give sodium bicarbonate only after adequate ventilation, chest compressions, and drug therapy fail to correct the acidotic state. Sodium bicarbonate is rarely a first-line drug in cardiac arrest situations; it is preferentially given based on results of arterial blood gas analysis when acidosis is severe. If a client has been in arrest for a prolonged period and blood gas analysis is not available, sodium bicarbonate may be ordered as part of the ongoing resuscitation attempt. The standard initial intravenous dose of sodium bicarbonate is 1 mEq/kg. The drug may be repeated at 0.5 mEq/kg every 10 min as needed.

Important nursing considerations relevant to sodium bicarbonate include careful monitoring of arterial blood gas analysis results. Sodium bicarbonate administration can lead to metabolic alkalosis. In addition, catecholamines such as epinephrine, norepinephrine, and dopamine should not be infused in the same site as sodium bicarbonate; catecholamines are inactivated by solutions containing sodium bicarbonate. Table 52–1 lists emergency cardiac drugs, their dosages, and indications.

PEDIATRIC IMPLICATIONS

If metabolic acidosis persists after attention has been directed at maintaining optimal ventilation and oxygenation, sodium bicarbonate may be given to the pediatric client in a 1-mEq/kg dose via the IV or intraosseous route. Subsequent doses of 0.5 mEq/kg may be given every 10 min if blood gases are not available. Sodium bicarbonate is hyperosmolar and should be diluted from an 8.4% solution (1 mEq/mL) to a 4.2% solution (0.5 mEq/mL) for infants younger than 3 months of age (see Chapter 13).

EMERGENCY DRUGS FOR NEUROSURGICAL DISORDERS

The neurosurgical drugs discussed in this section are commonly administered in emergency, trauma, and critical care settings. For maximum benefit, these agents must be given as early as possible when clinically indicated. Knowledge of proper administration techniques and guidelines enhances therapeutic effectiveness. These drugs are cross-referenced to the specialty chapters.

Mannitol

Mannitol is an osmotic diuretic used in the emergency and neurosurgical setting to treat cerebral edema and increased intracranial pressure, which may occur following head trauma, neurosurgery, and other types of intracranial pathology. Mannitol may be given as an intravenous bolus or via a continuous drip. The usual initial bolus dose of mannitol is 0.5 to 1.0 g/kg IV of a 25% solution. Subsequent dosing is highly variable and is influenced by serum osmolality. In general, mannitol is held when serum osmolality exceeds 310–320. Mannitol is highly irritating to veins. The nurse must use a filter needle when administering mannitol, because crystals may form in the solution and be inadvertently injected. In addition, the nurse should carefully assess the client's neurologic status, monitor laboratory studies, including serum osmolality, and keep accurate intake and

Table 52–1
Cardiac Emergency Drugs

GENERIC (BRAND)	ROUTE AND DOSAGE	USES AND CONSIDERATIONS
Adenosine (Adenocard)	A: Initially: 6 mg; then 12 mg in 1–2 min if needed; may repeat 12 mg × 1	Paroxysmal supraventricular tachycardia. *Pregnancy category:* C; PB: UK; $t\frac{1}{2}$: <10 sec.
Atropine sulfate	IV: ETT: 0.5–1 mg; can repeat up to 0.03–0.04 mg/kg or 3 mg *(max)*	Symptomatic bradycardia; asystole. *Pregnancy category:* C; PB: 60%–80%; $t\frac{1}{2}$: 2–3 h
Bretylium tosylate (Bretylol)	IV: Initially: 5 mg/kg; then 10 mg/kg q10–30 min up to 30 mg/kg total *(max)* over 24 h	Ventricular tachycardia, ventricular fibrillation. *Pregnancy category:* C; PB: 1%–6%; $t\frac{1}{2}$: 4–18 h
Diltiazem	IV: 0.25 mg/kg; repeat in 15 min at 0.35 mg/kg IV: drip 5–15 mg/h	Supraventricular tachycardia, atrial fibrillation and flutter. *Pregnancy category:* C; PB: 80%; $t\frac{1}{2}$: 2–5 h
Epinephrine	IV: ETT: 0.5–1 mg; may be repeated q5min	Asystole, ventricular fibrillation. *Pregnancy category:* C; PB: UK; $t\frac{1}{2}$: UK
Lidocaine	See Chart 52–1	
Magnesium sulfate	Dilute 1–2 g (2–4 mL of a 50% solution) in 10 mL of D_5W. Give IV push in cardiac arrest; over 1–2 minutes for ventricular tachycardia; for acute MI, 1–2 g diluted in 50–100 mL of D_5W given IV over 5–60 min followed by a continuous infusion of 0.5–1 g	Used for hypomagnesemia, treatment of ventricular tachycardia and ventricular fibrillation, and prevention of atrial and ventricular dysrhythmias after myocardial infarction Drug of choice for torsades de pointes. Rapid infusion can cause hypotension.
Morphine sulfate	IV: 1–3 mg q5–30 min	Chest pain, unstable angina, pulmonary edema. *Pregnancy category:* C; PB: 35%; $t\frac{1}{2}$: 2–2.5 h
Nitroglycerin (Nitrostat, Tridil)	SL: 0.3–0.4 mg IV: Drip: 10–20 μg/min, increased 5–10 μg/min q5–10 min (titrated)	Chest pain, angina, unstable angina, MI. *Pregnancy category:* C; PB: 60%; $t\frac{1}{2}$: 1–4 min
Procainamide HCl (Pronestyl)	IV: 20–30 mg/min; max: 17 mg/kg *Recognize end points:* • Hypotension • QRS widens >50% • Total dose of 17 mg/kg given Drip: 1–4 mg/min	PVCs, ventricular tachycardia, ventricular fibrillation, atrial dysrhythmias. *Pregnancy category:* C; PB: 20%; $t\frac{1}{2}$: 3–4 h
Sodium bicarbonate	IV: Initially: 1 mEq/kg; then 0.5 mEq/kg if needed	Metabolic acidosis. *Pregnancy category:* C; PB: UK; $t\frac{1}{2}$: UK.
Verapamil HCl (Isoptin, Calan)	IV: Age- and weight-dependent dosages; should not exceed 5 mg; repeat doses may be needed	Paroxysmal supraventricular tachycardia. *Pregnancy category:* C; PB: 90%; $t\frac{1}{2}$: 3–8 h

KEY: A: adult; ETT: endotracheal tube; IV: intravenous; PB: protein-binding; SL: sublingual; $t\frac{1}{2}$: half-life; UK: unknown.

output records to assess fluid volume status because diuresis may be substantial (see Chapters 13 and 38). Drug data for mannitol are presented in Chart 52–2.

Methylprednisolone

High-dose methylprednisolone (Solu-Medrol) may improve motor and sensory function in clients with traumatic spinal cord injuries from 6 weeks to 6 months after injury. A strict pharmacologic protocol must be followed. Methylprednisolone must be ad-

ministered in the following manner within 8 hours of acute spinal cord injury: a bolus dose of 30 mg/kg of client body weight is given intravenously over 15 min (mixed in 100 mL of normal saline solution); a maintenance infusion of 5.4 mg/kg/h is then initiated within 45 minutes of the bolus and continued for 23 hours if the injury is less than 3 hours old. If the injury is between 3 and 8 hours old, the maintenance infusion must run for 48 hours.

Contraindications include, allergy to the drug, penetrating trauma to the spinal cord or spinal lesions

Chart 52–2. Emergency Treatment of Neurosurgical States: Diuretic

MANNITOL

NURSING PROCESS

Assessment and Planning

Drug Name

Mannitol (Osmitrol)
Osmotic diuretic
Pregnancy Category: C

Dosage

A: IV: Initially 0.5–1.0 g/kg of 25% sol as a bolus
Highly individualized

Contraindications

Hypersensitivity, severe dehydration
Caution: Pregnancy, breast-feeding, current intracranial bleeding

Drug-Lab-Food Interactions

May *decrease* effectiveness with lithium

Interventions

Pharmacokinetics

Absorption: IV
Distribution: PB: Confined to extracellular space
Metabolism: $t\frac{1}{2}$: 100 min
Excretion: In urine

Pharmacodynamics

Decrease in Intracranial Pressure:
IV: Onset: 30–60 min
  Peak: 1 h
  Duration: 6–8 h
Diuresis: Onset: 1–3 h
  Peak: 1 h
  Duration: 6–8 h

Evaluation

Therapeutic Effects/Uses

To treat increased intracranial pressure, cerebral edema.

Mode of Action: Inhibition of reabsorption of electrolytes and water by affecting pressure of glomerular filtrate.

Side Effects

Temporary volume expansion, hypo/hypernatremia, hypo/hyperkalemia, dehydration, blurred vision, dry mouth

Adverse Reactions

Pulmonary congestion, fluid/electrolyte imbalances
Life-threatening: Convulsions

KEY: IV: intravenous; PB: protein-binding; $t\frac{1}{2}$: half-life; sol: solution.

below L2, human immunodeficiency virus (HIV) infection, severe infection, and a spinal cord injury more than 8 hours old. Relative contraindications include pregnancy and uncontrolled diabetes mellitus. Adverse effects include transient hypertension with administration of the loading dose and elevation of blood sugar during the infusion. The nurse must monitor vital signs and blood sugar and perform frequent and accurate neurologic assessments pertinent to spinal cord injury. Table 52–2 lists neurosurgical

emergency drugs and their dosages and indications (see Chapters 23 and 45).

EMERGENCY DRUGS FOR POISONING

Although there are numerous antidotes for specific types of poisoning, the drugs presented in this section are the most commonly prescribed agents in cases

Table 52–2
Neurosurgical Emergency Drugs

DRUG	DOSAGE	USES AND CONSIDERATIONS
Mannitol	See Chart 52–2	
Methylprednisolone (Solu-Medrol)	IV: bolus dose: 30 mg/kg in 100 mL NSS; then 5.4 mg/kg/h (23 h) or 48° for SCI > 3 h but <8 h old	For treatment of acute spinal cord injury (within 8 h of injury). *Pregnancy category:* C; PB: 80%–90%; $t_{\frac{1}{2}}$: 2–4 h. Contraindicated in penetrating spinal cord trauma.

KEY: *IV: intravenous; NSS: normal saline solution; SCI: spinal cord injury.*

of drug overdose and ingestion of toxic substances, with pertinent exceptions noted. Particular attention must be given to administration guidelines to achieve the best possible clinical outcome for the client. These drugs are cross-referenced to the specialty chapters.

Naloxone

Naloxone (Narcan) is classified as an opiate antagonist. It reverses the effects of all opiate drugs (common examples include morphine, meperidine, codeine, propoxyphene, and heroin) by competitively binding to opiate receptor sites in the body. Naloxone is indicated for individuals who have taken an overdose of opiate drugs, those experiencing respiratory or cardiovascular depression from therapeutic doses of opiates given in a health care setting, and those brought to the emergency department in a coma of unknown etiology (which may be drug-induced).

The typical dose of naloxone for actual or suspected opiate overdose in adults is 0.4 to 2 mg IV administered every 2 to 3 min until the client's condition improves to an acceptable level. If there is no improvement after 10 mg of the drug has been injected, nonopiate drugs or disease must be suspected. Although naloxone should be administered intravenously in emergency situations, it also may be given intramuscularly or subcutaneously if intravenous access is not obtainable.

Because most opiate drugs have a longer duration of action than naloxone, the nurse must monitor the client closely for signs and symptoms of recurrent opiate effects such as respiratory depression and hypotension. In this situation, naloxone administration may need to be repeated several times or a continuous IV infusion ordered. Naloxone has no major adverse effects but can precipitate withdrawal symptoms in clients addicted to opiate drugs. In addition, pulmonary edema has been reported following naloxone administration in clients who have had an overdose of morphine (see Chapter 17). Drug data for naloxone are presented in Chart 52–3.

Flumazenil

Flumazenil (Mazicon) is the reversal agent for the respiratory depressant and sedative effects of benzodiazepine medications (e.g., diazepam [Valium], midazolam [Versed], chlordiazepoxide [Librium]). It is administered to counteract the effects of benzodiazepines given as sedative or anesthetic agents, as well as to treat accidental or intentional benzodiazepine overdose. Flumazenil does not reverse the central nervous system (CNS) depressant effects of nonbenzodiazepine agents such as alcohol, opiates, and barbiturates. In addition, flumazenil may not reverse the amnesia induced by the benzodiazepine.

Flumazenil is given IV as an initial dose of 0.2 mg. Additional doses may be given over 30 sec every minute until the desired clinical response is achieved or until a total dose of 3 mg is given. In the event of re-sedation, doses of flumazenil may be repeated at 20-minute intervals (not to exceed 1 mg at a time) to a total hourly dose of no more than 3 mg IV.

Nursing considerations include careful assessment of respiratory rate and effort, blood pressure, and mental status. If the benzodiazepine is reversed too rapidly, patients may have emergent reactions in which they become agitated and confused, and have perceptual distortions. Because seizures are precipitated by benzodiazepine withdrawal, seizure precautions must be implemented for patients at risk (those with long-standing benzodiazepine use or abuse) or for those who have a known seizure disorder.

Ipecac Syrup

Ipecac syrup is an **emetic** (an agent used to induce vomiting of ingested poisons). It is a liquid, over-the-counter (OTC) medication that is taken orally. The standard dose of ipecac in children older than 1 year of age is 15 mL; in children older than 12 years and in adults, the dose is 15 to 30 mL PO followed by

Chart 52–3. Emergency Treatment of Poisoning

NALOXONE HCl

Drug Name *Naloxone HCl* (Narcan) Narcotic antagonist *Pregnancy Category:* B	**Dosage** IV/IM/SC: 0.4–2 mg; repeat every 2–3 min, as indicated
Contraindications Hypersensitivity, respiratory depression *Caution:* Opiate-dependent clients, cardiac disease, breastfeeding neonates of opiate-dependent mothers	**Drug-Lab-Food Interactions** Naloxone can precipitate withdrawal in a client dependent on narcotic analgesics *Lab:* Urine VMA, 5-HIAA, urine glucose

Assessment and Planning

Pharmacokinetics
 	
Absorption: IM/SC: Well absorbed
Distribution: PB: UK
Metabolism: t½: Adults 1–4 h; neonates: 1–3 h
Excretion: In urine metabolites
	Pharmacodynamics
	
	SC/IM: Onset: 2–5 min
	          Peak: UK
	          Duration: 1–4 h
	IV: Onset: 1–2 min
	          Peak: UK
	          Duration: 1–4 h

Interventions

NURSING PROCESS

Therapeutic Effects/Uses

To treat respiratory depression caused by narcotics; to treat narcotic-induced depressant effects and narcotic overdose.

Mode of Action: Blocks effects of narcotics by competing for the receptor sites.

Side Effects Negligible pharmacologic effect without narcotics in body	**Adverse Reactions** Nausea, vomiting, tremulousness, sweating, tachycardia, elevated blood pressure **Life-threatening:** Atrioventricular fibrillation, pulmonary edema (with overdose of morphine)

Evaluation

KEY: IV: intravenous; IM: intramuscular; SC: subcutaneous; PB: protein-binding; UK: unknown; t½: half-life.

---

adequate amounts of water to enhance the emetic effects (carbonated beverages may cause gastric distention; administration with milk decreases effectiveness). Administration of ipecac may be repeated once if vomiting has not occurred in 30 min.

Ipecac should be used with caution. The nurse should administer ipecac before activated charcoal (charcoal will inactivate ipecac). The nurse should also instruct clients and their family members to con-

tact a poison control center before taking or giving ipecac in the home setting; they should then seek medical attention immediately. The nurse must know the following contraindications to administration: cardiac disease or shock (ipecac is potentially cardiotoxic); unconsciousness or semiconsciousness or impaired gag reflex (may lead to aspiration of vomitus); and ingestion of petroleum products or corrosive agents such as acids or alkalis (aspiration of these chemicals is extremely harmful). If the client does not vomit within 20 min after two doses of ipecac syrup, gastric lavage is necessary; cardiotoxic effects can occur (e.g., cardiac dysrhythmias, hypotension, bradycardia, or fatal myocarditis). Other adverse effects include prolonged vomiting, diarrhea, and depression (see Chapter 41).

Activated Charcoal

Activated charcoal is prescribed for poisoning because it adsorbs ingested toxins in the gastrointestinal (GI) tract and prevents their absorption into the body. In cases of known or suspected poisoning, activated charcoal is prepared as a slurry and given orally or via a gastric tube. The dose is dependent on the amount of poison ingested; the minimum adult dose is 25 g. The pediatric dose is 1 g/kg.

Vomiting is a common adverse reaction, and the nurse should use activated charcoal with extreme caution in the client with an impaired gag reflex or altered level of consciousness because there is risk of aspiration. Activated charcoal should not be administered with milk products because they decrease its adsorptive properties. A cathartic is often ordered following administration of activated charcoal to speed elimination of the charcoal-toxin complex from the body. The client should be told that charcoal produces black stools (see Chapter 41).

Magnesium Sulfate/Magnesium Citrate

In poisoning, magnesium sulfate or citrate is given orally or via a gastric tube as a **cathartic,** an agent that speeds elimination of stool and evacuates the bowel. It is often prescribed following administration of activated charcoal, as described earlier. The typical oral dose of magnesium sulfate is 10 to 30 g administered in a glass of water. The oral dose of magnesium citrate is 100 to 300 mL. Cathartic action begins 1 to 2 h after ingestion. Cathartics are contraindicated in clients with bowel obstruction, abdominal pain, nausea, or vomiting. If the use of cathartics is prolonged, the nurse should monitor the client for dehydration and electrolyte imbalances.

Table 52–3 lists the emergency drugs for poisoning, their dosages, and indications (see Chapters 13, 41, and 47).

EMERGENCY DRUGS FOR SHOCK

Drugs may be required to elevate blood pressure and improve cardiac performance in various types of shock states. Therapeutic agents described in this section are indicated in conditions such as cardiogenic shock, neurogenic shock, septic shock, anaphylactic

Table 52–3
Emergency Drugs for Poisoning

DRUG	DOSAGE	USES AND CONSIDERATIONS
Flumazenil (Mazicon)	IV: Initial dose 0.2 mg. Additional doses every 1 minute as indicated. For re-sedation, may be repeated at 20-minute intervals to a total hourly dose of no more than 3 mg.	Reversal agent for benzodiazepine overdose; may precipitate seizures in patients with long-term use or abuse of benzodiazepines and those with seizure disorders; may precipitate emergent reactions.
Naloxone (Narcan)	IV, IM, SC: 0.4–2 mg, q 2–3 min if needed (also may be given via ETT) See Chart 52–3.	Opiate overdose; respiratory or cardiovascular depression from opiates; coma of unknown origin. *Pregnancy category:* C; PB: UK; $t_{\frac{1}{2}}$: 1–4 h (adults)
Ipecac syrup	A and C >12 y: 15–30 mL PO; can repeat in 30 min (see text for precautions) C >1 y: 15 mL PO	Emetic agent; to treat poisoning. *Pregnancy category:* C; PB: UK; $t_{\frac{1}{2}}$: UK
Activated charcoal	25–100 g PO C: 1g/kg PO	Poisoning; decreases absorption of ipecac, laxatives; onset <1 min. *Pregnancy category:* C; PB: NA; $t_{\frac{1}{2}}$: NA
Magnesium sulfate	PO: A: 10–15 g C: 2.5–10 g	Cathartic; poisoning. *Pregnancy category:* UK; PB: UK; $t_{\frac{1}{2}}$: UK
Magnesium citrate	PO: A: 100–300 mL C: 6–12 y: 30–100 mL	Cathartic; poisoning. *Pregnancy category:* UK; PB: UK; $t_{\frac{1}{2}}$: UK

KEY: ETT: endotracheal tube; IV: intravenous; NA: not applicable; PB: protein-binding; PO: by mouth; $t_{\frac{1}{2}}$: half-life; UK: unknown.

shock, and insulin shock. A noteworthy exception to the list of shock states is **hypovolemic shock** (shock resulting from loss of blood or fluid volume); drugs should not be used in an attempt to correct the hypotension associated with this condition. Administration of fluids or blood products or both is the only acceptable means to treat hypovolemic shock. These drugs are cross-referenced to the specialty chapters.

Dopamine

Dopamine (Intropin) is a sympathomimetic agent often used to treat hypotension in shock states that are *not* due to hypovolemia. Dopamine may also be used to increase heart rate (beta$_1$ effect) in bradycardic rhythms when atropine has not been effective. The dose range is 5 to 20 μg/kg/min. The actions of dopamine are dose-dependent: at low doses (1 to 2 μg/kg/min), dopamine dilates renal and mesenteric blood vessels, producing an increase in urine output (dopaminergic effect); at doses of 2 to 10 μg/kg/min, dopamine enhances cardiac output by increasing myocardial contractility and increasing heart rate (beta$_1$ effect) and elevates blood pressure through vasoconstriction (alpha-adrenergic effect). Alpha effects predominate at doses of 10 μg/kg/min and above: vasoconstriction of renal, mesenteric, and peripheral blood vessels occurs. Such vasoconstriction, although sometimes necessary to maintain adequate blood pressure in severe shock, can lead to poor organ and tissue perfusion, decreased cardiac performance, and reduction of urine output. The lowest effective dose of dopamine should be used. Clients must be weaned gradually from dopamine; abrupt discontinuation of the infusion can cause severe hypotension.

Dopamine is typically mixed as a concentration of 400 to 800 mg in 250 mL dextrose 5% in water and administered IV by a volumetric infusion pump for precision, preferably in a central vein. Continuous heart and blood pressure monitoring is essential. The nurse must carefully document vital signs and intake and output as ordered. Significant adverse effects include tachycardia, dysrhythmias, myocardial ischemia, nausea, and vomiting. The IV site must be assessed hourly for signs of drug infiltration: **extravasation** (escape into tissues) of dopamine can produce tissue necrosis that can necessitate surgical debridement and skin grafting. If extravasation occurs, the site should be injected in multiple areas with phentolamine (Regitine), 5 to 10 mg diluted in 10 to 15 mL of normal saline to reduce or prevent tissue damage (see Chapter 21). Drug data for dopamine are presented in Chart 52–4.

Dobutamine

Dobutamine (Dobutrex) is a sympathomimetic drug with beta$_1$-adrenergic activities. The beta$_1$ effects include enhancing the force of myocardial contraction (positive inotropic effect) and increasing heart rate (positive chronotropic effect). Dobutamine is indicated in shock states when improvement in cardiac output and overall cardiac performance is desired. Blood pressure is elevated only through the increase in cardiac output; dobutamine has no vasoconstriction effects and may produce a mild vasodilation. The usual IV dose range of dobutamine is 2 to 20 μg/kg/min administered via a volumetric infusion pump for precision. A typical concentration of dobutamine is 250 mg–1000 mg mixed in 250 mL of dextrose 5% in water or normal saline. Like dopamine, dobutamine administration should be tapered gradually as the client's condition warrants.

Continuous cardiac and blood pressure monitoring are required for clients receiving dobutamine infusions. Adverse effects are dose-related and include myocardial ischemia, tachycardia, dysrhythmias, headache, nausea, and tremors. The nurse must carefully monitor vital signs and intake and output and assess for any signs or symptoms of myocardial ischemia such as chest pain or development of dysrhythmias (see Chapter 21).

Norepinephrine

Norepinephrine (Levarterenol, Levophed) is a catecholamine with extremely potent vasoconstrictor actions (alpha-adrenergic effect). It is used in shock states, often when drugs such as dopamine and dobutamine have failed to produce adequate blood pressure. Like high-dose dopamine, the peripheral vasoconstriction that results has the potential to impair cardiac performance and decrease organ and tissue perfusion. In general, 4 to 8 mg of norepinephrine are added to 250 mL dextrose 5% in water or normal saline solution and infused at 2 to 12 μg/min for adults. Continuous cardiac monitoring and precise blood pressure monitoring are required. The drug must be tapered slowly; abrupt discontinuation can result in severe hypotension.

Nursing actions and considerations are the same as those for dopamine. Norepinephrine should not be used to treat hypotension in hypovolemic clients; fluid, blood, or both must be administered to restore adequate volume first. Adverse effects of norepinephrine include myocardial ischemia, dysrhythmias, and impaired organ perfusion. Extravasation of norepinephrine causes tissue necrosis; therefore, attention to the IV site is essential. If extravasation occurs, the area should be infiltrated with phentolamine, as described for dopamine (see Chapter 21).

Chart 52-4. Emergency Treatment of Shock

DOPAMINE HCl

NURSING PROCESS

Assessment and Planning

Drug Name

Dopamine HCl (Intropin)
Adrenergic
Pregnancy Category: C

Dosage

A: IV: Drip: 1–20 μg/kg/min (>10 μg/kg/min may be ordered if lower doses are ineffective)

Contraindications

Hypersensitivity, tachydysrhythmias, ventricular fibrillation, pheochromocytomas
Caution: Safety in children is not known

Drug-Lab-Food Interactions

Use within 2 wk of MAOIs may result in hypertensive crisis; concurrent IV administration of phenytoin may result in hypotension and bradycardia; sodium bicarbonate solutions inactivate dopamine—do *not* administer through the same IV line

Interventions

Pharmacokinetics

Absorption: IV
Distribution: PB: UK
Metabolism: t½: 2 min
Excretion: In urine

Pharmacodynamics

IV: Onset: 1–2 min
      Peak <5 min
      Duration: <10 min

Evaluation

Therapeutic Effects/Uses

To treat hypotension in shock states *not* caused by hypovolemia; to increase heart rate in atropine-refractory bradycardia. To increase urine output at a "renal dose" (<5 mg/kg/min).

Mode of Action: Stimulation of receptors to cause cardiac stimulation and renal vasodilation. Increase systemic vascular resistance at higher dose ranges.

Side Effects

Palpitations, tachycardia, hypertension, ectopic beats, angina, IV line site irritation, piloerection, nausea, vomiting

Adverse Reactions

Cardiac dysrhythmias, azotemia, tissue sloughing (from extravasation)
Life-threatening: MI, gangrene in extremities (from vasoconstriction)

KEY: IV: intravenous; MAOIs: monoamine oxidase inhibitors; PB: protein-binding; UK: unknown; t½: half-life; MI: myocardial infarction.

Epinephrine

Epinephrine is the drug of choice in the treatment of **anaphylactic shock,** an allergic response of the most serious type brought about by an antibody-antigen reaction. Anaphylactic shock can be fatal if prompt treatment is not initiated. Severe bronchoconstriction and hypotension resulting from cardiovascular collapse are its hallmarks. Epinephrine is also indicated for an acute, severe asthmatic attack.

Administration of epinephrine causes bronchodilation, enhanced cardiac performance, and vasoconstriction to increase blood pressure. In severe **asthma** and anaphylactic shock, epinephrine is given in a 0.2- to 0.5-mg dose range subcutaneously (SC) or intramuscularly (IM) for adults via a tuberculin syringe for accuracy (1:1000 solution). As an alternative, epinephrine can be given in a dose of 0.1 to 0.25 mg IV over 5 to 10 min (1:10,000 solution). Epinephrine administration can be repeated every 5 to 15 min if necessary.

The nurse must carefully monitor the client who receives epinephrine for tachycardia, cardiac dysrhythmias, hypertension, and angina. Clients who are given IV epinephrine must be on a cardiac monitor, with resuscitation equipment immediately available. Other adverse effects include excitability, fear, anxiety, and restlessness. In addition, the nurse should be alert to the possibility that the anaphylactic response may recur and necessitate repeated treatment. For this reason, steroids are commonly ordered and are slowly tapered over days to weeks to prevent recurrence. Examples of steroids are hydrocortisone sodium succinate, prednisone, and methylprednisolone. Client education should include strict avoidance of the agents responsible for the anaphylactic reaction and follow-up care with a physician. For some clients, such as those with severe allergic responses to bee stings, the physician may prescribe an epinephrine kit to be carried with the client for self-medication in the event of contact with the antigen. Proper client education regarding the use of the kit is essential (see Chapters 21 and 36).

Albuterol

Albuterol is a beta-adrenergic bronchodilator used to reverse bronchoconstriction in anaphylactic shock, asthma, and COPD. In emergency situations, it is administered via a nebulizer (adults: 0.5 mL of 0.5% inhalation solution in 2.5 mL saline). The nurse should assess breath sounds before and after administration; effectiveness is evidenced by relief of bronchospasm. In severe bronchospasm, wheezing may not be audible. As the bronchospasm is relieved, wheezing may become more pronounced, indicating that the drug is producing the desired therapeutic effect. Assessment of the patient's subjective feelings of respiratory distress before and after administration is especially important. Adverse effects of albuterol include tachycardia, tremor, nervousness, cardiac dysrhythmias, and hypertension.

Diphenhydramine Hydrochloride

Diphenhydramine (Benadryl), an antihistamine, is often administered with epinephrine in anaphylactic shock. This agent is effective for treating the histamine-induced tissue swelling and pruritus common to severe allergic reactions. The standard adult dose is 25 to 50 mg administered IV or deep IM. An oral form of the drug exists, but the parenteral form is preferred in emergencies. Adverse effects include drowsiness, sedation, confusion, vertigo, excitability, hypotension, tachycardia, GI disturbances, and dry mouth (see Chapter 35).

Dextrose 50%

Dextrose 50% is a concentrated, high-carbohydrate solution given to treat insulin-induced hypoglycemia or insulin shock. When insulin shock is known or suspected and the client's state of consciousness is impaired such that oral administration of sugar solutions is contraindicated, 50 mL of dextrose 50% is commonly ordered and given as an IV bolus. Dextrose 50% is highly irritating to veins and should be administered in a large peripheral or central vein whenever possible. Phlebitis can occur. Extravasation of the solution can cause tissue sloughing and necrosis. The nurse must monitor the client's blood sugar carefully; hyperglycemia is common, especially after rapid injection. Urine output should be accurately recorded, because osmotic diuresis can occur when blood sugar is elevated, and a hyperosmolar state can result. Client education must be centered on teaching about diabetes and insulin administration.

PEDIATRIC IMPLICATIONS
Glycogen stores in infants and children may be quickly depleted in stress states produced by severe illness. Because adequate amounts of glucose are essential to strong myocardial function, hypoglycemia must be corrected to provide the greatest chance for successful resuscitation. After determining that hypoglycemia is present by the finger- or heel-stick method of rapid blood glucose testing, dextrose 25% or less may be administered per physician order. Because glucose is supplied in a 50% concentration, it must be diluted 1:1 in sterile water before administration to reduce its osmolarity and prevent sclerosis of peripheral veins. The standard dose is 0.5 to 1.0 g/kg IV (see Chapter 46).

Glucagon

Glucagon is a hormone produced by the pancreas that elevates blood sugar by stimulating glycogen breakdown (glycogenolysis). Glucagon, like dextrose 50%, is indicated in the treatment of severe insulin-induced hypoglycemia or insulin shock. In an emergency when dextrose 50% is unavailable or cannot be administered intravenously, glucagon is an effective agent. Glucagon may be given subcutaneously, intramuscularly, or intravenously. The standard dose for adults and children is 0.5 to 1 mg, which can be repeated in 20 min for persistent coma. If the coma has not resolved after two doses, dextrose 50% should be administered. Adverse effects from glucagon are uncommon but can include nausea and vomiting. Glucagon can also be used as an agent to reverse the effects of beta blocker overdose. Table 52–4 lists the emergency drugs for shock, their dosages, and indications (see Chapter 46).

Table 52–4
Agents for Emergency Treatment of Shock

GENERIC (BRAND)	ROUTE AND DOSAGE	USES AND CONSIDERATIONS
Albuterol	A: nebulizer: 0.5 mL of 0.5% inhalation solution in 2.5 mL saline	Bronchoconstriction secondary to anaphylactic shock, asthma, and COPD. Tachycardia, tremor, nervousness, cardiac dysrhythmias, and hypertension
Dextrose 50%	A: IV: 50 mL C: 0.5–1.0 g/kg IV of a D 25% sol	Insulin shock; severe hypoglycemia; *Pregnancy category*: C; PB: UK; $t_{\frac{1}{2}}$: UK
Diphenhydramine (Benadryl)	IM/IV: 25–50 mg	Anaphylactic shock; acute allergic reaction. *Pregnancy category*: C; PB: 98%–99%; $t_{\frac{1}{2}}$: 3–8 h
Dobutamine (Dobutrex)	IV: Drip: 2–10 μg/kg/min	Low cardiac output. Effects anatagonized by beta blockers. *Pregnancy category*: C; PB: UK; $t_{\frac{1}{2}}$: 2 min
Dopamine HCl (Intropin)	See Chart 52–4	
Epinephrine	SC/IM: 0.2–0.5 mg (1:1000 sol) IV: 0.1–0.25 mg (1:10,000 sol) Intratracheal: 0.1 mg/kg q3–5 min	Anaphylactic shock; severe acute asthmatic attack. Hypertensive crisis with MAOIs; increased dysrhythmias with cardiac glycosides. *Pregnancy category*: C; PB: UK; $t_{\frac{1}{2}}$: UK
Glucagon	SC/IM/IV: 0.5–1 mg; may repeat × 1	Insulin shock; severe hypoglycemia; beta blocker overdose (reverses effects of beta blockers). *Pregnancy category*: B; PB: UK; $t_{\frac{1}{2}}$: 3–10 min
Norepinephrine (Levophed)	IV: Drip: 2–12 μg/min	Hypotension not responsive to other therapies. *Pregnancy category*: D; PB: UK; $t_{\frac{1}{2}}$: UK

KEY: *A: adult; IV: intravenous; IM: intramuscular; SC: subcutaneous; C: child; MAOIs: monoamine oxidase inhibitors; PB: protein-binding; $t_{\frac{1}{2}}$: half-life; UK: unknown.*

EMERGENCY DRUGS FOR HYPERTENSIVE CRISES AND PULMONARY EDEMA

A variety of pharmacologic agents may be prescribed to treat hypertensive crisis, generally defined as a diastolic blood pressure that exceeds 110 to 120 mmHg, and pulmonary edema. Three of the most commonly prescribed drugs are discussed in this section. The drugs are cross-referenced to the specialty chapter.

Sodium Nitroprusside

Sodium nitroprusside (Nipride) is an intravenous agent used to reduce arterial blood pressure in hypertensive emergencies. The mechanism of action is immediate direct arterial and venous vasodilation. Antihypertensive effects end when sodium nitroprusside is discontinued; blood pressure increases as soon as drug administration is stopped. Continuous and accurate blood pressure measurement is required. In general, 50 mg of sodium nitroprusside is mixed in 250 mL dextrose 5% in water. The average dose range for adults and children is 0.5 to 8 μg/kg/min.

There are several important nursing considerations:

1. Sodium nitroprusside is rapidly inactivated by light; the IV bottle or bag must be wrapped with aluminum foil or another opaque material to protect the solution from degradation.

2. Although a faint brown tint is typical, blue or brown discoloration of the solution indicates degradation and necessitates that the solution be discarded.

3. When sodium nitroprusside therapy is prolonged, clients are at risk for toxicity resulting from elevated serum thiocyanate or cyanide levels (byproducts of drug metabolism). Signs and symptoms include metabolic acidosis, profound hypotension, dizziness, and vomiting. Serum thiocyanate levels should be monitored at least every 24 hours for clients receiving prolonged infusions of more than 3 μg/kg/min. Clients with renal insufficiency or failure are at a higher risk because the metabolites are excreted in the urine.

4. Clients should be placed on an oral antihyper-

Chart 52–5. Emergency Treatment of Hypertensive Crisis

SODIUM NITROPRUSSIDE

Drug Name

Sodium Nitroprusside (Nipride)
Pregnancy Category: C

Dosage

A: IV: Drip 0.5–8 µg/kg/min; begin at 0.1 mg/kg/min and titrate to desired effect up to 10 µg/kg/min

Contraindications

Hypersensitivity, hypertension (compensatory), decreased cerebral perfusion, coarctation of aorta
Caution: Increased intracranial pressure

Drug-Lab-Food Interactions

Antihypertensives, general anesthetics
Do not mix with any other drug in syringe or solution
Lab: Decrease in PCO_2, pH

Pharmacokinetics

Absorption: IV only
Distribution: PB: UK
Metabolism: $t\frac{1}{2}$: <10 min
Excretion: In urine

Pharmacodynamics

IV: Onset: 1–2 min
      Peak: Rapid
      Duration: 1–10 min

Therapeutic Effects/Uses

To treat hypertensive crisis; to produce controlled hypotension to reduce surgical bleeding; and to decrease systemic vascular resistance to improve cardiac performance.

Mode of Action: Stimulation of smooth muscle of veins and arteries; produces peripheral vasodilation.

Side Effects

Dizziness, headache, nausea, abdominal pain, sweating, palpitations, weakness, vomiting

Adverse Reactions

Thiocyanate toxicity: tinnitus, dyspnea, blurred vision, metabolic acidosis
Life-threatening: Severe hypotension, loss of consciousness, profound cardiovascular depression

Assessment and Planning
Interventions
Evaluation

NURSING PROCESS

KEY: IV: intravenous; PCO_2: partial pressure of carbon dioxide; PB: protein-binding; UK: unknown; $t\frac{1}{2}$: half-life.

tensive agent as soon as possible so that sodium nitroprusside can be tapered slowly (see Chapters 38 and 39). Drug data for sodium nitroprusside are presented in Chart 52–5.

Furosemide

Furosemide (Lasix) is classified as a loop diuretic that acts by inhibiting sodium and chloride reabsorption from the ascending loop of Henle. It promotes the renal excretion of water, sodium, chloride, magnesium, hydrogen, and calcium, and has a potassium-depleting effect. Furosemide also has peripheral and renal vasodilating effects that can lower blood pres-

sure. The main indications for use of furosemide as an emergency drug are acute pulmonary edema from left ventricular dysfunction and hypertensive crisis.

Furosemide is given as an initial bolus of 20 to 40 mg IV over 1 to 2 min. For clients who take furosemide on a regular basis, the effective dose may be much higher (up to 2 mg/kg). The vasodilatory effects occur *before* diuresis begins and act to lower blood pressure. Central venous pressure is reduced through a decrease in venous return to the heart from venodilation. Diuresis should start within 10 minutes of drug administration and may continue for approximately 6 h.

The most significant adverse effects are severe hypovolemia, dehydration, and electrolyte disturbances (hypokalemia, hypomagnesemia, hyponatremia, and hypochloremia). Patients on digitalis preparations are at an increased risk of digitalis toxicity from hypokalemia. The client's fluid and electrolyte status must be carefully assessed before and after furosemide administration, including auscultation of breath sounds for rales, strict surveillance of intake and output, and review of laboratory data when available. Electrolyte and careful fluid replacement may be required during furosemide therapy to prevent physiologic consequences. The nurse must also exercise caution in administering the drug to clients with sulfonamide

sensitivity because furosemide is a sulfonamide derivative and can produce an allergic reaction.

Morphine Sulfate

Like furosemide, morphine sulfate is also indicated for acute pulmonary edema because it produces venous vasodilation which decreases cardiac **preload** (the amount of blood returning to the right ventricle). The net effect is a decrease in pulmonary venous congestion. Morphine has been discussed previously in this chapter. Table 52–5 lists the emergency drugs for hypertensive crises and pulmonary edema, their dosages and considerations.

Table 52–5
Emergency Drugs for Hypertensive Crises and Pulmonary Edema

GENERIC (BRAND)	ROUTE AND DOSAGE	USES AND CONSIDERATIONS
Sodium nitroprusside (Nipride)	Refer to Chart 52–5.	
Furosemide (Lasix)	IV: initial bolus of 20–40 mg over 1–2 min, up to 2 mg/kg.	Acute pulmonary edema from left ventricular dysfunction; hypertensive crisis. *Adverse effects:* hypovolemia, dehydration, electrolyte disturbances
Morphine	IV: 1–3 mg q5–30 min	Pulmonary edema, chest pain, unstable angina, MI

KEY: IV: intravenous; MI: myocardial infarction.

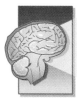

Critical Thinking in Action

J. S. is a 23-year-old male who was assaulted during a gang fight 1 h ago. He was stabbed in the back and suffered blows to the head with a baseball bat. The knife penetrated the spinal cord at the T4 level. At this time, J. S. opens his eyes spontaneously, is agitated, and does not follow commands. He moans and localizes to pain with his upper extremities only. His lower extremities exhibit no movement. His admitting diagnoses include penetrating spinal cord injury with paraplegia at the T4 level and a closed head injury with cerebral edema diagnosed by computed tomography (CT) scan at the trauma center.

J. S. is known to be an HIV-positive heroin addict. He also abuses oral Valium and other street drugs. His current vital signs are BP 88/56, HR 56, RR 24, temp 36°C. He has two functional IV catheters (one peripheral line in the right forearm and one central line in the left femoral vein), an oral gastric tube in place, and an indwelling urinary catheter.

1. On arrival to the trauma center, should J. S. have received supplemental oxygen based on his mechanism of injury? What type of oxygen device would be appropriate for J. S. upon initial presentation?
2. The physician orders 50 g of mannitol to be given now, IV push. On hand you have several 50-mL vials of "mannitol, 25%" solution. How many milliliters of mannitol will you need to draw up in the syringe to administer 50 g?

3. Describe the type of needle that must be used when administering mannitol and why. What size syringe should be used? Which IV line should be used to administer the mannitol to J. S.?

4. Based on the case study, what are the indications for mannitol administration? List at least three nursing considerations when giving mannitol.

5. J. S. has a T4 spinal cord injury with paralysis. Should methylprednisolone be administered within 8 h of injury in his case? Why or why not?

6. J. S. has a history of heroin and Valium abuse. List the reversal agents that could be used if the trauma team believes recent illicit drug use may be a contributing factor to his altered mental state. Would Ipecac syrup be indicated? Why or why not?

7. Because of J. S.'s spinal cord injury, he is exhibiting signs of neurogenic shock: bradycardia, warm skin, hypotension. What is the drug of choice that the nurse should keep at the bedside in case J. S. requires emergency treatment for symptomatic bradycardia? Name the drug, its mechanism of action, and dosing considerations.

8. The physician orders a dopamine infusion, 800 mg/250 mL D$_5$W, to be titrated to maintain systolic BP > 110 mmHg. Which IV site would be the best choice for a continuous dopamine infusion in J. S.? What is the consequence of dopamine extravasation? What is the treatment for dopamine extravasation?

9. What vital sign parameters must be monitored while J. S. receives dopamine? Name at least four adverse effects of dopamine.

Antibiotics are initiated to address the potential for infection in J. S.'s stab wound because it communicates with his spinal cord. Upon infusion of the antibiotic, a body-wide rash, swelling of the lips and tongue, wheezing, and hypotension develop.

10. What is happening to J. S.?

11. What are the drugs of choice to treat J. S.'s condition now?

12. How can the nurse evaluate the effectiveness of these drugs?

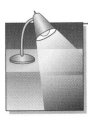

Study Questions

1. What is the minimum dose of atropine that should be given to an adult with bradycardia?

2. Explain the actions of epinephrine and diphenhydramine for clients in anaphylactic shock? How are these drugs administered in this situation?

3. What are the signs and symptoms of lidocaine toxicity?

4. List common adverse effects of bretylium.

5. What guidelines should be followed when administering ipecac syrup? What client and family educational points should be emphasized?

6. Why are activated charcoal and magnesium sulfate given for poisoning? List the actions of each.

7. In what poisoning situations should vomiting *not* be induced?

8. Compare and contrast dextrose 50% and glucagon.

9. For what class of drug overdose is naloxone effective? What important precautions must be taken?

10. Describe the protocol for administering methylprednisolone to a client with an acute spinal cord injury. Would you expect the drug to produce a noticeable effect immediately?

11. What are the emergency indications for mannitol in the neurosurgical setting? Describe pertinent nursing considerations for its administration.

12. List the adverse effects of isoproterenol and the pertinent nursing considerations and actions.

13. List the end points of procainamide administration.

14. What is the antidote for extravasation of both norepinephrine and dopamine? How should it be administered?

15. List the signs and symptoms of thiocyanate toxicity in clients receiving sodium nitroprusside.

16. Explain how dobutamine increases blood pressure as compared with dopamine.

17. Describe the dose-dependent effects of dopamine.

18. List relevant nursing considerations and actions when administering verapamil.

19. Discuss indications for adenosine. What are pertinent nursing considerations when administering adenosine?

20. Compare and contrast intravenous diltiazem and verapamil.

21. What is the maximum total adult dose of intravenous atropine for the treatment of bradycardia? Why will additional doses of atropine be ineffective?

22. List at least three contraindications to methylprednisolone administration in acute spinal cord injury.

23. What are the relevant nursing considerations when administering sodium nitroprusside?

24. After administering the initial dose of adenosine, the nurse observes a short period of asystole. Does this represent an adverse drug effect?

25. Describe how to administer sublingual nitroglycerin tablets to the client experiencing chest pain.

26. What teaching points should be emphasized when a client is discharged to home with a prescription for sublingual nitroglycerin?

27. Name the drug that is indicated to reverse significant respiratory depressant effects of morphine sulfate.

28. What is the typical dose range of intravenous morphine?

29. Describe how to dilute a 50% dextrose solution for safe administration to pediatric clients.

30. Name the reversal agent for benzodiazepine overdose and describe two key nursing considerations when administering this drug.

31. List the uses and indications for magnesium sulfate as they relate to clients with cardiac disorders.

32. Describe the mechanism of action for furosemide (Lasix) in relation to pulmonary edema and hypertensive crisis.

33. Name the drug of choice for hypoxemia.

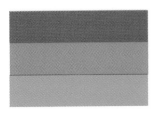

Generic Drugs with Corresponding Canadian Trade Drug Names*

GENERIC DRUG NAMES	CANADIAN TRADE/BRAND NAMES
Acebutolol	Monitan
Acetaminophen	Abenol, Atasol, Campain, Exdol, Robigesic, Rounox
Acetazolamide	Acetazolam, Apo-Acetazolamide
Acetohexamide	Dimelor
Acetylcysteine	Airbron
Albuterol	Novosalmol, Salbutamol
Allopurinol	Alloprin, Apo-Allopurinol, Novopurinol, Purinol
Aminophylline	Gorophyllin, Paladron
Aminosalicylate sodium	Parasal Sodium
Amitriptyline hydrochloride	Apo-Amitriptyline, Levate, Meravil, Novotriptyn, Rolavil
Amoxicillin	Apo-Amoxi, Amoxican
Amoxicillin clavulanate K	Clavulin
Ampicillin	Ampilean, Novo-Ampicillin, Penbritin
Ascorbic acid	Apo-C, Ce-Vi-Sol, Redoxon
Asparaginase	Kidrolase
Aspirin	Ancasal, Astrin, Entrophen, Novasen, Supasa, Triaphen-10
Atenolol	Apo-Atenolol
Atropine sulfate	Atropair
Bacampicillin hydrochloride	Penglobe
Benzalkonium chloride	Pharmatex
Benztropine mesylate	Apo-Benzotropine, Bensylate, PMS Benzotropine
Betamethasone	Beban, Betaderm, Betanelan, Betnesol, Betnovate, Celestoderm, Novobetamet
Bisacodyl	Apo-Bisacodyl, Bisco-Lax, Laxit
Bretylium tosylate	Bretylate
Carbamazepine	Apo-Carbamazepine, Mazepine, PMS Carbamazepine
Carbenicillin disodium	Pyopen
Cephalexin	Ceporex, Novolexin
Cephalothin sodium	Ceporacin
Chloral hydrate	Novochlorhydrate
Chloramphenicol	Novochorocap, Pentamycetin
Chlordiazepoxide hydrocholoride	Medilium, Novopoxide, Solium
Chlorphenesin carbamate	Mycil
Chlorpheniramine maleate	Chlor-Tripolon, Novopheniram
Chlorpromazine hydrochloride	Chlorpromanyl, Largactil, Novochlorpromazine
Chlorpropamide	Apo-Chlorpropamide, Chloronase, Novopropamide
Chlorprothixene	Tarasan
Chlorthalidone	Novothalidone, Uridon
Cimetidine	Novocimetine, Peptol
Cisplatin	Abiplatin
Clindamycin	Dalacin-C
Clofibrate	Claripen, Claripex, Novofibrate

Clonazepam	Rivotril
Clonidine hydrochloride	Dixarit
Clorazepate dipotassium	Novoclopate
Clotrimazole	Canesten
Cloxacillin sodium	Apo-Cloxi, Bactopen, Novocloxin, Orbenin
Codeine phosphate	Paveral
Colchicine	Novocolchine
Colestipol hydrochloride	Cholestabyl, Lestid
Co-trimoxazole	Apo-Sulfatrim
Cromolyn sodium	Fivent, Intal p, Rynacrom, Vistacrom
Cyanocobalamin	Anacobin, Bedoz, Cyanabin, Rubion
Cyclizine hydrochloride	Marzine
Cyclophosphamide	Procytox
Cyproheptadine hydrochloride	Vimicon
Danazol	Cyclomen
Dapsone	Avlosulfon
Dexamethasone	Deronil, Dexasone, Oradexon, Stress-Pam
Dextromethorphan	Balminil DM, Koffex, Ornex DM, Robidex, Sedatuss
Diazepam	Apo-Diazepam, Diazemuls, E-Pam, Meval, Novodipam, Vivol
Dicyclomine hydrochloride	Bentylol, Formulex, Lomine, Protylol, Viscerol
Diethylpropion hydrochloride	Nobesine
Diethylstilbestrol	Honval, Stilboestrol
Digitoxin	Digitaline, Purodigin
Dimenhydrinate	Apo-Dimenhydrinate, Gravol, Nauseatol, Novodimenate, Travamine
Dinoprostone	Prepidil Gel
Diphenhydramine hydrochloride	Allerdryl
Dipyridamole	Apo-Dipyridamole
Disopyramide	Rythmodan
Docusate sodium	Regulax
Dopamine hydrochloride	Revimine
Doxepin hydrochloride	Triadapin
Doxycycline hyclate	Doryx, Doxycin, Novodoxylin
Dyphylline	Protophylline
Econazole nitrate	Ecostatin
Epinephrine hydrochloride	SusPhrine, Eppy
Epinephrine racemic	Vaponefrin
Ergocalciferol	Ostoforte, Radiostol
Ergotamine tartrate	Gynergen
Erythromycin	Apo-Erythro Base, Erythromid, Novorythro, Ro-Mycin
Estradiol	Delestrogen
Estrogen, conjugated	C.E.S.
Estrogen, esterified	Climestrone, Neo-Estrone
Estrone	Femogen Forte
Ethambutol hydrochloride	Etibi
Ethopropazine hydrochloride	Parsitan
Fenfluramine hydrochloride	Ponderal
Ferrous fumarate	Neo-Fer-50, Novofumar, Palafer
Ferrous gluconate	Fertinic, Novoferrogulc
Ferrous sulfate	Novoferrosulfa
Flucytosine	Ancotil
Fluocinolone acetonide	Fluoderm
Fluocinonide	Lidemol, Lyderm, Topsyn
Fluoxymesterone	Ora T Estryl
Fluphenazine decanoate	Decanoate
Fluphenazine enanthate	Enanthate
Fluphenazine hydrochloride	Moditen HCl
Flurandrenolide	Drenison
Flurazepam	Apo-Flurazepam, Novoflupam, Somnol
Folic acid	Apo-Folic, Novofolacid
Furosemide	Fumide, Furomide, Luramide, Uritol
Gentamicin sulfate	Alcomicin, Cidomycin, Novosemide
Glyburide	DiaBeta, Euglucon
Griseofulvin, microsize	Grisovin-FP
Guaifenesin	Balminil, Resyl
Guanethidine sulfate	Apo-Guanethidine

Haloperidol	Haldol LA, Peridol
Heparin calcium	Calcilean, Calciparine
Heparin sodium	Hepalean
Hydrochlorothiazide	Apo-Hydro, Hydrozide, Neo-Codema, Urozide
Hydrocodone bitartrate	Hycodan, Robidone
Hydrocortisone	Cortamed, Cortiment, Rectocort
Hydroxocobalamin	Acti-B_{12}
Ibuprofen	Amersol
Imipramine hydrochloride	Impril, Novopramine
Indapamide	Lozide
Indomethacin	Indocid
Iodoquinol	Diodoquin
Isoniazid (INH)	Isotamine
Isosorbide dinitrate	Coronex, Novosorbide
Kaolin/pectin	Donnagel-MB, Kao-Con
Ketoprofen	Rhodis, Orudis E
Lactulose	Lactulax
Levothyroxine sodium (T_4)	Eltroxin
Lidocaine hydrochloride	Xylocard
Lithium carbonate	Carbolith, Duralith, Lithizine
Lorazepam	Apo-Lorazepam, Novolorazepam
Loxapine hydrochloride	Loxapac
Magaldrate	Antiflux
Meclizine hydrochloride	Bonamine
Mefenamic acid	Ponstan
Meperidine hydrochloride	Pethadol, Pethidine Hydrochloride
Meprobamate	Apo-Meprobamate, Novomepro
Mesalamine	Salofalk
Methohexital	Brietal
Methotrimeprazine	Nozinan
Methylclothiazide	Duretic
Methyldopa	Apo-Methyldopa, Dopamet, Novomedopa
Methyltestosterone	Metadren
Metoclopramide	Maxeran
Metoprolol	Apo-Metoprolol, Betaloc, Novometoprol
Metronidazole	Neo-Metric, Novonidazol, PMS Metronidazole
Miconazole	Monistat
Mineral oil	Kondremul, Lansoyl
Morphine sulfate	Epimorph, Statex
Naphazoline	Vasocon
Naproxen	Apo-Naproxen, Naxen, Novonaprox
Niacin (vitamin B_3, nicotinic acid)	Novo-Niacin, Tri-B3
Nifedipine	Adalat P.A., Apo-Nifed, Novo-Nifedin
Nitrofurantoin	Apo-Nitrofurantoin, Nephronex, Novofuran
Norethindrone acetate	Aygestin, Norlutate
Nylidrin hydrochloride	Arlidin Forte, PMS Nylidrin
Nystatin	Nadostine, Nyaderm
Omeprazole	Losec
Oxazepam	Ox-Pam, Zapex, Apo-Oxazepam, Novoxapam
Oxtriphylline	Apo-Oxtriphylline, Novotriphyl
Oxycodone	Supeudol
Oxymetazoline hydrochloride	Nafrine
Oxymetholone	Anapolon
Penicillin G potassium	Megacillin, NovoPen-G, P-50, Crystapen
Penicillin G procaine	Ayercillin
Penicillin G sodium	Crystapen
Penicillin V	Apo-Pen-VK, Nadopen-V, Novopen-VK
Pentamidine isethionate	Pentacarinat
Pentobarbital	Novopentobarb
Perphenazine	Apo-Perphenazine, Phenazine
Phenazopyridine	Phenazo, Pyronium
Phenazopyridine hydrochloride	Phenazo, Pyronium
Phentolamine mesylate	Rogitine
Phenylephrine, ophthalmic	Minims Phenylephrine
Pilocarpine hydrochloride	Pilocarpine, Milocarpine

Piroxicam	Apo-Piroxicant
Potassium chloride	Apo-K, Kalium Durules, Klong, Novolente K, Roychlor 10% and 20%, Slo-Pot
Potassium gluconate	Potassium Rougier, Royonate
Potassium iodide	Thyro-Block
Pramoxine hydrochloride	Tronothane
Prednisone	Apo-Prednisone, Winpred
Primidone	Apo-Primidone, Sertan
Probenecid	Benuryl
Procarbazine hydrochloride	Natulan
Prochlorperazine maleate	Stemetil
Procyclidine hydrochloride	Procyclid
Progesterone	Progestilin
Promethazine hydrochloride	Histantil
Propantheline bromide	Propanthel
Propoxyphene hydrochloride	642, Novopropoxyn
Propranolol hydrochloride	Apo-Propranolol, Detensol, Novopranol
Propylthiouracil (PTU)	Propyl-Thyracil
Protriptyline hydrochloride	Triptil
Pseudoephedrine hydrochloride	Eltor, Eltor 120, Pseudofrin, Robidrine
Psyllium hydrophilic mucilloid	Karasil
Pyrantel pamoate	Combantrin
Pyrazinamide	Tebrazid, PMS Pyrazinamide
Pyridostigmine	Mestinon, Regonol
Quinidine sulfate	APO-Quinidine, Novoquinidin
Quinine sulfate	Novoquinine
Reserpine	Novoreserpine, Reserfia
Rifampin	Rofact
Scopolamine	Transderm-V
Secobarbital	Novosecobarb
Silver sulfadiazine	Flamazine
Simethicone	Ovol
Sodium fluoride	Fluor-A-Day
Sotalol	Sotacor
Spironolactone	Novospiroton, Sincomen
Sucralfate	Sulcrate
Sulfasalazine	PMS Sulfasalazine, Salazopyrin, SAS-Enema, SAS Enteric-500, S.A.S.-500
Sulfinpyrazone	Antazone, Anturan, Apo-Sulfinpyrazone, Novopyrazone
Sulfisoxazole	Novosoxazole
Tamoxifen citrate	Nolvadex-D, Tamofen
Testosterone	Malogen
Testosterone enanthate	Malogex
Testosterone propionate	Malogen in oil
Tetracycline hydrochloride	Novotetra, Apo-Tetra, Tetralean
Theophylline	PMS Theophylline, Pulmophylline, Somophyllin-12
Thiamine HCl (vitamin B_1)	Bewon, Betaxin
Thioguanine (TG, 6-thioguanine)	Lanvis
Thioridazine hydrochloride	Novoridazine
Timolol maleate	Apo-Timol
Tolbutamide	Mobenol, Novobutamide
Tolnaftate	Pitrex
Trifluoperazine hydrochloride	Novoflurazine, Solazine, Terfluzine
Trihexyphenidyl hydrochloride	Aparkane, Apo-Trihex, Novohexidyl
Trimeprazine tartrate	Panectyl
Tripelennamine hydrochloride	Pyribenzamine
Valproic acid (divalproex sodium, sodium valproate)	Epival
Vinblastine sulfate	Velbe
Warfarin sodium	Warfilone

*Many of the trade or brand names are used in both the United States and Canada. This appendix lists selected trade or brand names that are specific to Canada.

Recommended Daily Allowances for Vitamins and Minerals During Pregnancy

NUTRIENT	RDA FOR PREGNANCY	USES AND CONSIDERATIONS
FAT-SOLUBLE VITAMINS		
A	4000 IU	Excessive intake can cause fetal bone malformations, cleft palate, renal anomalies, and eye/ear anomalies if above 10,000 IU/d. Toxic level in mother can result in liver damage RDA same as for nonpregnant state. Due to high toxicity potential, client should take only when prescribed during first trimester for a specifically identified deficiency. Check multivitamin bottle that vitamin A levels do not exceed 5000 IU.
D	10 μg/d	Excessive maternal amounts can yield excessive calcium levels in the fetus and cause cardiac defects (aortic stenosis). Avoid intake >25 μg/d due to toxic effects. Deficiency can affect fetal bone density and dental enamel and can cause neonatal hypocalcemia. Consider use in complete vegetarians, non-vitamin D fortified milk drinkers, those in northern latitudes in winter, and those with minimal sunlight exposure.
E	10 mg alpha-TE	Dietary sources should suffice; adequate amounts found in human milk (cow's milk level lower) for newborn.
WATER-SOLUBLE VITAMINS		
C	70 mg/d	The need for ascorbic acid is increased in pregnancy; however, dietary sources should suffice if the diet is nutritious and C-foods are available to help in the formation of collagen and are cooked in only small amounts of water to only a crisp-tender state, not held too long, and not reheated. Maternal plasma levels of this vitamin at term are twice as low as midway through pregnancy due to placental concentration of the vitamin with elevated fetal levels as an outcome. Deficiency can include premature rupture of fetal membranes and PIH. Excessive maternal intake may manifest in the neonate as a rebound form of scurvy with muscle weakness, capillary hemorrhage, and progressive demise. Neonates fed mainly cow's milk are at higher risk of vitamin C deficiency.

B$_1$ (thiamine)	1.5 mg/d	Requirement increased in pregnancy proportional to caloric increases needed for energy metabolism. Serves as a coenzyme. Deficiency can result in congenital beriberi, but no adverse effects have been associated with excess intake.
B$_2$ (riboflavin)	1.6 mg/d	Increased need during pregnancy proportional to caloric increases needed for both energy and protein metabolism. Deficiency can result in fissuring and dry scaling of the lips and corners of the mouth, dermatitis, skin changes in the genital areas, and anemias. No effects have been associated with excess intake.
B$_6$ (pyridoxine)	2.2 mg/d	Increased need during pregnancy proportional to protein intake. Serves as a coenzyme in amino acid metabolism; dietary sources should be adequate. Deficiency has been associated with seizures, dermatitis, and anemia. Excess consumption has been associated with gait disturbances and sensory neuropathy. Prior to pregnancy, oral contraceptive users may have lower storage levels of this vitamin.
B$_{12}$ (cobalamin)	2.2 μg/d	Deficiency rarely found in childbearing-age women. Serves as a coenzyme in protein metabolism, especially red blood cell formation. Deficiency most likely to be found in complete vegetarians; otherwise, dietary sources should be adequate. Inability to absorb vitamin results in pernicious anemia, with some women experiencing infertility as an outcome. Excess consumption not associated with negative pregnancy outcome.
Niacin	17 mg/d	Serves as a coenzyme in metabolism. Need known to increase slightly in pregnancy although little is known; dietary sources should be adequate.

MINERALS

Calcium	1200 mg/d	Increased need exists during pregnancy due to fetal skeleton mineralization, especially during the third trimester. Important for women under age 25 whose daily calcium intake is less than 600 mg. No evidence that pregnant women older than 35 years of age need special supplements of calcium. If maternal deficiency, fetal needs will be met through maternal bone demineralization. Deficiency may be related to PIH, while excesses two times or more above the pregnancy RDA may be associated with constipation and kidney stone development. Should be taken at mealtime to augment absorption and diminish interaction with iron supplements.
Phosphorus	1200 mg/d	Need increases during pregnancy but must be kept in ratio with calcium. If excessive intake from snack foods, cola drinks, processed meats, calcium absorption may be altered especially in presence of inadequate amounts of vitamin D and magnesium.
Magnesium	320 mg/d	Little known about this mineral in pregnancy except that it has a relationship to calcium and potassium levels and serves as a coenzyme in energy and protein metabolism.
Zinc	15 mg/d	Need increased in pregnancy especially for complete vegetarians and pregnant diabetics (due to altered zinc metabolism). Women with a specific zinc metabolism disorder causing severe deficiency may have high fetal mortality or malformations. Excessive intake may be related to prematurity and/or stillbirth. If iron supplementation is given above 30 mg/d for anemia, zinc supplementation is recommended due to interference with zinc absorption.

KEY: PIH: pregnancy-induced hypertension; >: greater than.
References: Brodsky, A. (1991). Nutrition and diet counseling. In Cohen, S. M., Kenner, C. A., and Hollingsworth, A. O., Maternal neonatal and women's health nursing (pp 451–479). Springhouse, PA: Springhouse Corp. Moore, M. C. (1991). Maternal and fetal nutrition. In Bobak, I. M., and Jensen, M. O., Essentials of maternity nursing (3rd ed) (pp 290–313). St. Louis: Mosby–Year Book, Inc. Martin, L. L., and Reeder, S. J. (1991): Essentials of Maternity Nursing (Chapter 9, Nutrition and Pregnancy, pp 172–203). Philadelphia: J. B. Lippincott Co.

Appendix C
Laboratory Tests Related to Drug Use

Test	Reference Values	
	ADULT	**CHILD**
Hematocrit (Hct)	Male: 40–54%; 0.40–0.54 SI units Female: 36–46%; 0.36–0.46 SI units	Newborn: 44–65%; 1–3 y old: 29–40%; 4–10 y old: 31–43%
Hemoglobin (Hb, Hgb)	Male: 13.5–18 g/dL Female: 12–16 g/dL	Newborn: 14–24 g/dL Infant: 10–15 g/dL Child: 11–16 g/dL
Red blood cells (RBCs)	Male: 4.6–6 mil/μL Female: 4–6 mil/μL	Newborn: 4.8–7.2 mil/μL Child: 3.8–5.5 mil/μL
RBC indices		
MCV	80–98 cu μ	Newborn: 98–108 cu μ Child: 82–92 cu μ
MCH	27–31 pg	Newborn: 32–34 pg Child: 27–31 pg
MCHC	32–36%	Newborn: 32–33% Child: 32–36%
RDW	11.5–14.5 Coulter S	
White blood cells (WBCs)	4500–10,000 μL	Newborn: 9000–30,000 μL 2 y old: 6000–17,000 μL
WBC differentials		
Neutrophils	50–70% of total WBCs	29–47%
Segments	50–65%	
Bands	0–5%	
Eosinophils	0–3%	0–3%
Basophils	1–3%	1–3%
Lymphocytes	25–35%	38–63%
Monocytes	2–6%	4–9%
Platelets	150,000–400,000 μL 0.15–0.4 $\times$ 10^{12}/L	Premature: 100,000–300,000 μL Newborn: 150,000–300,000 μL Infant: 200,000–475,000 μL Child: same as adult

KEY: *MCV: mean corpuscular volume; MCH: mean corpuscular hemoglobin; MCHC: mean corpuscular hemoglobin concentration; RDW: RBC distribution width.*

ELECTROLYTES

Electrolyte	Reference Values	
	ADULT	CHILD
Sodium (Na)	135–145 mEq/L 135–145 mmol/L (SI units)	Infant: 134–150 mEq/L Child: 135–145 mEq/L
Potassium (K)	3.5–5.3 mEq/L 3.5–5.3 mmol/L (SI units)	Infant: 3.6–5.8 mEq/L Child: 3.5–5.5 mEq/L
Calcium (Ca)	4.5–5.5 mEq/L or 9–11 mg/dL 2.3–2.8 mmol/L (SI units)	Newborn: 3.7–7 mEq/L or 7.4–14 mg/dL Infant: 5–6 mEq/L or 10–12 mg/dL Child: 4.5–5.8 mEq/L or 9–11.5 mg/dL
Ionized calcium (iCa)	2.2–2.5 mEq/L 4.25–5.25 mg/dL 1.1–1.24 mmol/L (SI units)	
Magnesium (Mg)	1.5–2.5 mEq/L 1.8–3.0 mg/dL	Newborn: 1.4–2.9 mEq/L Child: 1.6–2.6 mEq/L
Chloride (Cl)	95–105 mEq/L 95–105 mmol/L (SI units)	Newborn: 94–112 mEq/L Infant: 95–110 mEq/L Child: 98–105 mEq/L
Phosphorus (P) (Phosphate)	1.7–2.6 mEq/L or 2.5–4.5 mg/dL 0.78–1.52 mmol/L (SI units)	Newborn: 3.5–8.6 mg/dL Infant: 4.5–6.7 mg/dL Child: 4.5–5.5 mg/dL
Carbon dioxide (CO_2)	22–30 mEq/L	20–28 mEq/L

CARDIAC PROFILE

Test	Reference Values	
	ADULT	CHILD
Aspartate aminotransferase (AST, SGOT)	8–38 U/L (average range) 5–40 U/mL (Frankel) 4–36 IU/L 16–60 U/mL at 30°C 8–33 U/L at 37°C (SI units)	Newborn: 4 × adult level Child: same as adult
Creatine phosphokinase (CPK)	Male: 5–35 μg/mL, 30–180 IU/L, 55–170 U/L at 37°C (SI units) Female: 5–25 μg/mL, 25–150 IU/L, 30–135 U/L at 37°C (SI units)	Newborn: 65–580 IU/L at 30°C Male: 0–70 IU/L at 30°C Female: 0–50 IU/L at 30°C
CPK isoenzyme	CPK-MB: 0–6%	
Lactic dehydrogenase (LD, LDH)	100–190 IU/L, 70–250 U/L	Newborn: 300–1500 IU/L Child: 50–150 IU/L
LDH isoenzymes	LDH_1 14–26% LDH_2 27–37%	
Potassium (K)	3.5–5.3 mEq/L	*see* Electrolytes

KEY: CPK-MB: cardiac isoenzyme.

CORONARY (LIPOPROTEINS) PROFILE

| Test | Reference Values | |
	ADULT	CHILD
Lipids (total)	400–800 mg/dL 4–8 g/L (SI units)	
LDL	60–160 mg/dL, Low risk for CHD: <130 mg/dL	
HDL	29–77 mg/dL, Low risk for CHD: 46–59 mg/dL Very low risk for CHD: >60 mg/dL	

Cholesterol	Desirable: <200 mg/dL
	Moderate risk: 200–240 mg/dL
	High risk: >240 mg/dL
	Pregnancy: high risk but returns to normal
		Infant: 90–130 mg/dL
		2–19 y old:
		    Desirable: 130–170 mg/dL
		    Moderate risk: 171–184 mg/dL
		    High risk: >185 mg/dL

Triglycerides	12–29 y old: 10–140 mg/dL 30–39 y old: 20–150 mg/dL 40–49 y old: 30–160 mg/dL >50 y old: 40–190 mg/dL	Infant: 5–40 mg/dL 5–11 y old: 10–135 mg/dL
Phospholipids	150–380 mg/dL	
Glucose (fasting blood sugar)	Serum: 70–110 mg/dL Blood: 60–100 mg/dL	Newborn: 30–80 mg/dL Child: 60–100 mg/dL

KEY: LDL: low-density lipoproteins; HDL: high-density lipoproteins; CHD: coronary heart disease.

HEPATIC PROFILE

Test	Reference Values	
	ADULT	CHILD
Alkaline phosphatase (ALP)	42–136 U/L	Infant and Child <13 y: 40–115 U/L
ALP$_1$ isoenzyme	20–130 U/L	Older child 13–18 y: 50–230 U/L
Alanine aminotransferase (ALT/SGPT)	10–35 U/L; 4–36 U/L @ 37°C (SI units)	Infant: may be twice as high as adult Child: same as adult
Gamma-glutamyltransferase (GGT)	Male: 4–23 IU/L; 9-69 U/L @ 37°C (SI units) Female: 3–13 IU/L; 4–33 U/L @ 37°C (SI units) Values may differ among institutions	
International normalized ratio (INR)	2.0–3.0	
Lactic dehydrogenase (LDH/LD)	100–190 IU/L; 70–250 U/L	Newborn: 300–1500 IU/L Child: 50–150 IU/L

LDH isoenzymes
  LDH$_4$
  LDH$_5$
	
	8–16%
	6–16%	

Leucine aminopeptidase (LAP)	8–22 mU/mL, 12–33 IU/L	
5'Nucleotidase (5'NT)	<17 U/L	
Albumin	3.5–5 g/dL	
Protein	6–8 g/dL	Premature: 4.2–7.6 g/dL Newborn: 4.6–7.4 g/dL Infant: 6–6.7 g/dL Child: 6.2–8 g/dL
Bilirubin Total	 0.1–1.2 mg/dL; 1.7–20.5 μmol/L (SI units)	 Total, newborn: 1–12 mg/dL, 17.1–205 μmol/L (SI units) Total, child: 0.2–0.8 mg/dL
Direct	0.1–0.3 mg/dL 1.7–5.1 μmol/L (SI units)	
Prothrombin time (PT)	11–13 sec or 70–100% (depends on method and reagents used)	

RENAL PROFILE

Test	Reference Values	
	ADULT	**CHILD**
Albumin	3.5–5 g/dL	
Blood urea nitrogen (BUN)	5–25 mg/dL	Infant: 5–15 mg/dL Child: 5–20 mg/dL
Creatinine (Cr)	0.5–1.5 mg/dL 45–132.3 μmol/L (SI units)	Newborn: 0.8–1.4 mg/dL Infant: 0.7–1.7 mg/dL 2–6 y: 0.3–0.6 mg/dL; 24–54 μmol/L (SI units) 7–18 y: 0.4–1.2 mg/dL; 36–106 μmol/L (SI units)
Creatinine (urine)	Male: 20–26 mg/kg/24h 0.18–0.23 mmol/kg/24h (SI units) Female: 14–22 mg/kg/24h 0.12–0.19 mmol/kg/24h (SI units)	Similar to adult
Creatinine clearance (urine)	85–135 mL/min	
Electrolytes	*see* Electrolytes	
Glucose (FBS)	70–110 mg/dL (serum) 60–100 mg/dL (blood)	Newborn: 30–80 mg/dL Child: 60–100 mg/dL
Protein	6–8 g/dL	Infant: 6–6.7 g/dL Child: 6.2–8 g/dL
urine	0–5 mg/dL (random specimen) 25–150 mg/24h	
Uric acid	Male: 3.5–8 mg/dL Female: 2.8–6.8 mg/dL	Child: 2.5–5.5 mg/dL
urine	250–750 mg/24h (normal diet)	

KEY: FBS: fasting blood sugar.

THYROID PROFILE

Test	Reference Values	
	ADULT	**CHILD**
Calcitonin	Male: <40 pg/mL; <40 ng/L (SI units) Female: <25 pg/mL; <25 ng/L (SI units)	
Triiodothyronine (T₃)	80–200 ng/dL	Newborn: 90–170 ng/dL 6–12 y: 115–190 ng/dL
Thyroxine (T₄)	4.5–11.5 μg/dL 5–12 μg/dL (RIA) 1–2.3 ng/dL (thyroxine iodine)	Newborn: 11–23 μg/dL 1–4 mon: 7.5–16.5 μg/dL 4–12 mon: 5.5–14.5 μg/dL 1–6 y: 5.5–13.5 μg/dL 6–10 y: 5–12.5 μg/dL
Thyroid-binding globulin (TBG)	10–26 μg/dL	
T₃ resin uptake	25–35 relative % uptake	
Thyroid antibodies (TA)	Negative or <1:20 titer	
Thyroid-stimulating hormone (TSH)	0.35–5.5 μIU/mL, <3 ng/mL	Newborn: <25 μIU/mL

FEMALE REPRODUCTIVE PROFILE

Test	Reference Values	
	ADULT	CHILD
Estrogen	Early menstrual cycle: 60–400 pg/mL Midmenstrual cycle: 100–600 pg/mL Late menstrual cycle: 150–350 pg/mL Postmenopausal: <30 pg/mL Male: 40–115 pg/mL	
Estrogen (urine)	Female: Preovulation: 5–25 μg/24h Follicular: 24–100 μg/24h Luteal phase: 22–80 μg/24h Postmenopausal: 0–10 μg/24h Male: 4–25 μg/24h	
Estradiol (E_2)	Female: Follicular phase: 20–150 pg/mL Midcycle: 100–500 pg/mL Luteal phase: 60–260 pg/mL Male: 15–20 pg/mL	3–10 pg/mL
Progesterone	Preovulation: 20–150 ng/dL Midcycle: 250–2800 ng/dL	
Prolactin	Nonlactating female: 0–23 ng/dL Pregnancy: rise of 10–20 fold	
Follicle-stimulating hormone (FSH)	Female: Preovulation: 4–30 mU/mL Midcycle: 10–90 mU/mL Luteal phase: 4–30 mU/mL Postmenopausal: 40–250 mU/mL Male: 4–25 mU/mL	Child: 5–12 mU/mL
Follicle-stimulating hormone—urine (FSH-urine)	Female: Preovulation: 4–25 IU/24h Midcycle: 8–60 IU/24h Postmenopausal: 50–150 IU/24h Male: 4–18 IU/24h	Child: <10 IU/24h
Luteinizing hormone (LH)	Female: Follicular: 3–30 mIU/mL Midcycle: 30–100 mIU/mL Postmenopausal: 40–100 mIU/mL Male: 5–25 mIU/mL	Child: <10 mIU/mL
Pregnanediol (urine)	Female: Preovulation: 0.5–1.5 mg/24h Midcycle: 2–7 mg/24h Postmenopausal: 0.1–1 mg/24h Male: 0.1–1.5 mg/24h	Child: 0.4–1 mg/24h

URINALYSIS

Urine Content	Reference Values	
	ADULT	**CHILD**
Color	Light straw to dark amber	Light straw to dark yellow
Appearance	Clear	Clear
Odor	Aromatic	Aromatic
pH	4.5–8.0	4.5–8.0
Specific gravity (SG)	1.005–1.030 Average: 1.015–1.024	1.005–1.030
Protein	Negative 2–8 mg/dL	
Glucose	Negative	Negative
Ketones	Negative	Negative
RBC	1–2 per low-power field	Rare
WBC	3–4 per low-power field	0–4
Casts	Occasional hyaline	Rare

KEY: Units: mg: milligram; mEq: milliequivalent; L: liter; SI units: international system of units; g: gram; dL: deciliter; µL: microliter; cu µ: cubic micron; IU: international unit; mmol: millimole; ng: nanogram; pg: picogram; µg: microgram; µmol: micromole.

* Source: Tabular material adapted from Kee, J. L. (1999). Laboratory and Diagnostic Tests with Nursing Implications (5th Ed) Stamford, CT: Appleton & Lange.

References

Abbott, C. (1987). The impaired nurse. Part II: Management strategies. *Association of Operating Room Nurses, 46* (6), 1104–1115.

Abel, E. L., and Sokol, R. J. (1988). Alcohol use in pregnancy. In J. R. Niebyl (Ed.), *Drug use in pregnancy* (2nd ed) (pp 193–202). Philadelphia: Lea & Febiger.

Abel, E. L., and Sokol, R. J. (1988). Marijuana and cocaine use in pregnancy. In J. R. Niebyl (Ed.), *Drug use in pregnancy* (2nd ed) (pp 223–230). Philadelphia: Lea & Febiger.

Abernathy, E. (1987). Biological response modifiers. *American Journal of Nursing, 87* (4), 458–459.

Abraham, W. T., and Schrier, R. W. (1994). Body fluid volume regulation in health and disease. *Advanced Internal Medicine, 39,* 23–47.

Abu Gharbieh, P. (1998). Arab-Americans. In L. Purnell and B. Paulanka (Eds.), *Transcultural healthcare: A culturally competent approach* (pp 137–163). Philadelphia: FA Davis.

Alexander, S. E., and Aksel, S. (1990). Estrogen replacement therapy: Which regimen to choose? In R. C. Cefalo, *Clinical decisions in obstetrics and gynecology* (pp 226–278). Rockville, MD: Aspen Publishers.

Allen, J. E. (1993). Drug-induced photosensitivity. *Clinical Pharmacy, 12* (8), 580–584.

Alschuler, L., Benjamin, S., Duke, J., Duke, J., D'Epiro, N. (1997). Herbal medicine: What works, what's safe. *Patient Care, 31* (16), 49.

American Association of Colleges of Pharmacology/Eli Lilly and Company Geriatric Curriculum Project (1985). B. Ameer ed, *Pharmacy practice for the geriatric patient.* Carrboro, NC: Health Sciences Consortium.

American College of Obstetricians and Gynecologists (1994). *Antenatal corticosteroid therapy for fetal maturation.* ACOG Committee Opinion, No. 147. Washington, DC: ACOG.

American College of Obstetricians and Gynecologists (1995). Menopause: emerging issues. *ACOG Update: An Approved System for Continuing Medical Education, 21* (3), 1–9.

American Heart Association (1992). Guidelines for emergency cardiac care. *Journal of the American Medical Association, 268,* 16, October 28.

American Heart Association (1997). *Textbook of advanced cardiac life support.* Dallas, TX: American Heart Association.

American Journal of Nursing (1992). OSHA stiffens bloodborne rules, decrees free hepatitis B vaccine. *American Journal of Nursing, 92* (1), 82–84.

American Medical Association, Division of Drugs and Toxicology (1993). *Drug evaluations annual.* Chicago: American Medical Association.

American Society of Hospital Pharmacists (1995). *AHFS drug information.* Bethesda, MD: American Society of Hospital Pharmacists.

Amgen, Inc. (1991). *Neupogen (Filgrastim) product monograph.* Thousand Oaks, CA: Amgen, Inc.

Amgen, Inc. (1992). *Procrit: epoetin alpha for injections.* Product monograph. Thousand Oaks, CA: Amgen, Inc.

Aral, S. O., and Holmes, K. K. (1991). Sexually transmitted diseases in the AIDS era. *Scientific American, 264* (2), 62–68.

Association of Women's Health, Obstetrics, and Neonatal Nursing (AWHONN). (1993). *Cervical ripening and induction and augmentation of labor.* [Practice Resource], December.

Association of Women's Health, Obstetrics, and Neonatal Nursing (AWHONN), (1994). *Issues in contraceptive method selection.* Independent study, monograph, module 2, 4–30.

Asthma management (1998). *Postgraduate Medicine, 103* (3), 56–59.

Bachman, J. A. (1995). Management of discomfort. In I. M. Bobak, D. L. Lowdermilk, and M. D. Jensen. *Maternity nursing* (4th ed) (pp 221–245). St Louis: Mosby-Year Book, Inc.

Barbieri, R. L. (1991). The use of danazol as a treatment of endometriosis. In E. Thomas, and J. Rock (Eds.), *Modern approaches to endometriosis* (pp 239–255). Dordrecht, The Netherlands: Kluwer Academic Publishers.

Barnhart, E. R. (1998). *Physician's desk reference* (52nd ed). Oradell, NJ: Medical Economics Company.

Barkauskas, V., Stoltenberg-Allen, K., Baumann, L., and Darling Fisher, C. (1994). *Quick reference to health and physical assessment.* St Louis, CV Mosby.

Bartlett, J. G. (1998). *1998 medical management of HIV infection.* Baltimore: Port City Press.

Baylor College of Medicine (1995). Weighing the risks and benefits of hormone replacement therapy after menopause. *The Contraceptive Report, VI* (4), 4–14.

Bender, S. (1991). Personal communication. Letter from Professional Service Manager, Amgen, Inc. (February 20, 1991).

Benenson, A. S. (1990). *Control of communicable disease in man* (15th ed). Washington, DC: American Public Health Association.

Benson, M. D. (1994). *Obstetrical pearls: A practical guide for the efficient resident* (2nd ed). Philadelphia: FA Davis.

Berkowitz, G. S. (1988). Smoking and pregnancy. In J. R. Niebyl (Ed.), *Drug use in pregnancy* (2nd ed) (pp 173–191). Philadelphia: Lea & Febiger.

Besinger, R. E., and Niebyl, J. R. (1988). Tocolytic agents for the treatment of preterm labor. In J. R. Niebyl (Ed.), *Drugs used in pregnancy* (2nd ed) (pp 127–172). Philadelphia: Lea & Febiger.

Betz, C. L., and Poster, E. C. (1989). *Pediatric nursing reference.* St Louis: CV Mosby.

Biological Therapy Nurses of University of Chicago Hospital (1989). *Interleukin-2: A patient handbook.* Chicago: University of Chicago Hospital.

Blake, D. A., and Niebyl, J. R. (1988). Requirements and limitations in reproductive and teratogenic risk assessment. In J. R. Niebyl (Ed.), *Drug use in pregnancy* (2nd ed) (pp 1–9). Philadelphia: Lea & Febiger.

Bleck, T. P. (1990). Convulsive disorders: The use of anticonvulsant drugs. *Clinical Neuropharmacology, 13* (3), 198–209.

Blenner, J. L. (1991). Clomiphene-induced mood swings. *Journal of Obstetric, Gynecologic, and Neonatal Nursing, 20* (4), 321–327.

Blix, A. G. (1993). Environmental hazards. In S. Mattson, and J. E. Smith (Eds.), *NAACOG core curriculum for maternal newborn nursing* (pp 199–216). Philadelphia: WB Saunders.

Bobak, I. M. (1991). *Quick reference for maternity nursing.* St Louis: Mosby-Year Book, Inc.

Bobak, I. M., Jensen, M. O., and Zalar, M. K. (1989). *Maternity and gynecologic care: The nurse and the family* (4th ed). St Louis: CV Mosby.

Bobak, I. M., Lowdermilk, D. L., and Jensen, M. D. (1995). *Maternity nursing* (4th ed). St Louis: Mosby-Year Book, Inc.

Bond, L. (1993). Physiological changes. In S. Mattson, and J. E. Smith (Eds.), *NAACOG core curriculum for maternal newborn nursing* (pp 315–324). Philadelphia: WB Saunders.

Bortenschlager, L., and Zaloga, G. P. (1994). Vitamins. In B. Chernow (Ed.), *The pharmacologic approach to the critically-ill patient* (3rd ed) (pp 3–17). Baltimore: Williams & Wilkins.

Bozzette, S. A., Finkelstein, D. M., Spector, S. A., et al. (1995). Randomized trial of three antipneumocystis agents in patients with advanced human immunodeficiency virus infection. *New England Journal of Medicine, 332* (11), 593–639.

Brensilver, J. M., and Goldberger, E. (1996). *Water, electrolyte, and acid-base syndromes* (8th ed). Philadelphia: FA Davis.

Briggs, G. G., Freeman, R. K., and Yaffee, S. J. (1993). *Drugs in lactation.* Baltimore: Williams & Wilkins.

Briggs, G. G., Freeman, R. K., and Yaffe, S. J. (1994). *Drugs in pregnancy and lactation: A reference guide to fetal and neonatal risk* (4th ed). Baltimore: Williams & Wilkins.

Bristol-Myers Squibb Co. (1991). *Videx (didanosine) product* insert. Evansville, IN: Bristol-Myers Squibb Co.

Brogden, J. M., and Nevidjon, B. (1995). Vinorelbine tartrate (Navelbine): Drug profile and nursing implications of a new vinca alkaloid. *Oncology Nursing Forum, 22* (4), 635–646.

Brunner, B. (1998). *Information please almanac.* Boston: Houghton-Mifflin.

Bullock, B. L., and Rosendahl, D. P. (1988). *Pathophysiology: Adaptations and alterations in function* (2nd ed). Glenview, IL: Scott, Foresman.

Campinha-Bacote, J. (1998). African-Americans. In L. Purnell and B. Paulanka (Eds.), *Transcultural health care: A culturally competent approach* (pp. 53–73). Philadelphia: FA Davis.

Candesartan for hypertension (1998). *The Medical Letter, 40* (1040), 109, 110.

Cargill, J. M. (1992). Medication compliance in elderly people: Influencing variables and interventions. *Journal of Advanced Nursing, 17*, 422–426.

Cashion, K., and Johnston, C. L. A. (1995). Nursing care during the postpartum period. In I. M. Bobak, D. L. Lowdermilk, and M. D. Jensen. *Maternity nursing* (4th ed) (pp 463–503). St Louis: Mosby-Year Book, Inc.

Caudell, K., and Whedon, M. B. (1991). Hematopoietic complications. In Whedon, M. B. (Ed.), *Bone marrow transplantation: Principles, practice and nursing insights* (pp 135–151). Boston: Jones and Bartlett Publishers.

Caudle, P. (1993). Providing culturally sensitive health care to Hispanic clients. *Nurse Practitioner, 18* (12), 40–51.

Cefdinir—A new oral cephalosporin (1998). *The Medical Letter, 40* (1034), 85–87.

Centers for Disease Control and Prevention (1991). Guidelines for prophylaxis against *Pneumocystis carinii* pneumonia for children infected with human immunodeficiency virus. *Morbidity and Mortality Weekly Report, 40* (RR-2), 1–13.

Centers for Disease Control and Prevention (1991). Pelvic inflammatory disease: Guidelines for prevention and management. *Morbidity and Mortality Weekly Report, 40* (RR-5), 1–25.

Centers for Disease Control (1992). *1992 revised classification system for HIV infection and expanded AIDS surveillance case definition for adolescents and adults.* Draft of November 15, 1991. Atlanta: U.S. Department of Health and Human Services, Public Health Service, CDC.

Centers for Disease Control and Prevention (1993). Recommendations for the prevention and management of *Chlamydia trachomatis* infections, 1993. *Morbidity and Mortality Weekly Report, 42* (RR-12), 1–39.

Centers for Disease Control and Prevention (1994). Recommendations of the U.S. Public Health Service task force on the use of zidovudine to reduce perinatal transmission of human immunodeficiency virus. *Morbidity and Mortality Weekly Report, 43* (RR-11), 1–20.

Centers for Disease Control and Prevention (1993). Sexually transmitted diseases treatment guidelines. *Morbidity and Mortality Weekly Report, 42* (No. RR-14), 1–73.

Cerivastatin for hypercholesterolemia (1998). *The Medical Letter, 40* (1018), 13, 14.

Chameides, L., and Hazinski, M. F. (Eds.). (1994). *Textbook of pediatric advanced life support.* Dallas, TX: American Heart Association.

Chasnoff, I. J. (1990). Cocaine in pregnancy. In R. C. Cefalo (Ed.), *Clinical decisions in obstetrics and gynecology* (pp 336–337). Rockville, MD: Aspen Publishers, Inc.

Chasnoff, I. J. (1988). Drug use in pregnancy: Parameters of risk. *Pediatric Clinics of North America, 35* (6), 1403–1411.

Chasse, R. (1994). Diuretics, erythropoietin, and other medications used in renal failure. In B. Chernow (Ed.), *The pharmacologic approach to the critically-ill patient* (3rd ed) (pp 632–637). Baltimore: Williams & Wilkins.

Chernecky, C. (1991). *Cancer diagnostics and chemotherapy.* Philadelphia: WB Saunders.

Chernow, B. (Ed.) (1994). *The pharmacologic approach to the critically-ill patient* (3rd ed). Baltimore: Williams & Wilkins.

Chevalier, C. (1996). *The encyclopedia of medicinal plants* (pp 289–319). England: Dorling Kindersley.

Chiron Cetus Oncology Corporation (1994). Drug package insert for Proleukin. Emeryville, CA, The Chiron Corporation.

Choice of antibacterial drugs (1998). *The Medical Letter, 40* (1023), 33–42.

Clark, J., and Longo, D. (1986). Biological response modifiers. *Mediguide to Oncology, 6* (2), 1–5, 9, 10.

Clark, J., Queener, S., and Karb, V. (1990). *Pharmacologic basis of nursing practice* (3rd ed). St Louis: CV Mosby.

Colditz, G. A., Hankinson, S. E., Hunter, D. J., et al. (1995). The uses of estrogens and progestins and the risk of breast cancer in postmenopausal women. *New England Journal of Medicine, 332* (24), 1589–1593.

Coler, M. (1998). Brazilian-Americans. In L. Purnell and B. Paulanka (Eds.), *Transcultural health care: A culturally competent approach,* electronic chapter. Philadelphia: FA Davis.

Colfosceril (1995). *Drug evaluation monographs, 1974–1995.* Micromedex, Inc., 85, Aug 31, 1995.

Colucci, R. D., and Somberg, J. C. (1994). Treatment of cardiac arrhythmias. In B. Chernow (Ed.), *The pharmacologic approach to the critically-ill patient* (3rd ed) (pp 445–463). Baltimore: Williams & Wilkins.

Committee on Practice of NAACOG (1988). *OGN nursing practice resource: The nurse's role in the induction/augmentation of labor.* Washington, DC: Committee on Practice of NAACOG.

Community Program for Clinical Research on AIDS (1991). *The human immunodeficiency virus (HIV) and protocol synopses.* Wilmington: Mid-Atlantic Regional Education and Training Center, HIV Grant Program, Medical Center of Delaware.

Compendium of Pharmaceutical and Specialities (1998). (33rd ed). Canadian Pharmacists Association. Toronto: Webcom Limited.

Conte, J. E. (1995). *Manual of antibiotics and infectious disease* (8th ed). Baltimore: Williams & Wilkins.

Cotran, R. S., Kumar, V., and Robbins, S. L. (1994). *Robbins' pathologic basis of disease* (5th ed). Philadelphia: WB Saunders.

Craig, C. R., and Stitzel, R. E. (1997). *Modern pharmacology with clinical application* (5th ed). Boston: Little Brown.

Cummins, R. O. (Ed.). (1994). *Textbook of advanced cardiac life support.* Dallas, TX: American Heart Association.

Cunha, B. S., and Ortega, A. M. (1995). Antibiotic failure. *Medical Clinics of North America, 79* (3), 663–671.

Davies, K. (1990). Genital herpes: An overview. *Journal of Obstetric, Gynecologic, and Neonatal Nursing, 19* (5), 401–406.

Davis, J. R., and Sherer, K. (1994). *Applied nutrition and diet therapy for nurses* (2nd ed). Philadelphia: WB Saunders.

Deglin, J. H., and Vallerand, A. H. (1995). *Davis's drug guide for nurses* (4th ed). Philadelphia: FA Davis.

DeVane, C. L. (1995). Brief comparison of the pharmacokinetics and pharmacodynamics of the traditional and newer antipsychotic drugs. *American Journal of Health-Systems Pharmacology, 52* (3), S15–S19.

DHHS and The Henry J. Kaiser Family Foundation (1998). Panel on Clinical Practices for Treatment of HIV-Infection. Guidelines for the Use of Antiretroviral Agents in HIV-Infected Adults and Adolescents.

Diagnosing obstructive disorders (1998). *Postgraduate Medicine, 103* (4), 115–117.

Dickason, E. J. (1994). *Quick reference for maternal-infant assessment.* St Louis: Mosby-Year Book, Inc.

Dion, B. (1989). Hypertensive disorders in pregnancy. *International Journal of Childbirth Education, 4* (1), 29–30.

Dorr, R. T. (1992). *Hematopoietic colony stimulating factors.* Amgen Teleconference, February 21, 1992, Amgen, Inc.

Drug facts and comparisons (1998, updated monthly). St. Louis: J. B. Lippincott.

Drugs for pain (1998). *The Medical Letter, 40* (1033), 79–84.

Drugs for treatment of peptic ulcers (1997). *The Medical Letter, 39* (991), 1–4.

Dudjak, L. (1992). New roles of interferon-alpha. *American Journal of Nursing, 92* (2), 16.

Dutla, S. K., and Sood, R. (1994). Clinical pharmacology of drugs used in GI disorders of critically ill patients. In B. Chernow (Ed.), *The pharmacologic approach to the critically-ill patient* (3rd ed) (pp 614–628). Baltimore: Williams & Wilkins.

Ekbladh, L. (1995, June 7). *PMS*. Presentation given as one of series on women's health through sponsorship of Wilmington Hospital, Medical Center of Delaware, Wilmington, DE.

Engel, N. S. (1989). Anabolic steroid use among high school athletes. *The American Journal of Maternal/Child Nursing*, 14 (6), 417.

Engel, N. S. (1990). Update on cancer risks and oral contraceptives. *MCN: The American Journal of Maternal/Child Nursing*, 15 (1), 37.

Fehring, R. J. (1990). Methods used to self-predict ovulation: A comparative study. *Journal of Obstetric, Gynecologic, and Neonatal Nursing*, 19 (3), 233–237.

Finn, P. (1994). Addressing the needs of cultural minorities in drug treatment. *Journal of Substance Abuse Treatment*, 11 (4), 325–337.

Finnegan, L. P., and Wapner, R. J. (1988). Narcotic addiction in pregnancy. In J. R. Niebyl (Ed.), *Drug use in pregnancy* (2nd ed) (pp 203–222). Philadelphia: Lea & Febiger.

Fisher, D., and Knobf, M. T. (1989). *The cancer chemotherapy handbook* (3rd ed) (pp 366–386). Chicago: Year Book Medical Publishers, Inc.

Formulary and drug therapy guide, 1998–1999. Hudson, OH: Lexi-Comp, Inc.

Forrest, D. E. (1994). Common gynecologic pelvic disorders. In E. Q. Youngkin, and M. S. Davis (Eds.), *Women's health: A primary care clinical guide* (pp 241–280). Norwalk, CT: Appleton & Lange.

Freston, J. W. (1996). Insights on new paradigms in GI treatment. *The American Journal of Managed Care*, 11, Suppl, S32–S36.

Fry, S. T. (1989). Ethical issues in clinical research: Informed consent and risks versus benefits in the treatment of primary hypertension. *Nursing Clinics of North America*, 24 (4), 1033–1039.

Fujisawa (1990). *Adenocard (adenosine) for rapid bolus intravenous use*. Product insert No. 45514A. Deerfield, IL: Fujisawa.

Garner, C. H. (1994). The climacteric, menopause, and the process of aging. In E. Q. Youngkin, and M. S. Davis (Eds.), *Women's health: A primary care clinical guide* (pp 309–343). Norwalk, CT: Appleton & Lange.

Garner, C. H. (1994). Uses of GRH agonists. *Journal of Obstetrical, Gynecological and Neonatal Nursing*, 23 (7), 563–570.

Geissler, E. M. (1994). *Pocket guide to cultural assessments*. St Louis: Mosby-Year Book, Inc.

Gelone, S. (1995). *Therapy of opportunistic infections associated with the human immunodeficiency virus*. Philadelphia: Temple University Hospital.

Giamarellou, H. (1995). Empiric therapy for infections in the febrile, neutropenic compromised host. *Medical Clinics of North America*, 79 (3), 559–571.

Gill, P., Smith, M., and McGregor, C. (1989). Terbutaline by pump to prevent recurrent preterm labor. *MCN: The American Journal of Maternal/Child Nursing*, 14, 163–167.

Gilman, A. G., Goodman, L. S., and Gilman, A. (1991). *Goodman and Gilman's The pharmacologic basis of therapeutics* (8th ed). New York: Pergamon Press.

Gliashan, R. (1990). A randomized controlled study of intravesicular alpha 2b-interferon in carcinoma in situ of the bladder. *The Journal of Urology*, 144, 658–661.

Goldfien, A. (1995). The gonadal hormones and inhibitors. In B. G. Katzung (Ed.), *Basic and Clinical Pharmacology* (6th ed) (pp 608–636). Norwalk, CT: Appleton & Lange.

Goldzieher, J. W. (1994). Menopause: A deficiency disease. In J. A. Rock, S. Faro, N. F Gant, et al. (Eds.), *Advances in obstetrics and gynecology* 1 (pp 159–177). St Louis: Mosby-Year Book, Inc.

Gordon, S. (1994). Hispanic cultural health beliefs and folk remedies. *Journal of Holistic Nursing*, 12 (3), 307–322.

Gorman, C. (1998). Aspirin without ulcers. *Time* (July 13, 1998), 73.

Gravell, C. (1990). Progression of HIV infection in women: Asymptomatic state to frank AIDS. *NAACOG's Clinical Issues in Perinatal and Women's Health Nursing*, 1 (1), 20–27.

Green, M. R. (1991). *The role of colony-stimulating factors in chemotherapy-induced neutropenia*. Seattle, WA: Immunex Corporation.

Grepafloxacin—A new fluoroquinolone (1998). *The Medical Letter*, 40 (1019), 17, 18.

Griffin, J. E., and Wilson, J. D. (1992). Disorders of the testes and the male reproductive tract. In J. D. Wilson, and D. W. Foster (Eds). *Williams' textbook of endocrinology* (8th ed) (pp 799–852). Philadelphia: WB Saunders.

Groenwald, S., Frogge, M., Goodman, M., et al. (1990). *Cancer nursing: Principles and practice* (2nd ed). Boston: Jones and Bartlett Publishers.

Groopman, J. (1989). Clinical experience with hematopoietic growth factors. *Biotherapy and Cancer*, 2 (4), 1, 4, 5.

Gross, K. M., and Ponte, C. D. (1998). New strategies in the medical management of asthma. *American Family Physician*, 58 (1), 89–100.

Grothe, J. U. (1985). Nursing in research and clinical testing of drugs. Chapter 9 in Wiener, M. B., and Pepper, G. A., *Clinical pharmacology and therapeutics in nursing* (2nd ed). New York: McGraw-Hill.

Gullatte, M. M., and Graves, T. (1990). Advances in antineoplastic therapy. *Oncology Nursing Forum*, 17 (6), 867–876.

Gurevich, I. (1989) AIDS in critical care. *Heart and Lung*, 18 (2), 107–112.

Guyton, A. C., and Hall, J. E. (1997). *Human physiology and mechanisms of disease* (6th ed). Philadelphia: WB Saunders.

Haeuber, D. (1989). Recent advances in the management of biotherapy-related side effects: Flu-like syndrome. *Oncology Nursing Forum*, 16 (6), 35–41.

Haeuber, D., and Dijulio, J. E. (1989). Hematopoietic colony-stimulating factors: An overview. *Oncology Nursing Forum*, 16 (2), 247–255.

Hahn, M. B., and Jassak, P. T. (1988). Nursing management of patients receiving interferon. *Seminars in Oncology Nursing*, IV (2), 132–141.

Handbook of nonprescription drugs (1992). (10th ed). Washington, DC: American Pharmaceutical Association.

Haney, A. F. (1991). The pathogenesis and aetiology of endometriosis. In E. Thomas, and J. Rock (Eds.) *Modern Approaches to Endometriosis* (pp 3–19). Dordrecht, The Netherlands: Kluwer Academic publishers.

Hardman J. G., Limbird, L. E., Molinoff, P. B., and Ruddon, R. W. (1996). *Goodman and Gilman's The pharmacological basis of therapeutics* (9th ed). New York: McGraw-Hill.

Hardy, R. I., and Friedman, A. J. (1994). The role of gonadotropin-releasing hormone agonists in gynecology. In J. A. Rock, S. Faro, N. F. Gant, et al. (Eds.). *Advances in obstetrics and gynecology* 1 (pp 179–209). St Louis: Mosby-Year Book, Inc.

Harvey, C. J., and Burke, M. E. (1992). Hypertensive disorders in pregnancy. In L. K. Mandevill, and N. H. Troiano (Eds.). *High risk intrapartum nursing* (pp 147–164). Philadelphia: JB Lippincott.

Hatcher, R. A., Trussell, J., and Stewart, F., et al. (1994). *Contraceptive technology* (16th rev. ed). New York: Irvington Publishers, Inc.

Hayes, E. R., and Kee, J. L. (1996). *Pharmacology: Pocket companion for nurses*. Philadelphia: WB Saunders.

Hayes, J. E. (1982). Normal changes in aging and nursing implications of drug therapy. *Nursing Clinics of North America*, 17 (2), 253–261.

Hellerstein, D. K., and Lipshultz, L. I. (1993). Male infertility. In L. J. Copeland (Ed.), *Textbook of gynecology* (pp 347–368). Philadelphia: WB Saunders.

Henke-Yarbro, C. (Ed.), (1994). Management of patients receiving interleukin-2 therapy. *Seminars in Oncology Nursing*, 9 (3), Suppl. 1, 1–35.

Heslin, J. A. (1990). Guide to caffeine consumption. *Childbirth Educator*, 9 (2), 11, 36.

Higgs, D., Nagy, C., and Einhorn, L. (1989). Ifosamide: A clinical review. *Seminars in Oncology Nursing*, 5 (2) Suppl. 1 (May), 70–77.

Hillis, L. B. (1997). Low molecular weight heparins. *Advance for nurse practitioners*. October 1997, 53–56.

Hirsch, M. S. (1992). The treatment of cytomegalovirus in AIDS—more than meets the eye. *New England Journal of Medicine*, 326 (January 23, 1992), 264–266.

Hirschel, B., Lazzarin, A., Chorpard, P., et al. (1991). A controlled study of inhaled pentamidine for primary prevention of *Pneumocystis carinii* pneumonia. *New England Journal of Medicine*, 324 (April 18, 1991), 1079–1083.

HIV Digest (1991). Update: HIV infection among health care workers in 1991. *HIV Digest*, 1 (1), 1, 6. Publication of the Pennsylvania AIDS Education and Training Center.

Hobbs, C. (1998). *Handmade medicines—Simple recipes for herbal health*. Colorado: Interweave Press, Inc.

Hodgson, B. B., Kizior, R. J., *Saunders' Nursing Drug Handbook* 1999. Philadelphia: WB Saunders.

Hoechst-Roussel Pharmaceuticals, Inc. (1991). *Myeloid growth factors*. Somerville, NJ: Hoechst-Roussel Pharmaceuticals, Inc.

Hoechst-Roussel Pharmaceuticals (1991). *Prokine (Sargramostim)*, Product Monograph. Somerville, NJ: Hoechst-Roussel Pharmaceuticals, Inc.

Holgate, S. T., Bradding, P., and Sampson, A. P. (1996). Leukotriene antagonists and synthesis inhibitors: New directions in asthma therapy. *Journal of Allergy and Clinical Immunology*, 98 (1), 1–13.

Holmes, J., and Maglera, L. (1987). *Maternity nursing*. New York: Macmillan Publishing.

Hood, L. E. (1987). Interferon. *American Journal of Nursing*, 87 (4), 459–464.

Hostetler, J. (1993). *Amish society* (4th ed). Baltimore: The Johns Hopkins University Press.

Howards, S. S. (1995). Treatment of male infertility. *New England Journal of Medicine*, 332, (5), 312–317.

Immunex Corporation (1991). *Leukine (Sargramostim)*. Product Monograph. Seattle, WA: Immunex Corporation.

Intramuscular injections: A guide to sites and technique (1989). Philadelphia: Wyeth-Ayerst Laboratories.

Irbesartan for hypertension (1998). *The Medical Letter*, 40 (1019), 18, 19.

Irwin, M. M. (1987). Patients receiving biologic response modifiers: Overview of nursing care. *Oncology Nursing Forum*, 14 (6), Supplement, 32–37.

Irwin, R. P., and Nutt, J. G. (1992). Principles of neuropharmacology I. Pharmacokinetics and Pharmacodynamics. In H. L. Klawans, et al. (Eds.), *Textbook of clinical neuropharmacology and therapeutics* (2nd ed) (pp 1–28). New York: Raven Press.

Jackson, B., Strauman, J., Frederickson, K., et al. (1991). Longterm biopsychosocial effects of interleukin-2 therapy. *Oncology Nursing Forum*, 18 (4), 683–690.

Jassak, P. (1991). Knowledge deficit related to biotherapy. In J. McNally, E. Somerville, C. Miakowski, et al. (Eds.), *Guidelines for cancer nursing practice* (2nd ed). Philadelphia: WB Saunders.

Jawetz, E. (1995). Penicillins and cephalosporins. In B. G. Katzung (Ed.). *Basic and clinical pharmacology* (6th ed) (pp 680–692). Norwalk, CT: Appleton & Lange.

Johnson, J. (1997). Influence of race or ethnicity on pharmacokinetics of drugs. *Journal of Pharmacological Science*, 86 (12) 1328–1333.

Johnson, S. T. (1997). Antipsychotics. *RN*, August, 1997, 45–50.

Johnson, T. R. B., and Niebyl, J. R. (1988). Caffeine in pregnancy. In J. R. Niebyl (Ed.), *Drug use in pregnancy* (2nd ed) (pp 231–234). Philadelphia: Lea & Febiger.

Kaliner, M., Eggleston, P. A., and Mathews, K. P. (1987). Rhinitis and asthma. *JAMA*, 258 (20), 2851–2873.

Kee, J. L., and Paulanka, B. (1994). *Fluids and electrolytes with clinical applications* (5th ed). New York: John Wiley & Sons.

Kee, J. L. (1999), *Laboratory and diagnostic tests* (5th ed). Stamford, CT: Appleton & Lange.

Kee, J. L., and Hayes, E. R. (1990). Assessment of patient laboratory data in the acutely ill. *Nursing Clinics of North America*, 25 (4), 751–759.

Kee, J. L., and Marshall, S. M. (1996). *Clinical calculations* (3rd ed). Philadelphia: WB Saunders.

Kelley, W. N. (Ed.) (1992). *Textbook of internal medicine*. Vols. I and II (2nd ed). Philadelphia: JB Lippincott.

Keyler, D. E., VanDeVoort, J. T., Howard, J. E., et al. (1998). Monitoring blood levels of selected drugs. *Postgraduate Medicine*, 103 (3), 209–219.

Kimmel, D. C. (1990). *Adulthood and aging* (3rd ed). New York: John Wiley & Sons.

Kittler, P., and Sucher, K. (1989). *Food and culture in America*. New York: Reinhold.

Klawans, H. L., Goetz, C. G., and Tanner, C. M. (Eds.) (1992). *Textbook of clinical neuropharmacology and therapeutics* (2nd ed). New York: Raven Press.

Knudson, M. (1998). The hunt is on. *Technology Review*. January-February, 23–29.

Knuppel, R. A., and Drukker, J. E. (1986). Hypertension in pregnancy. In R. A. Knuppel and J. E. Drukker (Eds.), *High risk pregnancy: A team approach* (pp 362–398). Philadelphia: WB Saunders.

Koll, B. S., and Armstrong, D. (1995). Acquired immune deficiency syndrome (AIDS). In Rakel, R. E. (Ed.). *1995 Conn's current therapy* (pp 42–52). Philadelphia: WB Saunders.

Kuhn, M. M. (1991). *Pharmacotherapeutics* (2nd ed). Philadelphia: FA Davis.

Ladewig, P. W., London, M. L., and Olds, S. B. (1990). *Essentials of maternal-newborn nursing* (2nd ed). Redwood City, CA: Addison-Wesley Nursing.

LaGodna, G., and Hendrix, M. (1989). Impaired nurses: A cost analysis. *Journal of Nursing Administration*, 19 (9), 13–18.

Lauver, D., and Welch, M. B. (1990). Sexual response cycle. In C. I. Fogel and D. Lauver (Eds.), *Sexual health promotion* (pp 39–52). Philadelphia: WB Saunders.

Lehne, R. A. (1998). *Pharmacology for nursing care* (3rd ed). Philadelphia: WB Saunders.

Levin, R. H. (1991). Advances in pediatric drug therapy of asthma. *Nursing Clinics of North America*, 26 (2), 263–269.

Levy, R. (1993). *Ethnic and racial differences in response to medicines*. Reston, VA: National Pharmaceutical Council.

Levy, R. (1995). Multicultural medicine and pharmacy management: Part II: Compliance with medications. *Drug Benefit Trends*, 7 (4), 13–14, 24.

Levy, S. B. (1998). Multidrug resistance—A sign of the times. *New England Journal of Medicine*, 338 (19), 1376–1378.

Lieberman, J., Yunis, J., Egea, E., et al., (1991). HLA-B38, DR4, DQW3 and clozapine-induced agranulocytosis in Jewish patients with schizophrenia. *Archives of Psychiatry*, 47, 945–948.

Lipp, F. (1996). *Herbalism*. New York: Little, Brown and Co.

Lipson, J., and Haifizi, H. (1998). Iranians. In L. Purnell and B. Paulanka (Eds.), *Transcultural health care: A culturally competent approach* (pp 323–351). Philadelphia: FA Davis.

Lipton, S. A., and Gendelman, H. E. (1995). Dementia associated with the acquired immunodeficiency syndrome. *New England Journal of Medicine*, 332 (14), 934–940.

Lowdermilk, D. L. (1995). *Quick reference for maternity nursing* (2nd ed). St Louis: Mosby-Year Book, Inc.

MacLaren, A. (1994). *Maternal-neonatal nursing: Concepts and activities*. Springhouse, PA: Springhouse Corp.

Malinowski, J. S. (1989). Fetal well-being in preterm and post-term gestation. In J. S. Malinowski, C. G. Pedigo, and C. R. Philips (Eds.), *Nursing care during the labor process* (3rd ed) (pp 309–353). Philadelphia: FA Davis.

Malinowski, J. S. (1989). Labor stimulation. In J. S. Malinowski, C. G. Pedigo, and C. R. Phillips (Eds.), *Nursing care during the labor process* (3rd ed) (pp 158–184). Philadelphia: FA Davis.

Management of COPD (1998). *Postgraduate Medicine*, 103 (4), 131, 132, 136, 192.

Marshall, C. (1985). The art of induction/augmentation of labor. *Journal of Obstetric, Gynecologic, and Neonatal Nursing*, 14 (1), 22–28.

Martin, E. J. (1990). Module 5: Care of the laboring woman. In E. J. Martin (Ed.), *Intrapartum management modules: A perinatal education program* (pp 119–150). Baltimore: Williams & Wilkins.

Martin, L. L., and Reeder, S. J. (1991). *Essentials of maternity nursing*. Philadelphia: JB Lippincott.

Marcos, L., and Cancro, R. (1982). Pharmacotherapy of Hispanic depressed patients: Clinical observations. *American Journal of Psychotherapy*, 36 (4), 505–512.

Masten, Y. (1993). *The Skidmore-Roth outline series: Obstetric nursing*. El Paso, TX: Skidmore Roth Publishing, Inc.

Masters, W. H., Johnson, V. E., and Kolodny, R. C. (1988). *Human sexuality* (3rd ed). Glenview, IL: Scott, Foresman and Co.

Matocha, L. (1998). Chinese-Americans. In L. Purnell and B. Paulanka (Eds.), *Transcultural health care: A culturally competent approach* (pp 163–188). Philadelphia: FA Davis.

Matthews, H. (1995). Racial, ethnic, and gender differences in response to medicines. *Drug Metabolism: Drug Interaction*, 12 (2), 77–91.

Mattson, S. (1993). Ethnocultural considerations in the childbearing period. In S. Mattson, and J. E. Smith (Eds.), *NAACOG core curriculum for maternal newborn nursing* (pp 81–97). Philadelphia: WB Saunders.

McCance, K. L., and Huether, S. E. (1990). *Pathophysiology: The biologic basis for disease in adults and children*. St Louis: CV Mosby.

McCloskey, J. C., and Bulechek, G. M. (Eds.) (1992). *Iowa intervention project: Nursing interventions classification (NIC)*. St Louis: Mosby-Year Book, Inc.

McDonald, L. Y. (1994). Personal communication regarding IL-2 administration. Emeryville, CA, The Cetus Oncology Corporation.

McEvoy, G. K. (Ed.) (1998). *AHFS '98 drug information*. Bethesda, MD: American Society of Health-System Pharmacists.

McGregor, J. A. (1990). Trichomoniasis: A continuing challenge. In R. C. Cefalo (Ed.), *Clinical decisions on obstetrics and gynecology* (pp 289–295). Rockville, MD: Aspen Publishers, Inc.

McIntyre, A. (1992). *Herbs for common ailments*, New York: Fireside.

McIntyre, A. (1997). *The medicinal garden*. New York: Henry Holt.

McKay, M. (1990). Recurrent vulvar pruritus. In R. C. Cefalo (Ed.), *Clinical decisions in obstetrics and gynecology* (pp 296–298). Rockville, MD: Aspen Publishers, Inc.

McKenry, L. M., and Salerno, E. (1998). *Mosby's pharmacology in nursing* (20th ed.). St Louis: CV Mosby.

McKeon, V. A. (1993). Hormone replacement therapy: Evaluating the risks and benefits. *Journal of Obstetric, Gynecologic and Neonatal Nursing, 23* (8), 647–657.

McManus, M. T. (1990). Module 7: Induction and augmentation of labor. In E. J. Martin (Ed.), *Intrapartum management modules: A perinatal education program* (pp 235–258). Baltimore: Williams & Wilkins.

McMurdo, M. E. T., Jarvis, A., Fraser, C. G., and Ghosh, U. K. (1991). A novel approach to the assessment of drug compliance in the elderly. *Gerontology, 37*, 339–344.

Medical Center of Delaware (1995). *Formulary and drug therapy guide 1995–1996*. Hudson, OH: Lexi-Comp, Inc.

Meleis, A., and Meleis, M. (1998). Egyptian-Americans. In L. Purnell and B. Paulanka (Eds.), *Transcultural health care: A culturally competent approach* (pp. 217–243). Philadelphia: FA Davis.

Melone, L., Anderson-Drevs, K., Jassak, P., et al. (1991). A teaching booklet for patients receiving GMCSF-therapy. *Oncology Nursing Forum 18* (3), 593–597.

Miller, E. P., and Armstrong, C. L. (1990). Surfactant replacement therapy: Innovative care for the premature infant. *Journal of Obstetric, Gynecologic and Neonatal Nursing, 19* (1), 14–17.

Miller-Slade, D. (1994). Ask the experts: Is suppression of lactation in postpartum patients still an indication for the use of bromocriptine mesylate (Parlodel)? *AWHONN Voice, 2* (11), 11.

Minoff, H. (1990) HIV infection in pregnancy. In R. C. Cefalo (Ed.), *Clinical decisions in obstetrics and gynecology* (pp 34–36). Rockville, MD: Aspen Publishers, Inc.

Miranda, B., Spangler, Z., and McBride, A. (1998). Filipino-Americans. In L. Purnell and B. Paulanka (Eds.), *Transcultural health care: A culturally competent approach* (pp 245–273). Philadelphia: FA Davis.

Monahan, F. D., and Neighbors, M. (1998). *Medical-surgical nursing* (2nd ed.). Philadelphia: WB Saunders.

Monier, M., and Laird, M. (1989). Contraceptives: A look at the future. *American Journal of Nursing, 89* (4), 496–499.

Montelukast for persistent asthma (1998). *The Medical Letter, 40* (1031), 71–73.

Morbidity and Mortality Weekly Reports, May 15, 1998/Vol.47/No. RR-7.

Morbidity and Mortality Weekly Reports, August 5, 1994/Vol. 43/No. RR-11.

Moroso, G., and Holman, S. (1990). Counseling and testing women for HIV. *NAACOG's clinical issues in perinatal and women's health nursing, 1* (1), 10–19.

Moss, A. (1992). *HIV and AIDS: Management by the primary team*. Oxford: Oxford University Press.

Mott, S. R., and Fazekas, A. (1987). *Nursing care of children and families* (2nd ed.). Menlo Park, CA: Addison-Wesley Publishing Co.

Murphy, R. (1992). Infection in the compromised host. In S. T. Shulman, J. P. Phair, and H. M. Somers (Eds.), *The biologic and clinical basis of infectious diseases* (4th ed) (pp 394–405). Philadelphia: WB Saunders.

Nadler, J. L., and Rude, R. K. (1995). Disorders of magnesium metabolism. *Endocrinology and Metabolism Clinics of North America, 24* (3), 623–637.

National Institute of Allergy and Infectious Diseases (1998). *Understanding vaccines* (NIH Publication No. 98-4219). Washington, DC: US Department of Health and Human Services.

Nayduch, D., Lee, A., and Butler, D. (1994). High-dose methylprednisolone after acute spinal injury. *Critical Care Nurse, 14* (4), 69–78.

Neibyl, J. R., and Maxwell, K. D. (1988). Treatment of the nausea and vomiting of pregnancy. In J. R. Niebyl (Ed.), *Drug use in pregnancy* (2nd ed) (pp 11–20). Philadelphia: Lea and Febiger.

New triptans and other drugs for migraine (1998). *The Medical Letter, 40* (1037), 97–100.

Newman, V., Fullerton, J. T., and Anderson, P. O. (1993). Clinical advances in the management of severe nausea and vomiting during pregnancy. *Journal of Obstetric, Gynecologic and Neonatal Nursing, 22* (6), 483–490.

Newton, E. R. (1989). The use of mechanical dilators for cervical ripening. In R. H. Petrie (Ed.), *Perinatal pharmacology* (pp 303–312). Oradell, NJ: Medical Economics Books.

Nicolau, D. P., Quintiliani, R., and Nightingale, C. H. (1995). Antibiotic kinetics and dynamics for the clinician. *Medical Clinics of North America, 79* (3), 477–493.

Noble, S. L., Forbes, R. C., and Stamm, P. L. (1998). Diagnosis and management of common tinea infections. *American Family Physician, 58* (1), 163–174.

Nolan, L., and O'Malley, K. (1988). Prescribing for the elderly: Part II. *Journal of American Geriatrics Society, 38*, 245–254.

Noronha, S., and Arnason, B. G. W. Multiple sclerosis. In H. L. Klawans, *Textbook of clinical neuropharmacology and therapeutics* (2nd ed) (pp 287–296). New York: Raven Press.

Norton, B. A., and Miller, A. M. (1986). *Skills for professional nursing practice*. Norwalk, CT: Appleton-Century-Crofts.

Notterman, D. A. (1994). Pediatric Pharmacotherapy. In B. Chernow (Ed.), *The Pharmacologic Approach to the Critically-Ill Patient* (3rd ed) (pp 139–151). Baltimore: Williams & Wilkins.

Nowak, T. (1998). Vietnamese-Americans. In L. Purnell and B. Paulanka (Eds.), *Transcultural health care: A culturally competent approach* (pp 449–477). Philadelphia: FA Davis.

Nursing Drug Handbook (1994). Springhouse, PA: Springhouse Corp.

Nyerges, C. (1997). A better way to heal. *Mother Earth News, 161*, p. 22.

Olds, S. B., London, M. L., and Ladewig, P. W. (1996). *Maternal-newborn nursing: A family-centered approach*. Menlo Park, CA: Addison-Wesley.

Olin, B. R. (Ed.) (1994). *Drug facts and comparisons*. St Louis: Facts and Comparisons.

Oncology Nursing Society (1989). *Biologic response modifier guidelines: Recommendations for nursing education and practice*. Pittsburgh: Oncology Nursing Society.

Pedigo, C. G. (1989). Management of pain with drugs. In J. S. Malinowski, C. G. Pedigo, and C. R. Phillips (Eds.), *Nursing care during the labor process* (3rd ed) (pp 185–231). Philadelphia: FA Davis.

Pepping, P. B. (1994). Endometriosis: A nursing perspective. *Innovations in Women's Health Nursing, 1* (1), 2–8.

Pepping, P. B., and Fitzgerald, K. (1994). Treating endometriosis. *Innovations in Women's Health Nursing 1*, (1), 11–12.

Perry, P. J., Alexander, B., and Liskow, B. I. (1997). *Psychotropic drug handbook* (7th ed). Washington: American Psychiatric Press, Inc.

Perry, S. E. (1995). Nursing care of the newborn. In I. M. Bobak, D. L. Lowdermilk, and M. D. Jensen. *Maternity Nursing* (4th ed) (pp 361–405). St Louis: Mosby-Year Book, Inc.

Peter, G. (Ed.) (1997). *1997 Red book: Report of the committee of infectious diseases* (24th ed.). Elk Grove Village, IL: American Academy of Pediatrics.

Petree, B., and Mattson, S. (1993). Hypertensive states in pregnancy. In S. Mattson and J. E. Smith (Eds.), *NAACOG core curriculum for maternal-newborn nursing* (pp 412–433). Philadelphia: WB Saunders.

Phair, J. P., and Chadwick, E. G. (1992). Human immunodeficiency virus infection and AIDS. In S. T. Shulman, J. P. Phair, and H. M. Somers (Eds.), *The biologic and chemical basis of infectious diseases* (pp 380–393). Philadelphia: WB Saunders.

Phipps, W. J., Long, B. C., and Woods, N. F. (1995). *Medical-surgical nursing* (5th ed). St Louis: CV Mosby.

Porth, C. M. (1994). *Pathophysiology* (4th ed). Philadelphia: JB Lippincott.

Prendergast, M. R., Saxe, J. M., Ledgerwood, A. M., and Lucas, W. F. (1994). Massive steroids do not reduce the zone of injury after penetrating spinal cord injury. *Journal of Trauma*, 37 (4), 576–580.

Purnell, L. (1998a). The Purnell model for cultural competence. In L. Purnell and B. Paulanka (Eds.), *Transcultural health care: A culturally competent approach* (pp 7–52). Philadelphia: FA Davis.

Purnell, L. (1998b). Mexican-Americans. In L. Purnell and B. Paulanka (Eds.), *Transcultural health care: A culturally competent approach* (pp 371–395). Philadelphia: FA Davis.

Purnell, L. (1998c). Panamanian and Panamanian-American health beliefs and the meaning of respect afforded them by healthcare providers. *National Journal of Wellness*, 2(2), 17–27.

Purnell, L., and Counts, M. (1998). Appalachians. In L. Purnell and B. Paulanka (Eds.), *Transcultural health care: A culturally competent approach* (pp 107–136). Philadelphia: FA Davis.

Purnell, L., and Paulanka, B. (1998). In L. Purnell and B. Paulanka (Eds.), *Transcultural health care: A culturally competent approach.* Philadelphia: FA Davis.

Quetiapine for schizophrenia (1997). *The Medical Letter*, 39 (1016), 117–119.

Rainey, T. G., and Read, C. A. (1994). Pharmacology of colloids and crystalloids. In B. Chernow (Ed.), *The Pharmacologic Approach to the Critically-Ill Patient* (3rd ed) (pp 272–288). Baltimore: Williams and Wilkins.

Rakel, R. E. (Ed.). (1991). *Conn's current therapy 1991.* Philadelphia: WB Saunders.

Ramin, S. M., Maberry, M. C., and Cox S. M. (1993). Lower genital tract infections. In L. J. Copeland (Ed.), *Textbook of gynecology* (pp 505–516). Philadelphia: WB Saunders.

Rayburn, W. F., and Engdahl, K. L. (1989). Antiemetic agents for gestational nausea. In R. H. Petrie (Ed.), *Perinatal pharmacology* (pp 43–51). Oradell, NJ: Medical Economics Books.

Reiss, B. S., and Evans, M. E. (1990). *Pharmacologic aspects of nursing care* (3rd ed). Albany, NY: Delmar Publishers, Inc.

Repaglinide for type 2 diabetes mellitus (1998). *The Medical Letter*, 40 (1027), 55–58.

Rheinstein, P. H., and Albari, B. (1998). Significant FDA approvals in 1997. *American Family Physician*, 57 (11), 2865–2868.

Rittenberg, C., Grallo, R., and Rehmeyer, T. (1995). Assessing and managing venous irritation associated with vinorelbine tartrate (Navelbine). *Oncology Nursing Forum*, 22 (4), 707–710.

Robinson, W. (1988). Clinical use of colony-stimulating factors. *Mediguide to Oncology*, 8 (3), 1–4.

Roche Laboratories (1986). *Roferon-A in the treatment of hairy cell leukemia.* Nutley, NJ: Roche Laboratories.

Roche Laboratories (1987). *Roche oncology report #2: Tips on teaching self-administration techniques to the cancer patient.* Nutley, NJ: Roche Laboratories.

Rogers, A. (1990). Drugs and disturbed sexual functioning. In C. I. Fogel, and D. Lauver (Eds.), *Sexual health promotion* (pp 485–497). Philadelphia: WB Saunders.

Rogove, H. J., and Moore, K. A. (1993). *Critical Care Medicines: Handbook of intravenous pharmacotherapeutics.* Columbus, OH: Contemporary Critical Care Resources, Inc.

Romanczuk, A. N., and Brown, J. P. (1994). Folic acid will reduce risk of neural tube defects. *MCN: The American Journal of Maternal/Child Nursing*, 19 (6), 331–334.

Rowland, M., and Tozer, T. N. (1989). *Clinical pharmacokinetics: concepts and applications* (2nd ed). Philadelphia: Lea & Febiger.

Rudy, A. C., and Brater, D. C. (1994). Drug interactions. In B. Chernow (Ed.). *The pharmacologic approach to the critically-ill patient* (3rd ed) (pp 18–32). Baltimore: Williams & Wilkins.

Rudy, A. C., and Brater, D. C. (1994). Pharmacokinetics. In B. Chernow (Ed.), *The pharmacologic approach to the critically-ill patient* (3rd ed) (pp 3–17). Baltimore: Williams & Wilkins.

Sabet, L. (1998). Korean-Americans. In L. Purnell and B. Paulanka (Eds.), *Transcultural health care: A culturally competent approach* (electronic chapter). Philadelphia: FA Davis.

St. John's Wort (1997). *The Medical Letter*, 39, 1014, pp 107–108.

Santos, A. C., and Pedersen, H. (1989). Local anesthetics in obstetrics. In R. H. Petrie (Ed.), *Perinatal pharmacology* (pp 371–383). Oradell, NJ: Medical Economics Books.

Sautter, U. (1998). The new spice trade: A chemist's faith in garlic led to a big business in alternative medicine. Scientific credibility is key. *Time International*, 150, 32, p 48.

Scavone, J. M. (1994). Pharmacotherapy in the elderly. In B. Chernow (Ed.), *The pharmacologic approach to the critically-ill patient* (3rd ed) (pp 202–219). Baltimore: Williams & Wilkins.

Schad, R. F., and Rayburn, W. F. (1986). Antiemetics, iron preparations, vitamins, and OTC drugs. In W. F. Rayburn and F. P. Zuspan (Eds.), *Drug therapy in obstetrics and gynecology* (2nd ed) (pp 24–36). Norwalk, CT: Appleton-Century-Crofts.

Schwertz, D. W. (1991). Basic principles of pharmacologic action. *Nursing Clinics of North America*, 26 (2), 245–262.

Schwertz, D. W., and Buschmann, M. G. T. (1989). Pharmacogeriatrics. *Critical Care Nursing Quarterly*, 12 (1), 26–37.

Sekelman, J. (1998). Jewish-Americans. In L. Purnell and B. Paulanka (Eds.), *Transcultural health care: A culturally competent approach* (pp 371–395). Philadelphia: FA Davis.

Seligman, M. (1994). Bronchodilators. In B. Chernow (Ed.), *The pharmacologic approach to the critically-ill patient* (3rd ed) (pp 567–575). Baltimore: Williams & Wilkins.

Seymour, F. J. (1991). A new program for the management of the chemically impaired nurse in Delaware. Unpublished manuscript; an executive position paper.

Sharts-Engel, N. C. (1990). Syphilis in pregnancy: Centers for Disease Control guidelines. *American Journal of Maternal/Child Nursing*, 15 (6), 342.

Shattuck, J. C., and Schwarz, K. K. (1991). Walking the line between feminism and infertility: Implications for nursing, medicine, and client care. *Health Care for Women International*, 12 (3), 331–340.

Shaw, N. K. (1991). Pharmacotherapeutics for the obstetrical patient. In M. M. Kuhn (Ed.), *Pharmacotherapeutics: A nursing process approach* (2nd ed) (pp 326–356) Philadelphia: FA Davis.

Shaw, R. W. (1991). GrRH analogues in the treatment of endometriosis: Rationale and efficacy. In E. Thomas, and J. Rock (Eds.), *Modern approaches to endometriosis* (pp 257–274). Dordrecht, The Netherlands: Kluwer Academic Publishers.

Sibai, B. M., and Armon, E. A. (1989). Aspirin safety during pregnancy. In R. H. Petric (Ed.), *Perinatal pharmacology* (pp 53–60). Oradell, NJ: Medical Economics Books.

Simchak, M. (1989). Medications for labor pain. *International Journal of Childbirth Education*, 4 (4), 15–17.

Simpson, C., Seipp, D., and Rosenberg, S. (1988). The current status and future application of interleukin-2 and adaptive immunotherapy in cancer treatment: Seminars. *Oncology Nursing, IV* (2), 132–141.

Skidmore-Roth, L. (1994). *Nursing Drug Reference.* St Louis: CV Mosby.

Smith, K. V. (1993). Normal childbirth. In S. Mattson, and J. E. Smith (Eds.), *NAACOG core curriculum for maternal newborn nursing* (pp 255–283). Philadelphia: WB Saunders.

Some drugs that cause psychiatric symptoms (1998). *The Medical Letter*, 40 (1020), 21–24.

Sorting through *H. pylori* ulcer therapy options (1998). *Clinician Reviews*, 8 (6), 45–48.

Soules, M. R. (1990). Endometriosis: New facets of treatment for an old disease. In R. C. Cefalo (Ed.), *Clinical decisions in obstetrics and gynecology* (pp 208–212). Rockville, MD: Aspen Publishers, Inc.

Spector, R. E., (1991). Cultural diversity in health and illness (3rd ed). Norwalk, CT: Appleton & Lange.

Spratto, G. R., and Woods, A. L. (1999). *Nurse's drug reference.* New York: Delmar Publishers, Inc.

Steckler, J. (1998). German-Americans. In L. Purnell and B. Paulanka (Eds.), *Transcultural health care: A culturally competent approach* (electronic chapter). Philadelphia: FA Davis.

Stevens, D. A. (1995). Coccidioidomycosis. *New England Journal of Medicine*, 332 (16), 1077–1082.

Stockley, I. H. (1994). *Drug interactions* (3rd ed). Oxford: Blackwell Scientific Publications.

Stratton, P., and McGregor, J. A. (1993). Human immunodeficiency virus infection in women. In L. J. Copeland (Ed.), *Textbook of gynecology* (pp 576–585). Philadelphia: WB Saunders.

Streptococcal pharyngitis, assessment and treatment (1997). *Emergency medical abstracts*, 21 (12).

Swonger, A. K., and Matejski, M. P. (1991). *Nursing pharmacology* (2nd ed). Philadelphia: JB Lippincott.

Taylor, P. J., and Kredenster, J. V. (1993). Investigation of the infertile couple. In L. J. Copeland (Ed.), *Textbook of gynecology* (pp 261–275) Philadelphia: WB Saunders.

Theodore, W. H. (1990). Basic principles of clinical pharmacology. *Neurologic Clinics, 8* (1), 1–13.

Timmons, M. C. (1990). The use of estrogen replacement therapy. In R. C. Cefalo (Ed.), *Clinical decisions in obstetrics and gynecology* (pp 229–231). Rockville, MD: Aspen Publishers, Inc.

Tinkle, M. B. (1990). Genital human papillomavirus infection: A growing health risk. *Journal of Obstetric, Gynecologic, and Neonatal Nursing, 19* (6), 501–507.

Toremifene and letrozole for advanced breast cancer (1998). *The Medical Letter, 40* (1024), 43–46.

Tripp-Reimer, T., & Sorofman, B. (1998). Greek-Americans. In L. Purnell and B. Paulanka (Eds.), *Transcultural health care: A culturally competent approach* (pp. 301–322). Philadelphia: FA Davis.

Trissel, L. A. (1994). *Handbook on injectable drugs.* Bethesda, MD, American Society of Hospital Pharmacists.

Tucker, S. M. (1988). *Pocket nurse guide to fetal monitoring.* St Louis: CV Mosby.

Understanding lung medications: How they work—how to use them (1993). New York, American Lung Association.

Understanding the immune system (1991). N.I.H. Publication No. 88–529.

Upton, R. (1997). Herbal monographs push natural medicines into the 21st century. *The Journal of Alternative and Complementary Medicine, 3,* 4, pp 397–399.

USDA's food guide pyramid (April, 1992). Prepared by Human Nutrition Information Service. Home and Garden Bulletin.

U.S. Department of Health and Human Services. *Final regulations amending basic HHS policy for the protection of human subjects: final rule: 45 CFR 46. Federal register: rules and regulations 46* (No. 16, January 26, 1981): 8366–8392.

U.S. Department of Health and Human Services. *1992 revised classification system for HIV infection and expanded AIDS surveillance case definition for adolescents and adults.* CDC, November 15, 1991.

U.S. Department of Health and Human Services (1989). *Understanding the immune system.* Bethesda, MD: National Cancer Institute.

United States Pharmacopeia Drug Information (USP-DI) for the Health Care Professional (1998), Vol I, 18th ed. Rockville, MD, The US Pharmacopeial Convention, Inc.

U.S. Public Health Service Task Force on Antipneumocystis Prophylaxis for the Patient with Human Immunodeficiency Virus Infection (1992). *Recommendations for prophylaxis against Pneumocystis carinii pneumonia for adults and adolescents infected with human immunodeficiency virus.* Washington, DC: US Public Health Service.

Varivax (varicella virus vaccine live [Oka/Merck]) (product circular 7999906) (1997). West Point, PA: Merck.

Weiss, H. D. (1994). Parkinson's disease and other disorders of movement and tone. In B. Chernow (Ed.), *The pharmacologic approach to the critically-ill patient* (3rd ed) (pp 548–558). Baltimore: Williams & Wilkins.

Whaley, L. E, and Wong, D. L. (1995). *Essentials of pediatric nursing* (4th ed). St Louis: CV Mosby.

Wilcox, S. M., Himmelstein, D. U., and Woolhandler, S. (1994). Inappropriate drug prescribing for the community-dwelling elderly. *Journal of American Medical Association, 272* (4), 292–296.

Wilson, B. A., Shannon, M. T., and Stang, C. L. *Nurses Drug Guide 1999* Stamford, CT: Appleton & Lange.

Winter, M. E. (1994). *Basic clinical pharmacokinetics* (3rd ed). Vancouver, WA: Applied Therapeutics, Inc.

Woods, N. F., Olshansky, E., and Draye, M. A. (1991). Infertility: Women's experiences. *Health Care for Women International, 12,* 179–190.

Yarbro, C. (1989). Carboplatin: A clinical review. *Seminars in oncology nursing, 5* (2) Suppl 1 (May) 63–69.

Yasko, J., and Dudjak, L. (1990). *Biological response modifier therapy-symptom management.* Pittsburgh: Park Row Publishers.

Young, T. E., and Manqum, O. B. (1994). *NeoFax '94: A manual of drugs used in neonatal care* (7th ed). Columbus, OH: Ross Products Division, Abbott Laboratories.

Youngkin, E. Q., and Israel D. (1996). A review and critique of common herbal alternative therapies. *Nurse Practitioner 21* (10), 10, 39, 43–44, 49–52, 54–56, 59–62.

Yuen, B. H., Fluker, M., and Urman, B. (1993). Infertility: Medical management of ovulation induction. In L. J. Copeland (Ed.), *Textbook of gynecology* (pp 292–301). Philadelphia: WB Saunders.

Zaloga, G. P. (1994). Enteral nutrition in the critically ill. In B. Chernow (Ed.), *The pharmacologic approach to the critically ill patient* (3rd ed) (pp 1034–1046). Baltimore: Williams & Wilkins.

Zaloga, G. P., and Chernow, B. (1994). Insulin and oral hypoglycemics. In B. Chernow (Ed.), *The pharmacologic approach to the critically ill patient* (3rd ed) (pp 758–771). Baltimore: Williams & Wilkins.

Ziegler, M. G., and Ruiz-Ramon, P. F. (1994). Antihypertensive therapy. In B. Chernow (Ed.), *The pharmacologic approach to the critically ill patient* (3rd ed) (pp 405–425). Baltimore: Williams & Wilkins.

Zuspan, F. P., and Rayburn, W. F. (1986). Drug abuse during pregnancy. In W. F. Rayburn and F. P. Zuspan, *Drug therapy in obstetrics and gynecology* (2nd ed) (pp 37–52). Norwalk, CT: Appleton-Century-Crofts.

Index

Note: Page numbers followed by the letter t refer to tables.

SELECTED DRUG INTERACTIONS

Drug	Interacting With *
Aminoglycosides	Cephalosporins, ethacrynic acid, indomethacin
Aspirin	Acetazolamide, antacids, ethanol
Ciprofloxacin	Antacids, cyclosporine, iron supplements, sucralfate
Digoxin	Amiodarone, antacids, anticholinergics, captopril, cholestyramine, cyclosporine, diazepam, erythromycin, ethacrynic acid, furosemide, ibuprofen, kaolin, metoclopramide, penicillamine, prazosin, propafenone, quinidine, rifampin, tetracyclines, thiazides, verapamil
Lithium carbonate	ACE inhibitors, acetazolamide, anorexic agents, caffeine, fluoxetine, iodides, methyldopa, metronidazole, NSAIDs, tetracyclines, theophylline, thiazides, verapamil
Meperidine (Demerol)	MAO inhibitors, phenothiazines
Morphine	Cimetidine
Nifedipine	Cimetidine, ethanol
Phenothiazines	Anticholinergic agents, ethanol
Phenytoin	Cimetidine, disulfiram, ethanol, fluconazole, folic acid, isoniazid, nifedipine, omeprazole, phenylbutazone, rifampin, trimethoprim, valproic acid
Propranolol	Cigarette smoking, cimetidine, epinephrine, indomethacin
Sulfonylureas	Beta blockers, cimetidine, gemfibrozil, oxyphenbutazone, phenylbutazone, ranitidine
Theophylline	Allopurinol, barbiturates, caffeine, cigarette smoking, cimetidine, ciprofloxacin, disulfiram, erythromycin, mexiletine, phenytoin, propafenone, propranolol, rifampin
Tetracyclines	Antacids, iron supplements, oral contraceptives
Tricyclic antidepressants	Cimetidine, epinephrine, fluoxetine, nitrates (sublingual), MAO inhibitors
Valproic acid	Aspirin, azithromycin, clarithromycin, erythromycin
Warfarin	Amiodarone, aspirin, cimetidine, clofibrate, disulfiram, erythromycin, fluoroquinolones, glutethimide, griseofulvin, lovastatin, metronidazole, nalidixic acid, phenobarbital, phenylbutazone, rifampin, sulfamethoxazole, sulfinpyrazone, tamoxifen, thyroid

* Check drug references for the various effects of drug interaction.